Integrated

SECOND EDITION

Pharmacology

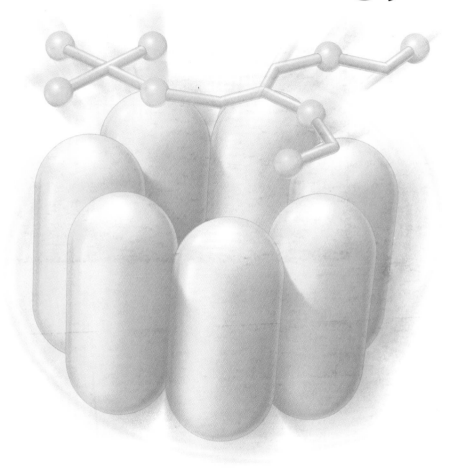

Commissioning Editor: **Louise Crowe**
Project Development Manager: **Ruth Swan**
Project Manager: **Colin Arthur**
Designer: **Marie McNestry**
Illustrators: **Mick Ruddy, Marion Tasker**

WWW. .com

The inter
medical
Have you

For s

- Free
- Onli favo
- Stud read
- Dow
- Win great prizes in our games and competitions

line resource
y involved in
cation

For instructors

- Download free images and buy others from our constantly growing image bank
- Preview sample chapters from new textbooks
- Request inspection copies
- Browse our reading rooms for the latest information on new books and electronic products
- Secure online ordering with prompt delivery, as well as full contact details to order by phone, fax or post

Log on and register FREE today

fleshandbones.com
– an online resource
for medical instructors
and students

fleshandbones.com

Integrated
Pharmacology

SECOND EDITION

Clive Page Professor of Pharmacology, Sackler Institute of Pulmonary Pharmacology, Guy's, King's and St Thomas' School of Biomedical Sciences, London, UK

Michael Curtis Reader in Pharmacology, Cardiovascular Research, Rayne Institute, St Thomas' Hospital, London, UK

Morley Sutter Professor of Pharmacology and Honorary Associate Professor of Medicine, Departments of Pharmacology, Therapeutics and Medicine, University of British Columbia, Vancouver, Canada

Michael Walker Professor of Pharmacology, Departments of Pharmacology and Therapeutics, University of British Columbia, Vancouver, Canada

Brian Hoffman Professor of Medicine, Stanford University School of Medicine and Geriatrics Research, Education and Clinical Center, Veterans Affairs Health Care System, Palo Alto, USA

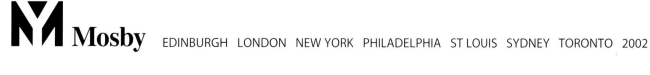
Mosby   EDINBURGH   LONDON   NEW YORK   PHILADELPHIA   ST LOUIS   SYDNEY   TORONTO   2002

MOSBY
An imprint of Harcourt Publishers Limited

© Mosby International Ltd 2002

M is a registered trademark of Harcourt Publishers Limited

The right of Clive Page, Michael Curtis, Morley Sutter, Michael Walker and Brian Hoffman to be identified as editors of this work has been asserted by them in accordance with the Copyright, Designs and Patents Act 1988

First published 2002

ISBN 0 7234 3221 X

British Library Cataloguing in Publication Data
A catalogue record for this book is available from the British Library

Library of Congress Cataloging in Publication Data
A catalog record for this book is available from the Library of Congress

Note
Medical knowledge is constantly changing. As new information becomes available, changes in treatment, procedures, equipment and the use of drugs become necessary. The editors, contributors and the publishers have taken care to ensure that the information given in this text is accurate and up to date. However, readers are strongly advised to confirm that the information, especially with regard to drug usage, complies with the latest legislation and standards of practice.

Printed in China

Preface

Integrated Pharmacology Second Edition continues with the unique approach of the First Edition, presenting drugs and their mechanism of action in the context of the diseases they are used to treat. The Second Edition has been thoroughly revised and expanded to comprehensively cover drug action at the molecular, cellular, tissue and organ levels.

The first section deals with the principles of drug action, and introduces concepts of how drugs exert their actions. It offers insights into how our overall knowledge and use of drugs is influenced by a range of factors including history and myth. An updated system of simple icons explains the main molecular and cellular actions of drugs. These are used in subsequent chapters, which deal with drug treatment of diseases within a framework of the body's systems. Each body system chapter addresses the common diseases affecting a system before comprehensively discussing the drug classes and specific drugs used to treat disease. The reader is also introduced to other increasingly important aspects of pharmacology, such as risk-benefit, pharmacoeconomics, and pharmacovigilance. In addition, the pertinent background biochemistry, physiology, and pathology are provided for each body system. New to this edition is a chapter on herbal medicines, which considers their widespread use and pharmacologic implications.

Throughout Integrated Pharmacology Second Edition, a color illustration program depicts pharmacology in a way that enhances understanding and memory. Key facts boxes, tables of adverse actions and drug interactions are used to explain and highlight important issues. At the end of the book is a self-assessment section comprising multiple choice questions and clinical vignettes.

Prescribing drugs is the endpoint of many contacts between physicians and their patients. For this reason, it is essential that students of medicine acquire a full and detailed understanding of pharmacology integrated with disease. We hope that this Second Edition helps make that understanding easier and will contribute towards training the next generation of physicians and other health care professionals who are faced with a quite bewildering number of drugs.

Integrated Pharmacology Second Edition has been designed for medical students, but will also be useful to other health care professionals, biomedical scientists and students interested in pharmacology, as it bridges the gap between fundamental mechanisms and the use of drugs to treat human disease.

The Editors hope that the readers of this Second Edition enjoy reading this book as much as we have enjoyed preparing it.

Acknowledgments

We would like to acknowledge the sterling efforts of our contributors who have helped us improve this Second Edition beyond our expectation. Our thanks also go to our colleagues at Harcourt for seeing this Second Edition through to completion and for keeping the editors on track! In particular, we would like to thank Louise Crowe for her continual support for this project, Ruth Swan who kept us all on schedule, Marie McNestry who is responsible for the page and cover design, and the excellent work of our illustrations team managed by Mick Ruddy.

Picture credits

Figures 14.1, 19.1, 21.1 and 21.3 adapted from *Human Histology*, 2nd edn, by Dr A Stevens and Professor J Lowe, Mosby International 1997.

Figures 16.1, 16.3, 16.7 and 16.8 adapted from *Immunology*, 4th edn, by Professor I Roitt, Dr J Brostoff and Dr M Dale, Mosby International 1996.

Chapter 24 image of eye courtesy of Dr P-M Bouloux, Department of Endocrinology, Royal Free Hospital, London, UK.

Contents

Contents

Contributors

Shlomo Abraham PhD
Department of Pharmacology
Israel Institute for Biological Research
Ness-Ziona, Israel

Fred Y Aoki MD FRCPC
Department of Medicine
University of Manitoba
Winnipeg, Canada

Teodor Bojanowski BEng MEng MD FRCSC
Division of Otolaryngology
University of British Columbia
Vancouver, Canada

Christopher John Bowmer BSc PhD
School of Biomedical Sciences
University of Leeds
Leeds, UK

Joseph Paul Eder MD
Dana-Farber/Harvard Cancer Center
and Harvard Medical School
Boston, Massachusetts, USA

R E Ferner MSc MD FRCP
West Midlands Centre for Adverse Drug Reaction Reporting
City Hospital
Birmingham, UK

Tommy W Gage DDS PhD
Division of Pharmacology
Baylor College of Dentistry
Dallas, Texas, USA

Keith Hillier BSc PhD DSc
Clinical Pharmacology and Division of Medical Education
University of Southampton
Southampton, UK

Zhuowei Hu MD PhD
Department of Medicine
Stanford University School of Medicine
Palo Alto, California, USA

Itsuo Iwamoto MD PhD
Department of Internal Medicine II
Chiba University School of Medicine, Japan

Akira Kaneko MD PhD
Department of International Affairs and Tropical Medicine
Tokyo Women's Medical University
School of Medicine
Tokyo, Japan
and
Department of Medicine
Unit of Infectious Diseases
Karolinska Institutet
Karolinska Hospital
Stockholm, Sweden

Robert Kerwin MA PhD MB Bchir DSC FRCPsych
Institute of Psychiatry and Maudsley Hospital
and Guy's, King's and St Thomas's School of Medicine and Dentistry
London, UK

Richard D Mamelok MD
Consultant, Clinical Research and Development
364 Churchill Avenue
Palo Alto, CA, USA

Ronald D Mann MD FRCP FRCGP FFPM
Southampton University
Southampton, UK

Jeffrey W Miller MD
Pfizer Global Research & Development
Groton, Connecticut, USA

Philip Moore BSc PhD
Division of Pharmacology and Therapeutics
Guy's, King's and St Thomas's School of Biomedical Sciences
King's College
London, UK

Robert J Naylor BPharm FRPharmS PhD DSc
The School of Pharmacy
University of Bradford
Bradford, UK

Toshimasa Nishiyama MD DMSc
Department of Public Health
Kansai Medical University
Osaka, Japan

Michael K Pugsley PhD
Department of Pharmacology
XOMA (US)
Berkeley, California, USA

David MJ Quastel MD PhD
Department of Pharmacology and Therapeutics
Faculty of Medicine
University of British Columbia
Vancouver, Canada

Craig R Ries MD FRCPC PhD
Department of Anesthesia
University of British Columbia
UBC Hospital, Vancouver, Canada

Jon Robbins BSc PhD
Division of Pharmacology and Therapeutics
School of Biomedical Sciences
King's College
London, UK

Nerys M Roberts FRCP MD BSc
Chelsea and Westminster Hospital
and Great Ormond Street Hospital
London, UK

Stuart Rosser MD FRCPC
University of Manitoba
Winnipeg, Canada

Stephen D Shafran MD FRCPC
Department of Medicine
University of Alberta
Edmonton, Alberta, Canada

Ollie Simons PhD
Department of Pharmacology
University of West Indies
Kingston, Jamaica

Daniel S Sitar PhD
Department of Pharmacology and Therapeutics
University of Manitoba
Winnipeg, Canada

Reza Tabrizchi PhD
Faculty of Medicine
Memorial University of Newfoundland
St. John's, Canada

Mike Travis BSc MB BS MRCPsych
Institute of Psychiatry and Maudsley Hospital
London, UK

John P Wade MD
Department of Rheumatology
University of British Columbia
Vancouver, Canada

Michael G Wyllie PhD
Director
URODOC Ltd
Kent, UK

Michael Stuart Yates BSc PhD
School of Biomedical Sciences
University of Leeds
Leeds, UK

The Editors would also like to thank contributors to the First Edition:

PG Adaikan PhD
Department of Obstetrics and Gynaecology
National University of Singapore
Singapore

Karl Erik Andersson MD PhD
Department of Clinical Pharmacology
University Lund Hospital
Sweden

Kathy Banner PhD
Discovery Biology
Pfizer UK

Graham E Bryce MD FRCSC
Division of Otorhinolaryngology
University of British Columbia
Vancouver, Canada

Richard Z Lin MD
Department of Medicine
University of New York
USA

John M Littleton PhD MD
Department of Molecular and Biomedical Pharmacology
University of Kentucky
USA

Ravinder Pabla PhD
Cardiovascular Research,
St Thomas' Hospital,
London UK

Sian Rees PhD
University Laboratory of Physiology
Oxford, UK

F Michelle Sutter MD FRCSC
Department of Surgery
University of British Columbia
Vancouver, USA

Catherine Wilson BPharm PhD DSc
Department of Obstetrics and Gynaecology
St George's Hospital Medical School
London, UK

1

Principles of Pharmacology

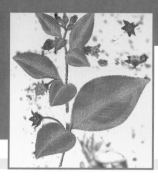

Chapter 1

Introduction

WHAT IS PHARMACOLOGY?

Pharmacology is the science that deals with the mechanism of action, uses, adverse effects, and fate of drugs in animals and humans

The word 'pharmacology' comes from the ancient Greek word for drug, *pharmakon*. It is the study of what biologically active chemical compounds do in the body, and how the body reacts to them.

The word 'drug' has many meanings, but is most commonly used to describe a substance used as a medicine for the treatment of disease. However, if the word drug is used to refer to any biologically active compound which is taken with the intent of producing a change in the body, then it includes:

- Familiar substances such as caffeine, nicotine, and alcohol.
- Other chemicals which are abused, such as cannabis, heroin, and cocaine.
- Food constituents such as vitamins, minerals and amino-acids.
- Cosmetics.

Pharmacology is not identical to pharmacy, which involves the manufacture, preparation and dispensing of drugs.

Pharmacology is concerned with the effects of drugs on living systems or their constituent components such as cells, cell membranes, cell organelles, enzymes and even DNA. As a result the effects of drugs can be studied at many levels of biological organization or complexity ranging from the interaction of drugs with large bio-molecules, such as enzymes, ion channels, or the receptors for neurotransmitters, hormones etc., to the effect of drugs on human populations. Pharmacologists therefore often identify themselves according to the level at which they study drugs. Thus there are pharmacologists

who label themselves as molecular, functional, system, or clinical pharmacologists.

A knowledge of pharmacology is essential in the practice of both human and veterinary medicine, where drugs are used to treat disease. The principles of pharmacology also apply to toxicology, where the effects of the chemicals of interest are harmful rather than therapeutic. Whether a drug is used for therapy, or as a poison, knowledge of its pharmacology is essential if it is to be used selectively for a defined purpose.

Ideally, all drugs should have a selective action, but often they do not. A selective action can be achieved if:

- A relatively high concentration of the drug can be obtained at the target cell, tissue, or organ where its action is required.
- The drug's chemical structure is such that it interacts selectively with the discrete molecule, cell, tissue, or organ at the location where it is to have its effect.

Pharmacologic terminology

As with all scientific disciplines, pharmacology has its own vocabulary. This includes terms such as pharmacodynamics, pharmacokinetics, pharmacotherapeutics, selectivity, selective toxicity, risk–benefit ratio, pharmacoepidemiology, pharmacoeconomics, toxicology, toxins, toxinology, poisons, and toxicity (see below).

Pharmacodynamics and pharmacokinetics

Pharmacodynamics describes the actions of a drug (qualitatively and quantitatively), i.e. what a drug does to the body; pharmacokinetics describes the fate of a drug (absorption, distribution, metabolism and distribution), i.e. what the body does to a drug. A knowledge of both pharmacodynamics and pharmacokinetics is essential to understand what drugs do, and how they do it.

Pharmacodynamics includes the measurement of responses to drugs and how response relates to drug dose or concentration

By examining the effects of a drug over a range of doses or concentrations (Fig. 1.1) it is possible to plot a 'dose (concentration)–response curve' which provides important pharmacodynamic information: the threshold effective dose, the therapeutic dose range, the maximum effect and the potency. Drug selectivity and safety can be determined by comparing dose–response curves for different types of response (therapeutic versus toxic, for example) and by comparing the dose–response curve for one drug against that for another drug.

 What is pharmacology?

- Pharmacology is the study of what drugs do, and how they do it
- A drug is a chemical usually used to treat disease
- Drugs are intended to have a selective action, but this ideal is seldom achieved
- There is always a risk of adverse effects as well as a benefit connected with using any drug
- A knowledge of pharmacology is essential for using drugs effectively in therapy

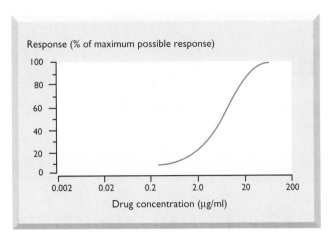

Fig. 1.1 A graph of a dose–response curve. This graph shows that the response to a drug increases with the logarithm to base 10 ($\log_{10}$) of its concentration. At low concentrations the rate at which a response develops is slow, the response then increases rapidly before reaching a maximum.

Pharmacologic definitions

- Pharmacodynamics is the study and measurement of drug effects
- Pharmacokinetics is the study of how the body absorbs, distributes, metabolizes, and excretes drugs
- Pharmacotherapeutics is the use of drugs to treat diseases
- Pharmacoepidemiology is the study of the effect of drugs on populations
- Pharmacoeconomics is the study of the cost-effectiveness of drug treatments

Pharmacokinetics is the study of how the body absorbs, distributes, metabolizes, and excretes drugs

Drug exposure may be deliberate, as when a medicine is prescribed to treat a disease, or inadvertent, as a result of intake of food, water or air.

The most common route of drug administration is by mouth (*per orem*) in the form of liquid, tablet or capsule. Drugs in liquid form are immediately available for absorption whereas tablets and capsules must first disintegrate, normally in the stomach, to allow the drug to dissolve in the gut fluids. The dissolved drug diffuses across the intestinal mucosa and so reaches the blood stream. The drug in solution in the blood passes through the liver to the heart, from where it is distributed via the blood to other parts of the body. It then diffuses out of the blood into the tissues. The total amount of drug presented to a particular region is proportional to the blood flow to that region. The rapidity with which a drug appears in a particular organ is thus dependent on blood flow and other factors special to that organ.

Depending on its nature, the absorbed drug may be metabolized or remain unchanged in the body. Metabolism often converts a drug into less active products (thereby limiting the drug's action). However some drugs are initially metabolized

from a less active (pro-drug) form to a more active metabolite. The liver is an important site for drug metabolism (see Chapters 4 and 21). Excretion occurs primarily via the kidney but may occur by other routes, such as the gut, sweat glands, or lungs (see Chapter 4).

Pharmacotherapeutics (pharmacotherapy)

Pharmacotherapeutics is the use of drug treatment to cure a disease, delay disease progression, alleviate the signs and/or symptoms of a disease, or facilitate nonpharmacologic therapeutic intervention; for example:

- Cure of an infection.
- Alleviation of pain and fever during infection.
- Avoidance of stroke by lowering blood pressure.
- Supplementation of insulin in type 1 diabetes mellitus.
- General anesthesia prior to and during major surgery.

Clearly, a knowledge of pharmacology is essential for the rational use of drugs. A knowledge of the disease being treated, and its pathology, are also required. A clinical pharmacologist is trained as both a physician and pharmacologist and often provides advice on the therapeutic use of drugs.

Selectivity

Pharmacotherapy is a scientific attempt to alter some physiologic or pathophysiologic process selectively by a drug in a way that benefits the recipient of the drug (Fig. 1.2). Due to similarities between a drug and certain molecular targets (such as receptors), usually a drug will interact strongly with some molecular targets and less strongly with others. A relatively selective drug would affect primarily only one target over a specific concentration range (the therapeutic range). However, if its therapeutic concentration range exceeds the window of selectivity, any drug can produce adverse effects.

The selectivity of a drug depends on:

- The chemical nature of the drug.
- The dose given and the route by which it is administered.
- Special features of the recipient, such as genetic make-up, age, and coexisting disease.

Selective toxicity

Selective toxicity is a term applied principally when drugs are used as chemotherapeutic (antimicrobial and anticancer) agents or pesticides (insecticides, antiparasitic agents, or herbicides). The aim is to kill the parasite or unwanted cells, but leave the host or environment relatively unharmed. The more closely the unwanted cell or parasite resembles the host, the more difficult it is to achieve selective toxicity. Therefore, although drugs can be relatively effective in their actions against bacteria, they are relatively nonselective in killing cancer cells.

Risk–benefit ratio

The phrase 'risk–benefit ratio' is used to describe the adverse effects of a drug in relation to its beneficial effects (Fig. 1.3). Whenever drugs are used the benefits from their use should be greater than the risks. What risk–benefit ratio is acceptable depends on the severity of the disease being treated. A greater risk would be accepted in the treatment of an otherwise fatal

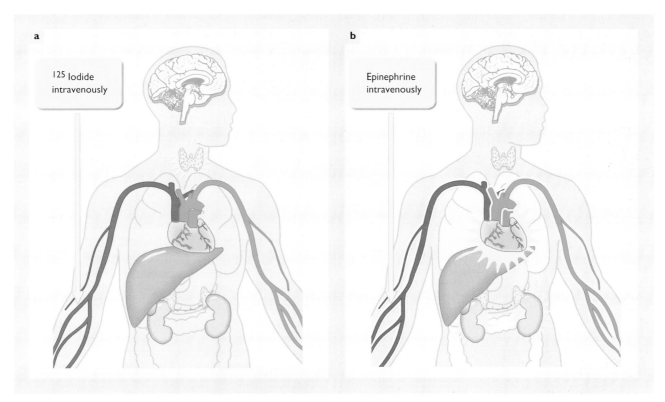

Fig. 1.2 Ideally, all drugs would have selective actions. However, complete selectivity is seldom achieved. (a) ^{125}I (radioactive) is selectively taken up by the iodide uptake system of the thyroid gland. Therefore, radioactivity is high in the thyroid and not elsewhere in the body. (b) Epinephrine has effects wherever its receptors (adrenoceptors) occur. For example, such receptors are present in the heart and blood vessels, so blood pressure and heart rate are raised. Adrenoceptors occur throughout the body and therefore the effects of epinephrine are widespread.

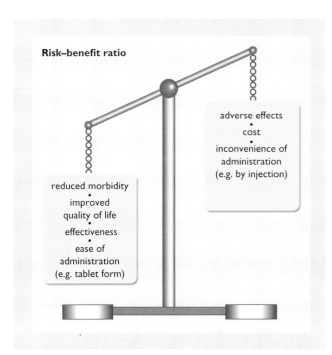

Fig. 1.3 Risk–benefit ratio. The beneficial effects of a drug should outweigh adverse effects. All drugs are capable of producing bad effects as well as the wanted good effects.

disease than in the treatment of a less serious one. All aspects of the use of a drug need to be considered, from basic (e.g. risk of death) to economic (e.g. cost per dose) to determine the risk–benefit ratio for any particular case.

To place risk–benefit ratios in an everyday setting, we must remember that each activity of everyday life, such as driving a car, skiing, flying or swimming, or even taking a shower, has an associated risk and our perception of these risks may be quite erroneous (see Fig. 6.2 in Chapter 6). Accurate information about the risks of a prescribed drug in relation to those of daily life is needed to keep the risks in perspective. This is obtained by studying the effects of the drug on large populations (see Chapter 6).

Pharmacoepidemiology and pharmacoeconomics

Pharmacoepidemiology is the study of both the beneficial and the adverse effects of a drug on large numbers of people, for example:

- The effect that widespread use of antibiotics in a community has on the type of pneumonia prevalent in that community.
- The influence of use of antihypertensive drugs on subsequent incidence of stroke in a population.

Similarly, it is also important to know the financial cost associated with the use of a drug. As a result the discipline of pharmacoeconomics has evolved. This is the study of the cost of medicines, taking into account:

- The financial cost of the disease involved.
- The retail cost of the drug, including marketing.

Pharmacoepidemiology is often linked to pharmacoeconomics since determining the financial costs of a drug usually involves studying large populations.

Toxicology, toxins, venoms, toxinology, poisons, and toxicity

Toxicity is injury or death produced by any substance when it is absorbed by a living organism. Poisons can be synthetic or naturally occurring: they are chemicals that kill or inhibit growth of living organisms including humans. Poisoning may be produced deliberately or accidentally. The latter is more common in children than adults.

Toxicology is the study of the harmful effects of drugs and other chemicals on humans, animals, or plants. The concepts of pharmacodynamics, pharmacokinetics, pharmacoepidemiology, and pharmacoeconomics apply to toxicology just as they do to pharmacotherapeutics. The only difference is that the endpoints differ: harm is the end-point in toxicology, and benefit that in pharmacotherapeutics.

Toxins and venoms are harmful substances produced by living organisms, both plants and animals (see Chapter 29). Toxinology is the scientific study of the actions of such compounds.

HISTORY OF PHARMACOLOGY

Magic, medicine and religion intertwined

The roots of pharmacology are entwined with the knowledge of herbal and other potions and their uses. Such knowledge was often the secret of the priest, holy man, or shaman in ancient societies, since the effects of such 'cures' and poisons were often viewed as magical. The person who knew about drugs and potions was respected, and often feared since intentional poisoning was not unknown.

 Understanding of drugs evolves in parallel with our understanding of disease

Despite the need to treat disease, knowledge of the mechanisms causing any disease is always limited. If a disease is believed to

---

Ancient and modern pharmacology

- Ancient civilizations used mixtures of magic, religion, and crude drugs to treat diseases. Drugs were often thought to be magical in their actions
- The drugs of antiquity mainly came from plant sources, or were obtained from animal parts or fluids
- Knowledge of drugs increased in parallel with knowledge of body function (anatomy, physiology, and biochemistry) and chemistry (especially organic chemistry)
- Modern drug development depends on intellectual cooperation between academia and industry

be caused by gods, spirits, or supernatural forces, then its treatment must invoke magic since supernatural causes can only be counteracted by supernatural means. In the past, therefore, drugs were often believed to be magical and, as such, were given magical names such as 'eye of the sun.'

The sources of drugs in ancient times were plants, minerals and animals. A frieze from Mesopotamia dated to the eighth century BC shows priests carrying a goat, mandrake flowers, and opium poppyheads. This illustrates the important combination of religion, plants, and animals in therapeutics as practiced by ancient peoples. Furthermore, such pictures confirm that the opium poppy was an ancient medicinal plant (Fig. 1.4).

Drug development in ancient civilizations

The earliest written record that specifically mentions drugs is the Egyptian Medical Papyrus (translated by Smith) dating from approximately 1600 BC, although it deals primarily with surgery and other treatments. The Ebers Papyrus, which dates from approximately 1550 BC, also lists some 700 remedies,

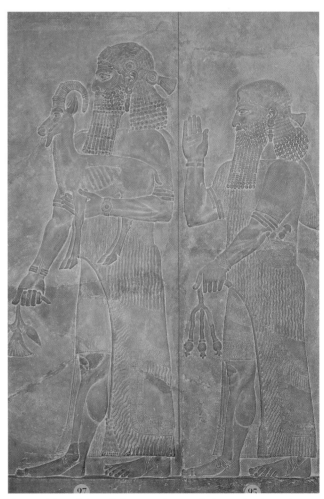

Fig. 1.4 The origins of pharmacology: religion, animals, and plants. A frieze from the palace of King Sargon II, in Kharasabad, Musée du Louvre, Paris, Antiquités Orientales. (Courtesy of Service de Documentation Photographique de la Réunion des Musées Nationaux, Chateau de Versailles.)

their preparation and use. Concoctions ranged from the occult, such as the thigh bone of a hanged man, to the familiar, such as preparations containing opium or castor oil. The latter two are still in use some 3500 years later!

Medicine and the use of drugs was evolving in China (as described in the *Shen Nung*) and India (Ayurvedic medicine) in parallel to their evolution in Ancient Egypt, but there was little Western contact with Asia at that time. For example, vaccination was practiced in India in 550 BC, but was only introduced into Western medicine some 2000 years later.

Ancient Greek culture contributed a great deal to the development of pharmacy and drugs. Hippocrates (460–377 BC) wrote on the ethics of medicine as well as on the causes of disease. The Greeks attributed disease to an imbalance of humors in the body, the humors being blood, phlegm, black bile, and yellow bile. This doctrine was elaborated by Galen (130–201 AD), a Greek physician, who practiced in Alexandria and in Rome. Galen's influence on medicines persisted right through to the 1500s, and can still be seen today in the use of herbal mixtures. The Romans organized and regulated the practice of medicine, including the use of drugs, but contributed little new knowledge to pharmacology. Theophrastus (372–287 BC) listed all that was then known about medicinal plants, and Dioscorides (57 AD), Nero's surgeon, used this list as his basis for a compendium of substances used as medicines – *materia medica* – which described nearly 500 plants and how to prepare remedies from them.

The Persians preserved Greek views of medicines and transmitted these to the Arabs when Persia was conquered. From approximately 700 to 1000 AD, the traditions of medicine and of pharmacy were maintained and developed by the Arabs, who regulated the practice of medicine and pharmacy and established apothecary shops, hospitals, and libraries. The Arabs built on the published works of Galen and introduced several new ways of preparing drugs. The English word 'alcohol' is from the Arabic word *al-kuhl* (Fig. 1.5). Paradoxically, the original meaning was 'all things very fine,' and referred to ground sulfides of lead and antimony used as eye make-up. The Arabs also introduced alchemy to Europe. Alchemy combined

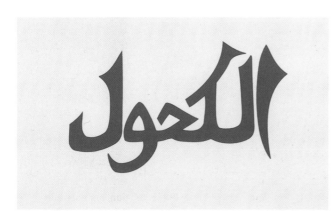

Fig. 1.5 The Arabic word *al-kuhl* or alcohol. It originally referred to one of the first ways of preparing drugs for external use and only later to ethanol and other alcohols.

Egyptian ideas, astronomy, astrology, and Greek natural philosophy, with Christian metaphysics, in an attempt to discover the origin and meaning of all things. Alchemy was the parent of chemistry and therefore an important ancestor of modern pharmacology.

Drug development since the Middle Ages

In the Middle Ages the practice of medicine and use of drugs in Europe was often centered on the monasteries. Many monasteries cultivated herbal gardens to provide a source for their drugs (see Chapter 30). Prior to the scientific age there was extensive documentation of herbs and their uses, some of which was of therapeutic usefulness. Unfortunately much of this information became confabulated and confused over time, and therefore rendered useless. Interestingly, where people used herbs as poisons for obtaining food, as with arrow poisons, their knowledge base remained intact over the years into modern times.

The grandfather of the science of pharmacology is generally agreed to be Paracelsus, who was born in 1493 in Switzerland. He was the son of a physician, traveled widely in Europe, and graduated as a doctor of medicine from Ferrara, Italy. Many of his writings were prescient. For example, he advised against use of the complicated mixtures that were common medications at that time, and urged that each drug (or plant) should be used alone. He wrote 'It is the task of chemistry to produce medicines for the treatment of disease since the vital functions of life are basically chemical in nature ... All things are poisons, for there is nothing without poisonous qualities. It is only the dose which makes a thing a poison.' These statements are still cornerstones of pharmacologic thought today, since it is now recognized that drugs are chemicals that alter biologic chemistry and that their selectivity is affected by the dose.

■ *Developments in pharmacology depended on the developing sciences of chemistry, pathophysiology, physiology, and botany*

The development of pharmacology depended on the increasing understanding of human physiology and disease processes (pathophysiology). Such understanding in turn depended on the application of scientific methods to these problems. In the 1600s there were many contributions to the understanding of physiology and diseases, including those of William Harvey (1578–1657), who introduced experimentation to demonstrate the circulation of blood, and Sydenham (1624–1689), who introduced classification into the study of diseases, their causes, and their treatment.

Developments in chemistry

The idea of using chemicals as drugs seems to have been first suggested by van Helmont (1515–1564), the discoverer of carbonic acid and the early scientist who introduced the term 'gas' into chemistry. The theory that an imbalance of body chemicals could cause disease was first proposed by the Dutch physician, Sylvius (1614–1672), while the physicist/chemist Boyle (1627–1691) was the first to demonstrate that drugs had an effect when given intravenously as well as by mouth. The activities and thoughts of chemists and physicians became closely linked.

Developments in botany

In the ancient, and recent past, most drugs came from plants, not from known chemicals (see Chapter 30). For example, the Egyptians used extracts from the opium poppy (see above). Plant use continued throughout history, and in the 1640s, cinchona bark, which contains quinine, was introduced into Europe from South America by the Jesuit priests of the Roman Catholic Church. It was used to treat fevers, often caused by malaria, a disease for which quinine is still used. However, one of the problems associated with the use of botanical material as medicines is the reliable identification of the plants. This was improved by the system of plant classification introduced by the Swedish botanist Linnaeus (1707–1778).

Several Swiss and French botanists such as Schröder (1641) and Lémery (1698) published more modern books on vegetable *materia medica*, in addition to those of the Ancient Egyptians, Babylonians, Indians, and Chinese. Medieval universities had established botanic gardens to learn more about medicinal plants. The botanic works of Haller (1708–1777), a physician in Berne and Göttingen who combined the study of both physiology and botany, were collected into a publication by Vicat in 1776, which in turn was translated into German by Hahnemann, the founder of homeopathy.

William Withering published an important treatise *An Account of the Foxglove and Some of its Medical Uses* in 1785. In this text he described observations made over a 10-year period on the

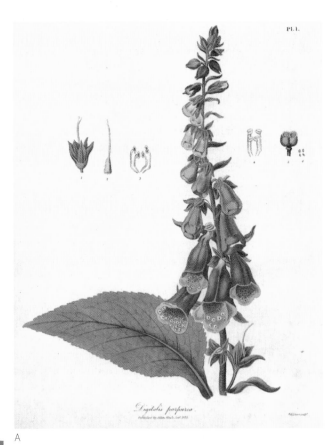

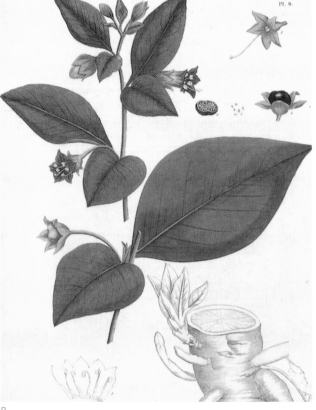

A

B

8

Fig. 1.6 Foxglove and deadly nightshade. These are the plant sources of digoxin and atropine, respectively. (Reproduced with permission from George Graves, Medicinal Plants, New York: Crescent Books. Copyright 1990 Bracken Books.)

therapeutic use of extracts of the foxglove (*Digitalis purpurea*) (Fig. 1.6). The principles he laid down at that time for the use of such digitalis extracts in the treatment of dropsy (swelling of the ankles and abdomen due to accumulation of extravascular fluid) are largely still valid today, although digoxin, a pure extract of the digitalis plant, is used these days.

Isolation of pure compounds

Progress in understanding plants, and the drugs they contain, was aided by the work of the Swedish chemist Carl Wilhelm Scheele (1742–1786). He produced pure chemicals, among them glycerin and malic acid, by processes such as crystallization. Scheele's work laid the foundation for the isolation of the first pure drug, morphine, by Sertürner (1783–1841) in 1805. Such advances led to pure substances, rather than crude extracts, being isolated and tested for their pharmacologic effects.

Developments in physiology

Understanding how and where drugs act requires a detailed knowledge of how the body functions (i.e. physiology and biochemistry). Such knowledge and understanding were advanced by the work of French physiologists, such as François Magendie (1783–1855), and his pupil Claude Bernard (1813–1878). Their techniques of investigation located the sites in the body where drugs act. Thus Claude Bernard, for example, had clearly demonstrated by 1856 that curare (an extract of a South American jungle dart poison) paralyzed skeletal muscle by acting selectively at nerve junctions.

Developments in pharmacologic concepts

Pharmacology uses information from physics, chemistry, and the biologic sciences to understand what drugs do, and how they do it. A few principles are, however, special to and underlie pharmacology, including:

- The concept first suggested by Felix Fontana (1730–1805) that in plant or other medicinal material there is an active principle that is responsible for its effect.
- The concept of a distinct relationship between the dose of a drug and its effect. This is attributed to Peter John Andrew Daries who postulated it in his doctoral dissertation of 1776, and Paracelsus also made an important contribution to this idea. The dose–response curve is the current expression of the concept (see Fig. 1.1). The mathematical formulation of dose–response curves is derived from the physicochemical mass-action construct of Langmuir, which was interpreted into a pharmacologic context by Clarke (1885–1941). The appropriate mathematic analysis for the relationship between dose and response is still evolving (see Chapter 4).
- The concept that structure–activity relationships (SAR) exist for drugs. The study of how chemical alterations to a basic chemical pharmacophore (the basic chemical structure which gives a pharmacologic effect) could alter the action of a drug began with James Blake (1815–1841). He systematically altered a series of inorganic salts and observed the resulting changes in pharmacologic effects. Paul Ehrlich (1854–1915) exploited this technique in his search for compounds that would selectively kill invading organisms– the search for a 'magic bullet.'
- The concept that most drugs must first bind to a receptor to produce their actions. This was first proposed by Langley in 1878 and extended by Ehrlich early in the twentieth century.

Modern drug development

Interactions between pharmacologic theories developed in academia and the pharmaceutical industry have been highly productive

The development of modern drugs was closely allied to the development of the dye industry in Germany, from which emerged the modern pharmaceutical industry. Many scientists have contributed to the development of drugs while working in industry, but only a few selected drugs and individuals can be mentioned here:

- Salicylic acid was synthesized from phenol in 1860 by Kolbe and Lautemann.
- Acetylsalicylic acid (aspirin) was synthesized from salicyclic in 1899 by Dreser.
- Prontosil, a therapeutically inactive dye which is transformed in the body to an antibacterial sulfonamide, was developed by Domagk in 1935.

Other sulfonamides were quickly synthesized following the discovery of Prontosil. This early success gave rise to a series of chemically related drugs developed by the pharmaceutical industry including: acetazolamide (a carbonic anhydrase inhibitor), thiazide diuretics developed by Karl Beyer, followed by the sulfonylurea oral hypoglycemics.

At the same time, academic pharmacology was making headway in the identification and classification of receptors. Such work had been initiated by Barger and Dale (1910) in industry and Gaddum (1933) in academia. Antihistamines were developed by Bovet (1944), while β adrenoceptor antagonists such as propranolol were developed by James Black (circa 1960). Later, around 1970, Black went on to develop H_2 antagonists such as cimetidine for the treatment of peptic ulcer, which became, for a time, the biggest-selling drug in the world.

Pharmacology is now using all the tools and knowledge of molecular biology to develop new drugs based on new insights into disease. These insights are often derived from studying cell function at a molecular level. Proving the effectiveness and safety of such drugs, however, still depends on studies involving experimental animals, individual patients and populations of patients. Thus one of the fascinations of pharmacology is how it spans the spectrum from molecules to the patient. When a chemical is found to affect a particular cellular function and thereby seems to have therapeutical potential, workers from many scientific disciplines including chemists, biochemists, physiologists, pharmacologists and clinicians must cooperate to investigate and develop that drug or a related compound.

Continued evolution of the drug development process

Drugs save lives and improve the quality of life for millions of people on a global scale. It has been estimated that drug

9

treatments have added 3–5 years to average life expectancy, and have revolutionized the treatment of many different diseases. However, today's pharmacologists are faced with the formidable task of finding novel drugs for the treatment of chronic diseases that pose significant health problems, such as cystic fibrosis, Alzheimer's disease, stroke, and acquired immunodeficiency syndrome (AIDS). Furthermore, although there are effective medications available for treatment of many diseases caused by micro-organisms, resistant strains of such organisms are developing all the time. There is, therefore, a continual need to develop even better drugs to treat infection.

It is estimated that, on average, 7–10 years are required to develop a new drug, from the first identification of a novel lead chemical compound through to the successful use in patients of a more effective chemical analog of the original pharmacophore, at a cost of US$250 million or more. As pharmacologists are involved in nearly every stage of this development process, pharmacology is an important branch of modern science.

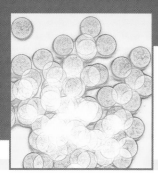

Chapter 2

Drug Names and Drug Classification Systems

INTRODUCTION

In this chapter the procedures used to name drugs, and those used to classify them, are discussed. There is always a need to name drugs unambiguously and to classify them according to a limited set of criteria, but unfortunately current methods are not especially systematic, nor scientific.

Drugs have to be named

Unfortunately any one drug can have many names. Thus a drug can have exact or abbreviated chemical names, official names and brand (commercial) names. The rules of chemical nomenclature laid down by IUPAC (International Union of Pure and Applied Chemistry) allow for the exact chemical description of a drug, but such systematic chemical names are very complex and hard to remember. Abbreviated chemical names are easier to use, but much less exact.

All new drugs intended for therapeutic use are given official (generic) names, but the different national committees for this purpose can give different official names to the same drug, although this happens less and less. Manufacturers (pharmaceutical companies) use brand names to describe their drugs. There can be more than one brand name for the same drug adding greatly to possible confusion. Currently the official (generic) name for a drug is usually suggested by the manufacturer, and often accepted by the appropriate national or international committee. If such committees act wisely, the generic name for a drug gives clues about the use or structure of the drug, and therefore contains elements of classification.

Drugs have to be classified

While the naming of a drug raises difficulties, classification is much more complex. There are many ways to classify drugs. They can be classified on the basis of chemical structure, mechanism of action, and/or effects produced. Classification is important since it gives order and structure to a science. Many sciences (e.g. chemistry, biochemistry, botany) have explicit universal rules for both classification and nomenclature. In pharmacology the attempt to develop a universal classification system continues, but it is by no means complete and thus the classification systems currently used in pharmacology are far from universal. There are many reasons for this. For example, pharmacology has been a recognized independent scientific discipline for over 100 years but there are still disagreements

Main factors for classifying drugs

- Pharmacotherapeutic actions (may be multiple)
- Pharmacologic actions (may be multiple)
- Molecular actions (both site and mechanism)
- Other factors (source and chemistry)

about the nature of pharmacology. Current methods of classification are often a confusion of systems, procedures, names, and implications. As a result the pharmacology student has to become familiar with extensive lists of drugs and their classifications, some of which may be contradictory and confusing. Existing schemes of drug classification are reviewed and discussed in this chapter.

WHAT IS A DRUG?

The first hurdle is to define a drug (see also Chapter 1):
- Webster's Dictionary defines a drug as 'a substance intended for use in the diagnosis, cure, mitigation, treatment, or prevention of disease.'
- Collins Dictionary gives the definition: 'any synthetic or natural chemical substance used in the treatment, prevention or diagnosis of disease,' and the Oxford Dictionary has a similar definition.

However defined, many chemically pure or impure substances are used by humans to produce changes in their own pathophysiology, or physiology for therapeutic or recreational use, or are given to other animals. Synonyms for drug include medicine, agent, compound, pharmacologic tool:
- 'Medicines,' originally plant or animal substances used to treat diseases (i.e. *materia medica*), are now therapeutically useful drugs.
- 'Agent' is often used as a collective noun for drugs of the same class, e.g., antitubercular, antihypertensive agents.
- 'Compound' denotes a chemical used for pharmacologic purposes, or a prototype drug, but not necessarily a therapeutic agent.
- 'Pharmacologic tool' means a pharmacologically active chemical or drug used for experimental purposes.
- 'Substances of abuse' are chemicals or pharmacotherapeutic drugs used for other than therapeutic purposes.

DRUG NAMES

As indicated above, a drug can have a variety of names. All drugs have at least two nonchemical names, an officially approved (generic) name, and a commercial (brand) name. While the generic name for a drug is often universal nowadays, the same drug can have many brand names, enforced by copyright laws worldwide. Generic names are not necessarily euphonious, but often have common roots and endings that provide clues as to pharmacotherapeutic use, or chemical class. Brand names are usually more catchy, euphonious and easier to remember, but contain little information.

All drugs available on prescription, and many over-the-counter nonherbal drugs, have a generic name. This name is the one which appears in official national pharmacopeias. Pharmacopeias were originally published as source books for *materia medica* (medical materials) and indicated the animal or plant source of individual drugs, manner of extraction, and a chemical or bioassay for determining the concentration of biologic activity. Since most of today's drugs are available in a pure form, modern pharmacopeias are concerned principally with pure generic drugs. Examples of variations in generic names include norepinephrine or levarterenol in the US and World Health Organization (WHO) versus noradrenaline in Europe and the UK; furosemide in the US versus frusemide in the UK, and cromolyn in the US versus cromoglycate in the UK.

There is greater harmonization today between the European Union, Japan, and the US in choosing generic names, and recent years have seen the increasing use of common roots and name endings consistent with classification. Examples include the endings:

- 'olol' for many β adrenoceptor antagonists.
- 'dipine' for Ca^{2+} channel blockers which chemically are dihydropyridines.
- 'tilide' for blockers of the delayed rectifier K^+ channel.

Examples of such roots and word endings can be found in Fig. 2.1.

▪ The generic name should be used in biomedical science and by physicians

When writing orders for drug treatment or prescriptions, use of the generic name causes less confusion and lessens the chance of error. In many countries use of the generic name in a prescription gives the dispensing pharmacist the right to dispense the cheapest form of the drug. Generic names must be used in scientific publications; it is the generic name that is the scientific and approved name. Although brand names are often easier to remember, generic names should be used wherever possible.

▪ In the commercial world, brand names for drugs will never follow a consistent pattern

A potential drug discovered by a pharmaceutical company research team is patented at some time during the discovery and development process. Depending on the country of patenting, this protection (which involves the right to be the

Common endings to official names which indicate the pharmacologic classification of a drug		
Ending	**Classification**	**Prototype for class**
-olol	β adrenoceptor blocking drug	Propranolol
-caine	Local anesthetic	Cocaine, procaine
-dipine	Calcium channel blocker of the dihydropyridine type	Nifedipine
-tidine	H_2 histamine receptor antagonist	Cimetidine
-prazole	Proton pump inhibitor	Omeprazole
-quine	Antimalarial drugs	Chloroquine
-ane	Halogenated hydrocarbon general anesthetics	Halothane
-zosin	α adrenoceptor blockers (not all)	Prazosin
-profen	One class of nonsteroidal anti-inflammatory drugs (NSAIDs)	Ibuprofen
-clovir	Antiviral (herpes)drugs	Acyclovir
-mycin	Macrolide/aminoglycoside antibiotics	Erythromycin/ streptomycin
-cycline	Teracycline-derived broad spectrum antibiotics	Tetracycline
-ium	Competitive neuromuscular blockers	Decamethonium (but the true pharmacologic protoype is *d*-tubocurarine)
-zolam, -zepam	Benzodiazepine sedatives	Diazepam

Fig. 2.1 Examples of common endings to official names which indicate the pharmacologic classification of a drug. There are no specific rules for such endings and so there are exceptions for particular drugs within a class. Therefore, such endings should be used only for guidance, and are not substitutes for proper research into a drug. It has to be remembered that although drugs may belong to a common classification, they can have very different pharmacologic, pharmacotherapeutic, and pharmacokinetic actions.

sole seller of the drug) will last for a number of years (e.g. 20 years). Drugs still under patent are usually marketed by the patenting manufacturer and will usually have one generic name and one brand name. However, once a patent expires, the generic name remains but brand names proliferate as different manufacturers become free to market the drug. Thus, there are many brands of acetylsalicylic acid, but only one Aspirin. The creation of brand names is one of the skills of marketing, and

Drug names

- The generic name for a drug should be used, if possible
- The existence of multiple brand names is confusing
- Generic names can vary between countries
- The generic name may provide a clue to the pharmacotherapeutic action and/or pharmacotherapeutic classification

pharmaceutical companies go to great lengths to find euphonious and catchy names for their drugs.

The official drug naming process generally proceeds as follows. A synthetic drug developed by a pharmaceutical company is first synthesized as a chemical compound with a code name, commonly letters and a number. The letters usually, but not in all cases, indicate the pharmaceutical company concerned. The number is sometimes just a numeric code, starting at one and often exceeding one million, or it may reflect somewhat more opaque procedures. There are no universal rules for compound numbering. The vast majority of coded compounds never become drugs and so generic names are only given when a compound is considered to have the potential to be a commercially viable drug. The company usually suggests generic names but such suggestions require approval and ratification by the appropriate national or international nomenclature committee. Nowadays, generic drug names use common root and group names to identify common pharmacologic actions.

DRUG CLASSIFICATION SYSTEMS

There are a number of ways of classifying drugs.

These approaches have arisen historically, and each has a different basis. It is difficult to decide which classification system to use, under what conditions. However classification systems for drugs are not exclusive, or even hierarchical. Thus, any one drug can be placed in a number of classes. For example, atropine can be classified as:

- A nonselective competitive antagonist at muscarinic receptors, i.e. a muscarinic antagonist on the basis of its molecular action.
- A parasympathetic antagonist, on the basis of its actions on the autonomic nervous system.
- An atropinic drug, as the prototype drug of its type.
- An antiulcer drug, because of its pharmacotherapeutic use in the treatment of peptic ulcer.
- A belladonna alkaloid, a naturally occurring drug from the plant, *Atropa belladonna*. (Extracts of *Atropa* were applied to eyes in medieval times to widen the iris in an attempt to beautify, thus *bella donna* or beautiful lady).

In the above examples the different classification systems provide information about atropine's source, chemical nature, pharmacologic actions, molecular mechanism of action, and pharmacotherapeutic use. Even new drugs are still classified in this complex manner, and not by means of a universal system, although IUPHAR (International Union of Pharmacology) and

WHO are currently attempting to provide universal drug classification systems.

The following is an attempt to summarize the present classification systems for drugs, which has some hierarchical features:

- Pharmacotherapeutic class refers to the clinical condition for which a drug is used. 'Pharmacotherapeutic' encompasses therapeutic actions or uses, whereas pharmacologic actions are not necessarily therapeutic.
- Pharmacologic class is based on a drug's mechanism of action. It also includes the type of pharmacologic action produced by the system which is responding to the drug, e.g. excitation, inhibition, block, agonism, antagonism, etc.
- Molecular mechanism of action is a subset of pharmacologic action. However, since this concerns how a drug interacts with its target molecule, it is a class in its own right.
- Chemical nature or source.

According to the above system, atropine would be classified as:

- An antimuscarinic (for its common spasmolytic and antiulcer actions) as a result of its pharmacotherapeutic actions.
- A muscarinic blocker, for its effects on cells and physiological processes.
- A competitive antagonist at M_1, M_2, and M_3 receptors, for its molecular mechanism of action.
- Solanaceous (from the plant family Solanaceae—potato, tobacco, deadly nightshade) or atropinic alkaloid, for its chemical nature and biological sources.

A systematic approach to classification would rely upon agreed definitions of drug actions, these definitions being selective, exclusive, precise, and clear-cut, in both pharmacotherapeutic and pharmacologic terms. These prerequisites are rarely met, either in medicine or pharmacology.

Pharmacotherapeutic classification

Pharmacotherapeutic classification can be difficult since the classification of disease is only precise if the pathology is understood, but not otherwise.

Pharmacotherapeutic classifications can be precise

Pharmacotherapeutic classifications can be broad as in antiviral, antibacterial and anticancer, or restrictive, as with neuromuscular blockers. The latter are used almost exclusively for producing skeletal muscle relaxation during surgery.

As an example of how classification by disease can be unambiguous, consider tuberculosis. In this disease, the causative organism is known (*Mycobacterium tuberculi*), well understood, and there is no confusion arising from the many possible clinical presentations of this infection. Thus, the classification of a drug as an antitubercular drug is appropriate for one used to treat such infections, and is inherently useful.

Pharmacotherapeutic classifications can be inconsistent and imprecise

On the other hand, the disease hypertension is only characterized by a blood pressure high relative to arbitrary normal levels. Some of the causes of hypertension are known, but most are not. As a result, the term 'essential hypertension' is used and so the classification 'antihypertensive drug' reveals only that a drug is, or has been, used to lower blood pressure.

Drug classification based on pharmacotherapeutic use may reveal little about the other actions (pharmacotherapeutic or otherwise) of a drug. Thus it is wrong to assume that drugs within a common pharmacotherapeutic classification share a common mechanism of action, or share the same adverse effects. However, in some cases drugs in the same pharmacotherapeutic class share similar pharmacologic and molecular mechanisms of action, but their effectiveness, toxicity, and adverse effects can be very different.

As indicated above, the major problem with pharmacotherapeutic classifications is imprecision because they are based on broad disease classes. A further example of imprecision is the pharmacotherapeutic classification 'antiarrhythmic' for a drug used to treat arrhythmias (disorders of heart rhythm). Disorders of heart rhythm have different anatomical locations, rates, mechanisms, and outcomes. Thus, 'antiarrhythmic' only classifies a drug as having been used to treat an arrhythmia, either clinically or experimentally, and implies nothing else about the drug.

From the above examples, it appears that pharmacotherapeutic classification might be improved by subclassification. For example, the general classification, antiviral, is useful but a subclassification, based upon the type of virus, is much more helpful. Subclassification is particularly useful for antibacterial and antiparasitic drugs, where a hierarchy of pharmacotherapeutic classification is useful.

The only inference that can be drawn from the pharmacotherapeutic classification of a drug is that the drug has been used, or is currently in use, for the disease condition indicated. It is clear that the pharmacology student must be careful in drawing conclusions from pharmacotherapeutic classifications. In addition, a knowledge of disease conditions, their classification and subclassification, is vital for appropriate use of pharmacotherapeutic classifications.

Pharmacologic classification

The word pharmacologic covers all actions of a drug other than the purely chemical. Pharmacologic actions are described by three elements: location, nature and type. Considering the first two elements, location encompasses all the levels of the body outlined below, and the nature of pharmacologic action refers to the overall actions of groups of drugs, such as anesthetic, antibiotic, antiarrhythmic, etc. Thus pharmacologic is an imprecise word covering actions from the molecular to those involving the whole organism, and pharmacotherapeutic actions. In the following, we consider pharmacologic actions as all those which are not pharmacotherapeutic, molecular or chemical.

Pharmacologic actions may be physiologic, as with 'sympathomimetic' drugs which mimic the effects of stimulation of the sympathetic nervous system, or the actions may be related directly to the receptor with which a drug interacts (see Chapter 3). For example, some sympathomimetic drugs are α adrenoceptor agonists because they activate α adrenoceptors to produce sympathomimetic actions, thereby pro-

ducing difficulties in differentiating between pharmacologic actions in general, and molecular actions in particular.

As will be discussed in full in Chapter 3, a useful hierarchy for considering the pharmacologic actions of a drug comprises its actions on:
- The whole body.
- Body systems (as in cardiovascular, renal, central nervous, and pulmonary).
- Body organs (as with the heart, liver, and kidney).
- Cells (as with cardiac, hepatic, and renal cells).
- Molecular targets (as with receptors, channels, and enzymes).

Each level can be considered as a different locus for drug action with a different description of mechanism of action.

Pharmacologic classification of a drug should include the type of action produced

It is obviously important to classify a drug on the basis of both the site at which the drug acts, and the type of action it produces. Pharmacology abounds with words used to describe drug actions and these are described in more detail in Chapter 3, which is concerned with the mechanisms of drug action. A short discussion is, however, included here with regard to drug classification.

Words used to describe the different types of pharmacologic action often come in pairs: inhibitor and activator, antagonist and agonist, depressant and excitant, direct and indirect. In these examples, each member of the pair is the antithesis of the other. Such terms help to classify the type of pharmacologic action produced by a drug, but are themselves often poorly defined. Furthermore, they are often everyday words, and thus liable to be used loosely.
- 'Inhibitor' is used for drugs that prevent or reduce physiologic, biochemical, or pharmacologic activity. Inhibition can be considered as happening at the level of: enzymes, neuronal, hormonal, and autacoid systems; of receptors; of ion channels, and even cell membranes, as well as organs or whole bodies.
- 'Activators' are opposite in action to inhibitors.

Thus almost any drug can be classified as being either an inhibitor, or an activator. One disadvantage is that inhibition in one situation may be activation in another. It is therefore possible to produce excitation at one site by inhibiting at another.

In a sense antagonist and agonist are related, in that an antagonist prevents an agonist from having its action since agonists are drugs which 'agonize' and thereby produce an action. If the terms are used precisely, both the agonist and antagonist should act on the same receptor. However the word antagonist can also be used loosely, as with calcium antagonist for a drug which blocks calcium channels.

The terms suppressant and excitant are less precise, and describe drugs which respectively decrease and increase activity in a body system, particularly the central nervous system.

Some responses to drugs are produced by a direct action on the tissue concerned, whereas others are produced indirectly, or secondarily to a direct action elsewhere. For example drugs can relax vascular smooth muscle by a direct action on the muscle itself, or secondarily via the release of a directly acting relaxant, or by inhibiting release or action of a contracting substance. Other examples include the secondary negative effects of beta blockers (e.g. propranolol) on cardiac contractility, by virtue of preventing the actions of the sympathetic system on the heart. Sympathomimetic amines directly increase heart rate via actions on the pacemaker cells controlling heart rate, whereas atropine can increase heart rate because, as a muscarinic antagonist, it antagonizes the action of parasympathetic nerves (via release of acetylcholine) on the heart.

Classification based upon the nature of pharmacologic actions

The nature of pharmacologic actions can be ill-defined. For example, anesthetic drugs by definition induce anesthesia or 'lack of feeling.' Both local and general anesthetic drugs achieve this, but at different sites and by different mechanisms. The ambiguity can be overcome by a subclassification into local and general anesthetics, but such subclassifications are not always possible. Furthermore, pharmacologic terms often have widely different meanings in different contexts and to different researchers.

Pharmacologic classifications can be precise

It is possible to obtain precise classifications if attention is paid to the above factors. For example, a drug that relaxes vascular smooth muscle can be classified pharmacologically as a smooth muscle relaxant, a vasodilator, and hypotensive. These classifications are related because arteriolar smooth muscle relaxation causes vasodilation and this, in the presence of a maintained cardiac output, lowers blood pressure (i.e. produces hypotension). The precision can, however, be further improved because vasodilation describes smooth muscle relaxation in arterioles and arteries, while venodilation refers to dilation of veins.

Classification based upon molecular action

If the exact biochemical, physiologic and pathologic role of one of the body's component biomolecules was understood, and a drug was known to interact with this molecule in a known manner, it would be possible to predict the pharmacologic and pharmacotherapeutic actions of that drug. The drug could then be unambiguously classified on the basis of the body molecule with which it interacted (bound to) and the type of interaction. Unfortunately this is not the case. As a result classification based upon the molecular action of a drug is still in its infancy and has to be supplemented by other classification systems.

The molecular method for drug classification depends on two factors:
- The target body molecule with which a drug interacts (e.g. receptor, enzyme).
- The nature of the binding between drug and the target molecule.

As discussed in more detail in Chapter 3, there are many molecular targets (receptors) at which drugs act to produce

pharmacotherapeutic and pharmacologic actions. These targets are mostly protein in nature and include receptors for hormones and neurotransmitters, ion channels, enzymes, and cell membrane transporter molecules. In many cases the chemical nature of such molecules is known, as are the sites at which drugs interact (e.g. the hydrolytic site on acetylcholinesterase, recognition site on β adrenoceptors).

Classification on the basis of molecular action is easy if a drug interacts with known receptors

There are many different receptors for neurotransmitters and hormones with which drugs interact, and by which drug actions can be classified. Such receptors are subdivided into different families, on the basis of their interaction with a related family of drugs, genetic and molecular structure, and the second-messenger mechanism linking them to cell responses. Other are classified on the basis of the endogenous molecules (e.g. neurotransmitter, hormone, autacoid) with which they interact. Thus, for example, there are two subfamilies of adrenoceptors for the neurotransmitter norepinephrine: α and β. These are further subdivided into subtypes (e.g., α_1, α_2, β_1, β_2). Similarly, ion channels are being identified together with their subtypes, while the structure of many enzymes is also known.

Drugs bind to a large number of molecular targets (receptors) using a limited number of mechanisms

A drug interaction with a molecular target almost invariably involves the drug selectively binding to a particular binding site. Binding may activate the target, inactivate it, or prevent it being activated by other drugs. With hormonal and neurotransmitter receptors, the terms agonist, partial agonist, and inverse agonist, respectively (see Chapter 3), are used for the three possibilities. They provide a good basis for classification. Subclassifications are possible, as with antagonists which act by different mechanisms, i.e. competitive, noncompetitive, reversible, or irreversible.

Analogous types of action occur with drugs which act on enzymes. Comparatively few drugs act on enzymes as substrates, but many drugs behave as enzyme inhibitors by binding to the active site to deny the endogenous substrate access to it (competitive inhibition). Inhibition can be competitive, noncompetitive, reversible, or irreversible. Classic examples are:
- Reversibly acting drugs such as neostigmine, which acts on the enzyme to inhibit acetylcholinesterase.
- Irreversible inhibitors such as the organophosphates (e.g. parathion), which covalently bind to acetylcholinesterase and thereby inhibit the enzyme.

Some drugs are classified as ion channel drugs

Some drugs act on ion channels (sites of selective ionic permeability) in the cell membrane to open these channels while other drugs prevent their opening. Such 'channel' drugs can be classified according to the channel type on which they act. The best-known ion channels are those for Na^+, K^+, and Ca^{2+}. Various subtypes of the basic channel type are recognized on the basis of their molecular structure and properties (e.g.

responsiveness to voltage or drugs). Drugs that inhibit opening are generally classified as ion channel blockers, or more loosely as antagonist. For example, verapamil, a Ca^{2+} channel blocker, is also referred to as a Ca^{2+} antagonist because at the physiologic level it antagonizes the actions of Ca^{2+}. The latter classification is, however, less acceptable since it confuses the mechanism of action, particularly as it has not been clearly established just how verapamil antagonism occurs in terms of binding to a receptor in the channel, probably a physiologically specific site. The term 'blocker' is probably more satisfactory in that it encompasses the idea that such drugs may block channels by physically occupying the pore in the channel through which ions travel. It is equally possible that such drugs disturb channel function by binding at a receptor site remote from the pore and allosterically disrupt channel function.

Drugs that open channels are known as channel activators or channel agonists. The neurotransmitter γ-aminobutyric acid (GABA) is a true agonist since it binds to a specific receptor on Cl^- channels and, in binding, opens the channel. Exogenous drugs are also capable of opening ion channels (e.g. K^+ channel openers such as cromakalim). These drugs bind to the adenosine triphosphate (ATP)-dependent K^+ channel, which opens in response to the binding, leading to vascular smooth muscle relaxation and blood vessel vasodilation.

Source (plant or animal) and chemical classifications of drugs

Although most drugs are totally synthetic in origin, discovered as a result of systematic and rational drug design, a few are still obtained from natural sources. The main natural source for drugs is the botanic world. When the source of a drug is the natural world both it, and related drugs, are often classified according to the species, genus, or family of the source. If such a drug is a small molecule containing nitrogen it is further known as an alkaloid. Alternatively, if the molecule contains amino acids it is often a polypeptide. Nature makes good use of the C17 hydrocarbon ring, the steroid ring found in cholesterol, and some of these steroids are the source of drugs. Both the source and chemistry of drugs of natural origin may be combined in classifying a drug, e.g. the digitalis glycosides, belladonna alkaloids. Digitalis glycosides are found in plants of the *Digitalis* genus (e.g. *Digitalis purpurea*), are chemically glycosides, and are therefore classified as digitalis glycosides, even when found in other species. Weak bases found in plants of the *Atropa* species are called belladonna alkaloids. One of these belladonna alkaloids, atropine, is named after the genus.

Classifications based on the chemical nature or source

Drugs can be classified on the basis of their chemistry. The chemical identity of most drugs is known with absolute

certainty and can be named and described explicitly according to the rules of IUPAC. By such rules atropine is endo(±)-a-(hydroxymethyl)benzeneacetic acid 8-methyl-8-azobicyclo [3.2.1.]oct-3-yl ester, and norepinephrine is 4-(2-amino-1-hydroxyethyl)-1,2-benzenediol. Such a name is not a classification, nor even a useful name, and thus exact chemical names are almost never used either to classify or name a drug. Instead, a variety of shorthand chemical names are used. This has resulted in a lack of consistency in naming drugs chemically, although the generic name often indicates a component chemical group.

A chemical group can be used to classify drugs which share a basic chemical structure and have similar pharmacologic profiles, for example, catecholamines include the neurotransmitters norepinephrine and dopamine, and the hormone epinephrine.

The term 'catechol' is the chemical description of a benzene ring containing two hydroxyl groups in the meta and para positions. Many catechols occur naturally, or have been synthesized, but few have biologic activity. The term 'amine' refers to their nitrogen group. Catecholamines are therefore molecules that chemically have a catechol moiety and an amine group, and this is a chemical description without biologic implications, but a pharmacologist uses the term to classify those molecules that have biologic activity or are metabolically related to the pharmacologically active catecholamines.

▪ *Many group names are used for classification according to chemistry*

Commonly used examples of chemically related group names include:

- Steroids. Many drugs contain a steroid group; some occur endogenously as hormones, while others are exogenous and synthetic in origin. Glucocorticosteroids, mineralocorticosteroids, sex hormones, and anabolic steroids are all steroids.
- Barbiturates (from barbituric acid).
- Benzodiazepines.
- Dihydropyridines.

Such groupings are useful classifiers both for official drugs, and for understanding the actions of chemically related drugs.

▪ *Care and experience are needed when inferring drug actions from their name or classification*

The above discussion illustrates that great care must be exercised in trying to make inferences from a drug's name or its classification. Such is the current state of naming and classifying drugs that erroneous conclusions can easily be drawn. Thus students of pharmacology have to acquire considerable knowledge and experience before they can navigate through current drug naming and classification systems.

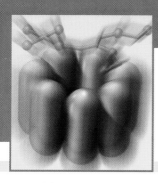

Chapter 3

General Principles of Drug Action

WHAT DOES A DRUG DO AND HOW DOES IT DO IT?

The purpose of this chapter is to illustrate how the mechanism of action of a drug may be understood by integrating the effects that take place at the molecular, cellular, tissue and system levels of biological function. Consequently, this chapter is subdivided according to these component processes, and explains how they are integrated. The main emphasis of the chapter is on drug actions at molecular and cellular levels since the specific actions of drugs on tissue and body systems are considered in each of the systems-based chapters.

Mechanism of action of drugs

Drugs act four different levels:

- **Molecular:** molecules are the immediate targets for most drugs.
- **Cellular:** biochemical and other components of cells participate in the process of transduction.
- **Tissue:** the function of heart, skin, lungs, etc. is then altered.
- **System:** the function of the cardiovascular, nervous, gastro-intestinal etc. system is then altered.

In order to understand the actions of a drug, it is necessary to know which molecular targets are affected by the drug, the nature of the effect, the nature of the transduction system (the cellular response), the types of tissue that express the molecular target, and the mechanisms by which the tissue influences the system. In view of this, it is important to consider mechanisms of action of drugs at each of the four levels of complexity.

The mechanisms of drug action at the four different levels can be illustrated using propranolol (a β adrenergic antagonist) as an example

Propranolol is a β adrenergic antagonist used to treat several diseases including angina pectoris, a cardiac condition resulting from localized ischemia (i.e. insufficient blood flow) in the heart:

- At the molecular level propranolol is a competitive and reversible antagonist of the action of epinephrine and norepinephrine on β adrenoceptors.
- At the cellular level, propranolol prevents β adrenergic agonism from elevating intracellular cyclic adenosine monophosphate (cAMP), initiating protein phosphorylation, Ca^{2+} mobilization and oxidative metabolism.
- At the tissue level, propranolol prevents β adrenergic agonism from increasing the contractile force of the heart and heart rate, i.e. it has negative inotropic and negative chronotropic effects.
- At a system level, propranolol improves cardiovascular function. It reduces the heart's β adrenergic responses to sympathetic nervous system activity thereby decreasing the requirements for blood flow in heart tissue. This reduced demand for blood flow is useful if blood supply is limited (by coronary artery disease).

The mechanism of drug action at the four different levels is also illustrated by rifampin, even though this drug acts on bacterial, rather than human tissue

The mechanism of action of any drug can be analyzed in the above manner, even if the drug does not act directly on human tissue in order to produce its beneficial actions. For example, rifampin is an effective drug in the treatment of tuberculosis:

- At the molecular level, rifampin binds to (and blocks the activity of) ribonucleic acid (RNA) polymerase in the mycobacterium responsible for tuberculosis.
- At a cellular level, rifampin inhibits mycobacterial RNA synthesis and thereby kills the mycobacterium.
- At a tissue level, rifampin prevents damage to lung tissue arising as a result of mycobacterial infection.
- At a system level, rifampin prevents the loss of lung function caused by tuberculosis.

Drugs may be classified on the basis of their molecular, cellular, tissue and system actions

Propranolol is always classified at the molecular level as a β adrenoceptor antagonist. However, its classification at the cellular, tissue and system level will depend on the condition that is being treated (e.g. angina versus hypertension).

Responses to a drug can be defined at molecular, cellular, tissue, and system levels

Since the mechanism of action of a drug can be defined at four levels of complexity, the responses to a drug can also be defined in the same manner (Fig. 3.1). Drugs that activate their molecular target are defined as agonists or activators (the exact term depending on the nature of the molecular target; see page 18). Drugs that prevent or inhibit the actions of agonists or activators, or deactivate a molecular target, are defined as antagonists, blockers or inhibitors. The latter do not directly produce a response at the cellular, tissue and system level, but may do so indirectly by virtue of blocking the molecular response to an endogenous or exogenous agonist or activator.

The four levels of drug action and drug classification		
Mechanism	**Definition**	**Response components**
Molecular	Interaction with the drug's molecular target	The drug target (e.g. receptor, ion channel, enzyme, carrier molecule)
Cellular	Transduction	The biochemicals linked to the drug target (e.g. ion channel, enzyme, G proteins)
Tissue	An effect on tissue function	Electrogenesis, contraction, secretion, metabolic activity, proliferation
System	An effect on system function	Integrated systems including linked systems (e.g. nervous system, cardiovascular system)

Fig. 3.1 The four levels of drug action and drug classification.

 Molecular drug targets include:

- Hormone and neurotransmitter receptors
- Enzymes
- Carrier molecules (symporters, or antiporters)
- Ion channels (ligand-gated or voltage-operated)
- Idiosyncratic targets (metal ions, surfactant proteins, gastrointestinal contents)
- Nucleic acids

MOLECULAR ACTIONS OF DRUGS

Characteristics of molecular targets

In order to produce an effect, a drug must first interact with its molecular target. The most common type of molecular target is known as a receptor. Other targets include ion channels, enzymes, and transport molecules. All of these are proteins. Molecular targets have specific characteristics that determine the nature of the responses to drugs: the molecular selectivity of drug action (which is determined by the similarity or divergence of structure of different molecular targets); the tissue selectivity of drug responses (in accordance with the distribution of the molecular target throughout the body); and the rapidity and persistence of the manifestation of cellular and tissue responses.

Receptors

A receptor is usually a protein molecular target for a drug (Fig. 3.2)

Hormone and neurotransmitter receptors differ from other types of molecular target because they usually do not have a definable biologic function like that of an enzyme (catalysis of a biochemical reaction) or an ion channel (movement of an

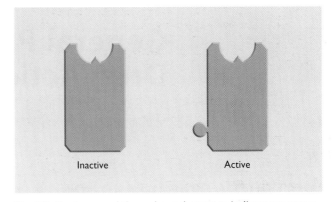

Inactive   Active

Fig. 3.2 The icon used throughout the text to indicate receptors.

ion). These receptors function simply to provide molecular communication between the agonist and the transduction process. Therefore, when activated (by an agonist) a receptor usually initiates a cellular response only when it is linked directly, or indirectly via specialized protein molecules such as guanylyl (G) nucleotide-binding proteins, to another cellular component such as an ion channel or enzyme. There are certain exceptions to this generalization that are discussed later.

Agonism is the molecular response to an agonist

Drugs and endogenous substances (hormones and neurotransmitters) that activate receptors are called agonists, and the molecular response is the production of the activated state of the receptor. This initiates the cellular response.

Many receptors have endogenous agonists. These are sometimes known as first messengers. This is because the interaction with their molecular target is the first message of intercellular communication (likewise the molecules that participate in the cellular response are sometimes known as second messengers).

An agonist that fully activates receptors is known as a full agonist (see the description of partial agonism, below, for further details).

In the absence of agonists, most receptors are in a rested state. However, even in the absence of an agonist, a receptor may convert temporarily, on a random basis, to an activated state. This produces a low-level cellular response. In the absence of an agonist, the rested state is favored. In contrast, the presence of an agonist shifts the equilibrium strongly in favor of the activated state.

The mathematical relationship between agonist concentration (A) and response is defined by binding to the receptor (R) with the response resulting from formation of an agonist–receptor complex (AR) that activates the receptor (R*). Therefore $A + R \leftrightarrow AR \leftrightarrow AR^*$. For some receptors, two molecules of agonist have to bind in order to produce activation ($A + A + R \leftrightarrow AAR \leftrightarrow AAR^*$). In contrast, for other receptors the reaction is $A + R + R \leftrightarrow ARR \leftrightarrow ARR^*$, i.e., binding of an agonist promotes the association of two inactive receptors into an activated homodimer. The mathematical basis of this relationship is discussed in more detail in Chapter 5. For all figures in the book, agonists are indicated by an icon (Fig. 3.3).

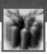

Fig. 3.3 The icon used throughout the text to indicate an agonist. Note, this icon has also been used in the book to indicate drugs that activate molecular targets, such as activators of enzymes.

Definitions

- Affinity is the tendency to bind receptors
- Efficacy is the relationship between receptor occupancy and the ability to initiate a response at the molecular, cellular, tissue or system level
- Intrinsic activity is the capacity of a single drug–receptor complex to evoke a response

Agonism

- Agonism is the production of a molecular and cellular response to an interaction between a drug (agonist) and a receptor that activates the receptor. The intrinsic activity of a full agonist is defined as equal to 1
- Partial agonism occurs when a drug interacts with a receptor to produce an average of less than 1 unit of molecular response. The average molecular intrinsic activity lies between 0 and 1
- Antagonism occurs when a drug interacts with a receptor to inhibit the action of an agonist. The molecular intrinsic activity is 0
- Inverse agonism occurs when a drug interacts with receptor to reduce its resting level of molecular activity. The molecular intrinsic activity is –1
- Partial inverse agonism occurs when a drug interacts with a receptor to reduce the resting level of molecular activity. The molecular intrinsic activity lies between 0 and –1

In most cells the maximum cellular response to an agonist is achieved when only a small proportion of its receptors are occupied. In other words, the number of receptors is usually much higher than that necessary for obtaining a maximum cellular response. The excess of receptors is usually referred to as 'spare receptors,' and is important because spare receptors increase the sensitivity of the cell to small changes in the concentration of agonist (see Chapter 5).

Partial agonism is the inefficient activation of a receptor resulting in an inefficient molecular and cellular response

A drug that activates a receptor in a relatively inefficient manner is a partial agonist. Conceptually, a partial agonist is a drug for which each interaction between it and the receptor produces a less than maximal molecular response, or randomly produces either a molecular response, or no response (a failed molecular response). In either case, the maximum cellular response to the partial agonist is less than the maximum cellular response to a full agonist acting on the same receptor, provided that there are no spare receptors. Partial agonists are required to interact with a large proportion of the receptor pool to produce a maximum cellular response, leaving only a small reserve of receptors, or none at all. If there are many spare receptors, it is possible for a partial agonist to elicit a maximum cellular response, although the partial agonist is said to have less efficacy than a full agonist in that it requires greater occupancy to elicit a maximal cellular response (see Chapter 5).

Inverse agonism is the initiation of an apparent cellular response by the prevention of spontaneous activation of a receptor

The molecular response to an inverse agonist is either:
- Deactivation of the activated receptor.
- Stabilization of receptors in an inactive conformation.

This is modeled as R ↔ R* and I + R* ↔ IR where R* is the activated state and I is an inverse agonist.

Antagonism is the prevention of the action of an agonist

Many drugs bind to a receptor and produce a drug–receptor complex that elicits no cellular response. Moreover, the occupancy of the receptor by the antagonist either prevents an agonist from binding, or prevents the agonist from evoking a molecular response when it binds to the receptor. Thus, antagonism can result from a variety of different molecular mechanisms. Mathematical descriptions of the effects of different types of antagonists are described in Chapter 5. Briefly, antagonism can be produced by:

- Binding of an antagonist to the same site on the receptor normally occupied by the agonist. The binding of the antagonist denies the agonist occupancy of the site (competitive antagonism).
- Binding of an antagonist to a site different from that normally occupied by the agonist (an allosteric site), resulting in a conformational change of the binding site for the agonist. This either prevents the agonist from binding, or prevents the bound agonist from eliciting a molecular response.

An antagonist that binds to its site only when the agonist is not bound, is called a noncompetitive antagonist. If the antagonist can bind to its site even when an agonist is bound, it is called an uncompetitive antagonist. The 'site' referred to here is often called a ligand binding site (where 'ligand' means agonist, antagonist, partial agonist, etc.).

Since antagonist binding can be reversible or irreversible, there are at least six possible types of antagonism, as shown in Fig. 3.4. The effects that an antagonist can have on the responses to an agonist are described mathematically in Chapter 5. Throughout the text antagonists will be shown using the icon in Fig. 3.5.

Physiologic antagonism is not a molecular action of an antagonist

Physiologic (or 'functional') antagonism is a term that is commonly used but misleading. In fact it describes the ability of an agonist (rather than an antagonist) to inhibit the response to a second agonist via activation of different receptors that are physically separate. This may occur if the receptors for the two agonists are linked to the same cellular response components

Six possible types of antagonism			
	Competitive	Noncompetitive	Uncompetitive
Reversible	✓	✓	✓
Irreversible	✓	✓	✓

Fig. 3.4 Six possible types of antagonism.

Fig. 3.5 The icon used throughout the text to indicate an antagonist. Note that this icon has also been used throughout the book to indicate drugs that block the activity of nonreceptor molecular targets, such as enzyme inhibitors.

but affect them differently, or are linked to different cellular response components that give rise to opposite tissue responses. A good example is the interaction between norepinephrine and acetylcholine in arterioles. Norepinephrine causes contraction and acetylcholine causes relaxation. It is obviously not helpful to describe norepinephrine as an acetylcholine antagonist, since one could equally describe acetylcholine as a norepinephrine antagonist, thereby rendering the terms agonist and antagonist interchangeable and, hence, meaningless. We suggest that the term 'antagonist' be used only to describe a drug that can inhibit the molecular response to an agonist, and the term 'functional antagonist' be avoided.

Classification of receptors

Drugs that act on receptors elicit a wide range of tissue and system responses for two reasons. The first is that different receptors are expressed discretely in different tissues. The other is that different types of receptor have very different types of structure and, hence, function. Therefore the cellular responses to receptor activation (transduction) vary considerably according to the structure of the receptor. Based on this there exist four types of receptor, referred to as receptor superfamilies (Fig. 3.6):
- G protein-coupled receptors
- DNA-coupled receptors
- Receptors that possess tyrosine kinase activity ('tyrosine kinase receptors')
- Receptor-operated channels (ROCs)

Tyrosine kinase receptors and ROC are different from the others since they do not require linkage to cellular transduction components to elicit a cellular response when activated by an agonist, meaning that the receptor molecule is more than simply a molecular link between the drug and transduction. A tyrosine kinase receptor is actually a membrane-bound enzyme that is 'switched on' by its agonists. A ROC is actually a specialized ion channel that is structurally distinct from the voltage-operated ion channel (VOC, see page 22) in that it has a highly stereoselective ligand binding site instead of a highly specialized voltage sensor region. In a ROC the ligand binding site and the channel are functionally distinct regions of a single molecule. The ROC is also known as a 'ligand-gated ion

The four receptor superfamilies

- Receptor-operated channel
- G protein-coupled
- Receptors that are enzymes (e.g. tyrosine kinase receptors)
- DNA-coupled receptors

channel.' The classification above acknowledges the conventional approach that refers to tyrosine kinase receptors, and ROCs, as 'receptors.'

G protein-coupled receptors

G proteins are transduction components (see page 22) and are shown as the icon in Fig. 3.7. G protein-coupled receptors are located in cell membranes and are composed of seven transmembrane helices (I–VII) (Fig. 3.8). In the rested state (no agonist present) the receptor is bound to a G protein that holds the receptor in an inactive conformation. The G protein itself is a complex of three subunits (α, β, and γ) and, in the rested state of the receptor, the three G protein subunits are bound together, and guanine nucleotide diphosphate (GDP) is tightly bound to the α subunit of the G protein. Agonist binding to the receptor causes a conformation change in the receptor. This causes a conformation change in the G protein that causes GDP to dissociate from the α subunit. This initiates the sequence of events that constitutes G protein-coupled receptor transduction. This is described fully in the section on transduction (page 23).

Interestingly, responses mediated by G protein-coupled receptors may wane with time, in spite of the continued presence of the agonist. This phenomenon has been called desensitization and is described in Chapter 5.

DNA-coupled receptors

Intracellular receptors that can interact with DNA exist for some molecules such as retinoic acid, corticosteroids, thyroid hormone, and vitamin D. These receptors are mainly composed of nuclear proteins. As a result, agonists have to pass through the cell membranes to reach this type of receptor. For example, steroids enter a cell and bind with a cytoplasmic receptor, which often has an inhibitory molecule bound to it, such as heat shock protein 90 (HSP_{90}). The molecular response is a receptor conformation change that causes dissociation of the receptor from the inhibitory molecule. The cellular responses to activation of DNA receptors are numerous and varied, and are discussed in the section on transduction.

Receptors that possess tyrosine kinase activity ('tyrosine kinase receptors')

Agonist action on tyrosine kinase receptors (Fig. 3.9) is involved in the regulation of growth, cell differentiation, and responses to metabolic stimuli. Endogenous agonists include insulin, epidermal growth factors, and platelet-derived growth factor. Agonists cause the receptor to change conformation and act as a tyrosine kinase enzyme (phosphorylating tyrosine residues in a wide variety of intracellular molecules).

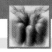

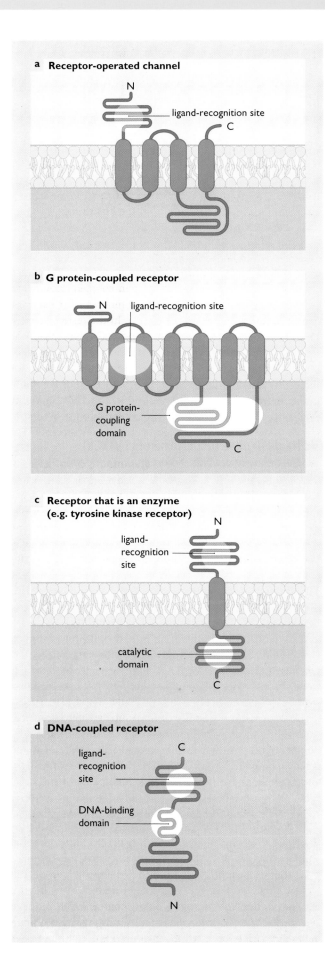

a Receptor-operated channel

b G protein-coupled receptor

c Receptor that is an enzyme (e.g. tyrosine kinase receptor)

d DNA-coupled receptor

Fig. 3.6 Schematic representation of the general structure of the four receptor superfamilies. (a) An extracellular binding domain is coupled to a hydrophobic α helical region of the protein that forms the membrane-spanning domain. Up to five subunits that have this general structure form a complex surrounding a central ion channel. This is best examplified by the nicotinic acetylcholine (ACh) receptor (see Fig. 3.10 for more detail). Typically, this type of receptor mediates the very fast action of neurotransmitters. C is the C terminal, and N the N terminal of the protein. (b) The ligand binding site is found within the α helices and the membrane-spanning domain is connected to an intracellular domain that couples to G proteins. This is a typical receptor structure for many hormones and slower-acting neurotransmitter systems that act via G protein-coupled transduction systems (e.g. ACh acting on muscarinic receptors on smooth muscle). The G protein coupling domain is the part of the receptor that interacts with the α subunit of the G protein to facilitate transduction following binding of an agonist to the binding domain. (c) The receptors for various growth factors and insulin have an extracellular ligand binding site linked directly to an intracellular catalytic domain that has either tyrosine kinase or guanylyl kinase activity when the ligand binding site is occupied by an appropriate agonist. These may be defined as tyrosine kinase receptors that are enzymes, although they are more commonly referred to as tyrosine kinase receptors. (d) The ligand binding site is linked to a DNA-binding domain. It is typified by the receptors for steroid and thyroid hormones. These may be defined as DNA-coupled receptors. (Adapted with permission from *Pharmacology*, 3rd edn, by Rang, Dale, and Ritter, Churchill Livingstone, 1995.)

Receptor-operated channels (ROCs)

The ROC is composed of subunits, each of which has four transmembrane domains. These domains form complexes of varying stoichiometry (Fig. 3.10). There are numerous different types of ROCs. Each possesses, as part of their structure, an extracellular ligand binding site that, when bound to an endogenous ligand (and certain drugs), initiates a conformation change in other parts of the ROC molecule that culminates with the opening of a central ion-selective pore. Passage of ions occurs only when the pore is open (the open 'state'). The molecular configuration of the channel therefore defines the state of the channel. The simplest model for channel behavior has three recognized states. They are:

- Rested (nonconducting, i.e. closed, but openable in response to an appropriate stimulus).
- Activated (open).
- Inactivated (i.e. closed and unable to open in response to what would be an appropriate stimulus for a rested state channel).

Some drugs have a molecular mechanism of action that involves modulation of the transition of the ROC between states (a process known as gating).

The ligand binding site in a ROC is commonly termed the 'receptor' (that operates the 'channel'). This makes the ROC semantically (as well as structurally and functionally distinguishable) from G protein-coupled and DNA-coupled receptors. Throughout this book ROCs are denoted by an icon that is different from those for other receptors, in recognition of this (Fig. 3.11).

It is important to note that the ROC is conventionally described as a 'receptor' as well as a 'channel' and a 'channel with a receptor site.' Thus, the nicotinic cholinergic 'receptor'

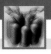

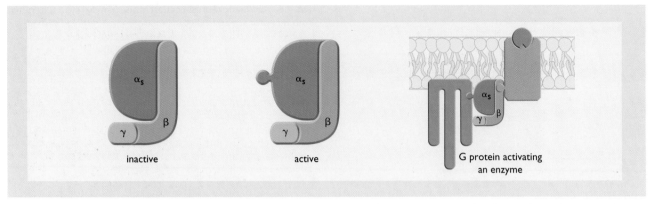

Fig. 3.7 The icon used throughout the text for the G protein in the inactive and active states. Note that the α_s subunit dissociates when the G protein is active (see Fig. 3.22) but, for simplicity, the icon for the active G protein is shown 'intact,' but with an 'appendage' (as for 'active' receptors, see Fig. 3.2). Also shown is the role the G protein plays in linking the receptor to the transduction cascade.

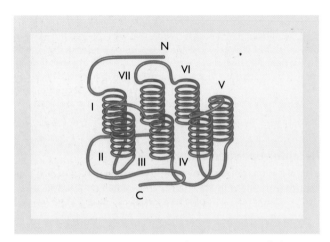

Fig. 3.8 Schematic representation of a G protein-coupled receptor. There are seven transmembrane helices (I–VII).

is actually a ROC (and, to add to the complexity, this ROC actually possesses two ligand binding sites).

In most cases a ROC agonist opens the channel, whereas an antagonist prevents the agonist from opening the channel, and an inverse agonist closes the open channel. ROCs include:

- The nicotinic ROC (activated by acetylcholine).
- The GABA$_A$ ROC.
- The glycine ROC.
- The 5-HT$_3$ ROC (activated by 5-hydroxytryptamine).
- The P$_{2x}$ ROC (activated by adenosine)

The nicotinic receptor is a ROC that exists as a tetramer with its two acetylcholine ligand binding sites on its external lip. Other ROCs show considerable homology with it. When two molecules of acetylcholine bind to the two ligand binding sites, the conformation of the ROC changes so that the channel component opens. This results in a sudden increase in permeability to Na$^+$ and K$^+$ ions which depolarizes the cell. There are several nicotinic ROC subtypes with small differences in composition, structure and tissue distribution. All are activated by acetylcholine, but certain drugs have selectivity for one or other subtype. Some drugs (e.g. hexamethonium) affect ganglionic nicotinic ROCs in preference to the skeletal muscle ROC, or vice versa (e.g. d-tubocurarine).

The GABA$_A$ ROC is a GABA-regulated Cl$^-$ channel with two ligand binding sites, one that binds GABA and another that binds a class of tranquillizer drugs, the benzodiazepines (see Chapter 14 on the nervous system). Agonist and antagonist binding to these sites results in a complex range of possible molecular responses. The GABA$_A$ ROC is found in many places in the central nervous system. Activation of this ROC generally causes hyperpolarization and this inhibits neuronal activity.

Voltage-operated channels (VOCs)

■ *The behavior of VOCs is modulated endogenously by membrane potential (voltage)*

VOCs share many properties in common with ROCs. VOCs, like ROCs are ion channels, but are 'operated' (gated) not by endogenous ligands but by voltage (although this functional distinction is not absolute, since some ROCs have a degree of voltage dependence). If the gating of an ion channel is normally controlled by membrane potential, the channel is classed as a VOC. Endogenous modulation of VOCs by biochemicals is normally only a minor feature of their behavior—most VOCs have no major endogenous modulators equivalent to acetylcholine (in its role as a nicotinic ROC agonist, for example). However, VOCs are the molecular targets for certain drugs that can alter VOC state shifts or VOC voltage-dependence (or simply cause channel block). Throughout this book VOCs are identified by the icon shown in Fig. 3.12.

VOCs constitute a family of molecular targets because of their gating mechanism, and because they all share a specific number of transmembrane domains and extracellular and intracellular components (Fig. 3.13). They are therefore structurally and functionally different from ROCs. A VOC drug target therefore possesses one or more ligand binding sites, a voltage sensor and a gating component. The gating component provides the molecular response, and is influenced by both the voltage sensor and the ligand binding site. The selectivity of VOCs to conduct different ions is determined by specific protein configurations within the channel pore.

■ *The cardiac Na$^+$ channel is an example of a VOC*

The cardiac Na$^+$ channel contains at least two voltage-operated gates that cause the VOC to open and close in response to

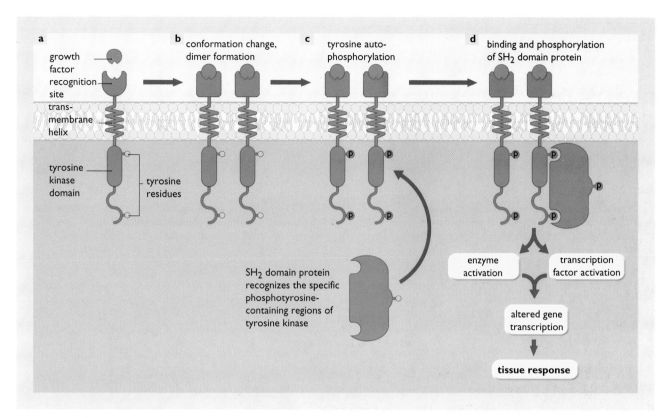

Fig. 3.9 Transduction mechanisms for tyrosine kinase receptors. (a) The binding of a growth factor to its receptor domain (b) leads to conformational changes resulting in dimer formation. This results in autophosphorylation of the tyrosine residues in the tyrosine kinase domain of the receptor (c). The specific phosphotyrosine-containing regions of the tyrosine kinase domain then bind the SH$_2$ domain which results in activation of various intracellular responses leading to the tissue response (d). (Adapted with permission from *Pharmacology*, 3rd edn, by Rang, Dale, and Ritter, Churchill Livingstone, 1995.)

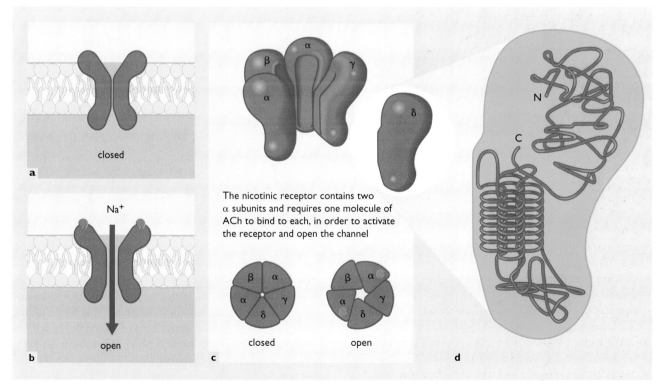

Fig. 3.10 The nicotinic acetylcholine (ACh) receptor-operated channel. The receptor-operated channel consists of five protein subunits (two α, and β, γ, and δ) all of which traverse the membrane and surround a central pore. ACh binds to the α subunits and the two ACh molecules must bind in order to open the channel (c). The complete structure of the δ subunit; a single subunit shown (d). C is the C terminal, and N the N terminal of the protein.

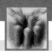

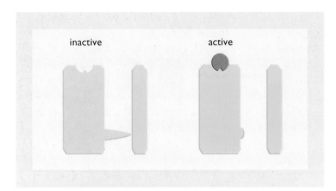

Fig. 3.11 Icon for receptor-operated ion channel. Note that in certain cases the inactive (agonist unbound) state is 'channel open' and the agonist closes the channel.

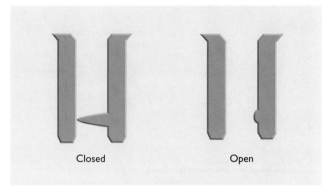

Fig. 3.12 The icon used throughout the text for a voltage-gated ion channel, showing the channel closed and open. Some channels have one and some two or three or more gates.

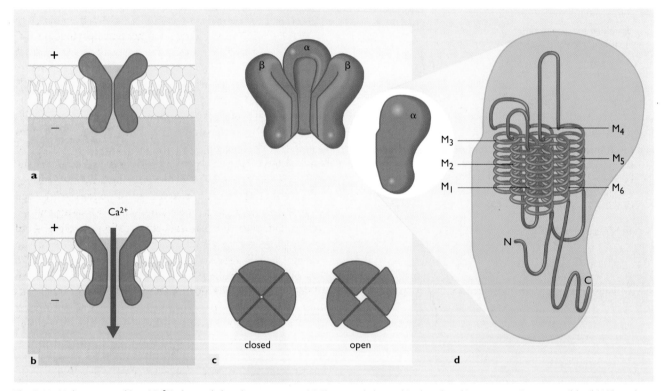

Fig. 3.13 Voltage-gated ion (Ca²⁺) channel showing structure. (a) The rested channel is closed and ion passage is not possible. (b) When the channel opens, ions move down their concentration and charge gradients. (c) Reorientation of two α and β subunits is responsible for channel opening. (d) The complete structure of one of the α subunits. M_1–M_6 refer to subunits of the channel.

changes in membrane potential. This process is known as voltage dependence. Thus:

- One gate (the fast gate) opens and closes quickly (in milliseconds).
- The other (the slow gate) opens and closes slowly (in tens of milliseconds).

During diastole, when the membrane potential is negative, the slow gate is open and the fast gate is closed. The net effect is that the channel is closed (nonconducting) but, because it can be activated, it is said to be 'rested' (Fig. 3.14). However, if the membrane potential becomes more positive, the fast gate opens very quickly, so both gates are open and the channel becomes

conducting and therefore is said to be in the 'activated' state. The slow gate then slowly closes in response to the change in membrane potential. As a result, if the membrane potential stays positive, the channel will, with time, become closed again, and unable to open in response to any stimulus ('inactivated'). Thus, VOCs that inactivate have the property of 'time dependence.'

Inactivation has an important effect. When the membrane potential repolarizes, the fast gate quickly closes while the slow gate requires further time to open. Thus both gates, and therefore the entire channel, are closed. If the membrane is suddenly depolarized (made positive) under these circumstances, the fast gate, which had rapidly opened before, will open again but

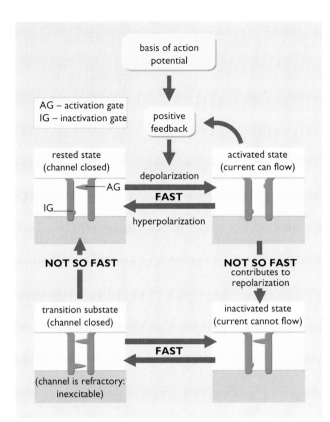

Fig. 3.14 Operation of inward currents in the heart. This is a simplified model showing two gates: one opens on depolarization and closes on hyper (re-)polarization, and the other functions in the converse mode. Transition from the rested to activated state, under the influence of depolarization, is fast and elicits a positive feedback. This is the basis of the action potential. Inactivation is time-dependent and results from a slower closure of a second gate at positive potentials. When the inactivation gate is closed (in the inactivated and transition substates), the cell is inexcitable. This transition contributes to repolarization. Transition from the slow voltage-dependent opening of the inactivation gate determines the refractory period (the period of inexcitability during the action potential).

the slow gate, which had closed during depolarization, will not open again, because it is opened by negative membrane potentials and not by depolarization. The VOC will therefore not open.

If the membrane potential remains negative, the slow gate will open slowly again (characterizing the time dependence of recovery of the channel). A second depolarization will now be able to open the channel again, because the fast gate will open before the slow gate has time to close again.

Drugs whose molecular mechanism involves modulation of VOCs may bind to a ligand binding site which is part of the channel. This ligand binding site can be described as a receptor. Some drugs (notably class I antiarrhythmics, see Chapter 18) can bind to a VOC and change its conformation so that it is fixed in the inactivated state all the while that the drug is bound to it.

The affinity of a drug for its ligand binding site may depend upon the state of the VOC

The apparent affinity of VOC-modulating drugs may depend on membrane potential, which determines the state of the VOC and the rate at which it cycles through its different states. This gives rise to the characteristic voltage and frequency dependence seen for the action of some drugs. There are two possible molecular explanations for such behavior:

- The affinity of the drug for its ligand binding site is determined by the state of the VOC.
- The access of the drug to its ligand binding site is determined by the state of the VOC.

It is possible to model the action of many VOC-modulating drugs by conceptualizing that the ligand binding site for the drug changes its conformation as the VOC changes state, hence changing the VOC's affinity for the drug. The simplest scenario is one in which a drug can bind to any one of the states of the VOC described above, and shown in Fig. 3.14. A drug therefore will bind to its ligand binding site preferentially when the VOC is in the rested state, the activated state, or the inactive state. A drug whose affinity is greatest for the activated state is therefore referred to as an activated state blocker.

If the ligand binding site is on an intracellular or intramembrane part of the VOC, and if the drug reaches this site through the open VOC, the drug will appear to be use-dependent in its action (an effect requiring the opening, or 'use' of the VOC). Highly lipid-soluble drugs do not necessarily need an open VOC to access their ligand binding site since they are able to easily move through the lipid bilayer of the cell membrane. Consequently their actions are less use-dependent.

It is difficult to discriminate between all the possible ligand binding sites within a VOC. As a result, a variety of terms are used to describe the actions of drugs on VOCs. The terms VOC blocker, agonist, antagonist and negative modulator have been used to describe drugs that modulate VOC function. The common terms most conventionally used (e.g. Na$^+$ channel blocker and Ca^{2+} antagonists) do not reflect the exact mechanism by which drugs modulate channel function.

Drug interactions with Na$^+$-selective VOCs (Na$^+$ channels)

Different types of Na$^+$ channels are found in neurons, cardiac muscle and skeletal muscle. They vary slightly in structure and protein composition. Drugs that impair Na$^+$ channel function are conventionally known as Na$^+$ channel blockers and, to a certain extent, can be used as tools in experiments to discriminate between the role of different types of Na$^+$ channel in health and disease. For example, tetrodotoxin (a toxin found in puffer fish, some salamanders, and one type of octopus) can block neuronal and skeletal muscle Na$^+$ channels at concentrations as low as 10 nM, but the concentration needed to block cardiac muscle Na$^+$ channels is 100 times higher.

Three types of drug that block Na$^+$-selective VOCs (Na$^+$ channels) are used therapeutically

Tetrodotoxin, class I antiarrhythmic drugs and local anesthetics block Na$^+$ channels:

- Tetrodotoxin has a molecular selectivity for neuronal channels, but is a highly charged molecule that does not cross the cell membrane.
- Class I antiarrhythmic drugs are used to treat certain forms of cardiac arrhythmia, and bind to an intracellular ligand binding site. There are three types of class I antiarrhythmic (class Ia, Ib, and Ic), defined according to the relative affinities and kinetics of binding and dissociation (called 'unbinding' in this context) with the VOC in its three states (see Chapter 18).
- Local anesthetics such as lidocaine and bupivacaine have little selectivity for the neuronal Na^+ channel, but when administered locally they have a preferential effect on sensory nerves (see Chapter 14 Drugs and the Nervous System). Some local anesthetics bind to the neuronal Na^+ channel at an intracellular ligand binding site, meaning that they must cross the cell membrane to block the channel.

Drug interactions with Ca^{2+}-selective VOCs (Ca^{2+} channels)

At least five types of Ca^{2+} VOC in the plasma membrane (L, T, N, P, Q) allow the entry of Ca^{2+} into cells. These VOCs can be found in many different types of tissue. The best characterized, and the most important (clinically) is the L (long-lasting) type. It is found in cardiac and smooth muscle. It opens during depolarization and then inactivates (more slowly than the Na^+ VOC) by voltage-dependent gating. The L-type VOC is blocked by a variety of clinically important drugs.

■ *There are three chemical classes of clinically important L-type Ca^{2+} channel blockers*

These classes are:
- Benzothiazepine derivatives (e.g. diltiazem).
- Phenethylalkylamines (e.g. verapamil).
- Dihydropyridines (e.g. nifedipine, amlodipine).

All L-type Ca^{2+} channel blockers have selective actions in vascular smooth muscle, but some are more selective than others

The 1,4-dihydropyridines (e.g. nifedipine) show marked selectivity for vascular smooth muscle in comparison with other tissue expressing L channels (notably cardiac tissue). Consequently, low doses cause vascular smooth muscle relaxation (vasodilation) without impairing cardiac output. This is the basis for the use of nifedipine in the treatment of high blood pressure. The main reason for this vascular selectivity is that vascular smooth muscle cells undergo sustained periods of depolarization (the basis of vasoconstriction) whereas cardiac tissue is depolarized relatively transiently (i.e. only during systole). Sustained depolarization maintains a high proportion of L channels in the activated and inactivated states compared with rested state. Nifedipine has relative selectivity for the activated and inactivated state of the L channel, associates (binds) relatively slowly during depolarization and dissociates (unbinds) relatively quickly when tissue repolarizes. Ca^{2+} channel blockers are also known as Ca^{2+} antagonists.

Verapamil (a phenethylalkylamine Ca^{2+} blocker) has different characteristics of L channel binding and as a consequence is less vascular-selective than the 1,4-dihydropyridines, and may block cardiac as well as vascular L channels, especially at high dosage. Unlike nifedipine, verapamil is therefore of value in the treatment of cardiac arrhythmias that involve the AV node (see Chapter 18). This is a good example of how tissue selectivity is determined by subtleties in molecular mechanism of action.

Drug interactions with K^+-selective VOCs (K^+ channels)

The opening of VOCs selective for K^+ results in the generation of outward-going (hyperpolarizing) currents. There are many types of K^+ channel, and they show great diversity in structure, characteristics of opening and closing, affinity for drugs and expression in different organs and tissues. This has major potential therapeutic implications for targeting of drugs for specific tissues and diseases. At least six different 'families' (with major structural differences) of K^+ channels have been identified, and each family contains several members (K^+ channels with minor variations in structure). It is not uncommon for a single type of tissue to express several different K^+ channels (e.g. there are more than 10 different types of K^+ channel in the heart).

The nomenclature for the K^+ currents associated with the different channels is confusing because it is largely determined by the tissue in which the current is observed. For example, the heart has a rapid Ca^{2+}-independent transient outward K^+ current that is called I_{to1}, and neuronal tissue has a K^+ current called I_A, but the channel responsible for both currents is actually the same. The nomenclature for K^+ channels is based upon the gene family, protein structure and voltage characteristics (K_v channels).

■ *K^+ channels and their associated currents vary in their dependence on voltage and time*

There are marked differences in dependence on voltage and time between different K^+ currents. For example, the rapid delayed rectifying K^+ current (I_{Kr}) is activated by depolarization and is time-dependent (it inactivates), whereas the inwardly rectifying K^+ current (I_{K1}) is activated by hyperpolarization and shows no time-dependent inactivation (Figs 3.15, 3.16). In the heart, the mixed properties of the different K^+ channels contribute to the unusual shape of the cardiac action potential.

Other VOCs

Although the majority of the scientific literature on ion channels has focused on cation (Na^+, Ca^{2+}, and K^+) channels, recently it has become more apparent that voltage-gated channels exist for anions, for example, Cl^-. Cl^- channels are found both peripherally and in the central nervous system (CNS). There are a variety of other ion channels with peculiar characteristics. Some are not selective for a single ion. For example, the channel responsible for the 'funny' current (I_f) in the heart allows the passage of both Na^+ and K^+.

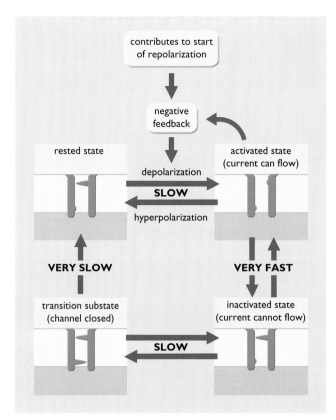

Fig. 3.15 Operation of the rapid delayed rectifier K⁺ current (I_Kr) found in the heart. The channel possesses two gates, and can thus cycle between four states. Depolarization shifts the channel state from rested to activated, allowing hyperpolarizing outward current to flow. This has a negative feedback influence on depolarization, thus contributing to the initiation of re-(hyper-)polarization. Time dependence occurs because of slow voltage-dependent transition to an inactivated state. This cycles, via a substate, to the basal state (rested). The relative speed of the state transitions (kinetics) is shown.

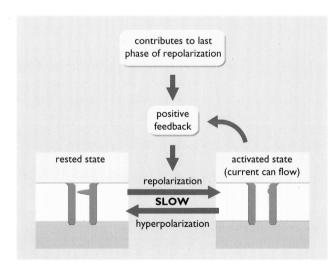

Fig. 3.16 Operation of the inward rectifier K⁺ current (I_K1) found in the heart. The channel possesses one gate and can thus cycle between two states only. Repolarization shifts the channel to the activated state. The K⁺ current that flows causes further repolarization so a positive feedback ensues. There is no inactivation because there is no second gate that closes after repolarization. However, the outward K⁺ current is reduced by intracellular Mg²⁺.

Transporters, symporters, antiporters and pumps

There is constant need for all cells to regulate internal concentrations of ions and molecules such as sugars and nucleic and amino acids. Their passage across cell membranes is facilitated by energy-independent carrier molecules (transporters, symporters and antiporters) and by energy-dependent pumps. All are oriented proteins that have one or more sites that bind weakly with one or more passengers (ion or molecule). This binding alters their conformation from a rested to an activated state. The change in conformation translocates the passenger across the membrane. In the case of pumps, the conformation change converts the protein into an enzyme that normally hydrolyzes ATP (the energy dependence of its activity), and ATP hydrolysis is necessary for the pump to translocate its passenger. Pumps and carriers can be molecular targets for certain drugs. Throughout this book, icons are used for energy-independent carriers (Fig. 3.17) and pumps (Fig. 3.18).

Energy-independent transporters, symporters and antiporters

Energy-independent carriers are called transporters (which move one type of ion or molecule in one direction), symporters

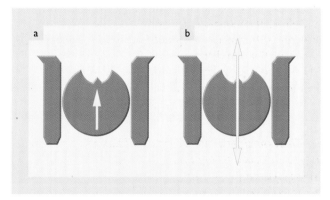

Fig. 3.17 The icon used throughout the text for an energy-independent carrier molecule (transporter, symporter or antiporter). (a) A transporter or symporter (characterized by unidirectional transport) here shown in its inactive state. (b) An antiporter (characterized by two-way transport) here shown in its activated state.

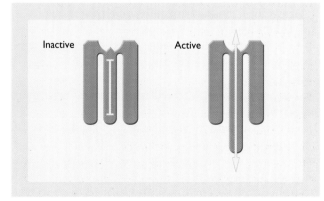

Fig. 3.18 The icon used throughout the text for a pump, showing the inactive and active states.

(which move two or more ions or molecules in one direction), or antiporters (which exchange one or more ions or molecules for one or more other ions or molecules). An example of an antiporter is the Na^+/Ca^{2+} exchanger, which normally extrudes Ca^{2+} out of the cell in exchange for Na^+ (although, in the heart, the direction of exchange may change during the cardiac cycle). The stoichiometry of this exchanger (ratio of ions exchanged) is three Na^+ to one Ca^{2+}. There are no therapeutically useful drugs that directly modulate this target, although digitalis modulates its activity indirectly.

Energy-dependent pumps

Energy-dependent carriers are called pumps. They are actually enzymes that, owing to their location and orientation in cell membranes, have the facility to translocate ions or other molecules through a central pore as a consequence of conformation changes that take place during the enzymatic hydrolysis of ATP (other enzymes that do not have this property represent another class of drug molecular target, and are described later).

▪ Na^+/K^+-dependent adenosine triphosphatase (ATPase) is a well-characterized membrane pump.

Its activity prevents Na^+ accumulation in nerve and muscle cells and the corresponding loss of K^+ that would otherwise occur as a consequence of the opening and closing of the ion channels that generate electrical activity in these cells. As Na^+ begins to accumulate as a result of Na^+ channel openings (action potentials), Na^+/K^+-dependent ATPase transfers Na^+ across the membrane to the extracellular fluid in exchange for K^+ ions from the extracellular fluid. The stoichiometry of this pump is two Na^+ for three K^+, meaning that the pump is electrogenic. The energy for this is supplied by the hydrolysis of ATP. This pump is an important molecular target for the heart drug, digitalis (see Chapter 18).

Enzymes

The cell and body fluids contain a large variety of enzymes, each of which is a potential molecular target for drugs.

Drugs can either mimic the enzyme's natural substrate (binding with the enzyme's substrate binding site, also known as its 'active' site) or bind with an allosteric site. Normally these molecular actions result in inhibition of enzyme activity. Thus, as seen with all molecular targets except some receptors, the molecular response is also the first step of the cellular response. The icon that is used throughout the book for drug target enzymes (that are not pumps) is shown in Fig. 3.19.

▪ Enzyme inhibition has characteristics similar to receptor antagonism

Drugs that bind with an enzyme at the substrate binding site are competitive inhibitors (in analogy with drugs that bind with a receptor at the ligand binding site, the competitive antagonists). However, other drugs can bind at a site separate from the substrate binding site. This can lead to enzyme inhibition via allosteric mechanisms, or by disruption of the enzyme's biochemical integrity. This is analogous to non- and

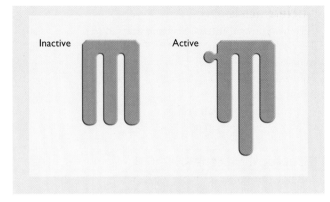

Fig. 3.19 The icon used throughout the text for an enzyme target showing the inactive and active states.

uncompetitive receptor antagonism (discussed on page 19 and in detail in Chapter 5).

▪ A typical example of an enzyme molecular drug target is acetylcholinesterase

Acetylcholinesterase is the enzyme responsible for degrading the neurotransmitter, acetylcholine. Acetylcholinesterase has a substrate binding site with two components, one of which binds to the esteratic moiety of acetylcholine and the other which binds to the charged anionic moiety. Once bound to the enzyme, acetylcholine then undergoes hydrolytic dissociation into its inert component molecules, choline and acetate. Some cholinester analogs of acetylcholine can bind with both components of the substrate binding site while other analogs bind with only one. In doing so, they inhibit the hydrolysis of endogenous acetylcholine. The interaction is competitive, and can be reversible or irreversible depending on the identity of the inhibitor. Organophosphates bind covalently with acetylcholinesterase at the esteratic component of the substrate binding site resulting in irreversible inhibition. These compounds have been used as nerve gases in chemical warfare and as insecticides (they can be an important cause of accidental poisoning). However, before organophosphates bind covalently there is an initial stage of reversible binding. Antidote drugs (e.g. pralidoxime) can prevent covalent binding during the reversible phase of organophosphorus poisoning by competing for binding, but late administration (after covalent binding is complete) achieves no benefit.

▪ Many anticancer drugs inhibit the activity of enzymes involved in protein and nucleic acid synthesis
(see Chapter 12)

Anticancer enzyme inhibitors include:

- Azathioprine, 6-mercaptopurine, and 6-thioguanine, which block with ribonucleotide synthesis from purines.
- 5-Fluorouracil and methotrexate, which act by blocking deoxyribonucleotides and 2′ deoxythymidylate synthesis.
- Cytarabine, which inhibits DNA polymerase and RNA synthesis.
- Doxorubicin, etoposide, amsacrine, and dactinomycin, which inhibit DNA replication and RNA transcription.

Nucleic acids

Certain types of anticancer drugs target nucleic acids, i.e., deoxyribonucleic acid (DNA) and ribonucleic acid (RNA), to achieve their effects. The cellular response (inhibition of DNA synthesis) is achieved by a variety of different molecular actions, for example:

- The bleomycins damage DNA and prevent its repair.
- Alkylating agents, mitomycin, and cisplatin cross-link DNA.

Structural macromolecules

Proteins (receptors, channels, symporters, etc.) are the most common molecular targets for drugs that act on cell membranes. However, certain drugs target structural macromolecules that do not have specialized ligand binding sites linked to transduction components. Therefore, by definition these drugs alter cell function indirectly by altering cell structure. Moreover the ligand binding sites usually consist of many repeated chemical motifs that require saturation by an equivalent number of drug molecules for an effect to be achieved. Thus, the typical effective concentration range for drugs that target structural macromolecules is millimolar (10–1000 fold higher than for most other types of drug).

In cell membranes (whether the plasma membrane or intracellular membranes including those surrounding cellular organelles such as the nucleus and mitochondria), the main structural component is a bilayer of phospholipids with a surrounding coat of glycoproteins. Other structural components include the cytoskeleton (a target for the anticancer drugs, colchicine and vinblastine).

Molecular targets not in mammalian cells
Chemical targets

Some drugs achieve their therapeutic effect without interacting directly with cells, for example:

- Chelating drugs, which act by binding to certain ions (such as Fe^{2+}, Fe^{3+} and Al^{3+}).
- Surfactants, which alter the surface physical properties of biologic fluids.
- Certain drugs used in the treatment of gastrointestinal disorders which adsorb substances in the gut and so alter the consistency and transit time of the bowel contents through the gastrointestinal tract.

Targets in or on bacteria, viruses, fungi, and parasites

In most cases of infection and infestation, therapeutic drugs act directly on the relevant organism (bacterium, virus, fungus, or parasite). The diverse molecular mechanisms of action of such drugs are conceptually identical to those of drugs that act on human tissue (i.e. modulation of receptors, enzymes) and are discussed in detail in Chapters 8, 9, and 10.

Summary of the mechanisms of drug action on receptors, ion channels, carriers and enzymes

The mechanisms of drug action on protein targets are sum-marized in Fig. 3.20. Examples of molecular targets for drug action are summarized in Fig. 3.21.

CELLULAR ACTIONS OF DRUGS (TRANSDUCTION)

The majority of drug molecular targets are linked by various biochemical mechanisms to cellular response components (G proteins, enzymes, ion channels, etc.). The operation of this linkage is known as transduction.

G protein-linked transduction

G proteins are molecules that are linked directly to a specific superfamily of receptors (described on page 20) or are linked indirectly to other drug molecular targets. The activated G proteins initiate (or suppress) many different cascades of cellular events that ultimately affect the function of ion channels, enzymes, DNA and other components of cells. Classic examples of this include the opening of K^+ channels in cardiac muscle following acetylcholine binding to muscarinic receptors, and the increased protein kinase activity following epinephrine binding to β adrenoceptors.

■ *G proteins consist of three subunits, α, β, and γ* (Fig. 3.22) *and act as on–off switches for cell signaling*
When an agonist activates a G protein-coupled receptor, a conformational change in the receptor leads to the activation of a G protein. Activation of G proteins involves the release of GDP and binding of GTP to its α subunit and the dissociation of this subunit from the $\beta\gamma$ subunit heterodimer. The α and $\beta\gamma$ subunits activate a number of effector molecules. The α subunit then hydrolyzes GTP to GDP, which in turn inactivates the α subunit, allowing it to reassociate with the $\beta\gamma$ complex, rendering the G protein inactive.

Stimulation or inhibition of G proteins results in modulation of the enzyme system responsible for producing the following other transduction components:

- Cyclic nucleotides.
- Diacylglycerol (DAG).
- Inositol phosphates.

For example, following β_1 agonism, a G protein is activated. This activates adenylyl cyclase, the enzyme that catalyzes the formation of cAMP. Transduction proceeds by cAMP activation, via protein kinases and phosphorylation, of enzymes whose types vary according to tissue.

There are many types of G protein in most cells. The α subtypes define the major properties of a G protein. For example, β adrenoceptors typically interact with G proteins having an α_s subunit which activates adenylyl cyclase.

Cyclic nucleotide-linked transduction

Of the transduction components linked directly to G proteins, the most widely distributed throughout the body is adenylyl cyclase. The cyclic nucleotide cAMP is synthesized from adenosine triphosphate (ATP) by the enzyme adenylyl cyclase. cAMP has diverse biologic actions.

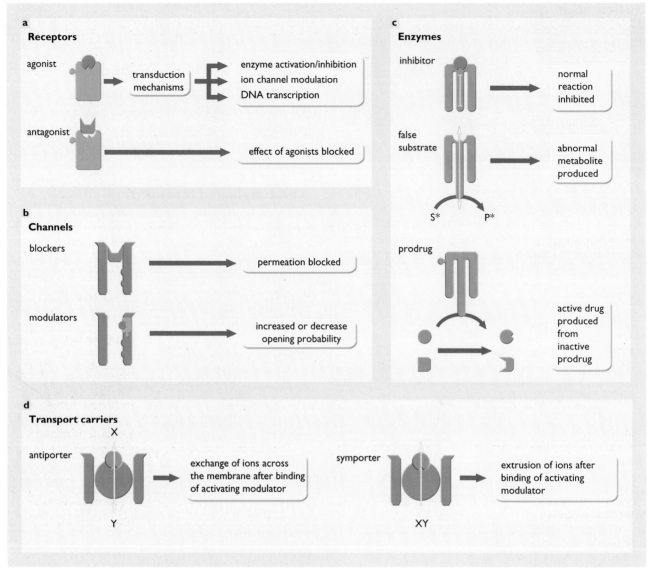

Fig. 3.20 Protein targets for drug action. These can be broadly divided into four classes. (a) Agonists can bind to receptors to initiate changes in transduction mechanisms, leading to a variety of cellular effects. Antagonists bind to receptors to block the effect of the agonist. (b) Drugs can block the passage of materials across channels or bind to components of the channel proteins to modulate the opening of ion channels. (c) Drugs can interact directly with the action of enzymes via a variety of mechanisms. S* and P* are false substrate and false product, respectively. (d) Drugs can bind to exchange proteins (antiporters) to move ions across the membrane. The direction of ion movement is shown by the direction of the arrow. Here, transporters are shown being activated by drugs, but note that some transporters are active at rest, and blocked by drugs. X and Y represent ions, which may have a positive or negative charge.

■ *cAMP has effects on energy metabolism, cell differentiation, ion-channel functioning, and contractile proteins*

cAMP phosphorylates intracellular proteins (many are enzymes) through the action of cAMP-dependent protein kinases. These protein kinases are activated by cAMP and phosphorylate the amino acids serine and threonine, using ATP as a source of phosphate (Fig. 3.23). Phosphorylation results in:

- Activation of hormone-sensitive lipase.
- Inactivation of glycogen synthase.
- Activation of phosphorylase kinase and therefore conversion

of inactive phosphorylase *b* to active phosphorylase *a* which results in increased lipolysis, reduced glycogen synthesis and increased glycogen breakdown.

- Activation of L-type Ca^{2+} channels and sarcoplasmic reticulum in cardiac cells by phosphorylation, so increasing Ca^{2+} currents and Ca^{2+} release, respectively.

Diacyl glycerol (DAG) and inositol 1,4,5-triphosphate (IP_3)-linked transduction

Many G proteins activate the DAG-IP_3 pathway.

One G protein, termed Gq, stimulates the activity of phos-

Some examples of molecular targets for drug action

Membrane receptors	Agonists	Antagonists
α_1 Adrenoceptor	Norepinephrine	Prazosin
α_2 Adrenoceptor	Norepinephrine	Yohimbine
β Adrenoceptor	Isoproterenol	Propranolol
Histamine (H_1 receptor)	Histamine	Terfenadine
Histamine (H_2 receptor)	Impromidine	Cimetidine
Opiate (μ-receptor)	Morphine	Naloxone
5-HT_2 receptor	5-HT	Ketanserin
Thrombin	Thrombin	Hirudin
Insulin receptor	Insulin	Not known

Intracellular receptors	Agonists	Antagonists
Estrogen receptor	Ethinyl estradiol	Tamoxifen†
Progesterone receptor	Norethindrone	Danazol
Glucocorticosteroid receptor	Budesonide	Mifepristone

Ion channels	Drugs that block channels	Modulators
Voltage-gated Na^+ channels	Lidocaine	
Voltage-gated Ca^{2+} channels	Dyhydropyridine	Dihydropyridines
Voltage-gated K^+ channels	4-aminopyridine	Ibutilide
ATP-sensitive K^+ channels	Glyburide	Lemakalim
		Sulfonylureas
GABA-gated Cl^- channels	Picrotoxin	Benzodiazepines
Glutamate-gated (NMDA) cation channels	Dizocilpine	Glycine

Enzymes	Inhibitors	False substrates
Acetylcholinesterase	Neostigmine	
	Organophosphate insecticides	
Choline acetyltransferase		Hemicholinium
Cyclo-oxygenase	Indomethacin	Eicosatetraenoic acid
Angiotensin-converting enzyme	Enalapril	
Carbonic anhydrase	Acetazolamide	
HMG-CoA reductase	Simvastatin	
Dopa decarboxylase	Carbidopa	Methyldopa
DNA polymerase	Cytarabine	Cytarabine
Enzymes involved in DNA synthesis	Azathioprine	
Enzymes of blood clotting cascade	Heparin	
Phosphodiesterase	Theophylline	

Carriers	Inhibitors
Choline carrier (nerve terminal)	Hemicholinium
Norepinephrine uptake 1	Tricyclic antidepressants
	Cocaine
5-HT uptake	Fluoxetine
Renal weak acid transfer	Probenecid
Na^+ pump	Digitalis
Na+/H+ exchanger	Amiloride

† Can act as a partial agonist in certain tissues.

Fig. 3.21 Examples of molecular targets for drug action. (GABA, γ-aminobutyric acid; 5-HT, 5-hydroxytryptamine; HMG-CoA, 2-hydroxy-3-methylglutaryl coenzyme A; NMDA, N-methyl D-aspartate)

pholipase C. This enzyme in turn leads to the production of DAG and IP_3 from the hydrolysis of polyphosphotide inosities. An alternative pathway involves activation of membrane phospholipase A_2 by G proteins, leading to the formation of DAG and phosphatidic acid. These transduction components have a diversity of actions.

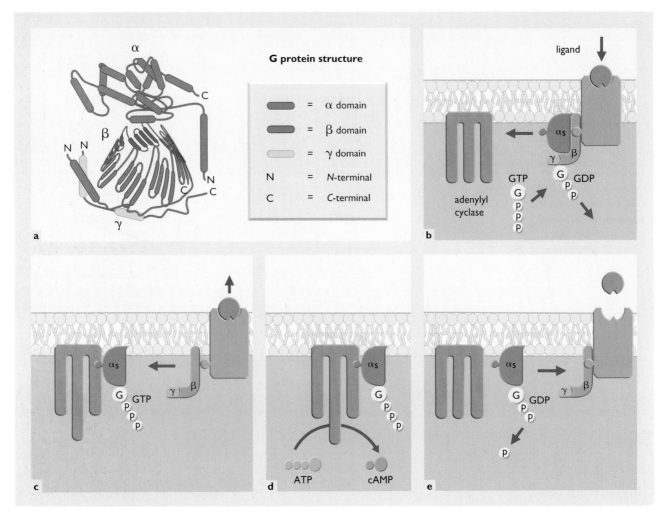

Fig. 3.22 Schematic representation of the activation of a G protein-coupled receptor. (a) The structure has several components. (b) The βγ complex serves to anchor the G protein to the membrane. Agonist binding to a G protein-coupled receptor promotes a conformation change in the receptor which in turn activates the G protein, leading to dissociation of the βγ heterodimer from its associated α subunit; in addition, bound GDP dissociates from the α subunit leading to binding of GTP to this protein. (c, d) The α–GTP complex subsequently interacts with a target protein (e.g. an enzyme such as adenylyl cyclase, or an ion channel). (e) The GTPase activity of the α subunit hydrolyzes the bound GTP to GDP, which allows the α subunit to recombine with the βγ complex.

IP_3 is not the only inositol phosphate produced in the cell by phospholipase. There appears to be a bewildering array of such compounds, which may have different functions. Inositol (1,3,4,5) tetraphosphate phosphate appears to facilitate the entry of Ca^{2+} into different cellular compartments (Fig. 3.23).

Ca^{2+}-linked transduction

Mobilization of intracellular Ca^{2+} is the common final link in the chain of events resulting from the production of many transduction components.

Ca^{2+} is involved in transduction in the following processes:
• Smooth muscle contraction.
• Increased rate of contraction and relaxation of cardiac myocytes.
• Secretion of transmitter molecules or glandular secretions.
• Hormone release.
• Cytotoxicity.
• Activation of certain enzymes.
Its mobilization is linked to the activity of other transduction

components. Ca^{2+} is stored on the membrane of endoplasmic reticulum of smooth muscle and is released when IP_3 acts on a specific ROC known as the IP_3 receptor.

DAG released by the actions of phospholipase C (and D) directly influences the activity of a membrane-bound protein kinase C, which is the enzyme responsible for phosphorylating serine and threonine and the subsequent change in activation state of more than 50 different proteins. There are at least six types of protein kinase C, each with its own substrate specificity.

Protein kinase C-linked transduction

Protein kinase C is an important component of transduction in the following processes:
• Modulation of the release of endocrine hormones and neurotransmitters.
• Smooth muscle contraction.
• Inflammation.
• Ion transport.
• Tumor promotion.

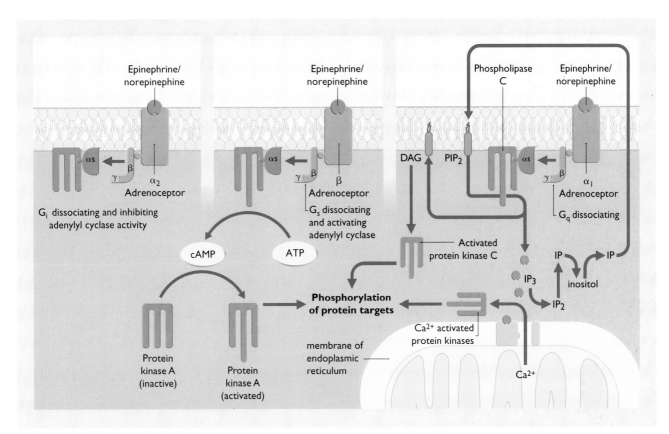

Fig. 3.23 Several types of transduction lead to phosphorylation of protein targets. cAMP and the phosphatidyl inositol cycle are important transduction components (second messengers). cAMP production increases in response to activation of many G protein-coupled receptors (e.g. α_2 or β_1 receptor activation by epinephrine). The central part of the figure shows this occurring in response to β adrenoceptor antagonism. Protein kinases (e.g. protein kinase A), activated by cAMP, are secondary transduction components participating in the cellular response. Certain types of agonism (e.g. α_2 adrenoceptor activation) lead to inhibition of cAMP production via activation of inhibitory G proteins (left panel of figure). The enzyme phospholipase C (located in the cell membrane) is activated by an agonist to produce the second messengers Ins $(1,4,5)$ P_3 (inositol triphosphate, IP_3) and diacylglycerol (DAG) (right hand panel). Intracellular IP_3 releases intracellular Ca^{2+} whereas DAG remains in the membrane where it activates protein kinase C. IP_3 undergoes sequential dephosphorylation by intracellular phosphatases (not shown) to give IP_2, IP and inositol which can then be incorporated into the membrane to form phosphatidyl inositol (PI), which, via ATP, is phosphorylated in steps to phosphatidyl inositol diphosphate (PIP_2). The recycling of IP_3 and DAG into phosphatidyl inositol is blocked by lithium, which depletes inositol lipids in the brain and is used as a drug in the treatment of manic depression (see Chapter 14).

 Actions of important G proteins

- G_s stimulates adenylyl cyclase and activates Ca^{2+} channels
- G_i inhibits adenylyl cyclase and activates K^+ channels
- G_q activates phospholipase C
- G_o inhibits Ca^{2+} currents
- G_t stimulates adenylyl cyclase in the eye
- G_{df} stimulates adenylyl cyclase in the nose

Transduction initiated by DNA-coupled receptors

Activation of DNA-coupled transduction involves a change in protein synthesis. For example, steroids displace HSP_{90} and the resulting steroid–receptor complex then translocates to the nucleus. Once in the nucleus and bound to the receptor, the steroid–receptor complex can recognize specific base sequences and activate specific genes. This is a slow process compared with that of the millisecond responses that are found in other forms of transduction (see Fig. 3.27).

- Glucocorticosteroids increase the production of lipocortin, which accounts for some of their actions as anti-inflammatory drugs (see Chapters 15 and 16).
- Mineralocorticosteroids increase the production of specific renal transport molecules involved in the renal tubular transport of Na^+ and K^+.

Transduction initiated by receptors with tyrosine kinase activity

The activation of tyrosine kinase receptors allows autophosphorylation of tyrosine residues, which serve as high-affinity sites for a variety of intracellular proteins. The tyrosine-phosphorylated receptor can then act as a platform for other proteins to bind to, leading to phosphorylation and the activation of pathways involving a cascade of other protein kinases. Many of the resultant signaling pathways are the same as those initiated by certain G proteins.

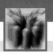

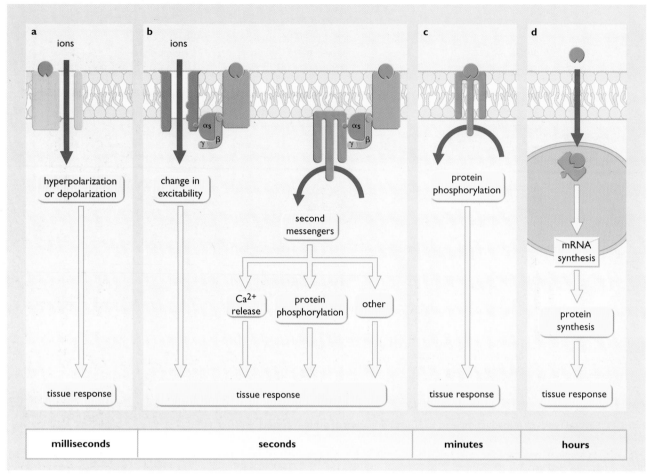

Fig. 3.24 Integration of molecular and cellular mechanisms. (a) Receptor-operated ion channel-linked transduction is very rapid. (b) G protein-linked transduction is rapid. (c) Enzyme and pump linked transduction is slow. (d) DNA-linked transduction is very slow.

Many tyrosine kinase receptors possess ligand binding sites for other proteins involved in signal transduction. One such binding site is termed SH_2. The binding of an inactive enzyme to SH_2 leads to a highly selective activation of the enzyme. Often the activated enzyme is involved in gene transcription. A series of protein kinases, IP_3 and Ca^{2+} may participate in the intermediary stages of transduction. Many growth factors act through this mechanism. There is therefore considerable interest in the possibility of finding drugs that interact with SH_2 or mimic SH_2 activity because they could have profound effects on growth and differentiation and, by implication, cancer, immunologic disease, and other disorders. Proteins involved in tyrosine kinase receptor transduction include the small G protein 'ras' (see Chapter 12).

Transduction initiated by ROCs

When a ROC initiates transduction, the events are triggered by a change in the membrane potential associated with an increase (or decrease) in the permeability of the ions that can pass through the ROC. Thus, transduction begins with the movement of charge. This results in depolarization or hyperpolarization of the membrane. The most common location of a ROC is the plasma membrane, but ROCs are also present in mitochondria and other intracellular organelles.

A change in membrane potential can directly modulate tissue function. In skeletal muscle, nicotinic ROC activation depolarizes the plasma membrane and, subsequently, the sarcoplasmic reticulum, which causes release of Ca^{2+} into the cytoplasm. This triggers muscle contraction.

Examples of integration of molecular and cellular mechanisms

Receptors and other molecular targets link to the cellular response components in the transduction cascade. Some examples of this integration of molecular and cellular mechanisms are described below. Characteristically, the speed of transduction, and production of the tissue response, are determined by the molecular target and by the mechanism of transduction (Fig. 3.24). The speed of this determines the onset of the tissue response. For example:

- Interaction of an agonist with a ROC produces rapid (milliseconds) cell hyperpolarization or depolarization.
- Interaction of an agonist with a G protein-coupled receptor may lead to one of many responses on a timescale of seconds.
- Interaction of a drug directly with an enzyme may lead to changes on a timescale of minutes.

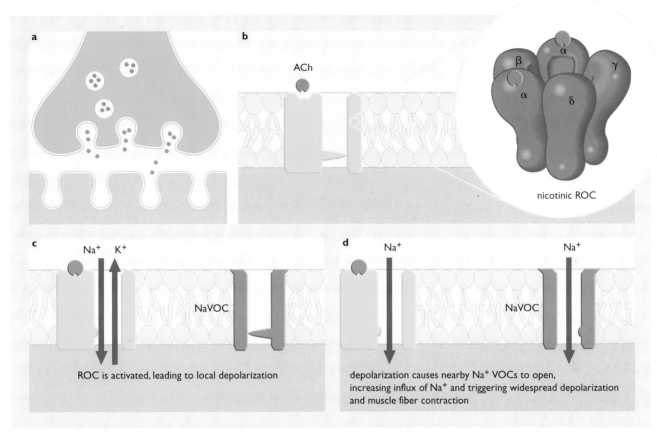

Fig. 3.25 Example of receptor-operated ion channel-linked transduction. (a) In response to an electrical impulse arriving at the nerve ending, vesicles of acetylcholine (ACh) fuse with the membrane of the nerve terminal, resulting in liberation of ACh into the synaptic cleft. (b) ACh binds to ligand-recognition sites within the α subunits of the ion channel (insert) leading to opening of the ion channel, allowing an influx of Na$^+$, causing local depolarization (c). This depolarization initiates transduction, causing voltage-operated channels to open in the adjacent regions of the membrane, increasing a further influx of Na$^+$ and thus triggering widespread depolarization and muscle fiber contraction (d).

- Interaction of a drug directly with DNA may lead to altered gene expression and the synthesis of a new protein over a period of hours.

Some examples of the integration between molecular and cellular responses are shown in Figs 3.25–3.27.

TISSUE AND SYSTEM ACTIONS OF DRUGS

Drugs have tissue and system actions that result from their molecular and cellular actions. Thus, in the case of some drugs we can now successfully explain their integrated molecular, cellular, tissue and system action. One example is tetrodotoxin. The molecular action of tetrodotoxin is to block Na$^+$ channels, with a diminishing order of potency in nervous tissue, skeletal muscle and cardiac muscle. Thus we are able to accurately predict tetrodotoxin's actions from cellular to tissue level. Since tetrodotoxin selects for Na$^+$ channels in nerves, low doses block peripheral nerves (sensory, autonomic and motor).

However it is difficult to predict tissue and system actions of new drugs on the basis of their molecular and cellular actions. This is because selectivity of action diminishes as one moves from molecular through cellular actions to actions at the tissue and system levels, as a consequence of cells and tissues reacting to the initial effects of the drug (homeostasis). Homeostasis is additionally altered by disease states. Thus we rarely have enough physiological and pathological knowledge to be able to predict exactly how molecular and cellular actions of new drugs will translate into tissue and systems actions.

Body systems are complex and under the control of many homeostatic inputs that respond to the initial tissue response and are perturbed by disease. The ultimate system response to any drug (or indeed any other bodily intervention) is therefore difficult to anticipate. Beyond the remit of pharmacology, but of therapeutic relevance, this is also a potentially poignant message for those who predict that diseases may one day be treatable by mutating (and altering the function) of specific individual cell components.

The concept of body systems is useful when considering mechanisms of action of drugs

The division of the body into various systems is somewhat arbitrary and subjective, but most pharmacologists accept that a systems approach is useful while recognizing that the whole body integrates all such systems. It is therefore possible to consider the action of drugs on the CNS separately from their actions on the cardiovascular or endocrine systems.

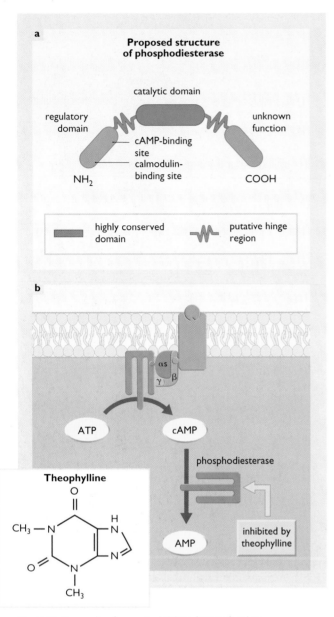

Fig. 3.26 Example of enzyme-initiated transduction.
Phosphodiesterase enzymes are involved in the metabolism of the cyclic nucleotides (e.g. cAMP). This family of enzymes is inhibited by theophylline. Inhibition leads to accumulation of cyclic nucleotides within cells. Note that cyclic nucleotides accumulate in response to the action of drugs on G protein-linked nucleotide cyclase enzymes.

As an example, the actions of some of the drugs used to treat high blood pressure can be explained solely in terms of their actions on the cardiovascular system (see Chapter 18). Obviously, actions on the cardiovascular system have implications for the rest of the body. However, when examining mechanisms of drug action it is reasonable for the sake of simplicity sometimes to consider only the target system itself and regard all other actions as a consequence of the effects on the target system.

This book is organized on the basis of body systems. Thus Chapters 13 to 25, inclusive, deal with drug actions on the component systems of the whole body. This 'systems' approach allows the reader to consider drugs from a quasi-pharmaco-therapeutic approach since the therapeutic actions of drugs often follow systems. Furthermore, many medical students now use the problem-based learning approach to study, which is generally systems-based.

THE FUTURE OF PHARMACOLOGY

Identification of molecular targets for drugs

Early identification of molecular targets involved the use of indirect techniques

The introduction of the receptor hypothesis (the notion that a drug interacts with a specific target to initiate its response) in the early part of the twentieth century initiated an interest in the structural and functional identification of molecular targets for drugs. For most of the last century indirect methods were used to identify and understand molecular targets and their function. In particular, the existence of receptor families, and their subtypes, had to be inferred from patterns of responses in a variety of different tissues to a variety of agonists, the inhibition of those responses by reversible and irreversible antagonists, and the manipulation of physical conditions, such as temperature. This was very successful in identifying the major known classes of receptors for neurotransmitters and hormones. It was easier to identify the existence of other molecular targets such as enzymes because they possess intrinsic biological activity.

Molecular biology has been very important in the development of molecular pharmacology

Developments in molecular biology are having major effects on pharmacology. The technique of ligand binding (see Chapter 5) has been important in locating and identifying molecular targets, allowing them to be purified and their amino acid sequence to be revealed. This has facilitated the cloning of genes for the molecular target, allowing the genetic code dictating the amino acid structure to be determined, and, by process of comparison, has identified how families of receptors are related. Identification of the DNA code for receptors allows immediate access to the mRNA carrying the message, and ultimately information about the turnover and expression of the receptor in question can be inferred. The findings have been remarkably consonant with the classical view (of specific molecular targets that allow selective binding to drugs). At the same time there has been a growth in our knowledge of intracellular transduction mechanisms for translating binding of a drug to a molecular target into a tissue response. The growth of this collection of knowledge and techniques, known as molecular biology, has initiated a third phase in our understanding of molecular targets and molecular mechanisms of drug action.

The discovery of new drugs

Techniques for discovering new drugs are highly (but not exclusively) dependent on the techniques of molecular biology

Pharmacology is the study of what drugs do, and how they do it. Consequently, pharmacology is also an important part of the drug discovery process. Almost all new drugs are discovered

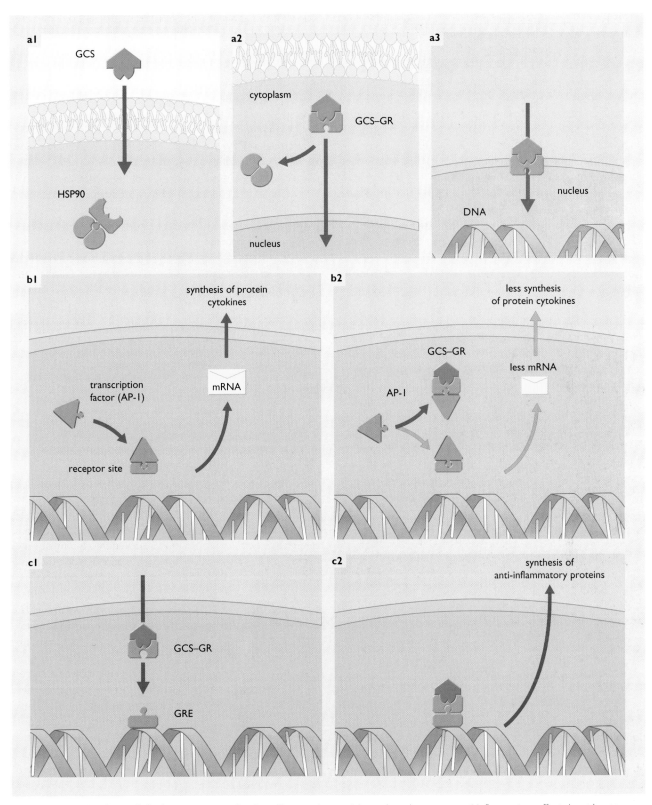

Fig. 3.27 Example of DNA-linked receptor transduction. Glucocorticosteroids are thought to exert anti-inflammatory effects by at least two distinct mechanisms. (a1) Glucocorticosteroids (GCS) cross the cell membrane and bind with receptors located in the cytoplasm (here bound in an inactive form to heat shock protein 90, HSP_{90}). (a2) First stage of transduction: dissociation of the glucocorticosteroid receptor complex (GCS–GR) from HSP_{90}. (a3) Next stage of transduction: translocation of GCS–GR into the cell nucleus. (b1) In some cells, the synthesis of a protein (e.g. pro-inflammatory cytokines) can be initiated by transcription factors acting on their own receptors. (b2) Once in the nucleus, GCS–GR binds to (and 'mops up') the transcription factor (e.g. AP-I), thereby reducing the amount of new protein synthesized. If this protein is a pro-inflammatory mediator (e.g. a cytokine), the net effect is to reduce inflammation. (c1) Alternatively, GCS–GR may bind with a glucocorticosteroid response element (GRE, a receptor on DNA). (c2) Binding of GCS–GR to the GRE inhibits the synthesis of proteins (e.g. anti-inflammatory lipocortins).

by pharmaceutical companies who require a constant stream of products in order to ensure their economic survival. The techniques of molecular biology are able to provide in a pure form the target biomolecules with which potential drugs can interact. These molecular targets can then be combined with suitable reporter systems that indicate whether ligands are agonists or antagonists. This type of technique, because of the large numbers of potential ligands that can be rapidly screened, is known as high-throughput screening (HTS). Current HTS can examine up to hundreds of thousands of chemical compounds in one day. This allows millions of compounds, of natural or synthetic origin, to be screened for binding and activation of a host of target molecules. This technique currently works best for hormone and neurotransmitter receptors, but is being expanded for enzymes and ion channels as well as for other molecular targets.

In addition to the large number of existing 'libraries' of ligands, there is a need for rapid methods for synthesizing new and novel compounds. Developments in synthetic organic chemistry, such as combinatorial chemistry, are capable of producing the large number of compounds required to meet the capacity of HTS. In addition HTS techniques are also being developed to screen potential drugs for desirable pharmacokinetic characteristics.

Combinations of HTS systems, therefore, allow identification of compounds which act on a known molecular target with sufficient potency, selectivity and appropriate pharmacokinetic behavior to suggest they might be given directly to humans to test their pharmacotherapeutic potential.

However, optimism that this approach will provide new drugs for every disease has yet to be justified by results. Why should this be? The reason is that we almost never have a clear understanding of the complete role of the currently available molecular targets in physiology and pathology and the complexity of the influence of homeostasis on the cellular cascades that they initiate.

Thus, while the molecular biologic approach to pharmacology provides fast routes to drug discovery, reliable assessment of therapeutic potential of new drugs still requires functional analyses of drug actions on isolated tissues, body systems and whole bodies (including animal models of the target disease). After all, the body is an integrated unit in which the whole is considerably more than the sum of the parts. Pharmacology is likewise integrated from molecular to cellular, tissue and system actions, and it is this integration that determines the therapeutic (and adverse) effects of drugs.

FURTHER READING

Lefkowitz RJ. G-proteins in medicine. *N Engl J Med* 1995; **332**: 185–187. [An excellent overview of the role of G proteins in health and disease.]

Robertson MJ, Dougall IG, Haper D, et al. Agonist–antagonist interactions at angiotensin receptors: application of a two-state receptor model. *Trends Pharmacol Sci* 1994; **15**: 364–369. [State-of-the-art discussion of receptor activation.]

The International Union of Pharmacological Committee on Drug Classification and Receptor Nomenclature (NC-IUPHAR) recommendations for individual receptors and ion channels. *Pharmacol Rev* 1991; **16**: 119–229. [The definitive classification for drug receptors and ion channels.]

Watson S, Girdleston D (eds) Receptor and ion channel nomenclature. *Trends Pharmacol Sci* (Suppl.). London: Elsevier; 1995. [A user-friendly guide to receptor and ion channel nomenclature.]

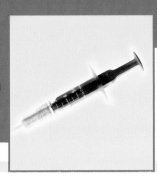

Chapter 4

Pharmacokinetic and Other Factors Influencing Drug Action

Drugs can be administered by a number of different methods such as the oral, intravenous and inhalation routes. Thus drugs must be in an appropriate form for a particular route (e.g. as a solution for intravenous injection). All drugs, other than those that are designed to act locally (topically), or are directly injected into the blood stream, are absorbed into the blood from their site of administration. Drug concentrations in body compartments (blood, tissues, etc.) increase by absorption and distribution and decrease as a result of metabolism and/or excretion. Absorption refers to the processes by which a drug enters the blood from its site of administration. Distribution refers to the processes by which a drug leaves the circulation and enters the tissues perfused by the blood. However, once a drug enters the tissues, it is possible for it to enter other cells, usually by diffusion, without using blood as the transport pathway. Metabolism refers to the processes by which tissue enzymes catalyze the chemical conversion of a drug to more polar forms (metabolites) that are usually more easily excreted from the body. Excretion refers to processes (renal excretion, etc.) that result in the removal of drug from the body. Alteration of any of the above processes (i.e. absorption, distribution, metabolism, and/or excretion) can modify a drug's actions.

DRUG DELIVERY

Drugs can be delivered in a variety of forms, including tablets, capsules, solutions, suspensions, modified release products, injectable solutions, ointments, creams, and suppositories. In addition, they may be given in the form of pro-drugs (a precursor of the active drug) that make use of the biologic characteristics of the host (e.g. metabolism) to liberate the pharmacologically active substance(s) in the body.

Drug formulation

Depending on the delivery system, a drug formulation can allow specific tissue sites to be selectively targeted, or systemic absorption of the drug to be avoided. Thus a drug's formulation, and the route of administration, determine its absorption and distribution. Some formulations are designed to deliver the drug only into the gastrointestinal tract in a convenient physical form (e.g. tablets, capsules, solutions, and suspensions). Liquid formulations of drugs are useful for adjusting the oral dose on an individual basis, and for those people who have difficulty in swallowing tablets or capsules.

A strategy for extending the activity of drugs that are rapidly metabolized or excreted from the body is to use a controlled-

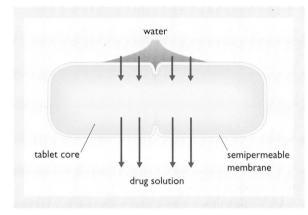

Fig. 4.1 A modified-release tablet. This tablet is coated with a membrane that is selectively permeable for water. Water passes into the core of the tablet and releases the drug solution through small holes in the membrane.

release formulation that only releases the drug slowly on its way through the gastrointestinal tract. Thus the period of delivery is prolonged. Tablets coated with a semipermeable membrane are an example of a newer controlled-release delivery system (Fig. 4.1). Several other formulation strategies can also be used for similar purposes. Thus plasma concentrations of a drug with time after dosing can be influenced by drug formulation. Such products include:

- Controlled-release theophylline for the treatment of asthma.
- Controlled-release verapamil for the treatment of hypertension.

■ *Drug absorption through the skin can be used to produce systemic effects*

An example of a delivery system for applying drug to the skin to produce systemic actions is shown in Fig. 4.2. The ideal properties of compounds for use in this type of delivery system include high potency and a relatively brief persistence in the body. High potency allows for a convenient size of delivery system while brief persistence ensures a prompt termination of drug effect once the delivery system is removed. Examples of this therapeutic approach include:

- Scopolamine skin patches for the prevention of motion sickness.
- Fentanyl skin patches for the treatment of chronic severe pain.
- Nicotine skin patches to help people trying to stop smoking tobacco.

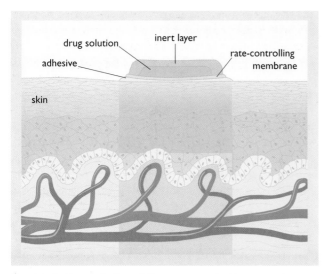

Fig. 4.2 A skin patch drug delivery system. In this system, drug solution diffuses through a membrane that controls the amount of drug delivered to the skin for subsequent absorption.

◼ *Topically applied drugs are usually used to produce a local therapeutic effect*

Topically applied drug-containing products include solutions, ointments, creams, suppositories, and aerosols. Sites to which they are applied include the eye, ear, skin, mouth, throat, lung, rectum, and vagina. However, both the skin and mucous surfaces are only relative barriers to the systemic absorption of drugs.

Routes for administering drugs

Most drugs are given by mouth—the oral route. A drug absorbed from the upper gastrointestinal tract is exposed to enzymes in the gut wall that can metabolize it. Absorbed drug then passes into the portal venous system that carries it to the liver, the major site for drug metabolism. Routes other than the oral route (e.g. rectal, sublingual, injection, application to the skin or mucosal surfaces, and inhalation) are considered if:

- A drug is unstable or rapidly inactivated in the gastrointestinal tract.
- The ability of a drug to be absorbed via the gastrointestinal tract, and to reach its required destination via the systemic circulation, is compromised as a result of drug loss due to metabolism by the intestine or liver, vomiting, or a disease state that may affect drug absorption.
- Therapeutic effects demand local administration, and systemic absorption would lead to adverse drug effects (e.g. local anesthesia).

Routes other than the oral route

The following routes bypass the gastrointestinal tract and can result in rapid action:

THE SUBLINGUAL ROUTE Absorption in the mouth through the buccal or sublingual mucosa bypasses exposure to the gastrointestinal tract and early exposure to the liver via the portal venous circulation. This route is useful for potent drugs that do not have a disagreeable taste. A classic example is sublingual nitroglycerin to rapidly relieve an acute attack of angina, or to provide prophylaxis against an impending attack.

THE SUBCUTANEOUS ROUTE Subcutaneous injection or implantation of a drug can slow its rate of absorption compared with intravenous and sublingual administration, and so extend its pharmacologic effect. An example is the subdermal implantation of progestins (e.g. norgestrel) as a method of contraception. In this case the formulation has the advantage of producing a depot of drug under the skin from which it slowly leaches into the circulation.

THE PARENTERAL ROUTE The most rapid route for drug administration is to inject it directly into the blood stream. This is usually accomplished intravenously. On rare occasions, intra-arterial injections are used. Alternative parenteral routes include subcutaneous, intramuscular, epidural, and intrathecal routes of injection. Antibiotics are sometimes given intramuscularly, and hormones are often administered subcutaneously. Absorption from these sites is usually rapid, and drugs bypass the gastrointestinal tract, thereby avoiding its metabolizing enzymes and those in the liver (presystemic metabolism) before reaching the systemic circulation. However, if drug absorption from an injection site is too rapid, it can be slowed by using:

- A vehicle in which the drug is formulated that binds the drug and slows its release from the injection site.
- A second drug in the vehicle so as to reduce blood flow at the injection site (e.g. the use of an α adrenoceptor agonist (vasoconstrictor) with a local anesthetic to prolong the local anesthetic's effect) (see Chapter 26).

THE RECTAL ROUTE Drugs can be placed in the rectum as a suppository. The exposure of drug to first-pass metabolism with this route is less than with the oral route because there is a limited portal blood flow system for the lower gastrointestinal tract compared with the upper gastrointestinal tract. However, rectal absorption can be inconsistent.

THE NASAL MUCOSA is also a useful site at which to administer drugs that undergo considerable presystemic elimination (e.g. by first-pass metabolism) when given orally. Nasal sprays can be used to deliver potent drugs for systemic effects (e.g. some hormones, and opioid analgesic drugs for the management of severe chronic pain). However, absorption from the nasal mucosa can also be inconsistent.

THE INHALATION ROUTE Vapors and gases (e.g. general anesthetics, Chapter 26) are well absorbed from the lung when inhaled. In addition, if the lung is the target of drug therapy, inhalation is often an appropriate method of drug administration, even for powders. The undesirable systemic effects of oral drugs used to treat reversible bronchoconstriction can be considerably reduced if the drug is inhaled, because the total dose can be reduced, and less of the administered dose reaches the systemic circulation. Examples of inhaled drugs include glucocorticosteroids and β_2 adrenoceptor agonists for the treatment of asthma. The proportion of a dose that reaches the site of action depends on the ability of the patient to coordinate inspiration with triggering of drug release from the canister. However, various new technologies are being introduced to facilitate such dosing. Interestingly, the majority of a dose administered by inhaler is usually swallowed.

FACTORS INFLUENCING DRUG ABSORPTION AND DISTRIBUTION

Absorption

Both the chemical and physiologic factors itemized in Fig. 4.3 can influence drug absorption.

▪ The diffusion rate of drugs through lipids usually determines their rate of absorption

Most drugs presently used are small organic molecules with a molecular weight less than 1000 that diffuse through biologic

Important chemical properties and physiologic variables affecting drug absorption	
Chemical properties	Chemical nature
	Molecular weight
	Solubility
	Partition coefficient
Physiologic variables	Gastric motility
	pH at the absorption site
	Area of absorbing surface
	Mesenteric blood flow
	Presystemic elimination
	Ingestion with or without food

Fig. 4.3 Important chemical properties and physiologic variables that influence drug absorption through cell membranes, including those of the gastrointestinal tract.

membranes in their uncharged form. This occurs because a major structural component of cell membranes is the lipid bilayer, and the uncharged drug form is far more lipid soluble than the charged form. However, some charged molecules are actively transported across membrane barriers (e.g. 5-fluorouracil and levodopa) by special transporter molecules (see Chapter 3). Since most drugs are either weak acids, bases, or are amphoteric in nature, the pH of the environment in which the drug disintegrates and dissolves will determine the fraction available in a non-ionized form that can diffuse across cell membranes. This fraction will depend on a drug's chemical nature, its pKa, and the local pH. The pKa of a drug is the pH at which 50% of the drug molecules in solution are ionized, and is described by the Henderson–Hasselbalch equation: For acidic (HA) drug molecules, $HA \Leftrightarrow H^+ + A^-$ where HA is the uncharged drug form, H^+ a proton, and A^- the anionic form. From this relationship the equation $pKa = pH + \log(HA/A^-)$ can be derived. The equation allows the ratio HA/A^- to be calculated for any pH value.

By analogy, for basic (B) molecules $BH^+ \Leftrightarrow B + H^+$ and the equation is $pKa = pH + \log(BH^+/B)$.

The pKa values, and hence fractions of ionized or non-ionized molecules, for different drugs at physiological pH (7.4) and other pH values, show how ionized fractions change with pH for acidic and basic drugs (Fig. 4.4). A useful summary of Fig. 4.4 is that a drug will exist in its ionized form when exposed to a pH opposite to its pKa. Therefore, acidic drugs are increasingly ionized with increasing pH (an increasingly basic environment), while basic drugs are increasingly ionized with decreasing pH (increasingly acidic environment).

▪ The site at which a drug is administered can alter its rate of absorption

The fraction of dissolved drug in its non-ionized form, and therefore its rate but not necessarily its extent of absorption, can depend on the pH at the site of administration. For

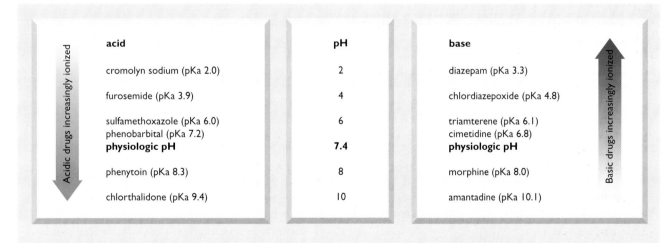

Fig. 4.4 The influence of pKa on the degree of functional group ionization in acidic and basic drugs relative to physiologic pH. The increasing depth of color in the arrows reflects increasing ionization relative to the physiologic pH of 7.4. Thus, for acidic drugs, the more basic the solution (the higher the pH) the greater is the proportion of drug that is ionized. Conversely, for basic drugs, the more acidic the solution (the lower the pH) the greater the proportion ionized. The extent of ionization is calculated from the Henderson–Hasselbalch equation (see text), relating pH and pKa to the fraction ionized.

example, in the stomach, where the pH is approximately 2.0, most dissolved acidic drugs will be non-ionized and therefore able to diffuse readily through the stomach lining to reach the blood stream. Conversely, most basic drugs will be almost completely ionized and will diffuse very slowly from the stomach into the blood stream.

▨ *The rate of diffusion of the non-ionized form of a drug across the membrane lipid bilayer depends on molecular size and lipid solubility*

The diffusion coefficient for a non-ionized molecule in lipid is inversely related to the square root of its molecular weight. This relationship indicates that if other confounding influences are disregarded, smaller molecules will diffuse more easily across membranes than larger molecules. However, since most drugs are of low molecular weight (below 600), molecular size is rarely the limiting factor in their absorption.

Lipid solubility is the second property of drugs that influences their diffusion across membranes. Lipid solubility is measured in terms of a drug's partition coefficient. The partition coefficient reflects the solubility of a drug molecule in a lipid solvent relative to its solubility in water, or physiologic buffer. Greater lipid solubility is reflected as a larger partition coefficient. This coefficient is determined only when the drug molecule is present at less than its saturation concentration in both phases. The higher the partition coefficient, the more rapidly a drug can diffuse across a lipid membrane. The therapeutic use of different barbiturates (central nervous system depressants) is related to their partition coefficients. Thus:

- Thiopental, with a pKa of 7.45 and a high partition coefficient (580), is used as a short-acting induction anesthetic by injection (see Chapter 26), because it rapidly enters brain tissue and therefore quickly induces anesthesia.
- Phenobarbital, with a similar pKa (7.20), but a low partition coefficient (3), is used primarily for the chronic treatment of epilepsy.

▨ *The route of administration can limit drug access to the systemic circulation*

As indicated previously, the route of administration can limit drug access to the systemic circulation. For example:

- A solution of drug administered as eye drops will have primarily local effects, although systemic effects may occur in some patients with potent drugs that are absorbed via the lacrimal ducts.
- Penicillin G is unstable in the acid environment of the stomach, and large oral doses are needed to compensate for drug decomposition at this site.
- Nitroglycerin is administered sublingually to allow rapid systemic absorption and to avoid its presystemic elimination through metabolism in the liver.

▨ *The rate of drug absorption after an oral dose can be a function of the rate of gastric emptying*

The rate of absorption from the gastrointestinal tract can be altered by retaining an acidic drug within the stomach, or

---

 Drug absorption

- Most drugs are well adsorbed from the gastrointestinal tract
- The site of absorption depends on the non-ionized fraction of drug in solution
- Gastric emptying can be accelerated by ingesting the dose with cold water
- Basic drugs ingested by mouth are poorly absorbed until they pass into the duodenum
- Modified-release dose forms prolong the duration of drug effect and allow for a more convenient dosage regimen

hastening passage of a basic drug into the small intestine. For example, in an empty stomach, a glass of water ingested together with a drug will accelerate gastric emptying and hasten exposure of the drug to the upper intestine with its higher pH and much larger surface area (absorptive surface). Accelerated gastric emptying also can be accomplished pharmacologically. The drug metoclopramide increases gastric motility and accelerates gastric emptying. Alternatively, a fatty meal, acid drinks, or drugs with anticholinergic effects will slow gastric emptying.

Distribution

A drug entering the blood stream will be distributed to different parts of the body at a rate that depends on various factors, including metabolism, excretion, and redistribution within the body. To reach extravascular tissue, a drug must first leave the blood stream. As indicated previously, most commonly used drugs have low molecular weights. As a result, they readily leave the circulation by being filtered through capillaries. However, the rate of such filtration may be modified by the extent to which a drug binds to plasma proteins such as albumin or α_1-acid glycoprotein.

▨ *Obesity can influence drug distribution*

Regardless of the route of administration, a drug will eventually reach all tissues at a rate that is proportional to blood flow (Fig. 4.5). At rest, blood flow to fat and muscle (measured in ml/kg tissue/min) is similar. With exercise, blood flow rises dramatically in muscle. Drugs accumulate to different amounts and at different rates in fat and muscle, depending on their lipid solubility. Thus differences in lean to fat tissue ratio for the same body weight can be expected to confound dose adjustment on the basis of total body weight for some drugs. Therefore drug doses are not always selected on the basis of total body weight, since the fat to lean ratio will influence plasma levels.

▨ *The concentration of free drug in the different fluid compartments of the body depends on the pKa of the drug and the pH of the fluid*

At equilibrium, the basis for calculating drug concentrations at a tissue site depends on the principle that the free concentration of non-ionized molecules will be equal on both

Total and weight-normalized tissue blood flow in an adult

Perfusion	Blood flow (ml/min)	Organ mass (kg)	Blood flow (ml/kg/min)
Cardiac output	5400	–	–
Myocardium	250	0.3	833
Liver	1700	2.5	680
Kidney	1000	0.3	3333
CNS	800	1.3	615
Fat	250	10.0	25
Other (muscle, etc.)	1400	55.0	25
Total		69.4	

Fig. 4.5 Total organ blood flow, organ weights and normalized blood flows for various organs in an adult human.

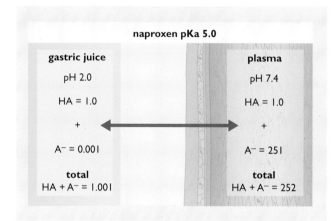

Fig. 4.6 **Distribution of an acidic drug.** The diagram shows the distribution of naproxen at equilibrium between gastric juice and plasma. Note that this acidic drug is concentrated in the circulation.

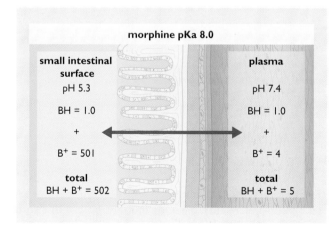

Fig. 4.7 **The distribution of a basic drug.** The diagram shows the distribution of morphine at equilibrium between the small intestinal tract cell surface and plasma. Note that this basic drug is concentrated in the small intestine, as opposed to plasma for the acidic drug in Fig. 4.6.

sides of the cell membrane. Figures 4.6 and 4.7 illustrate the distribution at equilibrium between two biologic environments for an acidic drug (naproxen) and a basic drug (morphine) and demonstrate that:

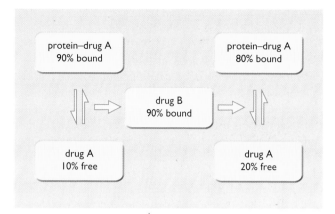

Fig. 4.8 **Protein binding and free fraction of drugs.** This diagram shows the outcome when one drug (A) is displaced from its protein binding site by addition of a second drug (B). The change in free fraction is considerable for highly bound drugs.

- Acidic drugs are likely to be concentrated in the circulation.
- Basic drugs concentrate in tissue outside of the circulation.

It should be noted that these examples refer only to the unbound fraction of drug dissolved in a specific biologic fluid or tissue. These examples are highly simplified, especially compared to the body as a whole under nonequilibrium conditions.

The binding of drugs to plasma proteins contributes to differences in total drug concentrations in different body compartments

Albumin is the most important plasma protein for binding acidic drugs. Competition for the binding sites on albumin can become clinically important for drugs that are more than 80% bound, and especially if binding exceeds 90%. In the presence of such a high degree of binding, any small change in the bound fraction will lead to a larger change in the free fraction, i.e. that fraction that exerts pharmacological effects (Fig. 4.8).

Many basic drugs are bound to a globulin fraction (i.e. α_1-acid glycoprotein). Interpretation of the clinical importance of this interaction is complicated because this protein is an acute-phase reactant in that its concentration fluctuates relatively rapidly and varies widely among people. The concentration of α_1-acid glycoprotein in plasma increases with age, inflammatory conditions, and with acute pathologic stress.

When a drug overdose is suspected, the most appropriate sample site in which to measure the drug depends on its chemical characteristics

Drugs that are acidic in nature will concentrate in the plasma, and as a result blood is an appropriate fluid to sample for acidic drugs. On the other hand, the stomach is a reasonable sampling site for basic drugs, regardless of the method of drug administration. Diffusion of basic drugs into the stomach results in their almost complete ionization in this environment. As a constant gradient remains, basic drugs concentrate in the stomach until there is distribution equilibrium of the non-ionized fraction. Ingesting bicarbonate to alkalinize the urine can prolong the actions of amphetamine. As a result of such alkalinization, an increasing fraction of urinary amphetamine is in the non-ionized form, and as such is readily reabsorbed across the luminal surface of the kidney.

◼ Anatomic and physiologic factors contribute to differential distribution of drugs in different biologic spaces

The anatomic and biochemical nature of the blood–brain barrier influences the ability of drugs to enter the brain. Diffusion out of brain capillaries is severely restricted by cellular zonulae, thereby increasing the barrier to drug diffusion into the brain. However, there are five brain regions where this barrier is absent; these are the pituitary gland, the pineal body, the area postrema, the median eminence, and the choroid plexus capillaries. The choroid plexus also contains transporters, which remove charged molecules from the cerebrospinal fluid (CSF). Normally, CSF contains no protein. As a result, the drug concentration in the CSF is similar to the free drug concentration in the blood.

◼ Unless shown otherwise, it should be assumed that all drugs cross the placenta and enter breast milk

Drugs diffuse across the placenta, but equilibrium between mother and fetus may be delayed because of the limited placental blood flow from the maternal circulation. Unless proven otherwise, it should be assumed that all drugs cross the placenta, and enter breast milk. The clinical importance of drugs in the placenta and in breast milk must be determined individually for each drug.

◼ That pharmacokinetic space into which a drug distributes is defined as the 'apparent volume of distribution'

The apparent volume of distribution is a calculated space and does not conform to an actual anatomic space. Its calculation is based upon the dose administered, and the resulting drug concentration in circulating plasma. Some molecules (e.g. ethanol) have an apparent volume of distribution that approximates the total body water (roughly 60% of body weight in non-obese young adults). With ethanol this might be unexpected since it is lipid soluble and expected to distribute into both water and lipid. Since water is the body's largest space, most ingested ethanol remains in the total body water. Some drugs have apparent volumes of distribution that considerably exceed body weight (Fig. 4.9). Such drugs are usually bases and their high apparent volume of distribution reflects extensive tissue binding. In this situation, almost all of the administered dose will be sequestered outside the circulation. Anatomic studies in animals demonstrate that basic drugs are often localized in specific organs of the body (e.g. the concentration of the antiviral drug amantadine in liver, lung, and kidney is several times that in blood).

Both the site of action of a drug, and the tissue mass in which it concentrates, are factors to consider when ascribing clinical importance to drug localization. The cardiac glycoside digoxin concentrates in muscle, and its apparent volume of distribution greatly exceeds body weight. Therefore the dose of digoxin needed to produce therapeutic plasma concentrations depends on the relative muscle weight to total body weight. In addition, it takes several hours to achieve equilib-

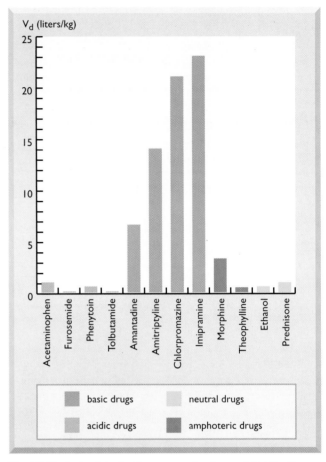

Fig. 4.9 Typical values for the apparent volume of distribution (V_d) for selected drugs. The large V_d values for basic drugs are explained by extensive tissue sequestration.

⚷ Drug distribution

- Drug distribution is based on the principle that the non-ionized concentration is the same throughout the body at equilibrium
- Charged drug molecules are effectively prevented from entering the brain by the blood–brain barrier except when the meninges are inflamed
- Basic drugs concentrate in the stomach because they are mainly ionized

rium between blood and muscle. Thus plasma digoxin concentrations do not readily relate to the inotropic response if distribution equilibrium has not occurred.

DRUG METABOLISM

Most drugs are metabolized before being lost from the body. Drug metabolism reactions have been broadly classified into phase 1 and phase 2 processes.

- **PHASE 1** reactions involve oxidation, reduction, and hydrolysis, reactions that provide a functional group to increase the polarity (and usually water solubility) of the drug. Such functional groups also provide a site suitable for phase 2 reactions.

- **PHASE 2** reactions involve conjugation or synthetic reactions in which a large chemical group is attached to the molecule. This process usually increases water solubility and facilitates excretion of the metabolite from the body.

The nature, function, and amount of drug-metabolizing enzyme varies among people, resulting in differing individual rates of drug disposition

The drug-metabolizing enzymes have broad substrate specificity. Enzyme specificity is relative rather than absolute. This means that one enzyme may catalyze the metabolism of many different drugs and that more than one enzyme isoform may be involved in the metabolism of the same drug. A common metabolic reaction is oxidation. During drug oxidation, an hydroxyl group is added to the drug substrate, or a short alkyl group (most commonly methyl) is removed. An example of such a metabolic pathway is the demethylation of theophylline to 1-methylxanthine. The primary enzyme responsible is cytochrome P-4501A2, but the reaction is catalyzed by the cytochrome P-450 isoforms 1A1 and 2D6 as well (see later, and Fig. 4.11).

Generally, drug-metabolizing enzymes occur in multiple forms, and inter-individual differences in their genetic expression can contribute to inter-individual differences in drug metabolism. The enzymes have been classified into families, subfamilies, and specific gene products. Furthermore, the degree of expression of such enzymes can be regulated at many levels. Some enzymes are expressed constitutively, in the sense that they are always present and active. Others are primarily expressed only when triggered by the presence of an exogenous chemical (e.g. drug, poison, and/or dietary factors). Gene mutations can result in deficient expression, or absence of a particular enzyme isoform. As a result, unexpected drug toxicity may occur with administration of a typically safe dose of a drug. Conversely, redundant genetic code may result in multiple copies of a particular drug-metabolizing enzyme. This situation is likely to result in resistance to typical therapeutic drug doses due to accelerated metabolism by excess tissue enzyme.

The activity of drug-metabolizing enzymes may be increased (induced) or inhibited

Many factors in the diet can influence the activity of drug-metabolizing enzymes, including the protein to carbohydrate ratio, plant foods containing flavonoids (e.g. cruciferous vegetables—cabbage, mustard, and cress), and barbecued foods, which are usually high in polycyclic aromatic hydrocarbons from burning charcoal.

Increased enzyme synthesis as a result of the presence of an exogenous chemical is referred to as 'induction' (Fig. 4.10). The induction process may be due to a combination of changes in nucleic acid transcription as well as translational and post-translational regulation. Induction can be produced by certain drugs, food constituents, alcohol, and smoking. When chronically ingested, some drugs (e.g. barbiturates, rifampin) induce

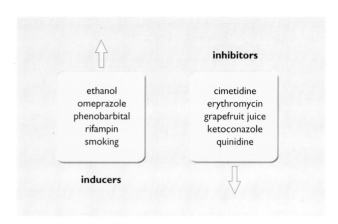

Fig. 4.10 Examples of enzyme inducers and enzyme inhibitors. The drugs shown are known to induce, or inhibit, the metabolism of other drugs administered concurrently.

their own metabolism as well as that of other drugs and endogenous substances. The tissue site where induction occurs may be determined by the nature of exposure to the chemicals responsible. Smokers induce expression of a particular isoform of the cytochromes P-450, primarily in the lungs and upper intestine.

Sometimes, two drugs will compete for metabolism by the same enzyme, resulting in a decreased rate of metabolism for one or both drugs. This process is referred to as 'inhibition' (see Fig. 4.10). One clinically important example of such an inhibition interaction is cardiac arrhythmias, or seizures, produced by theophylline when it is given concurrently with a macrolide-type antibiotic such as erythromycin.

Most tissues have the ability to metabolize specific drugs

Although the liver is justifiably regarded as the major site of drug metabolism, most tissues can metabolize specific drugs. Tissue specificity for drug metabolism depends on genetic regulation and expression of drug-metabolizing enzymes in particular tissues. Therefore selective tissue effects may result from a unique drug-metabolizing enzyme reaction at the relevant tissue site of action for a drug. For example, the kidney oxidizes the metabolite sulindac sulfide, the active cyclooxygenase inhibitor, back to sulindac, the parent pro-drug, thereby protecting the kidney from impaired function due to inhibition of cyclo-oxygenase by sulindac sulfide.

The loss of drug from plasma (elimination) occurs according to first order, zero order, and intermediate order kinetics

The concentrations of most drugs that occur in the body are considerably below those required to saturate the body's capacity to eliminate them. As a result the rate of loss of such drugs from the body is proportional to their concentration in the plasma (known as first order elimination kinetics), and the usual parameter used to reflect this process is their plasma half-life. Since the half-life is the time taken to lose half of the drug from the body, a drug with this disposition characteristic can be considered to be essentially completely removed from the circulation in five half-lifes. By two half-lifes, 75% of the drug

45

is lost (50% plus half the remaining 50% = 75%), 87.5% in three half-lifes, 93.75% in four, etc.

The concept of half-life is, however, inappropriate for a few drugs (e.g. ethanol) because their rate of elimination does not depend upon plasma concentration, unless the plasma concentration is very low, i.e. usually pharmacologically ineffective. The metabolism of ethanol is effectively saturated by a very low concentration resulting from ingestion of a small dose. The elimination of ethanol is best described on the basis of the loss of a constant amount of ethanol/unit time (zero order elimination). The average rate of removal of ethanol from the circulation is of the order of 120 mg/kg/h in social drinkers who ingest modest amounts infrequently. This average elimination rate is often reported in terms of change in blood alcohol concentration as 150 mg/L/h. This rate reflects removal of approximately one-half of a standard bottle of beer (5% v/v alcohol) per hour from a 70 kg male.

Other drugs (e.g. aspirin, phenytoin) show elimination characteristics that are intermediate between zero and first order kinetics. For such drugs, once the first order process is saturated, elimination kinetics approximate to zero order, and accordingly, plasma concentrations increase disproportionately with increasing dose since the elimination rate does not increase with dose for zero order processes. With such drugs, it is advisable to monitor plasma concentrations when changing a dose regimen, since relatively small changes in dose can lead to a disproportionate increase in plasma concentration and consequent toxicity.

Phase 1 metabolism

Oxidation is the most common pathway for phase 1 metabolism. Reduction and hydrolysis reactions, although important, occur considerably less often.

Oxidation

■ *Cytochromes P-450 form a superfamily of heme protein enzyme isoforms that catalyze oxidative metabolism of many substances, including drugs*

The process of drug oxidation involves both oxidation and reduction steps (see Fig. 4.12). Sites for oxidation vary considerably and have as a common physical property high lipid solubility.

Most oxidative metabolism of drugs is catalyzed by the cytochromes P-450, although other enzymes are also involved to a lesser extent. There are several hundred isoforms of the cytochromes P-450. Some are constitutive, while others are present only when synthesized in response to an appropriate stimulus, usually an exogenous chemical. Substrate specificity is a function of the cytochrome P-450 isoform, with specificity being relative rather than absolute. As a result, the absence of any particular isoform of cytochromes P-450 does not preclude a particular metabolic reaction. Genes for the cytochromes P-450 are found on several chromosomes.

A nomenclature for the cytochromes P-450 has been developed to help understand their inter-relationships:

• CYP—The capital letters 'CYP' indicate that the isoform is of human origin.

• CYP 'x' An Arabic numeral is next used to indicate the isoform family.
• CYP 'x' 'X' Subfamilies are designated by another capital letter.
• CYP 'x' 'X' 'x' A final Arabic numeral designates the individual gene product in the subfamily.

Designation of family and subfamily status relates to the degree of homology for the amino acid sequence of various P-450 isoforms. For example, the designation CYP1A2 refers to a human cytochrome P-450 isoform of the first family that is a member of the A subfamily of enzymes and is the second gene product assigned to that subfamily.

■ *Three families of the P-450 cytochromes have been identified as important for metabolizing a wide variety of drugs*

The three families of cytochromes P-450 that are important in metabolizing drugs are shown in Fig. 4.11, but only a few members have been identified as being important for drug metabolism. The CYP3A subfamily has been identified as the major constitutive form in human liver, and it contributes to the metabolism of a wide variety of drugs. This subfamily is also expressed in clinically significant amounts in tissues other than liver. The specific isoform CYP3A4 is responsible for intestinal metabolism (presystemic elimination) of many drugs that show poor bioavailability.

The isoform CYP2D6 has been associated with:
• The oxidative metabolism of many drugs including β adrenoceptor antagonists.
• Demethylation of tricyclic antidepressants.
• Demethylation of codeine to morphine.

Approximately 5–10% of Caucasians are deficient in the phenotypic expression of CYP2D6 as an autosomal recessive trait. Multiple mutations of CYP2D6 have been described. For example, an inability to demethylate codeine is associated with a lack of analgesic response to this drug. This is attributed to an inability to demethylate the administered codeine to the active drug, morphine.

CYP2E1 is a labile isoform induced by chronic alcohol consumption. CYP1A2 is important in the metabolism of theophylline and is induced by flavonoids and polycyclic aromatic hydrocarbons found in some diets. Knowledge of the metabolic constitution of a patient therefore has potential predictive value in determining whether a particular drug

Cytochrome P-450 families and the isoforms important to oxidative drug metabolism

Family	Isoform	Drug substrate
CYP1	CYP1A2	Theophylline
CYP2	CYP2D6	Codeine
CYP3	CYP3A4	Cyclosporine

Fig. 4.11 **Examples of the cytochrome P-450 families, and their isoforms, important for the oxidative metabolism of certain drugs.**

therapy is appropriate. Tests for the phenotypic expression of drug-metabolizing enzymes in individual patients are expected to be readily available in the future. Such information will be valuable for determining which specific drugs or drug classes should be free of problems with respect to drug oxidation. Caution is advised, however, in interpreting phenotypic expression of a gene product, since the former can be modulated by environmental and physiologic factors.

In order to function, cytochrome P-450 enzymes require the presence of the mixed function oxidase system

Cytochromes P-450 require the presence of molecular oxygen, NADPH cytochrome P-450 reductase, and NADPH in order to function. This combination of factors is referred to as the mixed function oxidase system. The cytochrome P-450 isoforms are present in considerable excess in this system in comparison with cytochrome P-450 reductase, the enzyme that contributes reducing equivalents to the oxidative reaction. The process by which cytochromes P-450 oxidize drug substrates is depicted in Fig. 4.12.

Oxidative reactions usually result in drug inactivation, but exceptions do occur and pro-drugs represent such an example

Pro-drugs are chemicals that are converted into pharmacologically active substances after absorption (e.g. the demethylation of codeine to morphine, Fig. 4.13). Sometimes drug oxidation results in the formation of an active metabolite with a duration of action that exceeds that of the administered drug (e.g. the conversion of diazepam to desmethyldiazepam).

When multiple drugs are administered concurrently, they can interact with the cytochrome P-450 isoforms to inhibit each other's rate of metabolism. As a result, pro-drugs may not be metabolized to active pharmacological entities and active drugs may not be removed at their expected rate. As a consequence, therapeutic failure or drug toxicity may result. Representative examples of such interactions are presented in Fig. 4.14.

Reduction

This metabolic reaction occurs occasionally at susceptible functional groups, such as nitro, keto or sulfoxide substituents. This process can result in activation or inactivation of drugs. Examples of important reductions include:

• Sulindac, a pro-drug whose sulfoxide group is reduced to produce sulindac sulfide. This metabolite is the active cyclo-oxygenase inhibitor used for the treatment of inflammation (see Chapter 16).
• Prednisone, a pro-drug that undergoes reduction of a ketone to an hydroxyl group to produce the active glucocorticosteroid prednisolone.

Hydrolysis

Hydrolysis can occur spontaneously owing to instability of substituent groups in the drug molecule. Esters are particularly liable to hydrolysis into their original acid and alcohol components. Also, many different types of esterase enzymes

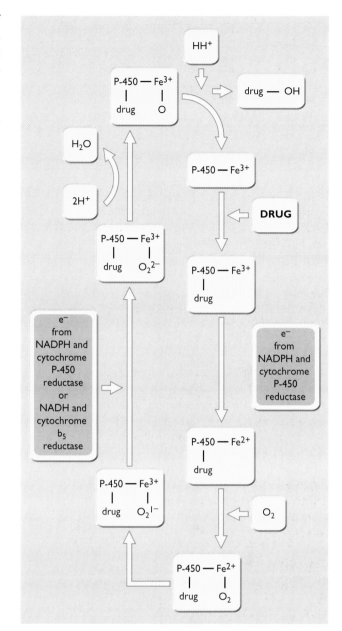

Fig. 4.12 The mechanism by which the mixed function oxidase system oxidizes a drug. The drug binds to the oxidized form of a specific cytochrome P-450 isoform. This complex then receives a single electron from NADPH via cytochrome P-450 reductase. The reduced complex then reacts with molecular oxygen, and a second electron is donated either via NADPH and cytochrome P-450 reductase, or NADH and cytochrome b_5 reductase. In the process, one atom of oxygen is released as water and the other is incorporated into the drug to produce the hydroxylated metabolite. This metabolic reaction also applies to dealkylation reactions in which short-chain alkyl groups (usually methyl) are removed from a drug and combined with oxygen to yield an aldehyde, which can be further oxidized or reduced.

are found in the body, and plasma esterases are important in the breakdown of many ester-containing drugs. Spontaneous hydrolysis in the absence of enzymes is seen with acetylsalicylic acid (aspirin), which is hydrolyzed to salicylic acid in the presence of moisture. Some therapeutic agents are administered

47

Drugs and pro-drugs and their clinically important active metabolites

Drug	Active metabolite
Allopurinol	Oxypurinol
Diazepam	Desmethyldiazepam
Imipramine	Desmethylimipramine

Pro-drug	Active metabolite
Codeine	Morphine
Prednisone	Prednisolone
Sulindac	Sulindac sulfide

Fig. 4.13 Examples of drugs and pro-drugs with clinically important active metabolites.

Examples of drugs and specific isoforms of cytochrome P-450 which require adjustment of medication to prevent metabolic interactions

Cytochrome P-450 isoform	Inhibitory drug	Major drugs affected by inhibition
CYP1A2	Fluvoxamine	Clozapine
		Haloperidol
	Cimetidine	Clozapine
		Propranolol
		Theophylline
CYP2D6	Amiodarone	Amitriptyline
	Fluoxetine	Codeine
	Cimetidine	Flecainide
	Quinidine	Propranolol
	Paroxetine	Thioridazine
CYP3A4	Cimetidine	Amiodarone
	Erythromycin	Astemizole
	Fluconazole	Carbamazepine
	Indinavir	Cyclosporine
	Omeprazole	Diazepam
	Sertraline	Fentanyl
		Simvastatin

Fig. 4.14 Examples of interactions between drugs and specific isoforms of cytochromes P-450 that require drug dose adjustment or a change in prescribed drug to prevent the metabolic interaction.

as pro-drugs that are hydrolyzed after ingestion. Examples of important hydrolyses include:
- Sulfasalazine is hydrolyzed into aminosalicylic acid and sulfapyridine by the bacterial flora in the lower gastrointestinal tract. It is these hydrolyzed substances that are believed to exert pharmacological effects.
- Bambuterol, a carbamate ester pro-drug of terbutaline, is concentrated in lung tissue where it is hydrolyzed by pseudocholinesterase to release the active β_2 adrenoceptor agonist terbutaline.

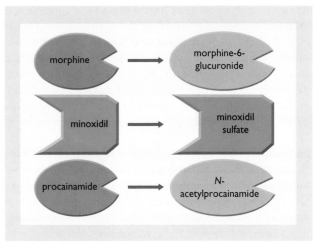

Fig. 4.15 Examples of conjugations that result in the production of active drug metabolites.

Phase 2 metabolism

Conjugation involves enzymatic attachment of chemical moieties to a drug, or a metabolite, resulting from phase 1 metabolism

Phase 2 reactions are also referred to as conjugation, and occur in a wide variety of tissues. They most often involve the enzyme-mediated attachment of hydrophilic moieties, such as glucuronic acid, sulfate, glutathione, and acetate, to a functional group on the parent molecule and/or to a metabolite generated by phase 1 metabolism. Glucuronic acid is first activated by combination with uridine diphosphate (UDP). The activated UDP–glucuronic acid is then transferred to the drug by a glucuronosyltransferase enzyme. Conjugates formed by such reactions are generally more hydrophilic than the parent drug, or its phase 1 metabolite, and as a result are more easily excreted by the kidneys. In general, conjugates are less pharmacologically active than the parent drug, but this is not always so (see below). Other conjugation reactions occur less often with substituents such as glycine, methyl groups, and the sugars, glucose and ribose. Examples of clinically important conjugation reactions are given in Fig. 4.15, with glucuronide conjugates being quantitatively the most important.

While conjugation usually increases water solubility, acetylation often results in metabolites with lower water solubility than the unconjugated precursor (e.g. as with the acetylation of sulfonamide antibiotics). Acetylation of a basic amine functional group converts the basic drug to a weak acid (amide). This chemical change has an effect on the distribution and elimination of the resulting metabolite.

Although conjugation reactions are usually considered to be inactivation processes, there are several notable exceptions, including:
- Acetylation of the antiarrhythmic drug procainamide results in the formation of acetylprocainamide, which is also antiarrhythmic (see Chapter 18), albeit with a different spectrum of ion channel blocking action than the parent drug.
- Morphine-6-glucuronide is an analgesic with a longer duration of action than the parent drug, morphine.

Impaired renal function has therapeutic and toxic implications with respect to both of the above metabolites.

Sulfate conjugation can also be an activation reaction. Minoxidil, an antihypertensive drug, must be sulfated at the N-oxide position in order to produce its vasodilator effect. Minoxidil also promotes hair growth but less potently than its sulfate metabolite. Variation in hair growth with minoxidil may therefore partly depend on a patient's ability to sulfate minoxidil at the hair follicle.

Multiple isoforms of the conjugating enzymes are being discovered and their relative specificities for various substrates and metabolites are being determined. At least two families and three subfamilies of glucuronosyl transferases, and multiple gene products for acetylation and sulfation, have been described.

The size of the dose of isoniazid, procainamide, and hydralazine depends on a patient's ability to acetylate these drugs. The faster the acetylation rate, the larger the dose that will be required to maintain therapeutic drug concentrations in the plasma. Phenotypic slow acetylators can appear to be rapid acetylators if certain drugs are ingested with ethanol. This has been demonstrated in humans who take procainamide or sulfamethazine concurrently with alcohol.

Deficiencies of one or more of the isoforms of conjugation enzymes are likely to influence the choice of drugs used to treat diseases. Thus, characterizing patients according to their ability to metabolize prototypical substrates has the potential for improving the individualization of drug therapy. Two clinically important examples include:

- Cancer patients with thiopurine methyltransferase deficiency require a 10–15 times reduction in their dose of 6-mercaptopurine to reduce the risk of severe hematopoietic toxicity.
- Cancer patients with deficiency in expression of the glucuronosyl transferase isoform UGTIA1 require dose reduction of the topoisomerase I inhibitor, irinotecan, to reduce the incidence of myelosuppression and diarrhea.

DRUG EXCRETION

Drugs are excreted from the body by several routes. These routes include the kidneys (urine), the intestinal tract (bile and feces), the lungs (exhaled air), breast milk, and sweat. However, excretion in urine and feces represent the most important routes for drug elimination.

Renal excretion

Renal excretion of drugs involves both filtration and secretion (see Chapter 17). Filtration occurs at the glomerulus of the kidney and secretion occurs along the nephron. The excretion of some drugs is impaired in the presence of renal disease. There is a wealth of data demonstrating that the renal excretion of many drugs correlates with the kidney's ability to excrete creatinine. If it is inconvenient or impossible to assess renal function directly by measuring a 24-hour creatinine clearance, renal function can be estimated using the widely accepted algorithm of Cockroft and Gault. These investigators established a relationship between patient age, weight and serum creatinine concentration ($C_{s,cr}$) from which creatinine clearance (Cl_{cr}) by the kidney can be estimated:

$$Cl_{cr} \text{ (ml/min)} = \frac{[(140 - \text{age}) \times \text{ideal body weight (kg)}]}{[0.8145 \times C_{s,cr} \text{ (\mumol/liter)}]}.$$

This equation applies to males. For females, the value for creatinine clearance is multiplied by 0.85.

Although renal creatinine excretion occurs both by filtration and secretion, the fraction excreted by each mechanism changes in favor of secretion as renal function decreases. It is likely that this relationship also applies to all drugs that are filtered and secreted by the kidney.

 There are various therapeutic strategies for increasing renal excretion of drugs

By virtue of the relationship between pKa and pH, the pH of the urine will determine the proportion of drug in its ionized state, and therefore the amount of filtered drug that cannot be reabsorbed by diffusion across the luminal surface of the nephron. For example, salicylic acid, which is a weak acid (pKa 3.0), is usually mostly metabolized before being excreted into the urine. However, as the urinary pH is increased, a higher fraction of the administered dose is lost in the urine. Indeed, treatment of salicylate intoxication can include alkalinization

 Drug metabolism

- Most drugs are metabolized before being eliminated from the body
- Drug metabolites are generally more polar than their parent compound
- The specificity of drug-metabolizing enzymes is relative rather than absolute
- The expression of drug-metabolizing enzymes differs between tissues
- Concurrent ingestion of two or more drugs can affect the rate of metabolism of one or more of them

Drug excretion

- Renal and fecal excretion are the most important routes for drug elimination
- Some drug conjugates are hydrolyzed in the lower gastrointestinal tract back to the parent compound and reabsorbed in a process referred to as enterohepatic circulation, which extends the duration of drug action
- For some drugs the fraction of the administered dose excreted unchanged by the kidney depends on the urinary pH
- Creatinine clearance can be used to assess any renal impairment and indicate whether drug doses need to be reduced if renal excretion is an important component of drug elimination

of the urine with oral or parenteral doses of bicarbonate to increase renal elimination of salicylic acid. This strategy can also be useful in the management of phenobarbital overdose.

Increasing urine flow also increases renal elimination of some drugs, since the contact time with the luminal surface is decreased, reducing the time for reabsorption of non-ionized molecules.

Gastrointestinal excretion

The removal of drugs from the gastrointestinal tract can be accelerated by the use of a polyethylene glycol electrolyte lavage solution. Large volumes of this solution can be ingested or placed in the gastrointestinal tract through a nasogastric tube to increase intestinal peristalsis and hasten excretion of unabsorbed drug via the rectum. The decreased transit time through the gastrointestinal tract associated with the induced diarrhea will decrease the absorption of nutrients, but in an acute situation this is not clinically important.

Enterohepatic circulation prolongs the pharmacologic effect

Some drug conjugates excreted in bile are hydrolyzed in the lower intestine to release the original drug substrate for reabsorption into the blood stream, and in consequence prolong their action. This recycling process is referred to as enterohepatic circulation. Examples of this process that are potentially clinically relevant include:

- The enterohepatic circulation of the sedative hypnotic drug lorazepam is due to hydrolysis of its glucuronide conjugate in the lower intestinal tract.
- The suggestion that failure of oral contraception can be due to inhibition of enterohepatic circulation following antibiotic therapy which removes the bacteria from the lower intestine that hydrolyze steroid conjugates. Thus steroid clearance is enhanced, and contraceptive failure is more likely.

Lung excretion

Volatile drugs are excreted by the lungs, although this route is only of major importance for general anesthetics that exist in gaseous or vapor phases. Such anesthetics are administered and lost via the lungs, providing for easily controlled anesthesia by adjusting the anesthetic concentration in the inhaled gas mixture. Excretion via the lung allows for monitoring of the end tidal concentration of expired anesthetic as a surrogate index of the level of anesthesia (see Chapter 26). Ethanol is excreted in small amounts by the lung. While this route of elimination is not quantitatively important for ethanol, it does provide a noninvasive method for estimating blood ethanol concentrations for legal purposes.

PHARMACOKINETICS

The analysis of the rate of all drug disposition factors (absorption, distribution, metabolism, and excretion) is termed pharmacokinetics. The word reflects the movement of drugs (*pharmaco*) into and out of the body.

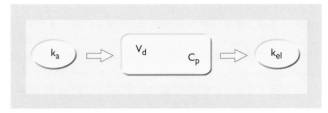

Fig. 4.16 Diagram of the one-compartment open pharmacokinetic model for drug disposition. The plasma concentration of a drug (C_p) is determined by the rate of drug absorption (k_a—rate constant for absorption), the apparent volume of drug distribution (V_d), and rate of drug elimination (k_{el}). When the drug is administered parenterally as a bolus, absorption is instantaneous.

The one-compartment model

In the simplest model, the body is considered to be a single uniform space (compartment) into which the drug of interest is administered, and from which it is eliminated (Fig. 4.16). In this model, it is assumed that the administered drug is immediately distributed throughout the space. If elimination is a first order kinetic process, the elimination rate is proportional to the plasma concentration, resulting in an exponential loss of drug. The mathematical equation for this exponential relationship is:

$$C_t = C_0 e^{-k_{el}t}$$

where C_t is plasma concentration at any time t, C_0 is the estimated initial plasma concentration at t = 0, k_{el} is the elimination rate constant, and e is the base for natural logarithms. By taking the logarithm of plasma concentration, the exponential process is reflected by a straight line (Fig. 4.17). The slope of the line in Fig. 4.17 is actually $k_{el}/2.303$, since the logarithmic transformation of plasma concentration data was to the base 10 rather than to base e. This presentation is used in the figure since base 10 semilogarithmic paper is the type

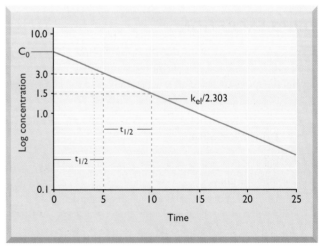

Fig. 4.17 A graph of the log of the plasma drug concentration versus time with a one-compartment open pharmacokinetic model for drug disposition after an intravenous dose. Extrapolation of the line (slope is k_{el}) to time 'zero' results in an estimate of the initial drug concentration (C_0) in the compartment if distribution were instantaneous.

of graph paper most commonly available. If the initial extrapolated drug concentration (C_0) in the compartment is divided into the administered dose, the theoretical volume needed to accommodate the drug dose is described. This space is defined as the apparent volume of distribution (V_d).

While the elimination rate constant tells us how quickly the drug is eliminated, a simple calculation using k_{el} gives the plasma half-life ($t_{1/2}$), a measure that is more commonly used, and better understood. The time for the drug concentration in plasma to decline by 50% is its $t_{1/2}$. Since the decline in logarithmic transformed drug concentration with time is linear, the $t_{1/2}$ will be constant, regardless of drug concentration. The k_{el} of a drug is related to $t_{1/2}$ by the equation:

$$t_{1/2} \times k_{el} = 0.693.$$

Since $t_{1/2}$ is related to the V_d, the $t_{1/2}$ value will not always reflect the ability of a body to eliminate a drug. The preferred kinetic term that indicates the body's ability to remove a drug from the circulation is plasma clearance (Cl_p), and is equal to $V_d \times k_{el}$. Clearance remains constant for most drugs if the elimination mechanisms are not modified by pathologic and/or physiologic factors.

Fig. 4.17 shows the fall in plasma concentration with time when the drug is administered parenterally. However, if the drug is given orally, it takes time to fill the space (absorption) and the drug disposition curve resembles that shown in Fig. 4.18. The shape of the plasma concentration versus time curve reflects the interaction of two first order processes that account for both entry (absorption) into, and exit (elimination) from, the single kinetic compartment. Calculation of V_d, $t_{1/2}$, k_{el}, and Cl_p is the same as after parenteral dose administration, but some of the derived parameters (V_d and Cl_p) will increase if there is significant presystemic drug elimination. This situation occurs because plasma drug concentrations are lower owing to presystemic elimination, and estimation of the initial drug concentration (C_0) is therefore lower. This simple model of a

single uniform space with first order kinetics serves remarkably well for the calculation of dosing regimens for most drugs.

The two-compartment model

For some drugs, the plot of the logarithm of plasma concentration versus time results in a curvilinear relationship (Fig. 4.19). To explain such observations, the simple one-compartment model needs to be expanded. The simplest expansion is to consider the body as two compartments (Fig. 4.20). Intuitively, it can be deduced that two linear processes could account for the curvilinear plot in Fig. 4.19. The two processes are known as the α and β phases and are characterized by their respective elimination rate constants (and half-lifes). In this model, the terminal linear phase (β) is not k_{el}. The β phase is a slower rate process than k_{el}. The greater the discrepancy between β and k_{el}, the larger the error is in assuming the validity of a one-compartment model. Fortunately, for most drugs, the discrepancy between β and k_{el} is not as great as interindividual differences in drug disposition. Therefore, as indicated above, in most cases the one-compartment open model serves as an acceptable clinical approximation for individualization of drug doses.

Obviously, both the one- and two-compartment models are oversimplifications of 'spaces' in the body into which drugs

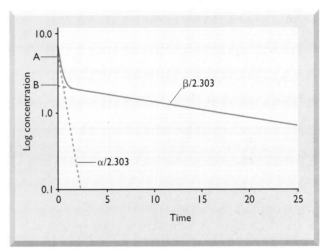

Fig. 4.19 A plot of log plasma drug concentration versus time for a two-compartment open model after an intravenous bolus dose. The terminal disposition rate constant is β and not k_{el}, and the decreasing plasma concentration with time reflects a more complex relationship between drug distribution and elimination. The initial more rapid decline in circulating drug concentration (α) primarily reflects redistribution of the drug to the peripheral compartment (V_p) (see Fig. 4.20) plus a modest component of elimination. The terminal, apparently linear, phase of plasma concentration versus time is a composite of drug elimination buffered by drug returning from V_p to the central compartment in which the drug distributes rapidly (V_c) to decrease the apparent rate of drug removal from the blood plasma. This phase is therefore referred to as the β phase. Extrapolation back to time zero provides an intercept (B). The extrapolated values of β are subtracted from the observed concentrations of drug at the same time after the dose and the residual values are plotted. A linear regression through these residual data points provides a slope (α) and a time zero intercept (A), that reflect drug distribution into V_p. If the discrepancy between β and k_{el} is large, a greater error will arise from assuming that a one-compartment model is valid.

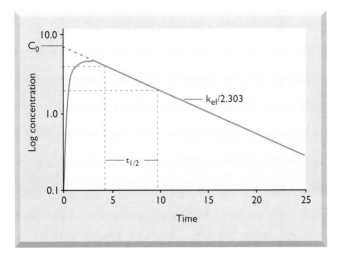

Fig. 4.18 A graph of log plasma drug concentration versus time for a one-compartment open pharmacokinetic model after an oral dose. The shape of the curve should be compared with the straight line in Fig. 4.17.

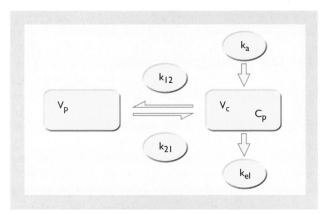

Fig. 4.20 Diagram of the two-compartment open pharmacokinetic model for drug disposition after a parenteral dose. With a bolus dose, k_a is instantaneous and is ignored in solution of the model. When the drug is administered by infusion, k_a is a zero order constant equal to the rate of drug infusion. There is a central compartment in which the drug distributes rapidly (V_c) and from which drug is eliminated, and a peripheral compartment into which the drug can distribute (V_p) and from which it can return to buffer the changing drug concentration in the central compartment when drug is eliminated (k_{el}, elimination constant).

 Time course of drug action

- Clinically it is more important to know the time course of drug action than the pharmacokinetics of drug concentrations. There may, or may not, be a linear or simple relationship between drug action (effector concentration) and blood concentration.

- The time required for drug effects to be expressed can be much longer than that for the drug to act at its molecular site since the response systems have their own time constraints.

- E.g. Beta blockers produce a very rapid slowing of heart rate whereas the anticoagulant effects of warfarin take days to develop.

are absorbed and from which they can be metabolized and excreted. When a discrepancy in modeling drug disposition becomes clinically evident for a particular drug its use has to be learned as a special case so as to account for the more complex disposition–effect relationship. Drugs that undergo dose-dependent disposition (e.g. phenytoin, aspirin) belong to this special category of more complicated relationships between dose, concentration, and pharmacologic effects.

The non-compartmental approach

A non-compartmental approach has been advocated to simplify the determination of pharmacokinetic parameters from which drug doses can be calculated. This approach borrows considerably from the one-compartment open model. In this approach, the area under the curve (AUC) of plasma concentration versus time is integrated, and the calculation of kinetic parameters is performed according to equations presented in Fig. 4.21. This method compensates somewhat for the extrapolation of drug

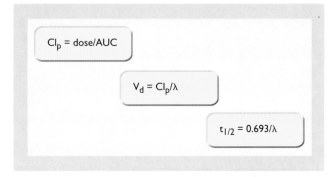

Fig. 4.21 Equations for pharmacokinetic drug disposition for non-compartmental conditions. The terminal disposition constant is renamed λ so that its interpretation is not prejudiced by either of the two models discussed in Figs 4.16–4.20. A new calculation is introduced which is called area under the plasma concentration versus time curve (AUC). Cl_p, plasma clearance; V_d, apparent volume of distribution, λ, terminal disposition rate constant.

concentrations to C_0 in the one-compartment model when no drug has yet been absorbed into the body after an oral dose.

Calculation of dosing

Most drugs are administered chronically. For drugs with first order elimination, the total amount in the body increases until the amount excreted is equal to the dose administered, i.e. a steady state plasma concentration is achieved. The time to steady state for such drugs depends only on the terminal elimination half-life. Simple calculation indicates that 94% and 97% of steady state are achieved after four and five elimination half-lives, respectively. For practical purposes, steady state is assumed to exist at this time (Fig. 4.22). The more frequently a drug dose is administered, the greater will be the amount of drug in the body at steady state, and the less the variation between its peak and trough plasma concentrations. The less frequently a drug dose is administered, the lower will be the amount of drug in the body at steady state, and the greater the variation between its peak and trough plasma concentrations. If the dose interval is longer than two terminal disposition half-lifes, drug

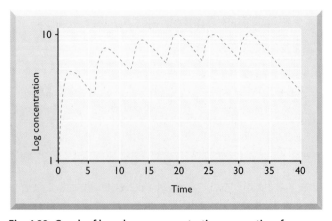

Fig. 4.22 Graph of log plasma concentration versus time for a drug administered by mouth every 6 hours for six doses when the drug's terminal·disposition half-life is 6 hours. The effective steady state occurs 24–30 hours (4–5 half-lifes) after starting the drug.

Pharmacokinetics

- Most drugs are eliminated from the body as a constant fraction of their plasma concentration (first order process)
- Time to steady state depends only on the rate of drug elimination
- Repeated doses result in significant drug accumulation when ingestion is more frequent than twice the terminal disposition half-life
- Practical time to steady state is 4–5 terminal disposition half-lifes
- The amount of a drug in the body at steady state depends on the frequency of ingestion and dose
- The plasma half-life of a drug does not reflect metabolic capacity if the apparent volume of distribution changes

accumulation with chronic ingestion is considered to be clinically unimportant.

A loading dose of drug can be given to achieve therapeutic drug concentrations rapidly

The loading dose of a drug is calculated on the basis of its V_d and the desired plasma concentration at steady state (C_{ss}):

Loading dose (mg/kg) = V_d (liters/kg) × C_{ss} (mg/liter)

When given intravenously, the loading dose is usually administered by infusion over a short period of time to reduce the risk of adverse effects associated with the presence of very high drug concentrations in the circulation. Maintenance doses are then based upon the Cl_p and the time interval between doses (t):

Maintenance dose (mg/kg) = Cl_p (liters/kg/h) × C_{ss} (mg/liter) × t (h).

AGE, SEX, AND ORIGIN

Age

Drug-metabolizing enzymes are deficient in the fetus and premature infants

The fetus is able to metabolize drugs early in its development, but the pattern of expression of drug-metabolizing enzymes differs from that of the adult, and fetal drug metabolism is usually less efficient. Drug-metabolizing enzymes are also deficient in premature versus full-term infants. Drug therapy in premature infants is therefore difficult, particularly when more than a single drug dose is administered. In addition, renal function is not fully developed in these babies, and as a result renal drug elimination is impaired (e.g. the diuretic response to loop diuretics, see Chapter 17).

Children metabolize many drugs more rapidly than adults

A few months after birth, the activity of the oxidative drug-metabolic pathways increases dramatically, such that by 2 years of age children can oxidize many drugs more rapidly than adults. The ability to conjugate drugs with glucuronic acid develops more slowly, and at different rates for different isoforms of glucuronosyl transferase. As an example, a greater fraction of an administered dose of acetaminophen is conjugated with sulfate in children than in adults. The frequency of drug administration may have to be altered to compensate for these special characteristics. As children approach puberty, the rate of drug metabolism approaches that of adults.

Changes associated with aging need to be considered when prescribing drugs for the elderly

Some of the changes that occur in the elderly and influence drug treatment include the following:

- Chronic diseases are more common in the elderly and are associated with the use of several drugs in a single individual. As a result, competition between drugs for cytochrome P-450 isoforms is much more likely to occur in the elderly.
- The concentration of serum albumin decreases with age, resulting in a reduced binding capacity for various drugs. This effect can result in saturation of the protein binding sites and an increase in the free fraction of drug in the circulation.
- Lean body mass decreases with age, and as a result the apparent volume of drug distribution may change for some drugs sufficiently to necessitate dose adjustments.
- Liver weight decreases with age and presystemic drug elimination may be reduced.

The expression of cytochrome P-450 enzyme isoforms appears to change with increasing age. This change is reflected as a reduced capability to oxidize drugs, and is seen mainly in elderly males. Available data indicate that induction of drug metabolism can be maintained or impaired in the elderly patient, depending on the drug considered.

Sex

Although some sex differences in drug disposition have been reported (e.g. a lower renal clearance of amantadine in women), the clinical importance of these observations remains to be explored.

Origin

Several differences in drug metabolism have been demonstrated for various human groups (Fig. 4.23). Differences with respect

Drug-metabolic pathways affected by racial origin		
Metabolic reaction	Caucasian	Asian
Acetylation	50% slow	5–10% slow
CYP2D6 oxidation	5–10% deficient	1% deficient
CYP2C18 oxidation	3–5% deficient	20% deficient

Fig. 4.23 Variations in drug-metabolic pathways in populations of humans of different origin. Deficiency in one metabolic pathway is not predictive for deficiency in other drug-metabolic pathways in the same population.

to acetylator phenotype and origin have been well documented. There are also differences in the expression of cytochrome P-450 isoforms. These differences need to be taken into account when drug therapy is considered for patients from such a previously identified group.

DRUG INTERACTIONS

The concomitant administration of drugs can be either beneficial or problematic in terms of interactions between drugs. These interactions can be pharmacokinetic and/or pharmacodynamic in nature. Examples of both beneficial and adverse drug interactions are presented below.

▌ *The concurrent use of levodopa and carbidopa for patients with Parkinson's disease produces a favorable drug interaction*

Carbidopa inhibits the conversion of levodopa to dopamine, but only in the peripheral tissues, since carbidopa does not cross the blood–brain barrier. As a result, orally administered levodopa is converted to dopamine only after it enters the brain, the site of the desired pharmacologic effect. In this instance, carbidopa eliminates or minimizes systemic adverse effects that would arise from the production of dopamine from levodopa in the periphery.

▌ *The hypotensive response of patients receiving a diuretic to treat hypertension can be impaired by concurrent administration of nonsteroidal anti-inflammatory drugs (NSAIDs)*

The renal function of some patients receiving diuretics to treat their hypertension is impaired, because NSAIDs block renal cyclo-oxygenase activity, thus decreasing prostaglandin synthesis in the kidney. Since prostaglandins help to maintain renal blood flow, inhibition of their production will often result in decreased renal elimination of waste products, sodium, and water. A consequence of this interaction is an increase in circulating blood volume and increased work for the heart, thus counteracting the antihypertensive response to the diuretic.

▌ *NSAIDs impair control of coagulation in patients on oral anticoagulant therapy*

Two mechanisms contribute to the interaction between anti-coagulants and NSAIDs:
- Inhibition of cyclo-oxygenase function by NSAIDs.
- Competitive displacement of oral anticoagulant from plasma protein binding by NSAIDs.

As a result, the anticoagulant effect produced by antagonism of vitamin K is increased by inhibition of platelet cyclo-oxygenase activity and inhibition of platelet aggregation as part of the clotting mechanism. Patients on oral anticoagulants should therefore be advised to use acetaminophen for analgesia instead of an NSAID.

▌ *Nutrient–drug interactions can interfere with drug efficacy*

Iron present in some multivitamin preparations can form complexes with certain chemical groups. For example, the catechol substituent on levodopa complexes with iron, resulting in a decrease in levodopa absorption, and decreased drug delivery to the brain. This interaction reduces the efficacy of levodopa in the treatment of Parkinson's disease. Another classical interaction between drugs and nutrients is complex formation of tetracycline antibiotics with Ca^{2+} in milk. This chemical complex results in reduced tetracycline absorption, and therefore decreased antimicrobial activity of the antibiotic. In contrast to the first two examples, ingestion of calcium channel blockers exhibiting high first-pass elimination with grapefruit juice will increase the fraction of the administered dose that reaches the peripheral circulation, and therefore their pharmacologic effect. The mechanism involves inhibition of the intestinal drug metabolizing cytochrome P-450 isoform CYP3A4. This interaction may result in hypotension, and other adverse effects associated with high plasma concentrations of calcium channel blocking drugs.

EFFECT OF DISEASE ON DRUG ACTION

The presence of a disease can have considerable effect on the choice of drug, its disposition, and the likelihood of increased inter-individual variation in drug response. In cases of kidney and liver disease, drug dose may have to be reduced in order to prevent toxicity due to impaired drug elimination by these organs. Usually, the most profound interactions will occur when the disease process affects organs involved in drug disposition. Some important examples of disease–drug interactions include:

- Cirrhosis and other liver diseases can impair the ability of the liver to metabolize drugs. This effect can lead to unpredictable drug accumulation and toxicity if hepatic impairment is not considered when the drug dose regimen is selected. Interestingly, the reserve capacity for phase 2 metabolic reactions seems to be preserved relative to that for phase 1. Therefore, in the presence of hepatic impairment it can be beneficial to choose a drug that is eliminated primarily by conjugation (phase 2). With respect to dose adjustment, there is as yet no consensus as to the biochemical marker that should be used. It is not clear that any one biochemical marker of liver function will reflect accurately the changing capacity of the drug-metabolizing enzymes in the diseased liver. If possible, monitoring of drug concentrations in patients with liver disease provides the best approach at present for adjustment of drug doses.
- In patients with renal disease, prostaglandins help to maintain residual renal function. The use of drugs that inhibit cyclo-oxygenase (e.g. NSAIDs) can lead to a rapid deterioration of residual renal function and consequently impaired drug excretion. Normally, when renal excretion is important for drug elimination, dose will be reduced based upon the directly measured or estimated creatinine clearance of the patient.
- Recent data suggest that intestinal CYP3A4 is suppressed in celiac disease, but is restored to normal with a gluten-free diet. Intestinal disease might therefore lead to variability in first-pass elimination of drugs metabolized by this isoform.

Variability of drug disposition

- The rate of drug disposition is most likely to be impaired in the very young and the very old
- Radical differences in the genetic expression of drug-metabolizing enzymes complicate the individualization of drug therapy
- Concurrent ingestion of multiple drugs increases the probability of drug interactions owing to the increased likelihood of inducing or inhibiting the drug-metabolizing enzyme systems responsible
- Drug doses should be modified if the patient has a disease that impairs the function of organs with an important role in drug metabolism and/or excretion

- Viral infections appear to suppress hepatic cytochromes P-450, perhaps as a result of interferon induction. A patient with a plasma drug concentration at the upper end of the therapeutic range can therefore suddenly show signs of drug toxicity during a viral infection.
- Achlorhydria (absence of stomach acid) is more common in the elderly. Lack of an acid pH in the stomach may affect the site of absorption of drug formulations with a pH-dependent coating.
- The choice of diuretic for a patient with cardiovascular disease can depend on whether the patient has osteoporosis. Hydrochlorothiazide is a diuretic that does not increase the renal elimination of Ca^{2+} and therefore is advantageous in this type of patient.
- β adrenoceptor antagonists are contraindicated in patients with asthma because these drugs increase bronchoconstriction. This interaction is due to the fact that circulating epinephrine in asthmatics helps to dilate their airways (see Chapter 19).

- Anticholinergic drugs can increase cognitive impairment in patients with Alzheimer-type dementia.

FURTHER READING

Benet LZ (ed.) *The Effect of Disease States on Drug Pharmacokinetics*. Washington, DC: American Pharmaceutical Association; 1976. [This classic monograph provides details on how diseases contribute to altered drug disposition.]

Cupp MJ, Tracy TS. Cytochrome P-450: new nomenclature and clinical implications. *Am Fam Physician* 1998; **57**: 107–116. [This review provides examples of important P-450 drug-metabolizing enzymes, their inducers and inhibitors, and relevant clinical cases to reinforce prescribing principles.]

Gaedigk A. Interethnic differences of drug-metabolizing enzymes. *Int J Clin Pharmacol Ther* 2000; **38**: 61–68. [This review summarizes our current understanding of the role of ethnic origin on the expression of some drug-metabolizing enzymes.]

Grymonpre RE, Mitenko PA, Sitar DS, Aoki FY, Montgomery PR. Drug associated hospital admissions in older patients. *J Am Geriatr Soc* 1988; **36**: 1092–1098. [This paper illustrates the role of multiple drug therapy as a contributing factor to hospital admissions.]

Johnson MD. Clinically significant drug interactions. What you need to know before writing prescriptions. *Postgrad Med* 1999; **105**: 193–222. [This review provides an indication of the current state of knowledge concerning drug interactions involving cytochrome P-450 isoforms.]

Rodighiero V. Effects of liver disease on pharmacokinetics. An update. *Clin Pharmacokinet* 1999; **37**: 399–431. [This review reflects our current state of knowledge concerning drug dose adjustment for patients with liver disease.]

Sitar DS. Human drug metabolism in vivo. *Pharmacol Ther* 1989; **43**: 363–375. [This review evaluates the contribution of factors alleged to cause variation of drug metabolism in man.]

Wolf RC, Smith G. Pharmacogenetics. *Brit Med Bull* 1999; **55**: 366–386. [This review illustrates the role of pharmacogenetics in the inter-individual variability in drug response and adverse drug reactions.]

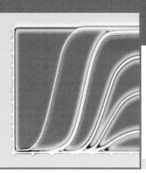

Chapter 5

Pharmacodynamics and the Measurement of Drug Action

THE RECEPTOR

Most drugs must bind to a receptor in order to produce their actions but there are exceptions as we will see later on. From the first studies of the effects of drugs on animal tissues in the late nineteenth century, it became evident that many drugs produce specific responses in specific tissues. That is:

- A drug that has profound effects on one type of tissue may have no effect on another type of tissue.
- A drug may have quite different effects on different tissues.

For example, the alkaloid pilocarpine, like the neurotransmitter acetylcholine (see Chapter 14), induces contraction of intestinal smooth muscle, but slows heart rate. To account for such differences, Langley (1852–1925) proposed in 1878, on the basis of studies of the effects of the alkaloids pilocarpine and atropine on salivation, that 'there is some "receptor" substance … with which both are capable of forming compounds …' Later, in 1905, when studying the action of nicotine and curare on skeletal muscle, he found that nicotine caused contractions only when applied to certain small regions of the muscle. He concluded that the 'receptive substance' for nicotine was confined to those regions, and that curare worked by blocking the combination of nicotine with its receptor.

Paul Ehrlich (1854–1915) appears to have independently developed the receptor concept, starting from the observation that many organic dyes selectively stain specific cell constituents. In 1885 he proposed that cells have 'side chains' or 'receptors' to which drugs or toxins must attach in order to produce their actions. Ehrlich was very influential in his time and is still remembered for his idea of the 'magic bullet,' a chemical compound constructed for its selective toxicity to, for example, an infectious organism, as well as for the synthesis of organic arsenicals that were effective in the treatment of syphilis. In the development of receptor theory, Ehrlich was the first to point out that the rapid reversibility of the actions of alkaloids implied that the 'combination' of such drugs with receptors did not involve strong (covalent) chemical bonds. Recent developments in molecular biology are rapidly clarifying the nature of drug–receptor binding at the molecular level. Today, a receptor is regarded as specific drug binding site on a biomolecule that acts as a target for a particular group of related drugs. When a binding site cannot be delineated from the rest of the molecular target, the whole complex is regarded as the receptor (see Chapter 3).

▇ Not all drugs have receptors

With drugs that target a known enzyme, the molecular target is the enzyme. The receptor for such drugs is that part on the enzyme that binds the drug. While the molecular targets for most drugs are proteins, it is now recognized that carbohydrates, lipids and other macromolecules can be targets for drugs. This view of receptors is more encompassing than a view in which receptors are those proteins mediating the actions of neurotransmitters, autacoids and hormones. As a binding moiety, receptors are identified and characterized by the techniques of molecular biology. However, for some types of drugs their actions are easily explained without the need for receptors. Drugs that do not act via a receptor include buffers (antacids) that reduce stomach acidity, bulk laxatives and chelating agents. At the other extreme are agents with obscure mechanisms of action which are characterized by the virtual absence of strict chemical specificity. The prime examples of this are the gaseous and volatile general anesthetics, including the inert gas xenon. For these anesthetics there is no evidence of a binding site, or a single molecular target. Nevertheless, it is possible anesthetics owe their pharmacologic effects to actions on an undiscovered membrane system (perhaps a voltage-gated ion channel) critical to normal neural function. Such a system would then be the molecular target for anesthetics.

▇ The classic receptor concept is very important for drugs that mimic or antagonize the actions of hormones, neurohormones, neurotransmitters, and autacoids

Drugs (including plant alkaloids, such as nicotine, curare, and atropine) that mimicked or antagonized the effects of

 Drugs and receptors

- Most drugs must first bind to a receptor in order to produce their pharmacologic actions. The drug–receptor complex is often very short-lived

- The activation produced by the agonist–receptor complex produces a response through an 'effector' or 'transduction system'

- Tissue responses are generally not directly proportional to the fraction of the total receptor pool which is complexed with agonist

- Maximum tissue responses can occur when only a fraction of the total receptor pool is complexed with agonist

neurotransmitters first led Langley to postulate the receptor idea. With such drugs, experimental study of how they act was originally limited to measuring their effects in whole animals and isolated tissues, for example, on blood pressure, heart rate, secretion, or commonly, contraction of intestinal, bronchial, vascular, or uterine smooth muscle. Such effects have long been recognized as indirect reflections of the interaction of drugs with their receptors. The receptor concept has led to the development of methods using such data to classify drugs in terms of the receptors upon which they act and to develop new drugs targeted to specific receptors.

Receptors are generally large proteins that contain a site which 'recognizes' drugs and binds them. This binding site is usually linked to a transduction system

In the last 20 years, there has been progress in the isolation and chemical characterization of receptors. It has become clear that many receptors are proteins or part of a protein. Such proteins have at least one distinct region to which drugs, both agonists and antagonists, bind. When an agonist binds, it produces a change that either directly induces a measurable response, such as an opening a channel, or changes the activity of an enzyme, or triggers a transduction chain that in its turn produces a measurable response. The link between the binding of agonist and transduction can be relatively direct, or involve second messengers and a chain of other proteins. Generally it is not the recognition site that is responsible for transduction but other regions of the same molecule, or even a separate molecule, such as the G proteins that are responsible for transduction and the ultimate cellular response. In addition, other parts of a receptor molecule can act as targets for a different type of drugs. Generally such drugs are not agonists, but inhibitors that are not 'competitive' antagonists, or they are drugs known as inverse agonists (see below and Chapter 3).

An active agonist–receptor complex produces a cellular response via 'transduction'

As indicated above the active agonist–receptor complex initiates transduction either locally at the membrane level or intracellularly. Examples of transduction systems are given in Chapter 3. It also seems to be generally accepted that, at least in most cases, the combination of an agonist with a receptor must lead to a conformational change in the latter so as to produce an active drug–receptor complex. This provides the basis for a model in which the different actions of agonists, partial agonists, and antagonists can be explained.

Many different classes of drugs may bind with a receptor. Such binding defines a drug as a 'ligand' for a receptor and the nature of the binding determines whether a drug is an agonist, an antagonist, partial agonist, or inverse agonist.

- If a ligand binds to a receptor and produces a molecular response (conformational change in the receptor), with subsequent cellular responses, it is an agonist.
- If a ligand binds to a receptor without initiating a molecular response leading to cellular and tissue responses, but competitively denies the agonists access to that receptor, the ligand is considered to be a competitive antagonist.

- Partial agonists are ligands which bind to a receptor but in such an inefficient manner that even high concentrations of drug are incapable of producing sufficient molecular responses to cause a maximum cellular response. Consequently the maximum tissue response to a partial agonist is less than with a 'full' agonist. A partial agonist thus can act as an antagonist to a full agonist.
- Inverse agonists that bind to receptors which, even in the absence of the agonist, exist in an activated state. This constant level of activation causes a 'background' level of transduction and cellular responses. When an inverse agonist binds to the activated receptor it inactivates it and therefore inhibits this background activation.

Tissue responses are not necessarily directly proportional to the molecular responses resulting from an agonist binding to its receptor

The relationship between tissue response and drug dose (concentration) is commonly called the dose–response relationship. This depends not only on the binding of agonist to receptor but also on transduction mechanisms which typically involve a series of biochemical/biophysical steps. In many cases, the tissue's effective maximum response to a drug is produced when only a small fraction of its receptors are occupied and have become active following conformational changes. This is exemplified at the skeletal neuromuscular junction (see Chapters 14 and 26). At this nerve–muscle junction there are about 30 million acetylcholine receptors. However, simultaneous activation of only 40,000 of these receptors is sufficient to elicit an action potential and maximum twitch of the muscle fiber. By using antagonists which bind irreversibly to receptors, or antibodies to the receptors, it is possible to determine what proportion of receptors needs to be occupied in order to produce a maximum response. The proportion of receptors not needed for the production of the maximal response is referred to as 'receptor reserve.'

Some tissues commonly have a 'receptor reserve' of a factor of more than 100, and some up to almost 10,000. That is, although reduction of available receptors in the presence of an irreversible antagonist always requires more agonist to produce a given response, the maximum attainable response to an agonist can remain virtually undiminished until only a small fraction of the original receptors remain. It therefore follows that tissue responses are not directly proportional to the fraction of receptors occupied and activated.

The practical consequence of 'receptor reserve' is that, for many agonists, the doses used clinically (or produced endogenously) activate only a very small fraction of receptors, even when the tissue response is quite large. As a result, the presence or absence of agonists scarcely changes the number of receptors occupied by a competitive antagonist. The effect of an antagonist, and how well its block can be surmounted by increasing the dose of agonist, is therefore essentially the same for an irreversible or a reversible antagonist. For example, blocking the enzyme acetylcholinesterase at the skeletal neuromuscular junction with a drug such as neostigmine effectively increases the amount of acetylcholine in the synaptic cleft and is equally effective in opposing the neuromuscular blockade produced by:

- Myasthenia gravis, where immune mechanisms destroy a large fraction of nicotinic receptors.
- A competitive nicotinic antagonist such as pancuronium (see Chapter 26).

As another example, adrenoceptor antagonism (see Chapter 14) may be produced clinically with:

- Phenoxybenzamine, whose irreversible actions on receptor actions are only overcome with the synthesis of new receptors.
- Phentolamine, a rapidly reversible competitive antagonist.

The decision as to which type of antagonist (reversible or irreversible) to use depends upon considerations such as the time course of action, and adverse effects of the drugs, rather than theoretical differences between competitive, irreversible, or noncompetitive antagonism. With these agents, theory predicts that a dose or concentration of the drug that effectively occupies or renders inactive, say, 90% of the receptors will reduce responses to endogenous or exogenous norepinephrine by about 90%, and the original response to exogenous norepinephrine may be obtained by increasing its dose tenfold. However, this will not be the case if there is little or no receptor reserve.

The quantitative analysis of mechanisms of drug action consists largely of interpreting dose–response curves

The quantitative analysis of mechanisms of drug action is important in the development of new drugs, where the aims are:

- To discover chemical agents that are specific in terms of the receptors with which they interact.
- To discover agents that are selective by virtue of their interaction with only one subtype of receptor.

Several principles are fundamental to an understanding of drug–receptor interactions and dose (concentration)–response curves. These principles, which apply to the majority of drugs used clinically and experimentally, are as follows:

- On any single cell in a tissue there are generally numerous receptors of any one type, and most cells contain many different types of receptor.
- When a drug is present, new drug–receptor complexes are continually created as the random movement of drug molecules leads to their collision with receptors that are not already occupied. The drug–receptor complexes are also continually breaking down randomly, thereby freeing receptors to combine again with the drug.
- Agonist–receptor complexes continually fluctuate between inactive and active conformations (the molecular response). The latter induce biophysical events such as the opening of ion channels, or biochemical events such as G protein activation that lead to a tissue response.
- The numbers of receptors expressed on a cell may change in pathologic conditions, and with chronic drug administration.

Two useful rules of thumb that may be added to these fundamental principles are:

- Submaximal tissue responses to agonists are proportional to the product of agonist dose (concentration) and the number of available receptors.
- Pharmacologic antagonists, in effect, reduce the number of available receptors to an extent that does not much depend upon how much agonist is present.

The fundamental principles listed above represent a view of how drugs act in linking empirical observations and experimental results to fundamental chemical and physicochemical events. The quantitative consequences of the theory are in many respects manifested in the binding of radioactively labeled ligands (drugs) to receptors isolated from tissues. As this kind of experiment is relatively easy to perform and understand, it is convenient to consider 'receptor binding,' before considering dose–response curves.

Receptor binding of drugs

A receptor can be considered as an entity that selectively and specifically binds ligands (drugs). When studying the binding of drugs to receptors it is usually sufficient to think of the receptor simply as an entity that can bind a variety of ligands. For the sake of simplicity it is postulated that a ligand binds selectively only to a single type of recognition site on the receptor, and not to other potential binding sites. This is postulated not only for a preparation of pure receptors, but also for the wide variety of complex macromolecules present in whole-tissue or broken-cell preparations.

The simplest model for reversible ligand binding to a receptor

The simplest possible model for reversible ligand binding to a receptor is one in which each molecule of ligand (L) can randomly collide with, and bind to, a molecule of receptor (R) in such a way as to form a ligand–receptor complex (LR). This complex can then break down at any moment to produce a free molecule of ligand and an unoccupied receptor. From basic kinetic theory (i.e. the law of mass action), the rate at which new LR complexes are formed at any given time is proportional to the concentration of L, written as $[L]$, and the concentration of free R, i.e. $[R]$. (Note the use of square brackets to indicate concentration.) At the same time the rate at which the ligand–receptor (LR) complex breaks down to L and R is proportional to the concentration of LR, i.e. $[LR]$. It is worth working through the mathematics of the binding interaction since doing so gives valuable insight into drug receptor–interactions.

At equilibrium, the rate at which new LR complexes are formed equals the rate at which LR complexes break down, thus:

$$K_L [LR] = [L] [R] \qquad \text{Eqn 1}$$

where K_L is the dissociation constant usually expressed as molar (M = gram molecules/L). The constant K_L depends upon physical factors such as temperature and, most importantly, the chemical nature of the interacting substances. In this simple model, K_L is the ratio of the off- to on-rate constants for binding to the receptor. It is worth noting that the same simple equation applies to more complicated models in which there are multiple conformations of R and LR. In the complex case K_L depends upon all the rate constants needed to describe the system. Nevertheless, regardless of how many conformations of R or LR exist, receptors may be considered in the two forms, R and LR, with K_L **[LR]** = **[L]** **[R]**. The alternative form of the equation is **[LR]** = **[L]** **[R]**/K_L.

■ *[LR] + [R] is a constant*

Since the total number of receptors is limited, the total concentration of **[LR]** + **[R]** is constant and designated **[R$_t$]**. Therefore:

$$[R_t] = [R] + [LR] = [R] (1 + [L]/K_L) \qquad \text{Eqn 2}$$

when **[LR]** is substituted by the term **[R]** **[L]**/K_L (see above). Further, combining this with K_L **[LR]** = **[L]** **[R]** gives

$$[LR]/[R_t] = ([L]/K_L)(1 + [L]/K_L) \qquad \text{Eqn 3}$$

with **[LR]**/**[R$_t$]** being the chance that any one R will at any moment be combined with L.

■ *Semilogarithmic plots are usually used for both binding studies and dose–response curves*

The graph of **[LR]** versus **[L]** for two ligands (A and B with very different K_L values) is shown in Fig. 5.1. It is notable that although both plots show the same initial linear rise with concentration, which gradually flattens to a maximum, it is inconvenient to use the same *x* axis for both A and B. In Fig. 5.2 the same information is plotted semilogarithmically, i.e. with **[LR]** versus the log of **[L]** rather than simply **[L]**. Besides allowing the data points for A and B to be easily plotted on the same axis, such a graph shows that both plots are essentially the same, differing only in their relative positions on the *x* axis. Such semilogarithmic plots are now usually used for both binding studies and dose–response curves, purely for convenience, although it is only with experience (or separate plots) that it can be seen that the beginning portions of the rising curves in Fig. 5.2 still represent **[LR]** rising in proportion to **[L]**. From the equation **[LR]** = **[R$_t$]** **[L]**/(**[L]** + K_L) given above, it follows that K_L is given by the value of **[L]** at which **[LR]** is just one half of **[R$_t$]**; the separation between the two parallel curves in Fig. 5.2 is simply the logarithm of the ratio of K_L values.

🗝 **General model of reversible ligand (drug) binding to receptors**

- Each molecule of ligand (L) can randomly collide with a molecule of receptor (R) in such a way as to form a ligand–receptor complex (LR)

- The LR complex can then break down at any moment to produce a free molecule of unchanged ligand (L), and an unoccupied receptor (R)

- At equilibrium, K_L **[LR]** = **[L]** **[R]** where K_L is the dissociation constant (Molar)

In a study of 'saturation' binding, tissue (or isolated receptor), samples are incubated with various concentrations of L where L is radioactively labeled (usually with ^{3}H), and then rapidly filtered and 'washed' to remove unbound ligand. The subsequent count of the retained radioactivity gives the total of how much ligand remains. Some of this is, however, simply ligand which is nonspecifically stuck in the interstices of the filter, or between cells or, perhaps, dissolved in the tissue lipid. This nonspecific, as opposed to specific, binding is illustrated in Fig. 5.3. The effect of nonspecific binding on binding that is

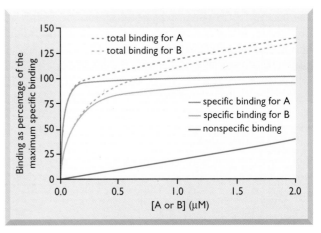

Fig. 5.1 Linear plots for specific and nonspecific receptor binding for the two ligands, A and B, which have K_L values of 0.01 (K_A) and 0.1(K_B) mM (microMolar), respectively, with specific and nonspecific binding. The *y* axis is binding (formation of AR or BR) expressed as a percent of maximum specific binding for A or B, respectively. The *x* axis is the concentration of A or B. Total binding is indicated with dashed lines. In this figure, it is assumed that nonspecific binding is proportional to **[A]** or **[B]** and does not saturate, but on the other hand that the specific binding for both A and B does saturate, and that the maximum specific binding is 100. Note the equal spacing on the concentration axis (i.e. it is linear), and that the intercept is 0,0. (μM = microMolar conc.)

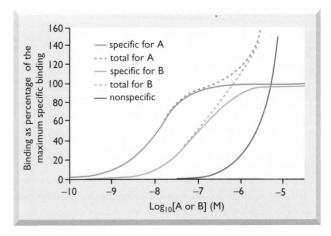

Fig. 5.2 Semilog plot of Fig. 5.1. Higher concentrations of A and B were studied for specific and nonspecific binding with conditions as in Fig. 5.1, with K_A = 0.01 mM and K_B = 0.1 mM. In this figure the *x* axis is now plotted on a $\log_{10}$ scale over a concentration range from 10^{-10} M to >10^{-5} M which is a more than 100,000-fold concentration range. The intercept of the *y* axis with the *x* axis is now 0, –10. (M = Molar conc.)

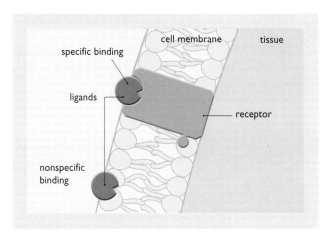

Fig. 5.3 Specific and nonspecific binding of ligands described in Fig. 5.1. The ligand is capable of binding with a receptor located within the cell membrane to form a LR complex. The ligand also binds in a nonspecific manner to the cell membrane.

expressed as a percentage of specific binding is shown in Figs 5.1 and 5.2.

Nonspecific binding, in contrast to specific binding, is unaltered by a relatively high concentration ('excess') of the same 'cold' (unlabeled) ligand in the incubation medium. Therefore, parallel experiments in the absence and presence of excess 'cold' ligand allow for subtraction of nonspecific from total binding so as to give specific binding. A plot of the specifically bound ligand, which we call '**B**' (which is the same as $[\mathbf{LR}]$), versus the log of the free ligand, '**F**' (which is the same as $[\mathbf{L}]$), then gives a characteristic sigmoid curve as shown in Fig. 5.2. Statistical curve-fitting procedures show whether data fit the theoretical receptor binding equation. If they do, the graph gives $\mathbf{B_{max}}$ (maximum possible **B**), which reflect $\mathbf{R_t}$, the amount of receptors in the tissue and K_d (i.e. the dissociation constant of the ligand), which is here the same as K_L.

In much of the older literature on binding, before inexpensive computers became readily available, the data obtained from such studies, were often plotted in terms of the 'Scatchard relation' from the equations $K_L[\mathbf{LR}] = [\mathbf{L}]\,[\mathbf{R}]$ and $[\mathbf{R_t}] = [\mathbf{R}] + [\mathbf{LR}]$ given above. Rearrangement of the equations gives the following:

$$K_L\,[\mathbf{LR}] = [\mathbf{L}]\,[\mathbf{R}] = [\mathbf{L}]\,([\mathbf{R_t}] - [\mathbf{LR}])$$

$$[\mathbf{LR}]/[\mathbf{L}] = ([\mathbf{R_t}] - [\mathbf{LR}])/K_L$$

Now if $[\mathbf{LR}]$ is **B**, $[\mathbf{L}]$ is **F** and K_L is K_d then

$$\mathbf{B}/\mathbf{F} = (\mathbf{B_{max}} - \mathbf{B})/K_d \qquad\qquad \text{Eqn 4}$$

where **B** is bound and **F** free and K_d is analogous to K_L.

Therefore, a plot of **B/F** (bound/free) versus **B** (bound) produces a straight line that extrapolates to the x axis at $\mathbf{B_{max}}$ and has a slope of $1/K_d$.

This type of mathematical approach has two problems:
- Esoteric considerations involved in dealing statistically with experimental errors.
- Insensitivity to a failure of data to fit the theoretical binding curve.

Binding data do not fit the expected curve if more than one kind of binding site for a ligand is present

A problem with binding studies arises when the tissue or receptor preparation being studied contains more than one kind of specific binding site for the chosen ligand. In this case, total binding fails to fit the theoretical binding curve for a single receptor, since two processes are at work.

It is also not uncommon to find that data for agonist binding do not fit the theoretical equation (i.e. $[\mathbf{LR}] = [\mathbf{R_t}]\,[\mathbf{L}]/([\mathbf{L}] + K_L)$) when tissue or cell preparations are used, presumably because the cellular response induced by the agonist–receptor interaction itself changes the molecular interaction between agonist and receptor, thereby changing agonist–receptor affinity.

Binding studies are more complicated when more than one ligand is present and competition between them can occur

Suppose that a receptor can bind either a molecule of ligand (L) or ligand (C), but not simultaneously (Fig. 5.4). Receptors now can exist in three forms:
- Free R, with a concentration of $[\mathbf{R}]$.
- LR with a concentration of $[\mathbf{LR}] = [\mathbf{R}]\,[\mathbf{L}]/K_L$.
- CR, with a concentration of $[\mathbf{CR}] = [\mathbf{R}]\,[\mathbf{C}]/K_C$ (where K_C is the dissociation constant of CR).

From the above, the following equation can be derived:

$$[\mathbf{R_t}] = [\mathbf{R}] + [\mathbf{LR}] + [\mathbf{CR}] \qquad\qquad \text{Eqn 5}$$

where $[\mathbf{R_t}]$ is the sum of all forms of R. Similar equations can be derived for $[\mathbf{LR}]$ and $[\mathbf{CR}]$.

A further series of useful equations can be derived by substitution.

An important feature of such equations is that, if $[\mathbf{L}]$ is high enough, most of the receptors will be in the form LR, despite C being present. Conversely, if $[\mathbf{C}]$ is high most of the receptors will be in the form, CR, despite L being present. Therefore C is said to 'compete' with L, and L with C. The competition arises simply because a single receptor site cannot bind both L and C simultaneously. Competition is mathematically equivalent to

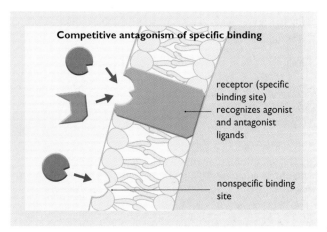

Fig. 5.4 Two different ligands 'competing' for binding to the specific binding site of a receptor.

multiplying the dissociation constant by $(1 + c)$ where c is the concentration of the competitor divided by its dissociation constant (i.e. $c = [C]/K_C$). It follows that the effect of any given concentration of competitor is to cause a parallel shift of the plot of [LR] versus log[L] (the dose–response curve) to the right on the x axis. The shift will be by a factor $\log(1 + c)$, where c is $[C]/K_C$ (Fig. 5.5).

This provides a method for experimentally determining the dissociation constant of a competitive molecule. At any given [C], the dose ratio (DR), which is the ratio of [L] values producing the same [LR] in the presence, and absence, of C is given by:

$$DR = 1 + [C]/K_C \qquad \text{Eqn 6}$$

Rearranging this gives:

$$(DR - 1)/[C] = 1/K_C$$

This method is less important in binding studies but of great importance in functional dose–response studies of agonist/antagonist–receptor interactions where the response to [LR] is measured, rather than its binding. Adding a competitive antagonist, C, in the presence of agonist L is equivalent to reducing the agonist concentration by the factor $(1 + [C]/K_C)$. This leads to a shift of the response–log[agonist] curve to the right. This shift is analogous to the shifts seen in Fig. 5.5. Therefore, original responses are restored by multiplying agonist doses by the DR, which is equal to $1 + [C]/K_C$.

In binding studies there is a way of calculating dissociation constants for a ligand that is not available in a radioactive-labeled form. All that is needed is another ligand which is radioactive, and which competes with the first. The appropriate mathematics suggests that [LR] in the presence of C follows a smooth displacement curve relative to what it is in the absence of C (Fig. 5.6), with a 50% reduction at a certain value of [C],

C_{50}, which gives K_C once K_L is known. To find K_L, C can simply be the same ligand as L, but in unlabeled form, so that K_C is the same as K_L (Fig. 5.7). The added concentration of C that displaces 50% of the label, C_{50}, is $K_L + [L]$ and $K_L = C_{50} - [L]$, [L] being the (constant) concentration of labeled ligand.

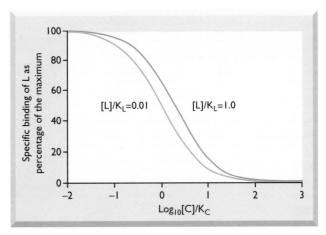

Fig. 5.6 Displacement of the binding of ligand (L) by a competitive antagonist (C). Two displacement curves are shown, one (in blue) where the occupancy is low, **[L]**/K_L = 0.01. The red curve is displacement of L from R when the ligand occupancy is high ($[L]$/K_L = 1.0). Note that the y axis shows the specific binding in terms of the maximum binding for low or high occupancy in the absence of C.

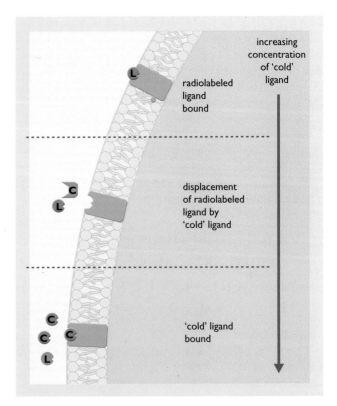

Fig. 5.7 A bound radiolabeled ligand (L) is displaced in an environment where the concentration of competitive antagonist (C) is high. Note that C can be the same drug as L where L is the radioactive form while C is the nonradioactive form. This concept of displacement is used to find K_L (compare with Fig. 5.6).

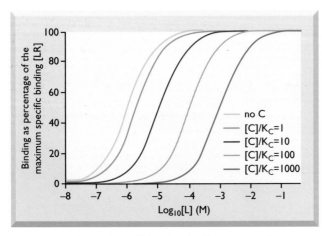

Fig. 5.5 Specific binding of ligand (L) in the presence of competitive antagonist (C), present in different concentrations such that [C]/K_C = 1, 10, 100, or 1000. As in Fig. 5.2 this is a semilogarithmic plot in which the x axis is expressed in $\log_{10}$ form. K_C is the dissociation constant for C. Note that the presence of C shifts the concentration–binding graphs for L to the right in a parallel manner. The amount of shift depends upon **[C]**/K_C with each 10-fold increase causing a log 1.0 (= 10) parallel shift. (M = Molar conc.)

In the 25 years since binding studies were begun, numerous experiments similar to those described above have been performed. Saturation binding curves have been used to establish the amount of receptor in a tissue, while displacement curves have been used to calculate dissociation constants for many drugs. In general, the displacement curves obtained correspond fairly exactly to the theoretical ones, as pictured in Fig. 5.6. Deviations sometimes occur with agonist ligands and the reasons for these deviations are subject to ongoing investigations. Displacement curves obtained experimentally also differ from the theoretical curves if the labeled ligand binds to more than one kind of receptor in the tissue preparation.

■ Not all antagonists are competitive

Not all drugs modify agonist binding in a competitive manner. The simplest reason for this occurrence is that a receptor contains more than one ligand-recognition site, and that binding at one site alters the affinity at another. This type of interaction is known as an allosteric interaction. It is characterized in saturation binding experiments by a half-maximal binding, denoted by L_{50b} (apparent K_L) value that can be varied continuously between two limits. At one extreme is the absence of the allosteric agent while at the other extreme virtually all receptors are bound to the allosteric agent. When the antagonist binds in this manner it is said to be non-competitive.

Another theoretical scenario is one where the antagonist can bind only to the ligand–receptor (LR) complex. This can occur only if the binding of L causes a change in conformation of the receptor (Fig. 5.8) such that it can now bind the antagonist. In such a case the antagonist may be termed an uncompetitive ligand (U). Because of the dynamics of the interaction between ligand (L), uncompetitive ligand (U), and receptors, the apparent affinity of the receptor for ligand L is increased in the presence of U. This essentially occurs because the form UR cannot exist and LUR must first dissociate to form LR and U before breaking down to form free R. So, in effect, L is trapped in the LRU form.

DOSE–RESPONSE CURVES

The relationship between the log of the dose (concentration) of an agonist drug and tissue response invariably follows a curve similar to those shown in Fig. 5.9, which in turn closely resemble the ligand–receptor binding curve shown in Fig. 5.2. The effect (**E**) might be either a tissue response or, less usually, the inhibition of spontaneous activity (e.g. slowing of heart rate by acetylcholine). Below a certain concentration of agonist (**[A]**), **E** is too low to measure, but at higher concentrations it becomes appreciable and rises with increasing agonist concentration (**[A]**) until at sufficiently high concentrations it can no longer be increased by raising **[A]**, and asymptotes to a maximum (**E_{max}**). A log (dose)–response curve can be conventionally characterized by three measures:

- **E_{max}**.
- The concentration of A (termed **[A_{50}]**), at which **E** is half of **E_{max}**.

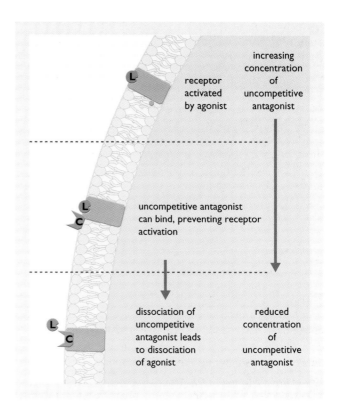

Fig. 5.8 This figure is analogous to Fig. 5.7, but in this case the antagonist is uncompetitive.

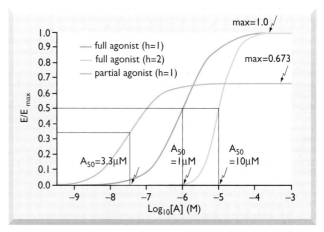

Fig. 5.9 Dose–response curves for different agonists (A) with various values for A_{50}, maxima, and slopes (h). Note that the response to agonist on the y axis is in the form **E/E_{max}**. Three agonists are shown; the higher the **A_{50}** concentration the more the curve lies to the right. For full agonists the maximum is the same whereas for partial agonists the maximum is lower. The higher the value of 'h' the steeper the slope of the dose–response curve. (M = Molar conc.)

- The slope parameter (Hill coefficient, h) which describes the steepness of the curve. It is obtained by fitting the **E − [A]** curve to another form of the dose–response equation, the logistic function:

$$E/E_{max} = [A]^h/[A]^h + A_{50}{}^h)$$

Eqn 7

Sometimes an agonist which is closely related chemically to another agonist, can have a lower E_{max}, despite both drugs

Dose (concentration)–response curves

- The relationship between the response to a drug and drug dose (concentration) is commonly called the dose–response curve.

- Quantitative analysis of drug action, and its mechanisms, is heavily dependent upon interpreting dose–response curves

- Semilogarithmic graphs (where the dose axis is expressed in log form) are usually used for dose–response curves

- Competitive antagonists shift dose–response curves for corresponding agonists in a parallel manner to the right

acting on the same receptor. For this reason, such an agonist is termed a partial agonist (Fig. 5.9).

Potency, intrinsic activity, and efficacy

Technically, the term potency refers to the A_{50} value. The lower the A_{50}, the less the concentration of drug required to produce 50% of maximum effect, and the higher the potency. E_{max} is referred to as intrinsic activity, or effectiveness. Therefore, agonist A might be more potent than agonist B even if it falls short of B's effectiveness (i.e. E_{max} for B is greater than for A). The term efficacy is often used loosely to mean effectiveness, but the term should be reserved in pharmacology for a technical meaning that is quite different as is explained below.

The relation between tissue response and concentration of agonist–receptor complex is often nonlinear

Since the typical log[A] versus response (E) curve is similar to the theoretical [LR] versus log[L] curve it was assumed (prior to 1956) that response E directly reflected the amount of agonist–receptor complex (AR). In particular, it was assumed that E/E_{max} was equivalent to $[AR]/[R_t]$. However, it is now clear that this is rarely the case, and that the relationship between E and [AR] is commonly nonlinear and may be complex.

Very often E_{max} merely reflects the capacity of the system to produce a response. For example, if A is an agonist which acts on a receptor to lower blood pressure, the maximum possible effect of A would be to lower blood pressure to 0 mmHg. Even when such a limitation to response does not apply, as shown by different agonists with different E_{max} values in the same tissue preparation, an E that is half of E_{max} is usually obtained with agonists at a value of $[AR]/[R_t]$ which is much less than 50%. Such conclusions have been reached because it has been possible to obtain good estimates of the dissociation constants for agonists using an analytic approach, based on the action of irreversible antagonists, first introduced by R. Furchgott in 1966. Of course, once an agonist's dissociation constant (K_A) has been obtained, a graph of E versus [A] can be translated into a graph of E versus $[AR]/[R_t]$, yielding information about the transduction system (cellular response) linking [AR] to E.

Competitive antagonists for endogenous agonists such as neurotransmitters, neurohormones, and autacoids

Competitive antagonists shift agonist dose–response curves to the right

Reversible competitive antagonists are usually termed competitive antagonists. The reversible aspect is understood since there is no difficulty in distinguishing between drugs whose effects are reversible in that their actions disappear upon being removed, and those whose effects are irreversible (i.e. maintained indefinitely). Such drugs are characterized by producing parallel shifts to the right of plots of **E** (effect or response) versus log[A], where A is an agonist (Fig. 5.10). Such a relationship arises automatically from the equation:

$$[AR] = [R_t] [A]/([A] + K_A (1 + [C]/K_C)) \qquad \text{Eqn 8}$$

Whatever the relationship between E (effect) and [AR], the inhibitory effect of a competitor (C), at any [A], can always be overcome, or nullified, by increasing [A] by the factor $(1 + [C]/K_C)$ which is the dose ratio (**DR**). In other words inhibition is surmountable at any level of response and E_{max} is not reduced. There is an easy way to check whether experimental results agree with the theory. Since $DR - 1 = [C]/K_C$ it follows that:

$$\log(DR - 1) = \log[C] - \log K_C \qquad \text{Eqn 9}$$

and when the latter relationship is plotted as shown in Fig. 5.11 it is known as the Schild plot. The intercept at $\log_{10}(DR - 1) = 0$ (where **DR** = 2) is the K_C value. By analogy with pH notation, the negative $\log_{10}$ of K_C is known as the pA_2. An alternative approach is shown in Fig. 5.12 where $(DR - 1)/[C]$ is plotted against log[C] when this ratio should remain constant ($= 1/K_C$) giving a straight line parallel to the x axis of the graph.

Sometimes the equation $(DR - 1) = [C]/K_C$ does not hold for some agonists even though antagonists are clearly com-

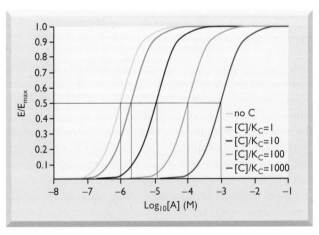

Fig. 5.10 Dose-response curves for an agonist (A) in the presence of competitive antagonist (C), at different concentrations such that [C]/K_C equals 1, 10, 100 or 1000. Compare this figure with Fig. 5.5. Note that the *x* axes are the same for both figures; however the *y* axis here is the ratio of the effects (**E**), produced by different concentrations of agonist, to the maximum effect (E_{max}).

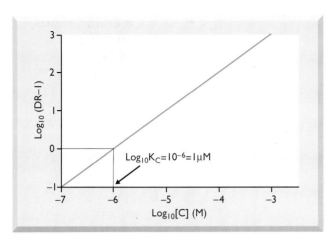

Fig. 5.11 Schild plot for a competitive antagonist (C). In this graph DR is the dose ratio, i.e. the value of A_{50} in the presence of a particular concentration of C divided by A_{50} in the absence of C. The data here are typical of that used to construct a Schild plot. The linear nature of this graph allows for easy estimation of K_c and the slope. Note that a wide range of concentrations of C can be studied.

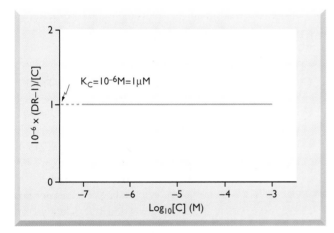

Fig. 5.12 A modified form of the Schild plot for a competitive antagonist (C). It can easily be inferred from this plot that for every increment in C there is a corresponding increment in dose ratio (**DR**).

petitive in that they produce parallel shifts to the right. Deviations from the equation can be expected if the receptor has more than one binding site for agonist, and the receptor is in its active form only when two or more agonist molecules are bound. An example of this situation is found with the nicotinic acetylcholine receptor in skeletal muscle (see Chapters 20 and 26). This classic receptor is now known to be part of a ligand-gated ion channel (see Chapter 3). This ion channel opens when two acetylcholine molecules are bound to receptors on one channel. That is the active receptor is of the form A_2R. If binding of only one molecule of competitor is sufficient to prevent receptor action, but simultaneous binding of 'n' molecules of A are necessary to produce E (i.e. the active receptor is of the form A_nR), the equation becomes $DR^n - 1 = [C]/K_c$.

Noncompetitive antagonists reduce E_{max}

When an antagonist (D) reduces E_{max} it is usually (and inaccurately) termed noncompetitive (Fig. 5.13). Such a response can arise from a variety of mechanisms such as uncompetitive antagonism (where the ARD complex is inactive), a mixture of uncompetitive and competitive antagonism, or from inhibition somewhere in the transduction chain. These forms of antagonism result in marked deviations from the straight-line plots for $\log(DR - 1)$ versus $\log[D]$, and $(DR - 1)/[D]$ versus $\log[D]$, seen with competitive antagonists. A good example of uncompetitive antagonism is ion channel blockade (see Chapter 3) in which the drug target is the ion channel that has been opened by an agonist.

Many clinically useful drugs are competitive antagonists for endogenous agonists such as neurohormones and autacoids, for example:

- Propranolol (beta adrenoceptors).
- Haloperidol (dopamine receptors).
- Naloxone (opioid receptors).
- Phentolamine (alpha adrenoceptors).
- Cimetidine (histamine H_2 receptors).
- Atropine (muscarinic receptors).
- Curare-like compounds (skeletal muscle nicotinic receptors).

In each of these cases the nature of the antagonism and effectiveness of the compounds (and K_d values) were established using the methods outlined above.

When used clinically, the effects observed with a competitive antagonist actually represent inhibition of responses to an exogenous or endogenous agonist. An example is the depression of endogenous histamine-mediated acid secretion in the stomach by cimetidine. Again, the dose–response curves are similar to those shown in Fig. 5.10 and are characterized by: (i) an E_{max}; (ii) a dose at which effect is half maximum (usually termed EC_{50}); and (iii) a slope parameter (h). As with dose–response curves for agonists, the exact form of such curves depends critically on the transduction system that links

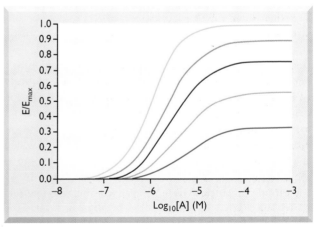

Fig. 5.13 Dose–response curves for an agonist (A) in the presence of different concentrations of a noncompetitive antagonist (D). This graph is analogous to that for a competitive antagonist shown in Fig. 5.11. Note the rightward shift of the dose–response curve with increasing concentrations of D and the fall in maximum.

the active agonist–receptor complex (AR*) to the tissue response, since for competitive antagonists each concentration of antagonist corresponds to a reduction of [A]. Nevertheless, it can be shown that the EC_{50} is generally close to the dissociation constant, K_d multiplied by $(1 + [A]/A_{50})$. That is, the EC_{50} is much the same, provided that the responses to the agonist are well below the maximum $([A] < A_{50})$. In general:

- Half-blockade of the agonist effect is associated with at least half-occupancy of receptors.
- Near-maximal effects of the competitive antagonist require that most receptors are bound by the drug.

This contrasts with what is found with most agonists, where near-maximal responses occur with a low receptor occupancy.

When a competitive antagonist is used to block the actions of an endogenous agonist (e.g. a neurotransmitter), it is sometimes found that the EC_{50} is much more than the K_d. The simple explanation for this is that [A] at the receptor site is usually high relative to A_{50}. Alternatively, the phenomenon may arise because physiologically [A] is far from constant and equilibrium-type equations do not apply.

Dose–response curves for noncompetitive antagonists representing inhibition of response to endogenous or exogenous agonist also resemble those shown in Fig. 5.13. Since these agents can act by a variety of mechanisms the only generalization that can be made is that, in contrast to competitive antagonists, the EC_{50} fails to rise in proportion to $1 + [A]/A_{50}$.

The actions of irreversible antagonists persist

As indicated by their name, irreversible antagonists are characterized by an antagonism that persists despite removal of the antagonist. Generally, irreversible antagonism produced by such a drug is less if a high concentration of agonist is present during incubation with the antagonist. This has led to the use of the confusing term 'irreversible competitive' to describe such antagonists. However, what is of primary importance is the irreversible nature of the inhibition caused by covalent chemical bonding that in effect removes functional receptors.

When irreversible antagonists were first developed, their effects on dose–response curves for agonists came as a surprise, since previously, pharmacologists had assumed that effect was directly proportional to [AR]. With irreversible antagonists it became clear that such drugs produced irreversible inhibition of responses to agonists in a manner consistent with the loss of a proportion of available receptors. However, contrary to expectation, despite such losses there was often little or no change in E_{max}. Typical results are illustrated in Fig. 5.14 where, at lower incubation times with an irreversible antagonist, curves are at first shifted in parallel manner with increases in A_{50} values and no reduction of E_{max}, a pattern similar to that seen with competitive blockade. After a sufficient period of incubation, E_{max} is reduced while the shifts in A_{50} are also reduced. The explanation for this phenomenon is that maximal responses normally require the activation of only a small fraction of receptors. The existence of far more receptors than is needed to produce a maximum response is often referred to as 'receptor reserve.'

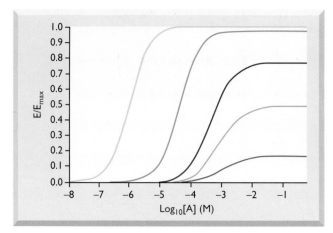

Fig. 5.14 Dose–response curves for an agonist (A) after increasing times of exposure to an irreversible antagonist. The more the curve is shifted to the right the longer the tissue has been incubated with the irreversible antagonist.

Receptor reserve implies that the A_{50} (the value of [A] for a half-maximum response) is less than K_A ([A] for occupation of 50% of receptors). Thus the ratio K_A/A_{50} is a reflection of receptor reserve, and that reserve varies for agonists acting on the same receptor. Therefore, changes in receptor reserve among closely related analogs of an agonist provide yet another method of characterizing receptors.

The simplest and most generally accepted explanation for differences (of what is technically called 'intrinsic efficacy') between agonists, is that only a particular conformation of the AR complex (say AR*) is 'active' in the sense that it produces a response. Agonists with low intrinsic efficacy (A_{50} close to K_A and little or no receptor reserve), which include partial agonists, have an AR that is seldom in the form AR*, while agonists with high intrinsic efficacy ($A_{50} \ll K_A$) have an AR mostly in the AR* form.

It was first recognized by Furchgott, that dose–response curves such as those shown in Fig. 5.14 contain the information needed to calculate the K_A of an agonist. The logic of his method is as follows; suppose an irreversible antagonist has been applied for a period of time sufficient to reduce E_{max}. The resulting change in dose–response curve is because $[R_t]$ has been reduced to a new value, say, $q[R_t]$. Now consider any level of response on the new curve. It corresponds to a particular receptor occupancy where:

$$[AR] = q[R_t] [A]/(K_A + [A]) \qquad \text{Eqn 10}$$

Before the antagonist was applied the same response occurred at $[A]_O$ from which:

$$[AR] = [R_t] [A]_O/(K_A + [A]_O) \qquad \text{Eqn 11}$$

However, since the responses are the same, [AR] must be the same leading to, after rearranging the equations:

$$1/[A]_O = (1/q - 1)/K_A + (1/q)/[A] \qquad \text{Eqn 12}$$

Each experimental observation in the new response–[A] curve gives a pair of values (i.e. [A] and $[A]_O$), and q and K_A can be obtained from a plot of $1/[A]_O$ versus $1/[A]$ (or $[A]/[A]_O$ versus $[A]$).

■ A simple model for efficacy was proposed by Stephenson

The simple model of efficacy introduced by Stephenson is useful for understanding how results such as those in Fig. 5.14 can arise. Suppose that AR produces a stimulus (S) which is proportional to [AR], and that response (E) is a function of S which is not limitless but saturates, then:

$$S = e[AR]/[R_t] \qquad \text{Eqn 13}$$

where e is a proportionality constant, called efficacy, that can vary from one agonist to another, and

$$E = E'S/(1 + S) \qquad \text{Eqn 14}$$

where **E** is effect and **E**′ represents a hypothetical maximum that would occur if **S** could be made infinite. If agonists vary in the fraction (**f**) of AR that is in an active conformation (AR*), e will be proportional to **f**. Also, with e defined as above, it must be proportional to $[R_t]$ (or $q[R_t]$ if some receptors are made inoperable). Intrinsic efficacy is $e/[R_t]$.

Combining the above two equations with that for agonist binding, and rearranging, gives:

$$E = E_{max}[A]/([A] + A_{50}) \qquad \text{Eqn 7}$$

where

$$E_{max} = E'e/(e + 1) \qquad \text{Eqn 15}$$

and

$$A_{50} = K_A/(e + 1) \qquad \text{Eqn 16}$$

Therefore, if e is initially large, say 1000, it can be greatly diminished by an irreversible antagonist 'removing' receptors before much reduction in E_{max} is seen, and all that occurs is an increase in A_{50}. However, once e is not much more than 1, or if e was close to 1 to start with, any (further) reduction of e causes E_{max} to diminish with relatively little increase in A_{50}, which can become, at most, the same as K_A.

On the basis of this model, agonists may be compared in terms of their relative e values, which are the same as relative intrinsic efficacies. The problem here is that the actual values of e obtained depend on the particular relationship assumed between **E** and **S**, that is, $E = E'S/(1 + S)$, which might or might not be true of any particular transduction system.

■ A partial agonist is an agonist of low intrinsic efficacy and e not much more than 1

From the above, a partial agonist can be seen simply as an agonist with low efficacy, with an e not much more than 1. Experiments with irreversible antagonists have shown that, in agreement with this theory, partial agonists are characterized by having A_{50} values close to K_A values and no receptor reserve. As already pointed out, the low e of a partial agonist relative to a full agonist may be explained simply on the basis that with a partial agonist only a small fraction of the AR complexes are in the active conformation (AR*).

■ When a full agonist is present at a high concentration, a partial agonist acts as an antagonist

Since a response to a partial agonist only occurs when receptor occupancy is high it becomes apparent that partial agonists act as antagonists of full agonists. Therefore, a partial agonist can be used therapeutically to block the effect of an endogenous agonist (e.g. norepinephrine) while at the same time producing a steady low level of receptor activation in the absence of a full agonist. A classic example of partial agonism is seen with certain beta blockers (e.g. pindolol) that are partial agonists rather than competitive antagonists. Pindolol becomes increasingly effective as a beta blocker as sympathetic nerve activity on the heart increases. Thus when sympathetic activity on the heart is low, pindolol can increase heart rate whereas the effect of sympathetic nerve activity on the heart is blocked. A classic beta-blocker drug never increases heart rate under any condition.

■ Drug responses change due to desensitization

Responses to drugs are often not fixed and constant over time, even though the concentrations of the drug at its receptor site may have reached steady-state values. In a variety of clinical situations, responses to a drug many wane over time. Many factors lead to loss in drug effects at an organ or system level, ranging from progression of the disease being treated (e.g. cardiac dysfunction) as well as physiologic adaptations (e.g. activation of the renin–angiotensin system in patients taking diuretics). When the loss in responsiveness to a drug occurs directly at the cellular level, this change in function is often termed desensitization. Many mechanisms have been found to contribute to desensitization, operating at transcriptional, translational, and protein levels of cellular regulation. These mechanisms may operate quickly (seconds to minutes) or relatively slowly, over the course of hours or days.

Mechanisms involved in rapidly developing desensitization have been extensively studied in molecular terms, especially for G protein-coupled receptors, and particularly β adrenoceptors. At the cellular level, stimulation of β adrenoceptors, with an agonist such as isoproterenol, leads to activation of adenylyl cyclase and a brisk rise in intracellular concentrations of the second-messenger cAMP. However, in many cells, the capacity of isoproterenol to activate adenylyl cyclase declines with time, leading to a fall in cAMP concentrations in the cell. Phosphorylation of β adrenoceptors, association of these receptors with other proteins, and changes in subcellular localization of the receptors, may all contribute to the diminished. ability of isoproterenol to activate cAMP accumulation.

Desensitization of β adrenoceptors (and other G protein-coupled receptors) can occur specifically due to the phosphorylation of agonist-bound receptors by a G protein-coupled receptor kinase (GRK). GRKs constitute a family of kinases. GRK2, originally known as bARK kinase, was discovered on account of its capacity to phosphorylate agonist-occupied β adrenoceptors. Agonist occupancy of these receptors leads to binding of a GRK to the receptor and its phosphorylation. This mechanism has been termed 'homologous' desensitization since it specifically involves agonist-occupied receptors. After being phosphorylated, the receptors bind a member of the arrestin protein family, leading to steric hindrance of interaction between these receptors and G proteins. The receptors may subsequently be sequestered away from the plasma membrane and move into the cell. Surprising new information suggests that the internalized receptors may contribute to novel mechanisms of β adrenoceptor signaling.

A second mechanism for receptor desensitization involves second-messenger feedback which can lead to desensitization of not only agonist-activated receptors but also different classes of receptors expressed in the same cell. This form of desensitization has been termed 'heterologous' desensitization, since the function of multiple types of receptors may simultaneously occur after activation of just one receptor type. The β adrenoceptors stimulate cAMP accumulation which leads to activation of protein kinase A; the activated catalytic subunit of protein kinase A can phosphorylate not only beta receptors, impairing their function, but also potentially phosphorylate a number of other receptors in the same cell with appropriate sites for phosphorylation by protein kinase A.

Physiologic antagonism

■ *Physiologic antagonists oppose the actions of agonists by mechanisms independent of the agonist–receptor interaction*

In the previous section, antagonist drugs that inhibit the actions of agonists were considered to produce their inhibition by virtue of acting in some manner on the same receptors as the agonists. However, drugs may antagonize the actions of agonists by other mechanisms.

■ *Drugs can oppose responses to other drugs by acting on different receptors*

It often happens that two drugs that act on different receptors have opposing actions on a tissue or organ. When this occurs, the drugs can be considered to be physiologic (functional) antagonists of one another. Obvious examples of such physiologic antagonism are epinephrine and acetylcholine, which respectively raise and lower heart rate, and glucagon and insulin, which respectively raise and lower blood glucose level.

A more subtle example is antagonism of neuromuscular blockade due to a nondepolarizing neuromuscular blocking drug, such as pancuronium, by an anticholinesterase, such as neostigmine (see Chapter 26). The dose–response curve for neuromuscular block versus dose of pancuronium is shifted by neostigmine in a noncompetitive fashion. This occurs because the two drugs act on quite different molecular targets, the nicotinic receptor for pancuronium and the enzyme acetylcholinesterase for neostigmine. Blockade of the activity of the enzyme can do no more than double the height of end-plate potentials and, as a result, an anticholinesterase cannot reverse neuromuscular blockade due to an excessive dose of pancuronium.

MEASURING RESPONSES AND PRACTICAL APPLICATIONS OF DOSE–RESPONSE CURVES

■ *Responses to drugs are measured in many different ways*

Drugs have their initial actions at a molecular level, usually by binding to their receptor. This ultimately results in cellular, tissue, organ or body system, whole body and population responses, all of which can be measured. Biochemical techniques are often used to measure intracellular responses to drugs, whereas the response of whole tissues and organs can also be measured using physical (electrical, optical, and mechanical) techniques, both *in vitro* (in glass) and *in vivo* (in life). For *in vitro* studies, the tissues and organs are isolated from the body and bathed with suitable physiologic buffers, generally in glass apparatus. When studies are made in intact animals and humans they are referred to as being *in vivo*.

In the above discussions the terms 'effect' and 'response' have been used synonymously but left undefined, because there are innumerable ways in which drugs act and in which their effects can be defined. However, it should always be borne in mind that, if given at sufficiently high concentrations, drugs have many measurable effects that may not be relevant to the clinical action of the drug.

Dose–response curves almost always appear similar to those shown in Fig. 5.9, the exceptions being those where the drug acts on more than one type of receptor. Below a certain dose or concentration, an effect is undetectable and as dose is increased the effect increases until a maximum effect is reached. The dose at which the effect is half-maximal is usually called the ED_{50} (effective dose 50%, i.e. that dose which produces a response equal to 50% of the maximum response to that drug). Similarly, the ED_{10} is the dose producing 10% of maximum response, ED_{25} produces 25%, ED_{75} 75%, etc. If the drug concentration [A] is known, the corresponding terms EC_{10}, EC_{25}, EC_{50}, etc. may be used.

The ratio ED_{75}/ED_{25} (or EC_{75}/EC_{25}) provides a simple measure of the steepness of the dose–response curve, which when measured exactly is 'h,' the Hill coefficient (see page 63) of the dose–response equation

$$E = E_{max}[A]^h / (EC_{50}^{\ h} + [A]^h)$$

This is another form of the dose–response equation in which [A] is drug concentration and h is theoretically expected to be

---

🔑 **Therapeutic ratio: an experimental index of risk versus benefit**

- The LD_{50} is the dose of a drug that is lethal to 50% of the animals tested
- The ED_{50} is the dose of a drug that is effective in 50% of the animals tested
- The ratio of LD_{50} to ED_{50} is the therapeutic ratio, an experimental measure of the usefulness of a drug
- Other therapeutic indices use nonlethal adverse effects to estimate risk versus benefit

the integer 1 or 2. It is notable that for drugs with 'h' more than 1.0 (EC_{75}/EC_{25} less than 9) responses increase steeply with dose which can be very dangerous. For example, with vapor general anesthesics, the depth of anesthesia may increase alarmingly with only a small increase in concentration of the vapor administered.

◾ Sometimes drug responses are all-or-nothing (quantal) in nature

In certain contexts the drug response measured is 'quantal' rather than 'graded'. That is, the response either occurs or it does not occur, as in cure or no cure, death or no death. With such quantal data, the response axis for the dose–response curve is expressed as a percentage of people, animals or cells, that respond, hence is known as a quantal dose–response curve. The classic quantal dose–response curve is a lethality curve in which the percentage of animals killed by a drug or poison is plotted for various doses. For such a curve, the dose that is lethal to 50% of animals is known as the LD_{50} (lethal dose 50%). Obviously the actual value of the LD_{50} for a particular drug depends upon the route of administration used, and the species in which the drug is tested. The LD_{50} is analogous to the ED_{50} which is the effective dose 50% (the dose which produces a desired effect in 50% of animals). The ratio of the two measures gives an estimate of the safety of a drug, the therapeutic ratio.

◾ Drugs are judged according to both their beneficial and adverse effects (benefit-to-risk ratio)

The 'therapeutic ratio,' a classic index of the safety of a drug is defined as the ratio LD_{50}/ED_{50}, as mentioned above. This index is useful but can be misleading if the log(dose)–response curve for desired effect is not parallel to the lethality curve, that is, they do not have the same slope 'h.' Some pharmacologists prefer to use ratios such as LD_{25}/ED_{75} or LD_{10}/ED_{90}, reflecting Ehrlich's early suggestion (circa 1900) that a drug is best judged by the ratio between its maximal tolerated dose and the minimal curative dose. Ratios involving estimation of lethal doses can only be determined using animals. However, other measures of toxicity can be used to estimate benefit–risk ratio. For example, the dose–response curve for beneficial effect can be compared with that for an adverse, but not lethal effect, and a therapeutic index, rather than the classic therapeutic ratio, calculated. The desire to reduce the use of animals for lethality testing has led to the increasing use of such indices. At a clinical level it is obviously important to try to compare dose–response curves for beneficial effects with those for adverse effects. Unfortunately the clinical information necessary to calculate reasonable indices is often not available. In the clinic only limited dose–response data can be obtained, since only a limited number of different doses can be given. Ethical considerations prevent further doses being given once an adverse effect has been encountered.

With quantal responses the steepness (h) of the dose–response curve directly reflects the variability in the population being tested. After all, for a lethality curve, if all animals were identical, they would all die at the same dose. There is extensive

statistical theory concerning how data of this kind should be treated (such as the use of 'probits') and the reliability of estimates of ED_{50}, LD_{50}, etc. However, quantal results can be fitted to a variant of the standard dose formula:

$$E/E_{max} = D^h/(LD_{50}^{\ h} + D^h) \qquad \text{Eqn 17}$$

where **D** is dose, with $E_{max} = 100\%$, and 'h' the slope co-efficient.

Occasionally, what appear to be graded responses in a tissue actually represents hidden quantal responses—what one measures is the sum of responses of many individual cells where each cell responds in an all-or-none fashion. This may sometimes provide an explanation of the steep dose–response curves encountered as, for example, when a neuromuscular blocking drug is used to inhibit nerve-induced contraction of skeletal muscle. Here individual neuromuscular junctions on skeletal muscle fibers are either blocked or not blocked by a given concentration of the drug, and single muscle fiber contractions are either present or absent. This contrasts with the situation in smooth muscle where contraction in each fiber is continuously graded with the dose of a drug.

◾ Dose–response relationships are fundamental to the discovery of receptors, development of new drugs and understanding drug actions

In research and drug development, the primary aim is to categorize drugs in terms of the receptors and biological systems with which they interact, and characterize their interactions with receptors; that is, whether they are agonists, partial agonists, or competitive, noncompetitive or irreversible antagonists. Here, the approach is to measure drug effects on a variety of enzyme systems and tissue preparations that contain receptors of different types. Thus a compound may be identified as an H_1 (histamine type 1 receptor) agonist if it acts in the same way as histamine in a preparation that both responds to histamine, and has its actions inhibited by an H_1 competitive antihistamine in a competitive manner. The unidentified active compound in a tissue extract is epinephrine if its potency relative to epinephrine is the same in preparations containing different proportions of adrenoceptors, and appropriate competitive antagonists shift dose–response curves to the unknown agent in the same way as they shift dose–response curves to epinephrine. If a drug or chemical compound has effects that cannot be explained in terms of actions on known receptors, a new receptor may have been discovered, and if the compound occurs naturally in tissues it may be a new autacoid. Historically, such work has led to most of our present understanding of how drugs act, as well as the discovery of endogenous transmitters and their receptors.

It is still common in pharmacological research to determine the effects of drugs in *vitro* by measuring specific responses from a smooth muscle preparation such as a piece of intestine, artery, vein, bladder, or uterus, etc. Such preparations characteristically respond to a variety of agents by contraction or relaxation, the response being graded with dose and fairly fast in onset and offset when the drug is added or removed, respectively. It is therefore possible to determine a dose–response relationship and its alteration by another drug in a matter of hours. The use of biochemical drug responses, such as accumulation or turnover of a second messenger, can often be even a more efficient measure of drug action, and is essential in cases when the drug being studied acts on receptors that are not present in tissue preparations which provide an easily measured physical response.

Clinical responses

Clinical responses to drugs are measured using a wide variety of techniques. These range from simple measurement of physiologic function (heart rate, blood pressure) to cure rates, or mortality, in populations of patients. In some cases the direct effects of a drug cannot be measured and therefore surrogate measures have to be used (see below). However, since the true aim of drug therapy is to cure or alleviate disease so as to improve both the quality and duration of life, increasingly attempts are being made to measure such effects directly. As noted previously, large numbers of patients are required to obtain such data, and clinical trials of new drugs are now sometimes designed to collect this. In addition, an alternative approach for new drugs entering the market is to monitor all prescriptions (up to some realistic limit) for fatal and adverse events (see Chapter 6).

Clinically, the use of any drug depends upon knowing the appropriate dose to use, which in turn depends upon dose–response curve data with respect to both desired and undesired (adverse) effects. Dose–response curves for a new drug are first obtained in isolated tissue preparations, then in experimental animals, and finally in humans. Generally, such determinations become more difficult and time-consuming the closer one approaches clinical reality. For example, the effect of a drug at a certain dose to diminish pain in people can be assessed using the visual analog pain scale in which a subject indicates the subjective pain experienced on a scale of 0 (no pain) to 10, the latter being maximal imaginable pain. However, the perception of pain varies with people, pain often fluctuates, and pain can arise from a variety of pathologic processes. As a result the determination of complete dose–response curves in man for a new analgesic against various kinds of pain would require hundreds of subjects and many person-years of investigator time. Such extensive studies are generally impractical. On the other hand, using experimental animals (rats or mice), pain reduction can be measured from the average time animals devote to licking a foot that has been injected by an agent that causes temporary inflammation. To obtain a dose–response relationship in this way may require 100–200 animals and several person-days of observation. Such an experiment would typically follow 'screens'—rather rough dose–response curves obtained with a variety of tissue preparations—to establish the absence of pharmacologic actions that could preclude the clinical use of the drug.

In view of the difficulty in obtaining any true dose–response relationship in the human, recourse is often made to 'surrogate' measures. For example, a permanently elevated blood pressure of unknown cause (essential hypertension) is statistically associated with increased morbidity and mortality. Therefore, the proper measure of an antihypertensive drug is the extent to which it reduces morbidity and mortality, versus the possibility of adverse effects. To assess an antihypertensive response to a drug according to such principles would require a prospective clinical trial involving thousands of subjects, followed over many years. The effects of antihypertensive drugs are therefore usually assessed in terms of their effectiveness and potency using the surrogate of blood pressure reduction, something which is fairly easy to measure. A dose–response relationship for true clinical effectiveness has not yet been obtained for most antihypertensives in common use, although increasing attention is being paid to whether they reduce mortality. Interestingly, despite the availability of many different antihypertensive drugs belonging to many different classes, comparatively few have been shown to reduce mortality in patients with essential hypertension.

Population effects

Different people respond in different ways to drugs. As a result procedures are needed to acquire data regarding the effects of drugs in the population, and experience has shown that data should be gathered according to some protocol, rather than during routine care.

Data gathered during phases II and III of clinical trials (Chapters 6 and 7) are an important source of information for assessing the effect of drugs in the population; they can be used not only to determine toxicity but also to maximize efficacy. One major problem associated with information obtained from pre-marketing studies, however, can be a lack of heterogeneity among the pool of patients taking the medication. This problem can be confounded further by differences in the severity of disease between different patients. However, these problems can be partly overcome by designing studies to incorporate a large patient base. Certainly in the long term, a continuous gathering of information about the actions of drugs in the population will serve a useful purpose in optimizing the dose to reduce toxicity and maximize the pharmacotherapeutic benefit (see Chapter 6).

Lifestyle needs to be taken into account when studying the effects of a drug in the population. For example, a patient who is a smoker defines a different population. In effect, this could mean that a physician prescribing a drug may need to shift from the population mean to accommodate individual patients. Therefore, such scenarios play an important role in the decisions that are made by physicians in writing prescriptions.

FURTHER READING

Black JW, Leff P. Operational models of pharmacological agonism. *Proc R Soc Lond [Biol]* 1983; **220**: 141–162. [Gives different perspectives on agonist–receptor dynamics.]

Kenakin T. The classification of drugs and drug–receptor antagonism. *Pharmacol Rev* 1984; **36**: 165–222. [Classification of receptors based on affinity of drugs.]

Pratt WB, Taylor P. *Principles of Drug Actions: The Basis of Pharmacology.* New York: Churchill Livingstone; 1990. [Introduction to the fundamentals of drug-receptor dynamics.]

Schild O. pA$_x$, and competitive drug antagonism. *Br J Pharmacol* 1949; **4**: 277–280. [Analysis of dose–response curves in the presence of antagonists.]

Stephenson RP. A modification of receptor theory. *Br J Pharmacol* 1956; **11**: 379–393. [An introduction of the concept of a response being a function of the stimulus.]

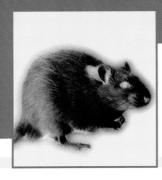

Chapter 6

Drug Safety and Pharmacovigilance

▥ *Drugs can damage health*

A drug is a chemical used to prevent, investigate, or treat disease, or to alter physiologic function (Fig. 6.1) while a medicine is a drug, or a mixture of drugs, combined with pharmacologically inactive substances, to make it stable, palatable, and useful for therapy. Drugs interact with tissues and organs and alter their function, but their effects are not always desirable. Any drug represents a hazard (i.e. has the potential to cause harm). The probability that a drug will cause some specified harm in any given circumstances is the 'risk' that it will cause that harm. This probability can be estimated by experiment or observation, or it can be estimated intuitively.

People are generally unable to estimate risk accurately, perceiving new and technical hazards as riskier than they are, while underestimating everyday and familiar hazards. Figure 6.2 illustrates the relationship between perceived risk and actual risk for 41 causes of death. The 'perceived risk' determines the way people behave, and can be manifest in what they say (the 'expressed risk'), or what they do (the 'revealed risk'). Patients are sometimes fearful of taking medicines (e.g. after a newspaper article discussing one particularly dramatic case of an adverse effect), but will happily continue smoking even though

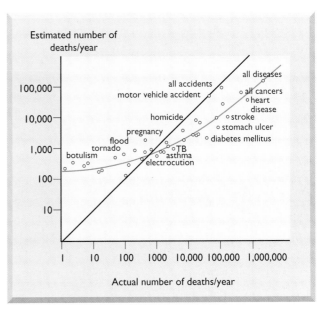

Fig. 6.2 Relationship between perceived frequency and the actual number of deaths/year for 41 causes of death. If the perceived and actual frequencies are equal, the data fall on the straight line. The points and the curved line fitted to them represent the average response. (Adapted with permission from *Judgment Under Uncertainty: Heuristics and Biases* by Kahneman, Slovic and Tversky, Cambridge University Press, 1982.)

in smokers the lifetime risk of a fatal illness due to tobacco is about 0.15 (15%). The risks perceived by doctors can also differ markedly from the true risks measured in well-designed studies. (It is interesting to compare this with the way we accept the cost–benefit ratio for travel by car. We gladly accept a real risk of death and injury for the benefit of convenient travel.)

PHARMACOTHERAPEUTIC DECISION-MAKING

Pharmacotherapeutic decisions are among the most difficult decisions in medical practice and are an integral part of medicine.

▥ *Why should the patient be treated, and with what drug?*

The physician's first pharmacotherapeutic task is to decide whether the patient has a condition that would benefit from drug treatment.

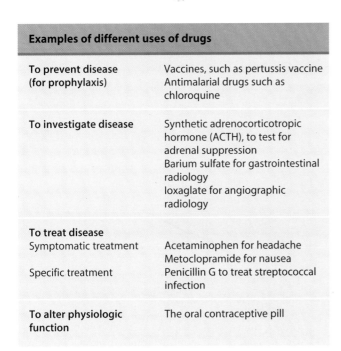

Examples of different uses of drugs	
To prevent disease (for prophylaxis)	Vaccines, such as pertussis vaccine Antimalarial drugs such as chloroquine
To investigate disease	Synthetic adrenocorticotropic hormone (ACTH), to test for adrenal suppression Barium sulfate for gastrointestinal radiology Ioxaglate for angiographic radiology
To treat disease Symptomatic treatment Specific treatment	Acetaminophen for headache Metoclopramide for nausea Penicillin G to treat streptococcal infection
To alter physiologic function	The oral contraceptive pill

Fig. 6.1 Examples of different uses of drugs.

If drug treatment is indicated, the physician then needs to consider its benefits and adverse effects, and decide whether the treatment should be prescribed. For example, acne can be treated effectively with the vitamin A derivative isotretinoin, but this drug can cause serious adverse effects including liver damage, increases in serum cholesterol concentration, and fetal malformation as a result of exposure in utero. It is therefore unsuitable for the treatment of mild acne. The physician also has to consider whether there are alternative treatments. For example, although the antibiotic chloramphenicol is an effective treatment of bacterial pharyngitis, it is avoided because it carries a risk of causing life-threatening bone marrow aplasia, once in 40,000 treatments, and penicillin V (phenoxymethyl-penicillin) is preferred.

What are the expected costs and benefits of treatment?

The doctor and, where possible, the patient, have to weigh up:
- The potential benefits of treatment to the patient.
- The risk of adverse effects to that particular patient.
- The health cost entailed if the treatment produces adverse effects.
- The financial cost of the treatment.

Usually, the benefits of treatment are benefits for an individual patient, such as freedom from pain. However, there are circumstances where the benefits accrue to society as a whole. For example, vaccines reduce the prevalence of disease in the community.

The costs fall on:
- The individual, who can suffer adverse effects.
- Society, if the government or insurance schemes pay for expensive drugs.

Recombinant enzymes used to treat the rare hereditary defect in β-glucosidase that causes Gaucher's disease cost around US$100,000/year/patient. Lipid-lowering drugs, which can significantly reduce the risk of dying from coronary heart disease for mildly hypercholesterolemic men who have never had a myocardial infarct, are also expensive, costing approximately US$300,000 per life saved. Such expense, and limited budgets, mean that a decision has to be made about whether spending so much money to benefit a single patient is warranted.

CONTROLLING DRUG SAFETY

Drug regulations are used in an attempt to ensure that drugs are reasonably free from adverse effects

Before a company can market a medicinal product, it has to demonstrate that the product is reasonably safe and effective according to governmental rules and regulations. These arose initially in the US, and later elsewhere, as a result of various drug misadventures. Regulation began in the US with the Food and Drug Administration (FDA) in 1906 and was strengthened there, and elsewhere, because of two major drug accidents (see also Chapter 7). The first of these episodes occurred in the late 1930s, when a company called Massengill dissolved the antibacterial drug sulfanilamide in ethylene diglycol (a sweet-tasting solvent) to make it palatable to children. Unfortunately,

the company failed to test ethylene diglycol for toxicity. Ethylene diglycol causes renal failure, and over 100 people, mainly children, died as a result. The subsequent outcry led to the effective regulation of medicines in the US through the FDA.

In Europe, the need for government regulation was recognized only later. The Medicines Act 1968 in the UK was passed in the aftermath of another drug disaster in 1961, involving thalidomide. This drug was marketed by the German firm Chemie Grünenthal as a safe alternative to barbiturate hypnotics, especially for pregnant women. However, it had been tested only perfunctorily in experimental animals for safety during pregnancy, and was subsequently found to cause severe fetal deformities when taken during the first trimester. The teratogenicity (toxicity to the fetus) of thalidomide led to an estimated 10,000 babies being born worldwide with phocomelia (a deformity in which the limbs are rudimentary stumps with malformed digits) in countries in which the drug had been widely used. It was little used in the USA because one FDA regulator (Dr Frances Kelsey) refused to allow the release of the drug, until more was known of its safety. As a result of such experiences, the regulatory authorities in most countries now insist on proof of efficacy, safety, and quality before licensing a drug for use (for further details see Chapter 7).

The assessment for possible toxicity of a new potential drug that has not previously been used for therapy involves the following studies (Fig. 6.3):
- In vitro toxicologic studies to test for genetic and biochemical toxicity.
- In vivo acute toxicologic studies in whole animals, involving physiologic systems (e.g. cardiovascular, central nervous, and gastrointestinal) and skin and mucosae (for acute irritancy and sensitization).
- In vivo studies of subacute and chronic toxicity in animals.
- In vivo studies of oncogenicity in animals.
- In vivo studies of developmental and reproductive toxicity in animals.
- In vivo studies of genetic toxicity in animals.

Acute studies investigate toxic effects occurring within hours or days of a single exposure. Chronic toxicity testing examines the effects of repeated doses given over weeks or months.

The human trials which follow the toxicity studies in animals are conducted in four phases known as phase I, phase II clinical trials, etc., and discussed in greater detail in Chapter 7.
- Phase I studies usually investigate the pharmacodynamics and pharmacokinetics in a small number of healthy volunteers and determine the maximum tolerated dose.
- Phase II studies are dose-ranging studies designed to find therapeutically effective and safe dosages, to characterize the drug's general clinical pharmacologic effects, and to expand the pharmacokinetic database in carefully selected volunteer patients. Often, these studies are carried out in special groups of patients who are at risk of adverse effects, such as those with renal failure.
- Phase III studies are extensive and carefully controlled clinical trials carried out in selected volunteer patients, including trials in special groups such as the elderly.

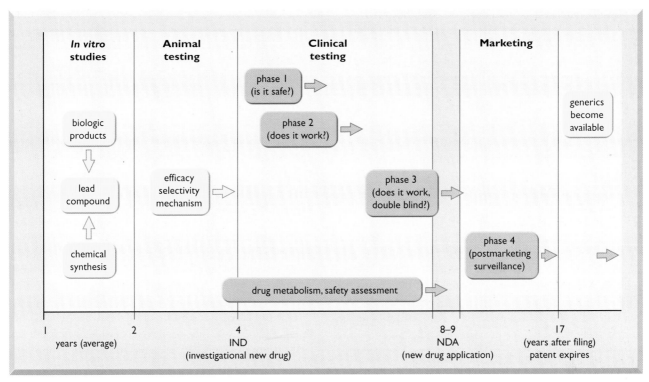

Fig. 6.3 The development and testing process required to bring a drug to market in the US. Some of the requirements may be different for drugs used in life-threatening diseases. (Adapted with permission from *Basic and Clinical Pharmacology, 6th edition* by Katzung, Appleton & Lange.)

- Phase IV studies involve post-marketing surveillance of treated patients and rely on spontaneous adverse reaction reports.

The most important test of a new drug is how safe it is in clinical use

A new drug, which is generally a new chemical entity (NCE), is known as an investigational new drug (IND) in the USA at this stage. It is usually given to approximately 1500 patients in pre-marketing clinical trials. This number of patients is far too small to detect uncommon or rare adverse events. However, increasing the number of patients studied prior to marketing would delay marketing of new drugs, thereby delaying the use of the potentially beneficial drugs by ill patients. A useful rule of thumb for gauging the possible occurrence of toxicity is the 'rule of three.' This states that if an event has not been observed in n patients, then it is 95% certain that the true frequency of the event in a larger population of patients lies somewhere between 0 and 3/n. Therefore, even if there is no fatal reaction to a drug among 1500 patients, the above statistics give a 5% chance it will cause up to one death among 500 treated patients.

Postmarketing surveillance is extremely important for ensuring drug safety

Rare and even fairly common adverse effects can be detected only after trials involving very large numbers of patients. Post-marketing surveillance ('pharmacovigilance'), particularly the spontaneous reporting of adverse reactions, is therefore useful

and necessary because many more patients receive a drug after it is marketed than during the pre-marketing phase I to III studies. It is inevitable that some drugs which are licensed subsequently prove to be less safe than is desirable. These drugs can then be removed from the market or their use restricted. Some drugs withdrawn from the market in the United States in the past 5 years are listed in the section below on Pharmocovigilance.

DETECTING ADVERSE DRUG REACTIONS

Adverse drug reactions frequently mimic ordinary diseases. Serious reactions tend to affect:

- Systems in which there is rapid cell multiplication (e.g. the skin, hematopoietic system, and lining of the gut).
- Organs in which drugs are detoxified and/or excreted (e.g. the liver and kidneys).

Typical examples of such serious reactions are toxic epidermal necrolysis, aplastic anemia, pseudomembranous colitis, hepatitis, and nephritis.

Adverse effects, especially uncommon ones, may be difficult to diagnose and a physician must always consider whether any effect associated with the use of a new drug is actually caused by the drug. However, since a general practitioner might work for a lifetime without seeing a case of aplastic anemia, the detection of both common and uncommon adverse drug reactions requires vigilance on the part of the patient, the physician and others involved in the drug treatment of patients, including the pharmacist and other health professionals.

◼ *Adverse reactions to drugs are most easily detected when they are dramatic, differ from natural disease, or are of rapid onset following the start of treatment.*

An anaphylactic reaction occurring within minutes of a penicillin injection and characterized by tissue edema, bronchospasm, and cardiovascular collapse is obviously an adverse drug effect. It is much more difficult to detect adverse effects that occur only after a long period of treatment or have an insidious onset. It is even more difficult to detect adverse effects that occur only after the drug has been discontinued. An example of a long-delayed adverse effect is the malignant disease that occurs in about 15% of patients previously treated with cyclophosphamide for lymphomas of childhood.

Adverse effects that mimic naturally occurring disease are more difficult to detect than those with unique features, especially if the adverse effect resembles a common or relatively innocuous disease. The defect of phocomelia is very obvious in its presentation of stunted or missing (seal-like) limbs and is extremely rare; therefore astute clinicians were relatively quick to associate phocomelia with taking thalidomide. In contrast, the increased risk of spina bifida in babies born to women taking the antiepileptic drug sodium valproate during pregnancy could be verified only by carefully designed clinical studies, since spina bifida is not uncommon.

◼ *If a specific adverse drug effect has a well recognized latency to onset, it can be anticipated and therefore detected more easily*

In deciding whether an adverse event that occurs with treatment is due to the drug, latency to the onset of the adverse event should be considered. Some adverse effects appear with a well-characterized latency, others less so, while obviously an adverse effect occurring before treatment cannot be due to the drug. Adverse effects may occur with characteristic latencies:

- Just after exposure (e.g. anaphylaxis to penicillin, intense vasodilation and hypotensive collapse after an injection of vancomycin—the syndrome known as l'homme rouge).
- A few days after exposure (e.g. serum sickness induced by snake antitoxins made from horse serum; an ampicillin rash in patients with infectious mononucleosis).
- Only after chronic treatment (e.g. iatrogenic Cushing's syndrome after weeks or months of treatment with glucocorticosteroids).
- After cessation of treatment (e.g. withdrawal syndromes from benzodiazepines or 5-hydroxytryptamine reuptake inhibitors).

⚷ **A drug is more probably responsible for an adverse effect:**

- If it is well recognized that the adverse effect occurs with the drug
- If the adverse effect is recognized as an adverse effect of a class of drugs and the suspect drug resembles this class (e.g. cough is an adverse effect associated with angiotensin-converting enzyme inhibitors)

- In subsequent generations (e.g. phocomelia with thalidomide, retinoid embryopathy).

Certain adverse effects, such as anaphylaxis and bone marrow aplasia, are characteristic adverse effects of drugs.

A drug is more probably the cause of a reversible event if the event disappears after the drug is stopped (de-challenge) and then reappears when the drug is restarted (re-challenge).

◼ *An alphabetic classification can be used to memorize the different types of adverse effects due to drugs*

The types of adverse effect seen with drugs are listed in Fig. 6.4. Most fit into this scheme, though some may fit into more than one category, and others are difficult to classify. The first two categories are fundamental. Type A (augmented pharmacologic) reactions are easily predicted from the known pharmacologic effects of a drug, while the risk of the reaction depends on the dose of the drug. Many, such as constipation with opiate analgesic agents, or throbbing headache with nitrate antianginal drugs, are a nuisance rather than a danger.

Type B (bizarre) adverse effects are unpredictable and often severe. Examples include anaphylaxis (which can result in a fatal cardiovascular collapse), renal and hepatic failure, and bone marrow suppression. Some of the more important type B reactions are given in Fig. 6.5.

◼ *Some patients are more susceptible than others to the adverse effects of a drug*

The benefits of any drug treatment must always be weighed against possible harm. Those who are particularly susceptible to adverse effects include the fetus, patients with pre-existing illnesses or genetic enzyme defects, patients who are already taking other drugs, and elderly patients.

Pregnant women

Treatment of pregnant women (and women at risk of pregnancy) must take into account the welfare of both the fetus and mother. Teratogenic drugs (those that are known to cause malformations to the fetus) must obviously be avoided. However, it is wise to regard all drugs as being potentially teratogenic. Therefore no drug should be prescribed to a pregnant woman, no matter how innocuous it may seem, unless:

- There is a clear need for it, and the drug is considered by the professions to be safe to the fetus.
- The mother is so ill that its use is justified even if the fetus might be harmed.

Pre-existing illnesses

Pre-existing illnesses such as liver or kidney disease can exacerbate or precipitate adverse drug effects. As a result of such conditions, a drug may be present in the body in a higher concentration, or for a longer period. Reduced metabolism or excretion makes patients more susceptible to type A (an augmented pharmacologic response to a standard dose) adverse effects. The adverse effects of some drugs are also more common in patients with organ failure. For example, the potassium-sparing diuretic amiloride is more likely to cause hyperkalemia

Type	Type of effect	Definition	Examples
A	Augmented pharmacologic effects	Adverse effects that are known to occur from the pharmacology of the drug, and are dose-related. They are seldom fatal and relatively common	Hypoglycemia due to insulin injection Bradycardia due to β adrenoceptor antagonists Hemorrhage due to anticoagulants
B	Bizarre effects	Adverse effects that occur unpredictably and often have a high rate of morbidity and mortality. They are uncommon	Anaphylaxis due to penicillin Acute hepatic necrosis due to halothane Bone marrow suppression by chloramphenicol
C	Chronic effects	Adverse effects that only occur during prolonged treatment and not with single doses	Iatrogenic Cushing's syndrome with prednisolone Orofacial dyskinesia due to phenothiazine tranquilizers Colonic dysfunction due to laxatives
D	Delayed effects	Adverse effects that occur remote from treatment, either in the children of treated patients, or in patients themselves years after treatment	Second cancers in those treated with alkylating agents for Hodgkin's disease Craniofacial malformations in infants whose mothers have taken isotretinoin Clear-cell carcinoma of the vagina in the daughters of women who took diethylstilbestrol during pregnancy
E	End-of-treatment effects	Adverse effects that occur when a drug is stopped, especially when it is stopped suddenly (so-called withdrawal effects)	Unstable angina after β adrenoceptor antagonists are suddenly stopped Adrenocortical insufficiency after glucocorticosteroids such as prednisolone are stopped Withdrawal seizures when anticonvulsants such as phenobarbital or phenytoin are stopped

Alphabetic classification of types of adverse drug effects

Fig. 6.4 An alphabetic classification of adverse drug effects.

Some important type B (bizarre) reactions

Adverse effect	Drug causes
Anaphylaxis	Penicillins and other antibacterial agents Foreign protein such as streptokinase or equine antirattlesnake vaccine Iodinated contrast media in radiology
Anaphylactoid reactions (nonimmunologic reactions resembling anaphylaxis, but occurring without prior exposure)	Angiotensin-converting enzyme inhibitors (angioedema) Intravenous N-acetylcysteine (urticaria and anaphylaxis) The solvent, polyethoxylated castor oil
Liver disease	Halogenated anesthetic gases such as chloroform, halothane, and enflurane (acute hepatic necrosis) Chlorpromazine, the oral contraceptive pill, and floxacillin (intrahepatic cholestasis) Minocycline (chronic active hepatitis)
Kidney disease	Nonsteroidal anti-inflammatory drugs (acute interstitial nephritis) Amphotericin (acute tubular necrosis) Angiotensin-converting enzyme inhibitors (vascular renal damage)
Bone marrow damage	The antithyroid drugs carbimazole, methimazole, and propylthiouracil Antibacterial agents such as chloramphenicol and co-trimoxazole Antirheumatic drugs such as gold salts and penicillamine

Fig. 6.5 Important type B (bizarre) reactions.

in patients with impaired kidneys because K^+ excretion occurs via the kidneys and therefore their capacity to eliminate K^+ is reduced. In patients with liver disease, the anticoagulant effect of warfarin can be greatly enhanced, because the warfarin is metabolized more slowly, and also because the ability of the liver to synthesize clotting factors is impaired. Pre-existing disease can predispose to adverse effects in other ways. For example, respiratory failure with sedatives such as diazepam is much more likely in patients with chronic obstructive pulmonary disease, whose respiratory drive is already reduced.

Genetically determined enzyme defects

As discussed in Chapter 4, the body contains many enzymes that metabolize drugs. Genetically determined deficits in such enzymes can make normally innocuous drug therapy hazardous, and sometimes lethal. An example of such a defect includes glucose-6-phosphate dehydrogenase (G6PD) deficiency, in its various forms, which is a chromosome X-linked recessive trait and therefore only occurs in males. Oxidants such as aspirin, primaquine, and dapsone can cause severe hemolysis in people with this deficiency, which is most common in people of Mediterranean, African, or South-East Asian origin.

Drug interactions

Drug interactions are an important clinical problem. They can be classified as:

- Pharmaceutical interactions in which there is a chemical or physical interaction between two or more drugs before they are absorbed into the body.
- Pharmacokinetic interactions where one drug alters the concentration of another via an interaction at the level of absorption, metabolism, distribution or elimination.
- Pharmacodynamic interactions in which the effects of two drugs given together differ from those of either drug given separately.

Pharmaceutical interactions

Pharmaceutical interactions include, for example, the chemical chelation of Fe^{2+} by tetracyclines, which makes both iron sulfate and tetracyclines less effective when given together than when given separately. This is because the concentration available for absorption of one is lowered by the presence of the other. Another example is the precipitation of calcium hydroxide which occurs when calcium gluconate is added to an intravenous infusion of sodium bicarbonate solution.

Pharmacokinetic interactions

Pharmacokinetic interactions are in practice the most important and potentially dangerous of all drug interactions. They include the important interactions that occur between drugs which are metabolized by the cytochrome P-450 (mixed function oxidase) enzyme system (see Chapter 4 for a discussion of this system) and drugs that inhibit it. For example, drugs such as the anticoagulant warfarin, theophylline (used in the treatment of asthma), and the antirejection drug cyclosporine are meta-bolized by cytochrome P-450. All the three drugs have a low therapeutic index (ratio between therapeutic concentration and toxic concentration; see Chapter 4) and therefore small changes in metabolism can provoke severe type A adverse effects. Drugs that inhibit cytochrome P-450 include the antibacterial agents erythromycin, co-trimoxazole and ciprofloxacin, the antifungal agents ketoconazole and fluconazole, and the H_2 receptor antagonist cimetidine. A small number of drugs can actually induce the production of cytochrome P-450 enzymes and, as a result, reduce the concentration of drugs metabolized by the enzyme system. Such enzyme inducers include the anticonvulsants phenobarbital and carbamazepine, and the antituberculous agent rifampin. Women on oral contraception who take these drugs need to take higher doses of estrogens than normal, otherwise the enhanced estrogen metabolism will leave them unprotected against pregnancy.

Renal excretion of one drug can be influenced by the presence of another. The classic example is the renal excretion of lithium, another drug with a low therapeutic index, which can be inhibited by thiazide diuretics.

Pharmacodynamic interactions

Anticholinergic drugs and levodopa are used to treat Parkinson's disease, with one drug reducing cholinergic activity and the other increasing dopaminergic activity. Both effects tend to improve the movement disorder, though both can also cause hallucinations and delirium. (For a fuller discussion see Chapter 14).

Pharmacovigilance

Pharmacoepidemiology is the study of the use and effects of drugs in large numbers of people, that is, the epidemiology of drugs. Pharmacoepidemiology uses the methods of epidemiology and is concerned with all aspects of the benefit–risk ratio for populations using particular drugs. Pharmacovigilance is a branch of pharmacoepidemiology. It is restricted to the epidemiologic study of drug-related events or adverse drug effects. In this context, 'events' are those recorded in the patient's notes during a period of drug monitoring. They may be due to the disease for which the drug is being given, an intercurrent disease or infection, an adverse reaction to the drug being monitored, the activity of a drug being given concomitantly, or a drug interaction.

Pharmacovigilance studies can be:

- Hypothesis-generating (e.g. to detect unexpected adverse drug effects of a recently-marketed drug).

Methods of pharmacovigilance

- Hypothesis-generating: spontaneous adverse drug effect reporting (yellow card in the UK)

- Hypothesis-generating and testing: prescription event monitoring (green form in the UK)

- Hypothesis-testing: case–control studies, cohort studies, randomized controlled clinical trials

- Hypothesis-testing (e.g. to prove whether any suspicions raised about a specific drug are justified).
- Both hypothesis-generating and hypothesis-testing.

Hypothesis-generating studies

It often happens in clinical practice that a patient becomes unwell while taking a medicine, and the doctor or pharmacist suspects that the 'adverse event' is due to the drug. In spontaneous reporting schemes, a health professional who suspects an adverse reaction is encouraged to notify a central agency of the suspicion. Such spontaneous reporting has led to the identification of many unexpected adverse drug effects.

This type of system was first introduced in the UK, as the 'yellow card' in 1964. A similar system for the reporting of adverse effects to drugs was established later by the FDA in the USA (Fig. 6.6). Similar systems are found throughout Europe, and in most developed countries. All these systems rely on voluntary reporting by the prescriber, or other health professional, if they consider an event to be an adverse effect due to drugs.

The great strengths of these schemes are:

- They are operated for all drugs throughout the whole of the drug's lifetime.
- They are an affordable method of detecting rare adverse effects.

Their main weaknesses are:

- Gross underreporting, since the system is voluntary.
- Bias due to sudden media interest in a particular drug.

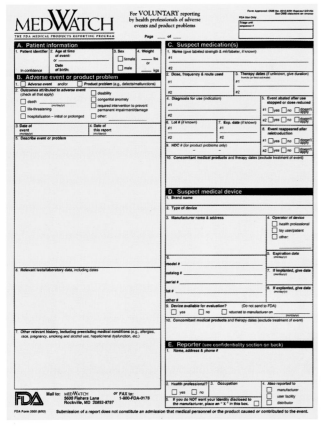

Fig. 6.6 The FDA MedWatch reporting card.

- The data provide only a numerator (i.e. the number of reports of each suspected reaction) but do not take into consideration how many patients have actually received the drug.

Nevertheless, these schemes are invaluable and it is essential that physicians fill in such drug report cards.

Spontaneous reporting has led to identification of many unexpected adverse effects, resulting in the withdrawal of a number of marketed drugs. Examples of drugs that have been removed from the UK market since 1972 because of adverse events reported under the yellow card system are shown in Fig. 6.7, and previously licensed drugs withdrawn from the US market between 1996 and 2000 are shown in Fig. 6.8.

Hypothesis-generating and hypothesis-testing studies

Adverse event monitoring related to prescriptions (prescription event monitoring; PEM) is an hypothesis-generating and testing process

Prescription event monitoring in the UK is an important technique which takes advantage of the way the country's National Health Service system is organized. It provides the denominator that is missing in the above systems. Dispensed prescriptions written by general practitioners are sent to a central Prescription Pricing Authority, which provides confidential copies of all prescriptions for newly introduced drugs that are being monitored, to a Drug Safety Research Unit. This Unit then sends a 'green-form' questionnaire (Fig. 6.9) to the general practitioner who wrote the original prescription. The green form is sent out 6 or 12 months after the first prescription. This procedure therefore provides the 'exposure data,' showing which patients have been exposed to the drug being monitored while the completed green forms provide the 'outcome data' detailing any events noted during the period of monitoring. The Drug Safety Research Unit can then follow up pregnancies, deaths, or events of special interest by contacting either the prescribing physician or other holders of the patient's medical record. So far 76 drugs have been studied and the average number of patients included in each study (the cohort size) has been about 10,500.

The strengths of the 'green form' method are:

- It provides a numerator (i.e. the number of reports) and a denominator (i.e. the number of patients exposed), both being collected over a precisely known period of observation.
- There is no interference with the physician's decision about which drug to prescribe for each individual patient. This avoids selection biases, which can make data interpretation difficult.

The main weakness of PEM in the UK is that only 50–70% of the green forms are returned. Attempts are now being made to establish PEM outside the UK.

Hypothesis-testing studies

Hypothesis-testing studies are used in the situation where previous data has led to the postulation of a specific hypothesis regarding a drug and adverse effects. The techniques used for this purpose include case–control and cohort studies. A

Drugs licensed since 1972 and withdrawn in the UK owing to toxicity

Product	Therapeutic class	Adverse reaction(s)	Type A/B reaction
Aclofenac	NSAID	Anaphylaxis	B
Polidexide	Hypolipidemic	Impurities	–
Nomifensine	Antidepressant	Hemolytic anemia	B
Fenclofenac	NSAID	Epidermal necrolysis	B
Feprazone	NSAID	Nephrotoxicity, GI toxicity	A
Benoxaprofen	NSAID	Photosensitivity, hepatotoxicity	A
Zomepirac	NSAID	Anaphylaxis	B
Indoprofen	NSAID	GI toxicity	A
Zimeldine	Antidepressant	Guillain–Barré syndrome	B
Suprofen	NSAID	Nephrotoxicity	A
Terodiline	Anti-incontinence	Ventricular tachycardia	A
Triazolam	Hypnotic	Psychiatric reactions	A
Temafloxacin	Antibiotic	Multi-organ toxicity	B
Centoxin	Antibiotic	Increased mortality	B
Remoxipride	Neuroleptic	Aplastic anemia	B
Flosequinan	Cardiac failure	Increased mortality	B
Metipranolol	Anti-glaucoma	Anterior uveitis	B

Fig. 6.7 Drugs licensed since 1972 and withdrawn in the UK, because of toxicity. The list shows that licensed drugs can be the cause of major unexpected adverse drug reactions and also demonstrates the importance of pharmacovigilance. (NSAID, nonsteroidal anti-inflammatory drug; GI, gastrointestinal.)

Licensed drugs withdrawn from the United States market 1996–2000

Drug	Use	Problem
Alosetron	Treating irritable bowel syndrome	Ischemic colitis
Phenylpropanolamine	Nasal decongestant	Hemorrhagic stroke
Troglitazone	Oral antidiabetic agent	Toxic to the liver
Cisapride	To increase gut motility	Arrhythmia
Grepafloxacin	Antibacterial	Severe cardiovascular events
Rotavirus vaccine	Protect against rotavirus diarrhea	Intussusception
Astemizole	Nonsedating antihistamine	Arrhythmia
Bromfenac sodium	Nonsteroidal anti-inflammatory	Severe hepatic failure
Mibefradil	Antihypertensive and anti-anginal	Potential for drug interactions
Terfenadine	Nonsedating antihistamine	Arrhythmia
Fenfluramine, dexfenfluramine	Anti-obesity agents	Heart valve disease
Chlormezanone	Sedative	Toxic epidermal necrolysis

Fig. 6.8 Licensed drugs withdrawn from the United States market, 1996–2000. Many of the drugs on the list have been withdrawn voluntarily by the manufacturers. This list shows that licensed drugs can be the cause of major unexpected adverse drug reactions and also demonstrates the importance of pharmacovigilance.

case–control technique will usually be chosen if there are only a few cases of the adverse effect and assembling a sufficiently large cohort of cases would be impossible. However, some pharmacoepidemiologists believe that the cohort technique provides more convincing results. In this context a cohort means a group of patients with a common demographic or statistical characteristic.

■ *Case–control studies compare cases of a disease with controls susceptible to but free of the disease*
Case–control studies are technically complex, but have been successfully used by government agencies and many academic units. The final results compare or relate the risks in the treated cases with the controls. The absolute risk can be determined

only in very special circumstances. Great care is needed in accurate diagnosis of the cases, and in data collection, so that potential biases are minimized or excluded, and marginal results are not over-interpreted. Clearly, a fairly small increase in the risk of a common serious condition such as breast cancer may be of far greater public health importance than a relatively large increase in very uncommon risk, such as primary hepatic carcinoma.

■ *Cohort studies follow up a large group of patients for long enough to assess the outcome of an exposure common to the cohort*
Comparative cohort studies include an unexposed control group. Again, potential biases can be a problem, but the

PLEASE RETURN THIS HALF OF THE FORM. Ref:

SEX	DATE OF BIRTH / /	WAS THIS DRUG EFFECTIVE? Yes☐ No☐
INDICATION FOR PRESCRIBING		PLEASE SPECIFY REASON FOR STOPPING THIS DRUG AND NAME OF DRUG(S) SUBSTITUTED
DATE PATIENT STARTED THIS DRUG / /		DATE PATIENT STOPPED THIS DRUG / /

DATE	DOSE mg/day	EVENTS WHILE TAKING THIS DRUG	DATE	EVENTS AFTER STOPPING THIS DRUG
		If there were **NO EVENTS ON DRUG** please tick this box. ☐		If there were **NO EVENTS OFF DRUG** please tick this box. ☐

IMPORTANT: PLEASE INDICATE ANY EVENT REPORTED TO CSM OR MANUFACTURER

Fig. 6.9 The data collection segment of the green form used for prescription event monitoring in the UK.

method, though usually expensive and time-consuming, has the advantage of revealing the absolute risk and not just relative risk.

■ Randomized controlled trials avoid biases

In randomized controlled trials one group of patients is divided into two in a strictly random order. One group is then exposed and the other is not exposed to the drug, so that the outcomes can be compared. However, although this method is resistant to biases, it has only a limited, but important, role as a pharmacoepidemiologic tool because most serious adverse effects are relatively uncommon. Appropriate randomized controlled trials can therefore become unmanageably large and expensive.

FURTHER READING

Davies DM, Ferner RE, de Glanville H (eds). *Davies's Textbook of Adverse Drug Reactions*, 5th edn. London: Chapman and Hall; 1998. [A textbook of adverse reactions arranged by disease.]

Dukes MNG, Aronson JK (eds). *Meyler's Side Effects of Drugs*, 14th edn. Amsterdam: Elsevier; 2000. [A textbook of adverse reactions arranged by drugs.]

Faich GA. US adverse drug reaction surveillance 1989–1994. *Pharmacoepidemiol Drug Safety* 1996. [This paper summarizes the North American experience of pharmacovigilance.]

Ferner RE. Hazards, risks and reality. *Br J Clin Pharmacol* 1992; **33**: 125–128. [A brief account of problems of risk related to pharmaceutical products.]

Rawlins MD. Pharmacovigilance: paradise lost, regained or postponed? *J R Coll Physicians (London)* 1995; **29**: 41–49. [A thoughtful account of the European experience.]

Stockley IH. Drug Interactions: *A Source-book of Drug Interactions, Their Mechanisms, Clinical Importance, and Management*, 5th edn. London: The Pharmaceutical Press; 1999. [An authoritative compendium of drug interactions.]

Useful websites
http://www.fda.gov/medwatch/index.html   United States Food and Drug Administration
http://www.eudra.org.emea.html   European Medicines Evaluation Agency
http://www.open.gov.uk/mcahome.htm   United Kingdom Medicines Control Agency

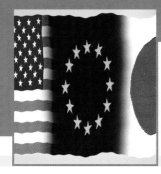

Regulation of Drug Use

■ *Drug regulation seeks to ensure efficacy, safety, and chemical purity*

Most drugs are sold for profit by pharmaceutical companies. Various methods have been developed to test whether a particular drug is effective and safe, and most national governments regulate both testing and approval for sale of drugs. Two distinct regulatory steps are generally recognized in this process: approval for clinical testing of a new drug; and approval for sale of a new drug. The main purposes of regulating drug approval are:

- To protect the public because of the conflict of interest between the need of pharmaceutical companies to make a profit, and the need of patients for medication that is likely to be of benefit.
- To apply standards of proof of efficacy, and adequate safety, so that practitioners can be assured that a drug has been tested sufficiently.
- To assure that manufacturing processes result in a predictable product with acceptable purity and constant physical properties.
- At a fourth level of regulation, to control the public's access to certain drugs, particularly those liable to abuse.

As discussed in Chapter 6 the regulation of drugs began in the United States with the Federal Pure Food and Drug Act (1906). This first drug Act was concerned only with drug purity, and was primarily passed in reaction to public disclosures of impurities and carelessness in the preparation of food and medicinal products. Later, the sulfanilamide tragedy led to the establishment of the Food and Drug Administration (FDA). The power of the FDA, and of regulatory authorities around the world, was expanded in the 1960s after the thalidomide tragedy in Europe. Laws were extended to require the demonstration of safety and efficacy in clinical trials prior to allowing the general availability of a new medicine.

It is not clear that such testing would have led to the discovery of the teratogenic effects of thalidomide prior to marketing, but as a general approach to evidence-based drug development the new requirements were scientifically sound and sensible. It is important to recognize that, although the rigorous establishment of safety and efficacy is a worthy goal of drug development and regulation, no system of regulation is guaranteed to prevent all harm that could come from a particular drug. Some effects are too rare to be detected in drug development programs involving only hundreds to some thousands of patients. Delaying approval of a drug until tens of thousands of people have been exposed could often result in many patients not getting a beneficial drug.

Drug development and regulation is thus an assessment of relative risk and benefit; quantitation of either is not absolute. Regulation will not prevent all ills resulting from the use of medication. It can only serve to obtain a certain degree of qualitative and quantitative rigor in establishing the risk and efficacy of a drug. Regulation has also led to a more uniform set of information that is readily available to clinicians who must assess the relative merits of a new drug compared with existing therapeutic agents. Although it is ultimately the responsibility of the prescribing physician or health professional to know what data support the use of a drug in a particular setting, and what the risks of such use are, an underlying assumption of regulation is that those authorized to prescribe need assistance in making choices.

Drug testing involves a progression from studies in animals to studies in humans. Since the 1990s, there has been great and continuing progress in making the requirements for drug development more uniform in the United States, Europe and Japan through harmonizing their different approaches. The International Conference on the Harmonization of Technical Requirements for Registration of Pharmaceuticals for Human Use (ICH guidelines) is an ongoing multinational attempt by authorities in drug development and regulation to evaluate scientific and technical aspects of the process of approving drugs. The effort is officially sanctioned by several bodies, including the European Commission of the European Union, the Ministry of Health and Welfare of Japan, the United States FDA, as well as several international scientific societies. Guidelines have been established, and mostly accepted by regulatory authorities, for principles of manufacture; methods to evaluate analytical procedures, chemical and physical stability of a product; conduct of preclinical and clinical trials and establishment of safety and efficacy. Thus regulatory bodies worldwide:

- Set the policy that defines what animal data are sufficient before human studies can start with a new drug.
- Enforce rules of manufacturing and purity for that drug so that the stated contents and amounts of a particular medication are accurate.
- To varying extents, limit what claims can be made about drugs in advertising and for what conditions the drug should be prescribed.

STAGES IN DRUG DEVELOPMENT

Several stages can be defined between the discovery of a new drug and the demonstration of its clinical efficacy and adequate safety (see Chapter 6 and particularly Fig. 6.3). The initial discovery stage usually involves deciding upon a therapeutic target (disease or condition) or a target molecule such as receptors, enzymes etc, and then finding a lead chemical compound, that is a compound with the characteristic actions of the required ideal new drug. In most drug discovery programs nowadays, a particular target molecule is chosen as a critical link in the disease process and small synthetic or natural chemicals are screened to determine whether they target this molecule, and therefore constitute a lead for further attempts to develop better compounds. Obtaining better compounds is an iterative process involving the synthesis of multiple chemical variants. Structure–activity relationship (SAR, or QSAR if quantitative) analysis is used to direct the production of new analogs for obtaining the required potency and efficacy (see Chapters 3 and 5).

Some analogs are subjected to extensive pharmacologic and toxicological studies to identify and characterize the drug candidates sufficiently to gain approval for testing in humans. After a series of clinical trials the data collected are submitted to regulatory authorities to secure approval for marketing the new drug. After approval, experiences with the drug in clinical practice are collected by a variety of methods in an exercise called postmarketing surveillance (see Chapter 6), an activity which is not as heavily regulated as the procedures that lead to approval.

Animal studies provide the justification for clinical trials

A profile of in vitro and in vivo pharmacologic effects of a drug forms the rationale for considering whether it is likely to have therapeutic value. These data are needed to justify investigating a new drug in humans since, without it, there would be no basis for anticipating benefit, or an acceptable risk of adverse effects. Preclinical drug development is the name given to in vitro and animal studies that are used to screen for particular molecular actions, test for cellular, tissue and system pharmacologic properties, and subsequently (using animal models of human disease) examine potential therapeutic effects. Ultimately, clinical studies cannot proceed unless a drug is shown to be safe and effective in a clinically relevant animal model of the targeted disease. However, the reliability of the data in predicting clinical outcome depends on the level of clinical relevance of the model. For example, models of pneumonia caused by *Staphylococcus aureus* are quite predictive. The infecting organism is the same in the model and in humans, and the animal's immunologic defenses against the bacteria and pulmonary pathology are very similar to those in humans. In contrast, animal models of rheumatoid arthritis only indirectly mimic the disease in man and are less predictive. Usually, the ability to develop models in animals is related to a basic understanding of the pathophysiology of a particular disorder. In the above examples, the immediate cause of the pneumonia is known whereas in rheumatoid arthritis the immediate precipitating cause is not known.

Animals also serve other purposes in drug development. They can be used to investigate the relationship between drug dose and plasma concentrations for both beneficial and toxic effects. This can guide initial dosing in humans so that the first

doses tested in people are not picked randomly. As part of the process, animals are given maximally tolerated doses in order that any potentially adverse effects are most likely to be revealed. Thus, in order to reveal any potential toxic effects, test animals receive a much greater total exposure to the drug than that expected in people. If the doses required for effectiveness in the animal model produce severe adverse effects this would preclude human studies. Animals are also used to screen for carcinogenic and teratogenic effects, but these tests require much longer exposure to the drug.

Human testing of drugs progresses through a series of clinical trials

Clinical trials begin after sufficient data have been generated to warrant testing a new drug in humans and the appropriate regulatory approval. The three phases of drug development have been denoted as phase I, phase II, and phase III. Phase IV has been defined as postmarketing surveillance and other post-approval clinical studies (see Fig. 6.3). These phases have been previously outlined in Chapter 6 but the following gives more detail.

Phase I comprises the first studies in humans, which are carried out under very close supervision and are usually open label or single blind (see Fig. 7.1 for terminology) to find the lowest dose that *cannot* be tolerated because of unacceptable, readily apparent acute toxicity. Further testing is carried out with doses less than this dose. Traditionally, these studies have been carried out in healthy young males, but increasingly the latter are being replaced by the type of patients who will eventually use the drug. Initial pharmacokinetic data can also be obtained at this phase.

Phase II begins after the tolerated dose range has been defined. These studies are carried out in patients for whom the new drug is deemed to have potential benefit. The major purpose is to gather evidence that the drug has the effects suggested by the preclinical evidence, i.e. that the drug is efficacious. Sometimes the end-point of phase II clinical trials is the actual goal of therapy, known as the definitive end-point; at other times a surrogate end-point is used. A surrogate end-point is one that is predictive, or thought to be predictive, of the definitive end-point. For example, a drug that is being tested in heart failure may have as its definitive end-point an improvement in exercise tolerance or in survival. A surrogate end-point for the same drug may be a decrease in peripheral vascular resistance with improved cardiac output. A drug that might be useful in preventing clotting following angioplasty might have as a surrogate end-point the inhibition of platelet aggregation, whereas the definitive end-point would be a reduction in re-stenosis. A surrogate end-point has most utility when its occurrence has been rigorously linked to the occurrence of the definitive end-point. Perhaps the most celebrated of all surrogate end-points is a reduction of blood pressure. The reason for treating hypertension is to reduce adverse cardiovascular events and renal failure, sequelae of the hypertension. Thus reduction of blood pressure is really a surrogate end-point for reduction in the consequences of hypertension.

Clinical trial terminology	
Term	Definition
Control	The established therapy (or a placebo if there is no established therapy) against which the efficacy of a new agent can be compared
Randomized	Patients entering the trial have an equal probability of receiving the test or control agent so that factors that could affect the outcome, other than the therapy being tested, are equally distributed in the experimental and control groups
Double blind	Neither the health professionals nor the patient know whether the patient is receiving the experimental or control agent, to avoid any bias about which therapy might be better
Single blind	The health professionals know which treatment a patient is receiving, but the patient does not know
Open label	The opposite of double blind. Both health professionals and patients know whether the drug is the experimental or the control agent and the dose that the patient is receiving
Parallel trial	At least two regimens are tested simultaneously, but patients are assigned only one therapy
Crossover trial	Patients receive each therapy in sequence and therefore serve as their own controls. For example, if therapy A is being tested against therapy B, some patients receive A before B and some receive B before A, so that the effect of the drug therapy, and not of the order in which each therapy is given, can be tested
Endpoint	This is measured to assess a drug's effect (e.g. blood pressure is the endpoint for testing an antihypertensive agent, while pain relief is the endpoint for testing an analgesic)
Surrogate endpoint	An outcome of therapy that predicts the real goal of therapy without being that goal (e.g. reduction in tumor size as a surrogate for survival)

Fig. 7.1 Clinical trial terminology.

Other purposes of phase II trials are to determine the pharmacokinetic profile of a drug, and to relate plasma concentrations to effects, if possible. The influence of hepatic and renal disease on the elimination of the drug from the body is also investigated, and pharmacokinetic and pharmacologic interactions of the new drug with other drugs liable to be co-administered can be explored. Phase II studies may be single or double blind and may be parallel or crossover in design, with patients being allocated randomly to treatment groups. In ethnically diverse populations, such as exist in the United States, pharmacokinetic studies are sometimes required to elucidate how various ethnic groups metabolize a drug. Ethnic identity is only a crude approximation of genetic classification. Perhaps in the future, a more elegant approach to predicting metabolic patterns and clinical outcomes will be employed to classify patients by genetic predisposition to metabolize drugs in particular ways. It may even be possible to predict which genotypes are most likely to benefit from a particular drug, or most likely to develop a toxicity.

Phase III consists of the definitive clinical trials that establish efficacy and safety of the new drug. Whenever possible, the trials are double blind, randomized, and controlled. They are almost always parallel in design. Statistical considerations must underpin the planning of design and size of all clinical trials, but especially phase III trials, so that valid conclusions can be made when the trials are completed. In addition, the population studied in phase III should approximate the target population for the drug. The trials should include patients with representative manifestations of the disease in question. The distribution of ethnic groups, men and women should mirror that in the diseased population. In recent years, more emphasis has been placed in studying pediatric patients as part of the initial application for approval. This is now required in the United States except in instances where such an effort would be absurd, such as in the study of a drug for Alzheimer's disease.

DRUG REGULATION FOR NEW DRUGS

■ *Drug regulation and approval proceeds by several steps*
Although practices vary from country to country, and continent to continent, drug regulations everywhere are aimed to ensure that marketed drugs are safe and effective. However, 'safe' and 'effective' are relative terms and require interpretation. Furthermore, the emphasis placed on either of the two aspects depends upon the intended medical use of an agent. Not unreasonably, toxicity is tolerated for drugs that have beneficial effects in otherwise fatal diseases for which there are few if any cures, for example AIDS and many cancers. However, the safety requirements for an analgesic for mild to moderate pain will be quite different: only minimal and nonmedically serious

adverse effects would be allowed. Also, some regulatory bodies give more weight to safety relative to efficacy than do others. Regulation also seeks to ensure that a drug product has adequate purity and that its chemical and physical characteristics are well described and can be reproduced in each manufactured batch.

As noted above, the process of 'harmonization' is underway to make the regulatory process more uniform, especially between the United States and Europe. Although there are differences in the details of the approval process and indeed, sometimes in the results of the process, the requirements and expectations are much more uniform than they were in the mid to latter third of the twentieth century. While this is not official policy, the European and American regulatory authorities in fact pay much attention to the activities and decisions of each other.

In the US, the Food and Drug Administration approves drugs

In the US a pharmaceutical company submits preclinical data to the Food and Drug Administration (FDA) in a document called an Investigational New Drug (IND) application. The FDA then gives or withholds permission to initiate clinical trials in humans. As clinical trials proceed, the pharmaceutical company keeps the FDA informed of progress and any adverse effect and/or toxicity. When phase III is completed, the company submits all preclinical and clinical data to the FDA in a New Drug Application (NDA). The FDA reviews the data and decides whether the data provide adequate documentation of safety and efficacy to support the use of the drug for a particular disease.

Sometimes, the FDA will seek the advice of independent advisory committees of clinicians possessing pertinent expertise. This most often occurs when a novel indication is sought, when a first representative of a new class of drugs is being considered, or when the results of a development program are not clear. The committees' deliberations are public events and may be observed by anyone who can get in the door. With or without an advisory committee, if the data so warrant, the FDA will then approve the drug. If the data are not adequate, the FDA will ask for additional clinical trials. Part of the approval process consists of writing a 'label.' The label provides details of the pharmacokinetics, efficacy and toxicity of the drug. In addition a summary of the main evidentiary clinical trials are described.

> **Information provided by the drug 'label' required for FDA approval in the US**
>
> - Data that support the approval
> - Pharmacologic actions of the drug
> - Indication (approved use) of the drug
> - A description of adverse effects
> - Instructions on dosing

The FDA also approves the manufacturing process, including the scientific standards for the chemical nature and formulation of the drug. Once an NDA is approved, the company may sell the drug. Although the FDA has the power to approve a drug for marketing for a particular indication, or set of indications, it does not have the power to regulate use once such approval is granted. Thus physicians may choose to use a drug for a nonapproved indication, so-called 'off-label use.' Often such use is warranted by strong evidence from clinical trials that, for one reason or another, have not been submitted to the FDA. For a drug with one approved indication, the results of clinical trials that would form the basis of an approval for a second indication are publicly available before the approval process runs its course. In these settings, such off-label use of a drug is perfectly reasonable. A prototypical example of appropriate off-label use was the early employment of propranolol for treating hypertension. This beta blocker was initially approved in the United States for angina. However, based both on pharmacologic considerations and clinical observations it was recognized that propranolol was effective in reducing blood pressure in hypertensive patients. The drug was widely used for this indication for many years before such use was approved. Some off-label use is, however, of dubious merit. It is the responsibility of the physician to know the data and to make judgements about what evidence supports expanding the scope of a drug's utility.

In Europe, drug approval is regulated by both centralized and decentralized processes that are aimed at producing more uniform practices across the member states of the European Union.

In Europe the regulation process has changed dramatically since the inception of the European Union (EU). With new procedures replacing the previous country-by-country approval process. As a result the prerequisites for approval have become uniform in the member states. However, the requirements to initiate trials in humans still differ from country to country. In general they are less restrictive than in the US. If a qualified clinical investigator deems that enough evidence has accumulated to justify testing in humans, the investigator is allowed to do so after summarizing the rationale for it. Regulatory authorities are notified that such testing is taking place, but they are less active than the FDA in actually approving such testing.

Once clinical drug development has been completed, a pharmaceutical company can proceed by either a centralized or decentralized (officially called mutual recognition) process, which ultimately results in more uniform practices across all member states. The process chosen by a pharmaceutical company depends on a combination of commercial and political considerations, as well as the kind of molecule being considered.

The centralized EU procedure

Under the EU centralized procedure, applications are submitted to the European Medicines Evaluation Agency (EMEA), which is responsible for administering the regulatory procedures and sending the application to the Committee on Proprietary Medicinal Products (CPMP). The CPMP, composed of representatives of all member states, appoints a rapporteur. The rapporteur is identified with a particular country and the staff of that country's drug regulatory agency are responsible for the initial review. When the review is complete the rapporteur prepares a report of the data and provides an opinion on whether approval is possible. The reports are then presented to the CPMP. The CPMP may request further information and pose questions that the sponsoring pharmaceutical company must answer. Finally, the CPMP formulates its opinion and a decision is made by majority vote, for or against approval. Approval by this centralized process entitles the pharmaceutical sponsor to sell the product throughout the member states of the EU. The EU 'label' is called the Summary of Product Characteristics, which is uniform in all member states. This label is much less detailed than the label of the United States, the latter presenting more details of the clinical trials that supported the application.

The mutual recognition (decentralized) EU procedure

In the decentralized EU procedure an application is made to one country, a so-called reference member state. The regulatory authority of that state reviews the data and makes a unilateral decision about whether to approve the application or not. If the reference member state approves the application, a report is sent to each of the member states in which the applicant would like to market the drug; these states can either accept the report, and therefore approve the application, or object to the report. In the case of objection, the applicant can choose to forgo approval in the rejecting state or to seek arbitration by the CPMP. The CPMP's decision is ultimately binding on all member states. Again, a uniform Summary of Product Characteristics is composed for all states in which the application is accepted.

While off-label use in Europe is possible, and sometimes occurs, it is much less prevalent than in the United States because payment for drugs in Europe is much more closely tied to the approval process than is payment in the United States.

In Japan, the approval process is carried out under the authority of the Ministry of Health and Welfare and the Central Pharmaceutical Affairs Council

Initiating clinical trials in Japan requires the approval of the Ministry of Health and Welfare (MHW). An application for approval is sent to the MHW after data have been assembled from clinical trials. The MHW acts as an administrative body and sends the data to the Central Pharmaceutical Affairs Council (CPAC) for review. The CPAC consists of experts in various disciplines such as medicine and pharmaceutical science, and recommends a course of action to the MHW, which implements the approval. In the last few years there have been several internal reviews of the Japanese testing and approval process. The barriers to data from non-Japanese patients have been somewhat penetrated, at least for phase II and phase III studies. Nevertheless, in practice, studies in Japanese patients are

> ### 🔑 Drug development is a lengthy process
>
> - The time taken from submitting an application for approval to receiving a decision can take from 6 months to many years, though 1–2 years is typical
> - The process of drug development, from discovery to approval, typically takes from 6 to more than 10 years

required on the grounds that the Japanese are sufficiently biologically and culturally different from the typical European or North American patient for a separate set of trials to be necessary. The underlying principle is the same as that which requires testing in minority ethnic groups versus the dominant population. Traditionally, the Japanese have not relied as heavily on controlled, blinded trials, although this may be changing with the effort towards harmonization.

The United States, Europe and Japan account for by far the most drug use in the world. However, drugs are regulated to one degree or another in most if not all countries. Some of these accept the same application made in Europe or the United States. Many of these countries make their own determinations based wholly or in large part on the decisions of the United States and Europe. Some accept these decisions outright while others remain more independent using the decisions as a point to consider, but by no means regarding them as binding or automatically acceptable.

DRUG REGULATIONS RELATING TO ACCESS TO DRUGS

The rules and regulations relating to access to drugs vary between countries, as does the implementation of those rules

All countries have regulations regarding the possession and prescribing of drugs, but these vary widely between different countries. In some countries the public has ready access to many drugs without needing a prescription. In other countries the sale and release of the same drugs is tightly controlled. This not only relates to which drugs can legally be sold as over-the-counter (OTC) medications, but also as to how regulations are applied. For example, vitamins and other herbal remedies are regulated as food products, not drugs, in many countries, including the United States. Thus extravagant and unsubstantiated claims can be made in advertising for herbs that would be illegal for medicinal products. There are, however, laws against adding modern drugs to herbal mixtures (a not uncommon practice).

Many drugs have the potential for abuse and are therefore tightly regulated

All countries have laws concerning the possession, sales and distribution of drugs that are abused, including narcotics, alcohol and tobacco. The latter two are, after all, drugs. The drugs most likely to be abused are those with central nervous system (CNS) actions, in particular the opiates (see Chapter 14), nicotine, CNS depressants such as barbiturates, and psychoactive drugs such as cocaine and lysergic acid diethylamide (LSD). The laws governing these agents vary both within countries (in particular the United States) and between countries. In addition to concerns about health, social acceptance of drug use and other moral concerns also affect policy. Both alcohol and cigarettes, the vehicle for delivering nicotine in a carcinogenic formulation to addicted consumers, have enormous medical and economic costs, but their purchase is only restricted on the basis of age. Meanwhile drugs whose possession is illegal, such as heroin, cause a large part of their damage because of unsterile methods of administration and criminal acts to secure illicit drugs. This is not to say that the primary effects of these drugs are benign. They are not.

Nevertheless, some very damaging drugs are tolerated by society and some are not. Some countries allow addicts to receive drugs on a regular basis at government controlled centers. In the Netherlands, cannabis is available in limited quantities in commercial establishments, the equivalents of cafes. A law recently passed in California allows for medicinal use of cannabis under defined circumstances. This law is being challenged by the Federal Government and is actively being adjudicated in the courts. There is active and lively debate regarding the success, or lack thereof, of the more punitive, legally based restrictions and punishments for drug possession. No matter what overall position one takes on the law, it is clear that both the cause and treatment of abusive self-administration of pharmacologically active agents have medical and psychological components.

FURTHER READING

Gogerty JH. Preclinical research evaluation. In: Guarino RA (ed.) *New Drug Approval Processes*. New York: Marcel Dekker; 1987, pp. 25–54. [A thoughtful discussion of issues in preclinical research as it bears on clinical drug development.]

Japan Pharmaceutical Reference, 3rd edn. Japan Medical Products International; 1993, pp. 14–34. [A description in detail of the requirements for approval for drugs in Japan.]

Mamelok RD. Drug discovery and development. In: *Clinical Pharmacology*, 4th edn. New York: McGraw-Hill; 2000, pp. 1289–1305. [A more detailed discussion of issues in demonstrating a drug's safety and efficacy.]

Useful websites

http://www.ifpma.org/ich1.html   For ICH guidelines: contains information on the process and details of the guidelines
http://www.fda.gov   For FDA: allows access to news about drug regulation, activities of FDA and information on regulations and guidelines issued by FDA
www.eudra.org/emea.html   For EMEA: provides information European regulations, CPMP opinions and deliberations, and links to many other relevant websites

2

Drug Action on Pathogens and Neoplastic Cells

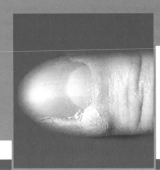

Chapter 8

Drugs and Viruses

BIOLOGY AND DRUG RESPONSIVENESS OF VIRUSES

Viral infections can involve any organ of the body. Most are asymptomatic. Symptomatic infection can range from a short benign illness such as the common cold to a protracted potentially lethal infection such as that caused by human immunodeficiency virus, type 1 (HIV-1).

◾ Viruses can be selectively inhibited by drugs

Selective inhibition of viruses by drugs depends upon either:

- Inhibition of unique steps in the viral replication pathways, such as adsorption of the virus to a cell receptor, penetration, uncoating, assembly, or release.
- Preferential inhibition of steps shared with the host cell, which include transcription and translation.

The potential therapeutic efficacy of an antiviral drug can be evaluated in vitro but such testing of viral susceptibility to drugs is less predictive than similar testing of bacterial sensitivity to antimicrobials. Lack of standardized in vitro testing and insufficient knowledge of pharmacokinetic–pharmacodynamic relationships preclude rigorous interpretations of associations between drug concentrations and their antiviral effect.

The development of resistance often limits the usefulness of these agents. Such antiviral resistance has been reported during therapy with all currently available antiviral drugs except ribavirin, trifluorothymidine, cidofovir and sorivudine. Drug resistance in viruses is due to development of nucleotide mutations but such viruses might still be susceptible to other antiviral drugs. The emergence of resistant strains sometimes can be minimized by using multiple drugs as in therapy for HIV-1 infection.

◾ Successful antiviral chemotherapy depends upon host immunocompetence

Currently available antiviral drugs are virustatic only. This contrasts with bacterial and fungal infections where cell-wall active agents such as the β-lactam antibiotics (e.g. penicillins) and antifungal agents (e.g. amphotericin B), respectively, are microbicidal and can produce a clinical cure with minimal contribution from the host's defense system.

◾ Symptoms and signs of viral infections are due to a variety of host responses

Host responses to viral infections range from acute inflammation (e.g. meningoencephalitis) to hypertrophy and hyperplasia (e.g. warts) and oncogenesis (e.g. human T-cell lymphotropic virus-1 leukemia).

The inflammatory response in cells usually terminates viral replication and leads to recovery from the infection. In contrast, an impaired host immune response can be associated with a prolonged and more severe illness. Occasionally, the normal host immune response is pathogenic and causes disease manifestations (e.g. dengue hemorrhagic fever). Rarely, virus replication causes little or no inflammatory reaction, but nevertheless the infection is fatal (e.g. rabies).

◾ Antiviral drugs are effective against some common viral infections

Antiviral chemotherapy is effective for infections caused by:

- Herpesviruses (HSV-1, HSV-2, HHV-8, VZV and CMV).
- Influenza A and B virus.
- Respiratory syncytial virus (RSV).
- Hepatitis B and C viruses (HVB and HVC).
- Papilloma viruses (HPV).
- The arenavirus of Lassa fever.
- Human immunodeficiency virus (HIV-1, HIV-2).

CLASSIFICATION OF ANTIVIRAL DRUGS AND THEIR SITES OF ACTION IN VIRAL REPLICATION

Antiviral drugs can be classified as nucleoside or non-nucleoside agents and according to their sites of action in the viral replicative cycle (Fig. 8.1). Some of the currently available agents have more than one site of action (e.g. ribavirin). Some agents are naturally occurring molecules (e.g. interferons). Antivirals that inhibit viruses other than HIV are presented in this list and discussed according to the step in the viral replicative cycle at which they act. These drugs and the viruses against which they are used are presented in Fig. 8.2. HIV inhibitors are discussed later.

INHIBITORS OF UNCOATING

Amantadine and rimantadine are the only two antiviral drugs which inhibit viral replication primarily by inhibiting uncoating of the virus. Amantadine was the first drug licensed for the prevention of influenza (1966) and its treatment (1976), followed by rimantadine in 1993.

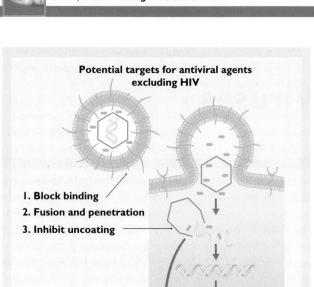

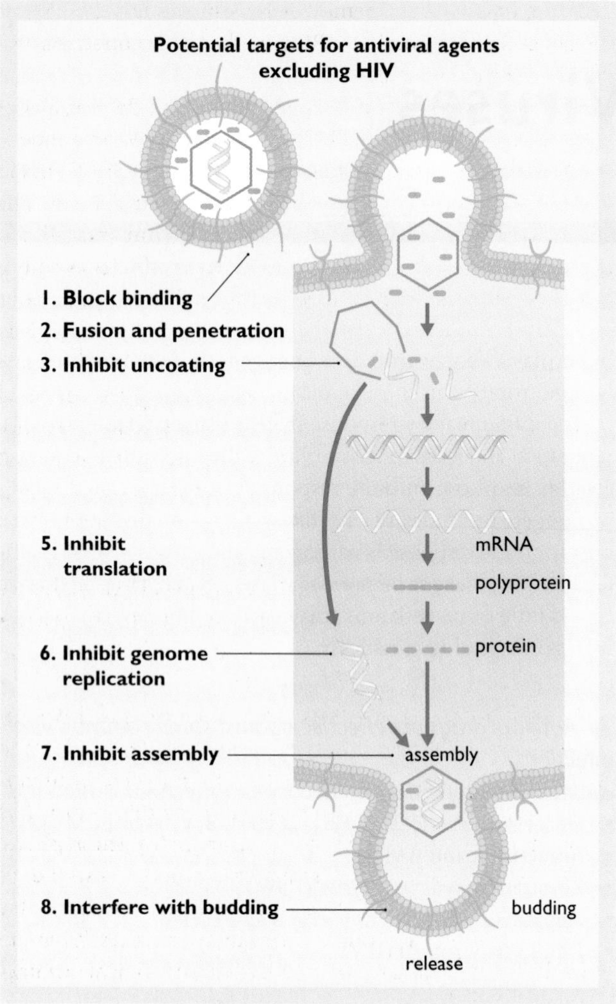

Potential targets for antiviral agents excluding HIV

1. **Block binding**
2. **Fusion and penetration**
3. **Inhibit uncoating**

5. **Inhibit translation**

6. **Inhibit genome replication**

7. **Inhibit assembly**

8. **Interfere with budding**

mRNA

polyprotein

protein

assembly

budding

release

Sites of action of antiviral drugs (other than HIV inhibitors)		
Viral replicative cycle step	Currently available drugs Nucleoside	Non-nucleoside
1. Adsorption		
2. Fusion & penetration		
3. Uncoating		Amantadine Rimantadine
4. Transcription		Interferons (IFN)
5. Translation		Fomivirsen
6. RNA or DNA replication	Acyclovir (ACV) Adenine arabinoside (ara-A) Cidofovir (CDV) Famciclovir (FCV) Foscarnet Ganciclovir (GCV) Penciclovir (PCV) Idoxuridine (IDU) Ribavirin Sorivudine Trifluorothymidine (TFT) Valacyclovir (VCV)	Foscarnet
7. Assembly		
8. Release and budding		Zanamivir Oseltamivir

Fig. 8.1 Currently available antiviral drugs and their site of action in the non-HIV replicative cycle.

Drugs used to treat common viral infections other than HIV						
Influenza (A, B)	Hepatitis (HBV, HCV)	Human papilloma virus (HPV)	Kaposi (HHV-8)	Cytomegalovirus (CMV)	Herpes viruses Simplex HSV-1, HSV-2	Varicella zoster (VZV)
A: Amantadine Rimantadine *A & B:* IFNs Ribavirin Zanamivir Oseltamivir	*B:* FCV Lamivudine *B & C:* IFNs *C:* IFNs + ribavirin	IFNs CDV	IFNs	CDV GCV Fomivirsen Foscarnet	ACV VCV PCV FCV Sorivudine Foscarnet *Topical:* Ara-A TFT IDU	Ara-A ACV CDV FCV PCV VCV Sorivudine

Fig. 8.2 Drugs used to treat common viral infections other than HIV.

CHEMISTRY Amantadine and rimantadine are tricyclic 10-carbon ring structures with an amine group on one pole. They are lipophilic, weak bases with a pKa of approximately 10.

MOLECULAR MECHANISM OF ACTION Both amantadine and rimantadine inhibit the replication of all known strains of

influenza A viruses in a variety of cells in culture and experimentally infected small animals. Influenza B and C viruses are not inhibited.

The two agents act similarly: they bind inside the ion-channel formed by the M2 transmembrane protein in the envelope of the virion. Binding creates a steric block, which prevents activation of the H⁺ ion-transport function of the channel, which normally acidifies the interior of the virion. The latter is essential for release of the RNA genome from the nucleoprotein complex, a process known as uncoating. Inhibition of uncoating prevents influenza virus replication.

Single nucleotide mutations in the M2 target site occur readily. These can obviate drug binding to the target site, confer shared drug-resistance on the virion and result in clinical treatment failure. Amantadine- and rimantadine-resistant mutants are susceptible in vitro to zanamivir and oseltamivir.

Amantadine was discovered serendipitously to possess antiparkinsonian activity (see Chapter 14). Rimantadine has no antiparkinsonian effect.

PHARMACOKINETICS Figure 8.3 shows selected pharmacokinetic parameters of amantadine and rimantadine in healthy young and old (>65 years) adults.

Amantadine or rimantadine are available only as oral formulations. Their pharmacokinetic characteristics are due to their high pKa and lipophilicity, with almost complete ionization in the low pH of the stomach and slow but relatively complete absorption from the intestine. They have a large apparent volume of distribution (AVD), which is approximately threefold greater for rimantadine than amantadine. They share similar trough plasma concentrations at steady state, both are cleared from plasma by first order processes, and their recommended doses are similar.

Amantadine is cleared almost exclusively by glomerular filtration and renal tubular secretion so that renal clearance exceeds creatinine clearance. Rimantadine undergoes extensive hydroxylation, conjugation and glucuronidation prior to renal excretion. Dose reductions are essential for safe use of amantadine in patients with renal disease. Rimantadine doses for patients with creatinine clearance less than 10 ml/min are recommended to be halved to 100 mg per day. Amantadine renal clearance is enhanced by urinary acidification; this may be of value in increasing removal from patients with an overdose of drug since hemodialysis removes less than 5% of the amantadine in the body. Rimantadine concentrations also are not affected by hemodialysis.

In severe, but not mild-to-moderate hepatic disease, a dose reduction of rimatadine to 100 mg per day is recommended.

Neurotoxicity, manifest as insomnia and tremors, occurs in 5–10% of healthy individuals given standard doses. The incidence of these adverse effects plus delirium and hallucinations is increased in persons with renal insufficiency unless doses are reduced. Similar adverse effects due to interactions have been described in patients receiving amantadine plus triamterene, hydrochlorothiazide or trimethoprim-sulfamethoxazole; this is attributed to inhibition of renal tubular amantadine secretion. Quinine and quinidine reduce amantadine renal clearance by 27 to 32% in male but not female adult volunteers. Amantadine does not alter acetaminophen disposition.

CLINICAL USES Amantadine and rimantadine are equieffective for the prevention and treatment of illness due to influenza A viruses. Prophylactic efficacy is approximately 70% and similar to that observed with influenza vaccine.

Treatment of influenza must be initiated within 2 days of onset of illness to be effective and is associated with rapid emergence of resistance. From 10 to 27% of treated immunocompetent individuals shed resistant virus within 4 to 5 days of initiation of therapy. Resistant strains are stable genotypically, transmissible, and cause disease that fails to respond to amantadine or rimantadine. These resistant strains are susceptible in vitro to zanamivir and oseltamivir but their successful use in individuals whose disease is due to amantadine- or rimantadine-resistant strains has not yet been reported.

Resistance may occur even more readily in immunocompromised patients treated with amantadine or rimantadine.

ADVERSE EFFECTS Both amantadine and rimantadine cause dose-related adverse effects.

Pharmacokinetic parameters of amantadine and rimantadine in healthy young and old (>65 years) adults				
Drug characteristic	Amantadine		Rimantadine	
	Young	Elderly	Young	Elderly
Relative oral bioavailability	62–93%	53–100%	75–93%	NA
Vd_{ss}, mean, L/kg at 200 mg/day	6	3.6	18	12
Plasma $t_{1/2}$, hours	15	26	29	37
Renal clearance, ml/min/70 kg	448	140	84	NA
Trough therapeutic plasma concentrations, mg/L) at dose of: 200 mg/day 100 mg/day	302 –	– 301	300 –	310 –
NA, not available				

Fig. 8.3 Selected pharmacokinetic parameters of amantadine and rimantadine in healthy young and old (>65 years) adults.

Amantadine doses of less than 100 mg/day cause no more adverse effects than placebo. The standard dose for young adults, 200 mg per day, causes mild, reversible central nervous system (CNS) adverse effects in 8–30% of subjects. Amantadine at 300 mg/day causes CNS adverse effects in about one-third of subjects, and 400 mg/day (twice the usual human dose) causes toxic effects in nearly all recipients. Amantadine cardiovascular adverse effects include livido reticularis in up to 90% of elderly patients.

Rimantadine is better tolerated than amantadine and tends to cause predominantly gastrointestinal (GI) adverse effects. Abdominal pain, nausea, vomiting and diarrhea occur in about 10% of rimantadine recipients.

INHIBITORS OF TRANSCRIPTION

Interferons

Interferons (IFNs) are a family of cytokines that evoke complex intracellular antiviral, antiproliferative, and immunomodulating effects. They are best known for their antiviral effect, which was first described in 1957 as the phenomenon of viral interference, that is, inhibition of the growth of a variety of viruses in cells by soluble mediators secreted by other infected cells of the same species. Three major classes of IFNs have been discovered which vary structurally, biologically and antigenically (Fig. 8.4).

IFNs are prepared by recombinant technology (rIFN-α, -β, and -γ) as well as by chemical synthesis (consensus IFN (CIFN)). rIFN-alpha consists of two species, 2a and 2b, that differ by a single amino acid. IFN-α and -β are the principal antiviral IFNs whereas IFN-γ is predominantly immunomodulatory. rIFN-α and rIFN-β are approved for treatment of chronic HBV, HCV, HPV and HHV-8 (Kaposi sarcoma) infections while rIFN-β is also efficacious for the therapy of multiple sclerosis. Being proteins, IFNs must be administered parenterally; for treatment of chronic HBV and HCV infection, subcutaneous self-administration three times weekly for 24 to 48 weeks is required.

Classification and characteristics of human interferons

Characteristics	Alpha (α)	Class Beta (β)	Gamma (γ)
Derivation	Leukocyte	Fibroblast	TH₁ lymphocyte
Number of species	> 23	1	1
Commercial formulation	rIFN-α-2b rIFN-α-2a C r met IFN-con 1	rIFN-β-1a rIFN-β-1b	IFN-γ

'r' indicates prepared by recombinant technology.
CIFN was developed by scanning the amino acid sequence of 11 natural IFN-α species and selecting the most frequently occurring amino acid at each of the corresponding positions.

Fig. 8.4 Classification and characteristics of human interferons.

Recently, IFN-α-2a modified by covalent attachment of a 40-kDa branched-chain polyethylene glycol moiety has yielded a slow-release formulation, administered by self-injection once weekly, that is more effective than IFN-2-alpha injected three times a week for treatment of chronic HCV infection with and without cirrhosis. This new agent is called pegylated-interferon, or PEG-IFN.

MECHANISM OF ACTION IFNs are rapidly synthesized and secreted by virus-infected cells as well as by cells stimulated by other pathogenic organisms, by cytokines (e.g. IL-I) and small molecules such as dsRNA. IFNs are not antiviral *per se* but rather stimulate a state of resistance to virus infection in uninfected cells. The state of resistance develops rapidly following binding of the IFN to cell surface receptors that are shared by IFN-α and IFN-β but differ for IFN-γ. IFN receptor binding activates Janus-activated kinases (JAK) that phosphorylate latent, constitutively expressed cytoplasmic proteins named signal transducers and activators of transcription (STATs); hence, the rapidity of the IFN-induced response. Phosphorylated STATs translocate to the nucleus and bind to cytokine response genes on chromosome 21 (IFN-α and IFN-β) or 6 (IFN-γ) and induce gene transcription. As a consequence, more than two dozen known proteins are synthesized that enhance cellular resistance by variably inhibiting entry, uncoating, transcription and/or protein synthesis of different viruses.

PHARMACOKINETICS The prolonged antiviral and other biological effects of IFNs are mediated by intracellular events and are not readily related to serum IFN concentrations or other conventional pharmacokinetic properties of these molecules. Following subcutaneous, intramuscular (i.m.) or intravenous (i.v.) injection, the bioavailability of IFN-α exceeds 80%. The bioavailability of IFN-β administered subcutaneously is only about 10% of that of rIFN-α because of slow diffusion through the lymphoid system and/or local catabolism by muscle lysosomal proteinases or tissue binding.

Systemic clearance is almost wholly due to renal elimination. The elimination half-life of IFN-α and -β is 2 to 4 h. Pegylation of IFN-α-2a slows absorption (T_{max} increased more than sevenfold), reduces systemic clearance and increases serum $t_{1/2}$ about 10-fold.

CLINICAL USES The following discussion is limited to studies of IFNs as antiviral agents. rIFN-α is efficacious after systemic administration for treatment of chronic HBV and HCV infections, for Kaposi sarcoma, caused by HHV-8, and, by intralesional injection, for therapy of condylomata acuminata (HPV skin infection). rIFN-β is efficacious for treatment of condylomata acuminata, by both systemic and intralesional injection, as well as for treatment of multiple sclerosis, although the biologic basis for the latter effect is unknown.

Many viruses are intrinsically resistant to IFNs. Higher doses of IFN are of limited value in overcoming resistance. Addition of ribavirin, however, augments the response of chronic HBV infection to IFN.

PEG-IFN 180 μg, subcutaneously once a week, is more

effective than IFN-α-2a, 6×10^6 units three times per week, for treatment of chronic HCV.

ADVERSE REACTIONS Studies in animals of human-derived IFNs are not generally informative since all IFNs are highly species-specific.

The adverse effects of IFNs result from their immuno-modulatory and antiproliferative effects. Such effects are common and generally mild and reversible, but can be severe, dose-limiting and not resolve for many months after discontinuation of therapy. Exogenous IFNs are antigenic and stimulate the development of circulating antibodies which can attenuate clinical responses to exogenous, but not necessarily to endogenous IFN.

Almost all patients treated with IFNs develop a flu-like syndrome characterized by fever (40 to 98%), fatigue or malaise (50 to 95%), myalgia (30 to 75%), chills (40 to 65%), headache (20 to 70%) and arthralgia (5 to 25%). These effects are probably mediated by stimulation of the synthesis of IL-I, the endogenous pyrogen, and other cytokines, may be prevented or attenuated by antipyretic analgesics, and diminish in severity after several weeks of therapy. However, fatigue may be profound, dose-limiting and even on cessation of therapy may last for months. Other major dose-limiting toxic effects of IFNs include myelosuppression causing neutropenia and thrombocytopenia in up to 70% of patients, and neurotoxicity (headache, irritability, anxiety, dizziness and neuropsychiatric disorders). Depression has been reported in up to 30% of patients and can be severe; delirium and psychosis may occur. Nausea, vomiting and diarrhea occur in up to 50% of patients. Anorexia and weight loss occurs in 25 to 65% of patients and can necessitate cessation of treatment. Hypo- and hypertension, chest pain and edema have been reported as well as cough, dyspnea and nasal congestion in up to one-third of patients. Proteinuria develops in up to 25% of patients. Serum creatinine increases in up to 10% of patients. Clinically important hyper- and hypothyroidism have been reported and are postulated to be due to induction of autoimmune thyroiditis or cross-reactivity of TSH with IFN receptors. Gynecomastia, loss of libido, abortion, skin rash and alopecia have been reported.

INHIBITION OF TRANSLATION

Fomivirsen

Fomivirsen is the first antisense therapy drug approved for clinical use in the USA. It is used to suppress cytomegalovirus (CMV) strains that are resistant to ganciclovir (GCV), cidofovir (CDV) and foscarnet.

CHEMISTRY Fomivirsen is a 21-nucleotide phosphorothioate antisense molecule that binds to complementary CMV mRNA transcripts which encode proteins that regulate immediate-early gene expression. Fomivirsen inhibits CMV replication by blocking translation.

PHARMACOKINETICS Fomivirsen is administered by intravitreal injection. Details of its pharmacokinetics in the eye are incomplete but it is catabolized over 7 to 10 days by exonucleases.

CLINICAL USES Fomivirsen is approved for the intravitreal treatment of CMV retinitis in AIDS patients who are intolerant of, not responsive to, or have contraindications to, other treatments.

ADVERSE EFFECTS Iritis, vitritis and increased ocular pressure have been reported in up to one-quarter of patients. Although fomivirsen is indicated for patients who have not responded to, or, are intolerant of cidofovir, there might be an increased risk of ocular inflammation in such patients.

Data on the oncogenicity and carcinogenicity of fomivirsen are not available.

INHIBITION OF RNA OR DNA GENOMIC REPLICATION

Acyclovir

Acyclovir (ACV) is the prototype for a family of synthetic nucleoside analogs widely used to prevent and treat infections caused by herpes simplex virus type 1 (HSV-1) and type 2 (HSV-2), varicella zoster virus (VZV) and cytomegalovirus (CMV). For her work in the discovery and development of ACV, Dr Gertrude Elion shared the Nobel Prize for Physiology and Medicine in 1988.

CHEMISTRY In addition to ACV, the other currently available members of this family include valacyclovir (VCV), penciclovir (PCV), famciclovir (FCV), ganciclovir (GCV) and cidofovir (CDV) (Fig. 8.5). They are all acyclic analogs of nucleosides and undergo intracellular phosphorylation to the active triphosphate nucleotide moiety. ACV-, PCV-, and GCV-triphosphate (TP) inhibit herpesvirus replication by competing with deoxyguanosine triphosphate (dGTP) for the viral DNA polymerase, while cidofovir-TP acts as a deoxycytidine TP (dCTP) substitute. In addition, they all interfere with viral DNA replication after incorporation into the elongating herpesvirus DNA chain by causing DNA chain termination. This occurs because absence of the 3'C and its OH group on the acyclic ribose molecule precludes formation of the 3'-5'-phosphodiester linkage needed to allow addition of the next nucleotide (Fig. 8.6).

ACV, VCV, PCV and FCV are discussed together because of their use primarily in patients with HSV and VZV infections. GCV and cidofovir are considered together because of their utility primarily for management of patients with CMV infection.

MECHANISM OF ACTION ACV is a potent and selective inhibitor of herpesvirus DNA replication. The antiviral action of ACV is

---

Pharmacologic bases for the selective inhibition of herpesvirus replication by acyclovir

- Selective concentration or trapping in infected cells due to avid phosphorylation by herpesvirus thymidine kinase
- Preferential affinity of acyclovir triphosphate for viral rather than cellular DNA polymerase

95

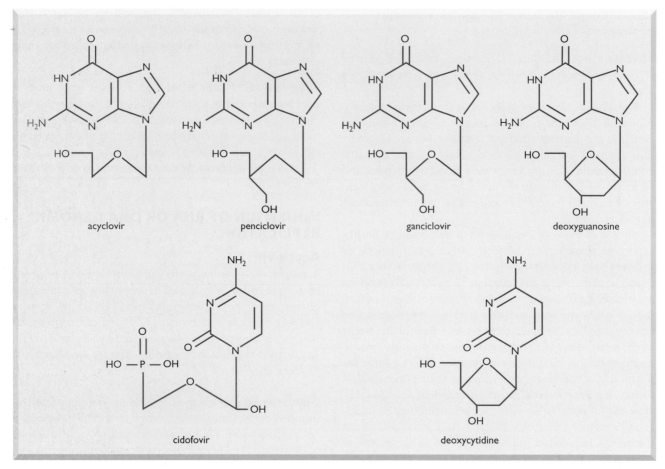

Fig. 8.5 Structures of deoxyguanosine and deoxycytidine analog inhibitors of herpesvirus DNA replication.

mediated by ACV-TP (Fig. 8.7). ACV-TP inhibits three steps in the replicative cycle: first, ACV-TP competitively inhibits viral DNA polymerase utilization of GTP; second, ACV-TP terminates elongation of the HSV DNA strand when incorporated as a guanosine analog substitute (Fig. 8.6). Third, viral DNA polymerase is inactivated by binding to ACV-TP on the DNA primer template. The DNA polymerases of CMV and EBV are less sensitive to the inhibitory effect of ACV-TP than those of HSV and VZV, accounting in part for the relative inefficacy of ACV for treatment of CMV and EBV infection. The selective effects of ACV on viral replication with minimal effects on host cell DNA replication are due to two factors: first, it is selectively concentrated in virus-infected cells due to the catalytic action of the virus-encoded thymidine kinase (TK) enzyme, and second, the active antiviral molecule, ACV-TP, has a higher affinity for HSV than cellular DNA polymerase, resulting in selective inhibition of the viral enzyme.

> **Mechanisms of action of the antiviral effect of acyclovir triphosphate**
>
> - Competitive inhibition of herpesvirus DNA polymerase
> - Viral DNA chain termination
> - Noncompetitive inhibition of herpesvirus DNA polymerase

PHARMACOKINETICS ACV is marketed as topical 5% cream and ointment, oral tablets and suspension, and intravenous formulations.

ACV is incompletely and slowly absorbed from the gastrointestinal tract (Fig. 8.8). Relative bioavailability is 13–21% of a 200 mg dose and declines with increasing doses. After intravenous injection, the pharmacokinetic characteristics of ACV are independent of dose and best fit a two-compartment open model. Elimination from plasma is a first order process.

ACV is widely distributed in the body so that herpesvirus infections in any organ can be effectively treated by oral or intravenous administration. It also crosses the placenta at all stages of pregnancy and is secreted into breast milk.

Approximately 80% of ACV is excreted unchanged in the urine. ACV renal clearance exceeds creatinine clearance, indicating that ACV is both excreted by glomerular filtration and renal tubular secretion. In anuric patients, clearance is reduced to approximately 30 ml/min/1.73m², and the elimination half-time increases to 20 hours. Oxidation yields the predominant metabolite, 9-(carboxymethoxy) methyl guanine. Less than 15% of ACV is normally cleared by this route. Dose reduction is recommended when creatinine clearance is less than 50 ml/min. Hemodialysis reduces ACV plasma concentration by 60% so that a supplemental dose of 50% of the standard dose is recommended after each hemodialysis treatment. Peritoneal dialysis is much less efficient in removing

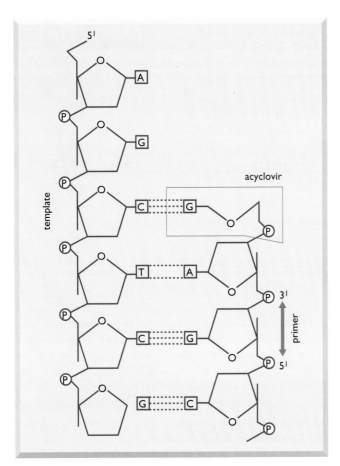

Fig. 8.6 Representation of acyclovir triphosphate termination of DNA chain elongation. Absence of the 3'-C molecule on the acyclic ribose molecule precludes formation of the 3'-5'-phosphodiester linkage needed to allow DNA chain elongation. (Adapted from Elion GB. Mechanism of action and selectivity of acyclovir. *Am J Med* 1982; Acyclovir Symposium: 7–13, with permission from Excerpta Medica Inc.)

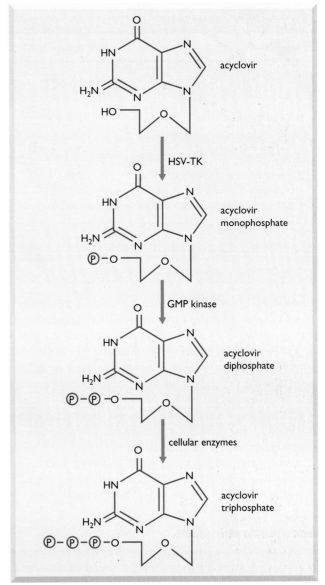

Fig. 8.7 Enzymatic conversion of acyclovir to its mono-, di-, and triphosphate forms. Herpes simplex virus thymidine kinase (HSV-TK) avidly catalyzes the formation of acyclovir monophosphate. Cellular kinases convert the monophosphate to the di- and triphosphate forms. Acyclovir triphosphate is the active antiviral moiety. (Adapted from Elion GB. Mechanism of action and selectivity of acyclovir. *Am J Med* 1982; Acyclovir Symposium: 7–13, with permission from Excerpta Medica Inc.)

ACV so that no dose supplementation is needed for such patients. No dose reduction is required for patients with hepatic disease.

Little ACV is absorbed into the systemic circulation after topical application of the cream and ointment formulations. ACV penetration into the deeper layers of the epidermis, where HSV replicates to cause recurrent cold sore and genital herpes, is poor, but greater for the cream than the ointment preparations. Poor epidermal penetration accounts for part of the relative ineffectiveness of topical ACV for treatment of recurrent cold sore and genital HSV infection.

CLINICAL USES ACV inhibits the replication of HSV, VZV, CMV and EBV in infected cells but has no effect on latent infection. ACV is used for prophylaxis and treatment of a wide range of HSV and VZV infections in both immunocompetent and immunocompromised patients. ACV is more effective than placebo in immunocompetent subjects with HSV genital, orolabial, corneal, hand (whitlow) infection, encephalitis and neonatal infection. HSV encephalitis and neonatal HSV infection are treated intravenously. ACV is efficacious in patients with chickenpox and herpes zoster. ACV decreases recurrence of

orolabial and genital HSV infection in immunocompetent individuals.

In immunocompromised patients, ACV is effective for treatment of mucocutaneous (orolabial and anogenital) HSV infection as well as herpes zoster.

ACV-resistant HSV and VZV strains of virus can develop but usually only after prolonged use of ACV and in immuno-compromised patients. Resistance arises largely through the selection of strains that do not synthesize thymidine kinase (thymidine kinase-negative; TK⁻). Occasionally, strains emerge whose resistance is due to reduced affinity for TK or reduced

97

Pharmacokinetic parameters of oral acyclovir, valacyclovir, penciclovir and famciclovir

Parameter	Acyclovir	Valacyclovir	Penciclovir	Famciclovir
Bioavailability	13–21%	54%	5%	77%
Vd_{ss}, L/1.73 m²	47	47	112	112
Renal clearance, ml/min/1.73 m²	250–280	250–280	415–530	415–530
Half-life, mean (range), hours	3.0 (1.5–6.3)	3.0 (1.5–6.3)	(2.2–2.3)	(2.2–2.3)
Urinary excretion of unchanged drug	80%	80%	50–60%	50–60%

Fig. 8.8 Selected pharmacokinetic parameters of oral acyclovir, valacyclovir, penciclovir and famciclovir.

affinity for viral DNA polymerase. Infections caused by ACV-resistant strains respond to intravenous foscarnet.

ADVERSE REACTIONS ACV is remarkably well tolerated and safe. Rapid intravenous administration of ACV can cause a rise in creatinine due to renal tubular lumen obstruction by ACV crystals. Accordingly, it must be administered over no less than 60 min. The other dose-related adverse effect of ACV is neurotoxicity (lethargy, confusion, tremor, hallucinations, delirium, seizures and coma), particularly in patients with renal insufficiency receiving standard doses of ACV intravenously. Nephrotoxic and neurologic side effects are reversible on discontinuation of ACV therapy. Hemodialysis might be useful in severe cases. Extravasation of ACV during intravenous administration can cause cellulitis and blistering, probably related to the alkaline pH (9–10) of the solution.

Adenine arabinoside

Adenine arabinoside (ara-A), a nucleoside analog, was the first antiviral drug safe enough to allow parenteral administration (for treatment of HSV and VZV infections). Due to its poor aqueous solubility and the attendant need for large volumes of intravenous fluid and relative inefficacy, it has been supplanted by acyclovir. However, it continues to be used as a safe and effective topical treatment for HSV keratitis.

CHEMISTRY AND MOLECULAR MECHANISM OF ACTION Ara-A is an analog of adenosine that is metabolized by cellular kinases to its antiviral triphosphate nucleotide. Ara-A-TP inhibits viral DNA polymerase preferentially and is incorporated into both elongating cellular and viral DNA strands, resulting in chain termination. The antiviral effect is augmented further by its hypoxanthine metabolite, which acts synergistically with the parent molecule. HSV TK⁻ strains resistant to acyclovir are sensitive in vitro to ara-A.

PHARMACOKINETICS Little ara-A is absorbed systemically from the 3% ara-A ointment applied to the eye. During intravenous infusion, ara-A is rapidly converted to ara-hypoxanthine by adenosine deaminase. As a result, only the metabolite is measurable in plasma. The serum half-life is 3–4 h; 50% of a dose of ara-A is recovered in urine as hypoxanthine arabinoside and a very small amount as parent drug.

CLINICAL USES Intravenous ara-A has been generally replaced by ACV because of the large volumes of fluid required for ara-A administration intravenously and their therapeutic equivalence.

For HSV keratitis, topical ara-A is as effective as tri-fluorothymidine and better than idoxuridine.

ADVERSE EFFECTS Topical ara-A 3.0% ophthalmic ointment is less toxic than topical idoxuridine.

Intravenous ara-A causes a range of neurotoxic but reversible symptoms including hallucinations, ataxia, tremor; IFN administered concomitantly may intensify these adverse effects.

Ara-A is mutagenic and carcinogenic in vitro.

Cidofovir

Cidofovir (CDV) is an acyclic phosphonate analog of cytidine. It exhibits broad spectrum inhibitory activity against all human herpesviruses and several other DNA viruses. These include HSV-1 and -2, VZV, CMV, EBV, HHV-6, -7 and -8, and human papilloma (HPV) and polyoma and adenoviruses. CDV is approved for intravenous therapy of CMV retinitis in AIDS patients.

CHEMISTRY Inside virus-infected and uninfected cells, CDV is phosphorylated to mono- and di-phosphate nucleotides by cellular kinases. Accordingly, phosphorylated CDV metabolite concentrations in infected and uninfected cells are similar. Since CDV itself is a phosphonate, CDV-DP functions as a TP antiviral molecule. CDV-DP has a prolonged intracellular half-life of 13 to 65 hours. A metabolite, CDV-phosphate-choline, has a half-life of 87 hours and may serve as an intracellular reservoir for CDV-DT.

MECHANISM OF ACTION CDV-DP inhibits viral DNA synthesis by both inhibiting viral DNA polymerase and acting as an alternate substrate for it in competition with the natural substrate, dCTP. Incorporation of CDV-DP into the growing viral DNA chain reduces the rate of viral DNA synthesis; incorporation of two consecutive CDV-DP terminates chain elongation.

PHARMACOKINETICS The oral bioavailability of CDV is less than 5%. CDV injected intravenously has a terminal half-time of about 2–3 hours. The drug distributes widely throughout the body, although penetration into CSF and the eye has not been well characterized. Elimination is via the kidney by both glomerular filtration and renal tubular epithelial cell secretion.

CLINICAL USES CDV administered intravenously once a week for 2 weeks with probenecid and concomitant intravenous saline hydration prevents CMV retinitis progression in AIDS patients. The therapeutic effect is comparable to that observed with intravenous GCV.

Topical CDV may have potential utility for treatment of HPV skin infection, while intralesional CDV has shown promise for treatment of laryngeal and respiratory papillomatosis. In vitro studies indicate that CDV inhibits replication of papovavirus infection. Thus, intravenous CDV may have potential value for treatment of progressive multifocal leucoencephalopathy, a progressive, fatal opportunistic infection in immunocompromised individuals, particularly those with advanced HIV.

ADVERSE REACTIONS CDV is mutagenic, embryotoxic, gonado-toxic, teratogenic and carcinogenic in animals. In several species, intravenous CDV causes dose-dependent nephro-toxicity, which is the principal dose-limiting effect of the drug. Proximal convoluted renal tubular epithelial cell necrosis can be prevented by concurrent probenecid administration and is at least partially reversible on drug discontinuation.

Increased serum creatinine has been observed in 10% of intravenous CDV recipients and proteinuria in 45%. Ocular hypotony occurred in 12% of treated patients and anterior uveitis or iritis in 7%. Neutropenia occurred in 25%.

The nephrotoxic effects of intravenous CDV can be intensified by concomitant administration of other potentially nephrotoxic drugs. Therefore, the following agents should be avoided during intravenous CDV therapy: aminoglycoside antibiotics, pentamidine, amphotericin B, foscarnet, nonsteroidal anti-inflammatory drugs and ionic, hypertonic radiographic contrast dye.

Famciclovir and penciclovir

Famciclovir (FCV), which has no antiviral activity, is the pro-drug of penciclovir (PCV), a potent and selective inhibitor of herpesviruses comparable in vitro, and, clinically, to ACV.

MOLECULAR MECHANISM OF ACTION PCV, like ACV, must undergo phosphorylation to PCV-TP, the antiviral molecule. As in the case of ACV in herpesvirus-infected cells, the initial monophosphorylation of PCV is catalyzed by herpesvirus TK. PCV-TP acts as an alternate substrate for dGTP in the synthesis of viral DNA by viral DNA polymerase. Whereas incorporation of ACV-TP immediately causes chain termination, incorporation of PCV-TP allows some limited incorporation (3 PCV-TP) before chain elongation is arrested. PCV-TP acts as a potent inhibitor of HBV polymerase-reverse transcriptase.

PHARMACOKINETICS FCV is administered as oral tablets and PCV, as a topical cream. Only 5% of orally administered PCV is

absorbed, whereas the oral bioavailability of PCV from FCV is 77%.

Elimination from plasma is a first order process with a mean plasma half-life of 2 h in persons with normal renal function. PCV is 75% excreted into urine and 25% into feces.

In patients with renal dysfunction, PCV clearance is reduced in direct proportion to the reduction in renal function. In patients with creatinine clearance of 7 to 39 ml/min, the PCV elimination mean half-life is 10 h. It is recommended that the dose be progressively decreased in patients with renal insufficiency.

CLINICAL USES FCV is licensed for the treatment of first episode and recurrent genital HSV infection and herpes zoster in immunocompetent and immunocompromised adult patients. Topical 4% PCV cream minimally reduces the duration of recurrent orolabial HSV infection and shortens healing time compared with placebo.

FCV reduces HBV DNA and transaminase levels in patients with chronic HBV infection and appears to be more effective when combined with interferon for such patients. PCV-resistant HBV variants have been demonstrated in liver transplant patients receiving chronic FCV therapy. Resistance is due to altered DNA polymerase.

Foscarnet

Foscarnet is trisodium phosphonoformate, a pyrophosphate analog. Foscarnet inhibits the replication of HSV, VZV, CMV, EBV, and HHV-6 and -8, as well as HIV and HBV, but clinical use is limited to CMV and some HSV infections.

MECHANISM OF ACTION Foscarnet directly inhibits viral DNA polymerase and HIV reverse transcriptase. Unlike nucleoside antiviral drugs, foscarnet does not undergo intracellular metabolism. Foscarnet binds to and blocks the pyrophosphate binding site of viral polymerase, thereby inhibiting cleavage of pyrophosphate from deoxyribonucleotide-TP and blocking viral DNA synthesis.

PHARMACOKINETICS Oral bioavailability averages about 10%, too low to permit oral therapy. After intravenous infusion, foscarnet plasma concentration declines triexponentially as first order processes with successive half-lifes of 0.5, 3 and

---

 Properties of foscarnet, the only available non-nucleoside herpesvirus inhibitor drug

- Antiviral effect does not require intracellular metabolism
- Directly inhibits herpesvirus DNA polymerase
- Particularly valuable for treating nucleoside-resistant herpes simplex virus, varicella zoster virus, and cytomegalovirus infection
- Requires intravenous administration
- Causes reversible, but serious, multiple organ toxicity

18 hours. The drug is widely distributed throughout the body so that intravenous foscarnet is effective therapy for infection of all organs caused by susceptible viruses.

Doses must be reduced progressively with increasing degrees of renal dysfunction, beginning with even minor reductions in creatinine clearance. Foscarnet is not metabolized. No dose adjustment in the presence of liver disease is deemed to be necessary.

CLINICAL USES Intravenous foscarnet is approved for treatment of CMV retinitis in AIDS patients and acyclovir-resistant mucocutaneous HSV infections. Compared with intravenous GCV for treatment of CMV retinitis in AIDS patients, foscarnet controls retinitis but also increases survival, presumably due to an antiretroviral effect.

Foscarnet appears to be effective for treatment of GCV-resistant CMV infection plus other CMV infections in HIV patients, particularly gastrointestinal, pulmonary, central nervous system and radicular neurologic infections. Foscarnet may be effective for prevention of CMV disease in bone marrow transplant recipients but established CMV pneumonia in these patients is unresponsive.

Resistance to foscarnet, demonstrable *in vitro*, occurs uncommonly during treatment but is associated with clinical treatment failure. Resistance is associated with point mutations in the DNA polymerase in herpesviruses and the reverse transcriptase of HIV. Foscarnet-resistant CMV infections may respond to GCV or cidofovir therapy.

ADVERSE REACTIONS Nephrotoxicity, manifest as proteinuria, rising serum creatinine and, occasionally, acute tubular necrosis, is the principal dose-limiting adverse effect of intravenous foscarnet therapy. Approximately one-third of patients exhibit increases in serum creatinine. The incidence of acute renal failure has declined recently, because of attention to adequate hydration, dose reduction effected promptly in the face of rising serum creatinine concentration, and avoidance of concomitant nephrotoxic drugs.

Metabolic perturbations are common. Hypo- and hypercalcemia and hypo- and hyperphosphatemia attributed to chelation to foscarnet deposited in bone, plus hypomagnesia, are reported in 10 to 44% of patients and necessitate a low rate of drug administration. Hypocalcemia may cause paresthesias, tetany and seizures.

CNS adverse effects including headache, irritability and hallucinations occur in up to 10% of subjects. Gastrointestinal adverse effects such as nausea, vomiting and diarrhea are reported in 30 to 50% of patients. Painful subpreputial ulcers attributed to deposition of urine with foscarnet in high concentration in this area have been described in up to 10% of male patients. Anemia in 20 to 50% of AIDS patients and granulocytopenia are attributed to myelosuppression.

Ganciclovir

Ganciclovir (GCV) is an analog of ACV which is equally potent as an inhibitor of HSV, VZV and EBV *in vitro*. However, it is 10- to 100-fold more active than ACV in inhibiting CMV replication *in vitro*. GCV is the first antiviral drug with demonstrated efficacy in CMV disease.

MOLECULAR MECHANISM OF ACTION GCV as GCV-TP inhibits viral DNA synthesis. Phosphorylation of GCV within herpesvirus-infected cells is initiated by viral kinases. In HSV- and VZV-infected cells, viral TK catalyzes the initial monophosphorylation step. CMV does not possess a TK enzyme. However, a kinase encoded on the UL97 region of the CMV genome subserves this kinase function. Conversion of GCV-MP to -DP and -TP is catalyzed by cellular kinases. In uninfected cells, cellular kinases appear to convert GCV to its -TP nucleotide metabolite.

GCV-TP is a competitive inhibitor of dGTP incorporation into DNA. It preferentially inhibits viral more than host cell DNA polymerase. Incorporation of GCV-TP into viral DNA does not result in obligate chain termination as occurs with ACV-TP incorporation. Rather, short subgenomic CMV DNA fragments are synthesized which cannot be packaged into virions. Incorporation of GCV-TP into host cell DNA results in radiomimetic adverse effects on bone marrow, gastrointestinal mucosa and spermatogenesis.

PHARMACOKINETICS GCV is available as a parenteral formulation for intravenous injection, capsules for oral administration and as a slow-release system for intraocular implantation. Recently, a valine ester oral pro-drug of GCV, valganciclovir, has been developed.

GCV administered orally is poorly bioavailable. Elimination from plasma is a first order process. GCV distributes widely throughout the body so that intravenous therapy can be used to treat CMV disease in any organ. Almost 100% of an administered dose is excreted as unchanged drug in the urine. The plasma half-time in patients with normal renal function is 2 to 4 hours; it increases in direct proportion to declining renal function.

GCV is 60% bioavailable from valganciclovir. GCV is marketed as capsules for oral administration. Bioavailability from capsules ranges from 3 to 7%; food increases absorption by 20%. Intravitreal GCV implants release drug at a rate of approximately 1 μg per hour over 5 to 8 months. They are efficacious for suppression of CMV retinitis in AIDS patients but do not prevent CMV disease in the other eye or extraocular CMV disease.

CLINICAL USES GCV is indicated for the treatment and prevention of CMV diseases in immunocompromised patients. These include retinitis in AIDS patients, AIDS-related gastrointestinal and other organ disease and CMV disease in transplant recipients. In immunocompromised transplant patients, CMV primary infection and reactivation of latent infection cause morbidity and mortality and the use of GCV in such patients is warranted. Intravenous GCV reduces the risk of CMV disease in CMV seronegative recipients of heart, liver and lung transplants from CMV seropositive donors.

It is probable that valganciclovir will replace oral and, perhaps, intravenous GCV for some indications.

ADVERSE REACTIONS The vast majority of GCV adverse effects are dose-related. Myelosuppression is the principal dose-related side effect of intravenous GCV therapy with neutropenia observed in about 40% and thrombocytopenia in 15 to 20% of treated AIDS patients. These effects are usually reversible within 1 to 2 weeks of discontinuing therapy. Gonadal toxicity, based on preclinical toxicologic studies, is expected after intravenous GCV therapy in both genders but no clear evidence confirming this expectation is currently available. Renal impairment due to obstruction of renal tubules by crystallization of GCV has been reported in 20% of bone marrow transplant patients given intravenous GCV for 4 months. Confusion, abnormal mentation and seizures rarely have been reported. Oral GCV 1000 mg t.i.d. causes diarrhea, nausea and vomiting in 3 to 13% of recipients compared with 0 to 7% of recipients of intravenous GCV.

RESISTANCE GCV resistance associated with CMV treatment failure and in vitro resistance occurs in 8% of CMV isolates from AIDS patients after 3 or more months of continuous therapy. Resistance is mostly due to point mutations in the genome of the UL97 gene and less commonly to point mutations in viral DNA polymerase.

Most resistant isolates retain susceptibility to foscarnet and cidofovir.

Idoxuridine

Idoxuridine (IDU) is 5-iodo-2′-deoxyuridine. Its topical use in treatment of HSV keratitis in 1962 marked the first demonstration of the efficacy of a drug for treatment of a viral infection.

CHEMISTRY AND MOLECULAR MECHANISM OF ACTION IDU is an analog of thymidine. It resembles acyclovir in being preferentially converted to a monophosphate nucleotide by viral TK with subsequent synthesis of di- and triphosphate nucleotides by cellular kinases. ID-TP is incorporated into both viral and mammalian DNA.

Such DNA is more susceptible to breakage and altered viral proteins may result from faulty transcription, resulting in inhibition of viral replication and adverse effects on rapidly proliferating mammalian cells. It also inhibits DNA polymerase but does not cause chain termination.

Resistance of HSV to IDU develops readily in vitro as well as in patients. Resistance is due to the same mechanisms as mediate acyclovir resistance in HSV.

PHARMACOKINETICS Little IDU is absorbed after topical administration so no systemic effects are observed. Any IDU absorbed is metabolized to 5-iodouracil, uracil and iodide which are devoid of antiviral activity.

CLINICAL USES IDU 0.1% ophthalmic solution is administered as one drop onto the cornea every hour during the day and every 2 h at night. Frequency of administration is halved once definite improvement is observed on fluoroscein staining.

Treatment is continued to a maximum of 21 days to minimize corneal epithelial dystrophy.

ADVERSE EFFECTS Inflammation of the tissues of the eye due to cytotoxic effects of IDU or to allergic reactions can occur. Burning upon instillation and, punctate keratitis, eyelid edema and irritation occur in 2 to 10% of patients.

Ribavirin

Ribavirin is a guanosine analog with inhibitory activity against several RNA and DNA viruses. It is approved for the aerosol treatment of severe RSV infection in neonates and infants with associated pulmonary, cardiac and immune deficiency disorders. Oral ribavirin combined with interferon therapy has recently been approved for treatment of chronic HCV infection. Intravenous ribavirin reduced the mortality rate in patients with severe Lassa virus infection from 76% to 32%.

MECHANISM OF ACTION Ribavirin is taken up by infected and uninfected cells and phosphorylated by cellular kinases to mono-, di- and triphosphate nucleotides. Ribavirin-MP is a potent inhibitor of inosine monophosphate dehydrogenase. The resulting inhibition blocks synthesis of dGTP and therefore nucleic acid synthesis. Ribavirin-TP can inhibit RNA polymerase of influenza viruses and inhibit dGTP-dependent 5′-capping of mRNA as well. Additional mechanisms of action probably operate so that ribavirin in vitro inhibits a variety of RNA viruses (ortho- and paramyxo-, arena-, bunya-, RNA tumor, and retroviruses) as well as some DNA viruses (herpes, adeno-, and pox viruses).

PHARMACOKINETICS Ribavirin is effective for treatment of a limited number of viral infections when administered intravenously, by mouth and by inhalation as an aerosol.

Oral biovailability of ribavirin averages 45%. Absorption of ribavirin administered as aerosol depends on the concentration and duration of exposure and particle size. For lower respiratory tract infection, a special generator is required to produce particles 1 to 5 microns in diameter that are suspended and do not settle on the walls of the tracheobronchial tree. Such aerosols deliver 70% of inhaled drug to the lungs.

After intravenous injection, the ribavirin plasma concentration declines in at least three phases with successive half-lifes of 2, 18–36 and 22–64 hours. The apparent volume of distribution at steady state, 647 liter (range 378–1138 liter), is extremely large and appears to be due to sequestration in erythrocytes (where ribavirin concentration is ninefold greater than in plasma) and perhaps other cells. Ribavirin is eliminated by both hepatic metabolism (65%) and renal excretion (35%). Only 4% of drug is excreted unchanged in urine.

CLINICAL USES Ribavirin delivered by aerosol to neonates and infants with RSV lower respiratory infection complicating bronchopulmonary, cardiac or immunodeficiency diseases, shortens the duration of pulmonary RSV shedding and improves selected clinical parameters.

101

Oral ribavirin in patients with chronic HCV infection does not reduce serum HCV RNA concentration but reversibly reduces fatigue, serum transaminase levels and hepatic inflammation by an unknown mechanism. Concomitant therapy with IFN-α significantly increases the clinical and virologic response rate in such patients so that combined ribavirin–IFN-α is currently the standard treatment for chronic HCV infection.

Ribavirin intravenously or by mouth reduces mortality in patients with Lassa fever. Intravenous ribavirin reduces mortality and the risk of renal failure in patients with hemorrhagic fever with renal syndrome. The efficacy and safety of intravenous ribavirin for treatment of hantavirus pulmonary syndrome is under investigation. It is not useful in HIV infections.

ADVERSE EFFECTS Ribavirin accumulation in erythrocytes, which are poor in triphosphatases, is associated with a shortened erythrocyte lifespan and mild to moderate anemia due to extravascular hemolysis. Hemoglobin falls 20 to 30 g per liter; rarely transfusions and interruption of therapy are required. Aerosolized ribavirin can cause mild conjunctival irritation. Bronchospasm is uncommon even in asthmatics, but airway narrowing due to precipitation of ribavirin on the tracheobronchial mucosa may occur. Anemia is not observed with aerosol therapy.

Ribavirin is not mutagenic in bacteria but may be carcinogenic, embryotoxic and gonadotoxic in animals. Accordingly, ribavirin use is relatively contraindicated for treatment of infection in pregnant patients. Pregnant personnel should not be involved in ribavirin aerosol administration.

Sorivudine

Sorivudine is a pyrimidine nucleoside analog that can inhibit VZV in vitro at concentrations more than 1000-fold lower than those required with acyclovir. It is equivalent to acyclovir against HSV-1 but inactive against CMV and HSV-2, the latter being due to the lack of affinity of HSV-2 thymidine kinase for sorivudine.

MECHANISM OF ACTION Sorivudine is converted to its active triphosphate form by sequential phosphorylation, which is initially mediated by viral thymidine kinase. Sorivudine triphosphate competitively inhibits viral DNA polymerase but is not incorporated into viral DNA.

PHARMACOKINETICS Sorivudine oral bioavailability is approximately 75%. Most of the drug is eliminated unchanged into the urine.

CLINICAL USES Studies have demonstrated the efficacy of sorivudine in healthy adults with chickenpox and HIV-1-infected adults with shingles. Sorivudine is licensed for VZV infections.

ADVERSE EFFECTS Tolerance to sorivudine is good: mild nausea, vomiting and diarrhea, and occasional elevations in hepatic enzymes are observed. Fatal myelosuppression occurred in patients treated concurrently with sorivudine and 5-fluorouracil, probably due to sorivudine inhibition of the metabolism of 5-fluorouracil, which then accumulated to marked myelotoxic levels.

Trifluorothymidine

Trifluorothymidine (trifluridine or TFT) is a fluorinated analog of thymidine that is approved for topical treatment of HSV keratitis.

CHEMISTRY AND MOLECULAR MECHANISM OF ACTION Structurally, TFT differs from IDU in that the iodine atom is replaced by a methyl radical possessing three fluorine atoms. TFT is converted by cellular thymidine kinase to the antiviral metabolite, TFT-TP, that is incorporated into both HSV and mammalian cell DNA, as is IDU-TP, with similar antiviral and cytotoxic effects.

PHARMACOKINETICS TFT enters corneal epithelial cells (like IDU) by diffusion. Little TFT is absorbed systemically after topical administration to the eye.

TFT is hydrolyzed to 5-carboxy-2′-deoxyuridine, which has no antiviral activity.

CLINICAL USES A 1.0% ophthalmic solution is 80 to 95% effective in HSV keratitis, compared with 75 to 80% for IDU.

ADVERSE EFFECTS See IDU. TFT administered systemically is mutagenic and teratogenic in animals.

Valacyclovir

Valacyclovir (VCV) is the L-valyl ester of ACV with oral bioavailability three- to fourfold greater than that of ACV, independent of dose. It was licensed 12 years after ACV.

CHEMISTRY During absorption, VCV undergoes extensive and rapid first-pass metabolism to ACV and L-valine. VCV hydrolysis is mediated by hepatic and possibly intestinal mitochondrial VCV hydrolase.

PHARMACOKINETICS Only an oral tablet formulation of VCV is marketed. Bioavailability is about 50% of an oral dose and is not affected by food. The ACV plasma concentration over 24 h after a single oral VCV dose of 1000 mg is similar to that after intravenous ACV doses of 5 mg/kg q8 h.

The pharmacokinetic characteristics of ACV from VCV are identical to those of ACV itself (Fig. 8.8).

CLINICAL USES The enhanced oral bioavailability of ACV produced from VCV has permitted development of regimens that are more effective and more convenient than those using ACV. For example, in immunocompetent adults, VCV 1 g t.i.d. was more effective than ACV 800 mg five times per day in herpes zoster, as measured by zoster-associated pain or post-herpetic neuralgia. It is also approved for once-daily suppression of frequently recurring genital herpes, whereas ACV must be ingested at least twice daily.

ADVERSE REACTIONS In patients with advanced HIV infection treated with VCV, thrombotic microangiopathy developed in some recipients whereas none was observed in those receiving ACV.

INHIBITORS OF VIRUS RELEASE

Zanamivir and oseltamivir carboxylate (hereafter, oseltamivir) are sialic acid analog inhibitors of influenza neuraminidase that were recently licensed for the prevention and treatment of influenza A and B infection. Their licensure capped five decades of study that began in 1945 with the discovery of enzymatic activity on the surface of influenza viruses that removed virus receptors from the surface of erythrocytes. That enzyme, and, those receptors, are now known as neuraminidase and sialic acid, respectively. The design of potent and selective inhibitors of neuraminidase quickly followed delineation of its crystal structure in 1983.

CHEMISTRY Zanamivir and oseltamivir are potent, selective, competitive inhibitors of influenza virus neuraminidase. Other viral and mammalian neuraminidases require 80,000 to 1,000,000 times greater concentration for inhibition. The enzymatic pocket of influenza neuraminidase is highly conserved among influenza A and B viruses and both drugs inhibit all known subtypes of influenza A virus as well as influenza B. Neither drug is toxic to cells in culture (>10 mM).

MECHANISM OF ACTION Zanamivir and oseltamivir interfere with influenza A and B virus replication by inhibiting viral neuraminidase. Neuraminidase catalyzes the cleavage of the β-ketosidic bond linking a terminal neuraminic acid residue to the adjacent oligosaccharide moiety of sialic acid. Neuraminidase activity is essential for release of daughter virions from infected cells by cleaving terminal sialic acid residues from the cell membrane envelope on the budding virion. Neuraminidase inhibition causes aggregation and clumping of virions at the cell surface resulting from binding of hemagglutinin (protruding from the lipid envelope of virions) to persisting sialic acid residues on adjacent virions.

PHARMACOKINETICS Zanamivir oral biovailability is <5% so that for clinical use, it must be delivered to the target organ, the ciliated columnar epithelial cells of the tracheobronchial tree by oral inhalation as a micronized powder. Of inhaled zanamivir, 80% is deposited in the oropharynx and 10 to 15%, uniformly, in the lungs; 15 to 20% of inhaled drug is absorbed. Zanamivir persists in the lower respiratory tract for up to 24 h. This probably explains the efficacy of orally inhaled zanamivir as twice daily doses for therapy and once daily doses for prophylaxis.

Oral oseltamivir phosphate is readily absorbed from the intestine and is converted by hepatic esterases to oseltamivir. At least 75% of an oral dose reaches the systemic circulation as oseltamivir. Less than 5% of an oral dose of oseltamivir phosphate is recovered in urine as unchanged drug. Elimination of zanamivir and oseltamivir are first order processes with similar plasma elimination half-lifes of 1.5 to 1.8 hours.

Excluding the nervous system, oseltamivir distributes widely throughout the body including sites in the respiratory tract such as the middle ear where influenza viruses may replicate.

In patients with creatinine clearance less 30 ml/min, oseltamivir doses should be halved even though the drug has little toxic potential. Zanamivir absorption after oral inhalation is so minor that renal function need not be considered during its administration.

CLINICAL USES Both zanamivir and oseltamivir appear to be comparably effective in accelerating resolution of influenza symptoms. Both reduce the duration and severity of illness by about 25 to 35% compared with placebo when therapy is initiated within 2 days of onset of symptoms.

Both drugs are 75 to 80% effective for preventing influenza illness compared with placebo. For both prophylaxis and therapy, there are substantial data from studies in healthy adults ill with influenza A virus infection, but fewer data exist on the efficacy of these agents in subjects infected with influenza B virus, or in unhealthy patients, such as those with advanced age, or chronic cardiopulmonary, metabolic or renal disease.

Resistance to both zanamivir and oseltamivir is due to alterations in the hemagglutinin or in the neuraminidase. The former results in amino acid substitutions near the receptor binding site of the hemagglutinin, which reduces affinity for sialic acid, reducing binding and aggregation of daughter virions, even in the presence of neuraminidase inhibitor drugs. The second type of resistance involves amino acid substitutions at positions 119 and 227 that reduce affinity of the drugs for the enzyme and diminished inhibition of neuraminidase activity. In clinical use, zanamivir resistance has not been demonstrated in immunocompetent individuals. Oral oseltamivir therapy has been associated with recovery of resistant viruses in 1 to 2% of subjects. These levels of emergence of resistance are markedly less than those observed during therapy of patients with influenza with amantadine or rimantadine. Amantadine- and rimantadine-resistant strains are susceptible to neuramindase inhibitor drugs in vitro.

ADVERSE REACTIONS Orally inhaled zanamivir has been well tolerated. However, individual case reports suggest that in individuals with influenza, both with and without underlying bronchopulmonary disease, bronchospastic respiratory distress can be triggered by zanamivir therapy.

From 5 to 10% more subjects ingesting oseltamivir experience nausea and vomiting compared to placebo.

INHIBITORS OF HIV REPLICATION

Pandemic HIV-1 infection has led to an intensive search for antiviral agents to control this disease. Three different classes of drugs have been demonstrated to be effective in the treatment of HIV-1 disease:
- Nucleoside reverse transcriptase inhibitors (NRTI).
- Non-nucleoside reverse transcriptase inhibitors (NNRTI).
- Protease inhibitors (PI).

Treatment with antivirals delays the onset of AIDS-defining illnesses or death, and leads to improvements in surrogate markers of treatment outcome, i.e. CD4-positive T-lymphocyte counts and plasma viral load. Single- and dual-agent regimens have been associated with high of disease progression and viral resistance to drugs, therefore, three or more drugs are now used concurrently to treat HIV infection. Efforts to induce virus suppression with three antivirals and then maintain the effect with only two drugs have also yielded unacceptably high relapse rates. Generally, drug combinations are chosen from two or more of the currently available classes.

NUCLEOSIDE REVERSE TRANSCRIPTASE INHIBITORS (NRTIs)

Zidovudine (ZDV, AZT) a thymidine analog, is the prototypic NRTI. It was the first antiviral agent approved for the treatment of HIV infection. It inhibits HIV-1, HIV-2, human T-cell leukemia/lymphoma virus-1, and other mammalian retroviruses.

The six agents of the NRTI class (Fig. 8.9) share the following characteristics:

- They require intracellular conversion by cellular enzymes to the corresponding triphosphate nucleotides for activation.

Nucleoside reverse-transcriptase inhibitors (NRTIs) of HIV						
	Zidovudine (ZDV, AZT)	**Didanosine (ddI)**	**Stavudine (d4T)**	**Lamivudine (3TC)**	**Abacavir**	**Zalcitabine (ddC)**
Analog	Thymidine	Adenosine	Thymidine	Cytidine	Guanosine	Cytidine
Recommended dose	200 mg t.i.d., or 300 mg b.i.d.	Body weight >60 kg: 200 mg b.i.d. or 400 mg o.d. <60 kg: 125 mg b.i.d. or 250 mg o.d.	>60 kg: 40 mg b.i.d. <60 kg: 30 mg b.i.d.	150 mg b.i.d.	300 mg b.i.d.	0.75 mg t.i.d.
Formulation	100 mg capsules 300 mg tablets Intravenous solution 10 mg/ml Oral solution 10 mg/ml Combivir: AZT 300/3TC 150	25, 50, 100, 150 and 200 mg buffered tablets 125, 200, 250 and 400 mg enteric-coated capsules	20, 30, 40 mg tablets Oral solution 1 mg/ml	150 mg tablets Oral solution 10 mg/ml	300 mg tablets Oral solution 20 mg/ml	0.375, 0.75 mg tablets
Oral bioavailability (%)	65	30–40	82–86	85	83	70–90
Effect of food	NS*	Decreases 55% with food	NS	NS	NS	NS
Intracellular half-life, hours	3	25–40	3.5	12	3.3	3
CSF concentrations (% of serum)	15–20	19–21	9	15	18	20
Elimination	Renal, after glucuronidation in liver	Renal	Renal	Renal	Hepatic (alcohol dehydrogenase/ glucuronyl transferase)	Renal
Incidence of adverse effects (%)	Anemia (1–7) Neutropenia (2–31) Headaches (12–18) Nausea (4–26) Myopathy (6–18)	Pancreatitis (5–9) Peripheral neuropathy (2–20) Diarrhea (15–28)	Peripheral neuropathy (13–24)	None significant	Hypersensitivity syndrome (3–5) Rash (3–5)	Peripheral neuropathy (10–30) Stomatitis (2–17) Rash (10–20)
NS, not significant						

Fig. 8.9 Nucleoside reverse-transcriptase inhibitors (NRTIs) of HIV.

Characteristics of nucleoside reverse transcriptase inhibitors (NRTIs) of HIV-1 replication

- Activated intracellularly by phosphorylation by cellular kinases
- Triphosphate forms competitively inhibit reverse transcriptase
- Incorporation into HIV-1 DNA causes chain termination
- Resistant strains emerge with variable facility

Main dose-limiting toxic effects of nucleoside inhibitors of HIV-1 reverse transcriptase

Drug	Main toxic effect
Zidovudine	Myelosuppression
Didanosine	Pancreatitis and peripheral neuropathy
Zalcitabine	Peripheral neuropathy
Stavudine	Peripheral neuropathy
Lamivudine	None

- All lose antiretroviral activity due to the development of mutations in the reverse transcriptase: amino acid substitutions in the RT protein result in decreased affinity of the enzyme for the NRTI. The rate of emergence of resistance and its degree vary for different drugs.
- Selectivity is attributable to the greater affinity of NRTI-triphosphate for reverse transcriptase than for cellular DNA polymerases.

Mechanism of action

The retrovirus HIV must initially create a proviral DNA copy of its RNA genome in order to replicate. An HIV-specific enzyme, reverse transcriptase (RT), draws from the infected cell's pool of deoxynucleosides (thymidine, guanosine, adenosine, cytidine) to synthesize the complementary DNA chain. The NRTIs are dideoxy-nucleoside analogs. They lack a second hydroxyl group, essential for the addition of subsequent bases to the growing DNA strand, and their incorporation by RT thus terminates the elongation of the DNA chain. They also have a competitive, inhibitory effect on RT itself.

Pharmacokinetics

The NRTIs are well absorbed orally. Didanosine is acid-labile, and must be administered in buffer-containing tablets. The divalent cations in the buffer can interfere with the absorption of other medications. A newer, enteric-coated preparation of didanosine should not carry the same risk of drug interaction, but might require an empty stomach for absorption.

Elimination of NRTIs from the plasma is rapid, and serum half-lifes vary from 1 hour for stavudine to 3 or 4 hours for lamivudine. Depletion of intracellular NRTI nucleotides is slower, making extended dosing intervals possible. All NRTIs except abacavir are excreted in the urine. Urinary excretion of zidovudine occurs after glucouronidation in the liver, while other NRTIs are excreted unchanged. Dose reductions for dialysis-dependent renal failure range from 50% for zidovudine, stavudine, and zalcitabine, to 80 to 90% for lamivudine and didanosine. NRTI metabolism does not depend on the cytochrome P-450 system. NRTIs are not highly protein-bound, and they penetrate the CNS in significant, though varying, concentrations.

Clinical uses

In multi-drug regimens, zidovudine can delay HIV disease progression and prolong survival, and has been used success-fully in the treatment of HIV-associated dementia. When administered to pregnant women from the second trimester onward, and to their infants for the first 6 weeks postpartum, zidovudine can reduce the risk of vertical (mother to infant) HIV transmission by about two-thirds, from 25 to 8%.

Adverse effects

As a class, NRTIs have been rarely associated with hepatic steatosis (fatty liver) and lactic acidosis. These, and other NRTI adverse effects such as myopathy (AZT) neuropathy (d4T, ddC) and pancreatitis (ddI), are thought to arise from inhibition of mitochondrial DNA polymerases and subsequent mitochondrial dysfunction.

Abacavir has been associated with an idiosyncratic adverse effect termed a 'hypersensitivity reaction.' It most often occurs within the first 6 weeks of treatment (> 85%), and includes: fever, rash, sore throat; cough or other respiratory symptoms; nausea, vomiting, or other gastrointestinal symptoms. The drug must be stopped permanently; re-challenge has been associated with fatal cardiovascular collapse. Other agent-specific toxicities are listed in Fig. 8.9.

NON-NUCLEOSIDE REVERSE TRANSCRIPTASE INHIBITORS (NNRTIs)

NNRTIs have been developed over the past decade. Three agents, nevirapine, delavirdine and efavirenz (Fig. 8.10) are currently available, derived from different chemical classes.

Mechanism of action

NNRTIs inhibit HIV replication by binding to a hydrophobic pocket of reverse transcriptase (RT) which leads to a conformational change in the enzyme, and its subsequent inactivation.

Agents of the NNRTI class share the following characteristics:
- They are potent inhibitors of HIV-1, but not of HIV-2, other retroviruses, or cellular DNA polymerases.
- They do not require intracellular phosphorylation for their antiviral activity.
- The presence of a single RT mutation at position (amino acid) 103 confers cross-resistance to all currently available NNRTIs.

Pharmacokinetics

The NNRTIs have excellent oral bioavailability. They are highly protein-bound, and have reasonable penetration into the CNS

Non-nucleoside reverse transcriptase inibitors of HIV			
	Nevirapine	**Delavirdine**	**Efavirenz**
Recommended dose	200 mg b.i.d. or 400 mg o.d. (Dose escalates over 2 weeks)	400 mg t.i.d., or 600 mg b.i.d.	600 mg o.d.
Forms available	200 mg tablets	100 mg tablets	200 mg tablets
Oral bioavailability (%)	> 90	85	42
Effect of food	NS	NS	NS (but avoid high-fat meal: may increase absorption 50%)
Serum half-life, hours	25–30	5.8	40–55
Elimination	Hepatic: cytochrome P-450	Hepatic: cytochrome P-450	Hepatic: cytochrome P-450
Incidence of adverse effects (%)	Hepatitis (3–8)	Headache (3–11)	Central nervous system symptoms (52 total, 6 severe)
NS, not significant			

Fig. 8.10 Non-nucleoside reverse transcriptase inhibitors (NNRTIs) of HIV.

proportional to the free plasma concentrations of each drug. They are metabolized by the cytochrome P-450 system, and have variable inducing/inhibiting effects on this system.

Clinical uses

When used in combination with NRTIs, NNRTIs are potent inhibitors of HIV replication. Their effects are comparable to those of NRTI/protease inhibitor regimens (see below). They are used for the treatment of antiretroviral drug-naive individuals, or those in whom protease inhibitor-based regimens have failed. Nevirapine, when given in single doses to pregnant women during labor, and to their infants in the early postpartum period, has been shown to reduce the risk of vertical (mother to infant) HIV transmission by about 40%.

Adverse effects

Maculopapular rashes are a major side effect of this class, occurring in about 20% of patients treated with nevirapine, 10 to 20% of those receiving delavirdine, and 5 to 10% of subjects on efavirenz, and require discontinuation of treatment in 7%, 5%, and 1% of patients respectively. Mild to moderate rashes may be treated symptomatically with antihistamines. Nevirapine has been associated with severe hepatitis, and regular monitoring of hepatic enzymes is recommended. Efavirenz has a unique neuropsychiatric adverse effect profile, including symptoms of dizziness, lightheadedness, impaired concentration, agitation, and abnormal dreams. These symptoms appear most often in the first few days of treatment, and usually lessen or resolve within 2 to 4 weeks.

PROTEASE INHIBITORS (PIs)

The first of the six PIs (Fig. 8.11) approved for prescribing was saquinavir, in 1995, but its efficacy was limited by poor bioavailability. The development of ritonavir and indinavir launched the era of highly active antiretroviral therapy (HAART).

Agents of the PI class share the following characteristics:
- They bind competitively to the aspartic proteases of HIV-1 and HIV-2, preventing the post-translational breakdown of viral polyprotein into the components required for viral assembly and budding.
- They do not require intracellular activation for their effects.
- Marked resistance develops through an accumulation of mutations with amino acid substitutions at both the active enzymatic site and other regions. Viruses with mutated proteases seem less fit than wild-type viruses.

Certain PIs (saquinavir, ritonavir, indinavir, and amprenavir) are peptidomimetic, and exhibit structural similarity to the cleavage sites of the HIV polyproteins. Others (nelfinavir) are nonpeptidomimetic. Amprenavir is a sulfonamide compound.

Pharmacokinetics

The oral absorption of ritonavir, indinavir, nelfinavir and amprenavir is between 60 and 80%. That of saquinavir is approximately 10%. Cerebrospinal fluid (CSF) penetration is limited, although recent data suggest that indinavir may achieve clinically significant concentrations in the CNS.

All PIs are metabolized via the cytochrome P-450 system, and important drug interactions occur (see below).

Protease inhibitor (PI) drugs for the treatment of HIV infection

	Saquinavir	Ritonavir	Indinavir	Nelfinavir	Amprenavir	Lopinavir-ritonavir
Recommended dose	SGC 1200 mg t.i.d. HGC*	600 mg b.i.d.	800 mg t.i.d.	750 mg t.i.d., or 1250 mg b.i.d.	1200 b.i.d.	400 mg lopinavir/100 mg ritonavir b.i.d.
Formulation	200 mg capsules	100 mg capsules Oral solution 80 mg/ml	200, 333, 400 mg capsules	250 mg tablets Powder for solution, 50 mg/g	300 mg tablets Oral solution 20 mg/ml	133 mg lopinavir/33 mg ritonavir
Oral bioavailability, (%)	HGC 4 SGC: not available	Not available	65	20–80	83	Approx. 80
Effect of food	Increases absorption	Increases absorption	Decreases absorption substantially	Increases absorption	Avoid high-fat, otherwise no effect	Increases absorption (decreases 30–40% if fasting)
Serum half-life, hours	1–2	3–5	1.5–2	3.5–5	3.3	5–6
Elimination	Hepatic: cytochrome P-450	Hepatic: cytochrome P-450	Hepatic: cytochrome P-450	Hepatic: cytochrome P-450	Hepatic: cytochrome P-450	Hepatic: cytochrome P-450
Incidence of adverse effects (%)	Elevated hepatic transaminases (2–6)	Circumoral paresthesias (3–6) Taste perversion (5–15) Hypertriglyceridemia (2–8) Elevated hepatic transaminases (5–6)	Nephrolithiasis (3–5) Increased indirect bilirubin (10) Hair, skin, nail changes	(Class effects)	Rash (18 total, 6 severe)	(Class effects)

SGC, soft-gel capsule
*HGC, hard-gel capsule: use only if combined with cytochrome P-450 inhibitor (e.g. ritonavir). NS, not significant

Fig. 8.11 Protease inhibitor (PI) drugs for the treatment of HIV infection.

> **Characteristics of current protease inhibitors that inhibit HIV-1 replication**
>
> - Interfere with post-translational processing of HIV-1 precursor proteins
> - Combination treatment with nucleoside reverse transcriptase inhibitor drugs produces additive antiviral effects
> - Combination therapy with nucleoside reverse transcriptase inhibitor drugs reduces the incidence of resistance
> - Well tolerated

Clinical uses

PIs, in combination with NRTIs (and with NNRTIs) are potent inhibitors of HIV-1 and HIV-2 replication, and their use seems to improve survival and allow fewer hospitalizations for HIV-infected individuals. In clinical trials, rates of complete suppression of viremia of 80% or better have been achieved for up to 3 years. In clinical practice, results have been less impressive, with 1-year rates of continued virologic suppression of the order of 50 to 60%, possibly because of problems of drug toxicities and adherence to therapy.

Adverse effects

The principal side effects of PIs are gastrointestinal, with nausea affecting 3 to 30% of patients (highest for ritonavir and amprenavir) and diarrhea of varying severity in 5 to 30% of cases (highest for ritonavir and nelfinavir). Other agent-specific adverse effects are listed in Fig. 8.11.

Increasingly, a syndrome of lipodystrophy—comprising peripheral fat wasting, central fat accumulation, hyperlipidemias, and insulin resistance, in variable combinations and proportions—is being observed with long-term PI use. Elements of this syndrome can appear in the absence of PI use, and an NRTI-mediated mitochondrial toxicity has been suggested as a contributor to the syndrome.

CYTOCHROME P-450 INTERACTIONS
(see Chapter 4)

All currently available antiretroviral protease inhibitors and NNRTIs are metabolized (oxidized) in the cytochrome P-450 system. These agents serve both as substrates for this metabolic pathway and as P-450 inducers or inhibitors.

The HIV-1 protease inhibitors all function as P-450 inhibitors, and the strength of their inhibition may be ranked as follows: ritonavir (most potent), indinavir, lopinavir, nelfinavir, amprenavir, saquinavir. Of the NNRTIs, delavirdine is a P-450 inhibitor, nevirapine is a P-450 inducer, and efavirenz has mixed effects. Certain medications should not be administered concurrently with the protease inhibitors (or other P-450 inhibitors) because of the risk of toxic adverse effects related to drug accumulation (Fig. 8.12). Concurrent use of potent P-450 inducers (e.g. rifampin, certain anticonvulsants, dexamethasone) with PIs and NNRTIs should be avoided.

The potent P-450-inhibitory effects of ritonavir have been used therapeutically to block the metabolism of other protease inhibitors, thereby improving PI pharmacokinetics. For example, ritonavir 100 mg administered with indinavir 800 mg, each

Examples of drugs metabolized by cytochrome P-450 enzymes, with clinically important adverse interactions when administered concomitantly with antiretroviral protease inhibitor drugs, and alternative agents

Drug class	Representative agents	Alternative
Nonsedating antihistamines	Terfenadine, astemizole	Loratidine, cetirizine, fexofenadine
Calcum channel blockers (dihydropyridines)*	Bepridil	(Other antihypertensive/antianginals)
Anti-arrhythmics*	Amiodarone, propafenone, quinidine, flecainide	(Monitor effects closely)
Antihyperlipidemics	Lovastatin, simvastatin	Atorvastatin, pravastatin
Gastrointestinal motility agents	Cisapride	Metoclopramide
Psychoactive agents*	Bupropion, clozapine, pimozide	SSRIs, haloperidol, respiridone
Benzodiazepines	Midazolam, triazolam, diazepam	Lorazepam, oxazepam
Ergot derivatives	Ergotamine, dihydroergotamine	(Other migraine drugs)

*Principal risk is with concurrent ritonavir use

Fig. 8.12 Examples of drugs that are metabolized by cytochrome P-450 enzymes. Clinically important adverse drug interactions are caused when these are administered concomitantly in standard doses with antiretroviral protease inhibitor drugs. Alternative agents that obviate the risk of an adverse reaction are also listed.

twice daily, increases the trough levels (fourfold) and the AUC (area under the curve) of the latter drug, reduces the number of pills needed and makes food restrictions unnecessary. Similar effects apply to the proprietary fixed-drug combination of lopinavir–ritonavir. Other pharmacokinetically enhanced combinations which have either proven effective or are currently being evaluated include: saquinavir 400 mg–ritonavir 400 mg b.i.d., indinavir 800 mg–ritonavir 200 mg b.i.d., amprenavir 600 mg–ritonavir 100 mg b.i.d.

FURTHER READING

Balzarini J et al. Biochemical pharmacology. In: Merigan TC, Bartlett JG, Bolognesi D (eds) *Textbook of AIDS Medicine*. Baltimore: Williams and Wilkins; 1999, pp. 815–859. [Covers the biochemistry and detailed pharmacology of the major classes of antiretroviral agents.]

Coen DM. The implications of resistance to antiviral agents for herpesvirus drug targets and drug therapy. *Antiviral Res* 1992; **12**: 245–264. [A useful review of the data concerning resistance to herpesvirus drugs and strategies for treating infection caused by such viruses.]

Dollery CT, Boobis A, Rawlins M, Thomas S, Wilkins (eds) *Therapeutic Drugs*, 2nd edn. Edinburgh: Churchill Livingstone; 1999. [Additional encyclopedic review of drugs, including antiviral agents].

Hayden FG. Antiviral agents. In: Mandell GL, Bennett JE, Dolin R (eds) *Principles and Practice of Infectious Diseases*. New York: Churchill Livingstone; 1995, pp. 411–449. [Comprehensive, authoritative text on antiviral drugs for the practitioner.]

Max B, Sherer R. Management of the adverse effects of antiretroviral therapy and medication adherence. *Clin Infect Dis* 2000; **30**: S96–116. [Review of individual antiretroviral agents and their toxicities.]

Whitley RT, Gnann JW Jr. Acyclovir: a decade later. *N Engl J Med* 1992; **327**: 782–789. [A comprehensive review of the mainstay of our therapeutic armamentarium for herpesvirus infections.]

Useful websites
http://www.aidsmap.com/about/bhiva/bhivagol.asp BHIVA Writing Committee on behalf of the BHIVA Executive Committee. British HIV Association (BHIVA) guidelines for the treatment of HIV-infected adults with antiretroviral therapy. [British guidelines for the treatment of HIV infection.]
http://www.medscape.com/medscape/HIV/ClinicalMgmt/CM.drug/public/toc-CM.drug.html C, Piscitelli SC. Managing drug–drug interactions in HIV disease. [Review of drug metabolism, including mixed-function oxidases.]
http://hivatis.org/trtgd/ns.html Adult Panel on Clinical Practices for Treatment of HIV Infection (Department of Health and Human Services (DHHS) and the Henry J. Kaiser Family Foundation). Guidelines for the use of antiretroviral agents in HIV-infected adults and adolescents. [The North American guidelines for the treatment of HIV infection.]

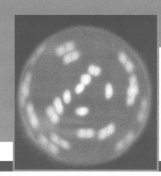

Chapter 9

Drugs and Bacteria

■ *Bacterial infections are exceedingly common and cause substantial morbidity and mortality*

Bacterial diarrhea is a leading cause of infant mortality worldwide, and tuberculosis a very frequent cause of death due to infection. Antibacterial drugs are among the most important therapeutic discoveries of the twentieth century and have dramatically changed the course of many illnesses, reducing mortality (e.g. of bacterial meningitis and bacterial endocarditis) and morbidity. On the other hand, antibiotics are now among the most overprescribed agents, partly because many of them have excellent safety profiles. As a result, overuse of antibiotics is a significant contributing factor to the growing international problem of antibiotic resistance by a variety of bacteria.

■ *In practice, the term antibiotic has become synonymous with antibacterial agent*

Strictly speaking, antibacterial drugs are classified as antibiotics, chemotherapeutic or synthetic agents, and semisynthetic agents, depending on whether they are:

- Byproducts of micro-organisms (antibiotics).
- Entirely synthesized in the laboratory (chemotherapeutic or synthetic agents).
- A hybrid of the two (semisynthetic agents).

In practice, the term antibiotic has become synonymous with antibacterial agent, and this more liberal definition of antibiotic will be used throughout this chapter.

MECHANISM OF ACTION

■ *The ideal antibiotic interferes with a vital function of bacteria without affecting host cells*

Antibiotics are said to possess selective toxicity because they interfere with a vital function of bacteria with minimal effect on host cells. In devising antibiotics, scientists attempt to identify functions that are specific for the bacterium as potential targets. For example, bacteria possess cell walls, whereas mammalian cells do not. Accordingly, drugs that interfere with the production of the bacterial cell wall are toxic to bacteria, but harmless to the host. Similarly, the bacterial ribosome (70S) is sufficiently different from eukaryotic ribosomes (80S) for sites on the bacterial ribosome to be good targets for antibacterial drugs. Figure 9.1 shows the sites of action of the major types of antibiotics. Because of their selective toxicity, many antibiotics have a high therapeutic index (i.e. ratio of toxic dose to therapeutic dose).

■ *Whether an antibiotic inhibits or kills bacteria depends on its concentration*

The activity of a given antibiotic against a given bacterium can be readily measured in the laboratory. By exposing a standard inoculum of a bacterium to a range of concentrations of an antibiotic, the lowest concentration of the drug that inhibits bacterial growth can be determined. This is called the minimum

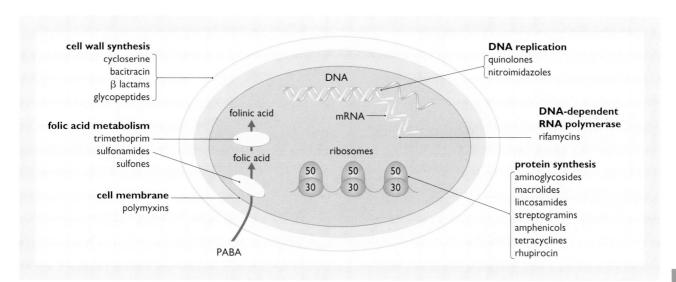

Fig. 9.1 Sites of action of different types of antibiotic agent. (PABA, para-aminobenzoic acid.)

inhibitory concentration (MIC). As the concentration of anti-biotic is increased above the MIC, a concentration is eventually reached that will actually kill the bacterium (technically a 3 $\log_{10}$-fold or 99.9% reduction in the inoculum). The lowest concentration of antibiotic required to kill the bacterium is known as the minimum bactericidal concentration (MBC). Often, the MBC is 2–8 times that of the MIC. Antibiotics for which achievable blood concentrations regularly exceed the MBC of common pathogens are classified as bactericidal antibiotics, whereas antibiotics whose blood concentrations readily exceed the MIC but do not usually exceed the MBC are classified as bacteriostatic antibiotics. However, categorizing antibiotics as predominantly bacteriostatic or bactericidal is imperfect since there is a unique relationship between each bacterium and each antibiotic. For instance, penicillin, which is classically considered a bactericidal antibiotic, is nearly always bactericidal against streptococci, but is bacteriostatic against enterococci. Similarly, chloramphenicol, which is classically considered bacteriostatic, is bacteriostatic against most Enterobacteriaceae, but is bactericidal against most strains of *Haemophilus influenzae*.

Antibiotics may act together synergistically, antagonistically, or indifferently

Occasionally, two or more antibiotics are used together against the same pathogen. In the laboratory it is possible to categorize the relationship between two or more antibiotics against one bacterium as synergistic, antagonistic, or indifferent, depending on the effect of the drug combination on the growth of the bacterium compared with that of each drug alone (Fig. 9.2):

- If the combination of drugs markedly increases the anti-bacterial effect above that of the most active drug, the combination is synergistic.

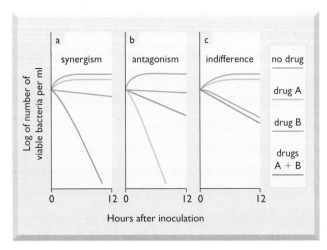

Fig. 9.2 Bacterial growth curves showing synergism, antagonism, and indifference of two antibiotics, A and B, against three different organisms. In (a) the combination is synergistic because it exerts a significantly greater antibacterial effect than the more active drug alone. In (b) the addition of drug B significantly reduces the antibacterial effect of drug A and therefore, the combination is antagonistic. In (c) the antibacterial activity of the combination is essentially the same as that of the more active drug, and the combination is therefore classified as indifferent.

- If the combination results in less inhibition of bacterial growth than the most active agent alone, the combination is antagonistic.
- If the combination is neither synergistic nor antagonistic, it is indifferent.

In practice, most combinations are indifferent.

The clinical relevance of *in vitro* synergism and antagonism is generally unknown. However, both important synergistic and antagonistic combinations have been demonstrated clinically.

- The success rate of treating enterococcal endocarditis with a combination of penicillin plus aminoglycoside is signi-ficantly greater than that using penicillin alone, highlighting the relevance of synergy.
- The combination of penicillin and tetracycline for treating bacterial meningitis is associated with significantly higher mortality than when using penicillin alone, and is an example of antagonism *in vivo*.

Killing by bactericidal drugs can be concentration-dependent or time-dependent

Killing of bacteria by some bactericidal drugs (e.g. amino-glycosides and fluoroquinolones) is concentration-dependent, whereas that by others (e.g. β lactams and glycopeptides) is time-dependent. Concentration-dependent killing implies a greater bactericidal activity with higher concentrations of antibiotic. With time-dependent killing, there is little or no enhancement of bactericidal activity with drug concentrations above the MBC; rather, the killing depends on maintaining the concentration of antibiotic above the MBC for as much of the dosing interval as possible.

Normal bacterial replication is often delayed after an antibiotic has been stopped

When bacteria are exposed to an antibiotic at concentrations above the MIC and the antibiotic is then removed from the medium, bacterial replication often does not resume normally (as if no antibiotic were present) for a variable period of time (usually measured in hours) after removal of the antibiotic. This phenomenon is called the postantibiotic effect (PAE). The PAE does not occur with all bacterium–drug combinations but when it is present its duration is often concentration-dependent. In other words, the higher the concentration of antibiotic to which the bacterium has been exposed, the longer the duration of the PAE. Aminoglycosides and fluoroquinolones consistently demonstrate a PAE against Gram-negative bacteria, whereas β lactams, with the exception of carbapenems, do not. However, β lactams do demonstrate a modest PAE against Gram-positive bacteria. Figures 9.3 and 9.4 show concentration-dependent and time-dependent killing of Gram-negative bacteria illustrating PAE in the former but not the latter.

The postantibiotic effect provides a rationale for pulse dosing antibiotics

Pulse dosing refers to the administration of relatively large doses of antibiotic to produce peak blood concentrations far higher than the MIC or MBC of the causative organism at dosing intervals longer than several serum half-lifes of the drug.

For example, crystalline penicillin G has a serum half-life of about 30 minutes and yet it is usually administered every 6 hours (i.e. every 12 half-lifes). This dosing schedule is markedly different to that used with most other drugs (e.g. anticonvulsants), which are generally given no less frequently than every serum half-life. There are a variety of reasons why pulse dosing is effective with antibiotics.

- The therapeutic index of most antibiotics is high and it is often possible to achieve high peak serum concentrations without significant toxicity.
- Some antibiotics demonstrate concentration-dependent killing and therefore it is desirable and more efficacious to achieve high peak serum concentrations.
- It is often possible to maintain the serum antibiotic concentration above the MIC of the pathogen for the entire dosing interval, despite dosing relatively infrequently relative to the serum half-life (Fig. 9.5).
- Even if the serum antibiotic concentration does fall below the MIC for part of the dosing interval, the PAE may prevent bacterial multiplication during the brief time when the serum antibiotic concentration falls below the MIC before the next antibiotic dose (Fig. 9.6).
- Except for very immunocompromised patients, antibiotics are not the only defense against bacterial infection. The host immune system plays an active role in combatting the infection. Indeed, before the antibiotic era many people did survive bacterial infections, although their recovery was generally slower and associated with more complications than with antibiotic treatment.

Properties of antibacterials

Pharmacologic characteristics of selected antibacterials are listed in Fig. 9.7.

Antibiotic spectrum of activity

An antibiotic may have a broad or narrow spectrum of activity

Antibiotics that are active against many bacterial species are referred to as broad spectrum antibiotics, whereas those that

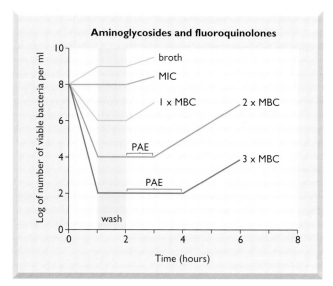

Fig. 9.3 Concentration-dependent bactericidal action and the postantibiotic effect (PAE). Time–kill study in broth containing various concentrations of an antimicrobial agent that shows concentration-dependent bactericidal action. A PAE on the residual organisms is present after washing these organisms and resuspending them in antibiotic-free broth. (MBC, minimum bactericidal concentration; MIC, minimum inhibitory concentration.)

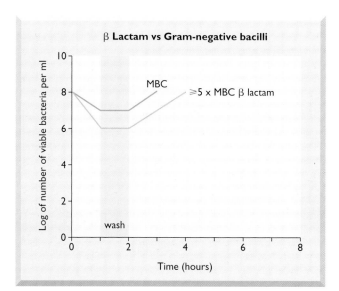

Fig. 9.4 Time-dependent bactericidal action. Time–kill study in broth containing various concentrations of a β lactam that shows time-dependent bactericidal action against a Gram-negative bacillus. There is no postantibiotic effect (PAE) on the residual organisms after washing and resuspending in antibiotic-free broth. (MBC, minimum bactericidal concentration.)

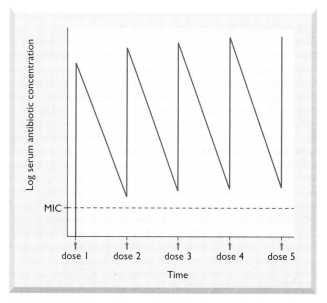

Fig. 9.5 Pulse dosing of an antibiotic. In this example, the antibiotic is very active against the pathogen and the serum antibiotic concentration remains above the minimum inhibitory concentration (MIC) at all times, despite infrequent dosing. Maintaining the serum antibiotic concentration above the MIC at all times is desirable if there is no postantibiotic effect (PAE).

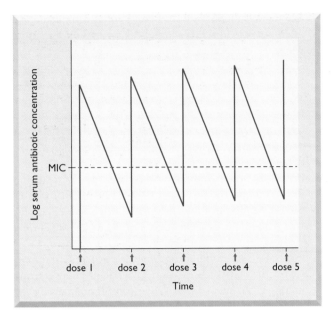

Fig. 9.6 Pulse dosing of an antibiotic. In this example, the peak serum antibiotic concentration following each dose is well above the minimum inhibitory concentration (MIC), but the serum antibiotic concentration falls below the MIC for the latter part of each dosing interval. If there is a postantibiotic effect (PAE), there is no harm in allowing the serum antibiotic concentration to fall below the MIC for a small proportion of the dosing interval.

are active against only a few species are termed narrow spectrum agents. However, this distinction is somewhat arbitrary.

Antibiotic resistance

Antibiotic resistance is classified as either innate or acquired

Innate resistance refers to an intrinsic resistance based on the mechanism of the drug. For example, anaerobic bacteria lack the oxygen-dependent transport mechanism required for aminoglycosides to enter the bacterial cell and therefore they are innately resistant to aminoglycosides.

Acquired resistance refers to the acquisition of a resistance gene in a bacterium that is not innately resistant to a particular antibiotic. There is no antibiotic against which acquired resistance has not developed, at least in some bacterial species.

The major stimulus for the development of acquired antibiotic resistance is the use of the antibiotics themselves, as such use exerts selective pressure on the bacteria to develop resistance to survive. However, the probability of developing resistance does appear to depend upon both the specific drug and the specific bacterium involved. In some instances, a single mutation in the bacterial genome is sufficient to result in clinically significant resistance. In others, multiple mutations are needed for phenotypic resistance.

Properties of selected antibacterials

Drug	Routes of administration	Oral bioavailability (%)	Clearance route	Serum half-life (normal renal function), (hours)	Comments
Standard penicillins					
Penicillin G	i.v., p.o.	20	Renal	0.5	Avoid oral use: acid-labile
Penicillin V	p.o.	65	Renal	0.5	Preferred to penicillin G for oral use
Aminopenicillins					
Ampicillin	i.v., p.o.	40	Renal	1.0	Amoxicillin is preferred for oral use
Amoxicillin	p.o.	80	Renal	1.0	
Antistaphylococcal penicillins					
Nafcillin	i.v., p.o.	35	Hepatic	0.5	Low oral absorption
Oxacillin	i.v., p.o.	30	Mainly renal	0.5	Low oral absorption
Cloxacillin	i.v., p.o.	50	Mainly renal	0.5	Intravenous formulation not available in US
Dicloxacillin	p.o.	60	Mainly renal	0.5	Better oral absorption than oxacillin or nafcillin
Floxacillin	p.o.	70	Mainly renal	0.5	Highest oral absorption of antistaphylococcal penicillins
Ureidopenicillins					
Piperacillin	i.v.	Not used	Renal	1.0	Active against *Pseudomonas aeruginosa*
First-generation cephalosporins					
Cefazolin	i.v.	Not used	Renal	1.5	
Cephalexin	p.o.	>95	Renal	1.0	

Properties of selected antibacterials (Continued)

Drug	Routes of administration	Oral bioavailability (%)	Clearance route	Serum half-life (normal renal function), (hours)	Comments
Second-generation cephalosporins					
Cefuroxime	i.v., p.o.	40	Renal	1.5	Active against *Haemophilus influenzae* Oral formulation is cefuroxime axetil
Cefoxitin	i.v.	Not used	Renal	1.0	Active against *Bacteroides fragilis*
Third-generation cephalosporins					
Cefotaxime	i.v.	Not used	Renal	1.5	Has active metabolite
Ceftazidime	i.v.	Not used	Renal	1.5	Active against *Pseudomonas aeruginosa*
Ceftriaxone	i.v.	Not used	Renal and hepatic	7.0	
Carbapenems					
Imipenem–cilastatin	i.v.	Not used	Renal	1.0	Can precipitate seizures
Meropenem	i.v.	Not used	Renal	1.0	Can be used to treat bacterial meningitis
Tetracyclines					
Tetracycline	p.o.	75	Renal	9	Contraindicated in pregnancy and children <8 years
Doxycycline	i.v., p.o.	95	GI tract	18	Contraindicated in pregnancy and children <8 years
Minocycline	p.o.	95	GI tract	18	Contraindicated in pregnancy and children <8 years Most lipophilic tetracycline
Macrolides					
Erythromycin	i.v., p.o., topical	25	Hepatic	1.8	Phlebitic i.v. formulation
Clarithromycin	p.o.	5	Hepatic	6	Active metabolite
Azithromycin	i.v., p.o.	35	GI and hepatic	68	Highly concentrated intracellularly
Quinolones					
Norfloxacin	p.o.	40	Renal	3	Used for UTI only
Ciprofloxacin	p.o., i.v.	75	Renal	4	Very active against aerobic Gram-negative bacilli; Weak Gram-positive activity
Levofloxacin	p.o., i.v.	>95	Renal	7	Active against most *Streptococcus pneumoniae*
Gatifloxacin	p.o., i.v.		Renal	8	Broad spectrum fluoroquinolone
Moxifloxacin	p.o.	85	Hepatic > renal	12	Broad spectrum fluoroquinolone
Miscellaneous Gram-positive antibiotics					
Vancomycin	i.v., p.o.	Minimal	Renal	5	Active only against Gram-positive bacteria; oral vancomycin is used only to treat *Clostridium difficile* colitis
Quinupristin–dalfopristin	i.v.	Not used	Hepatic	8.5	Active against Gram-positive cocci, including phlebitic VRE
Linezolid	i.v., p.o.	≥95	Hepatic	5.5	Active against Gram-positive cocci, including VRE

Properties of selected antibacterials (Continued)

Drug	Routes of administration	Oral bioavailability (%)	Clearance route	Serum half-life (normal renal function), (hours)	Comments
Other antibiotics					
Chloramphenicol	i.v., p.o., topical	80	Hepatic	3	Myelotoxic
Metronidazole	i.v., p.o., topical	>95	Hepatic	10	
Trimethoprim	p.o.	80	Renal	11	Used mainly for UTI in patients allergic to sulfonamides
Trimethoprim–sulfamethoxazole	p.o., i.v.	85	Renal	1	
Nitrofurantoin	p.o.	45	Renal	0.3	Does not achieve systemic levels; for UTI only
Clindamycin	i.v., p.o., topical	90	Hepatic	2.5	
Gentamicin	i.v., topical	Not used	Renal	2.5	Active only against aerobic Gram-negative bacteria; nephrotoxic, ototoxic

i.v., intravenous; p.o., by mouth; GI, gastrointestinal; UTI, urinary tract infection; VRE, vancomycin-resistant enterococci.

Fig. 9.7 Properties of selected antibacterials.

The three main biochemical mechanisms of acquired resistance are as follows:

- Reduced bacterial permeability, which results from changes in the cell membrane of Gram-negative bacteria (see below).
- The production of bacterial enzymes that alter the structure of the antibiotic. These enzymes may be hydrolytic (e.g. β lactamases) or nonhydrolytic (e.g. aminoglycoside-modifying enzymes).
- Alteration in the target site, where a single mutation where the antibiotic normally binds can be sufficient to produce clinically significant drug resistance (e.g. methicillin-resistant staphylococci).

Reduced bacterial permeability

There are significant differences between the structure of the cell wall and membrane of Gram-positive and Gram-negative bacteria

Gram-positive bacteria contain many layers of peptidoglycan beneath which lies the cell membrane, and there is no appreciable barrier to the entry of antibiotics (Fig. 9.8). In contrast, Gram-negative bacteria possess an outer membrane that contains copious amounts of lipopolysaccharide, as well as an inner membrane which is the true cytoplasmic membrane. The inner

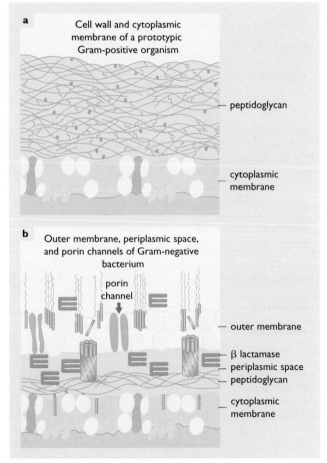

Fig. 9.8 Structure of the bacterial cell wall and membrane.
(a) Gram-positive bacterium. (b) Gram-negative bacterium. Note that only Gram-negative bacteria possess an outer membrane, which provides an additional obstacle to the entry of antibacterial drugs.

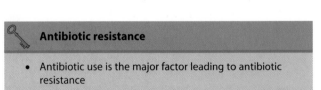

Antibiotic resistance

- Antibiotic use is the major factor leading to antibiotic resistance
- The three main mechanisms of antibiotic resistance are reduced bacterial permeability, enzymatic alteration of antibiotics, and altered target site

membrane is covered by considerably fewer layers of pepti-doglycan than are present in Gram-positive bacteria and is separated from the outer membrane by the periplasmic space. The outer membrane consists of a phospholipid bilayer with aqueous channels formed by outer membrane proteins termed porins. Gram-negative bacteria therefore present a challenge to the entry of drugs, favoring those that are lipophilic or aqueous drugs of low molecular weight, which can enter via the porin channels. Alterations in porin proteins or outer membrane lipopolysaccharides can result in resistance due to reduced permeability to antibiotics. Alterations in the bacterial cell membrane that lead to decreased permeability to one antibiotic will often result in decreased permeability to other antibiotics and consequently, multi-drug resistance.

SELECTING ANTIBIOTIC THERAPY

Antibiotics can be used either prophylactically or therapeutically. In either case, the same basic principles apply. Bacterial, host, and drug factors must all be considered (Figs 9.9, 9.10).

Bacterial factors

Antibacterial therapy is effective only for bacterial infections. It is therefore important to restrict the use of antibiotics to those situations where bacterial infection is either known to be present or is highly probable. The all-too-common practice of prescribing antibiotics for infections that are probably viral is to be discouraged because it is ineffective, unnecessarily costly, generates unnecessary adverse effects, and contributes to global antibiotic resistance.

Once a bacterial infection is confirmed or is suspected, it is important to identify the infecting organism(s) in order to make a rational antibiotic choice. If the identity of the infecting organism(s) is not known, as is often the case when antibiotic therapy is started, it is usually possible to make a reasonable guess about the likely pathogen(s) based on statistical probabilities. For example:

- Urinary tract infection in sexually active premenopausal women is due to *Escherichia coli* in approximately 85% of cases.
- Cellulitis of an arm or leg is usually due to either *Streptococcus pyogenes* or *Staphylococcus aureus*.

To make an informed guess about the likely pathogen(s) it is important to know:

- The site of infection.
- Whether the infection is community-acquired or nosocomial (hospital-acquired).
- Details about the host, including age, underlying illness, and/or other predisposing factors.
- The usual susceptibility trends in the local hospital or community setting (e.g. penicillin-resistant pneumococci are highly prevalent in Spain and South Africa, but much less prevalent in Scandinavia).

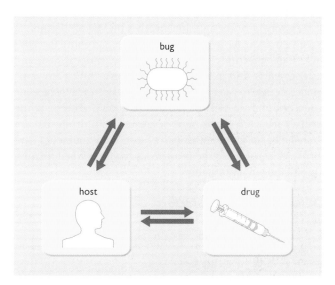

Fig. 9.9 Triangle depicting the classic bidirectional three-way interaction between a microbial pathogen ('bug'), an antimicrobial agent (drug), and the host, whose immune function is a major determinant of the outcome of an infection.

The bacterial, host, and drug factors that must be considered when selecting antibiotic therapy		
Bug factors	**Host factors**	**Drug factors**
Identity of pathogen(s)†	Site of infection	Activity against pathogen(s)†
Susceptibility of pathogens†	Allergies Renal function Hepatic function Neutropenia Digestive tract function Other underlying diseases Concomitant medication Pregnancy Desired route of administration	Ability to get to site of infection Potential for drug interactions Available routes of administration Dosing frequency (for outpatients) Taste (for liquid formulations) Stability at different temperatures (for liquid formulations) Cost

† Often not known at the start of therapy.

Fig. 9.10 The bacterial, host, and drug factors that must be considered when selecting antibiotic therapy.

In selected instances, it is appropriate to start antibiotic therapy without carrying out laboratory studies to identify the pathogen (e.g. most cases of cellulitis). In other cases, particularly those where the pathogen(s) cannot be reliably predicted or in patients with severe illness, appropriate specimens should be collected before starting antibiotic therapy. The microbiology laboratory can then identify the pathogen(s) and carry out in vitro antibiotic susceptibility testing so that the therapy can be modified to the most appropriate regimen. Usually susceptibility results are not available until 48–72 h after a specimen has been collected for culture.

Host factors

Many host factors need to be considered before selecting an antibiotic for a given infection.

■ *One of the most important host factors is the site of the infection*

It is essential that the antibiotic reaches the site of infection at a concentration above the MIC in all cases, and above the MBC in certain infections such as meningitis, endocarditis, and osteomyelitis, and in neutropenic patients. Only a few antibiotics are able to enter the central nervous system in therapeutic concentrations to treat meningitis or a brain abscess, while urinary tract infections must be treated with drugs that are excreted by the kidney in an active form. Many antibiotics have difficulty penetrating the prostate, as required when treating chronic bacterial prostatitis.

Other important host factors

Other important host factors include:
- Drug allergies, since certain antibiotics are relatively allergenic.
- Renal and hepatic function, since antibiotics are cleared by either the kidney or the liver.
- Concomitant medications, since some antibiotics are involved in drug interactions.
- Age, since certain antibiotics are contraindicated in neonates (sulfonamides, ceftriaxone), children (tetracyclines and fluoroquinolones), and pregnant women.

■ *A decision must be made about the route of administration*

In general, the oral route is preferred when it is possible. Parenteral therapy is necessary if the digestive tract is nonfunctional, the patient has hypotension, therapeutic drug concentrations are required immediately (e.g. in life-threatening infections), or no oral drugs are absorbed in adequate amounts to achieve therapeutic concentrations at the site of infection. The topical route is appropriate for selected local infections (e.g. bacterial conjunctivitis).

Drug factors

■ *Several important drug factors must be taken into account before selecting an antimicrobial agent to treat a bacterial infection*

These include:
- Its activity against the pathogen(s), though such information may not be known when the treatment needs to be started.
- Its ability to reach the site of infection in a therapeutic concentration. This requires a knowledge about whether the drug should be bactericidal or bacteriostatic against the known or suspected pathogen, since bactericidal activity is required for certain infections.
- Its available routes of administration and whether they are appropriate for the patient.
- Its adverse effect profile and whether this could affect underlying illnesses or result in drug interactions.
- Its dosing frequency, as acceptance of a drug in the outpatient setting is increased with dosing frequencies of two or fewer doses per day.
- When a liquid formulation is required (predominantly in young children), whether the taste is acceptable, as well as whether it is stable at various temperatures. Some antibiotic suspensions require refrigeration to remain stable.
- Its cost, recognizing that the true cost of therapy is not merely the cost of the medication itself, but also includes the cost of administration, monitoring, and complications, including treatment failures and the cost of retreatment.

MAJOR ANTIBIOTICS

Antibiotics that inhibit bacterial cell wall synthesis

■ *The bacterial cell wall is an obvious target for antibiotics*

As mycoplasmas, chlamydiae and rickettsiae lack a cell wall they are innately resistant to antibiotics that inhibit bacterial cell wall synthesis. The two most important classes of antibiotics that inhibit bacterial cell wall synthesis are β lactams and glycopeptides. The topical antibiotic bacitracin and the second-

Host factors influencing the choice of an antibiotic
• Site of infection
• Renal and hepatic function
• Age
• Drug allergies
• Required route of administration

Drug factors influencing the choice of an antibiotic
• Activity against the pathogen
• Ability to reach the site of infection
• Available routes of administration
• Adverse effect profile
• Dosing schedules
• Taste (for suspensions)
• Cost

line oral antituberculous agent cycloserine also inhibit this step.

β Lactams

β Lactam antibiotics possess a four-member nitrogen-containing β lactam ring and interfere with bacterial cell wall synthesis, principally by inhibiting the cross-linkage of the peptide side chains of the bacterial cell wall. These antibiotics are mainly bactericidal and exhibit time-dependent killing. Most are eliminated unchanged by the kidney, so they are suitable for treating urinary tract infections. β Lactams have a high therapeutic index, with the main adverse event being allergic reactions, most commonly a pruritic erythematous maculopapular rash. Rarely, beta lactams cause anaphylaxis. They are considered safe for use in pregnancy.

There are three principal mechanisms of β lactam resistance:
- The most important is enzymatic hydrolysis of the β lactam ring by β lactamases. This mechanism occurs in staphylococci, gonococci, enterobacteriaceae, and *Bacteroides fragilis*. There are many β lactamases, which differ in their substrate specificity.

- The second most important mechanism of resistance is alteration of the target sites, called penicillin-binding proteins. Alteration in a specific penicillin-binding protein is the principal mechanism of resistance in methicillin-resistant staphylococci, as well as penicillin-resistant pneumococci.
- A third mechanism of resistance is through reduced permeability in Gram-negative cell membranes.

There are four subclasses of β lactams: penicillins, cephalosporins, carbapenems, and monobactams (Fig. 9.11).

PENICILLINS Penicillin was discovered by Alexander Fleming in 1928 as a byproduct of *Penicillium notatum*, from which its name originates. Penicillins consist of a β lactam ring fused to a five-member, sulfur-containing thiazolidine ring. Modification of the side chain at position six of the β lactam ring results in drugs with different antibacterial and pharmacologic properties. There are four classes of penicillins: standard penicillins, antistaphylococcal penicillins, aminopenicillins, and antipseudomonal penicillins (Fig. 9.12).

■ *The standard penicillins are benzylpenicillin, known as penicillin G, and phenoxymethylpenicillin, known as penicillin V*

Penicillin V (Fig. 9.13) is significantly more stable in the presence of acid than penicillin G and is therefore the preferred form of penicillin when oral administration is appropriate. Penicillin G is reserved for parenteral therapy.

In addition to crystalline penicillin G, which is used for intravenous therapy, there are two repository forms of penicillin G, which are used exclusively for intramuscular use:

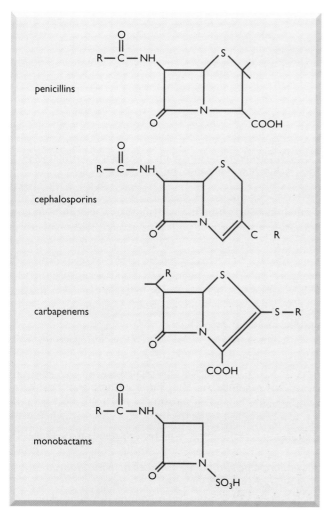

Fig. 9.11 Basic chemical structures of the four main classes of β lactam antibiotics. R denotes sites where chemical substitutions are made to create individual drugs.

Classification of penicillins	
Standard penicillins	Crystalline penicillin G (i.v.) Penicillin V (p.o.) Aqueous procaine penicillin G (i.m.) Benzathine penicillin G (i.m.)
Antistaphylococcal penicillins	Methicillin (i.v.) Nafcillin (i.v.) Isoxazolyl penicillins (i.v. or p.o.) Oxacillin Cloxacillin Dicloxacillin Floxacillin
Aminopenicillins	Ampicillin (i.v. or p.o.) Amoxicillin (p.o.)
Antipseudomonal penicillins	Carboxypenicillins Carbenicillin (i.v.) Ticarcillin (i.v.) Ureidopenicillins Piperacillin (i.v.) Azlocillin (i.v.) Mezlocillin (i.v.)

Fig. 9.12 Classification of penicillins. The four classes of penicillins are standard penicillins, antistaphylococcal penicillins, aminopenicillins, and antipseudomonal penicillins. (i.m., intramuscular; i.v., intravenous; p.o., oral)

119

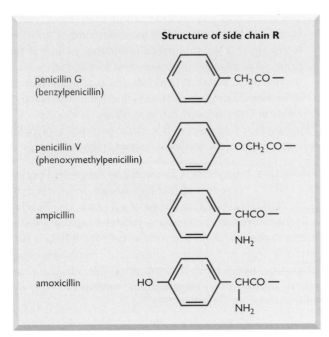

Fig. 9.13 Chemical structure of the side chain at position six of the β lactam ring of the standard penicillins and aminopenicillins.

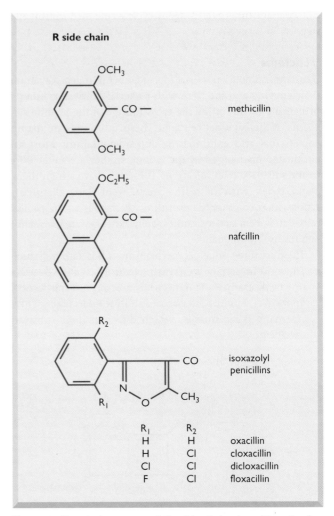

Fig. 9.14 Chemical structure of the side chain at position six of the β lactam ring of the antistaphylococcal penicillins.

- Aqueous procaine penicillin G (APPG) is a mixture of procaine and penicillin. The procaine delays the absorption of the penicillin, resulting in therapeutic blood concentrations for approximately 12 h.
- The other repository penicillin is benzathine penicillin G, which contains penicillin G and an ammonium base. Benzathine penicillin G results in low but detectable serum concentrations of penicillin G for up to 1 month and is principally used in the treatment of syphilis, excluding neurosyphilis. It is also used to prevent recurrences of rheumatic fever.

Penicillin remains the drug of choice for streptococcal and meningococcal infections, syphilis, and infections due to *Pasteurella multocida*, although there is some resistance in streptococci, notably *S. pneumoniae*, and meningococci in some parts of the world.

Penicillin is useful in combination with an aminoglycoside in the treatment of infections due to enterococci and *Listeria monocytogenes*. It also remains an important drug in the treatment of dental infections, including actinomycosis, since most oral bacteria are susceptible to penicillin.

When penicillin G is given in a large dosage intravenously, cerebrospinal fluid concentrations are adequate for treating neurosyphilis and meningitis due to susceptible strains of *S. pneumoniae* and *Neisseria meningitidis*.

Antistaphylococcal penicillins are stable to staphylococcal β lactamase

Shortly after the introduction of penicillin into clinical use, most strains of staphylococci became resistant to penicillin by producing penicillinase (β lactamase). Subsequently, several penicillins were developed that are stable to the staphylococcal β lactamase (Fig. 9.14). The first of these antistaphylococcal

penicillins was methicillin, a drug that is seldom used now because it is associated with a relatively high incidence of allergic interstitial nephritis. Instead, either nafcillin or one of the isoxazolyl penicillins is preferred. The isoxazolyl penicillins are based on the parent drug oxacillin. The substitution of a chlorine atom, two chlorine atoms, and a chlorine plus a fluorine atom, in place of hydrogen, results in cloxacillin, dicloxacillin, and flucloxacillin, respectively.

Nafcillin and isoxazolyl penicillins are used to treat staphylococcal infections, but are not active against methicillin-resistant strains. The antimicrobial activity of the four isoxazolyl penicillins is similar, but they differ in their oral absorption, with oxacillin being considerably less well absorbed than the other three. Nafcillin, which is not an isoxazolyl penicillin, is not well absorbed orally and is reserved for parenteral use (Fig. 9.7).

Aminopenicillins have enhanced activity against aerobic Gram-negative bacilli

The addition of an amino group on the penicillin side chain results in the aminopenicillins, which have enhanced activity against aerobic Gram-negative bacilli but, like standard penicillins, are not stable to staphylococcal β lactamase. Specifically, aminopenicillins are active against many strains of E. coli, Proteus mirabilis, and approximately 70% of H. influenzae strains. Amino-penicillins are active against some strains of Salmonella and Shigella species. They are also slightly more active than penicillin G against enterococci and L. monocytogenes, but both drugs are only bacteriostatic against these organisms without the addition of an aminoglycoside.

The two most important aminopenicillins are ampicillin and amoxicillin (see Fig. 9.13). Ampicillin is preferred for intra-venous therapy and amoxicillin for oral therapy because of its better oral bioavailability.

Aminopenicillins are used for community-acquired respiratory tract infections because of their activity against S. pneumoniae and H. influenzae. Amoxicillin can be used to treat uncomplicated urinary tract infection, but trimethoprim–sulfamethoxazole is generally preferred, owing to its greater efficacy. Intravenous ampicillin is often used in conjunction with gentamicin in the treatment of infections due to enterococci and L. monocytogenes. Large intravenous doses of ampicillin result in cerebrospinal fluid concentrations that are adequate to treat meningitis due to susceptible strains of S. pneumoniae, N. meningitidis, and H. influenzae.

Antipseudomonal penicillins are extended spectrum aminopenicillins

The antipseudomonal penicillins are best thought of as extended spectrum aminopenicillins, since they generally possess the same spectrum of activity as aminopenicillins plus additional activity against aerobic Gram-negative bacilli including Pseudomonas aeruginosa. They are not stable against staphylococcal β lactamase.

There are two subclasses of antipseudomonal penicillins, based on the chemical structure of the side chain: carboxy-penicillins and ureidopenicillins (Fig. 9.15). The carboxypenicillins are carbenicillin and ticarcillin, while piperacillin, mezlocillin and azlocillin are ureidopenicillins. The ureidopenicillins have generally replaced carboxypenicillins, owing to their broader spectrum of activity and lower sodium content. Piperacillin is also active against anaerobic bacteria, including B. fragilis.

The antipseudomonal penicillins are used parenterally in clinical settings where infection due to P. aeruginosa has either been confirmed or is suspected.

CEPHALOSPORINS The first cephalosporin was discovered in 1945 by Giuseppe Brotzu from the mold Cephalosporium acremonium. Cephalosporins consist of a β lactam ring fused to a six-member sulfur-containing dihydrothiazine ring. Individual cephalosporins are created by side-chain substitutions at position seven of the β lactam ring and position three of the dihydrothiazine ring (see Fig. 9.11).

Cephalosporins are traditionally classified into first-, second-, and third-generation drugs based on their spectrum against aerobic Gram-negative bacilli, which increases from first to

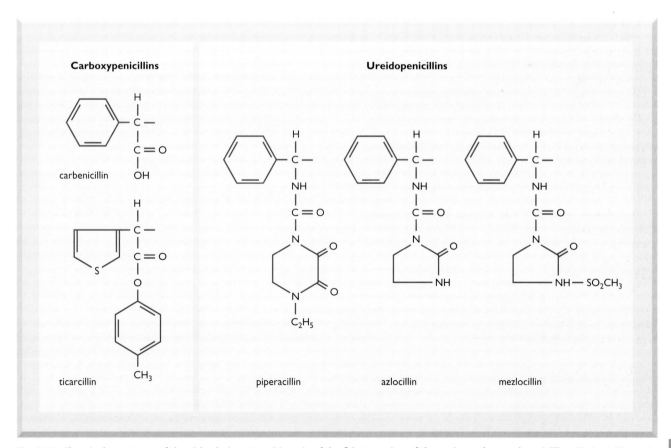

Fig. 9.15 Chemical structures of the side chains at position six of the β lactam ring of the antipseudomonal penicillins. Carbenicillin and ticarcillin are carboxypenicillins whereas piperacillin, azlocillin and mezlocillin are ureidopenicillins.

third generation (Fig. 9.16). In addition, the antistaphylococcal activity decreases from first to third generation, although there is no loss in antistreptococcal activity. Virtually all cephalosporins are stable to staphylococcal β lactamase and all have activity against aerobic Gram-negative bacilli superior to that of aminopenicillins. Unlike penicillins, cephalosporins are not active against either enterococci or *L. monocytogenes* but, like antistaphylococcal penicillins, they are not active against methicillin-resistant staphylococci.

Although cephalosporins are structurally related to penicillins, there is only approximately 10% cross-allergenicity between the two families of drugs. Accordingly, cephalosporins can often be safely used in individuals with penicillin allergy. In general, cephalosporins should be avoided in patients who have shown IgE-mediated penicillin allergy, but can usually be safely used in patients with non-IgE-mediated allergic reactions to penicillin such as a maculopapular rash.

First-generation cephalosporins are useful for skin and soft tissue infections

First-generation cephalosporins are active against streptococci, staphylococci, *E. coli*, *P. mirabilis*, and *Klebsiella pneumoniae*. They are useful in skin and soft tissue infections since these are usually due to *Streptococcus pyogenes* and/or *S. aureus*, and are commonly used as prophylaxis against infection following surgical procedures. First-generation cephalosporins are also used as alternatives to penicillins in penicillin-allergic individuals to treat infections that would otherwise be treated with penicillin

Classification of cephalosporins

First generation	Cefadroxil (p.o.), cefazolin, cephalexin (p.o.), cephalothin, cephapirin, cephradine (i.v./p.o.)
Second generation with *Haemophilus influenzae* activity	Cefaclor (p.o.), cefamandole, cefonicid, ceforanide, cefprozil (p.o.), cefuroxime, cefuroxime axetil (p.o.)
Second generation with *Bacteroides fragilis* activity	Cefmetazole, cefotetan, cefoxitin
Third generation	Cefotaxime, ceftriaxone, ceftizoxime, cefoperazone, moxalactam
Third generation with *Pseudomonas aeruginosa* activity	Ceftazidime, cefepime
Oral broad-spectrum	Cefixime, cefpodoxime proxecil

Fig. 9.16 Classification of cephalosporins. This classification was based on their spectrum of activity against aerobic Gram-negative bacilli, which increases from first to third generation. The drugs are available only parenterally unless indicated otherwise. (i.v., intravenous; p.o., oral)

First-generation cephalosporins

• Are active against streptococci and staphylococci but not enterococci

• Are active against most *Escherichia coli*, *Proteus mirabilis*, and *Klebsiella pneumoniae*

G, an aminopenicillin, or an antistaphylococcal penicillin. Cefazolin is the most frequently used parenteral agent.

There are two subtypes of second-generation cephalosporins
The two subtypes of second-generation cephalosporins are:
• Those with activity against *H. influenzae*.
• Those with activity against *B. fragilis*.

Second-generation cephalosporins with activity against *H. influenzae* are active against strains of *H. influenzae* whether or not they produce β lactamase, which inactives aminopenicillins. However, they do not achieve adequate concentrations in the cerebrospinal fluid to kill *H. influenzae* reliably, unlike third-generation cephalosporins. Otherwise, their activity is similar to that of first-generation cephalosporins. These drugs are commonly used in the empiric treatment of community-acquired respiratory tract infections in which either *S. pneumoniae* or *H. influenzae* may be a pathogen (e.g. sinusitis, otitis media, pneumonia). These drugs are also useful for the empiric treatment of a variety of infections in children in which streptococci, *S. aureus*, and *H. influenzae* may be pathogens except for meningitis.

Second-generation cephalosporins with activity against *B. fragilis* are generally used in the treatment of mixed aerobic–anaerobic infections, which are usually intra-abdominal, but are occasionally ischemic skin and soft tissue infections, such as infected lower limb cutaneous ulcers in people with diabetes mellitus.

Third-generation cephalosporins have markedly increased activity against aerobic Gram-negative bacilli
Compared with first- and second-generation cephalosporins, third-generation cephalosporins have markedly increased activity against aerobic Gram-negative bacilli, particularly Enterobacteriaceae and *H. influenzae*. They are stable to the β lactamase that can be produced by *H. influenzae* and *N. gonorrhoeae*, and to many of the β lactamases produced by Enterobacteriaceae, with the important exception of the type I chromosome-mediated inducible cephalosporinase, which may be produced by *Enterobacter cloacae*, *E. aerogenes*, *Citrobacter freundii*, *Serratia marcescens*, and *P. aeruginosa*. Therefore it is generally recommended that third-generation cephalosporins are not used as monotherapy for infections due to these pathogens.

In general, third-generation cephalosporins have reduced activity against *S. aureus* compared with first- and second-generation cephalosporins. A few third-generation cephalosporins, particularly ceftazidime, are active against *P. aeruginosa*.

An important property of the third-generation cephalosporins is that they achieve adequate concentrations in cerebrospinal fluid to be bactericidal against Enterobacteriaceae and the three major bacterial meningeal pathogens (i.e. *S. pneumoniae*, *N. meningitidis*, and *H. influenzae*).

Third-generation cephalosporins are important drugs for treating bacterial meningitis. They are also useful for treating serious infections such as nosocomial pneumonia due to aerobic Gram-negative bacilli, particularly when aminoglycosides are contraindicated.

Oral extended spectrum cephalosporins can be used to treat Enterobacteriaceae infections resistant to other oral β lactams

Over the last few years, a variety of oral extended spectrum cephalosporins have become available. These drugs are sometimes called oral third-generation cephalosporins, but have considerably less activity against aerobic Gram-negative bacilli than parenteral third-generation cephalosporins. None of the oral agents is active against *P. aeruginosa* and some (cefixime, ceftibuten) are inactive against *S. aureus*. These drugs can provide an oral option for treating infections due to Enterobacteriaceae resistant to other oral β lactams.

CARBAPENEMS Carbapenems consist of a β lactam ring fused with a five-member carbon-containing penem ring (see Fig. 9.11). The carbapenems currently available in the US are imipenem and meropenem.

Carbapenems have the broadest spectrum of all available antibiotics

Carbapenems are stable to most β lactamases and active against streptococci, staphylococci, Enterobacteriaceae, *P. aeruginosa*, *Haemophilus* species and anaerobic bacteria, including *B. fragilis*. Carbapenems are active against many strains of *Enterococcus faecalis*, but not against other species of *Enterococcus*. Like cephalosporins, they are not active against *L. monocytogenes* or methicillin-resistant staphylococci.

Imipenem is broken down in the kidney by a human β lactamase called dehydropeptidase-1 to a nephrotoxic metabolite. It is therefore always co-administered with the drug cilastatin, which is a specific inhibitor of the renal β lactamase. The commercial preparation contains a fixed ratio of imipenem to cilastatin. Meropenem is not broken down by renal dehydropeptidase and does not require concomitant cilastatin. Imipenem can cause seizures in susceptible individuals, particularly those with concomitant renal insufficiency. Meropenem, but not imipenem, can be used to treat bacterial meningitis. Carbapenems are particularly useful for treating infections due to bacteria resistant to other antibiotics. Because of their very broad spectrum of activity, they are also used to treat polymicrobial infections instead of using two or more other antibiotics.

MONOBACTAMS The name monobactam is short for monocyclic β lactam. Monobactams consist of a single ring structure, the β lactam ring, attached to a sulfonic acid group (see Fig. 9.11).

The only available monobactam is aztreonam

The only available monobactam is aztreonam, which is active only against aerobic Gram-negative bacilli including *P. aeruginosa*. Unlike other β lactams, it has no activity against Gram-positive bacteria. Aztreonam also lacks activity against anaerobes. It is available only for parenteral use.

A novel property of aztreonam is that it is essentially nonallergenic and can be used in individuals with penicillin and cephalosporin allergy.

β LACTAMASE INHIBITORS Several specific inhibitors of bacterial β lactamases have been developed for clinical use, specifically the agents clavulanate, sulbactam, and tazobactam. These drugs contain a β lactam ring (Fig. 9.17), but none has clinically useful intrinsic antibacterial activity. They act by covalently binding bacterial β lactamase, allowing β lactam drugs that would otherwise be destroyed by the β lactamase to exert their antibacterial effect. None of the β lactamase inhibitors is available for use on its own. They are only available in a fixed-dose combination with a penicillin (Fig. 9.18).

The β lactamase inhibitors inhibit most of the important bacterial β lactamases, including those produced by staphylococci, gonococci, *H. influenzae*, *B. fragilis*, and some Enterobacteriaceae. However, they do not inhibit the type I chromosome-mediated

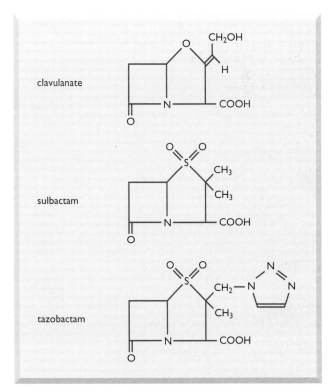

Fig. 9.17 Chemical structures of three β lactamase inhibitors: clavulanate, sulbactam, and tazobactam. Note that all three contain a β lactam ring, but none has significant antibacterial activity clinically alone. They are used in combination with aminopenicillins and antipseudomonal penicillins.

Fig. 9.18 Penicillin–β lactam inhibitor combinations. β Lactamase inhibitors are not available for use on their own, but are available in fixed-dose combinations with a penicillin. (i.v., intravenous; p.o., oral)

inducible cephalosporinase, which can hydrolyze all cephalosporins, including third-generation cephalosporins.

Penicillin–β lactamase inhibitor combinations are useful for polymicrobial infections where the use of a single commercial product (albeit containing two drugs) may obviate the need for two or more agents. In practice, they are most frequently used in the treatment of intra-abdominal infections, bite-wound infections and infected cutaneous ulcers.

Glycopeptides

■ *Glycopeptides are high molecular weight drugs consisting of sugars and amino acids*

Vancomycin is currently the only glycopeptide available in the US, but teicoplanin is available in parts of Europe. Vancomycin is a predominantly bactericidal antibiotic that inhibits bacterial cell wall synthesis by covalently binding to the terminal two D-alanine residues at the free carboxyl end of the pentapeptide, thereby sterically hindering the elongation of the peptidoglycan backbone (Fig. 9.19). In contrast, β lactams inhibit a later stage of cell wall synthesis by blocking the cross-linkage of pentapeptide side chains. Owing to its high molecular weight,

vancomycin is unable to penetrate the cell membrane of Gram-negative bacteria and its activity is confined to Gram-positive bacteria.

Vancomycin is not absorbed from the digestive tract and is therefore used intravenously for most indications, but can be given by mouth to treat intestinal infection due to *Clostridium difficile*. When infused rapidly, vancomycin causes histamine release, resulting in an erythematous rash that is usually confined to the neck and upper trunk. This phenomenon is called the red neck syndrome and can be mistaken for allergy. It is prevented if vancomycin is infused slowly. Vancomycin is excreted unchanged by the kidney.

Because vancomycin does not contain a β lactam ring and binds to peptide side chains rather than to penicillin-binding proteins, vancomycin is unaffected by β lactamase production or penicillin-binding protein alteration. It is therefore useful in the treatment of b-lactam-resistant Gram-positive infections. Acquired vancomycin resistance is uncommon, is usually confined to *E. faecium*, and due to an altered target (pentapeptide side chain).

THERAPEUTIC INDICATIONS Vancomycin is useful in the treatment of infections caused by streptococci, staphylococci, enterococci, *Corynebacterium jeikeium* and *C. difficile*. It is the drug of choice for infections caused by methicillin-resistant staphylococci and high-level penicillin-resistant pneumococci. Vancomycin is frequently used as an alternative to β lactams in patients with serious β lactam allergy as there is no cross-reactivity between vancomycin and β lactams.

Vancomycin is very effective orally in the treatment of *C. difficile* enteritis, though metronidazole is usually preferred for this indication because of its markedly lower cost.

Vancomycin enters the cerebrospinal fluid in concentrations that are close to the MBC of streptococci and staphylococci, but clinical experience with vancomycin in the treatment of bacterial meningitis is limited. Vancomycin should not, therefore, be used in the treatment of meningitis unless the pathogen is resistant to third-generation cephalosporins and chloramphenicol.

Antibiotics that inhibit bacterial cell membrane functioning

Polymyxin B and polymyxin E (also known as colistimethate) are octapeptides of high molecular weight that injure the plasma membranes of Gram-negative bacteria, resulting in a bactericidal effect. Because of their considerable toxicity when given systemically, their use is mainly confined to topical therapy of infections due to aerobic Gram-negative bacilli. Colistimethate is used intravenously only to treat serious infections due to aerobic Gram-negative bacilli resistant to all other systemic agents.

Antibiotics that inhibit bacterial protein synthesis

Several major classes of antibiotics act principally by inhibiting bacterial protein synthesis (Fig. 9.20). These drugs exhibit selective toxicity by inhibiting bacterial protein synthesis to a

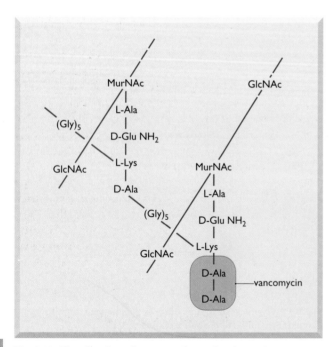

Fig. 9.19 Site of action of vancomycin on the elongating peptidoglycan polymer in bacterial cell walls.

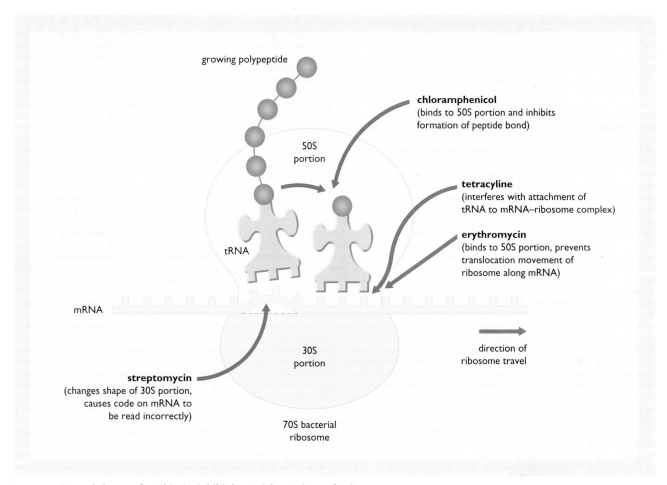

Fig. 9.20 Several classes of antibiotics inhibit bacterial protein synthesis.

much greater extent than they inhibit host cell protein synthesis, as a result of binding to specific bacterial targets. Most of these drugs are predominantly bacteriostatic, except for the amino-glycosides and oxazolidinones, which are bactericidal.

Aminoglycosides

Aminoglycosides consist of two or more amino sugars linked by glycosidic bonds to an aminocyclitol ring. They enter bacterial cells via an oxygen-dependent transport system, which is not present in anaerobic bacteria or streptococci. Accordingly, anaerobes and streptococci are innately resistant to amino-glycosides. Once inside the bacterial cell, aminoglycosides bind irreversibly to sites on the ribosome, inhibiting protein synthesis. There is also at least one other mechanism of action that is not currently understood, which probably accounts for their bactericidal activity.

Aminoglycosides are active against aerobic Gram-negative bacilli, staphylococci, and mycobacteria. Although they are not intrinsically active against either enterococci or L. monocytogenes, the addition of an aminoglycoside to penicillin G, ampicillin, or vancomycin is often synergistic and usually results in bactericidal activity.

The two principal mechanisms of acquired bacterial resist-ance to aminoglycosides are:

- Reduced bacterial permeability caused by alterations in the bacterial cell membrane.
- Production of a variety of aminoglycoside-modifying enzymes.

Aminoglycoside-modifying enzymes, which are non-hydrolytic, add acetyl, adenyl, or phosphoryl groups to the aminoglycoside, rendering them incapable of reaching their target sites on the bacterial ribosome. Each aminoglycoside-modifying enzyme has a different substrate specificity and may modify only some aminoglycosides. Accordingly, bacteria may be resistant to one aminoglycoside and not to another.

The aminoglycosides available in the US are listed in Fig. 9.21.

Aminoglycosides are not absorbed from the digestive tract and must be used parenterally to obtain a systemic effect. They are excreted unchanged by the kidney and are suitable for treat-ing urinary tract infections. They do not enter the cerebrospinal fluid in therapeutically relevant concentrations, except in neonates.

Aminoglycosides have two major toxicities

The two major toxicities of aminoglycosides are nephrotoxicity and ototoxicity (both auditory and vestibular). The risk of these toxicities is both dose- and duration-dependent. Nephrotoxicity

Aminoglycosides currently available in the US, their route of administration, and their use

Agent	Routes	Comment
Streptomycin	i.m. (i.v.)	For tuberculosis, plague, tularemia, severe brucellosis, some gentamicin-resistant enterococci
Neomycin	p.o.	Used to reduce the load of Enterobacteriaceae in the bowel and to treat hepatic encephalopathy, or with erythromycin as prophylaxis in elective colorectal surgery
Paromomycin	p.o.	For certain intestinal protozoa
Kanamycin	i.v./i.m.	Rarely used, owing to bacterial resistance
Gentamicin	i.v./i.m.	The 'workhorse' aminoglycoside; used for Enterobacteriaceae, *Pseudomonas aeruginosa*, enterococci
Netilmicin	i.v./i.m.	Similar to effect of gentamicin against Enterobacteriaceae and *P. aeruginosa*; poor synergistic activity against enterococci
Tobramycin	i.v./i.m.	Similar to effect of gentamicin against Enterobacteriaceae; more active than gentamicin against *P. aeruginosa*; poor synergistic activity against enterococci
Amikacin	i.v./i.m.	Aminoglycoside least affected by aminoglycoside-modifying enzymes; good activity against Enterobacteriaceae and *P. aeruginosa*; the most active against mycobacteria; poor synergistic activity against enterococci; the most expensive aminoglycoside

Fig. 9.21 Aminoglycosides currently available in the US, their route of administration, and their use. (i.m., intramuscular, i.v., intravenous; p.o., oral)

is more common, but is usually mild and reversible. Ototoxicity is often permanent (see Chapter 25). Because aminoglycosides are more toxic than most other antibiotics and must be given parenterally, their use is largely limited to serious infections due to Enterobacteriaceae and *P. aeruginosa*, and usually limited to the hospital setting. Aminoglycosides are also used in conjunction with penicillin, ampicillin, or vancomycin in the treatment of serious infections due to enterococci and *L. monocytogenes*. Because of their potential toxicity, serum aminoglycoside concentrations are often monitored, but toxicity can occur even with 'ideal' serum concentrations.

■ *Gentamicin is the most frequently used aminoglycoside*
Gentamicin is the most active aminoglycoside for synergy against enterococci (i.e. it is the 'workhorse' aminoglycoside). Tobramycin is usually more active than gentamicin against *P. aeruginosa*, but no more active against Enterobacteriaceae, and unlikely to be synergistic against enterococci. Ophthalmic preparations of gentamicin and tobramycin are available.

■ *Streptomycin can be used as part of a multi-drug regimen for tuberculosis*
Not only can streptomycin be used as part of a multi-drug regimen for the treatment of tuberculosis, but it is also the drug of choice in plague and tularemia, although recent evidence suggests that gentamicin is equally effective for these two infections. Streptomycin demonstrates synergy with penicillin, ampicillin, or vancomycin in the treatment of a few enterococcal strains for which gentamicin does not. Streptomycin plus doxycycline is used to treat brucellosis.

THERAPEUTIC INDICATIONS Amikacin is the aminoglycoside least susceptible to aminoglycoside-modifying enzymes and is sometimes active against bacteria that are resistant to other aminoglycosides.

Neomycin is no longer used parenterally because of its lower efficacy and greater toxicity than other aminoglycosides. It can be used orally to reduce the intestinal load of Enterobacteriaceae (without a systemic effect) in the treatment of hepatic encephalopathy, or, in combination with erythromycin, as a prophylactic regimen to reduce the incidence of wound infection following elective colorectal surgery.

Kanamycin is rarely used, owing to acquired resistance.

Paromomycin, which is related to neomycin, is used only orally to treat intestinal protozoal infections.

Macrolides, lincosamides, and streptogramins
Macrolides, lincosamides, and streptogramins (MLS drugs) are chemically unrelated but possess similar mechanisms of action, resistance, and antimicrobial activity. They reversibly bind to the 50S ribosomal subunit and so block the translocation

Aminoglycosides

- Are not absorbed orally
- Are active aerobic Gram-negative bacilli
- Demonstrate concentration-dependent killing
- Cause nephrotoxicity and ototoxicity (their major adverse effects)

reaction. Although classically considered as bacteriostatic antibiotics, they are bactericidal against specific isolates. The principal mechanism of acquired resistance is a specific mutation in the ribosomal ribonucleic acid (RNA) of the 50S ribosomal subunit. Resistance to one member of the MLS class does not necessarily imply resistance to others.

Macrolides are named after the macrocyclic lactone ring that forms the nucleus for these drugs

The prototypic macrolide is erythromycin, which is available in different salts. In recent years, several newer macrolides have been introduced in the US, including clarithromycin, azithromycin, and dirithromycin. Other macrolides are available in Europe and Asia. Macrolides are usually given orally, although intravenous forms of erythromycin and azithromycin are available, and erythromycin lotion can be used in the treatment of acne vulgaris. Macrolides are metabolized in the liver and do not penetrate the cerebrospinal fluid in therapeutically relevant concentrations.

Erythromycin is active against streptococci, staphylococci, Bordetella pertussis, Corynebacterium diphtheriae, Campylobacter jejuni, Mycoplasma pneumoniae, Ureaplasma urealyticum, Legionella species and Chlamydia species. Erythromycin and dirithromycin have weak activity against H. influenzae, but both clarithromycin and azithromycin have considerably better activity against this organism. Macrolides are not active against Enterobacteriaceae, P. aeruginosa, or Mycoplasma hominis.

Macrolides are used primarily in the treatment of respiratory tract infections. They are alternatives to penicillin for treating streptococcal pharyngitis, especially in patients who are allergic to penicillin.

Macrolides are the drugs of choice for community-acquired pneumonia as they are active against pneumococci, M. pneumoniae, C. pneumoniae and Legionella species. In cases where infection may be due to H. influenzae, clarithromycin or azithromycin are preferred. Erythromycin is:

- The drug of choice for the treatment of pertussis.
- Equivalent to penicillin in eradicating the carrier state in diphtheria.
- The drug of choice for legionnaires' disease.
- Equivalent to tetracycline in the treatment of M. pneumoniae infections.
- The co-drug of choice for C. jejuni enteritis.
- The drug of choice for treating infections due to Chlamydia trachomatis in pregnancy, when tetracyclines are contraindicated.

Macrolides can be used as an alternative to β lactams for mild skin and soft tissue infections due to S. pyogenes and S. aureus.

Erythromycin causes gastrointestinal adverse effects

Erythromycin is probably the single most poorly tolerated oral antibiotic, owing to dyspepsia, nausea and vomiting. It interacts with motilin receptors to increase gastrointestinal motility and has been used successfully in the treatment of diabetic gastroparesis. The newer macrolides clarithromycin and azithromycin produce less severe gastrointestinal adverse effects than erythromycin, and may be suitable for individuals who have demonstrated gastrointestinal intolerance to erythromycin.

Erythromycin and clarithromycin interact with other drugs

Erythromycin elevates serum theophylline concentrations when given concomitantly. In combination with the nonsedating histamine-H_1 antagonists astemizole or terfenadine, or the promotility drug cisapride, erythromycin and clarithromycin can lead to significant prolongation of the QT interval in the electrocardiogram. This can result in the torsades de pointes variant of ventricular tachycardia, which can be fatal.

Clarithromycin and azithromycin are more active than erythromycin against some pathogens

Clarithromycin and azithromycin, but not dirithromycin, are more active than erythromycin against H. influenzae and are more appropriate choices for the empiric treatment of respiratory tract infections if H. influenzae is a possible pathogen.

Both clarithromycin and azithromycin are active against Mycobacterium avium complex, an important pathogen in patients with acquired immunodeficiency syndrome (AIDS). Clarithromycin is useful in the treatment of most other nontuberculous mycobacteria. It is also very active against Helicobacter pylori and is routinely used in a multi-drug regimen to treat duodenal ulcer caused by H. pylori. Azithromycin is active against C. trachomatis and is the only drug that can cure C. trachomatis urethritis and cervicitis in a single dose.

KETOLIDES Recently, a series of modified macrolides have been synthesized in which the cladinose at position 3 of the macrolactone ring has been replaced by a keto group. These modified macrolides are called ketolides, and the first agent in this class is telithromycin. The major difference between ketolides and macrolides is that ketolides are much more resistant to the principal mechanism of MLS resistance in Streptococcus pneumoniae, so that the majority of macrolide-resistant pneumococci remain susceptible to ketolides. Otherwise, ketolides are similar to the newer macrolides clarithromycin and azithromycin.

LINCOSAMIDES Lincomycin and clindamycin are the two available lincosamides. Lincomycin is named after Lincoln, Nebraska where it was first isolated from the mold Streptomycin linconensis. The replacement of an hydroxyl group by a chlorine atom led to clindamycin. Since clindamycin has greater activity and superior oral bioavailability, it has supplanted lincomycin in clinical use.

Clindamycin is active against streptococci, staphylococci, and anaerobic bacteria, including B. fragilis. It is also active against Mycoplasma hominis, but not M. pneumoniae or U. urealyticum. It has no useful activity against enterococci or aerobic Gram-negative bacilli. Clindamycin is also active against several protozoa.

Clindamycin can be given either orally or intravenously. There is also a topical solution for the treatment of acne vulgaris and a vaginal cream for the treatment of bacterial vaginosis. Clindamycin is metabolized by the liver and does not penetrate the cerebrospinal fluid.

Clindamycin is an important antibiotic in the treatment of anaerobic infections, particularly in mixed aerobic–anaerobic infections where it is usually used in combination with other antibiotics. It can also be used as an alternative to β lactams in people who are allergic to β lactams, particularly if the oral route is appropriate.

Clindamycin is associated with a higher risk of *Clostridium difficile* enteritis than other antibiotics.

STREPTOGRAMINS Streptogramins consist of a natural combination of two chemically unrelated groups of molecules, referred to as groups A and B. Pristinamycin is such a combination, which has been available in Europe for many years as an oral antistaphylococcal agent, but it is not available in the US.

Quinupristin–dalfopristin (Synercid) is an intravenous streptogramin consisting of a 30:70 ratio of quinupristin to dalfopristin, which was introduced into clinical use in the late 1990s. This combination is active against staphylococci (including methicillin-resistant staphylococci), streptococci (including penicillin-resistant pneumococci), and *Enterococcus faecium* (but not most *Enterococcus faecalis*). Quinupristin–dalfopristin is rapidly cleared by nonrenal mechanisms, but there is a long post-antibiotic effect against the target organisms *Staphylococcus aureus*, *Streptococcus pneumoniae* and *Enterococcus faecium*, so that twice-daily dosing is clinically effective. Its major toxicity is infusion-related phlebitis, which can be avoided if the drug is administered via a central venous catheter.

The major clinical indication for quinupristin–dalfopristin is the treatment of infections due to vancomycin-resistant *Enterococcus faecium*, and as an alternative to vancomycin in the treatment of infections due to methicillin-resistant staphylococci.

Tetracyclines

Tetracyclines are moderately broad spectrum, primarily bacteriostatic antibiotics that have a nucleus of four fused cyclic rings (Fig. 9.22), hence the name tetracyclines. Specific agents are derived from substitutions at positions five, six, and seven of the tetracycline nucleus.

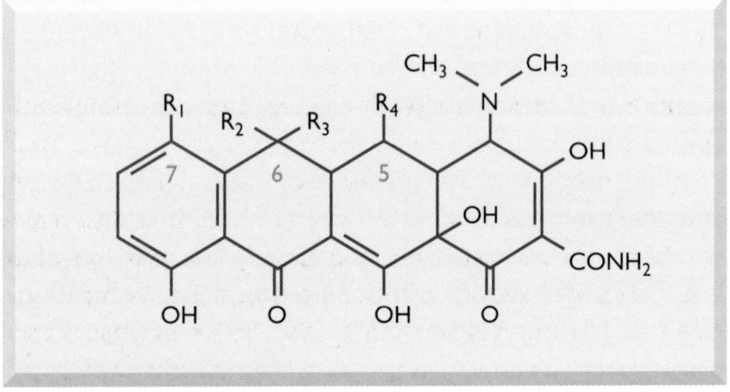

As tetracyclines are concentrated intracellularly, they are useful for intracellular infections. They are excreted mainly by the kidneys and do not achieve therapeutic concentrations in cerebrospinal fluid. They are usually used orally but intravenous preparations are available, as well as a topical formulation for acne vulgaris.

Of the six tetracyclines commercially available in the US, only three are used with any frequency: tetracycline, doxycycline, and minocycline. Tetracycline is a short-acting drug that is usually administered four times daily, whereas both doxycycline and minocycline have long half-lifes, allowing once- or twice-daily administration.

Tetracyclines reversibly bind to the 30S ribosomal subunit in such a manner that they block the binding of transfer RNA to the messenger RNA–ribosome complex, preventing the addition of new amino acids to the growing peptide chain (see Fig. 9.20). Acquired tetracycline resistance is usually due to changes in the transport mechanism, resulting in a lack of tetracycline accumulation within the bacterial cell.

▪ *Tetracyclines are chelated by divalent or trivalent cations* Absorption is therefore markedly decreased when these drugs are taken orally in conjunction with calcium-, magnesium-, and aluminum-containing antacids, dairy products, calcium supplementation, or sucralfate.

Although tetracyclines are active against a wide variety of bacteria, the important organisms against which they are consistently active include chlamydiae, mycoplasmas, spirochetes (including those that cause leptospirosis, Lyme disease, and relapsing fever), rickettsial infections, *Legionella* species and *Brucella* species. Tetracyclines, particularly minocycline, are also effective in the treatment of acne vulgaris.

Tetracyclines have a strong affinity for developing bone and teeth, to which they give a yellow–brown color. They are therefore contraindicated in pregnant and breastfeeding women, as well as in children under eight years of age.

Amphenicols

Chloramphenicol (Fig. 9.23) is the only amphenicol available in the US. The related drug, thiamphenicol, is available in parts of Europe. Chloramphenicol is a relatively broad spectrum, predominantly bacteriostatic antibiotic that reversibly binds to the 50S ribosomal subunit to prevent the attachment of the amino acid-containing end of transfer RNA to the peptide chain (i.e. it blocks peptidyl transferase) (see Fig. 9.20).

Acquired chloramphenicol resistance results from either:
• Reduced bacterial permeability.

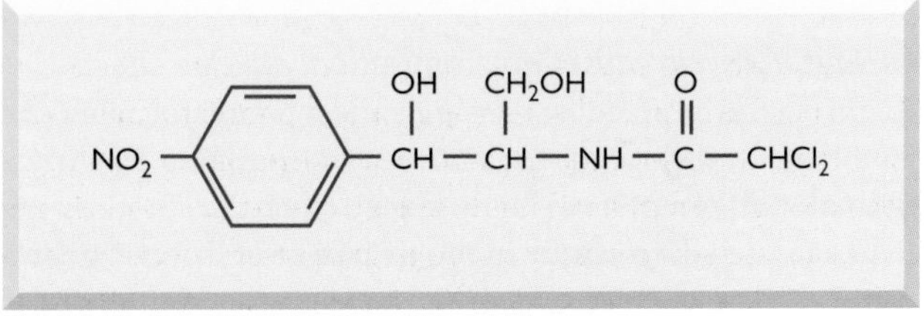

Fig. 9.22 Chemical structure of tetracylines. Substitutions at positions five, six, and seven result in different drugs, including the three common agents tetracycline, doxycycline, and minocycline.

Fig. 9.23 Chemical structure of chloramphenicol.

- Production of the chloramphenicol-modifying enzyme, chloramphenicol acetyltransferase.

Chloramphenicol is available both orally and parenterally as well as in a topical ophthalmic preparation.

▓ Chloramphenicol's main adverse effect is hematologic

Chloramphenicol exerts a dose-dependent myelosuppression, which is common and reversible. Approximately 1 in 30,000 recipients develop irreversible aplastic anemia. Although this idiosyncratic reaction is rare, it is the major reason why chloramphenicol is seldom used in developed countries. Chloramphenicol is more widely used in developing countries because of its low price, broad spectrum of activity, and efficacy in enteric fever. Chloramphenicol enters the cerebrospinal fluid in therapeutically effective concentrations for the three principal bacterial meningeal pathogens (i.e. S. pneumoniae, N. meningitidis and H. influenzae), but not for Enterobacteriaceae. Chloramphenicol also enters brain parenchyma in concentrations sufficient to be useful in the treatment of brain abscess.

▓ Chloramphenicol is conjugated in the liver to its inactive glucuronide

Neonates are less able to conjugate chloramphenicol; this sometimes results in high serum chloramphenicol concentrations, with resultant toxicity. Such toxicity is manifest as the gray baby syndrome, which is characterized by abdominal distension, vomiting, cyanosis, and circulatory collapse. If chloramphenicol must be used in neonates, serum concentrations need to be monitored closely.

THERAPEUTIC INDICATIONS Chloramphenicol is seldom used in developed countries, but:

- Is an acceptable alternative for the treatment of bacterial meningitis, particularly in patients with cephalosporin allergies.
- May be used in the treatment of brain abscess or enteric fever, although a variety of Salmonella strains around the world are resistant to chloramphenicol.
- Is an alternative to tetracycline for the treatment of Rocky Mountain spotted fever.

Oxazolidinones

Oxazolidinones are the newest class of antibiotics for use in humans. They are entirely synthetic. They inhibit bacterial protein synthesis at a very early step, preceding the interaction of transfer RNA and the 30S ribosome with the initiator codon. The only oxazolidinone antibiotic currently available is linezolid, which is available in both oral and intravenous formulations. Because of its unique mechanism of action, there is no cross-resistance with other classes of antibiotics.

Linezolid is active against most important aerobic Gram-positive cocci, including staphylococci (including methicillin-resistant staphylococci), streptococci (including penicillin-resistant pneumococci) and Enterococci—both E. faecalis and E. faecium, including vancomycin-resistant enterococci. Linezolid has complete oral bioavailability and a long serum half-life. Clearance is nonrenal. Because of its high cost, linezolid is reserved for the treatment of infections due to susceptible Gram-positive cocci, which cannot be treated with other agents. Its principal use is for the treatment of vancomycin-resistant enterococci, and as an alternative to vancomycin for methicillin-resistant staphylococci.

Antibotics that inhibit bacterial deoxyribonucleic acid synthesis
Quinolones

▓ The quinolones are synthetic antibiotics that consist of a nucleus of two fused six-membered rings

The first drug of this class was nalidixic acid, which was of limited clinical value because of its relative inactivity and the rapid emergence of resistance. The addition of a fluorine atom at position six of the quinolone nucleus markedly enhances activity against Gram-negative bacteria and led to a new generation of drugs known as fluoroquinolones (Fig. 9.24).

Quinolones inhibit bacterial deoxyribonucleic acid (DNA) gyrase, the enzyme responsible for supercoiling, nicking, and sealing bacterial DNA. Acquired resistance may develop through either decreased permeability or alterations in DNA gyrase.

Fluoroquinolones are predominantly bactericidal, exhibit concentration-dependent killing, and are renally excreted. Most have excellent oral bioavailability. They penetrate the prostate in therapeutically useful amounts. Although cerebrospinal fluid concentrations appear to be therapeutic, there is very little clinical experience in the use of quinolones for meningitis and their use is not recommended for bacterial meningitis. Like tetracyclines, fluoroquinolones are chelated by divalent and trivalent cations.

Fluoroquinolones are perhaps the best tolerated of all oral antibiotics, although more expensive than most.

Fluoroquinolones are highly active against aerobic Gram-negative bacilli including Enterobacteriaceae, Haemophilus species, Moraxella catarrhalis and, in the case of ciprofloxacin, P. aeruginosa. They are active against some mycobacteria, including most strains of M. tuberculosis. 'Older' fluoroquinolones, such as norfloxacin and ciprofloxacin have weak activity against streptococci and staphylococci, and no activity against anaerobes. Some of the newer fluoroquinolones have been called 'respiratory fluroquinolones' because of improved activity against Streptococcus pneumoniae, including penicillin-resistant strains. Such fluoroquinolones include levofloxacin, gatifloxacin and moxifloxacin. Gatifloxacin and moxifloxacin are also active against anaerobic bacteria.

THERAPEUTIC INDICATIONS Fluoroquinolones are useful in the treatment of infections due to aerobic Gram-negative bacilli that are not susceptible to less expensive agents. In many instances, they will be the only oral agents active against certain aerobic Gram-negative bacilli, particularly P. aeruginosa, in which case fluoroquinolones can obviate the need for parenteral therapy. Of the currently available agents, ciprofloxacin is the most active against Gram-negative bacteria and the most commonly used. It is available in oral, parenteral, and ophthalmic formulations. The 'respiratory fluoroquinolones' can be used in the treatment of pneumonia, and may be particularly useful in

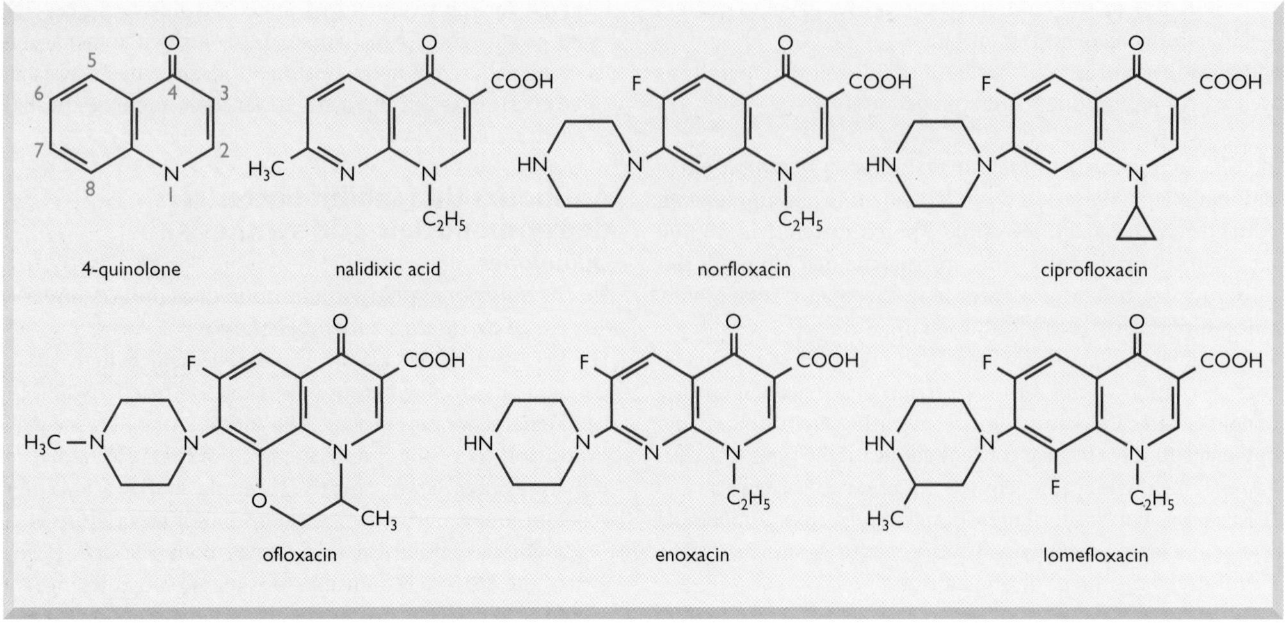

Fig. 9.24 Chemical structure of quinolone antibiotics. Note the fluorine atom at position six in the agents other than nalidixic acid. These drugs are fluoroquinolones and are much more active against aerobic Gram-negative bacilli than nalidixic acid.

🔑 Ciprofloxacin

- Is the most commonly used fluoroquinolone
- Has excellent oral bioavailability
- Is very active against aerobic Gram-negative bacilli
- Is not active against anaerobes
- Has only limited activity against streptococci and staphylococci

---

regions where there is a high prevalence of penicillin-resistant *Streptococcus pneumoniae*.

ADVERSE EFFECTS Some quinolones, including ciprofloxacin, increase serum concentrations of theophylline when given concomitantly. In addition, as fluoroquinolones cause cystic lesions in the articular cartilage of growing animals, they are relatively contraindicated in children and pregnant women.

Nitroimidazoles

Nitroimidazoles are well absorbed, predominantly bactericidal agents with antimicrobial activity restricted to strict anaerobes and certain protozoa. They can enter most bacteria but only susceptible organisms produce nitroreductase, which is needed to reduce these agents to the short-lived cytotoxic intermediates that bind to DNA and inhibit its synthesis. Aerobic bacteria are innately resistant owing to their lack of nitroreductase activity. Acquired resistance can develop as a result of either:
- Decreased uptake of the drug.
- Decreased nitroreductase production.

▪ *Metronidazole is the only nitroimidazole currently licensed in the US*

Both oral and intravenous preparations of metronidazole are available, with the oral form having close to 100% bioavailability. A topical formulation is available for the treatment of acne rosacea. Metronidazole achieves therapeutic concentrations in both cerebrospinal fluid and brain parenchyma.

Metronidazole is active against most anaerobic bacteria, but has greatest activity against Gram-negative anaerobes including B. *fragilis*. It has no activity against aerobic bacteria. It is also very effective in the treatment of three important protozoal infections: giardiasis, amebiasis, and trichomoniasis.

THERAPEUTIC INDICATIONS Metronidazole is useful in the treatment of a variety of anaerobic infections including bacterial vaginosis, which is the most common cause of abnormal vaginal discharge. In bacterial vaginosis, the bacterial flora of the vagina, which is normally dominated by *Lactobacillus* species, is replaced by an abnormal polymicrobial flora comprising predominantly anaerobes.

Metronidazole is usually considered the drug of choice for C. difficile enteritis.

In addition to its use against specific micro-organisms, metronidazole is useful in hepatic encephalopathy and in Crohn's disease, particularly with perianal involvement.

▪ *Metronidazole should be used with caution in pregnant women*

As metronidazole is mutagenic in bacteria and causes tumors in rodents, it should be used with caution in pregnant women, and its use in the first trimester should be avoided wherever possible. However, there is no evidence to date of human carcinogenicity.

Antibiotics that inhibit bacterial ribonucleic acid synthesis

Rifamycins

▪ *Rifamycin antibiotics inhibit bacterial RNA synthesis by inhibiting DNA-dependent RNA polymerase*

Acquired resistance is usually due to a mutation in the DNA-dependent RNA polymerase. Two rifamycin derivatives are currently available: rifampin and rifabutin. A third rifamycin, rifapentine, which has a very long serum half-life, is being developed.

The rifamycins are all metabolized in the liver and impart an orange color to most body fluids, especially urine.

RIFAMPIN Rifampin was originally developed for the treatment of tuberculosis and remains a mainstay of antituberculous therapy. It is also useful in the treatment of several non-tuberculous mycobacterial infections, particularly M. leprae (the cause of leprosy), M. kansasii, and M. marinum.

Rifampin is usually used orally, but an intravenous formulation is also available.

Rifampin must never be used alone for the treatment of mycobacterial infections, since acquired resistance will usually develop; it must be used in combination with at least one other antimycobacterial drug. Rifampin achieves concentrations in the cerebrospinal fluid adequate to treat tuberculous meningitis.

Rifampin is also active against a number of conventional bacteria, notably staphylococci, N. meningiditis, H. influenzae, and *Legionella pneumophila*. It is:

- The drug of choice for eliminating the nasal carriage state of N. meningiditis, H. influenzae type b, and S. aureus.
- Sometimes used as a second antistaphylococcal agent in combination with a β lactam or vancomycin in the treatment of serious staphylococcal infections, particularly endocarditis and osteomyelitis.
- Sometimes added as a second agent to erythromycin in the treatment of severe legionnaires' disease.

Rifampin may cause hepatotoxicity, a 'flu-like' syndrome, or fever (drug fever).

▪ *Rifampin is a potent inducer of hepatic microsomal enzymes*

Rifampin is a potent inducer of hepatic microsomal enzymes. As a result, the metabolism of many other drugs is increased. Such drugs include glucocorticosteroids, oral contraceptives, quinidine, phenytoin, barbiturates, theophylline, clarithromycin, ketoconazole, itraconazole, cyclosporine, and warfarin.

RIFABUTIN Rifabutin is active against most strains of M. tuberculosis, including 30% of the strains that are resistant to rifampin. It is significantly more active than rifampin against M. avium complex and is effective as a single agent in the prevention of M. avium complex bacteremia in patients with AIDS. It is also useful as part of a multi-drug combination in the treatment of established M. avium complex infection.

Although there is much more clinical experience with rifampin, rifabutin is useful in the treatment of tuberculosis as part of a multi-drug regimen.

Rifabutin is available only as an oral formulation.

In comparison with rifampin, rifabutin causes less hepatic microsomal enzyme induction, so the magnitude of the drug interactions (see above) are less than those that occur with rifampin.

Rifabutin can cause a reversible uveitis, particularly when it is used in combination with clarithromycin, which is known to increase the serum concentration of both rifabutin and rifabutin's biologically active metabolite. The antifungal drug fluconazole and the human immunodeficiency virus (HIV) protease inhibitors indinavir and ritonavir also increase serum rifabutin concentrations.

Antifolates

▪ *Folates are necessary cofactors in the synthesis of purines, and consequently of DNA*

Although mammalian cells can use exogenous preformed folate, bacteria must synthesize their own from para-aminobenzoic acid (PABA). The folate synthetic pathway is outlined in Fig. 9.25. This pathway can be antagonized at two steps, by inhibition of either dihydropteroate synthetase (DHPS) or dihydrofolate reductase (DHFR).

Sulfonamides

Sulfonamides were developed in the 1930s as the first modern anti-infective drugs. These agents compete with PABA

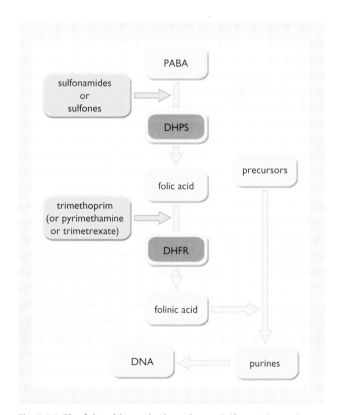

Fig. 9.25 The folate biosynthetic pathway. Sulfonamides and sulfones compete with para-aminobenzoic acid (PABA) for dihydropteroate synthetase (DHPS). Trimethoprim and the antiprotozoal drugs pyrimethamine and trimetrexate inhibit dihydrofolate reductase (DHFR).

(Figs 9.25, 9.26) for DHPS, thereby inhibiting folate synthesis. Their effect is bacteriostatic. Acquired resistance can occur as a result of:

- Decreased permeability.
- Increased PABA production.
- Altered DHPS for which the drugs lack affinity.

Although many sulfonamides were once produced, the use of sulfonamides alone is no longer recommended, owing to the relatively high rates of bacterial resistance and the availability of superior antibiotics. Few laboratories routinely perform susceptibility testing of clinical isolates to sulfonamides alone. However, sulfonamides can be used alone in the treatment of infections due to Nocardia species, since the addition of a DHFR antagonist does not improve the activity against these organisms. Ophthalmic preparations of sulfacetamide are useful in the treatment of bacterial conjunctivitis.

■ Sulfonamides are perhaps the most allergenic of antibiotics

Sulfonamide allergy is most frequently manifest as a diffuse pruritic maculopapular rash. The risk of an allergic reaction with sulfonamides is substantially greater in people infected with HIV. Rarely, sulfonamides can cause Stevens–Johnson syndrome or toxic epidermal necrolysis, both of which are life-threatening desquamating skin disorders. Of all the drugs that can cause toxic epidermal necrolysis, sulfonamides carry the highest risk.

Sulfones

Sulfones are synthetic agents related to sulfonamides and also compete with PABA for DHPS. The only commercially available sulfone is diaminodiphenyl sulfone (DDS), which is better known as dapsone.

Dapsone is active against most strains of M. *leprae*, but few conventional bacteria. It is used as part of a multi-drug regimen for the treatment of leprosy. It can also be used in the prevention and treatment of *Pneumocystis carinii* pneumonia and in the treatment of some noninfectious skin diseases such as dermatitis herpetiformis.

There is only partial cross-allergenicity between sulfonamides and sulfones.

Dihydrofolate reductase inhibitors

Of the three DHFR inhibitors available to treat human infections (i.e. trimethoprim, pyrimethamine, and trimetrexate), only trimethoprim is useful for bacterial infections. Trimethoprim is a bacteriostatic agent and is active against many Enterobacteriaceae. It is excreted unchanged in the urine and, as it enters the prostate in therapeutic concentrations, it is useful in the treatment of chronic bacterial prostatitis. Trimethoprim can be used alone in the treatment of urinary tract infection and may be useful in individuals who are allergic to sulfonamides. More often, trimethoprim is used in combination with sulfamethoxazole (see below).

Trimethoprim–sulfamethoxazole

Trimethoprim and sulfamethoxazole block two different steps of the folate biosynthetic pathway. When used in combination, their antibacterial effect is often synergistic and bactericidal. Both drugs are excreted unchanged by the kidney. Because they have similar serum half-lifes, their relative concentrations remain fairly constant. The combination trimethoprim–sulfamethoxazole (TMP–SMZ), sometimes called co-trimoxazole, is active against most Enterobacteriaceae, H. *influenzae*, and many strains of streptococci and staphylococci. At concentrations achievable in the urine, TMP–SMZ inhibits many enterococci. TMP–SMZ is also very active against P. *carinii*. It is not active against P. *aeruginosa* or anaerobic bacteria. Although it does penetrate the cerebrospinal fluid, there is only limited experience with its use in meningitis, and therefore other agents are preferred for this indication.

TMP–SMZ is available in both oral and intravenous formulations.

THERAPEUTIC INDICATIONS TMP–SMZ:
- Is a very important drug for the treatment of urinary tract infection, and is usually the drug of choice for urinary tract infections caused by susceptible bacteria.
- Can also be used to treat infections caused by susceptible organisms at other body sites.
- Is the drug of choice for the prevention and treatment of P. *carinii* pneumonia.
- May be useful for acute exacerbations of chronic bronchitis, shigellosis, and enteric fever.

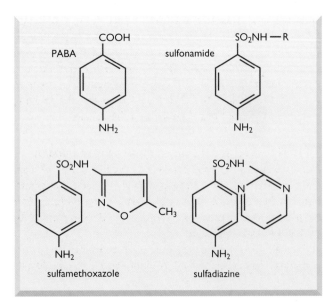

Fig. 9.26 Chemical structures of para-aminobenzoic acid (PABA) and sulfonamides. Note the similarity between PABA and sulfonamide drugs, which compete for the same bacterial enzyme, dihydropteroate synthetase (DHPS).

Miscellaneous antibacterial drugs
Nitrofurantoin

Nitrofurantoin is a synthetic nitrofuran and is used exclusively for the treatment of urinary tract infection. Its mechanism of action is unknown. It is active against most Enterobacteriaceae and enterococci, but not *P. aeruginosa*.

Nitrofurantoin is available only as an oral formulation. It is almost completely absorbed, after which approximately two-thirds are rapidly metabolized in the tissues with about one-third excreted unchanged in the urine. Blood concentrations of nitrofurantoin are very low and inadequate to treat infection, but urinary and renal concentrations are relatively high and sufficient to treat urinary tract infections. Nitrofurantoin does not enter the prostate in adequate concentration to treat chronic bacterial prostatitis. Because the activity of nitrofurantoin is reduced in an alkaline pH, it is not suitable for treating urinary tract infections due to *Proteus* species since this genus produces urease, which reduces urea to ammonium, thereby alkalinizing the urine.

Nitrofurantoin may be useful in the treatment of urinary tract infections in patients who have allergies and/or intolerance to both sulfonamides and β lactams, but trimethoprim alone and fluoroquinolones are also options for such patients. Nitrofurantoin should never be used to treat a urinary tract infection if there is any possibility of a concomitant bacteremia, because of its lack of therapeutic serum concentrations.

ADVERSE EFFECTS With prolonged use, nitrofurantoin can cause peripheral neuropathy and pulmonary fibrosis.

Mupirocin

Mupirocin is a unique agent, binding to bacterial isoleucyl-tRNA synthetase and preventing incorporation of isoleucine into the protein chains of the bacterial cell wall. It is available only as a topical formulation and is active against streptococci and staphylococci, with predominantly bactericidal activity. Acquired resistance is uncommon and due to altered isoleucyl-tRNA synthetase.

Mupirocin ointment is useful in the treatment of impetigo, folliculitis, secondarily infected burns, infected lacerations, and infected skin ulcers, as well as for eradicating nasal carriage of *S. aureus*.

Antimycobacterial drugs

The rifamycins, aminoglycosides, fluoroquinolones, dapsone, and the two newer macrolides, clarithromycin and azithromycin noted above, all have a role to play in the treatment of mycobacterial infections. There are three additional agents with activity restricted to mycobacterial infections that are important first-line drugs in the treatment of *M. tuberculosis* infection: isoniazid, pyrazinamide, and ethambutol (Fig. 9.27).

Isoniazid

Isoniazid (isonicotinic acid hydrazine, INH) is a critical drug in the treatment of tuberculosis. Mycobacteria differ from conventional bacteria in having a cell wall that contains large quantities of lipid. One of the most important lipid constituents of mycobacteria is mycolic acid. Isoniazid inhibits the synthesis of mycolic acid and is predominantly bactericidal against *M. tuberculosis*. It has relatively poor activity against non-

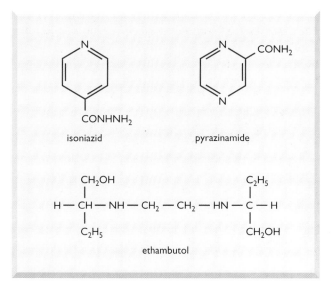

Fig. 9.27 Chemical structures of isoniazid, ethambutol, and pyrazinamide. All these agents are first-line drugs for the treatment of tuberculosis.

tuberculous mycobacteria. Isoniazid is well absorbed orally and is metabolized in the liver by acetylation. It achieves concentrations in the cerebrospinal fluid sufficient to treat tuberculous meningitis.

Isoniazid is a cornerstone drug in the treatment of tuberculosis

In general, the treatment of active tuberculosis requires a combination of isoniazid plus rifampin, plus at least one other antimycobacterial drug until susceptibility results are available. Most experts choose to start with four antimycobacterial drugs pending susceptibility results, to minimize the risk of acquired resistance. In addition, an important principle of modern antituberculous therapy is the use of directly observed therapy whereby the ingestion of every dose of antituberculous medication is witnessed by a health care worker.

Individuals with positive tuberculin skin tests (indicative of tuberculosis infection) in whom active tuberculosis is excluded are treated with isoniazid alone (i.e. INH preventive therapy) to prevent the development of active tuberculosis.

Isoniazid causes hepatitis and peripheral neuropathy

Isoniazid causes hepatitis, the risk of which increases with age and underlying liver disease. It may also cause a peripheral neuropathy, particularly in malnourished individuals. This peripheral neuropathy can be prevented or reversed by pyridoxine administration.

Isoniazid can also cause drug fever and increases serum concentrations of phenytoin when administered concommittently.

Pyrazinamide

Pyrazinamide (PZA) is a synthetic analog of nicotinamide with bactericidal activity against *M. tuberculosis*, and is commonly used together with isoniazid and rifampin as a first-line agent. It is

133

a pro-drug that must be converted by pyrazinamidase present in M. *tuberculosis* to pyrazinoic acid, which acts against intracellular organisms. It is not useful for other mycobacterial species. PZA is available only as an oral formulation and is metabolized in the liver.

Pyrazinamide can be hepatotoxic and cause hyperuricemia

PZA can be hepatotoxic but, curiously, there is no increased hepatotoxicity of a regimen consisting of isoniazid, rifampin, and PZA compared with a regimen of isoniazid and rifampin without PZA. PZA also causes hyperuricemia, but rarely leads to acute gouty arthritis.

Ethambutol

Ethambutol is an oral drug and is bacteriostatic against M. *tuberculosis* and several other slow-growing mycobacteria. Its precise mechanism of action is not known, but it is believed to inhibit bacterial RNA synthesis. It is primarily excreted by the kidneys.

Ethambutol is never used alone, but is used in combination with other drugs in the treatment of disease due to M. *tuberculosis* and several nontuberculous mycobacterial species, particularly M. *avium* complex, M. *kansasii*, and M. *marinum*.

Ethambutol can cause retrobulbar neuritis

Ethambutol is usually very well tolerated, but a unique toxicity is retrobulbar neuritis, which is usually manifest first as red–green color blindness and later as reduced visual acuity. The risk of this adverse effect is both dose- and time-dependent. Baseline and serial visual acuity and color perception tests should be performed when long-term ethambutol therapy is anticipated.

Other antituberculous drugs

In cases of multi-drug-resistant M. *tuberculosis* or if there are allergies, intolerance, or contraindications to the use of the main antituberculous drugs, second-line antituberculous drugs may need to be used. These include:

* Capreomycin and viomycin, which are parenteral polypeptide antibiotics.
* Ethionamide, an oral drug that is chemically related to isoniazid.
* Cycloserine, an oral drug that inhibits cell wall synthesis but causes considerable central nervous system toxicity.
* Para-aminosalicylic acid, an oral PABA analog that inhibits DHPS and is similar to sulfonamides and sulfones.
* Clofazimine, an oral agent, that has a role in the treatment of leprosy.

Antibiotics of choice

The principles of antibiotic selection have been outlined in the first part of this chapter. Bacterial, host, and drug factors all need to be taken into account. Two patients infected with the identical organism may require different antibiotics because of:

* Differences in the site of infection.
* Drug allergies.
* Underlying illness.
* Concomitant drug therapy.
* Age.
* Pregnancy status.

In the absence of allergies, pregnancy, underlying illness, and potential drug interactions, there are often accepted antibiotics of choice for common bacterial infections, and the appropriate antibiotic choices for selected common pathogens are presented in Fig. 9.28.

Drugs of choice and alternatives for selected common bacterial pathogens

Bacterium	Drug(s) of choice	Alternatives	Comments
Streptococcus species	Penicillin	A first-generation cephalosporin Erythromycin Clindamycin Vancomycin	Some strains are penicillin-resistant, especially a growing proportion of *S. pneumoniae* Erythromycin is only for mild infections Vancomycin is only for serious infections Certain fluoroquinolones are active against *S. pneumoniae*
Enterococcus species	Penicillin or ampicillin plus gentamicin	Vancomycin plus gentamicin Quinupristin–dalfopristin Linezolid	There are some strains for which streptomycin is synergistic but gentamicin is not Some strains are resistant to synergy with any aminoglycoside Some strains are resistant to vancomycin (VRE)
Staphylococcus species	An antistaphylococcal penicillin	A first-generation cephalosporin Vancomycin	Vancomycin is required for methicillin-resistant strains Rifampin is occasionally used to eradicate the nasal carriage state
Neisseria meningitidis	Penicillin	A third-generation cephalosporin Chloramphenicol	Rare strains are penicillin-resistant

Drugs of choice and alternatives for selected common bacterial pathogens

Bacterium	Drug(s) of choice	Alternatives	Comments
Neisseria gonorrhoeae	Cefixime	Ciprofloxacin A third-generation cephalosporin	Some strains are fluoroquinolone-resistant (especially in Asia)
Bordetella pertussis	Erythromycin	TMP-SMZ (trimethoprim–sulfamethoxazole)	Other macrolides are also active *in vitro*
Pasteurella multocida	Penicillin	A first-generation cephalosporin	
Haemophilus influenzae	Aminopenicillin	Cefuroxime A third-generation cephalosporin Chloramphenicol	Approximately 30% are aminopenicillin-resistant; therefore aminopenicillins should not be used empirically in serious infections until susceptibility results are available Rifampin is used to eradicate the nasal carriage state
Enterobacteriaceae in urine	TMP–SMZ	Ciprofloxacin Gentamicin	β Lactams are less effective than TMP–SMZ or fluroquinolones for the treatment of urinary tract infection
Enterobacteriaceae in cerebrospinal fluid	A third-generation cephalosporin	Meropenem TMP–SMZ	In neonates only, aminoglycosides are equivalent to third-generation cephalosporins Experience with TMP–SMZ in meningitis is limited
Enterobacteriaceae elsewhere (blood, lung, etc.)	Gentamicin or a third-generation cephalosporin or ciprofloxacin	TMP–SMZ Carbapenems	Two-drug therapy is sometimes used in serious infection Monotherapy with a third-generation cephalosporin should be avoided if the pathogen is *Enterobacter cloacae, E. aerogenes, Serratia marcescens* or *Citrobacter freundii*
Pseudomonas aeruginosa	Antipseudomonal penicillin plus aminoglycoside	Ceftazidime Ciprofloxacin A carbapenem	Two-drug therapy recommended except for urinary tract infection
Bacteroides fragilis	Metronidazole or clindamycin	A carbapenem A penicillin–β lactamase inhibitor	*B. fragilis* is usually involved in polymicrobial infections; therefore another antibiotic active against Enterobacteriaceae is often required
Mycoplasma pneumoniae	A macrolide (e.g. erythromycin)	A tetracycline	Although tetracyclines are as effective as macrolides, the latter are recommended because of better activity against *Pneumococcus*, which can mimic this infection
Ureaplasma urealyticum	A tetracycline	Erythromycin	A few strains are tetracycline-resistant
Mycoplasma hominis	A tetracycline	Clindamycin	Erythromycin is not active against *M. hominis*
Chlamydia trachomatis	A tetracycline	Azithromycin Erythromycin	Azithromycin is the only therapy effective in a single dose Erythromycin is used in pregnancy
Rickettsial species	A tetracycline	Chloramphenicol	
Listeria monocytogenes	Ampicillin plus gentamicin	Vancomycin plus gentamicin	
Legionella species	A macrolide	A tetracycline A fluoroquinolone	Rifampin is occasonally used as a second agent in severe cases
Clostridium difficile	Metronidazole	Vancomycin (oral)	

Drugs of choice and alternatives for selected common bacterial pathogens (Continued)

Bacterium	Drug(s) of choice	Alternatives	Comments
Mycobacterium tuberculosis	Isoniazid plus rifampin plus pyrazinamide plus ethambutol	Streptomycin A fluoroquinolone Ethionamide Cycloserine Viomycin Capreomycin	Directly observed therapy (DOT) is recommended Isoniazid is used alone for treatment of latent tubercular infection
Mycobacterium avium complex	Clarithromycin plus ethambutol ± rifabutin	Ciprofloxacin Amikacin	
Mycobacterium leprae	Dapsone plus rifampin ± clofazimine	Clarithromycin	Thalidomide is useful for erythema nodosum leprosum

Fig. 9.28 **Drugs of choice and alternatives for selected common bacterial pathogens.**

Adverse effects of antibiotics
• *Nearly all can cause* Clostridium difficile *enteritis*
• *Aminoglycosides can cause irreversible aplastic anemia and the gray baby syndrome*
• *Sulfonamides can cause a skin rash, Stevens–Johnson syndrome, and toxic epidermal necrolysis*
• *Tetracycline can discolor the teeth if given to children under 8 years of age*

FURTHER READING

Kaye D (ed.) Antibacterial therapy: in vitro testing, pharmacodynamics, pharmacology, new agents. *Infect Dis Clin N Am* 1995; **9(3)**: 463–810. [Essentially a small textbook on antibacterial therapy.]

Levy SB. *The Antibiotic Paradox: How Miracle Drugs are Destroying the Miracle*. New York: Plenum Publishing; 1992. [A more detailed account written for the educated layperson about global antibiotic resistance.]

Levy SB. Confronting multidrug resistance. A role for each of us. *JAMA* 1993; **269**: 1840–1842. [A brief overview of the problem of global antibiotic resistance.]

Mandell GI, Bennett JE, Dolin R (eds) *Mandell, Douglas and Bennett's Principles and Practice of Infectious Diseases*, 5th edn., New York: Churchill Livingstone; 2000. [An excellent and comprehensive textbook for the discipline of infectious diseases.]

Neu HC. The crisis in antibiotic resistance. *Science* 1992; **257**: 1064–1073. [This article gives a historic overview of the most common types of antibiotic resistance over time.]

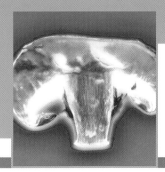

Chapter 10

Drugs and Fungi

BIOLOGY OF FUNGI

Fungi differ from higher plants in their structure, reproduction, and nutrition. They lack chlorophyll, leaves, true stems, and roots, reproduce by spores, and live as saprophytes or parasites. The method of sexual reproduction of most pathogenic fungi is unknown (i.e. they are Fungi Imperfecti). Fungi that infect skin (dermatophytes) are classified according to their predominant ecologic site (Fig. 10.1).

Relatively few species of fungi are pathogenic and pathogenicity results from:
- Mycotoxin production.
- Allergenicity.
- Tissue invasion.

Zoophilic (Fig. 10.1) species tend to cause highly inflammatory skin reactions in humans, while anthropophilic species produce mild chronic lesions. The reactions are site-dependent and altered by the host's immune status. Opportunistic pathogens are important causes of disease in immunosuppressed patients.

MANAGEMENT OF FUNGAL INFECTIONS

Most fungi are not affected by antibacterial drugs. There are few specific antifungal agents and the use of many of these is restricted by their relative toxicity.

■ *The diagnosis of systemic fungal infection must be established before starting treatment because many systemic antifungal treatments have significant adverse effects*

Certain fungi causing skin lesions, including *Microsporum* (e.g. *M. canis*, *M. audouinii*, *M. distortum*), produce brilliant green fluorescence under Wood's ultraviolet light, while *Trichophyton schoenleinii* causes a paler green fluorescence of infected hair (Fig.

10.2). Wood's light can also be used to diagnose pityriasis versicolor as the scales usually fluoresce yellow.

Superficial skin mycoses can be diagnosed by microscopy and culture of skin scrapings, plucked (not cut) hairs, or nail clippings, while systemic mycoses can be diagnosed by microscopy and culture of pus, exudate, tissue biopsy, feces, urine, sputum, spinal fluid, or blood. If possible, specimens should be inoculated directly onto the media.

Serologic tests are mainly available only in specialist laboratories, but help establish the diagnosis of many mycoses (Fig. 10.3). Skin tests are useful diagnostically only if a patient has recently visited an endemic area for the first time, but may be of value for sporotrichosis and *Aspergillus* hypersensitivity. Positive tests have no diagnostic value in ringworm and candidal infections and are of limited significance in histoplasmosis and coccidioidomycosis.

General measures for infected patients

Spread of infection must be minimized (e.g. children should stay away from school until treatment is established (*M. canis*) or until there is no fluorescence and the hair has regrown (anthropophilic species), and topical treatment should be used. Schoolchildren should be screened with Wood's ultraviolet light and scalp massage techniques for early diagnosis and treatment.

Advice regarding a likely source of infection can be given if the species of fungus is known (e.g. treatment of infected pets or prophylactic antifungal dusting powder after swimming).

Preventive measures should be taken for patients at high risk (e.g. frequent oral toilet, adequate denture care, and careful

Classification of fungi according to site of origin	
Origin	Name
Soil	Geophilic
Animals	Zoophilic
Human skin	Anthropophilic

Fig. 10.1 Classification of fungi according to site of origin.

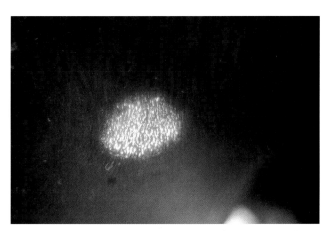

Fig. 10.2 Tinea capitis. Note the characteristic fluorescence under Wood's light. (Courtesy of Dr Richard Staughton.)

Availability and usefulness of serologic tests in diagnosing fungal infections		
Serologic test useful	Serologic test useful for deep-seated infection	Serologic test useful, but not widely available
Histoplasmosis	Candidiasis	Sporotrichosis
Coccidioidomycosis	Cryptococcosis	Mycetoma
Blastomycosis		Nocardiosis
Aspergillosis (sometimes)		Chromomycosis
		Zygomycosis

Fig. 10.3 Availability and usefulness of serologic tests for diagnosing fungal infections.

attention to drying and ventilation of skin fold areas in the seriously ill can help prevent candidiasis).

Specific antifungal treatment

The three main classes of antifungal medicines are the polyene macrolides, the antifungal azoles, and the allylamines (Fig. 10.4).

Polyene macrolide antibiotics

AMPHOTERICIN B This antifungal antibiotic is produced by *Streptomyces nodosus*. It binds to ergosterol in the fungal cell membrane (Fig. 10.5) with the formation of 'amphotericin pores' (Fig. 10.6), resulting in a loss of macromolecules and ions from the fungus, and irreversible damage.

Amphotericin is poorly absorbed from the gastrointestinal (GI) tract and is therefore effective orally only for GI fungal

Antifungal medicines and their routes of administration		
Drug class	Drug name	Routes of administration
Polyene macrolides	Amphotericin B	T, I, P
	Nystatin	T (O for GI tract only)
	Natamycin	T
	Candicidin	T
Azoles Imidazoles	Clotrimazole	T
	Miconazole	T, I
	Ketoconazole	T, O
	Isoconazole	T
	Tioconazole	T
	Econazole	T
	Sulconazole	T
	Terconazole	T
	Oxiconazole	T
	Butoconazole	T
Triazoles	Fluconazole	O
	Itraconazole	O
Allylamines	Naftifine	T
	Terbinafine	T, O
Other	Griseofulvin	O
	Amorolfine	T
	Flucytosine	O

Fig. 10.4 Antifungal medicines and their routes of administration. (GI, gastrointestinal; I, intravenous; O, oral; P, parenteral; T, topical)

infections. Given parenterally, it is highly protein-bound (90%) and penetration into body fluids and tissues is poor. Toxicity is common and a test dose needs to be administered and subsequent administration closely supervised with monitoring of

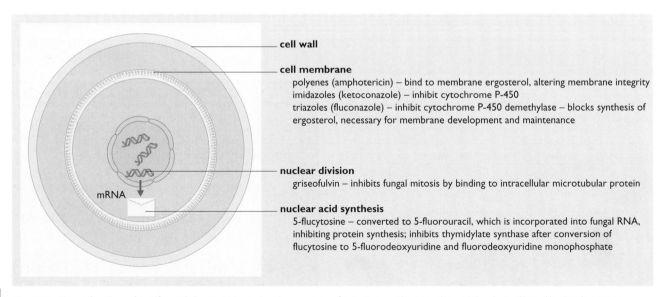

cell wall

cell membrane
polyenes (amphotericin) – bind to membrane ergosterol, altering membrane integrity
imidazoles (ketoconazole) – inhibit cytochrome P-450
triazoles (fluconazole) – inhibit cytochrome P-450 demethylase – blocks synthesis of ergosterol, necessary for membrane development and maintenance

nuclear division
griseofulvin – inhibits fungal mitosis by binding to intracellular microtubular protein

nuclear acid synthesis
5-flucytosine – converted to 5-fluorouracil, which is incorporated into fungal RNA, inhibiting protein synthesis; inhibits thymidylate synthase after conversion of flucytosine to 5-fluorodeoxyuridine and fluorodeoxyuridine monophosphate

mRNA

Fig. 10.5 Sites of action of antifungal drugs. (Adapted with permission from *Human Pharmacology: Molecular to Clinical* by Brody, Larner, Minneman, and Neu, Mosby-Year Book Inc., 1994.)

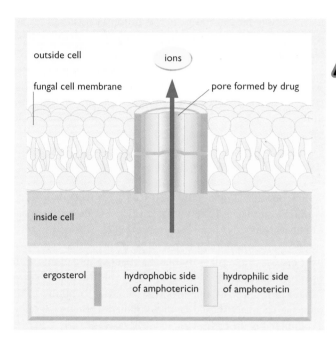

outside cell

ions

fungal cell membrane

pore formed by drug

inside cell

| ergosterol | hydrophobic side of amphotericin | hydrophilic side of amphotericin |

Fig. 10.6 Mechanism of action of polyene antifungal agents.
Binding to ergosterol damages the membrane with leakage of ions and irreversible fungal cell damage. (Adapted with permission from *Human Pharmacology: Molecular to Clinical* by Brody, Larner, Minneman, and Neu, Mosby-Year Book Inc., 1994.)

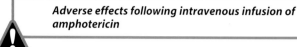

Adverse effects following intravenous infusion of amphotericin

- Fever
- Chills
- Hypotension
- Vomiting
- Dyspnea
- Headaches
- Thrombophlebitis at the site of injection
- Renal toxicity is invariable, but treatment can be continued to a creatinine concentration of 200 μmol/liter

liver and renal function, electrolytes and blood counts. The drug should be administered by slow infusion since there is a risk of arrhythmias. Prophylactic antipyretics or corticosteroids should not be co-administered except to treat anaphylactic reactions which can rarely ensue. The drug is also nephrotoxic and neurotoxic. In addition pain and thrombophlebitis can occur at the injection site.

Binding to cholesterol (e.g. on red blood cell membranes) may account for some of amphotericin's adverse effects.

Amphotericin is excreted in the urine over several days. Only 2–3% of the blood level is achieved in the cerebrospinal fluid (CSF) after intravenous injection, so intrathecal (or intracisternal) injection is necessary for fungal meningitis.

Use of amphotericin encapsulated in liposomes has reduced its toxicity. It can also be complexed with sodium cholesteryl sulfate. These newer infusions are indicated for severe systemic fungal infections and invasive candidiasis where amphotericin alone is contraindicated due to its renal toxicity.

Intravenous amphotericin for the Treatment of systemic fungal infections (see the section on Treatment indications, below) must be given cautiously. An initial dose is administered with careful monitoring, and then a slow infusion, with gradual increases in dose until there is a therapeutic response. Daily treatment often has to be continued for 6–12 weeks. Longer-term treatment on alternate days (this is sufficient once a steady state is achieved) is often needed to maintain blood levels.

Amphotericin resistance can develop if the fungus alters the amount of ergosterol on its membrane or modifies its structure so that the drug binds less avidly.

Topical amphotericin is used to treat mucosal candidiasis.

NYSTATIN This is a polyene macrolide with a similar mechanism of action to amphotericin. It is stable when dry, but quickly disintegrates on contact with water or plasma. It is not absorbed from skin, mucous membranes, or the GI tract, and orally administered nystatin is excreted in the feces. It is too toxic for parenteral administration. Its clinical use is limited to topical applications for the skin and mucous membranes (buccal and vaginal), and oral administration to suppress *Candida* in the lumen of the gut in infants and those with impaired immunity. Resistance to nystatin does not develop *in vivo*, but some *Candida* species are not susceptible.

NATAMYCIN is a polyene antifungal agent used as a 5% ophthalmic suspension.

CANDICIDIN is a polyene antibiotic used topically for vaginal candidiasis.

Antifungal azoles

Imidazoles and triazoles:

- Inhibit fungal lipid (especially ergosterol) synthesis in cell membranes.
- Interfere (Fig. 10.5) with fungal oxidative enzymes (primarily the 14a-demethylase microsomal P-450-dependent enzyme), resulting in accumulation of 14a-methyl sterols, which may disrupt the packing of acyl chains of phospholipids, inhibiting growth and interfering with membrane-bound enzyme systems.

Triazoles have greater selectivity against fungi than imidazoles, and cause less endocrine disturbance.

These agents are available mainly for topical use; clotrimazole is too toxic to use systemically. Intravenous miconazole can be used for disseminated mycoses, but is limited by its adverse effects (vomiting, hyponatremia, hyperlipidemia, thrombophlebitis, hematologic disturbances).

KETOCONAZOLE was the first orally active azole antifungal agent. It is less toxic and less effective than amphotericin. However it has been associated with fatal hepatotoxicity and should not be used for superficial fungal infections. It is well

| **Adverse effects of ketoconazole** |

- *Nausea*
- *Vomiting*
- *Photophobia*
- *Skin rashes*
- *Hepatotoxicity*
- *Mild elevation of hepatic enzymes (5–10%)*
- *Symptomatic hepatitis is rare, but progressive fatal hepatotoxicity reported with high doses so liver function tests required at regular intervals*
- *Gynecomastia and reduced libido*
- *Menstrual irregularities (10% of women)*
- *High dose ketoconazole should be avoided in patients with tuberculosis, histoplasmosis, paracoccidioidomycosis, and AIDS*

absorbed (but see interactions below), although CSF concentrations are low; it is largely protein-bound, and is metabolized by the liver. Ketoconazole is indicated for:

- Serious chronic resistant mucocutaneous candidiasis (1–2 weeks; 4–10 months for mucocutaneous candidiasis).
- Resistant dermatophyte infections (3–8 weeks).
- Systemic infections, particularly disseminated blastomycosis, but not fungal meningitis.

Liver function needs to be monitored clinically and biochemically. Ketoconazole should be avoided in pregnancy breastfeeding mothers and patients with porphyria. It has important drug interactions (see below).

FLUCONAZOLE (a bistriazole) is indicated for the treatment of local and systemic candidiasis and cryptococcal infections. It is more readily absorbed from the GI tract than ketoconazole and penetrates the blood–brain barrier, producing CSF concentrations 50–80% of those in the blood. It is excreted by the kidneys unchanged, so its half-life is considerably prolonged in renal insufficiency.

Skin, genital and mucosal candidiasis; cutaneous dermatophyte infections; pityriasis versicolor and invasive candidiasis can be treated with fluconazole. It can be used for systemic infections including cryptococcal meningitis, although relapse is common. It has a role in prophylaxis of fungal infection in immuno-compromised patients following cytotoxic chemotherapy or radiotherapy, and in preventing relapse of cryptococcal meningitis in AIDS.

Adverse effects include vomiting, diarrhea and rashes (including Stevens–Johnson syndrome). Thrombocytopenia and transient abnormalities of hepatic function are also described, but there seem to be no endocrine effects. Animal studies suggest that it is teratogenic.

ITRACONAZOLE is a synthetic dioxolane triazole. It is useful in the treatment of oropharyngeal and vulvovaginal candidiasis, pityriasis versicolor, tinea corporis and tinea pedis. It can be

used for systemic infections such as histoplasmosis and can be used in aspergillosis, candidiasis and cryptococcosis where other antifungal drugs are inappropriate or ineffective.

Absorption from the GI tract is incomplete, but increases when it is taken with food. It is 99% protein-bound and is concentrated in tissues such as lung, liver, and bone, but has limited CSF penetration. It is excreted by the liver and has one active metabolite with a half-life of 20–40 hours, which is also excreted by the liver. In neutropenic patients, a loading dose should be given for the first 4 days and a maintenance dose of 400 mg is often required to achieve adequate serum levels.

Itraconazole is generally well tolerated, though nausea, vomiting, headaches, abdominal pain, and transient increases in hepatic enzymes have been reported. Liver function tests should be monitored if it is given to patients with a history of liver disease. Bioavailability may be reduced in patients with renal impairment, and blood levels should be measured in patients with AIDS and neutropenia where absorption can be reduced. The drug should be discontinued if patients develop a peripheral neuropathy.

RESISTANCE TO THE AZOLE DRUGS This is rare, but resistant *Candida* strains have been recovered from patients with chronic mucocutaneous candidiasis and AIDS.

IMPORTANT INTERACTIONS OF AZOLE DRUGS These drugs will:

- Increase the phenytoin, oral hypoglycemic, anticoagulant and cyclosporine plasma concentrations (by inhibition of P-450).
- Increase simvastatin myotoxicity.
- Increase antihistamine and cisapride (no longer marketed) cardiotoxicity.

Azole absorption is reduced by antacids, cimetidine or rifampin, and increased by thiazide diuretics.

Allylamines

NAFTIFINE IS AN ALLYLAMINE NAPHTHALENE DERIVATIVE FOR TOPICAL USE. It inhibits the enzyme squalene epoxidase and decreases ergosterol synthesis.

TERBINAFINE IS THE FIRST ORALLY ACTIVE ALLYLAMINE. It prevents ergosterol synthesis by inhibiting squalene epoxidase, resulting in squalene accumulation, which leads to membrane disruption and cell death (Fig. 10.7).

Terbinafine is well absorbed, and is concentrated in the dermis, epidermis, and adipose tissue (because it is lipophilic). It is secreted in sebum and appears in the stratum corneum hours after oral administration. It also diffuses from the nail bed, penetrating distal nails within 4 weeks. It is metabolized in the liver and the inactive metabolites are excreted in the urine. It is effective mainly against dermatophytes. Clinical trials show impressive clinical and mycologic cure and relapse rates (Fig. 10.8).

Terbinafine is well tolerated. Nausea, abdominal pain, and allergic skin reactions can occur, but are often mild. Loss of taste has been reported. Terbinafine concentrations are increased by cimetidine and reduced by co-administration with rifampin.

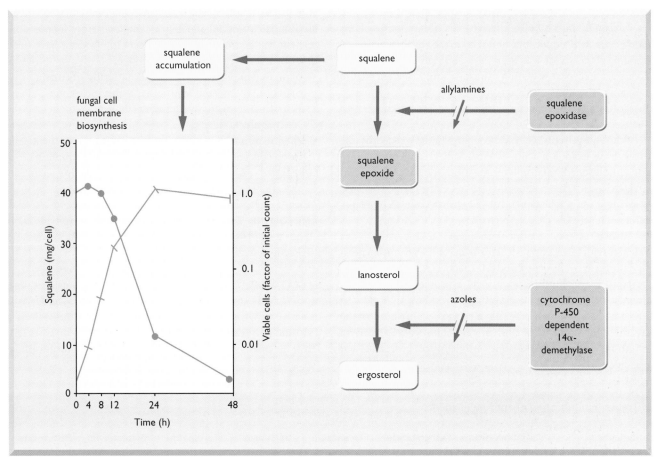

Fig. 10.7 Terbinafine inhibits squalene epoxidase, resulting in the accumulation of squalene inside the fungal cell. This accumulation of squalene (red line) correlates with cell death (blue line). (Adapted with permission of Blackwell Science Ltd. from Ryder NS, *Clin Exp Dermatol* 1989; **14**: 98–100.)

Effectiveness of terbinafine

Infection	Dosage	Clinical cure (%)	Mycologic cure (%)	Relapse rate (%)
Tinea unguium	250 mg 12 wks		81–88	
Tinea pedis	250 mg 2 wks	87	78	Low 6/52 later
Tinea corporis/cruris	250–500 mg	85	92	
Onychomycosis (hands)	250–500 mg	85	95	80% cure at 3–12 month follow-up
Onychomycosis (toes)	250–500 mg	80	80	
Candidiasis	500 mg 4 wks	70	80	

Fig. 10.8 Effectiveness of terbinafine.

Other antifungal agents

GRISEOFULVIN This was the original, orally active, antifungal agent. It is isolated from *Penicillium griseofulvum*. Its mechanism of action is not established, but it probably interferes with microtubule function or nucleic acid synthesis and poly-merization. It inhibits dermatophyte growth, but has no effect on the fungi producing deep mycoses or on *Candida* species. Absorption varies according to the preparation, but micro-particle preparations are better absorbed, peaking 1–3 hours after ingestion. Serum concentrations decrease after 30 hours.

141

It is concentrated in actively metabolizing cells of the skin and passes rapidly into fully keratinized cells, reaching the outermost cells in 8 hours, but is not thought to bind firmly to keratin. Since sweat transports griseofulvin in the stratum corneum, excessive sweating can cause rapid clearance from the skin. Griseofulvin is metabolized in the liver to 6-demethyl griseofulvin, which is then excreted via the kidneys and perhaps bile.

Although griseofulvin has been largely superseded by the azole drugs in adult practice, it remains the treatment of choice for childhood dermatophyte infections (10 mg/kg in two divided doses). The treatment schedules are prolonged because the drug is fungistatic rather than fungicidal. Long-term relapse rates are high (40–70% for toenails).

Adverse effects are uncommon, but a hypersensitivity reaction with fever, skin rash, leukopenia and a serum sickness-like illness is well recognized. Headaches are common, and irritability and nightmares can be a problem, but usually improve on continuing the drug. If not, the dose can be reduced for a few days and then gradually increased, giving most of the treatment at night. Griseofulvin can cause light sensitivity eruptions and petechial rashes, and has also been associated with urticarial rashes, which settle despite continuing treatment. Hepatotoxicity, peripheral neuritis, bone marrow suppression, proteinuria and estrogen-like effects in children have been described, and griseofulvin is teratogenic.

Griseofulvin resistance can develop during treatment. Griseofulvin interacts with other drugs including:
- Warfarin, increasing warfarin metabolism and reducing the anticoagulant effect.
- Phenobarbital, with simultaneous treatment reducing the blood concentration of griseofulvin after oral administration.

Griseofulvin exacerbates porphyria, and reportedly precipitates or exacerbates systemic lupus erythematosus.

AMOROLFINE This is a recently introduced antifungal, available as a nail lacquer, that is fungicidal for dermatophytes and has some activity against molds.

FLUCYTOSINE This agent is active orally and interferes with nucleic acid synthesis by inhibiting thymidylate synthetase. It is active only in cells able to transport it into the cell via a cytosine permease and convert flucytosine to 5-fluorouracil. This is then metabolized by uridine monophosphate

Treatment indication of antifungal agents							
Infection	Amphotericin B	Ketoconazole	Fluconazole	Itraconazole	Terbinafine	Griseofulvin	Flucytosine
Dermatophytes		x		x	x	x	
Pityrosporum		x		x			
Candidiasis	xC	x	x	x	x		x
Aspergillus	x	x		x			x
Blastomycosis	x	x		x			
Coccidioidomycosis	x	x					
Cryptococcosis	xC	x	x				x
Histoplasmosis	x	x		x			
Paracoccidioidomycosis	x	x		x			x
Chromoblastomycosis							
Sporotrichosis	x			x			
Mucormycosis	x						x
Torulopsis							
Pseudoallescheriasis		x					
Zygomycosis		x					

Fig. 10.9 Treatment indication of antifungal agents. (C, amphotericin B used in combination with flucytosine)

pyrophosphorylase and can be incorporated into RNA or metabolized to 5-fluorodeoxyuridylic acid, a potent thymidylate synthetase inhibitor. DNA synthesis is disrupted as a result.

The clinical usefulness of flucytosine is limited by the rapid development of resistance, which is partly delayed by co-administration of amphotericin B. Proposed mechanisms include loss of the permease for cytosine transport or decreased uridine monophosphate pyrophosphorylase or cytosine deaminase activity.

Flucytosine is well absorbed and penetrates the CSF (60–80% of serum levels). It is excreted largely unchanged in the urine, so the dose should be reduced in renal impairment.

Adverse effects include hepatotoxicity (enzyme abnormalities occur in about 5% of patients, but are usually reversible), enterocolitis, hair loss, and bone marrow suppression. Blood counts should be monitored weekly. Uracil reduces bone marrow suppression without reducing antifungal efficacy. The plasma concentration should be monitored.

Treatment indications of antifungal agents

A summary of the effectiveness of antifungal agents is shown in Fig. 10.9.

Neutropenia and suspected fungal infection

Antifungal treatments must be started in any neutropenic patient with a fever resistant to antibiotics before knowing the nature of the fungal infection. Amphotericin B is the drug of choice and the full therapeutic dose should be achieved within 24 hours because treatment of established candidiasis or aspergillosis in such patients is often unsuccessful. Furthermore, fungal infections often reactivate with subsequent periods of neutropenia. Empirical amphotericin treatment before antileukemic treatment may be justified, and needs to be continued until the neutrophil count recovers.

Prophylaxis

Fluconazole can be used prophylactically against candidiasis in neutropenic patients, but ketoconazole is not recommended for transplant recipients because it interferes with cyclosporine concentrations. Itraconazole seems to afford some protection against aspergillosis and candidiasis, but absorption is a problem. It is recommended in units without high-efficiency particulate air filters, and should be used in preference to fluconazole for patients who remain neutropenic for more than 3 weeks.

Nonspecific treatment of fungal infections

A variety of topical preparations are available for skin infections and can be effective if used regularly.

Compound benzoic acid ointment (Whitfield's ointment) is effective, but less acceptable cosmetically, than some newer preparations. It must be diluted by 50% for use in the scrotum and groin (in emulsifying ointment). Antiseptic paints such as Castellani's paint, undecenoate fatty acids and their salts, benzoyl peroxide, salicylic acid, ciclopirox olamine, iodochloroxolamine, triacetin, haloprogin and tolnaftate are alternatives for dermatophyte infections. Contact dermatitis is a rare adverse effect with all these treatments, and irritant dermatitis can pose problems, especially in patients with raw skin and fissures.

Selenium sulfide 2.5% in a detergent base is widely used for pityriasis versicolor. It stains clothing and can be irritant, but is considerably cheaper than topical azoles. Alternatively, 20% sodium hyposulfite solution and 50:50 propylene glycol in water can be used over the long term to prevent relapses.

Saturated potassium iodide solution given orally remains the treatment of choice for lymphocutaneous sporotrichosis.

FURTHER READING

Bickers DR. Antifungal therapy: potential interactions with other classes of drugs. *J Am Acad Dermatol* 1994; **31**: S87–90. [A useful review of the clinically relevant interactions of commonly used antifungal drugs with other drug classes.]

Bjorkholm M. Chemoprophylaxis of fungal infections in neutropenic patients. *Ann Oncol* 1994; **5**: 571–574. [A review of the prevention of fungal infections in neutropenic patients.]

Filler SG, Edwards SG. When and how to treat serious candidal infections: concepts and controversies. *Curr Clin Top Infect Dis* 1995; **15**: 1–8. [A review of the treatment of candidal infections.]

Finlay AY. Global overview of Lamisil. *Br J Dermatol* 1994; **43**: 1–3. [An extensive review of the clinical trial data with terbinafine.]

143

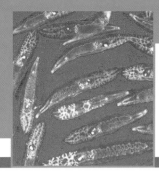

Chapter 11

Drugs and Parasites

Parasitism is a type of symbiosis between two organisms. The parasite is generally the smaller of the two and is usually metabolically dependent on its host. The term parasite is generally reserved for protozoa, helminths, and arthropods.

Treatment of protozoan and helminthic diseases is complicated by the variable structure and metabolism of the different forms of these organisms during their life cycle
Knowledge of the biochemistry and molecular biology of protozoa and helminths has recently expanded and new compounds to treat these diseases are being developed.

PROTOZOAN DISEASES

Protozoa are small, unicellular and are among the simplest organisms of the animal kingdom. Parasitic protozoa can replicate within the host's body and are usually divided into four subphyla according to their type of locomotion:

- Sarcodina (amebae) are characterized by ameboid movements producing pseudopods (e.g. *Entamoeba histolytica*).
- Mastigophora (flagellates) are characterized by flagella producing a whip-like motion (e.g. *Giardia lamblia*, *Trichomonas vaginalis*, *Trypanosoma* spp. and *Leishmania* spp.).
- Ciliophora (ciliates) are characterized by cilia to produce movement (e.g. *Balantidium coli*).
- Sporozoa typically have no locomotor organs in the adult stage (e.g. *Plasmodium* spp., *Toxoplasma gondii*. *Pneumocystis carinii*).

The ten major tropical diseases defined by the United Nations Development Program–World Bank–WHO Special Program for Research and Training in Tropical Diseases (TDR)

- Parasitic malaria—protozoan
- Parasitic schistosomiasis—helminthic
- Parasitic lymphatic filariasis—helminthic
- Parasitic African trypanosomiasis—protozoan
- Parasitic leishmaniasis—protozoan
- Parasitic Chagas disease—protozoan
- Parasitic onchocerciasis—helminthic
- Tuberculosis—bacterial
- Leprosy—bacterial
- Dengue—viral

Malaria

Malaria is a protozoan disease that is usually transmitted by mosquitoes
Malaria is the most important parasitic disease in tropical medicine. Worldwide there are 200 million malaria cases each year and 2 million deaths due to malaria. It is endemic in more than 100 countries in Africa, Asia, Oceania, Central and South America, and certain Caribbean islands, and approximately 60% of the world's population live in these countries.

There are four species of malaria parasites (Plasmodia)
Malaria is usually transmitted by anopheline mosquitoes and rarely by congenital transmission, transfusion of infected blood, or the use of contaminated syringes. It is caused by four species of plasmodial parasites:

- *Plasmodium falciparum*, is widely distributed, results in the most severe infections, and is responsible for nearly all malaria-related deaths (Fig. 11.1a).
- *P. vivax*, is also widespread and causes more benign disease than do *P. malariae* and *P. ovale* (Fig. 11.1b).
- *P. malariae* is also widespread.
- *P. ovale* is confined mainly to Africa.

The clinical features of infection depend on the species of the parasite and the immunologic status of the patient
Acute falciparum malaria is a potentially fatal disease, and nonimmune travelers to malarious areas risk severe attacks. Acute malaria occurs where exposure is limited or seasonal and where the collective immunity is relatively low. In these circumstances it can occur in epidemic proportions and affect all age groups in the endemic community. Complications include cerebral malaria, hypoglycemia, pulmonary edema, acute renal failure, and massive intravascular hemolysis. Chronic repeated infection often leads to splenomegaly and progressive anemia (Fig. 11.1c). There is a particularly high risk of death among untreated pregnant women with falciparum malaria, especially where transmission is intermittent. The fetus is inevitably exposed to the effects of placental insufficiency.

Infants born to immune mothers living in holoendemic areas are unlikely to acquire malaria for several months after birth, largely owing to the passive transfer of maternal antibodies across the placenta. Thereafter, they are subject to severe and recurrent acute potentially fatal attacks during infancy and early childhood. From the age of 5 years until adulthood, the severity and frequency of these attacks decrease as immunity develops.

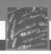

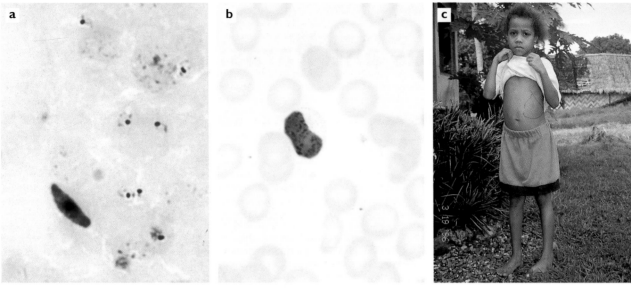

Fig. 11.1 Malaria. (a) *Plasmodium falciparum*, ring forms and a gametocyte. Giemsa thick smear. (b) *P. vivax*, a mature trophozoite in an enlarged erythrocyte. Giemsa stain, thin smear. (c) A schoolgirl with anemia and splenomegaly, Vanuatu, the Southwest Pacific.

Clinically significant malaria is uncommon among adults (other than pregnant women and immunocompromised individuals) who have always lived in areas of high transmission.

◼ Antimalarial drugs target different phases of the malarial life cycle

The malarial life cycle is as follows:

- Sporozoites are produced in the mosquito vectors from sexual forms of the parasite and migrate to the salivary glands (sporogony).
- Once injected into the human blood stream, the sporozoites rapidly penetrate the parenchymal cells of the liver, where they transform and grow into large tissue schizonts containing considerable numbers of merozoites (exo-red blood cell schizogony).
- The large tissue schizonts begin to rupture after 5–20 days, depending upon the species, and the released merozoites invade circulating red blood cells and rapidly multiply within the red cells.
- The host red blood cells rupture, releasing the merozoites, which then invade and destroy more red blood cells in the same way.

The four species of malaria

- *Plasmodium falciparum* causes the most severe infection; its resistance to antimalarial drugs is a major problem
- *P. vivax* causes more benign disease, as do *P. malariae* and *P. ovale*
- *P. vivax* and *P. ovale* have relapsing forms that are harbored in the liver
- *P. ovale* is mainly confined to Africa

- Some merozoites develop into male and female gametocytes, so the infected human becomes a reservoir of infection for mosquitoes and completion of the transmission cycle is assured.

The destruction of the red blood cells and the release of the waste products of the parasites produce the episodic chills and fever that characterize the disease. Certain tissue forms of *P. vivax* and *P. ovale* persist in the liver for many months and even years (hypnozoites) and are responsible for the relapses that are characteristic of these forms of malaria. Such latent forms are not generated by *P. falciparum* or *P. malariae*. Recrudescence of these infections results from persisting blood forms in inadequately treated or untreated patients.

◼ The chemotherapy used to treat malaria depends on the infecting parasite, the drug's bioavailability, metabolism, and adverse effects, and the host's immunity

The effectiveness of a chemotherapeutic agent in treating malaria depends on the interactions between the malaria parasites, the antimalarial drugs, and the human host. The choice of drug therefore depends on:

- The species of infecting parasite and its stage of development. Parasite resistance is becoming a worldwide problem. There are also differences in drug effectiveness between strains of the same species in different geographic areas.
- The drug's metabolism; this may be controlled by genetic factors (e.g. cytochrome P-450 enzymes), which are often different between geographical populations.
- The balance of a drug's adverse effects against its beneficial effects.
- The host's immunity, since people with a degree of immunity as a result of prolonged exposure to the infection can be cured or protected much more easily than those who have not, and may respond to lower drug doses.

■ *Antimalarial drugs are classified according to where they act in the life cycle of the malaria parasite.*

Antimalarial drugs have a selective action on the different phases of the parasite's life cycle (Fig. 11.2) and may be classified as:

- Tissue schizontocides, which act on exo-red blood cell forms in the liver.
- Blood schizontocides, which attack the parasite in the red blood cell, thereby preventing or terminating the clinical attack.
- Gametocytocides, which are drugs that destroy the sexual forms of the parasite (gametocytes) in the blood to prevent transmission.
- Hypnozoitocides, which kill the dormant hypnozoites of *P. vivax* and *P. ovale* in the liver and are used as antirelapse drugs.
- Sporontocides, which interrupt the development of the sporogonic phase in mosquitoes that have fed on gametocyte carriers so that the mosquitoes cannot transmit the infection.

There are no drugs available that act against sporozoites in the blood.

■ *Antimalarial drugs are used to protect against or cure malaria or to prevent transmission*

PROTECTIVE (PROPHYLACTIC) USE To prevent clinical attacks, antimalarial drugs are used before infection occurs or before it becomes evident, and the aim is to prevent the occurrence of any of its symptoms:

- Suppressive prophylaxis involves the use of blood schizontocides to prevent acute attacks of malaria.

- Causal prophylaxis involves the use of tissue schizontocides to prevent the parasite from becoming established in the liver.

CURATIVE (THERAPEUTIC) USE refers to the use of drugs to act against established infection. It consists of suppressive treatment of the acute attack, usually with blood schizontocides. Radical treatment of the dormant liver forms with hypnozoitocides is needed for relapsing malaria.

PREVENTION OF TRANSMISSION refers to eradication of infection in mosquitoes using either gametocytocides or sporontocides. This is important for controlling malaria in endemic areas.

■ *Several chemical groups of antimalarial compounds are in general use*

The actions of antimalarial drugs are summarized in Fig. 11.3.

Antimalarial drugs
4-Aminoquinolines

Chloroquine and amodiaquine are active against blood schizontocides and are thought to act by:

- Being concentrated in the parasite's lysosomes where hemoglobin is being digested.
- Inhibiting the polymerization of toxic hemin into insoluble hemozoin (malaria pigment).

They are gametocytocidal against *P. vivax*, *P. malariae*, and *P. ovale*, but not against *P. falciparum*.

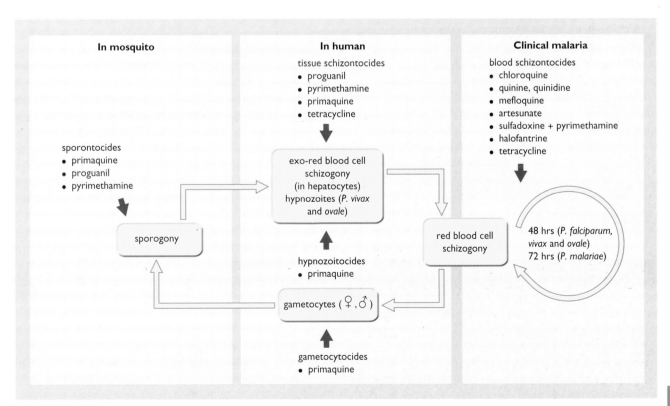

Fig. 11.2 Antimalarial drugs act at different stages of the malaria parasite's life cycle.

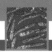
Antimalarial drugs and their mechanisms of action

Class	Drug (International generic name)	Pharmacodynamics					
		Against sporozoites	Tissue schizontocide	Hypnozoitocides	Blood schizontocide	Gametocytocide	Sporontocide
4-Aminoquinolines	Choloroquine	–	–	–	+	vmo	–
	Amodiaquine	–	–	–	+	vmo	–
Arylaminoalcohols							
Quinoline methanols	Quinine	–	–	–	+	vmo	–
	Quinidine	–	–	–	+	vmo	–
	Mefloquine	–	–	–	+	vmo	–
Phenanthrene methanol	Halofantrine	–	–	–	+	–	–
Antifolates							
Type 1	Sulfadoxine	–	–	–	+	–	–
	Dapsone	–	–	–	+	–	–
Type 2	Proguanil	–	f	–	+	–	+
	Chlorproguanil	–	f	–	+	–	+
	Pyrimethamine	–	f	–	+	–	+
8-Aminoquinolines	Primaquine	–	+	+	±	+	+
Antibiotics	Tetracycline	–	f	–	+	–	–
Quinghaosu	Artemisinin	–	–	–	+	+	–

Fig. 11.3 Antimalarial drugs and their mechanisms of action.
(–, no effect; ±, slight effect; +, marked effect; f, effective against *P. falciparum*; vmo, effective against *P. vivax, P. malariae*, and *P. ovale*)

CHLOROQUINE is the most widely prescribed antimalarial drug in the tropics. If the malaria parasite is susceptible to it, it is invaluable for curative use because it acts rapidly, and it is useful for suppressive prophylaxis.

Chloroquine is rapidly absorbed after ingestion and therapeutic blood concentrations are reached within 2–3 hours. It is slowly eliminated from the body. The kidney is the main route of elimination. Chloroquine is predominantly excreted unchanged (about 50%), and 50% of chloroquine is metabolized in the liver, mostly by oxidation via the cytochrome P-450 sytem.

Immediate adverse effects include nausea, vomiting, headache, uneasiness, restlessness, blurred vision, hypotension, and pruritus. It is considered to be relatively safe for use in pregnancy.

A resistant strain of *P. falciparum* transports chloroquine out of its food vacuole more rapidly than susceptible strains. Ca^{2+} channel blockers (e.g. verapamil and nifedipine) suppress the efflux of chloroquine and, if given with chloroquine, could theoretically allow effective therapy against chloroquine-resistant strains. Recently the molecular genetic base of chloroquine resistance has been described.

AMODIAQUINE is similar to chloroquine in many ways, but appears to retain some activity against chloroquine-resistant strains of *P. falciparum*. However, this advantage is usually short-lived, and one of its metabolites, a quinoneimine, produces toxic hepatitis and potentially lethal agranulocytosis. Its use is now discouraged.

Arylaminoalcohols

The quinoline methanols (quinine, quinidine, and mefloquine) and the phenanthrene methanol (halofantrine) are blood schizontocides that are effective only on the blood stages of the malaria parasite engaged in digesting hemoglobin. They are used to treat acute disease because of their rapid effect on the blood stages.

QUININE AND QUINIDINE are alkaloids extracted from the bark of the cinchona tree. They remain the drug of choice for the treatment of severe and complicated malaria and should always be given by rate-controlled infusion. Quinine is considered to be relatively safe in pregnancy.

Mild adverse effects are common, notably cinchonism (i.e. tinnitus, hearing loss, nausea, uneasiness, restlessness, and blurring of vision), though hypoglycemia is the most serious frequent adverse effect.

MEFLOQUINE is structurally similar to quinine and is a long-acting blood schizontocide that is effective against all malarial species including multi-drug-resistant *P. falciparum*. It can also be used for suppressive prophylaxis. It is available only in tablet form.

Adverse effects include nausea, vomiting, abdominal colic, sinus bradycardia, sinus arrhythmia, and postural hypotension. Serious but relatively rare adverse effects are acute psychosis and a transient encephalopathy with convulsions. It has been suggested that mefloquine may cause fetal abnormalities when taken during the first trimester of pregnancy.

HALOFANTRINE is another synthetic antimalarial drug that is active against multiresistant *P. falciparum*. Its oral bioavailability is poor and variable, but can be increased if it is taken with a fatty meal. There is no parenteral preparation.

Halofantrine is usually well tolerated, with minor and reversible events such as nausea, abdominal pain, and diarrhea. However, it has been shown to prolong the electrocardiographic QTc interval at the standard recommended dose and there have been rare reports of serious, sometimes fatal, ventricular arrhythmias.

Antifolates (see also Chapter 9)

The sulfonamides (sulfadoxine, sulfalene, and co-trimoxazole), a sulfone (dapsone), the biguanides (proguanil and chlorproguanil), and a diaminopyridine (pyrimethamine) are drugs that affect parasite folate metabolism and are divided into two groups:

- The sulfonamides and dapsone are known as type 1 antifolate drugs. They compete for the enzyme dihydropteroate synthetase (DHPS), which is found only in the parasites.
- The biguanides and the diaminopyrimidines are known as type 2 antifolate drugs since they specifically inhibit malaria dihydrofolate reductase (DHFR) (Fig. 11.4).

Since both type 1 and type 2 antifolates inhibit all growing stages of the malaria parasite, these drugs are used for causal prophylaxis and treatment, and are also sporontocides as they prevent the growth of sporogonic stages in the mosquito. Mixtures of type 1 and type 2 antifolates are used in the treatment of chloroquine-resistant *P. falciparum* infections.

SULFADOXINE has a long half-life of 120–200 hours. It is less effective against *P. vivax* than against *P. falciparum*. It is synergistic in combination with pyrimethamine in a ratio of 20:1, though as the combination acts only on the late red blood stages, it seems to have a much slower action than chloroquine. This combination may cause systemic vasculitis, Stevens–Johnson syndrome, or toxic epidermal necrosis in patients who are hypersensitive to sulfonamide, and should preferably not be given in late pregnancy, during lactation, or to newborn infants because of the theoretical risk of provoking kernicterus.

SULFALENE has a half-life of 65 hours and it is often used in combination with pyrimethamine.

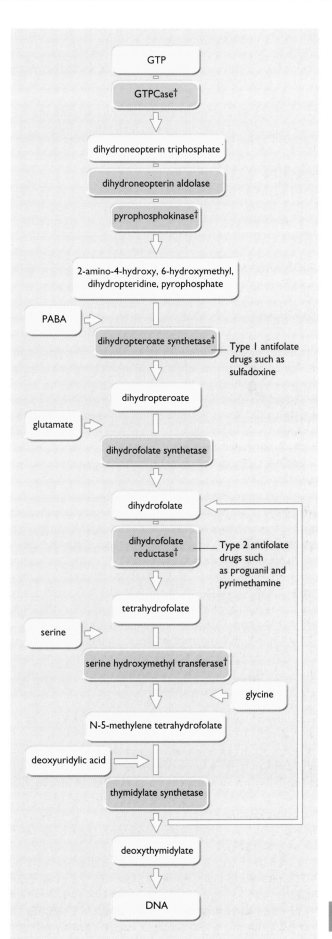

Fig. 11.4 Sites of action of antifolate drugs. Synthesis of DNA from guanosine triphosphate (GTP) by malaria parasites. The enzymes indicated with a dagger have been detected in malaria parasites, the others are presumptive. (GTPCase, GTP cyclohydrolase; PABA, para-aminobenzoic acid) (Adapted from Warhurst DC, *Parasitology Today* 1986; **2**: 58–59, with permission from Elsevier Science.)

DAPSONE has a half-life of 25 hours. It is mainly used in combination with pyrimethamine as the chemoprophylactic drug maloprim. This combination is often prescribed for travelers from the UK and Australia.

CO-TRIMOXAZOLE (TRIMETHOPRIM AND SULFAMETHOXAZOLE) is an antibacterial combination with significant antimalarial activity.

PROGUANIL (and the analog chlorproguanil, which has a considerably longer half-life) are metabolized in the liver into the active metabolites, cycloguanil and chlorcycloguanil, respectively, which are strong DHFR inhibitors. There appear to be two groups in the population, in whom this metabolism by the hepatic enzyme cytochrome P-450 (CYP) 2C19 is either extensive or poor. Poor metabolizers represent 3–6% of Europeans and Africans, and 13–23% of Asians. An unprecedentedly high prevalence (71%) of CYP2C19-related poor metabolizer genotype individuals, and of poor metabolism of proguanil was reported on islands of Vanuatu in eastern Melanesia. A study in Vanuatu also suggested that the parent compound, proguanil, has significant intrinsic efficacy against falciparum and vivax malaria independent of the metabolite cycloguanil.

Proguanil has a half-life of 11–20 hours. It has a slow schizontocidal action on the red blood cell forms of malaria parasites, but is highly effective against the exo-red blood cell forms in the liver and has sporontocidal effects on *P. falciparum*.

Because of its safety, proguanil (200 mg/day) is widely prescribed in combination with chloroquine (300 mg/week) as a causal prophylactic agent. This combination can be used in pregnancy. Proguanil given alone is no longer recommended for the treatment of malaria, but recently there has been renewed interest in its use in combination with sulfones, sulfonamides, or atovaquone.

PYRIMETHAMINE has a half-life of 95 hours. It is used only in combination with sulfonamides or sulfones for treatment and prophylaxis, as resistance to it is now widespread.

Unfortunately, *P. falciparum* seems to undergo spontaneous mutations of its *dhfr* gene, usually as a result of drug pressures, which convey resistance to pyrimethamine and/or cycloguanil. Resistance to sulfadoxine is the result of point mutations of the *dhps* gene. Both pyrimethamine and sulfadoxine are eliminated from the body slowly and, after a standard combination dose, plasma concentrations are initially high enough to kill most *P. falciparum* strains. Unfortunately, thereafter, drug concentrations fall slowly, and only sensitive strains are killed; this provides a powerful selection pressure for emergence of resistant strains.

8-Aminoquinolines

PRIMAQUINE is particularly active against the nongrowing stages of malaria (i.e. gametocytes and hypnozoites). It is currently the only drug available as a gametocytocide for *P. falciparum* and as a hypnozoitocide (antirelapse) for *P. vivax* and *P. ovale*.

Adverse effects include acute intravascular hemolysis in people with glucose-6-phosphate dehydrogenase (G6PD)

deficiency (a hereditary deficit of this red blood cell enzyme), but severe hemolysis is unusual.

Primaquine can cross the placenta and is excreted in breast milk and should not, therefore, be used during pregnancy or lactation. A single dose of 30–45 mg base is adequate for eliminating gametocytes of *P. falciparum*, but 15 mg base is given daily for 14 days to kill the hypnozoites and achieve a radical cure of *P. vivax* and *P. ovale* malaria.

TAFENOQUINE, a congener of the 8-aminoquinoline primaquine, is being developed. It has a better therapeutic index than primaquine and much slower elimination (its half-life is about 14 days). The former property might make tafenoquine a safer drug, but its therapeutic role has yet to be established.

Antibiotics

These drugs (i.e. tetracycline, doxycycline, clindamycin, see Chapter 9) have a slow but marked action on the red blood cell stages of malaria. They are all inhibitors of ribosomal protein synthesis:

- Tetracycline has proved a useful addition to quinine in the treatment of multi-drug-resistant *P. falciparum*.
- Doxycycline is used as a suppressive prophylactic, especially in areas where mefloquine resistance is now common, such as Thailand and Cambodia, but may have a photosensitizing effect in some individuals.

Tetracyclines should not be used in pregnant or lactating women or children under 8 years of age, because they may produce ossification disorders of developing bones and teeth.

Clindamycin is a synthetic derivative of lincomycin and has proved effective in the treatment of uncomplicated falciparum malaria. It may also be used for treatment in combination with quinine.

ARTEMISININ AND ITS DERIVATIVES Artemisinin (quinghaosu) is a sesquiterpene lactone extracted from the herb *Artemisia annua* (sweet wormwood), which has been used in China as an antipyretic for over 2000 years. The active component was isolated and characterized in 1971. Its peroxide (trioxane) configuration is responsible for its antimalarial activity. It has been used successfully both by mouth and as suppositories, but several semisynthetic derivatives have been developed. Artemisinin derivatives in common use include: artemether, artesunate and dihydroartemisinine (which is also the principal metabolite of artemether and artesunate).

All drugs in this class produce central nervous toxicity in laboratory animals at high dose.

Clinical trials of artemisinin and its derivatives (artemether, which is an intramuscular preparation, and artesunate, which is available as an oral and intravenous preparation) suggest that they are rapidly acting blood schizontocides against malaria parasites including multiresistant strains of *P. falciparum*, but recrudescences are common. They have an important potential in the treatment of severe and complicated malaria, including cerebral malaria. In a recent trial in Thailand, artesunate tablets combined with mefloquine proved more effective for the treatment of multiresistant *P. falciparum* than artesunate or

Antiparasitic actions of antimalarial drugs

- 4-Aminoquinolines such as chloroquine are concentrated in the parasite's lysosomes where hemoglobin is being digested
- Arylaminoalcohols such as quinine and mefloquine act on parasites digesting hemoglobin
- Antifolate drugs such as sulfadoxine, pyrimethamine, and proguanil affect parasite folate metabolism
- Antibiotics such as tetracycline inhibit parasite ribosomal protein synthesis
- Primaquine is particularly active against the non-growing stages (i.e. gametocytes and hypnozoites)
- Artemisinin and its derivatives have a peroxide (trioxane) configuration that is responsible for its action

Serious adverse effects of antimalarial drugs

- *Chloroquine and proguanil: mainly mild adverse effects; may be relatively safe in pregnancy*
- *Amodiaquine: lethal agranulocytosis*
- *Quinine: hypoglycemia; appropriate in pregnancy with severe malaria*
- *Mefloquine: acute psychosis and a transient encephalopathy with convulsions*
- *Halofantrine: electrocardiographic prolongation of the QT interval*
- *Sulfadoxine and pyrimethamine: Stevens–Johnson syndrome*
- *Primaquine: acute intravascular hemolysis in people with glucose-6-phosphate dehydrogenase deficiency*
- *Tetracycline: damages development of bones and teeth in children under 8 years of age*
- *Artemisinin: relatively safe to date*

mefloquine alone. Artemisinin and its derivatives have a significant effect on gametocytogenesis. Studies in the Thailand and Myanmer border suggest that artemisinin-based drugs may reduce transmission and, consequently, the spread of resistant strains. Artemisinin derivatives are now among the most promising drugs for malaria chemotherapy because of their novel molecular structure, rapidity of action, and relative safety to date.

New antimalarial drugs

ARTEMETHER–LUMEFANTRINE During treatment with two drugs, the chance of a mutant resistant to both drugs emerging can be calculated from the product of the individual per-parasite mutation rates. The artemisinin derivatives reduce the parasite biomass by around 4 logs for each asexual cycle. This rapid reduction has a major theoretical role when artemisinin derivatives are combined with another antimalarial drug: the parasite population available to develop mutations to the second drug is markedly reduced.

Lumefantrine was synthesized in the 1970s by the Academy of Military Medical Sciences, Beijing. It is a slowly eliminated oral antimalarial drug as a solution in linoleic acid. However, there is marked variation in its pharmacokinetic parameters, indicating poor bioavailability. The fixed-ratio combination of lumefantrine with artemether is close to registration for the treatment of uncomplicated P. falciparum infections and represents the combination therapy approach to treatment.

ATOVAQUONE–PROGUANIL The antimalarial potential of the naphthoquinones was recognized in the mid-1940s. The most interesting compound in this group is now hydroxynaphthoquinone (atovaquone), which clears resistant P. falciparum parasites. Atovaquone alone has an unacceptably high recrudescence rate, but its fixed-ratio combination with proguanil may prevent this.

CHLORPROGUANIL–DAPSONE represents new uses for old drugs and is one of the possible alternatives to sulfadoxine–pyrimethamine. The former combination is eliminated more rapidly than the latter, offering the possibility of lower selection pressure for resistance. Furthermore, chlorproguanil–dapsone retains activity against parasites with mutations of the dhfr gene at positions 108, 51 and 59. This combination is effective for uncomplicated malaria in Africa.

PYRONARIDINE is a mannich base that was synthesized in 1970 at the Institute for Parasitic Diseases, Shanghai. Although it is structurally similar to amodiaquine, it may have a different mechanism of action and differing toxicity. The current oral formulation is effective against multiresistant P. falciparum and well tolerated, but its oral bioavailability is low.

The main adverse reactions of the oral formulation include headache, dizziness, gastrointestinal disorders, and transient electrocardiographic changes.

Parasite resistance to antimalarial drugs

P. falciparum was noted to be resistant to chloroquine in 1959 in Thailand and in Colombia in 1960, and the rapid worldwide spread of chloroquine-resistant falciparum malaria has posed serious problems. The problem of chloroquine resistance has been further complicated by the increasing prevalence of parasite resistance to the combination of sulfadoxine–pyrimethamine and quinine. There are also mefloquine-resistant strains of P. falciparum in South-East Asia and some African countries. However, despite the extensive spread of chloroquine-resistant strains of P. falciparum and the recent emergence of chloroquine-resistant P. vivax in Papua New Guinea, chloroquine is still the most widely used antimalarial drug in the world; there is nevertheless a need for alternative antimalarials.

The resistance of the parasites to antimalarials ranges from a minimal loss of effect, detected only by delayed recrudescence, to a high level of resistance, at which the drug has no suppressive effect. In 1967 the WHO proposed a grading system based on the response of P. falciparum parasites to normally recommended doses of chloroquine (Fig. 11.5). This

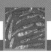

rashes, edema, and anemia. Later, there is invasion of the central nervous system (CNS) with meningoencephalitis leading to apathy, lethargy, and somnolence. Untreated patients ultimately die from malnutrition, intercurrent infection, or deepening coma.

African trypanosomiasis is treated with suramin, pentamidine isethionate, melarsoprol, or eflornithine. If there are no CNS changes, suramin or pentamidine isethionate are the drugs of choice during the early stage of infection, while melarsoprol was until recently the only substance that could be used to treat patients with CNS involvement. Recent studies, however, have shown that eflornithine may be preferable for T. gambiense CNS disease.

SURAMIN After intravenous administration, suramin binds to plasma proteins and persists at low concentrations for as long as 3 months. It does not penetrate into the CNS and is therefore restricted to the treatment of early acute disease. The mechanism of its action is uncertain, but inhibition of many enzymes is probably important because it is a polyanion that readily complexes with proteins.

Suramin causes a variety of adverse effects. Direct adverse effects that call for immediate withdrawal of treatment include rare cases of potentially fatal collapse during the first injection, heavy albuminuria, stomal ulceration, exfoliative dermatitis, severe diarrhea, prolonged high fever, and prostration. Less serious symptoms include anorexia, malaise, polyuria, urticaria, paresthesia, and hyperesthesia.

Suramin is also active against adult Onchocerca volvulus.

PENTAMIDINE ISETHIONATE Pentamidine isethionate is a diamidine compound and is administered intravenously. It is highly tissue-bound, excreted slowly, and does not penetrate into the CNS. Some interactions, such as selective adherence to the DNA of trypanosomal kinetoplasts and inhibition of ribosomal RNA polymerase, may be important to its mechanism of action.

Adverse effects include tachycardia, nausea, rash, hypotension, hypoglycemia or insulin-dependent diabetes mellitus due to direct pancreatic damage, and reversible renal failure.

Pentamidine isethionate may also be used to treat Pneumocystis carinii pneumonia.

MELARSOPROL Melarsoprol is a trivalent arsenical compound and is administered intravenously to treat CNS trypanosomiasis. Arsenicals react with sulfhydryl groups and therefore bind to proteins. It may inactivate pyruvate kinase, a critical enzyme in the metabolism of trypanosomes. It is largely metabolized to nontoxic pentavalent compounds and is excreted in the urine and feces within a few days.

The most serious adverse effect of melarsoprol is encephalopathy, which is fatal in about 6% of patients. Other severe adverse effects include myocardial damage, renal failure, hepatotoxicity, and hemolysis in people with G6PD deficiency. Less serious adverse effects include hyperthermia, urticarial rashes, headache, diarrhea, and vomiting.

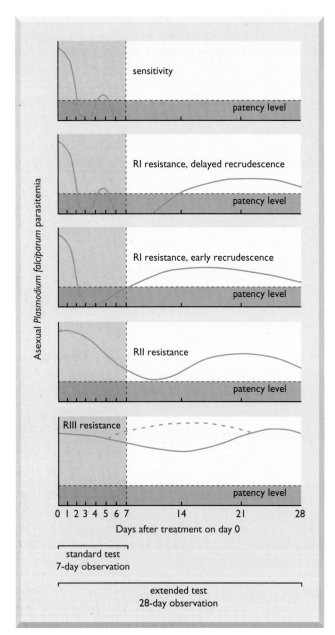

Fig. 11.5 The response of malaria parasites to chloroquine. The diagram shows degrees of response ranging from sensitivity to the highest resistance (RIII). (Adapted with permission from *WHO Technical Report Series No. 529*, by WHO Scientific Group, 1973.)

grading is also used for other blood schizontocides and other species of human malaria.

African trypanosomiasis (sleeping sickness)

■ *African trypanosomiasis is a protozoan disease transmitted by tsetse flies*

Two subspecies of *Trypanosoma brucei* (*T. brucei gambiense* and *T. brucei rhodesiense*) cause African trypanosomiasis, which is a serious health risk to at least 50 million people in sub-Saharan Africa. The early acute disease is a systemic illness characterized by hemolymphatic involvement with intermittent fever, skin

EFLORNITHINE Eflornithine (DL-d-difluoromethylornithine) is a relatively new agent for the treatment of African trypanosomiasis in patients with CNS involvement. Polyamine synthesis in *T. brucei* and *Leishmania* species, as in mammalian cells, is initiated by ornithine decarboxylase (ODCase). Eflornithine inhibits this enzyme. Its therapeutic use is based on the evanescence of human ODCase (which has a half-life of less than 1 hour) compared with that of trypanosomal ODCase (which has a half-life of more than 6 hours). Human cells are capable of regenerating ODCase after eflornithine is eliminated. Eflornithine hydrochloride can be given either intravenously or orally, and 80% is excreted unchanged in the urine. The ratio of cerebrospinal fluid to serum concentrations ranges from 0.09 to 0.45.

Adverse effects of eflornithine hydrochloride are usually mild and reversible. They include anemia, thrombocytopenia, vomiting, diarrhea, and a transient loss of hearing. It is a safer drug than suramin, pentamidine isethionate, or melarsoprol.

American trypanosomiasis (Chagas disease)

■ *American trypanosomiasis is a protozoan disease transmitted by the Triatominidae family of insects, blood transfusion, organ transplantation, and congenital infection*

American trypanosomiasis is caused by *Trypanosoma cruzi* and affects approximately 16–18 million people and a variety of animals in Central and South America. Many people with the infection have no clinical manifestations. The infection starts with an acute parasitemic phase lasting a few weeks and continues with a chronic lifelong phase. *T. cruzi* multiplies in the amastigote phase in body tissues, particularly the heart muscles. Life-threatening manifestations in the acute phase include myocarditis and meningoencephalitis. Chronic sequelae include myocardial damage and intestinal tract involvement.

■ *American trypanosomiasis is treated with nifurtimox or benznidazole*

Both nifurtimox and benznidazole are useful drugs in the treatment of acute American trypanosomiasis. The value of therapy in the chronic phase is not clear.

Nifurtimox reduces the duration of symptoms in the acute phase of American trypanosomiasis and decreases the associated mortality due to myocarditis and meningoencephalitis. It is well absorbed after oral administration and extensively metabolized; little is excreted in the urine. Metabolic reduction of the nitro group yields a nitro anion radical. In the presence of oxygen, the nitro compound is regenerated with the production of superoxide, which is toxic to the parasite and host.

Adverse effects of nifurtimox are frequent, dose-related, and reversible. They include nausea, vomiting, gastric pain, anorexia, vertigo, myalgia, convulsions, and polyneuritis.

BENZNIDAZOLE is another nitroimidazole derivative used in the treatment of acute American trypanosomiasis. Its efficacy and toxicity are similar to those of nifurtimox, but its mechanism of action is unclear.

Leishmaniasis

■ *Leishmaniasis is a group of protozoan infections of the viscera, skin, and mucous membranes transmitted by sandflies*

Leishmaniasis is caused by protozoa of the *Leishmania* species. It is estimated that approximately 12 million people are infected worldwide.

■ *Leishmaniasis is treated with pentavalent antimonial compounds*

Leishmaniasis is usually responsive to pentavalent antimonial compounds. Patients who have relapsed and become unresponsive to antimonials alone have been successfully treated with antimonials combined with allopurinol, pentamidine, or amphotericin B.

Pentavalent antimony

Meglumine antimoniate or sodium stibogluconate are two forms of antimony used to treat leishmaniasis. Their efficacy varies according to the leishmanial species, the geographic area, and the nutritional status and immunocompetence of the host. The pentavalent antimonials are relatively well tolerated. Dose-related electrocardiographic changes are T-wave inversion and prolonged QT intervals. Nausea, anorexia, malaise and lethargy are uncommon, except when high doses (more than 20 mg/kg/day of sodium stibogluconate) are administered.

Other protozoan diseases

Amebiasis

Amebiasis is caused by *Entamoeba histolytica*, which is a protozoan parasite and is worldwide in distribution. It is usually transmitted from person to person through cyst-contaminated food and drink or hands, and may also be transmitted by sexual contact. There are two groups of parasites that can not be distinguished morphologically: a pathogenic parasite (*E. histolytica*) and a nonpathogenic parasite (*E. dispar*). The clinical features of intestinal amebiasis due to *E. histolytica* infection range from mild diarrhea to fatal dysentery. The stools are usually soft, have a foul smell, and are often mucopurulent and bloody (i.e. look like strawberry jelly).

> ⚠️ **Serious adverse effects of drugs for trypanosomiasis and leishmaniasis**
>
> - *Suramin: fatal collapse, heavy albuminuria, stomal ulceration, exfoliative dermatitis, severe diarrhea, prolonged fever, prostration*
> - *Pentamidine: hypotension, hypoglycemia, insulin-dependent diabetes mellitus, reversible renal failure*
> - *Melarsoprol: encephalopathy, myocardial damage, renal failure, hepatotoxicity, hemolysis in people with glucose-6-phosphate dehydrogenase deficiency*
> - *Eflornithine: usually mild and reversible adverse effects*
> - *Nifurtimox: myalgia, convulsions, and polyneuritis*
> - *Pentavalent antimony: relatively well tolerated*

153

Amebic liver abscess is most frequently seen in extraintestinal amebiasis. Clinical manifestations commonly include right hypochondrial or epigastric pain, fever, chills, anorexia, and weight loss. Liver aspiration is a useful diagnostic and therapeutic procedure. The aspirated pus, which looks like anchovy paste or chocolate milk, is mixed with blood and necrotic liver tissue. Pleuropulmonary amebiasis, amebic brain abscesses, and amebic skin ulcers are sometimes seen.

▓ Drugs used to treat amebiasis are metronidazole, tinidazole, or dehydroemetine

Metronidazole and tinidazole are contraindicated in people with known hypersensitivity or chronic alcohol dependence, and in early pregnancy. If dehydroemetine is used, the heart rate and blood pressure should be carefully monitored and treatment should be stopped immediately if tachycardia, severe hypotension, or electrocardiographic changes develop.

METRONIDAZOLE (see Chapter 9) is a nitroimidazole derivative with antiprotozoan activity. It also has antibacterial activity against all anaerobic cocci and both anaerobic Gram-negative bacilli and anaerobic spore-forming Gram-positive bacilli. Its mechanism of action is inhibition of DNA synthesis and degradation of existing DNA, and therefore it is potentially teratogenic.

Adverse effects of metronidazole are usually mild, but headache and gastrointestinal symptoms are common. More serious reactions are stomatitis, leukopenia, peripheral neuritis, and ataxia. When taken with alcohol it can cause abdominal pain, vomiting, flushing, and headache.

Metronidazole is given at a daily dose of 30 mg/kg divided into three portions, for 5–10 days.

TINIDAZOLE is also a nitroimidazole derivative that has recently been developed as an antiprotozoan drug. Its mechanism of action is the same as that of metronidazole, but its adverse effects are less severe.

Tinidazole is given at a daily dose of 2 g, divided into two portions for 2–3 days.

DEHYDROEMETINE Emetine is an alkaloid extracted from ipecac. Dehydroemetine is a derivative of (and is less toxic than) emetine. Following intramuscular injection it is widely distributed in body tissues.

Dehydroemetine has been one of the most widely used drugs in the treatment of severe invasive intestinal amebiasis, amebic liver abscess, and other extraintestinal types of amebiasis.

Adverse effects primarily involve:
- The neuromuscular system, producing weakness (e.g. dyspnea and muscular pain).
- The gastrointestinal tract.
- The heart and cardiovascular system, producing hypotension, precordial pain, tachycardia, and dysrhythmias (e.g. flattening and inversion of the T wave and prolongation of the QT interval).

Dehydroemetine should not, therefore, be used unless the nitroimidazoles are ineffective or contraindicated. Injections should always be given intramuscularly.

Giardiasis

Giardiasis is an infection caused by the flagellated protozoon *Giardia lamblia*. It is transmitted through cyst-contaminated water or food and occurs worldwide, particularly where sanitation is poor. The infection is usually asymptomatic, but moderate to heavy infection usually causes anorexia, nausea, malaise, abdominal muscle cramps, vomiting, abdominal distension, and diarrhea. The clinical signs and symptoms of chronic infection are those of a malabsorption syndrome, with weight loss, steatorrheic stool, and debility.

Giardiasis is treated with either metronidazole or tinidazole.

Toxoplasmosis

Toxoplasmosis is a protozoan infection caused by *Toxoplasma gondii*. It occurs worldwide, but is particularly common in warm humid areas. The sexual reproduction of *T. gondii* takes place in the intestinal epithelium of the cat, which is its final host. Toxoplasmosis is transmitted to humans in several ways, for example through:
- The feces of infected cats (transmitted via oocysts).
- Ingestion of infected raw meat, usually pork (transmitted via cysts).
- Transplacental transmission, to cause congenital toxoplasmosis.

The most common clinical manifestation is cervical lymphadenopathy, but other clinical features are fever, malaise, lymphadenopathy, atypical lymphocytosis, and myalgia. The infection has serious implications in immunocompromised hosts. Congenital infections are generally severe and can result in a fatal syndrome characterized by hydrocephalus, hepatosplenomegaly, icterus, mental retardation, and chorioretinitis.

Toxoplasmosis is treated with pyrimethamine, which is normally used in combination with sulfadiazine (see also previous section on Malaria). Pyrimethamine and sulfadiazine are inhibitors of folate metabolism that kill the tachyzoites but do not eradicate encysted organisms. A combination of pyrimethamine and sulfadiazine is particularly effective because both drugs penetrate the cerebrospinal fluid in therapeutically active concentrations. Pyrimethamine alone has been used to treat toxoplasmic encephalitis in patients who are hypersensitive to sulfadiazine. In adults, the daily dosage is 2–4 g of sulfadiazine, along with 50 mg of pyrimethamine. The dose of pyrimethamine should be halved after 3 days and treatment should continue for 30 days. Since pyrimethamine is an inhibitor of folic acid, leukocyte counts should be checked at least twice a week.

Adverse effects of pyrimethamine are anorexia, abdominal cramps, vomiting, ataxia, tremor, and seizures. It can induce thrombocytopenia, granulocytopenia, and a megaloblastic anemia due to folic acid deficiency at the high dosage needed to treat toxoplasmosis. Adverse effects of sulfadiazine are nausea, vomiting, diarrhea, headache, and occasionally hypersensitivity reactions (e.g. Stevens–Johnson syndrome). Both pyrimethamine and sulfadiazine are contraindicated in people with known hypersensitivity, or severe hepatic or renal dysfunction, and in the first 3 months of pregnancy.

Four major signs of congenital toxoplasmosis

- Retinochoroiditis
- Hydrocephalus
- Intracranial calcification
- Psychomotor disorders

Trichomoniasis

Trichomoniasis is a flagellate protozoan disease caused by *Trichomonas vaginalis*. It is sexually transmitted and is the commonest protozoan infection in the world. *Trichomonas* species have only a trophozoite stage, which multiplies by longitudinal binary fission and is transmitted from host to host. The infection can be asymptomatic in men, but usually causes vaginitis, cystitis, and cervicitis in women.

Drug treatment of trichomoniasis is with metronidazole or tinidazole.

Pneumocystosis

Pneumocystosis is caused by *Pneumocystis carinii*, which has previously been classified as both a protozoan parasite and a fungus. Recently, several studies have reported *P. carinii* as being an organism more closely related to fungi than protozoans. *P. carinii* is a common cause of opportunistic infection in patients who are immunocompromised, as with HIV or malnourishment. *P. carinii* pneumonia is the most frequent immediate cause of death in patients with AIDS. The typical clinical manifestations are severe respiratory symptoms (e.g. dyspnea, tachypnea, cough, and cyanosis).

■ *Drug treatment of pneumocystosis is trimethoprim–sulfamethoxazole or pentamidine isetionate*

TRIMETHOPRIM–SULFAMETHOXAZOLE Most cases of *P. carinii* pneumonia respond to trimethoprim–sulfamethoxazole given in a high daily dosage. These two drugs have a similar anti-protozoan spectrum and independently inhibit different steps in the enzymic synthesis of tetrahydrofolic acid (See Chapter 9).

Adverse effects of trimethoprim–sulfamethoxazole are common and include nausea, vomiting, glossitis, and skin rashes. Hypersensitivity reactions can be severe (e.g. Stevens–Johnson syndrome), while agranulocytosis, aplastic anemia, and thrombocytopenic purpura may also occur. Trimethoprim–sulfamethoxazole is contraindicated in people with known hypersensitivity and severe renal dysfunction.

PENTAMIDINE ISETHIONATE is a diamidine compound with antiprotozoan activity (see section on Trypanosomiasis), and appears to be an effective treatment for *P. carinii* infection. The recommended dose is 4 mg/kg/day for 14 days, either by slow intravenous infusion over at least 60 minutes or by intra-muscular injection.

Adverse effects of pentamidine isethionate include nephro-toxicity, which is common and usually completely reversible.

Other common adverse effects are hypotension, hypoglycemia, and syncope, which occur after rapid intravenous infusion. Pentamidine isethionate is contraindicated in people with known hypersensitivity and severe renal dysfunction.

HELMINTHIC DISEASES

The helminths are large multicellular organisms with complex tissues and organs. Helminth is derived from the Greek word *helmins* and means worm. The three groups of helminths that parasitize humans are:
- Nematoda (roundworms).
- Trematoda (flukes).
- Cestoda (tapeworms).

Nematode (roundworm) infections
Ascariasis

■ *Ascariasis is caused by an intestinal nematode and is acquired by ingesting contaminated vegetables and drinking-water*

Ascariasis is caused by *Ascaris lumbricoides* and is the most prevalent helminthic infection in the world. It is acquired by ingesting mature eggs in contaminated vegetables and drinking-water. The adult worm usually lives in the small intestine, but can migrate to the main bile duct, gall bladder, and pancreatic duct, or can penetrate the small intestinal wall, resulting in erratic infection. The clinical manifestations include a dull upper abdominal pain, loss of appetite, nausea, vomiting, and abdominal distension.

■ *Ascariasis is treated with pyrantel pamoate or piperazine*

PYRANTEL PAMOATE is a broad spectrum anthelmintic and is the drug of choice for treating ascariasis. It is also used to treat *Enterobius vermicularis*, and hookworm infections. It is a depolarizing neuromuscular-blocking agent and inhibits cholinesterase, causing respectively a spastic paralysis and slow contracture of these worms. Pyrantel pamoate is poorly absorbed from the gastrointestinal tract and most of the drug is excreted in the feces.

Adverse effects of pyrantel pamoate are usually rare when it is used in normal doses. It is usually given as a single dose of 5–10 mg/kg.

PIPERAZINE is highly effective against *A. lumbricoides* and *E. vermicularis* infections. It blocks the neuromuscular junction and causes a flaccid paralysis in *A. lumbricoides*. Piperazine is rapidly absorbed after oral administration.

Adverse effects of piperazine are occasional dizziness and an urticarial reaction. It is contraindicated in people with known hypersensitivity, epilepsy, or a renal or hepatic disorder. Piperazine is given as a single dose of 30–80 mg/kg or as divided doses amounting to 50–80 mg/kg in total.

Pyrantel pamoate and piperazine have antagonistic effects and should not be used together.

155

Hookworm infection

Hookworm disease is also one of the most common helminthic infections. It is caused by *Ancylostoma duodenale* (Old World hookworm) or *Necator americanus* (New World hookworm). *A. duodenale* occurs predominantly in temperate zones such as the Mediterranean basin, the Middle East, northern India, China, and Japan, while *N. americanus* occurs in the tropical and subtropical areas of Africa, Asia, and the Americas. The adult worms live in the human intestine as bloodsuckers. The life cycles of both are similar, but the penetration sites by infective larvae (filariform) are different. Old World hookworm larvae penetrate the oral mucosa, whereas New World hookworm larvae penetrate the skin. The major symptoms of infection are related to iron deficiency anemia and a loss of plasma protein.

■ *Hookworm infection is treated with pyrantel pamoate*

PYRANTEL PAMOATE is reported to be more effective against *A. duodenale* than against *N. americanus* and the anthelmintic action of this drug is discussed above. A single dose will decrease the number of worms harbored, but complete cure may require several courses of treatment.

ENTEROBIASIS (OXYURIASIS, PINWORM INFECTION) Enterobiasis is a worldwide infection caused by *E. vermicularis* and is the most common helminthic infection in the developed countries of the northern hemisphere, especially among schoolchildren. The parasite rarely causes serious complications. The major clinical symptom is pruritus ani.

Enterobiasis is normally treated with pyrantel pamoate.

Strongyloidiasis

Strongyloidiasis (*Strongyloides stercoralis* infection) has a worldwide distribution, and is found particularly in tropical and subtropical areas. The infective form (filariform larvae) can penetrate through intact skin and cause an itchy erythema at the point of penetration. These larvae are carried in the blood to the lung and the sputum contaminated with these larvae is swallowed. The larvae then enter the small intestine, penetrate the mucosa, and mature into adult worms. The fertilized female discharges partially embryonated eggs. Larvae are excreted in the stools and some may penetrate the mucous membrane of the lower bowel and the anal skin (autoinfection).

The host immune mechanism and the parasite reproductive mechanism remain in balance so that neither is seriously affected. If this balance is disrupted, massive numbers of larvae can penetrate into all parts of the body (hyperinfection).

■ *Strongyloidiasis is treated with albendazole or thiabendazole, but these should not be given to pregnant women*

ALBENDAZOLE is a benzimidazole derivative that is highly effective in treating strongyloidiasis and is considered to be the drug of choice. It is thought to exert its anthelmintic effect by blocking glucose uptake, depleting their glycogen stores and decreasing the formation of ATP in susceptible helminths, and studies have shown that it has vermicidal, ovicidal, and larvicidal activity. Less than 5% is absorbed after oral admin-istration. A 3-day course of 400 mg once daily is normally prescribed.

Albendazole is well tolerated by both adults and children over 2 years of age, though gastrointestinal discomfort and headache have been reported. It has, however, shown a teratogenic and embryotoxic potential experimentally, and should not therefore be given to pregnant women.

THIABENDAZOLE is a benzimidazole derivative that inhibits the helminth-specific mitochondrial fumarate reductase system of various helminths. It is rapidly absorbed from the gastrointestinal tract and treatment with two divided doses of 50 mg/kg/day for 3 days is very effective against strongyloidiasis. It should be taken for at least 5 days to treat hyperinfection of strongyloidiasis.

Thiabendazole is associated with a high incidence of acute adverse effects such as vertigo and gastrointestinal discomfort (e.g. nausea, a loss of appetite, and vomiting). It also has a teratogenic and embryotoxic potential experimentally and should not be given to pregnant women. Ivermectin can be used as an alternative drug.

Infection with nematode larvae

Visceral larva migrans (toxocariasis), angiostrongyliasis, and trichinosis are examples of infection with nematode larvae:

- Visceral larva migrans is a syndrome caused by the migration of the larvae of *Toxocara canis* in the viscera. Most patients are infected with only a small number of larvae and are usually asymptomatic. The infection is frequently associated with eosinophilia.
- Trichinosis is much more common in Europe and America than in Africa and Asia and is caused by *Trichinella spiralis*. The initial phase of the infection can cause transient gastro-intestinal complaints such as nausea, diarrhea, vomiting, and abdominal pain. The phase of muscle invasion by the larvae typically causes the triad of myalgia, palpebral edema, and eosinophilia.
- Angiostrongyliasis is caused by *Angiostrongylus cantonensis*. Approximately 2000 cases have now been reported in the Asian Pacific area. The major clinical manifestations of cerebral angiostrongyliasis are eosinophilic meningitis with peripheral eosinophilia.

These infections are all treated with thiabendazole for at least 1–2 weeks.

Filariasis (Bancroftian filariasis, Brugian filariasis, loiasis)

Bancroftian filariasis and Brugian filariasis are caused by *Wuchereria bancrofti* and *Brugia malayi*, respectively, and have different geographic distributions:

- Bancroftian filariasis occurs in tropical areas (e.g. Central Africa, South America, India, southern China).
- Brugian filariasis is restricted to Indonesia, the Malay peninsula, Vietnam, southern China, central India, and Sri Lanka.

Both Bancroftian and Brugian filariasis are referred to as lymphatic filariasis since the organisms are found in the lymphatic system and are diagnosed mainly by detecting microfilariae in the peripheral blood.

- Loiasis is caused by the African eye worm (*Loa loa*). It is endemic only to the rainforest areas of central and west Africa. The major clinical features (fugitive swelling or Calabar swelling) result from the continuous migration of the adult worm into subcutaneous tissues.

Diethylcarbamazine is used to suppress and cure infections with W. bancrofti, B. malayi and Loa loa

DIETHYLCARBAMAZINE kills both the microfilariae and the adult worms of Bancroftian and Brugian filariasis and loiasis. A total cumulative dosage of 72 mg/kg is needed to eliminate *W. bancrofti* infections, but a lower dosage is recommended for treating *B. malayi*.

Adverse effects of diethylcarbamazine are anorexia, nausea, headache, and vomiting. They are not severe and usually disappear within a few days despite continued therapy.

Onchocerciasis (river blindness)

Onchocerca volvulus is the parasite that causes river blindness and is common in all parts of West and Central Africa, particularly along the rivers of the savanna in south Sahara.

Ivermectin has replaced diethylcarbamazine as the drug of choice to treat onchocerciasis

IVERMECTIN immobilizes *Onchocerca volvulus* by producing a tonic paralysis of the peripheral muscle system (Fig. 11.6). It is given as a single oral dose of 0.15–0.20 mg/kg every 6–12 months.

Adverse effects are generally not reported with ivermectin, although a mild ocular irritation, transient nonspecific electrocardiographic changes, and somnolence have been reported. An immediate inflammatory reaction resulting from the death of microfilariae (Mazzotti reaction) can be severe.

Trichuriasis and capillariasis

Trichuriasis (whipworm disease) is distributed worldwide, but is most prevalent in tropical and subtropical areas. It is caused by *Trichuris trichiura*. The eggs are usually stained with bile and are barrel-shaped, and transparent bipolar mucoid plugs in the feces are characteristic and diagnostic features. Patients with mild infection are usually asymptomatic, but may have gastrointestinal symptoms such as abdominal pain, diarrhea, nausea, anorexia, anemia, rectal prolapse, weakness, and cachexia.

Intestinal capillariasis is caused by *Capillaria philippinensis* and is reported in the Philippines, Thailand, Japan, and Iran. Symptoms include watery stools, malaise, anorexia, nausea, and vomiting.

Both trichuriasis and capillariasis can be treated by albendazole (as described above) or by mebendazole.

MEBENDAZOLE is a benzimidazole derivative that inhibits glucose transport. Its site of action is cytoplasmic microtubules and intestinal cells of nematodes, where it binds to the colchicine receptor on tubulin dimers (Fig. 11.7). The small amounts absorbed after oral ingestion are extensively metabolized within the liver to inactive moieties.

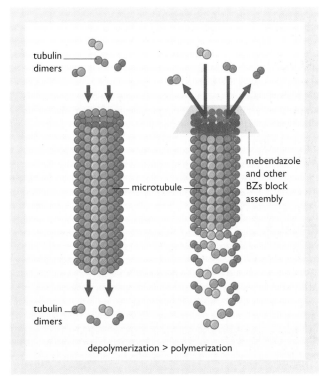

Fig. 11.7 Mechanism of action of mebendazole and other benzimidazoles (BZs). Microtubules are polar, with polymerization continually occurring at one end and depolymerization at the other. These drugs bind with high affinity to a site on the tubulin dimer, so preventing polymerization. Depolymerization leads to complete breakdown of the microtubule. (Adapted with permission from Brody, Larner, Minneman and Neu, *Human Pharmacology Molecular to Clinical*, Mosby-Year Book Inc.; 1994.)

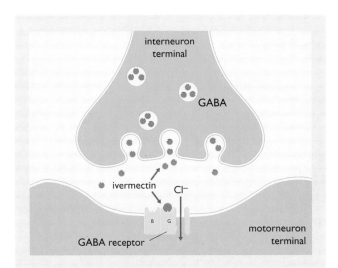

Fig. 11.6 Interaction between the nematode synapse and ivermectin. Potentiation of γ-aminobutyric acid (GABA) results in an influx of Cl⁻ and motor neuron hyperpolarization. Ivermectin also potentiates GABA release, which may explain its anthelmintic mechanism of action by causing worm paralysis.

Trematode infections
Schistosomiasis (bilharziasis)

Schistosomiasis is caused mainly by *Schistosoma japonicum*, *S. mansoni*, and *S. haematobium*, the type depending on the geographic location:

- *S. japonicum* infection is endemic to China, the Philippines, Thailand, Laos, and the Indonesian island of Celebes.
- The endemic area of *S. mansoni* infection includes the Middle East, Africa, and South America.
- The endemic area of *S. haematobium* infection includes Africa and the Middle East.

Infected snails are the intermediate hosts for fresh water transmission.

S. japonicum and *S. mansoni* primarily involve the liver, spleen and gastrointestinal tract, whereas *S. haematobium* affects the genitourinary tract.

Schistosomiasis is treated with praziquantel

PRAZIQUANTEL is highly active against a broad spectrum of trematodes, including all species of schistosomes pathogenic to humans. At the lowest effective concentrations it increases muscular activity, and this is followed by contraction and spastic paralysis. At slightly higher but still therapeutic concentrations, it causes vacuolization and vesiculation of the tegument of susceptible parasites (Fig. 11.8). It is given at a daily dose of 50 mg/kg divided into three portions after meals for 2 days only.

Praziquantel is well tolerated and safe when given in one to three doses during the same day for single or mixed infections with all species of *Schistosoma*. Adverse effects include abdominal discomfort, nausea, headache, and dizziness, and may occur shortly after administration. It is preferable to delay treatment of pregnant women until after delivery, though praziquantel has not been reported to be mutagenic, teratogenic, or embryotoxic.

Clonorchiasis and opisthorchiasis

Clonorchiasis is caused by *Clonorchis sinensis* and is endemic to China, Taiwan, Hong Kong, Japan, and Korea. Opisthorchiasis is caused by *Opisthorchis viverrini*, which is distributed in Thailand, Laos, and Kampuchea, and *O. felineus* in Russia and Central and Eastern Europe. Most infections are asymptomatic in the acute stage, but may sometimes cause acute signs and symptoms including chills, fever, epigastric discomfort, hepatosplenomegaly, and eosinophilia. In the chronic stage, patients often have nonspecific gastrointestinal symptoms, including nausea, vomiting, a loss of appetite, and abdominal pain. The most frequent complication is recurrent cholangitis. These diseases are also a common cause of pancreatitis.

Clonorchiasis and opisthorchiasis are treated with praziquantel, 50–75 mg/kg, divided into three portions, after meals for 2 days.

Paragonimiasis

Paragonimiasis is caused by a lung fluke of a variety of *Paragonimus* species, most commonly *P. westermani*. However, many other pathogenic species have been reported:

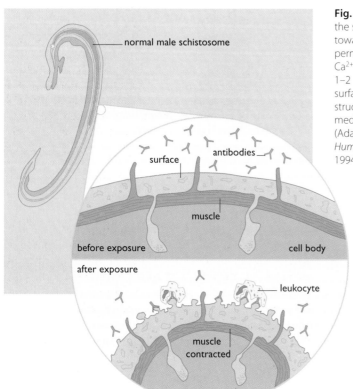

normal male schistosome

antibodies

surface

muscle

before exposure

cell body

after exposure

leukocyte

muscle contracted

Fig. 11.8 Mechanism of action of praziquantel. Before exposure the schistosome is unaffected by the numerous antibodies directed towards its surface. Exposure to praziquantel increases membrane permeability to certain monovalent and divalent cations, particularly Ca^{2+}, inducing an influx of Ca^{2+} into the schistosome tegument within 1–2 seconds. The resultant change in permeability of the schistosome surface towards external ions causes small holes and balloon-like structures to form, making the schistosome vulnerable to antibody-mediated adherence of host leukocytes, killing the schistosome. (Adapted with permission from Brody, Larner, Minneman and Neu, *Human Pharmacology Molecular to Clinical*, Mosby-Year Book Inc.; 1994.)

- In Asia, *P. skrjabini, P. hueitungenesis, P. heterotrema, P. philippinensis* and *P. miyazakii.*
- In Latin America, *P. kellicotti, P. mexicanus, P. ecuadoriensis* and *P. calilensis.*
- In Africa, *P. africanus* and *P. uterobilateralis.*

Paragonimiasis is contracted by ingesting infected uncooked crustaceans, which are the second intermediate host of *Paragonimus.* In Japan, flesh meat of wild boars (the paratenic host of *P. westermani*) is a source of infection.

The major clinical manifestations of paragonimiasis are pulmonary signs and symptoms (e.g. pleural pain, dyspnea, bloody sputum, cough). Complications include pleural effusion, pneumothorax, pulmonary abscess, and empyema. Eosinophilia is common. Chest radiographs may show diffuse infiltration and nodular or ring shadows. Ectopic migration of the parasites has been reported in practically all internal organs. The most important complication is cerebral paragonimiasis. It is most frequently encountered in children in Japan and Korea.

Paragonimiasis is treated with praziquantel as a daily dose of 50–75 mg/kg, divided into three portions for 3 days, or bithionol.

BITHIONOL is used in a dosage of 50 mg/kg divided into two or three portions after meals on alternate days for a total of 10–15 doses. Its mechanism of action is inhibition of respiration of the parasite mitochondria.

Adverse effects of bithionol are common and are generally mild and transient, but the symptoms are occasionally severe (e.g. anorexia, diarrhea, nausea, vomiting, dizziness, headache, and abdominal cramps).

Fascioliasis

Fascioliasis is caused by *Fasciola hepatica, F. gigantica* and other *Fasciola* sp. (Japanese large liver fluke). It occurs worldwide, is common in cows, goats, and horses, and is endemic in Europe, South and Central America, Africa, and Asia. *F. gigantica* has been reported mainly in Africa. After ingestion these worms incidentally infect the biliary system of humans, and freshwater plants such as watercress, lettuce, and alfalfa, and cow's liver have been reported as sources of infection. The worms are harbored in intrahepatic bile ducts and patients with fascioliasis usually have hepatomegaly, fever, and eosinophilia.

Fascioliasis was previously treated with bithionol at a dose of 50 mg/kg divided into three portions after meals on alternate days for a total of 10–15 doses or praziquantel at a dose of 75 mg/kg divided into three portions for 7 days. Recently, triclabendazole, a benzimidazole derivative, has been found to be more effective than bithionol or praziquantel in the treatment of fascioliasis. Triclabendazole is given in a single dose of 10 mg/kg.

Fasciolopsiasis

Fasciolopsiasis is caused by *Fasciolopsis buski* and the endemic areas of this disease are eastern China, Taiwan, Thailand, Vietnam, Laos, India, and Indonesia. People become infected by eating contaminated aquatic plants, and the parasite then lodges in the duodenum and jejunum. Most infections are asymptomatic, but clinical signs and symptoms such as fever, eosinophilia, generalized edema, intestinal obstruction and malnutrition can occur in severe infection.

Fasciolopsiasis is treated with praziquantel at a dose of 50–75 mg/kg divided into three portions for 3 days.

Heterophyiasis

Heterophyiasis is caused by the members of the family Heterophyidae (e.g. *Heterophyes heterophyes* and *Metagonimus yokogawai*). *H. heterophyes* is found mainly in Egypt, the Mediterranean basin, and Japan, while *M. yokogawai* is most common in the Far East and is contracted by eating raw fish. These two parasitic infections are asymptomatic, though severe infection may produce gastrointestinal signs and symptoms (e.g. colic, abdominal tenderness, and diarrhea).

Heterophyiasis is treated with praziquantel at a dose of 50 mg/kg divided into three portions for 1–2 days.

Cestode infections

Large intestinal tapeworms (except *Taenia solium*)

Taeniasis saginata is caused by adult *Taenia saginata*, which is known as the beef tapeworm, and humans are the definitive hosts. The adult worms are 5–8 m long and are made up of 1000–2000 proglottides. *T. saginata* is distributed worldwide. The adult worm is harbored in the small intestine of the host, and the gravid proglottides are expelled. Taeniasis saginata is common in Ethiopia and in Mexico, and relatively common in South America and East and West Africa. It rarely produces severe clinical features, but must be distinguished from taeniasis caused by *T. solium.*

Diphyllobothriasis is caused by the adult *Diphyllobothrium latum*, which is known as the fish tapeworm. The infection is seen in most parts of the world (e.g. in many European countries, the Near East, Siberia, Japan, and North America). People can become infected by eating poorly cooked fillets of salmon, trout, and pike, which are intermediate hosts. The adult worm is the longest tapeworm that infects man, measuring 4–10 m in length. Most patients are asymptomatic, but in Finland some patients with this disease are anemic owing to a lack of vitamin B_{12}.

These large tapeworm infections can be treated with praziquantel, niclosamide, or Gastrografin.

PRAZIQUANTEL Before the treatment, the patient is given an laxative electrolyte solution (e.g. GoLytely, a polyethylene glycol lavage solution) to reduce the quantity of feces in the intestinal lumen. Praziquantel then is given as a single dose of 10 mg/kg. Magnesium sulfate is taken as a rapid-acting laxative to expel the tapeworm 2–3 hours after the praziquantel.

NICLOSAMIDE has an anthelmintic action, stimulating oxygen uptake at low concentrations and blocking glucose uptake at higher concentrations. When the parasite dies, the scolex is released from the intestinal wall and the worms are digested. Niclosamide is a safe drug because very little is absorbed from

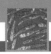

the gastrointestinal tract. On the day of treatment, the patient is fasted until treatment. The adult dose is 2 g as a single dose. Children weighing more than 34 kg are given 1.5 g, while those weighing 10–34 kg are given 1 g, and those under 10 kg, 0.6 g. The tablets should be chewed thoroughly before swallowing and washed down with a little water. Post-treatment purges to expel the worm are not necessary because the scolex and proglottides may be digested by the effect of this drug.

Adverse effects of niclosamide are not severe, though mild gastrointestinal disturbances can occur.

GASTROGRAFIN is a water-soluble contrast material for the gastrointestinal tract that has recently been shown to have an anthelmintic effect on intestinal tapeworm (*T. saginata*, *D. latum*, *Diplogonoporus grandis*). Its mechanism of action has not been reported. A laxative solution such as GoLytely is used to decrease the volume of feces in the intestine before Gastrografin treatment. Gastrografin (300 ml) is injected through a duodenal tube inserted through the mouth until the tip reaches the duodenal flexure. Under fluoroscopic monitoring, the tapeworms are evident as radiolucent shadows descending in the intestine treated with Gastrografin. When the parasites reach the rectum, the patient is encouraged to defecate.

Taeniasis solium and cysticercosis cellulosae

Taeniasis solium is also caused by *T. solium* (pork tapeworm). The adult lives in the human intestine, like *T. saginata* and *D. latum*. Adult *T. solium* possesses 800–900 proglottides and measures approximately 2–3 m in length. Taeniasis solium has a worldwide distribution. Cysticercosis is caused by the larvae of *T. solium* (*C. cellulosae*), which live subcutaneously in the muscle, orbit and brain. Most cases result from ingestion of food and water contaminated with the eggs of *T. solium*. Taeniasis solium and cysticercosis occur in Latin America, Eastern Europe, India, Pakistan, Indonesia, China, and Korea. The clinical manifestations of cerebral cysticercosis depend on the location of the cyst.

▪ *Drugs used to treat taeniasis solium and cysticercosis include Gastrografin, praziquantel, and albendazole*

Gastrografin is the drug of choice for taeniasis because it does not cause any damage to the worm and therefore dangerous live eggs of *T. solium* are not released into the intestinal lumen. The anthelmintic action and dose for therapeutic use of Gastrografin are as described above for the treatment of diphyllobothriasis.

Cysticercosis must be treated after the Gastrografin treatment for taeniasis solium. Praziquantel and albendazole are also useful. Praziquantel is administered in a daily dose of 75 mg/kg, divided into three portions, for 7 days. After a further 7 days, it is given again at the same dose. Prednisolone (15 mg daily divided into three portions) should be given throughout the treatment period to prevent or reduce allergic reactions that may result from the destruction of the cysticerci.

ALBENDAZOLE is a good choice for treating cysticercosis and hydatid disease. Albendazole is absorbed from the gastrointestinal tract and is rapidly and extensively metabolized in the liver. It is recommended that it be taken on an empty stomach when it is used against intestinal parasites, but with a fatty meal when used against tissue parasites. Two 7-day courses of 10–15 mg/kg/day divided into three portions are separated by treatment-free periods of 7 days. Prednisolone should be given throughout the treatment period to reduce allergic reactions.

Adverse effects of albendazole include transient gastrointestinal discomfort and headache.

Echinococcosis (hydatid disease)

▪ *Echinococcosis is caused by the larval forms of the tapeworms* Echinococcus granulosus *and* E. multilocularis *and is acquired by ingesting the eggs*

E. granulosus is found worldwide and echinococcosis (cystic hydatid disease) is seen in East Africa, the Mediterranean littoral, South America, the Middle East, Australia, India, and Russia. *E. multilocularis* is the second most common species. Echinococcosis from *E. multilocularis* (alveolar hydatid disease) occurs in Canada, Central Europe, Siberia, Alaska, and northern Japan. The adult worms of *E. granulosus* and *E. multilocularis* measure 2–7 mm and 1.2–4.5 mm in length, respectively. The scolex of these worms possesses four suckers and a rostellum with two rows of hooklets.

The adult worms live in the small intestine of a final host (e.g. dog, fox, wolf). Humans are the intermediate hosts and ingest the eggs excreted by an infected final host. The clinical manifestations depend on the size of the cyst (*E. granulosus*) and the degree of infiltration (*E. multilocularis*) in the liver, lung, and other organs. Echinococcosis from *E. multilocularis* resembles carcinoma in its ability to metastasize and is frequently fatal.

Surgery is still the treatment of choice for operable cases of echinococcosis. Chemotherapy with albendazole can be effective, given as four 30-day courses of 10–15 mg/kg/day divided into three portions separated by treatment-free periods of 15 days.

Hymenolepiasis

Hymenolepiasis is caused by *Hymenolepis nana* (the dwarf tapeworm) and *H. diminuta*. *H. nana* is the smallest tapeworm that infects humans; it measures 1–4 cm, and commonly infects children in tropical and subtropical regions. The infection is acquired by ingesting eggs in food and water. Autoinfection and rapid reproduction increase the worm population in malnourished or immunocompromised children, who experience gastrointestinal manifestations including nausea, vomiting, diarrhea, and abdominal pain.

H. diminuta is a common parasite of rats and mice that occasionally infects humans. The adult worm measures 20–60 cm in length. Its life cycle requires an intermediate host (fleas) and final host (rats and mice). People acquire the infection by accidentally ingesting infected fleas.

Treatment is with praziquantel administered as a single dose of 10–25 mg/kg. Niclosamide can be used alternatively:
- On 7 consecutive days for *H. nana* infections, using 2 g on the first day and 1 g on the remaining 6 days.

- For *H. diminuta* infections, as for large intestinal tapeworms (i.e. a single dose of 2 g).

Some antiparasitic drugs and diseases for which they are used are summarized in Fig. 11.9.

Drugs and parasitic infections in which they are used

Drug	Infection(s)	Drug	Infection(s)
Albendazole	Strongyloidiasis Trichuriasis and capillariasis *Taenia solium* and *Cysticercus cellulosae* infection Echinococcosis (hydatid disease)	Pentamidine isethionate Piperazine Praziquantel	African trypanosomiasis Pneumocystosis Ascariasis (roundworm) Schistosomiasis (bilharziasis)
Amodiaquine	Malaria		Clonorchiasis and opisthorchiasis
Antibiotics (clindamycin, tetracycline, doxycycline)	Malaria		Paragonimiasis Fasciolopsiasis
Artemisinin	Malaria		Heterophyiasis
Atovaquone–proguanil	Malaria		Diphyllobothriasis
Benznidazole	American trypanosomiasis (Chagas disease)		Taeniasis saginata Hymenolepiasis
Bithionol	Paragonomiasis, Fascioliasis	Primaquine Pyrantel pamoate	Malaria Ascariasis (roundworm)
Chloroquine	Malaria		Hookworms (*Ancylostoma* or *Necator* spp.)
Co-trimoxazole	Malaria		Enterobiasis (oxyuriasis, pinworm infection)
Dapsone	Malaria		
Dehydroemetine	Amebiasis		
Diethylcarbamazine	Filariasis	Pyrimethamine–sulfadiazine	Malaria Toxoplasmosis,
Eflornithine	African trypanosomiasis		
Gastrografin	*Taenia saginata* and *T. solium*	Pyronaridine	Malaria
Halofantrine	Malaria	Quinidine	Malaria
Ivermectin	Onchocerciasis (river blindness)	Quinine	Malaria
Mebendazole	Trichuriasis and capillariasis	Sodium stibogluconate	Leishmaniasis
Mefloquine	Malaria	Sulfadoxine	Malaria
Meglumine antimoniate	Leishmaniasis	Sulfalene	Malaria
Melarsoprol	African trypanosomiasis	Suramin	African trypanosomiasis
Metronidazole	Amebiasis Giardiasis Trichomoniasis	Tafenoquine Thiabendazole	Malaria Strongyloidiasis, nematode larval infections
Niclosamide	Taeniasis saginata Hymenolepiasis	Tinidazole	Amebiasis Giardiasis
Nifurtimox	American trypanosomiasis (Chagas disease)		Trichomoniasis
		Triclabendazole	Fascioliasis

Fig. 11.9 **Drugs and parasitic infections in which they are used.**

FURTHER READING

Djimdé A, Doumbo OK, Cortese JF et al. A molecular marker for chloroquine-resistant falciparum malaria. *N Eng J Med* 2001; **344**: 257–263. [The latest understanding of the molecular mechanism of chloroquine-resistant malaria.]

Kaneko A, Taleo G, Kalkoa M et al. Malaria eradication on islands. *Lancet* 2000; **356**: 1560–1564. [An example of antimalarial drug use for prevention of transmission in endemic areas.]

Karbwang J, Harinasuta T. *Chemotherapy of Malaria in Southeast Asia.* Bangkok: Mahidol University; 1992. [A useful publication for explaining the clinical pharmacology of antimalarials.]

Marr JJ. Antiprotozoal and antihelminthic chemotherapy. In: Hoeprich PD, Jordan MC, Ronald AR (eds) *Infectious Diseases*, 5th edn. Philadelphia:

J.B. Lippincott Company; 1994, pp. 289–298. [An explanation of the chemotherapy of trypanosomiasis and leishmaniasis.]

Sherman IW (ed.) *Malaria: Parasite Biology, Pathogenesis, and Protection.* Washington: American Society for Microbiology; 1998. [This book describes the latest scientific advances in malaria diseases and antimalarial drugs.]

Strickland GT (ed.) *Hunter's Tropical Medicine and Emerging Infectious Diseases*, 8th edn. Philadelphia: W.B. Saunders; 2000. [This textbook describes general aspects of tropical and parasitic diseases and their treatment.]

Warrell DA. Treatment and prevention of malaria. In: Gilles HM, Warrell DA (eds) *Bruce-Chwatt's Essential Malariology*, 3rd edn. London: Edward Arnold; 1993, pp. 164–195. [This book discusses the general principles of malaria chemotherapy.]

White NJ. Preventing antimalarial drug resistance through combinations. *Drug Resist Updates* 1998; **1**: 3–9. [This paper provides a theoretical basis for combination therapy.]

Winstanley PA. Chemotherapy for falciparum malaria: the armoury, the problems and the prospects. *Parasitol Today* 2000; **16**: 146–153. [The latest review of malaria chemotherapy with many useful references.]

World Health Organization. *Management of Uncomplicated Malaria and the use of Antimalarial Drugs for the Protection of Travellers: Report of an Informal Consultation, Geneva, 18–21 September 1995. WHO/MAL/96.1075.* Geneva: WHO; 1996. [Practical information about major antimalarial drugs.]

World Health Organization. *WHO Model Prescribing Information: Drugs Used in Parasitic Diseases.* Geneva: WHO; 1990. [This publication provides practical and clinical information on essential drugs in the treatment of parasitic infections.]

World Health Organization, *Triclabendazole and Fascioliasis—A New Drug to Combat an Age-old Disease, Factsheet N-191.* Geneva: WHO; 1998.

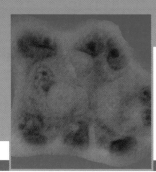

Chapter 12

Drugs and Neoplasms

Numerous diverse agents are used for the treatment of cancer. In order to understand the pharmacology of cancer treatment, certain fundamental aspects of the pathophysiology of cancer and issues relating to its treatment need first to be considered.

TUMORIGENESIS

Tumors are neoplastic growths ('new growths') of cells. Benign tumors do not spread or metastasize from their original site. Malignant tumors, which are also known as cancers, spread or metastasize by:

• Direct extension into surrounding tissues.
• Via the lymphatic system.
• Via the blood (hematogenously).

Cancer is an increasing mass of abnormal cells derived from a single normal cell as a result of clonal expansion that invades surrounding normal tissues and spreads throughout the body via the lymphatic system or the blood. The growth of a cancer is known as carcinogenesis or tumorigenesis and is a multistep process (Fig. 12.1).

Cancer in an individual may be initiated by extrinsic factors (e.g. chemical carcinogens) and by a genetic predisposition. For most cancers, there is an apparent interaction between the two. However, the nature and extent of the interaction vary between individuals. Data from twins suggests that genetic factors contribute approximately 42% of the relative risk of prostate cancer, 35% of colorectal cancer and 25% of breast cancer, with a lesser contribution to other types of cancer.

Extrinsic factors that contribute strongly to carcinogenesis include bacteria such as *Helicobacter pylori*, viruses such as Epstein–Barr, human papilloma or hepatitis B and C, fungi, such as those producing aflatoxins, and chemicals such as benzene.

Oncogenes are DNA sequences that code for the key proteins involved in tumorigenesis. They were first isolated from viruses

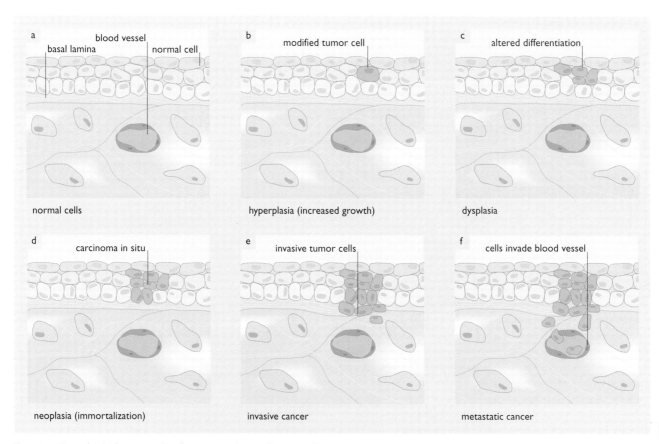

Fig. 12.1 Hypothetical progression from normal to malignant cells.

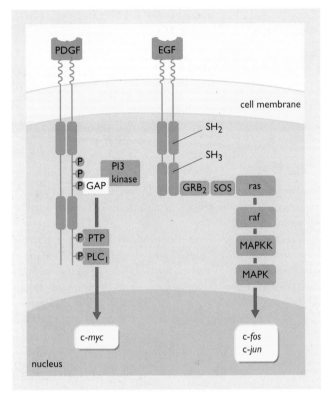

Fig. 12.2 Two schemes showing how extracellular growth factors stimulate cancer cell proliferation. Overexpression of any of these cellular homologs of oncogenes or a mutation that produces constitutive activation may contribute to enhanced growth. (EGF, epidermal growth factor; PI3, phosphoinositol-3-kinase; GAP, GTP-ase activating protein; GRB$_2$, G (protein)-related protein B$_2$; MAPK, mitogen-activated protein kinase; MAPKK, mitogen-activated protein kinase kinase; PDGF, platelet-derived growth factor; PLC, phospholipase C; PTP, phosphotyrosine phosphatase; ras, raf, cellular signal transducers; *c-fos, c-jun, c-myc*, inducers of DNA synthesis)

that caused cancers in laboratory animals and are overexpressed in cancer cells. Oncogenes can code for growth and mitogenic factors and therefore cancer cells can stimulate their own proliferation (Fig. 12.2).

Functional growth factor receptors can be expressed constitutively on the surface of cancer cells, but other growth factors may be needed to initiate expression and activation of some receptors.

Proliferative pathways are normally linked to antiproliferative pathways, leading to feedback control of proliferation. Some oncogene products can inhibit proliferation. Oncogene mutations or overexpression can shift the balance between stimulation and suppression of proliferation. In tumorigenesis, the balance is shifted in favor of proliferation.

Proliferation is also controlled by a separate set of tumor suppressor genes, which act via the cell cycle. Mutations or loss of tumor suppressor genes, such as *p53* in the Li–Fraumeni syndrome or *rb* in retinoblastoma, predisposes individuals and families to an increased risk of cancer.

Proliferation is balanced by cell death. The growth of a population of cancer cells, a tumor, is the net result of proliferation and cell death. Apoptosis is an energy-requiring process by which cells undergo a choreographed process of

cell death. Apoptosis may be the direct result of receptor binding (*Fas* and its ligand in lymphocytes) or release of cytochrome C into the cytoplasm after disruption of the mitochondrial membrane by lethal intracellular events. There are pro-apoptotic proteins, such as Bad and the caspases, which are balanced by antiapoptotic proteins like Bcl-2. Overexpression of Bcl-2 may result from oncogene expression and has been associated with transformation to cancer.

Loss of normal genomic DNA replication is critical to cancer development

Cancer cells can propagate only when the normal capacity to recognize and repair mutations in the genome is lost. Individuals and families with mutations in DNA repair genes are prone to cancer, for example:

- DNA repair genes to repair mismatched base pairs are mutated in hereditary nonpolyposis colon cancer.
- DNA repair to helicases is absent or defective in xeroderma pigmentosum, a genetic disease characterized by defective repair of ultraviolet radiation damage.

p53 may have a crucial role in the cellular response to DNA damage or mutation. Normally, *p53* arrests cells before DNA replication to allow repair to take place and also initiates apoptosis (programmed death of obsolete or damaged cells). Loss of normal *p53* function allows flawed DNA to replicate and the survival of flawed cells.

Cancer cells are immortalized cells

Every cell in the body, except for the germ cell of the gonads, is programmed for a finite number of cell divisions before senescence. This cellular program is the telomere. Telomeres are at the ends of the chromosome and must pair and align at mitosis. They are produced and maintained by an enzyme, telomerase, in germ cells and embryonic cells. This enzyme loses its function during normal development. A portion of the telomere is therefore lost with each cell division and such telomeric loss serves as a cellular clock. Cancer cells re-express telomerase, which allows them to proliferate endlessly. Loss of the normal cell cycle controls imposed by *rb* and *p53* facilitate the re-emergence of telomerase expression. As many as 95% of cancer cells express telomerase, making it a potential target for therapeutic intervention.

Once established and proliferating, cancer invades through the basement membrane and into adjacent connective tissue

Cancer cells express collagenases and plasminogen activators and move through the supporting tissues along the path of least resistance.

🔑 **Characteristics of cancer**
• Increased proliferation
• Loss of regulatory proteins
• Genomic instability
• Immortalization

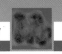

Angiogenesis is essential to supply nutrients and is stimulated by fibroblast growth factor and vascular endothelial growth factor. Collagen, vitronectin, and fibronectin expression promotes cell scaffolding and may aid in attachment at sites of metastasis. Many of the essential components of this complex process are provided by the normal tissues, which can unwittingly contribute to their own demise. The processes of invasion and metastasis are less important in leukemias and lymphomas (blood cancers).

Invasion and metastasis are often well advanced before there are clinical symptoms and the cancer is detected. Pharmacologic therapies are required once a cancer has spread overtly or microscopically beyond its site of origin and has become a systemic disease.

Expert histologic diagnosis is an essential component of cancer chemotherapy

The histologic diagnosis of some tumors is essential to establish whether the objective of therapy is palliation or cure, for example:

- If a non-Hodgkin's lymphoma (NHL) has a low-grade favorable histologic subtype it is incurable, but its growth is relatively indolent. Treatment is therefore conservative, with one chemotherapeutic agent rather than aggressive multiagent chemotherapy.
- If a NHL has an intermediate- or high-grade histologic subtype it has a rapidly fatal natural course, but is often cured by multiagent chemotherapy, while single-agent or less intensive regimens have no effect.
- Extensive, even metastatic, small-cell lung cancer can be cured with multiagent chemotherapy, but nonsmall-cell lung cancer at the same stage is incurable.
- Histologic typing in acute leukemia to show whether it is lymphoblastic or nonlymphoblastic determines the choice of chemotherapeutic agents and the outcome.

Staging is the accurate determination of the extent of tumor spread by local invasion and lymphatic and hematogenous metastases

There is a staging system for each histologic type of cancer based upon its clinical and anatomic characteristics, and the use of biochemical, cytologic, and molecular biologic determinants increases accuracy. Accurate staging serves two purposes:

- It allows precise comparisons between patients and patient groups for a more accurate evaluation of the effectiveness of treatment.
- It is a guide for deciding which treatment to use for an individual patient.

Patients with an early stage of cancer and a favorable prognosis may require less intensive treatment (e.g. less extensive surgery and/or avoidance of chemotherapy). This reduces short-term morbidity and long-term adverse effects, which have become apparent as the treatment of cancer has become increasingly effective and more patients, especially children, survive. Long-term consequences of anticancer drugs include infertility, growth retardation, and second malignancies.

PRINCIPLES OF CELL PROLIFERATION AND CHEMOTHERAPY

A knowledge of the basic processes of cellular proliferation is essential to understand the mechanisms of action of anticancer drugs. Cells in a tissue are in one of the following three stages:

- Actively dividing (cycling).
- Differentiating (dying).
- Dormant (can actively divide if cellular environmental conditions allow).

Four distinct cell cycle phases are recognized: the S, G_1, G_2, and M phases (Fig. 12.3). The activity of replicative enzymes such as thymidine kinase, DNA polymerase, dihydrofolate reductase, ribonucleotide reductase, RNA polymerase II and topoisomerases I and II is increased during the S-phase. Control of a G_2–M checkpoint to allow DNA repair or completion of replicative DNA synthesis is a crucial element in cell cycle control. The G_1 phase may be virtually absent, as in embryonic cells, or so prolonged that it produces dormancy (G_0).

Techniques for measuring cell cycles include the use of tritiated thymidine (^{3}H-TdR)-uptake pulse labeling to determine the fraction of cells actually synthesizing DNA. The S phase can also be measured by using a cell sorter to identify chromosome number (i.e. 2n, 4n). These measurements are used clinically in the staging of breast cancer.

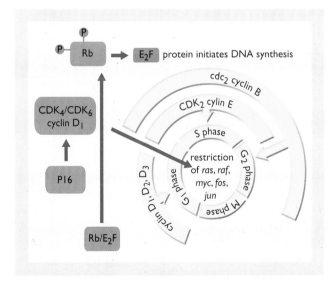

Fig. 12.3 The cell cycle and some of the important regulatory proteins. The S phase refers to the active synthesis of DNA and lasts approximately 12–18 hours. The G_2 phase lasts 1–8 hours and the DNA complement is 4n (twice the normal number of chromosomes). Mitosis (M) lasts about 1–2 hours. The duration of the G_1 phase is variable, and the late G_1 phase is associated with an increase in DNA synthesis enzymes. The complex regulation of the restriction point for the start of S phase involves cyclins and CDKs (cyclin-dependent kinases), which continue to regulate the CDKs through the entire cell cycle. (cdc$_2$, cell division cycle protein 2, an essential controlling gene for cell cycle progression; ras, raf, myc, fos, jun, cellular homologs of viral oncogenes involved in cellular proliferation; Rb, retinoblastoma protein; E$_2$F, a transcription factor)

165

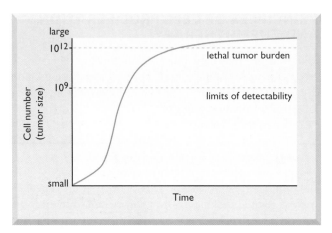

Fig. 12.4 Gompertzian kinetics, not logarithmic growth, best describes cancer cell growth. There is a low growth rate in very small and very large tumors, while intermediate-sized tumors grow exponentially.

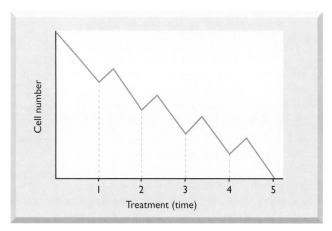

Cell kinetics of leukemia and bone marrow

Cell type	Labeling index (%)	Cell cycle time (h)
Acute leukemia	3–12	48–72
Chronic myelogenous leukemia	6–25	48–72
Chronic lymphocytic leukemia	0–1	48–72
Normal myeloblasts	32–75	16–24
Normal myelocytes	18–25	16–24

Fig. 12.5 Cell kinetics of leukemia and bone marrow.

Fig. 12.6 Log kill hypothesis. A drug or drug combination can kill a constant fraction of cancer cells. Certain cells survive each treatment by chance alone and are sensitive to subsequent treatments.

■ *Cancer cell populations do not grow in a linear manner with time*

The growth of a tumor population is best described by Gompertzian kinetics characterized by slow linear growth at the smallest and largest tumor sizes, with exponential growth in between (Fig. 12.4).

Growth retardation and cell loss correlates with cytologic and spatial factors. Proximity to blood vessels and access to oxygen are important determinants of cell viability and growth and have a significant therapeutic impact on:

• Radiation therapy, where oxygen is an essential intermediate.
• Chemotherapy, where many drugs target multiplying cells.

■ *The dose-limiting toxicity of anticancer drugs on normal tissue is often directly related to its rate of growth*

Normal tissues can be divided into different types on the basis of their cell proliferation kinetics:

• Rapidly proliferating tissues (labeling index (LI) >5%) include the bone marrow, gut mucosa, reproductive organs, and hair follicles.
• Slowly proliferating tissues (LI <1%) include the trachea, bronchial epithelium, liver, kidney, and endocrine organs.
• Nonproliferating tissues in adults include skeletal muscle, heart, bone, and nerve tissue.

The bone marrow is commonly the organ most sensitive to the antiproliferative effects of cancer chemotherapy.

■ *Different tumors have different labeling indexes and doubling times*

A comparison of the growth kinetics of normal bone marrow granulocytes and leukemic cells (Fig. 12.5) shows that the rate of cell proliferation in leukemia is less than in normal bone marrow. However, the cell population in leukemia expands because cell proliferation exceeds cell maturation and death. Solid tumors typically have a much lower fraction of actively growing cells. The LI is 1–5% in slow-growing adenocarcinomas, but up to 30% in Burkitt's lymphoma, testicular carcinoma, Ewing's sarcoma, NHL, and subclinical breast cancer.

Doubling times are 30–70 days in Hodgkin's disease, osteosarcoma, and fibrosarcoma, while slow-growing adult carcinomas with doubling times longer than 70 days include lung cancer, colon and gastrointestinal cancers, and advanced breast cancer. The slower rate of growth results from the presence of many nonproliferating cells and a high rate of cell death.

■ *Several fundamental principles of clinical cancer therapy are determined by cell proliferation kinetics*

The log kill hypothesis postulates that drugs kill a constant fraction of tumor cells (related to the log number of cells) and not a constant number of cells (Fig. 12.6). A proportion of cells in a cancer can survive a course of treatment by chance without being specifically drug resistant. Therefore, each drug or combination of drugs has a certain cytotoxic capacity. As a result, combination therapy is more likely to provide a cure than single-drug therapy.

The log kill varies with cell growth rate and so there is a progressive decrease in log kill in the late stages of tumor growth when cells stop cycling. Early recurrences of slow-growing tumors occur because the log kill is small. Late

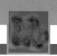

recurrences of rapidly growing tumors may occur despite effective treatment if too few courses of treatment are given. This is referred to as the period of risk.

Some cancer therapies kill cells at specific phases of the cell cycle

Certain classes of intervention (i.e. antineoplastic drugs and radiotherapy) show phase-specific lethality.

In cancer chemotherapy there are several characteristic curves of dose versus cell survival (Fig. 12.7). In exponential curves, the proportion of surviving cells is exponentially related to the dose of the intervention. As the dose increases, the cell kill increases. Such interventions are not cycle- or stage-specific (i.e. they kill cells anywhere in the cell cycle, even resting cells) and include:

- 5-Fluorouracil, cisplatin, glucocorticosteroids, nitrogen mustard, and melphalan.
- Radiotherapy.

Cyclophosphamide and other alkylating agents are active in all cells, but have increased activity in cells at the G_1–S boundary.

Phase-specific survival curves show a plateau with no increase in kill at higher doses. Further kill can be obtained, however, by increasing the exposure time, but not the dose. Drugs producing this type of curve are:

- The antimetabolic cytotoxic drugs such as cytarabine, thioguanine, and hydroxyurea, which are active only in the S phase.
- Methotrexate, doxorubicin, epipodophyllotoxin, and vinca alkaloids, which have maximum lethal toxicity during the S phase.

- Bleomycin, which has maximum activity in the G_2 and M phases.

Cytotoxic drugs block the cell cycle

All cytotoxic anticancer drugs can interfere with progression of cells through the cell cycle, leading to synchronization and slowing of rapidly proliferating cells. This results in decreased sensitivity to S-phase drugs.

Cytotoxicity is proportional to the total drug exposure

The pharmacokinetics of cancer chemotherapeutic agents can be complex, and cytotoxicity is proportional to the total drug exposure (area under the curve (AUC)), and not the peak plasma concentration of drug (Fig. 12.8). The drug has first to penetrate into individual cancer cells and then to interact with its molecular target. As this interaction is often reversible, at least initially, a cytotoxic concentration must be maintained at this time. In addition, the number of individual interactions between a drug and target molecules needed to kill a single cell can be enormous. It is estimated that 1 million molecules of cisplatin must bind to the DNA of a single cell to kill it.

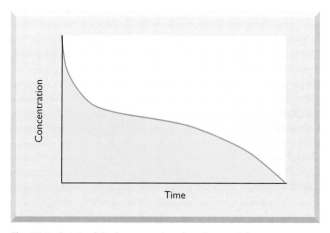

Fig. 12.8 Cytotoxicity is proportional to the total drug exposure or area under the curve (shaded).

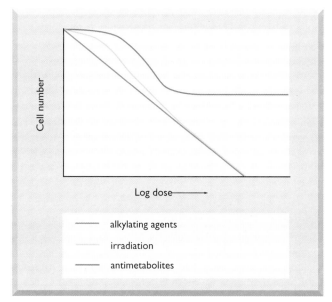

Fig. 12.7 Cycle-specific drug lethality. For noncycle-dependent agents like irradiation or alkylating agents, increasing dose produces increasing cell kill. For cycle-specific agents, like antimetabolites, which kill only actively growing cells, increasing doses have a plateau effect as cell growth slows with chemotherapy. Prolonging the duration of exposure will increase the cell kill.

Principles of cytotoxic cancer therapy
- Drugs kill a constant fraction, not a constant number, of cells
- Cells may have discrete periods of vulnerability to cytotoxic drugs
- Cytotoxic drugs slow the progression of cells through the cell cycle
- Cytotoxic drugs are not selectively toxic toward cancer cells
- Cytotoxicity is proportional to total drug exposure

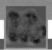
PRINCIPLES OF COMBINATION CHEMOTHERAPY

Combinations of anticancer drugs were introduced because it was found that single agents did not produce significant remissions or cures except for choriocarcinoma.

Drugs used for combination therapy should:
• Be effective when used alone.
• Preferably produce a high fraction of a 'complete response' (defined as a 100% kill of cells in a tumor) rather than a partial response (e.g. less than a 50% kill).
• Have different biochemical mechanisms of action to attack a tumor containing a heterogeneous population of cells.
• Not have similar adverse effects, otherwise the dosage will need to be reduced, resulting in a loss of the added benefit of the combination.

Tumors are heterogeneous in a variety of ways, including drug sensitivity, as a result of their unstable generic make-up. Most drug resistance is innate for the tumor type. It may become clinically apparent when sensitive clones in the tumor are killed and the resistant clones propagate and become dominant. Curability is proportional to the tumor cell number and, in accordance with the Goldie–Coldman hypothesis, there is a greater probability of (drug-resistant) mutations in a larger population of cells (Fig. 12.9).

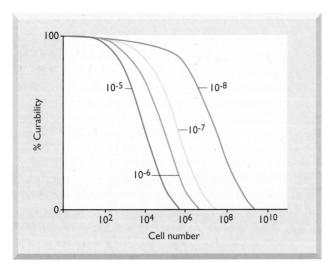

Fig. 12.9 The Goldie–Coldman hypothesis. For an intrinsic rate of mutation to drug resistance, the chances of drug failure (incurability) increase with size of the tumor (10^{-5} to 10^{-8} indicate mutation rate per cell division, i.e. 10^{-5} is one mutation per 100,000 divisions).

Principles of combination chemotherapy

• Drugs used have individual anticancer actions, nonoverlapping toxicity, and different mechanisms of action
• Optimal dose and schedule regimens used
• Shortest possible dosing interval

Benefits of combination therapy over single interventions

• Increases maximum cell kill and decreases toxicity
• Kills cells in tumors with heterogeneous cell populations
• Reduces the chances of development of resistant clones

LATE COMPLICATIONS OF CANCER CHEMOTHERAPY

Gonadal dysfunction

The cancer therapies most likely to produce gonadal dysfunction are alkylating agents (and irradiation), and this is dose-related.

About 80% of males with Hodgkin's disease treated with MOPP (mechlorethamine, vincristine, procarbazine, and prednisolone) become oligo- or azoospermic, and about 50% recover within 4 years. Procarbazine is the principal cause.

In females, amenorrhea, vaginal atrophy, and endometrial hypoplasia are dose- and age-related. Irreversible changes and menopause due to ovarian failure are more likely with increasing age. Alkylating agents (and irradiation) are the most common causes.

Gonadal dysfunction is less severe and more reversible in prepubertal children, but boys at puberty appear to be more susceptible than any other patient group.

Carcinogenesis

Carcinogenic chemicals and some therapeutic drugs can cause cancer. One common factor in their mechanism of action is interaction with DNA.

Testing for environmental and occupational carcinogens involves examining the capacity of an agent to produce mutations in bacteria (Ames test) or to produce sister chromatid exchanges (translocations of genomic sequences from one chromosome to its identical, diploid counterpart) in cultured mammalian cells. Clinical proof of carcinogenesis is difficult to establish.

Drugs have high, low, or unknown risks of producing malignancies, and anticancer drugs are the drugs most commonly associated with drug-induced cancer (Fig. 12.10).
• The alkylating agents are particularly implicated in hematopoietic malignances, and those used in low daily doses for prolonged periods are most likely to produce leukemia, characteristically 3–7 years after treatment begins.
• Ovarian cancer treated with chemotherapy is followed by an approximately 27-fold increase in acute nonlymphocytic leukemia (ANLL).
• Breast cancer treated with melphalan is followed by an up to sevenfold increase in ANLL.
• Myeloma treated with melphalan is followed by an approximately 214-fold increase in ANLL at 50 months (17.4% of the total incidence), but there is no increase in ANLL after 20 years of follow up in patients with breast cancer treated with a combination of cyclophosphamide, methotrexate, and 5-fluorouracil (CMF).

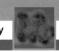

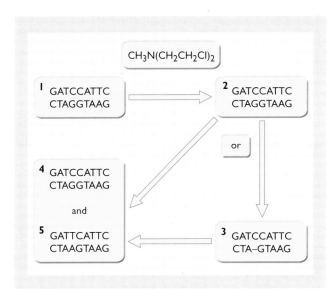

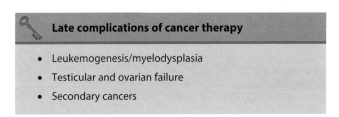

Fig. 12.10 Carcinogenesis or leukemogenesis occur because drugs, especially the alkylating agents, cause permanent genetic mutations. This is exemplified by the G to A transition shown. (1) Correct base pair sequence (hypothetical). (2) Alkyl adduct binds to guanine (white). (3) Spontaneous loss of the adducted guanine (depurination), producing a strand break. (4) Repair/removal of the alkyl adduct and return to correct base pair sequence. (5) G to A transition producing a mutation. A mutation in a proto-oncogene or tumor suppressor gene would confer a proliferation to that cell and its clonal progeny.

Late complications of cancer therapy

- Leukemogenesis/myelodysplasia
- Testicular and ovarian failure
- Secondary cancers

An increased incidence of early leukemias (ANLL less than 2 years after treatment) with a different chromosomal translocation at 11q23 has been noted in patients treated with drugs acting on topoisomerase II, such as etoposide and doxorubicin.

RESISTANCE TO CHEMOTHERAPY

If a cancer is incurable, some fraction of the cancer cells must be resistant to treatment. Resistance that is clinically apparent at the time of initial treatment because the majority of cells in the tumor are resistant is called *de novo* resistance. If the treatment initially kills nonresistant cells in the tumor, resistance is said to be acquired.

De novo resistance can be *de novo* genetic (i.e. the cells are initially inherently resistant), or can arise because drugs are unable to reach the target cells because of permeability barriers such as the blood–brain barrier (i.e. the cancer cells reside in pharmacologic 'sanctuaries').

Mechanisms of generic resistance to cytotoxic drugs

- Abnormal transport
- Decreased cellular retention
- Increased cellular inactivation (binding/metabolism)
- Altered target protein
- Enhanced repair of DNA damage
- Altered processing

De novo genetic resistance is a property of an individual cell and is transferable to its progeny

One widely studied form of genetic resistance produces abnormal transport mechanisms, resulting in either decreased cellular uptake or increased cellular efflux at the cell membrane level. The substrates for such transporters are primarily natural products like plant alkaloids, and include anthracyclines, epipodophyllotoxins, vinca alkaloids, and paclitaxel. Multiple drug resistance arises from a single mutation or amplification of the *mdr 1* gene. The *mdr* gene is a member of the functionally diverse ABC transmembrane superfamily of transport proteins and ion channels, including the membrane resistance protein (MRP) and cystic fibrosis genes.

Many drugs are retained in cells after alteration or activation, for example after the kinase addition of phosphate groups to nucleosides (cytarabine) or polyglutamation of methotrexate. Absent or diminished levels of these enzymes decrease the cellular retention of these drugs and may confer *de novo* resistance.

Pharmacologic sanctuaries include the inaccessible compartments of the blood–brain barrier and the testes

Pharmacologic sanctuaries can occur in solid tumors because their blood supply and diffusion (and therefore drug delivery) are limited by the palisading effect (cells piling up in successive rows) that occurs in tumors. Inappropriate H^+ concentrations (pH) can also confer resistance, as extracellular acidosis in a tumor will ionize some drugs (e.g. doxorubicin) and decrease their cross-membrane movement into cells.

Acquired resistance never develops in non-cancerous cells

Acquired resistance is an imprecise term. It fails to distinguish between the unmasking of innate genetic resistance in the initial heterogeneous tumor that becomes evident only as sensitive cells are killed off, and acquired genetic resistance that is actually induced by the chemotherapy itself, or emerges spontaneously during treatment. Acquired resistance never develops in noncancerous cells and is therefore a property of the unstable mutable genome of transformed cancer cells. In clinical terms, acquired resistance means that the therapeutic ratio (the ratio between the minimum therapeutic and toxic doses) is not constant.

169

Multiple acquired drug resistance is expressed as a dominant phenotype. Gene transfer can confer drug resistance to cells. The amount of P-glycoprotein of 170 kDa (P-GP 170) found on the surface of multiple drug resistance cells correlates with the degree of resistance. The expression of this protein may be increased by oncogenes like *ras* or mutant *p53*.

Membrane resistance protein is a 190,000 kDa ATP binding plasma membrane protein that can confer acquired multi-drug resistance similar to the P-GP 170 MDR protein. Decreased uptake due to deletion or altered kinetics of a transport mechanism, as in methotrexate and melphalan resistance has been described in experimental tissue culture.

Increased intracellular metabolism produces acquired resistance (Fig. 12.11). Enzymes inactivate many drugs by chemical processes such as oxidation, deamination, and reduction, and their enhanced activity may inactivate drugs. For example, aldehyde dehydrogenase oxidizes cyclophosphamide to inactive metabolites and cytidine deaminase inactivates cytarabine.

Altered intracellular concentrations of target protein may result in acquired resistance (see Fig. 12.11):

- An increased concentration of target protein by gene amplification, such as dihydrofolate reductase amplification in methotrexate-resistant cells, may exceed the capacity for drug uptake and binding.
- Decreased topoisomerase concentrations reduce DNA damage and alter cytotoxicity caused by drugs that use topoisomerase I or II as the essential intermediate in producing DNA damage and lethality.
- Compartmentalization of target proteins away from the site of cytotoxic interaction can also produce resistance.

Altered target proteins are frequently encountered in highly resistant tumor cell lines. Mutations in the amino acid sequence of target proteins may change the active site and decrease or abolish drug binding, as in topoisomerase I (camptothecins) and II (etoposide), dihydrofolate reductase (methotrexate), and thymidylate synthetase (5-fluorouracil).

Mutation to a doubly resistant phenotype is stepwise. If there are two effective therapies, resistance may be prevented or delayed by alternating the treatments.

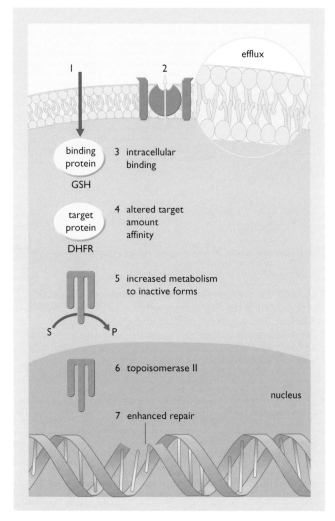

Fig. 12.11 Diagram showing several possible mechanisms of drug resistance. The classical biochemical view. Resistance can occur because of: (1) decreased uptake; (2) rapid efflux via membrane transport proteins; (3) increased intracellular binding to glutathione (GSH); (4) an altered target protein, either an increased amount or decreased binding affinity; (5) inactivation by intracellular detoxifying enzymes; (6) altered topoisomerase II, either a decreased amount or reduced affinity for a drug; and (7) enhanced repair of DNA damage. (DHFR, dihydrofolate reductase)

ANTINEOPLASTIC DRUGS (Fig. 12.12)

DRUGS DIRECTLY INTERFERING WITH DNA

Alkylating agents

History

Paul Ehrlich developed the first rationally designed anticancer agent, methyl nitrosourea, in 1898. Sulfur mustard gas was used as chemical vesicant on the western front in the 1914–1918 war. It caused severe skin burns on contact and pulmonary edema when inhaled. The United States Army developed a derivative, nitrogen mustard, in 1943. When accidental exposure was noted to produce lymphopenia, the agent was administered to patients with malignant lymphoproliferative disorders with resultant partial or complete resolution, albeit transiently, of the disease. A new therapeutic age was entered.

Mechlorethamine (nitrogen mustard), melphalan, cyclophosphamide, chlorambucil, and ifosfamide are in widespread clinical use. Aziridines, such as thiotepa, epoxides (dibromodulcital), and alkyl alkane sulfonates such as busulfan are less frequently used. The nitrosoureas such as carmustine, lomustine, and semustine are highly lipophilic and easily cross the blood–brain barrier and can therefore be used to treat brain tumors.

Antineoplastic drugs

Drugs that interact with DNA

Direct acting
- Alkylating agents: mechlorethamine hydrochloride, cyclophosphamide, ifosfamide, melphalan, chlorambucil, uracil mustard
- Nitrosoureas: lomustine, carmustine, streptozotocin
- Miscellaneous: thiotepa, busulfan, dacarbazine (DTIC), pipobroman, procarbazine, cisplatin, carboplatin, altretamine

Indirect acting
- Anthracyclines: doxorubicin HCl, daunorubicin HCl, idarubicin HCL, epirubicin, mitoxantrone HCl
- Topoisomerase-acting: etoposide, teniposide, topotecan, irinotecan
- Miscellaneous: bleomycin, dactinomycin, plicamycin

Antimetabolites
- Methotrexate, trimetrexate, fluorouracil, floxuridine, capecitabine, cytarabine, gemcitabine
- Mercaptopurine, thioguanine, fludarabine, cladribine, pentostatin
- Hydroxyurea

Drugs that interact with tubulin
- Depolymerizing agents: vincristine sulfate, vinblastine sulfate, vinorelbine, estramustine phosphate
- Polymerizing agents: paclitaxel, docetaxel

Hormones
- Estrogens: diethylstilbestrol, estradiol
- Antiestrogens: tamoxifen
- Aromatase inhibitors: anastazole, letrozole aminoglutethimide, testolactone
- Gonadotrophin-releasing hormone partial agonists: leuprolide, goserelin
- Antiandrogens: bicalutamide, flutamide
- Progestins: medroxyprogesterone acetate, megesterol acetate
- Androgens

Miscellaneous
- Interferons
- Levamisole HCl
- Asparaginase
- Mitotane
- Phosphotyrosine kinase inhibitors

Radiopharmaceuticals
- Sodium iodide (NaI), [131]I
- Sodium phosphate, [32]P
- Strontium nitrate, [89]Sr

Fig. 12.12 Antineoplastic drugs.

Streptozocin is a monofunctional alkylating agent with no bone marrow toxicity, but it destroys the β cells of the pancreas, causing diabetes mellitus.

Mechanism of action

The molecular mechanism of action of alkylating agents is alkylation with nucleophilic substitution of DNA. All alkylating

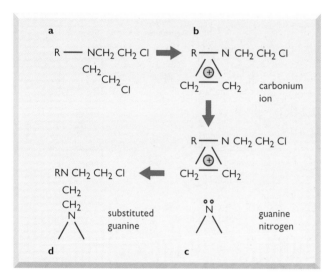

Fig. 12.13 Formation of a reactive carbonium ion (b) from an alkylating agent such as nitrogen mustard (a), and intermediate SN$_1$ nucleophilic attack of a guanine nitrogen (c, d). The resulting adduct can cause the base to hydrolyze and produce an apurinic site, cause a change in base pair formation by tautomerization with a resulting mutation, or a second adduct can bond to another base and make a covalent cross-link. This reaction requires SN$_1$ and depends only on the concentration of drug.

agents produce covalent bonding of alkyl (saturated carbon atoms) group(s) to cellular molecules and have reactive electrophilic intermediates, which bind to nucleophiles such as DNA (Fig. 12.13).

MECHLORETHAMINE serves as a prototype and like all alkylating agents is a pro-drug. Drug decomposition occurs spontaneously at physiologic pH and chloroethyl-diazonium or carbonium ions alkylate DNA or protein. The molecular mechanism of action is alkylation with nucleophilic substitution (SN$_1$ or SN$_2$) of DNA, preferentially the [7]N-guanine, [6]O-guanine, and [3]N-cytosine (see Figs 12.13, 12.14).

Sites of alkylation are widespread and include proteins (enzymes, cell membranes) and nucleotides, accounting for adverse as well as therapeutic effects. All O and N atoms of purines and pyrimidines are preferred substrates, such as [6]O-guanine, [7]N-guanine, [3]N-cytosine, [3]N-thymidine, and [1]N-adenine.

Bifunctional alkylating agents produce more DNA damage than monofunctional agents. Formation of interstrand crosslinks (ISCs) correlates best with cytotoxicity. Some evidence suggests that these ISCs may preferentially alkylate transcriptionally active genomic regions. ISCs prevent DNA replication and RNA transcription. Monofunctional adducts produce single-strand DNA breaks as a result of depurination by endonucleases or spontaneously. Tautomerization of adducted bases produces mismatched base pairing, which is a major cause of mutations and possible carcinogenesis/leukemogenesis in normal cells.

Cellular uptake of alkylating agents is by active transport into cells via physiologic transporters (for nitrogen mustards) or passively for nitrosoureas. For example mechlorethamine uses the choline transporter, melphalan the L-glutamine transporter, and cisplatin the methionine transporter.

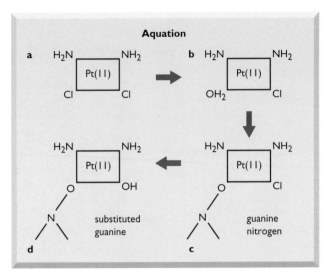

Fig. 12.14 An SN$_2$ reaction of cisplatin on a guanine nucleotide after aquation. Cisplatin (a) loses a Cl$^-$ and bonds to water (b), this OH$_2$ group then bonds to an electron-rich nitrogen molecule and displaces the OH$_2$ group to form a covalent bond (c). Since cisplatin is bifunctional, cross-links may be formed and, since the reaction rate depends on both the concentration of cisplatin and a neutrophile (d), it is an SN$_2$ kinetic reaction. (Pt (11), platinum)

Pharmacokinetics

The alkylating agents, except for cyclophosphamide, have very short half-lifes in plasma. Clearance is rapid as a result of spontaneous decomposition (mechlorethamine), hydrolysis and metabolism (cyclophosphamide). Mechlorethamine has a half-life of 10 minutes. Melphalan gives variable blood levels when taken orally owing to poor absorption (~30%), and a half-life of 1.8 hours when given intravenously. Chlorambucil is well absorbed orally (50%) with a half-life of 1.5–3 hours. Alkylating agents are generally unaffected by even significant impairment of hepatic and renal function.

CYCLOPHOSPHAMIDE is the most widely used alkylating agent. The plasma half-life is the longest of any alkylating agent except the closely related ifosfamide. It has rare nonmyelosuppressive toxicities and the myelosuppression is brief, predictable and noncumulative. It is available as intravenous or oral (100% bioavailability) formulations. Cyclophosphamide peak levels are dose-dependent (500 nM with 60 mg/kg).

Cyclophosphamide is a pro-drug that requires oxidation to active 4-hydroxycyclophosphamide in the liver via the hepatic microsomal cytochrome P-450 (CYP 450) system. This is followed by the spontaneous reversible formation of aldophosphamide in the blood, and then a reaction to yield phosphoramide mustard, the active alkylating form of the drug intracellularly and in the blood. Of all the metabolites of cyclophosphamide, 4-hydroxycyclophosphamide has the highest therapeutic index. The parent drug has a half-life of 3–10 hours whereas the half-life for its alkylating activity is 8 hours. Concurrent and/or repeated administration of some drugs including cyclophosphamide itself can increase total drug exposure by induction of CYP-450 enzymes and increase both activation and inactivation of cyclophosphamide.

Ifosphamide has a half-life of 15 hours; this is longer than that of cyclophosphamide, and it increases at higher doses (4–5 g/m^2). Stearic hindrance to the hydroxylation of the chloroethyl side chains is clinically important for the activation (ring hydroxylation) of ifosfamide.

Resistance

Resistance to alkylating agents has several causes:
- Membrane transport may be decreased (e.g. for melphalan, cisplatin).
- The drug may be bound by glutathione (GSH) via GSH-S-transferase or metallothioneins in the cytoplasm and inactivated.
- The drug may be metabolized to inactive species (e.g. by enzymes such as aldehyde dehydrogenase I, or the chloroethyl groups of the active binding residues of cyclophosphamide or melphalan may be hydroxylated).

Adverse effects

Myelosuppression (decrease in normal host erythrocytes, leukocytes, and platelets) is the dose-limiting adverse effect for all alkylating agents. Nausea and vomiting are common as are teratogenesis and gonadal atrophy, although in the latter cases these are variable, according to the drug, its schedule, and route of administration. Treatment also carries a major risk of leukemogenesis and carcinogenesis. Other adverse effects include:
- Alopecia with cyclophosphamide.
- Interstitial pneumonitis with the nitrosoureas and busulfan.
- Renal and bladder toxicity with cyclophosphamide and ifosfamide.

People with genetic defects in DNA repair, such as ataxia–telangiectasia, Fanconi's anemia, Bloom's syndrome, and xeroderma pigmentosa are highly sensitive to DNA-damaging agents. Prior radiation or prior exposure to alkylating agents may enhance the myelosuppression.

Nitrosoureas
Carmustine

Cumulative and delayed myelosuppression, as well as damage to other organs limits the use and usefulness of the nitrosoureas in current practice. The lipophilic nature of carmustine allows excellent CNS penetration and it remains a mainstay of treatment in brain tumors. The chloroethyl-diazonium reactive

---

Characteristics of alkylating agents

- Directly damage DNA
- Have a broad spectrum of antitumor activity and immunosuppression
- Active against proliferating and nonproliferating cells
- Cause dose-limiting myelosuppression
- Are genotoxic and associated with an increased risk of leukemogenesis

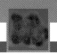

group binds to DNA and is responsible for the cytotoxic and myelosuppressive effects. An isocyanate byproduct is thought to produce the pulmonary toxicity and fibrosis. Carmustine is given intravenously, although oral availability is good. Lomustine and semustine are orally available (~60%). Nitrosureas have peak levels of 5 mM with a distribution phase of 5 minutes and a serum half-life of 70 minutes.

Miscellaneous alkylating agents
Procarbazine
MECHANISM OF ACTION Procarbazine is not itself cytotoxic or mutagenic, but is activated in the liver to an azo intermediate, which is converted to alkylating azoxy compounds. The main molecular mechanism of action is DNA alkylation (although methylation, free radical-mediated damage, and inhibition of DNA and protein synthesis may be additional mechanisms). The cellular mechanism of action is chromatid breakage and translocation, and the tissue mechanism of action is termination of cell cycle progression due to the secondary cellular action, which is inhibition of the G_1–S phase transition.

PHARMACOKINETICS Procarbazine is almost 100% absorbed when given orally, and peak plasma levels occur in 1 hour. Procarbazine and its metabolites are cleared from plasma within 2 hours, and the parent drug has a half-life of 7 minutes. Phenytoin and phenobarbital increase both the clearance and antitumor effect of procarbazine by accelerating production of its cytotoxic metabolites.

RESISTANCE develops rapidly to procarbazine and may be due to nucleic acid synthesis to replace adducted bases, which is more rapid during active DNA synthesis.

ADVERSE EFFECTS Procarbazine inactivates monoamine oxidase, causing hypertensive crises with tyramine-containing foods (e.g. cheese, red wine). It also has an 'Antabuse' effect, causing severe nausea with ethanol. Nausea and vomiting are significant. Myelosuppression occurs following oral, but not intravenous, administration. Neurotoxicity is worse with intravenous therapy owing to higher peak levels and includes somnolence, confusion, mood changes, and paresthesias, which may respond to pyridoxine. Allergic reactions have also been noted. Procarbazine is an alkylating agent in which dose modification for hepatic or renal insufficency may be necessary.

Dacarbazine
Dacarbazine is a pro-drug that is metabolized in the liver to release a methyldiazonium ion, which is the active alkylating product. It has poor cerebrospinal fluid (CSF) penetration and is therefore of no use for central nervous system (CNS) cancers. Its major adverse effects are severe nausea and vomiting. The β half-life is 40 minutes and oral absorption is variable. Fifty percent is excreted in the urine and dose modification for hepatic or renal insufficency may be necessary.

Altretamine
Altretamine (hexamethylmelamine) is a pro-drug that is activated in the liver. It is only available in an oral form, although oral absorption is variable. Peak levels occur 0.5–1 hours after dosing and the first two half-lifes are 0.5 hours and 5–10 hours. It is highly protein-bound. Its major adverse effects are nausea and vomiting, and myelosuppression occurs in 50% of all patients. Neurotoxicity, 1–3 months after treatment, includes mood changes and paresthesias.

Platinum compounds
In 1968, it was observed that electric currents through platinum electrodes caused filamentous growth in bacteria, which is a sign of inhibited DNA synthesis. Within 3 years, cisplatin was in clinical trials. Cisplatin revolutionized the treatment of testicular cancer, moving cure rates from 5–15% to 70–90% for metastatic disease. It is an important component of treatment for ovarian, bladder, head and neck, and lung cancers.

Cisplatin
Cisplatin (dichloro-diamino-cis platinum II) requires the replacement of Cl^- with water (aquation) for activation. Activation is slow (2.5 hours) and only the cis enantiomer is cytotoxic.

MECHANISM OF ACTION Cisplatin binds to guanine in DNA and RNA, and the interaction is stabilized by hydrogen bonding. The molecular mechanism of action is unwinding and shortening of the DNA helix. Although ISCs occur (10% of all adducts), the cellular mechanism of action, cell inactivation, appears to be principally due to the formation of intrastrand links (75–80%). A relationship exists between the number of cross-links, ability to repair cross-links, and cytotoxicity.

RESISTANCE to cisplatin may involve DNA repair similar to that which removes the cyclobutane dimers formed on interaction of DNA with ultraviolet light.

PHARMACOKINETICS Cisplatin is inactivated in blood and intracellularly by covalent interaction with the sulfhydryl groups in glutathione and metallothioneins. Protein binding to tissue, blood cells, and plasma proteins also inactivates cisplatin. Cisplatin is filtered by glomeruli and actively secreted in the proximal convoluted tubules. Approximately 25% of a dose is excreted within 24 hours, and 90% in the urine. The α, β, and λ half-lifes are 30 minutes, 60 minutes, and 24 hours. Cisplatin is not orally bioavailable.

ADVERSE EFFECTS The major adverse effect of cisplatin is renal toxicity with renal tubular damage and necrosis, similar to that seen with heavy metals. Protective procedures to avoid this involve hydration and diuresis. Myelosuppression, usually thrombocytopenia, is less common. If there is adequate renal protection, peripheral neuropathy becomes dose-limiting. Ototoxicity with hearing loss, allergic reactions, severe nausea, and vomiting are common. Cisplatin should not be administered if renal clearance of creatinine is <60 ml/min.

Carboplatin

Carboplatin is an analog of cisplatin with the same mechanism of cytotoxicity. It was developed to be less nephrotoxic and less likely to cause vomiting. The intracellular DNA adduct is identical to cisplatin. Like cisplatin, no metabolism occurs and carboplatin is excreted by the kidneys. Knowing the creatinine clearance enables dosing on a precise AUC (total drug exposure) basis, rather than on a mg/m² basis. Drug half-lifes are similar to cisplatin. Carboplatin is myelosuppressive.

AGENTS INDIRECTLY DAMAGING DNA

Anthracyclines

DOXORUBICIN AND DAUNORUBICIN have a wide spectrum of usefulness in cancer chemotherapy, which is second only to the usefulness of alkylating agents. Doxorubicin is effective against:

- Non-Hodgkin's lymphoma.
- Hodgkin's disease.
- Acute leukemias.
- Carcinomas of the breast, lung, stomach, and thyroid.
- Sarcomas.

Doxorubicin is used to treat solid tumors, and in leukemia daunorubicin is sometimes used because it causes less mucositis. Doxorubicin is a pro-drug. The active metabolite idarubicin is effective against leukemia and is itself used therapeutically because it can be given orally. Anthracyclines have a unique cumulative cardiotoxicity. Free-radical quinones cause peroxidation of the sarcoplasmic reticulum, with loss of high-affinity Ca^{2+} binding sites and the release of Ca^{2+} into the cytoplasm. Excess intracellular Ca^{2+} is toxic, resulting in the disruption of actin and myosin and uptake of Ca^{2+} into the mitochondria to displace ATP (P), resulting in a loss of contractility, death of cells and, later, thinning of the heart wall. This toxicity may be blocked by the iron chelator, desrazoxane. Epirubicin is less cardiotoxic than other anthracyclines and is widely used in Europe. It is particularly effective in breast cancer. Anthracycline cytotoxicity does not depend on the dosing regimen.

MECHANISM OF ACTION Anthracyclines and anthracenediones intercalate with DNA and bind avidly to nuclear chromatin, forming a ternary complex of drug intercalated into DNA and topoisomerase II (Top II) to produce strand cleavage. This is their molecular mechanism of action. The Top II-mediated mechanism is probably the most important.

Free radical formation via electron reduction is a second cytotoxic mechanism. All anthracyclines are quinones capable of producing free radicals, which damage membranes, proteins, and lipids. Glutathione and catalase can detoxify the free radical quinones, and lack of catalase in cardiac tissue is the basis for anthracycline cardiotoxicity. Complexes of iron and anthracycline bind tightly to cell membranes to cause spontaneous membrane destruction. Recently, activation of a ceramide synthetase pathway that produces apoptotic cell death has been described. The relevance of this to the beneficial effects of these drugs in cancer treatment is not certain.

RESISTANCE Mechanisms include:

- p-Gp 170/*mdr* gene glycoprotein-mediated drug efflux.
- Altered Top II concentrations.
- A mutant topoisomerase II.
- Increased glutathione concentration.
- Increased glutathione peroxidase activity (this enzyme detoxifies free radicals).
- Decreased glucose-6-phosphate dehydrogenase concentration.

PHARMACOKINETICS Anthracyclines and anthracenediones diffuse passively into cells in the non-ionized form. The compounds become charged and are prevented from diffusing into cells if there is extracellular acidification, which is common with solid tumors. The long terminal half-life of doxorubicin, 30 hours, accounts for the lack of schedule-dependency for therapeutic purposes. Prolonged infusions or weekly schedules are less cardiotoxic than bolus infusions administered monthly. Except for idarubicin, all anthracyclines are available intravenously only. Doxorubicin is a potent radiation sensitizer. Heparin binds the daunosamine sugar and increases clearance. Doxorubicin decreases paclitaxel clearance.

ADVERSE EFFECTS of anthracyclines include myelosuppression, mucositis, and stomatitis, especially with doxorubicin, and with a continuous infusion rather than bolus schedule. Cardiac toxicity, a particular and potentially lethal problem, causes heart failure. Factors increasing the risk of heart failure include pre-existing heart disease, hypertension, and cardiac radiation therapy. Cardiac toxicity is a function of peak dose concentration, and continuous infusions or weekly dosing decrease the risk. Desrazoxane, an iron chelator, decreases cardiotoxicity. Anthracyclines cause extensive and severe soft tissue necrosis if extravasated.

Idarubicin

Idarubicin is effective against acute leukemia and breast cancer. It has the same mechanism of action and resistance as doxorubicin, and its oral bioavailability is 30%. Its effectiveness depends on its metabolism to an active metabolite, 13-epirubicinol.

Idarubicin is less cardiotoxic than doxorubicin.

Mitoxantrone

Mitoxantrone is an anthracenedione that is less cardiotoxic than anthracyclines. Its molecular mechanism of action is interaction with Top II and DNA, resulting in its cellular mechanism of action of producing breaks in DNA strands. Mitoxantrone does not produce free-radical generation. The mechanisms of resistance to mitoxantrone are the same as for doxorubicin.

ADVERSE EFFECTS of mitoxantrone include extravasation injuries, alopecia, and nausea, and dose-limiting myelosuppression. Overall, the adverse effect profile is much more favorable than that for anthracyclines, especially with respect to cardiotoxicity. However, cardiotoxicity is seen in patients who have previously been treated with doxorubicin. Cardiotoxicity is less frequent, but just as severe, than with anthracyclines.

Topoisomerase-active drugs

Topoisomerases I and II are nuclear enzymes that cleave one (Top I) or two (Top II) strands of DNA, to allow DNA strand passage to unwind DNA and relieve torsional stress and to decatenate intertwined segments of DNA (Top II only). Top I and/or Top II are necessary for DNA replication and RNA transcription. Top II is necessary for the completion of mitosis. Top II plays a crucial role in the tertiary structure of chromatin. Two isoforms have been isolated. The predominant isoform, Top IIα, is tightly cell cycle-regulated (increased in S phase and increased further in M phase). Top IIα and especially Top I can be elevated in neoplastic cells independently of increased proliferation.

Topoisomerases form a covalent bond with DNA through a tyrosine transester linkage. Drugs stabilize this transient intermediate, preventing religation of the DNA strands. The exact molecular mechanism of cytotoxicity is uncertain, since enzyme inhibition is fully reversible. Possible cellular mechanisms include:

- Inappropriate recombination of topoisomerase-bound DNA strands (sister chromatid exchange (SCE)).
- Apoptosis due to unreplicated DNA or unrepaired DNA strand breaks, and/or decreases in mitotic promotion factor (MPF), which is a complex of two proteins, a cyclin and cdc2 (p34), a phosphokinase, which phosphorylates other proteins to regulate the passage into mitosis.

Etoposide and teniposide

Structurally, etoposide and teniposide are semisynthetic epipodophyllotoxins, which are derivatives of podophyllotoxin, a tubulin-binding extract of the mandrake plant (*Mandragora officinarum*).

MECHANISM OF ACTION The molecular mechanism of action of epipodophyllotoxins is the ability to stabilize transiently a 'cleavable complex' of Top II and DNA, which is reversible after drug withdrawal (Fig. 12.15). Top II is a necessary intermediary since the drugs do not interact directly with DNA. Although the cellular mechanism of cytotoxicity is unclear, there is a linear relationship between drug concentration, double-strand DNA breaks, and cytotoxicity.

RESISTANCE Mechanisms of resistance include increased levels of pGp 170 and *mdr* gene amplification/overexpression with enhanced efflux, an enhanced capacity to repair DNA strand breaks, decreased Top II levels (with a collateral increase in Top I), and altered (mutant) topoisomerase II enzymes capable of religating the separated DNA strands despite the presence of drug.

PHARMACOKINETICS Since 95% of these drugs are protein-bound, penetration into the CNS (5%) and ascites is poor. Oral absorption (approximately 50%) of an ingested dose is adequate, but marked variability occurs between patients. A divided course over many days provides therapeutic efficacy superior to single or weekly doses. Daily oral etoposide for

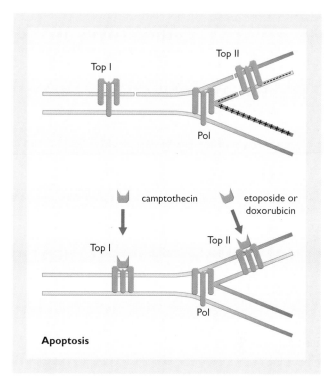

Fig. 12.15 Sites of action of camptothecin and etoposide or doxorubicin. They stabilize the normally transient covalent cleavage in replicating DNA produced by topoisomerase I (Top I) and/or topoisomerase II (Top II), which produces a double-strand DNA break by collision with the DNA replication apparatus of DNA polymerase a (leading strand 5'→3') and polymerase d (lagging strand 3'→5') (Pol).

21 days is significantly more effective than other single agent regimens.

ADVERSE EFFECTS include myelosuppression, especially neutropenia, which is dose-limiting, and oral mucositis. Toxicity depends on the regimen. A unique form of acute nonlymphocytic leukemia, with a translocation of the AML1 gene at the 11q23 locus, has occurred after treatment with prolonged and high total cumulative doses of etoposide.

Camptothecin and derivatives

MECHANISM OF ACTION Camptothecin (Fig. 12.16) is a plant alkaloid derived from a Chinese tree, *Camptotheca accuminata*. It was first introduced in clinical trials in the 1970s, but it was then abandoned because it lacked clinical efficacy and caused severe hemorrhagic cystitis. Interest was renewed 15 years later with the discovery that the molecular target of camptothecin is Top I, which is highly expressed in neoplastic tissues. All Top I inhibitors have an intact lactone E ring. Hydrolysis of the lactone to produce a carboxylate inactivates the drug. Multiple analogs, as well as camptothecin itself, are now in clinical trials. As S phase-specific agents (cellular mechanism of action), camptothecins have to be present in the cell over a prolonged period.

Common properties of the camptothecins include:
- Activity in a wide variety of epithelial cancers.
- A high degree of binding to serum albumin (>80%).

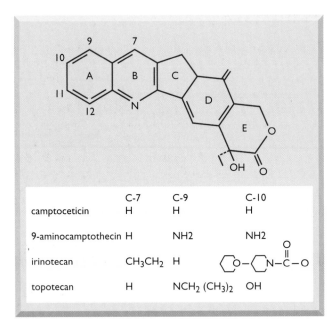

	C-7	C-9	C-10
camptoceticin	H	H	H
9-aminocamptothecin	H	NH2	NH2
irinotecan	CH₃CH₂	H	O—⟨⟩—N—C—O
topotecan	H	NCH₂ (CH₃)₂	OH

Fig. 12.16 Chemical structures of the camptothecins, which act on topoisomerase I. The lactone E ring must be intact for topoisomerase I interation. Substitutions at C-7, -9 and -10 increase water solubility. The C-10 substitution of irinotecan is hydrolyzed to OH. This metabolite, called SN-38, is 200 times more active than the parent drug.

- Severe reversible myelosuppression.
- Marked interpatient variability in pharmacokinetics.
- Significant schedule-dependency (activation is greater with a divided dose schedule).

Camptothecins have a wide spectrum of activity in solid tumors, including nonsmall-cell lung cancer (NSCLC), small-cell lung cancer (SCLC), and colon, cervical, and ovarian cancers. They are also effective against leukemias and lymphomas.

RESISTANCE Mechanisms of resistance include:
- Decreased Top I levels.
- An altered/mutant topoisomerase that cannot bind the drug or one that can religate in the presence of camptothecin.
- Enhanced membrane efflux via p-Gp 170 for water-soluble analogs such as topotecan (see Fig. 12.16), which is a semisynthetic water-soluble camptothecin analog.

IRINOTECAN (CPT-11) (see Fig. 12.16) is a pro-drug and is cleaved by ubiquitous carboxylesterases to a metabolite (SN-38), a significantly more effective Top I inhibitor. The protein binding of SN-38 (<60%) is much less than most camptothecins. Irinotecan causes a particularly severe diarrhea, which is responsive to octreotide and preventable with high-dose loperamide. Less frequently it causes severe myelo-suppression, which is not related to serum drug levels, but is associated with weekly dosing schedules. Conjugation to glucuronides via UDP glycosylases is a major mechanism of metabolism and enterohepatic recirculation may account for excessive toxicity and plasma pharmacokinetic variability in patients.

Miscellaneous
Bleomycins
The bleomycins are a family of complex glycopeptides isolated from a *Streptomyces*, which avidly chelate metals. Bleomycin A_2 is the major bleomycin used clinically. Bleomycin is used to treat Hodgkin's disease, NHL, and testicular, cervical, head, and neck cancers. Its inclusion in regimens for the chemotherapy of germ cell cancers results in an increased cure rate.

MECHANISM OF ACTION All active bleomycin compounds bind reduced iron (Fe^{2+}), so their molecular mechanism of action is not directed towards tissue. Their cellular mechanism of action is to produce single- and double-strand DNA breaks. Such breaks are reflected as DNA chromosomal gaps, deletions, and fragments. These result from a secondary molecular mechanism of action in which free-radical formation from Fe^{2+}–bleomycin–oxygen forms an intercalated complex between DNA strands. Intercalation of drug into DNA is the initial step, before Fe^{2+} is oxidized, and oxygen is reduced to the radicals $\cdot O_2^-$ or $\cdot OH$. DNA cleavage occurs after the inter-calated bleomycin complex is assembled and DNA strand-breaking absolutely requires oxygen.

PHARMACOKINETICS Bleomycins are large cationic molecules and penetrate cell membranes poorly via a bleomycin-binding membrane protein. Internalized bleomycins are either trans-located to the nucleus or hydrolyzed by bleomycin hydrolase, a cysteine protease present in normal and malignant cells, but found in decreased concentrations in lung and skin.

ADVERSE EFFECTS Bleomycin toxicity is confined to the lungs and skin. Pulmonary toxicity is the major problem and is manifest as subacute or chronic interstitial pneumonitis and, at a later stage, fibrosis.

Dactinomycin
Dactinomycin (actinomycin D) has significant anticancer actions against solid tumors in children, such as Wilms' tumor, Ewing's tumor, neuroblastoma, rhabdomyosarcoma, and choriocarcinoma.

MECHANISM OF ACTION Structurally, dactinomycin is two symmetric polypeptide chains attached to a phenoxazone ring. The molecular mechanism of action is intercalation of the phenoxazone ring perpendicular to the long axis of DNA while the peptide chains lie in the minor groove. The resulting cellular mechanism of action is inhibition of RNA and protein synthesis by prevention of chain elongation. Dactinomycin enters cells by passive diffusion. Drug resistance is associated with increased expression of p-gP/mdr.

ADVERSE EFFECTS of dactinomycin include nausea, vomiting, mucosal ulceration, dose-limiting myelosuppression, and dermatologic manifestations. Dactinomycin is a severe vesicant and a radiation-sensitizing agent, and can produce severe radiation 'recall injury.'

Mitomycin C

Mitomycin C has significant theoretical appeal because it is selectively toxic to hypoxic cells, a major problem in solid tumors. Mitomycin C has widespread but limited clinical usefulness in the treatment of a broad range of solid tumors, including those of the gastrointestinal tract, breast, lung, head, neck, and bladder, and gynecologic tumors. It is synergistic with 5-fluorouracil and with radiotherapy. Experimentally, initial trials with mitomycin C were disappointing because of severe cumulative bone marrow, pulmonary, and renal toxicity. However, it can be used in combination with other agents using an intermittent schedule.

MECHANISM OF ACTION The mechanism of action of mitomycin C depends on bioreductive alkylation under anaerobic, reducing conditions as it needs to be reduced at quinone sites to form unstable intermediates, which react monofunctionally at the guanine ^2N position. It is therefore a pro-drug. About 10% of adducts can form ISCs. Free-radical formation under aerobic conditions (a second basis for pro-drug activity) may lead to single-strand DNA breaks, or these may result from unsuccessful alkylation repair.

RESISTANCE The mechanisms of resistance to mitomycin include:
- Decreased bioactivation.
- Increased DNA repair.
- Increased p-gP/mdr gene product expression.

PHARMACOKINETICS Mitomycin C is used intravenously since oral absorption is erratic. Impaired liver or renal function does not change its pharmacokinetics.

ANTIMETABOLITES

Amethopterin, an analog of folic acid, has been in use since 1948 when it was first demonstrated that folate antagonists could induce complete (but transient) remissions of childhood acute leukemia. Sidney Farber at the Boston Children's Hospital had noted megaloblastic changes in the bone marrow of children with leukemia and surmised that exacerbating depletion of folate stores could stop the proliferation of leukemic cells. This is an example of rational target selection in cancer therapy, as distinct from the empiric (but invaluable) approach demonstrated with the alkylating agents.

Methotrexate

MECHANISM OF ACTION The molecular mechanism of action of methotrexate (Fig. 12.17) is inhibition of the enzyme dihydrofolate reductase.

Folates are one-carbon cofactors in purine and pyrimidine biosynthesis and include:
- Pteridine.
- Para-aminobenzoic acid.
- Glutamate complexes.

Polyglutamates are more efficient cofactors because they are retained longer in the cells. The tetrahydro (reduced) folates are the active forms and the essential role of dihydrofolate reductase is to maintain a supply of reduced folate cofactors. Dihydrofolate and formyl dihydrofolate, which accumulate after inhibition of dihydrofolate reductase, directly inhibit folate-dependent enzymes.

Methotrexate is actively transported via a ^5N-methyl tetrahydrofolic acid (reduced folate) system through the cell membrane into the cytoplasm, where it binds and inactivates

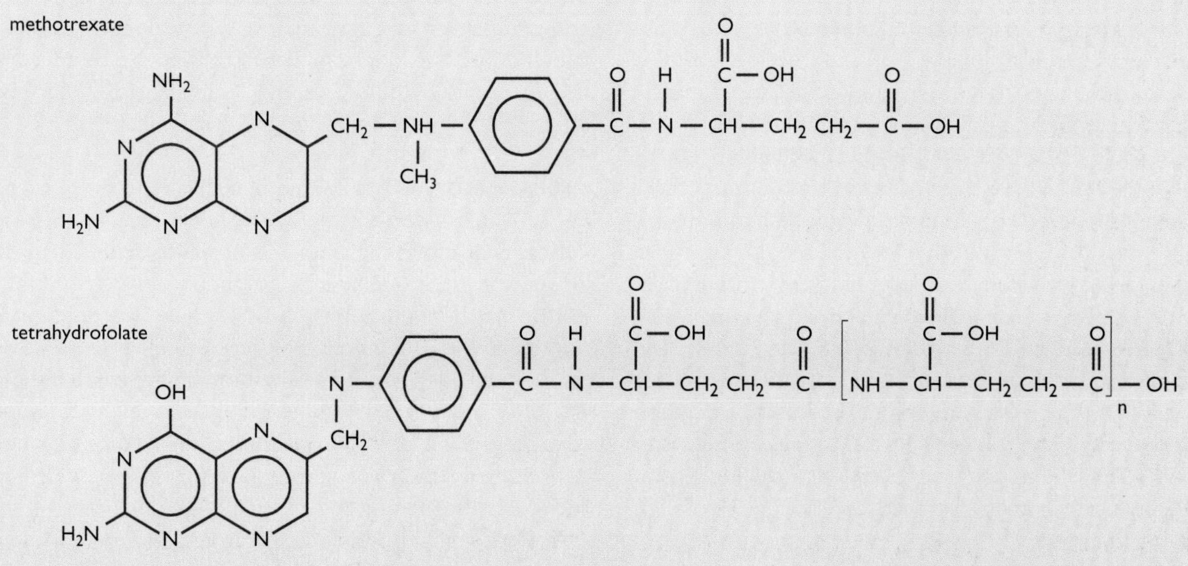

Fig. 12.17 Chemical structure of methotrexate and tetrahydrofolate. Methotrexate is an analog of tetrahydrofolate and binds to dihydrofolate reductase. The NH_2 group at position 4 converts methotrexate from a substrate to a tight binding inhibitor of dihydrofolate reductase.

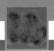

dihydrofolate. Free methotrexate competes with increased concentrations of dihydrofolate (from decreased thymidylate synthase activity) to inhibit dihydrofolate reductase. The cellular mechanism of action is a reduction in the availability of thymidylate synthase.

Methotrexate also has effects on purine synthesis, where 10-formyl dihydrofolate is a necessary cofactor in two steps of *de novo* purine synthesis. The required intracellular concentration of methotrexate for inhibiting pyrimidine synthesis is 1×10^{-8} M, while that for inhibiting purine synthesis is 1×10^{-7} M. In general, cytotoxicity is directly proportional to the duration of exposure, although increased drug concentrations may overcome resistance and increase cytotoxicity.

RESISTANCE Multiple mechanisms have been described for methotrexate resistance. These include:
- Decreased membrane transport.
- Decreased affinity of dihydrofolate reductase for methotrexate.
- Increased concentration of dihydrofolate reductase.
- Decreased polyglutamation due to decreased folate polyglutamyl synthase.
- Decreased thymidylate synthesis.

PHARMACOKINETICS Oral absorption of methotrexate is good but variable. Poor absorption correlates with increased relapses in childhood acute lymphocytic leukemia. It has three half-lifes (5 minutes, 2–3 hours, 8–10 hours), and the latter two are prolonged if there is impaired renal function or fluid accumulation. Re-emergence of methotrexate into the blood from pleural effusions or ascites, produces a prolongation of drug exposure which increases toxicity. Methotrexate penetration into the CNS is poor, with a plasma:CSF concentration ratio of 31:1. The major mechanisms of metabolism are by intracellular conversion to polyglutamates and 7-hydroxylation in the liver. Elimination is via unchanged drug in the urine. Methotrexate dose should be reduced in proportion to any decrease in creatinine clearance. Special attention should be given to its use in patients with effusions of any kind and the elderly, where decreased creatinine clearance, as a result of decreased muscle mass, may occur with a normal serum creatinine.

High doses of methotrexate have been used clinically to overcome the limited transport of methotrexate into cancer cells. Higher intracellular concentrations of methotrexate can partially overcome resistance due to increased dihydrofolate reductase or altered dihydrofolate reductase affinity for methotrexate. This increases intracellular polyglutamate formation and so increases the duration of drug action. The efficacy of high doses of methotrexate compared with conventional doses is, however, uncertain, and 'rescue' is required using a reduced folate source, 5-formyl tetrahydrofolic acid (leucovorin). Thymidine and blockade of cell cycle progression with l-asparaginase have also been tried to allow the use of high doses of methotrexate.

ADVERSE EFFECTS Myelosuppression and mucositis are the major adverse effects of methotrexate. CNS damage is most severe when methotrexate is given intrathecally with irradiation

Characteristics of antimetabolites

- Mimic essential cellular 'metabolites'
- Usually effective against actively proliferating cells
- Have common toxicities of myelosuppression and mucositis
- Are teratogenic, but not usually leukemogenic

and may manifest as one of the following:
- Chemical arachnoiditis, which is characterized by headache, fever, and nuchal rigidity, and is the most common and most acute adverse effect. It may be due to additives in the diluent (benzoic acid in sterile water).
- Subacute CNS toxicity, which occurs 2–3 weeks after administration and is characterized by motor paralysis, cranial nerve palsy, seizures, and coma.
- Chronic demyelinating encephalitis, which produces dementia and spasticity with cortical thinning, enlarged cerebral ventricles, and cerebral calcifications.

The latter two adverse effects may be worsened by radiotherapy.

Cirrhosis and portal vein fibrosis result from prolonged oral use. Chemical hepatitis is reversed by choline administration.

Trimetrexate

Trimetrexate is a methotrexate analog that enters cells by diffusion. It is therefore active against reduced folate-transport mutants and polyglutamation-deficient mutants that are resistant to methotrexate. It is also used to treat *Pneumocystis carinii* pneumonia.

Pyrimidine analogs
Fluorinated pyrimidines (5-fluorouracil)

5-Fluorouracil (Fig. 12.18) was developed by Charles Heidelberger in 1957 on the basis of an observed increased uracil incorporation into rat hepatomas. Despite its long history in the clinic, fluorouracil and its analogs continue to be effective as the optimal scheduling, dosing, and usage are continually refined with resultant significant clinical benefit.

MECHANISM OF ACTION 5-Fluorouracil is a pro-drug that must be activated (ribosylated, phosphorylated) to 5-fluoro-deoxyuracil monophosphate. The molecular mechanism of action of 5-fluoro-deoxyuracil monophosphate is inhibition of thymidylate synthase (Fig. 12.19). RNA incorporation of 5 fluoro-deoxyuracil monophosphate corresponds to cytotoxicity in many cell lines. Thymidine alone cannot reverse all the effects of 5-fluoro-deoxyuracil monophosphate, which also impairs precursor rRNA processing and polyadenylation of nuclear RNA. Incorporation of 5-fluorouracil into DNA also produces base pair mismatching and faulty mRNA transcripts.

5-Fluorouracil is rapidly taken up into cells, where a series of phosphorylases and kinases act upon it. Fluorouracil deoxyribose is activated in one additional step by thymidine kinase. Activation is complex and interdependent, with many sites at which resistance can develop.

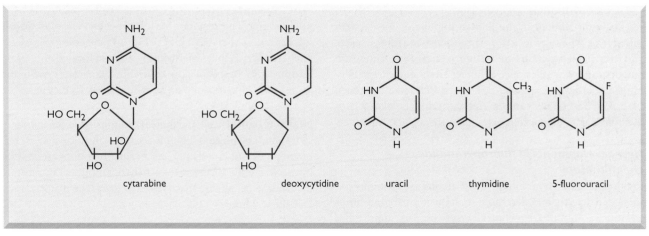

Fig. 12.18 Chemical structures of cytarabine, deoxycytidine, uracil, thymidine, and 5-fluorouracil. Like methotrexate, cytarabine and 5-fluorouracil are analogs of nucleotides which are taken up and actuated by normal cellular processes. However, because of a unique feature, they become inhibitors of DNA synthesis rather than building blocks of DNA. There are many potential sites of resistance because of the complex biochemistry.

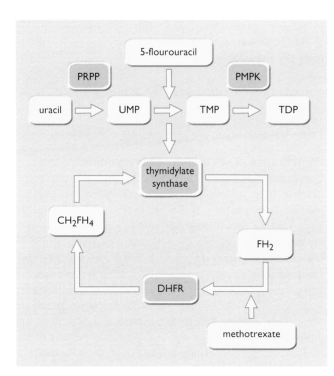

Fig. 12.19 The thymidine pathway showing the inhibition of thymidylate synthase by 5-fluorouracil. Methotrexate and 5-fluorouracil both act to decrease the synthesis of thymidine. (DHFR, dihydrofolate reductase; CH_2FH_4, methylene tetrahydrofolate, the donor of a methyl group to uracil; FH_2, dihydrofolate; PMPK, pyrimidine monophosphate kinase; PRPP, phosphoribosyl pyrophosphatase; TDP, thymidine diphosphate; TMP, thymidine monophosphate; UMP, uracil monophosphate)

PHARMACOKINETICS The primary half-life is 6–20 minutes. 5-Fluorouracil is metabolized intracellularly to nucleotide forms and catabolized to dihydrofluorouracil by the enzyme dihydropyrimidine dehydrogenase (DPD) in the liver. More than 90% of the drug is metabolized and <5% renally excreted. Oral absorption of 5-fluorouracil is poor as a result of first-pass metabolism in the gut and liver by DPD. An intravenous loading dose rapidly produces steady-state levels. With increasing dose there is nonlinear pharmacokinetic behavior as hepatic metabolism is saturated and total body clearance decreases, producing ever-higher plasma levels. Intra-arterial administration allows selective drug delivery to liver metastases where a first-pass metabolism by the tumor reduces systemic drug levels, and adverse effects.

Combination chemotherapy

5-Fluorouracil has been used in combination with many drugs in the treatment of solid tumors.

Methotrexate increases 5-fluorouracil triphosphate formation and increases cytotoxicity. Thymidine inhibits 5-fluorouracil degradation and thereby increases its half-life. Infusion of thymidine triphosphate, a feedback inhibitor of ribonucleotide reductase, increases 5-fluorouracil triphosphate incorporation into RNA. Inhibitors of *de novo* purine synthesis such as pyrazofurin, L-phosphonoacetyl-l-alanine, and allopurinol increase 5-fluorouracil triphosphate production.

Leucovorin increases the inhibition of thymidylate synthase, which requires reduced folate cofactors to form a tight ternary complex with 5-fluorouracil. Leucovorin increases the cytotoxicity in 5-fluorouracil-insensitive tumors by stabilizing the ternary complex, slowing the reversibility of the reaction, and increasing deoxythymidine monophosphate (dTMP). Leucovorin doubles the effectiveness of 5-fluorouracil in the treatment of colon and breast cancers. 5-Fluorouracil significantly prolongs survival when used in the treatment of locally advanced rectal and pancreatic cancers.

ADVERSE EFFECTS 5-Fluorouracil produces reversible myelosuppression, mucositis and diarrhea as its major toxicities. These vary in severity depending on the dose and schedule used and the presence of other drugs. Very prolonged infusions cause palmar erythema and desquamation. Lacrimal duct stenosis and cerebellar ataxia at high doses (due to inhibition of the tricarboxylic acid cycle in the cerebellum) are rarely encountered.

179

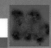

Dihydropyrimidine dehydrogenase (DPD) activity is normally distributed in the human population and certain individuals with activity <5% are at increased risk for severe and even fatal reactions to 5-fluorouracil. DPD saturation kinetics can reduce clearance at higher levels and DPD activity in the gut limits oral absorption. Elevated DPD levels have been identified in certain tumors and the rapid breakdown of 5-fluorouracil in these cells may confer therapeutic resistance.

New developments in fluoropyrimidine chemotherapy

Continuous intravenous infusions of 5-fluorouracil demonstrate increased activity and decreased toxicity compared to bolus administration but are technically difficult. Two approaches taken recently are the inhibition of degradative enzymes to prolong exposure to 5-fluorouracil, and the synthesis of orally available drugs.

UFT combines tegafur, a 5-fluorouracil pro-drug, and uracil. Tegafur is converted in the liver to 5-fluorouracil by thymidine/uridine phosphorylase. Uracil is added in a 4:1 ratio as a competitive substrate for DPD to enhance oral absorption and prolong the half-life of 5-fluorouracil. Diarrhea is the dose-limiting toxicity in the 14-day and 28-day schedules and myelosuppression with the 5-day schedule. UFT has comparable activity to 5-fluorouracil in colorectal cancer and other cancers.

CAPECITABINE is a pro-drug of 5-fluorouracil that requires a complex activation. The first step is hydrolysis by carboxylesterases (predominantly in the liver) to form 5′-deoxy-5-fluorocytidine. Cytidine deaminase then removes the C-amine, producing 5′-deoxy-5-fluorouridine. Pyrimidine nucleoside phosphorylase (PNP) produces the actively antineoplastic drug, 5-fluorouracil. PNP has been identified at higher levels in certain tumors and this may confer some selectivity. Oral absorption of capecitabine is rapid and the 6-week b.i.d. dosing schedule produces plasma 5-fluorouracil levels similar to those obtained with intravenous administration of 5-fluorouracil at 300 mg/m²/day. Hand-foot syndrome, diarrhea, and stomatitis are the dose-limiting toxicities.

S1 is an oral 5-fluorouracil preparation of tegafur and 5-chloro-2,4-dihydroxy-pyridine (CDHP) and oxonic acid. CDHP is a DPD inhibitor. Oxonic acid is an inhibitor of orotate phosphoribosyl transferase which decreases 5-fluorouracil conversion to fluorouracil monophosphate (FUMP) and its incorporation into RNA. A 28-day cycle shows promising clinical activity and comparable toxicity to the other oral formulations described above.

Cytarabine

Cytarabine (cytosine arabinoside, also known as ara-C) is a nucleoside analog of cytosine. It is a pro-drug that requires phosphorylation to produce the active monophosphate product, ara-CMP and subsequently the triphosphate (ara-CTP). The molecular mechanism of action of ara-CMP is ultimately via

ara-CTP competition with cytosine triphosphate for DNA polymerases. The resultant cellular mechanism of action is incorporation of ara-CTP into DNA. This produces cytotoxicity. The secondary cellular mechanism of action is premature chain termination. Resistance to cytarabine correlates with the decreased formation and/or retention of ara-CTP.

PHARMACOKINETICS Cytarabine is deaminated in the intestines so it cannot be given orally. It is actively transported across cell membranes and rapidly phosphorylated in a stepwise fashion by deoxycytidine kinases to the active triphosphate. Deamination by cytidine deaminase inactivates the drug. The major plasma half-life is 2 hours.

ADVERSE EFFECTS of cytarabine include myelosuppression, which is dose-limiting, severe, and reversible. Cholestatic jaundice and mucositis are less common. Cerebellar dysfunction due to a loss of cerebellar Purkinje cells occurs in up to 30% of patients treated with a high-dose regimen >3 g/m² for six or more twice daily doses. This occurs more frequently in elderly patients with renal insufficiency and the syndrome is usually irreversible.

COMBINATION CHEMOTHERAPY Synergism, due to decreased DNA repair, has been reported with cyclophosphamide, cisplatin, carmustine, and thiopurines.

Gemcitabine (2′-2′, difluorodeoxycytidine)

Gemcitabine is a cytidine analog. It has activity in pancreatic, ovarian, lung, and breast carcinomas where cytarabine is inactive. Gemcitabine is 5–8 times more active in vitro against solid tumors than cytarabine and is similar in that it is deaminated, activated by deoxycytidine kinase, and inhibits DNA synthesis. However, while it is less effective as a DNA chain terminator than cytarabine, it is much less easily removed when incorporated into DNA. It also inhibits ribonucleotide reductase. The triphosphate, dFdCTP, has a much longer intracellular retention time than cytarabine and its feedback inhibition of cytidine deaminase prevents removal of the activated species. Gemcitabine is active throughout the cell cycle (not S phase-specific like cytarabine) and active against resting/noncycling cells. Gemcitabine demonstrates cytotoxic synergy with platinum compounds and ionizing radiation.

PHARMACOKINETICS The drug is not extensively protein-bound (V_d = 6–31 liters/m²) and equilibrates poorly with tissues during short infusions (<1 h) but increases with prolonged infusions, suggesting a deep compartment. The clearance is moderate to high suggesting extensive metabolism by the liver and other tissues (46–66 liters/h/m²). The half-life is 11–25 minutes for infusions ≤1 h. This increases for longer infusions and with repeated dosing. The major metabolite is difluoro-deoxyuracil (91–98%) which is renally excreted. Gemcitabine does not require modification where there is renal impairment. Myelosuppression is the major toxicity of gemcitabine, which is otherwise well tolerated.

5-Azacytidine

Structurally and functionally, 5-azacytidine is an analog of cytosine. It is chemically unstable and after phosphorylation to a triphosphate is incorporated into RNA and DNA (its molecular mechanism of action) where it cleaves spontaneously. This cleavage product prevents cytosine methylation. Hypomethylation of cytosine occurs preferentially in actively transcribed regions of DNA. Unlike cytarabine, it is phosphorylated by uridine–cytidine kinase. It is inactivated by cytidine deaminase. Azacytidine is under investigation for its potential to modify gene expression and produce terminal differentiation in undifferentiated malignant cells.

Hydroxyurea

Hydroxyurea was first synthesized over 100 years ago. Its use is limited to chronic myelogenous leukemia, myeloproliferative diseases, hypereosinophilic syndrome, and intracerebral leukostasis in acute leukemia. It may be mildly synergistic with radiotherapy in cervical cancer. Hydroxyurea can increase fetal hemoglobin (hemoglobin F, $\alpha_2\gamma_2$) in sickle-cell disease, through stochastic increases in F stem cell number or survival. This decreases the frequency and severity of painful sickle-cell crises (microvessel ischemia and infarcts, especially in bone) and decreases the incidence of cerebral ischemic events.

MECHANISM OF ACTION The molecular mechanism of action of hydroxyurea is inhibition of ribonucleotide reductase. As a result, its cellular mechanism of action is inhibition of S-phase cells and synchronization of cells at the G_1–S interface. The effects of hydroxyurea are reversed by deoxyribonucleotides. Hydroxyurea rapidly enters the CSF and ascitic fluid and is therefore effective for CNS cancer.

ADVERSE EFFECTS Leukopenia is a common adverse effect. Hydroxyurea is very short-acting and rapidly reversible. A lichen planus-like skin change has been noted.

Purine antimetabolites

The purine analogs, 6-mercaptopurine and 6-thioguanine, were derived from research by Hitching and Elion into inhibitors of purine metabolism as a treatment for hyperuricemia and gout in the 1940s and 50s. Their research was later recognized with the award of the Nobel Prize in Medicine in 1988.

MECHANISM OF ACTION The general cellular mechanism of action is a reduction in purine levels in tumor cells. This is achieved in a variety of ways:

*   The ribonucleotide 6-mercaptopurine inhibits *de novo* purine biosynthesis. Its molecular mechanism of action is inhibition of glutamine 5-phosphoribosylpyrophosphate aminotransferase, the first step in purine synthesis, by negative feedback through mimicking a purine nucleoside (see Fig. 12.20). 6-Mercaptopurine also inhibits the interconversion

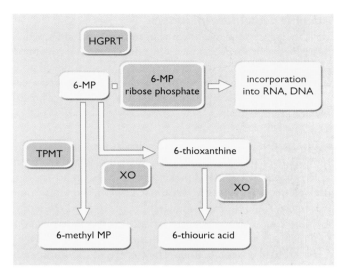

Fig. 12.20 The purine nucleoside pathway. 6-Mercaptopurine (6-MP) is activated to the triphosphate to be incorporated into DNA and RNA or to produce negative feedback on *de novo* purine synthesis. Metabolism is via xanthine oxidase (XO) to thiouric acid (allopurinol can interfere with this reaction and produce excessive toxicity), and via methylation and desulfuration to 6-methylpurine. One in 300 people lack thiopurine methyltransferase (TMPT) and can have excessive toxicity to the usual clinical dose. (HGPRT, hypoxanthine guanine phosphoribosyltransferase)

of inosinate to adenylate, and inosinate to xanthylate, the precursor to guanylate.
*   Azathioprine, a widely used immunosuppressant, is a pro-drug of 6-mercaptopurine.
*   6-Thioguanine, when converted to the active form thioGMP, inhibits glutamine 5-phosphoribosylpyrophosphate amino-transferase and inosinic acid dehydrogenase.

PHARMACOKINETICS Metabolic alterations are the major source of removal and renal clearance is minor at conventional doses. This changes drastically with high intravenous doses, where renal clearance may be 20–40%. 6-Mercaptopurine is approximately 50% orally absorbed. The half-life is approximately 50 minutes (range 20–60) in adults, but less (approximately 20 minutes) in children. 6-Mercaptopurine is metabolized via xanthine oxidase. Allopurinol can interfere with metabolism and result in toxicity (dose is decreased to 25%). 6-Thiaguanine is incompletely absorbed, with a half-life of approximately 90 minutes (range 25–240). Deamination and oxidation produce the major metabolites.

Thiopurine S-methyltransferase (TPMT) catalyzes the S-methylation of thiopurines such as 6-mercaptopurine and 6-thiaguanine. TMPT activity is genetically polymorphic with 1 in 300 persons deficient in TMPT as an autosomal recessive. At standard doses, TMPT-deficient individuals experience hematopoietic toxicity due to excess accumulation of thiopurines.

TOXICITY Myelosuppression, mucositis and teratogenesis occur. Reversible cholestatic jaundice occurs with 6-mercaptopurine.

Adenine deaminase inhibitors

New analogs designed as adenine deaminase inhibitors, which decrease *de novo* purine synthesis by phosphoribosyl pyrophosphatase (PRPP) via accumulation of dATP, have produced good results in previously refractory diseases such as hairy cell leukemia, chronic lymphocytic leukemia, and Waldenström's macroglobulinemia.

FLUDARABINE is the 2-fluoro derivative of ara-A-5′-monophosphate. Fludarabine is dephosphorylated in serum with increased cellular uptake and conversion to the triphosphate form which inhibits DNA polymerase and ribonucleotide reductase. Fludarabine is activated by deoxycytidine kinase and catabolized by adenine deaminase (ADA), to which it is relatively resistant. F-ara A levels in blood have a terminal half-life of 10 hours. The toxicity is predominantly severe reversible myelosuppression. Severe defects in cellular immunity (with lowered CD4 counts) occur, especially when combined with corticosteroids.

2-CHLORODEOXYADENOSINE (2-CDA) is a purine analog resistant to ADA which accumulates intracellularly as 2-cDA-TP with feedback inhibition of purine synthesis. 2-CDA is preferentially retained in leukemic cells (chronic lymphocytic leukemia, hairy cell leukemia, and ANLL). The major clinical toxicities are neutropenia and suppression of cell-mediated immunity. It is administered as a 7-day infusion or more recently as a five times daily bolus infusion.

DEOXYCOFORMICIN (PENTOSTATIN) has an α half-life of 10 minutes and a β half-life of 5 hours, with 80–100% being excreted in the urine in 24 hours. Major toxicities are dose-related, with profound immunosuppression due to T-cell cytolysis, somnolence and coma, and decreased renal function in 30–40% of patients.

TUBULIN-BINDING AGENTS

Vinca alkaloids

Vincristine, vinblastine, vindesine, and vinorelbine are all alkaloids derived from the periwinkle plant (*Vinca rosea*).

MECHANISM OF ACTION The cellular mechanism of action of vinca alkaloids is the prevention of microtubule assembly, causing cells to arrest in the late G_2 phase by preventing formation of mitotic filaments for nuclear and cell division. They achieve this by the molecular mechanism of action of binding to and inactivating tubulin. Their basic structure is a complex alkaloid of vindoline and catharanthine, differing by only one or two substituents for each alkaloid, but producing widely varying spectra of activity and toxicity.

Vinca alkaloids enter cells by nonsaturable energy-independent membrane transport and then bind to tubulin. This inhibits microtubule assembly. Tubulin polymerizes to form microtubules and is important in mitosis, transport, and cell structure (Fig. 12.21). Very low concentrations induce a

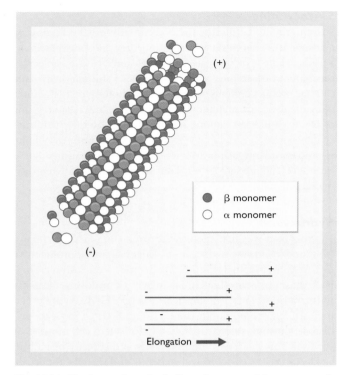

Fig. 12.21 The formation of tubulin polymers and the process of tubulin migration. The polymers are made up of α and β monomers and the process of tubulin migration involves elongation at a (+) end and shortening at a (–) end. Vinca alkaloids decrease the association rate at the (+) end and prevent polymerization of a and b dimers. Toxanes stabilize multimers and prevent dissociation at the (–) end, resulting in increased polymerization. Either effect on the dynamic equilibrium is cytotoxic.

metaphase arrest. Although the alkaloids act throughout the cell cycle, they are especially effective in the late S phase or G_2–M. The cytotoxic dose is low and is selective for transformed lymphocytes.

Experimental work suggests that prolonged exposure to vincristine is necessary to achieve maximal cytotoxicity and so continuous infusions are now being evaluated in lymphomas.

RESISTANCE to vinca alkaloids involves mutations in tubulin-binding sites.

ADVERSE EFFECTS Sensory and motor peripheral neuropathies are characteristic adverse effects of all vinca alkaloids. Autonomic neuropathy after a high single dose and hepatic failure have been reported. Toxicity is cumulative and its severity is dose-related. The spectrum of neurotoxicity and additional toxicities varies between the alkaloids:

- Vincristine is the most neurotoxic, followed by vindesine and then vinblastine, with vinorelbine being the least neurotoxic.
- Vinblastine is the most myelotoxic, followed by vindesine and then vinorelbine. Vincristine is not myelosuppressive.
- All cause mild alopecia, but this is more severe with

vinblastine and vindesine than for vincristine and vinorelbine.

- All induce the syndrome of nephrogenic inappropriate antidiuretic hormone action.
- All cause equally severe local extravasation injury.

L-Asparaginase decreases hepatic metabolism and increases toxicity, so vinca alkaloids should be given 12–24 hours before L-asparaginase.

Paclitaxel

Paclitaxel is a complex diterpine taxane originally isolated from the bark of the Western yew by Wall and colleagues in 1958. Purification and formulation problems resulted in a 25-year delay before paclitaxel went into clinical trials.

Taxanes enhance all aspects of tubulin polymerization, an action that is the opposite to that of vinca alkaloids, but they are also cytotoxic, emphasizing the dynamic importance of tubulin polymerization as a target for cytotoxic drugs. Taxanes stabilize tubulin polymers and do not prevent polymerization.

A low concentration of paclitaxel increases both the microtubule number and the formation of bundles, changes cell shape, and produces mitotic arrest in actively dividing cells. Altering the microtubule ↔ tubulin equilibrium by irreversible polymerization of tubules is the major mechanism for the antineoplastic actions of the taxanes.

PHARMACOKINETICS It is insoluble in water and therefore is emulsified in cremophor, which can induce a severe anaphylactic reaction. Paclitaxel has a biphasic plasma disappearance with half-lifes of 20 minutes and 6–8 hours. Paclitaxel is hepatically metabolized by the CYP450 3A4 isoenzyme to inactive species. This produces the potential for interaction with a host of other agents which share this pathway.

Taxanes act as a substrate for multi-drug resistance-mediated cellular efflux. At appropriate concentrations cremophor itself can inhibit the P-gP/mdr efflux pump. Alterations in tubulin itself may reduce or even prevent taxane binding or, in vitro, produce a mutant tubulin that requires a taxane for normal polymerization kinetics.

ADVERSE EFFECTS Anaphylactic reactions due to cremophor are frequent and can be controlled by pretreatment with a glucocorticosteroid and antihistamine. Major adverse effects of paclitaxel are neutropenia and neuropathy, particularly with 24-hour infusion.

Interactions have been reported with several antineoplastic agents. These have occurred only with the prolonged (24-hour) infusion. There is an increased incidence and severity of mucositis when doxorubicin is used before paclitaxel than when paclitaxel is used before doxorubicin.

DOCETAXEL is derived from the leaves of the European yew. It has similar antineoplastic properties, although differences may exist in certain cancers (e.g. breast). There is a decreased incidence of allergic reactions but increased incidence of edema and effusions.

HORMONES

The manipulation of hormone levels in the treatment of cancer dates from the nineteenth century. In 1896, Beatson in Edinburgh used bilateral oöphorectomy to palliate pain from breast cancer metastasized to bone in premenopausal women. In 1952, the American surgeon Huggins and colleagues were able to accomplish this in postmenopausal women by bilateral adrenalectomy. In 1941, Huggins and Hodges had demonstrated regression of prostate cancer metastasis by bilateral orchiectomy or estrogen administration.

Steroid hormones are ultimately derived via synthetic pathways from cholesterol. Their synthesis in vivo and mechanism of action are described in Chapter 15.

In breast cancer, hormonal therapy is significantly influenced by the expression of estrogen receptors (ER) and progesterone receptors (PR) on the tumor cells. Patients with ER-positive tumors are more than fivefold more responsive than ER-negative patients. Quantitative ER/PR analysis (by immunocytochemistry or competitive radiolabeled displacement) increases the predictive value of the test, as greater receptor density on tumors increases the probability of response.

A significant body of evidence supports the concept that a substantial portion of the benefit of adjuvant combination chemotherapy in premenopausal women with breast cancer results from chemotherapy-induced menopause.

Estrogens

Knowledge of the role of estrogens as a promoter for breast cancer growth dates from observations in the nineteenth century on the effects of menstrual cycle on breast cancer. It is seemingly a paradox that high doses of estrogens can have an antineoplastic effect. Diethylstilbestrol (DES) poduces regressions in breast cancer equivalent to antiestrogens but with significantly more toxicity, especially venous thromboembolism. The mechanism is uncertain. Proposed mechanisms include the down-regulation of estrogen receptors, direct cytotoxic effects related to perturbations of the cell cycle, and effects on chromosome stability. Estrogen therapy of breast cancer is of historical interest only, having been replaced by antiestrogens and aromatase inhibitors. DES is still used in prostate cancer only, as a cost-saving measure.

DES is well absorbed orally, the initial half-life is 1.5 hours and the terminal half-life is 24 hours. Metabolism occurs through aromatic hydroxylation of the ethyl side chains, which may be carcinogenic. DES is four times more potent than estradiol at suppressing follicle-stimulating hormone (FSH). A 1 mg dose produces daily plasma concentrations of 1–2 ng/ml.

Ethinyl estradiol is 20 times more potent than DES. It has a half-life of 24 hours. The metabolism is via glucuronidation. The usual daily dose is 1 mg t.i.d. for breast cancer.

Antiestrogens

TAMOXIFEN Tamoxifen is one of the most important drugs in the treatment of breast cancer. It offers significant palliation and tumor regressions in advanced metastatic disease in ER-positive women, provides potentially curative benefit in the

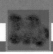

adjuvant setting in ER-positive women, and has been used to prevent breast cancer in women at high risk for the disease. It is a synthetic triphenyl ethylene.

Tamoxifen has properties of a mixed estrogen antagonist and agonist. Tamoxifen blocks estrogen activation of the ER and promotes its tight association, preventing repetitive signaling. This results in decreased transforming growth factor alpha (TGF-α), mid-G$_1$ arrest, decreased cell proliferation, antagonism of the effect of insulin-like growth factor 1 (IGF-1), and increased TGF-β, an antiproliferative protein. While decreasing breast epithelial proliferation, tamoxifen increases endometrial proliferation, reduces or prevents the mineral loss in bone associated with estrogen withdrawal, and maintains the favorable hepatic cholesterol profile seen in menstruating women.

Tamoxifen undergoes hepatic metabolism to 4-hydroxytamoxifen (50-fold more potent in ER affinity than tamoxifen), tamoxifen N-oxide, and N-desmethyltamoxifen (both equipotent as tamoxifen). The α half-life is 4–14 days and the β half-life is >7 days. Steady-state levels are achieved only after 4–12 weeks. Elimination is via glucuronide conjugation and biliary excretion. The clinical dose is 20 mg daily. Tamoxifen is continued until progression in advanced disease and for 2–5 years in the adjuvant setting. In advanced disease with progression on tamoxifen, discontinuing the agent may produce tumor regressions. One theory is that imbalances in the intracellular ratio of *cis:trans* species of 4-hydroxytamoxifen may produce estrogenic stimulation promoting tumor growth.

There is a small incidence of endometrial cancers and venous thrombosis associated with tamoxifen use. It will produce anovulation in premenopausal women, with resulting menopausal symptoms in some.

Aromatase inhibitors

Postmenopausal women have persistent circulating estrogen levels as a result of conversion of adrenal androstenedione and testosterone to estrone in peripheral tissues. Aromatase is a heme-containing enzyme that hydroxylates steroids at the C-19 position. Aromatase has been assigned to the CYP450 C19 family. In premenopausal women, enzyme (aromatase) activity in the ovary is stimulated in the theca cells by follicle-stimulating hormone (FSH) activity and substrate (androstenedione) levels in granulosa cells, by luteinizing hormone (LH) such that estradiol levels increase tenfold at ovulation. In two-thirds of breast cancer patients, there is increased aromatase activity, perhaps responsible for local estrogen levels that may be 4–5-fold higher in transformed than in untransformed cells.

Aminoglutethimide, originally developed as an anticonvulsant, was discovered to inhibit steroid 18-hydroxylation and cleavage of cholesterol side chains, and produced symptoms and signs of glucocorticoid deficiency. This observation was applied to breast cancer to deprive tumor cells of secondary sources of estrogen. Hydrocortisone was co-administered. Approximately one-third of all patients, and 50% of ER-positive patients, responded to aminoglutethimide. Among patients who were already responsive to tamoxifen, 50% responded to amino-

glutethimide compared with 25% of nonresponders. Rashes, fever, and lethargy were major toxicities. Because of its inhibition of CYP450 hydroxylation, interaction occurs with many agents including warfarin and theophylline. The initial half-life of 12 hours decreased to 7 hours after 6 weeks of therapy because of enzyme induction.

Second- and third-generation aromatase inhibitors have been developed. Suicide agents compete for and alkylate the active site. Exemestane is such an agent. It is orally available, and has activity comparable to aminoglutethimide with fewer adverse effects. Anastrazole and letrozole are third-generation nonsteroidal competitive inhibitors of the CYP450 hydroxylation steps. Both show comparable activity to progestational agents as second-line therapy with a survival advantage and a superior toxicity profile. Anastrazole and letrozole are comparable to tamoxifen as first-line therapy, with a lower incidence of venous thromboembolism. Both are available as a single daily oral formulation.

Testolactone has little current use.

Androgens

Androgens have limited clinical use in cancer today. Androgen activity in breast cancer is similar to that of estrogens, perhaps for the same mechanistic reasons. Virilizing effects and hepatic toxicity make them unacceptable to most patients. Fluoxymesterone is the most widely used agent. Danazol has use in hematology in aplastic anemia and congenital anemias.

Antiandrogens

Antiandrogens have a role in the therapy of prostate cancer. Flutamide is a pure antiandrogen, which interferes with activated androgen receptor (AR) complex formation in target cells and thus inhibits DNA synthesis in the prostate. The parent drug undergoes extensive hepatic metabolism. The plasma half-life of the major hepatic metabolite is 6 hours. Flutamide is valuable in preventing 'flare,' during the initial testosterone surge induced by gonadotrophin partial agonists (see below). Randomized clinical trials have failed to substantiate earlier claims of a survival benefit when combined with orchiectomy or gonadotrophin partial agonists. A syndrome of 'rebound regression' of progressive prostate cancer growth may be observed following withdrawal of flutamide. The mechanism is uncertain; androgen hyper-responsiveness or mutations in the AR, which utilize flutamide as a positive effector, have been proposed. Bicalutamide has similar activity. Adrenal steroid inhibitors aminoglutethimide and ketoconazole have potential for benefit in refractory cancers.

Progestins (see Chapter 15)

The mechanism of anticancer action of progestins is uncertain. Direct cytotoxicity, suppression of gonadotrophin-releasing hormones (FSH, LH, and ACTH), decrease in ER levels and production of growth inhibitory factors have been proposed, but support for each hypothesis is weak. Therapeutically, progestins are equivalent or nearly so to antiestrogens and aromatase inhibitors.

Medroxyprogesterone acetate (MPA) is used to treat breast and endometrial cancer. It is usually administered intramuscularly. The α half-life is 1 hour and the β half-life is 4 hours. It is extensively metabolized in the liver; 30–40% is excreted in the urine as metabolites.

Megestrol acetate is a synthetic progestin. It is orally available, extensively metabolized in the liver, but 60–80% excreted in the urine, including 10–12% of the parent compound. The half-life is 4 hours.

Progestins have the undesirable effects of weight gain, pedal edema, hirsutism, sweating, hyperventilation, and Cushingoid fat distribution. These often cause progestins to be second-line drugs from the perspective of patient preference in spite of their therapeutic level. The increased appetite caused by progestins is widely exploited as treatment for cancer cachexia.

Luteinizing hormone-releasing hormone agonists and Gonadotropin-releasing hormone agonists

Luteinizing hormone-releasing hormone (LHRH) stimulates the release of FSH and luteinizing hormone (LH) and is normally pulsatile (see Chapter 15). The clinically useful LHRH agonists produce a constant release of synthetic peptide, which results in the down-regulation of LHRH receptor number and uncoupling of the signal transduction mechanism. This produces desensitization to the gonadotropins with resultant castrate levels of testosterone in men and estrogen in women. However, there is an initial surge of hormone levels prior to the cessation of sex steroid production. The resultant involution of hormone-sensitive tissues, such as prostate and breast, via apoptosis, is responsible for the antineoplastic effect.

The oral bioavailability of LHRH agonists is poor because of peptide hydrolysis. Intranasal administration is convenient but again bioavailability is low (1–2%). The most widely used clinical routes of administration are subcutaneous or intramuscular. Native LHRH has good (75–90%) bioavailability. The plasma pharmacokinetics vary depending on the formulation, injection site, volume, blood flow, local proteolysis, and antibody formation. The clinically used compounds are co-polymers of glycides and esterified amides. They degrade and gradually release the active peptides over 28 to 80 days. The potency of goserelin is 100 times that of the native LHRH. The α and β half-lifes of native LHRH administered subcutaneously are approximately 5 and 40 minutes. Subcutaneous leuprolide has a half-life of 3 hours and for subcutaneous goserelin the half-life is 5 hours.

Leuprolide produces responses equivalent to DES or orchiectomy in men with prostate cancer. Premenopausal women treated with goserelin have responses equivalent to those produced by tamoxifen.

The adverse effects are identical with those of castration. Men and women experience loss of libido, hot flashes, losses of muscle mass, weight gain, gastrointestinal disturbances, and loss of bone mineral density. Men become impotent; women experience vaginitis, breast atrophy, and emotional lability. Because of the partial agonist effects, there may be transient exacerbations of bone pain in patients with osseous disease.

Glucocorticoids

Glucocorticoid hormones have been used in cancer therapy since the 1950s. They are integral components of curative therapy for acute lymphoblastic leukemia, non-Hodgkin's lymphoma, and Hodgkin's disease. Glucocorticoids have essential roles in the prevention of allergic reactions (taxanes), emesis control, relief of intracranial hypertension or spinal cord compression in neurologic complications, and pain relief. (See Chapter 15 for a complete description.)

MISCELLANEOUS AGENTS

Interferons

Interferons (IFNs) are a family of proteins with chemical, antigenic, and biologic variability (see Chapter 8). The genes that code for IFN-α and -β reside on chromosome 9, have approximately 30% amino acid homology, and share a single cell surface receptor. The IFN-α alleles produce proteins with approximately 90% amino acid homology. IFN-γ is located on chromosome 12, has minimal sequence homology with IFN-α and -β, and has a unique receptor. There are about 2000 IFN receptors per cell and they are present on every kind of normal and malignant cell type.

The mechanism of action of the IFNs in cancer is not known precisely. Postulated mechanisms include a direct cytostatic effect via the action of 2′-5′-oligoadenylate synthetase (2-5A synthetase, which stimulates the ribonuclease activity of IFNs) on cellular messenger or ribosomal RNAs, prolongation of the cell cycle, or oncogene modulation. Indirect mechanisms of immune activation to increase host defenses include enhanced major histocompatibility complex (MHC) expression, increased tumor-associated antigen expression, Fcγ expression, increased numbers of intercellular adhesion molecules (thereby increasing immune recognition), and the increase in the number and activity of immune effector cells (cytotoxic T cells, helper T cells, natural killer cells, and antigen presenting cells). IFN-α has antiangiogenic effects on tumor endothelial cells through inhibition of basic fibroblast growth factor.

As proteins, the IFNs must be given parenterally. IFN-α is given intramuscularly, with injections of 5×10^6 to 50×10^6 units producing peak plasma concentrations of 200–2000 pg/ml within 4–6 hours. Immunologic activation studies in patients have not conclusively demonstrated a dose–response curve for all parameters, perhaps reflecting the individual variability of the response and the low patient numbers. The duration of biologic action may be detected for 24–72 hours for IFN-α. Clinical responses correlate in some studies with the induction of 2-5A synthase in leukemia, lymphoma, carcinoid tumors, and breast cancer, suggesting that individuals capable of responding to IFNs may have a better clinical result than nonresponders.

The toxicities of pharmacologic doses of IFN include fever, chills, malaise, myalgia, headache, fatigue, weight loss, anorexia, neutropenia, and hepatic transaminase elevation. The acute toxicities have rapid (8 hours) tachyphylaxis, but fatigue, anorexia, and mental slowing are dose-limiting with chronic use.

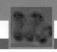

In cancer, their role is uncertain. In the adjuvant treatment of melanoma, one large cooperative trial showed a modest (10%) survival advantage but other trials were negative in the same setting. IFNs have shown activity in hairy cell leukemia and chronic lymphocytic leukemia, only to be supplanted by the purine analogs. Similarly, the role of IFNs in maintaining remissions (with hydroxyurea) in chronic myelogenous leukemia will probably be replaced by the *bcr-abl* tyrosine kinase inhibitor imatinib.

L-asparaginase

L-asparagine is nonessential amino acid formed from the transamination of l-aspartic acid from glutamine by the enzyme l-asparagine synthetase. The enzyme is present in all tissues but often lacking in malignant lymphocytes. L-asparaginase, derived from either E. coli or Erwinia, hydrolyzes asparagine to aspartic acid and ammonia. L-asparaginase has significant activity in childhood acute lymphocytic leukemia and is a component of standard induction and consolidation therapy.

The mechanism of action is depletion of l-asparagine, leading to the inhibition of protein synthesis. Asparagine donates an amino group in the synthesis of glycine, so depletion of glycine levels may contribute to cytotoxicity.

The affinity for asparagine of the E. coli or Erwinia enzyme is approximately 1×10^{-5} M, less than the 4×10^{-5} M plasma concentrations in man. This affinity accounts for the modest selectivity of this particular enzyme. The agent is given intramuscularly or intravenously; the former produces lower peak levels but may be less immunogenic. Clearance is another factor in determining efficacy and the E. coli asparaginase has a half-life of 14–22 hours. The half-life falls markedly with antibody production, a significant factor in clinical usage. Levels rise proportionally with increased doses and the remission rate may be higher with doses of 6000 IU/m^2 than 3000 IU/m^2. Asparagine levels may be undetectable for a week after therapy. A recent modification, the addition of polyethylene glycol, increases the half-life to 14 days by decreasing clearance without a change in the volume of distribution.

The toxicities of asparaginase are considerable. Hypersensitivity reactions occur in up to 40% of patients receiving single-agent asparaginase but in only 20% when it is administered in combination therapy with glucocorticoids and 6-mercaptopurine. The hypersensitivity usually occurs after several doses and in successive cycles. The reaction may be only urticaria, but may be severe with laryngospasm or rarely, serum sickness. Fatal reactions occur in <1% of the cases of hypersensitivity reactions. Changing the source of enzyme is the appropriate initial step.

Toxicity can occur as a result of protein synthesis inhibition. Despite prolongation of prothrombin and partial thromboplastin times, clotting, not bleeding, is a more frequent adverse occurrence. Decreases in the anticoagulant proteins antithrombin III, protein C, and protein S are responsible. Elevated hepatic transaminase levels occur due to fatty metamorphosis; pancreatitis, and nausea and vomiting also occur. Neurologic complications, with confusion or stupor, may be due to elevated ammonia or to lowered levels of asparagine.

Mitotane

Mitotane (o,p-DDD0), which chemically is 1,1-dichloro-2-(o-chlorophenyl)-2-(p-chlorophenyl) ethane, is an oral agent which has direct cytotoxic effects on the zona fasiculata and zone glomerulosa of the adrenal gland, and prevents formation of 17-hydroxycorticosteroids. It is biotransformed by the CYP450 system to an acyl chloride which combines with binucleophils in the adrenal cortical cells. The dose is titrated against urinary cortisol/17-hydroxycorticoteroid levels in adrenal cortical cancer. Responses of up to 33% have been observed. Exogenous cortisol and occasionally mineralocorticoids must be given.

Imatinib

Imatinib is a 2-phenylaminopyrimidine agent selectively inhibiting the *c-abl* tyrosine kinase. The development of imatinib over 14 years is likely to become a paradigm for cancer therapeutic development in the future.

Chronic myelogenous leukemia (CML) has a characteristic chromosomal translocation, 9:22. This places the cellular homologue of the feline Abelson leukemia virus tyrosine kinase downstream from the break point cluster region, *bcr*, and results in the unregulated expression of the fusion p210Bcr-Abl oncogene, which functions as a cytoplasmic protein kinase. Bcr-Abl is necessary and sufficient to produce CML, although additional chromosomal aberrations develop in the later stages of the disease. Imatinib interferes with the binding of ATP to the tyrosine kinase site on *abl*. Imatinib produces hematologic remission in virtually 100% of interferon-refractory patients with the accelerated phase of CML. Nearly 30% of patients have disappearance of the Philadelphia chromosome/9:22 translocation. Imatinib has activity against two tyrosine receptor kinases, c-kit and PGDF (platelet derived growth factor). C-kit mutations occur in 70% of patients with gastrointestinal stromal tumors (GIST, a sarcoma arising from the myenteric neurons of Cajal). Imatinib produces significant responses in this otherwise refractory sarcoma.

The usual dose is 400–800 mg/day. Oral absorption is 98%. The peak plasma level after a 400 mg dose is 2.3 μg/ml and the steady state levels, 0.72 μg/ml, exceed the necessary cytotoxic level in plasma. The half-life is 12–18 hrs. 70% of a dose is eliminated in the feces, 20% unchanged. 13% is excreted in the urine, 5% unchanged. The N-desmethylpiperazine metabolite is as active as the parent drug and has a half-life of 40 hrs. Metabolism is via CYP450 3A4. This makes for possible interaction with other CYP450 3A4 substrates such as the erythromycins, azole antifungal agents, cyclosporine, and anticonvulsants, such as phenytoin. Toxicities include elevations of bilirubin/hepatic transaminases (1.5%), rashes and fatigue (each approximately 35%).

RADIOPHARMACEUTICALS

Radiation has been used therapeutically in cancer medicine since the first years of the twentieth century. Then as now, the predominant mode of delivery is by external beam irradiation, which is beyond the scope of this book. However, irradiation

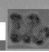
can be delivered via soluble chemical isotopes in a small number of specific instances. The potential for more widespread use of radioisotopes has increased with the advent of monoclonal antibody therapy as a method of molecular targeting of specific cell types.

Sodium phosphorous ^{32}P has been used for decades to treat malignant effusions, without reproducible benefit. ^{32}P is still used in the treatment of polycythemia vera, although its leukemogenic potential makes it an option in only a small number of patients. ^{32}P is a β-emitter (produces an ionizing electron), with a half-life of 14.3 days. It is taken up into bone as inorganic phosphorous and provides local irradiation. The single dose is 4 mCi, which may be repeated at 3–4-month intervals, up to about 16 mCi as a lifetime dose. The toxicities are myelosuppression, some of which is intended, and leukemogenesis.

^{89}Strontium chloride is used for the treatment of painful bony metastases in prostate and breast cancer. Strontium substitutes for calcium in bones. ^{89}Strontium is a β-emitter, with a half-life of 50 days. The half-life in metastatic bone (>50 days) is greater than in normal bone (14 days) and the uptake in metastatic bone is tenfold greater than in normal marrow. The onset of response is 7–12 days, with a peak at 6 weeks, and a duration of 3–12 months. Clearance is into bone. In metastatic bone cancer, 80–90% of the dose remains in bone at 100 days, with renal clearance of the remainder of the dose. In healthy patients, 80% will be cleared by renal (65%) and hepatic (33%) mechanisms. The usual dose is 40 uCi/kg or a fixed dose of 40 miCi. Bone marrow suppression is the major adverse effect and the dosing interval should be 3 months or greater.

^{131}Iodine is used for the treatment of thyroid cancer. Thyroid tissue avidly takes up inorganic iodine and organifies it into thyroid hormone. After surgery, well-differentiated thyroid cancers with adverse prognostic factors are treated with radioiodine ablation. ^{131}Iodine is a low-energy γ (photon)-emitter with a radioactive half-life of 8.04 days. Sodium iodide is rapidly cleared from the blood with half-lifes of 40 minutes, 9 hours, and 60 hours. Following ^{131}I treatment, patients have lifelong thyroid hormone replacement.

^{131}I is a component of the monoclonal antibody tositumomab. ^{131}I-tositumomab is a murine monoclonal antibody directed at the lymphoid cell surface marker CD20 (B1), which is expressed on many transformed lymphocytes in Hodgkin's disease and non-Hodgkin's lymphoma. ^{131}I-tositumomab treatment produces complete or partial regression of refractory diseases in up to 60–90% of patients whose tumors express CD20. The uptake of a 2.5 mg/kg dose is 0.01% per gram of tumor tissue in CD20-positive patients, and 0.002% in CD20-negative patients. ^{131}I-tositumomab has a half-life of 36–48 hours. The dose of irradiation delivered to the tumor is in the order of 10–92 Gy (280–800 mCi), which exceeds the dose to the lung (6.5–30 Gy), bone marrow (1–6.4 Gy), and total body (1–5.7 Gy). Bone marrow suppression is the major

Specific cytotoxic drug interactions

- Procarbazine inhibits monoamine oxidase
- Allopurinol inhibits 6-mercaptopurine metabolism
- Barbiturates and cimetidine increase activation of cyclophosphamide
- Cisplatin and doxorubicin enhance paclitaxel toxicity when given before paclitaxel
- Asparaginase inhibits the metabolism of vinca alkaloids

General principles of cancer chemotherapy administration

- Allow for full recovery of myelosuppression before resuming dosing, though this may not apply for aggressive leukemias and lymphomas
- Avoid concomitant administration of platelet-inhibiting drugs
- Avoid drug interactions involving cytochrome P-450 metabolism
- The dose of certain drugs needs adjustment if there is hepatic and renal impairment
- There is no evidence that hematopoietic cytokines given to ameliorate myelosuppression improve outcome, but they markedly increase costs

toxicity, but transient pneumonitis has been observed as the lung receives the highest radiation dose of any normal tissue. Reactions to the murine protein include fever, serum sickness, anaphylaxis, and the development of tositumomab-neutralizing human antimouse antibodies (HAMA).

FURTHER READING

Chabner BA, Longo DL. *Cancer Chemotherapy and Biotherapy*, 3rd edn. Philadelphia: Lippincott Williams and Wilkins; 2001. [This is the most comprehensive and current textbook on cancer pharmacology.]

DeVita VT Jr, Hellman S, Rosenberg SA. *Cancer: Principles and Practice of Oncology*, 5th edn. Philadelphia: Lippincott Williams and Wilkins; 1997. [Excellent review of the principles of cancer pharmacology and major chemotherapeutic agents. The remainder of the book is an excellent guide to clinical cancer medicine.]

Lodish HF, Berk A, Zipursky L, Matsudaira P, Baltimore D, Darnell J. *Molecular Cell Biology*, 4th edn. New York: W.H. Freeman and Co., Scientific American Books; 2000. [Superbly illustrated, expertly written text on molecular biology. The best in the field.]

Perry MD. *The Chemotherapy Source Book*, 3rd edn. Baltimore: Lippincott Williams and Wilkins; 2001. [Very good review of cancer pharmacology with guides to the treatment of various malignant diseases.]

Skeel RT. *Handbook of Cancer Chemotherapy*, 5th edn. Philadelphia: Lipincott Williams and Wilkins; 1999. [Very good short pocket size text with excellent practical information.]

Drug Action on Body System Targets

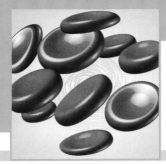

Chapter 13

Drugs and the Blood

PHYSIOLOGY OF THE HEMATOPOIETIC SYSTEM

Blood is a suspension of cells in plasma, which is a solution of proteins and salts. The cells of the blood are red blood cells (erythrocytes), white blood cells (leukocytes) and platelets.

- Erythrocytes are anuclear cells containing hemoglobin and carry oxygen from the lung to all the tissues where it is exchanged for carbon dioxide.
- Leukocytes (neutrophils, monocytes, lymphocytes, and others) defend the body against micro-organisms that enter the body from the environment.
- Platelets form plugs with coagulation proteins in the plasma to stop leaks from blood vessels (Fig. 13.1).

All blood cells are derived from hematopoitic stem cells

Blood cells originate in the bone marrow except during an early part of fetal life. The bone marrow provides the hematopoietic microenvironment to support the process of hematopoietic self-renewal and differentiation. These stem cells self-replicate and exist in very small numbers in the bone marrow and blood. Although each stem cell has a great capacity for self-renewal, as a group, hematopoietic stem cells are relatively quiescent and only a minuscule fraction are proliferating and differentiating at any one time to replenish the lost blood elements.

Hematopoietic growth factors and cytokines control hematopoiesis

Hematopoietic stem cells give rise to hematopoietic progenitor cells. Compared with stem cells, these cells have a decreased capacity for self-renewal and are more committed to differentiating into a particular blood cell type. With each generation, the descendants of the progenitor cells differentiate further into more mature cells with a more limited lifespan and become restricted to a particular blood cell lineage. Ultimately, the

Normal concentrations (mean ± SD) of hemoglobin and hematocrit

| | Hemoglobin | | Hematocrit |
	g/dl	(mmol/liter)	%
Prepubertal child	12.5 ± 1.5	(7.37 ± 0.93)	38 ± 4
Male adult	15.4 ± 1.8	(9.56 ± 1.12)	44 ± 5
Female adult	13.5 ± 2.0	(8.38 ± 1.24)	38 ± 5

Hematocrit in third trimester for pregnant women may be as low as 30%

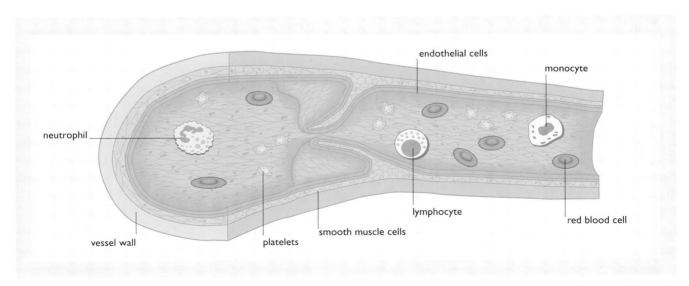

Fig. 13.1 Blood vessel and the blood cells. The blood vessel wall and its surrounding smooth muscle cells are lined by endothelial cells, which provide a nonthrombotic surface for smooth blood flow. White blood cells, including neutrophils, monocytes, and lymphocytes, interact with the blood vessel cells to defend the body against microbial invasion. Red blood cells carry oxygen to end organs. Platelets plug leaks in the blood vessels to prevent blood loss.

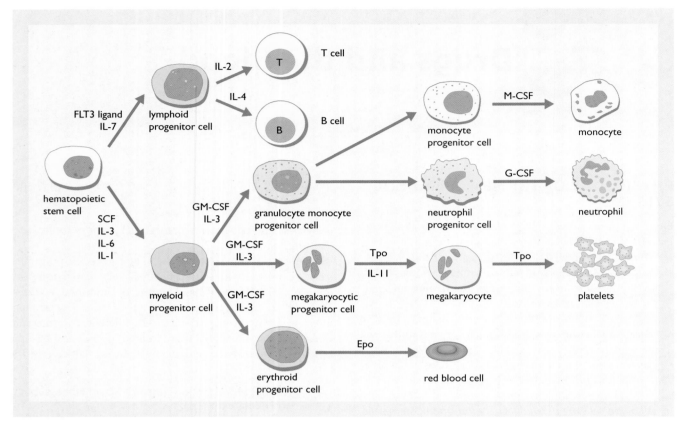

Fig. 13.2 Hematopoiesis and hematopoietic growth factors. Hematopoietic stem cells have a high regenerative potential, but with each generation the descendant cells acquire lineage-specific characteristics and decreased proliferative capacity. Growth factors including Epo, G-CSF, GM-CSF, IL, M-CSF, SCF, and Tpo are needed for regulating each step of hemopoiesis. (Epo, erythropoietin; FLT3, C-FMS-like tyrosine kinase; G-CSF, granulocyte colony-stimulating factor; GM-CSF, granulocyte–macrophage colony-stimulating factor; IL, interleukin; M-CSF, macrophage colony-stimulating factor; SCF, stem cell factor; Tpo, thrombopoietin)

process ends with mature cells, which have no further capacity to divide and give rise to red cells, leukocytes, and platelets.

This maturation process is controlled by hematopoietic growth factors and cytokines that activate the appropriate growth factor or cytokine receptors leading to cell differentiation and proliferation. Many of these have been purified and cloned. Some have been produced by recombinant technology and are used as protein therapeutics for a variety of disorders, as discussed later (Fig. 13.2).

DRUGS USED FOR DISEASES OF THE BLOOD

This chapter describes the pharmacologic agents that are useful in the treatment of three important dysfunctions of the blood: anemia, thrombosis, and bleeding.

- Anemia is a below-normal concentration of circulatory hemoglobin. Its symptoms result from the decreased oxygen-carrying capacity of red blood cells.
- Thrombosis is the formation of unwanted clots in blood vessels, which blocks the delivery of blood to end organs or the return of blood to the heart.
- Bleeding disorders result from failure of the hemostatic system to form clots and to stop leaks in the blood vessels.

Drugs used to treat these disorders are shown in Fig. 13.3. Several hematopoietic growth factors, that have become standard therapeutic agents for hematologic or nonhematologic disorders, are also discussed in this chapter.

ANEMIA AND AGENTS USED TO TREAT ANEMIA

Anemia is a reduction in the red blood cell mass. When the hematocrit value is less than 40% (less than 37% in women), or when the blood concentration of hemoglobin falls below the established mean by more than two standard deviations, a person is anemic. Anemia causes similar signs and symptoms, such as pallor, shortness of breath, and fatigue, regardless of underlying etiologies because they all result from the decreased capacity of hemoglobin to carry oxygen.

Based on the ability of bone marrow to produce red blood cells, by measuring the number of young red blood cells (reticulocytes) in the blood, causes of anemia can then be classified into two categories:

- A low reticulocyte count and therefore a hypoproliferative anemia; the bone marrow is not making an adequate number of red blood cells.

Drugs used to treat blood disorders

Drugs for anemia	Iron Deferoxamine Vitamin B$_{12}$ Folate Hydroxyurea
Hematopoietic growth factors	Erythropoietin (Epo) Granulocyte colony stimulating factor (G-CSF) Granulocyte-macrophage colony stimulating factor (GM-CSF) Oprelvekin (Interleukin-11, IL-11) Thrombopoietin (Tpo)
Antiplatelet agents	Irreversible COX inhibitor (aspirin) Reversible COX inhibitors (some NSAIDs) ADP antagonists (ticlopidine, clopidogrel) GPIIb/IIIa antagonists (abciximab, eptifibatide, tirofiban) Dipyridamole
Anticoagulants	Inhibitor of coagulant factor formation (warfarin) Indirect inhibitor of thrombin (heparin, LMWH (enoxaparin)) Direct inhibitor of thrombin (hirudin (lepirudin))
Thrombolytics	Streptokinase APSAC Urokinase Tissue plasminogen activator (tPA) Reteplase
Procoagulants	Coagulant factor concentrates Desmopressin (DDAVP) Vitamin K ε Aminocaproic acid (EACA) Aprotinin Topical hemostatics (thrombin, collagen, absorbable gelatin, oxidized cellulose)

Fig. 13.3 Drugs used to treat blood disorders. (COX, cyclo-oxygenase; ADP, adenosine diphosphate; APSAC, anisoylated plasminogen–streptokinase activator complex; NSAIDs, nonsteroidal anti-inflammatory drugs; LMWH, low molecular weight heparin)

- A high reticulocyte count and therefore a hemolytic anemia, in which there is increased peripheral destruction of red blood cells despite increased production by the bone marrow.

Hypoproliferative anemias can be further subdivided according to the size of the red blood cells as seen under the microscope, as follows:

- Microcytic (small red blood cells).
- Normocytic (normal size red blood cells).
- Macrocytic (large red blood cells).

Figure 13.4 lists the etiologies of anemia according to these criteria.

Causes of anemia

Hypoproliferative	
Microcytic	Iron deficiency Anemia of chronic disease Sideroblastic anemia
Normocytic	Anemia of chronic disease Endocrine anemia Bone marrow failure
Macrocytic	Vitamin B$_{12}$ deficiency Folic acid deficiency Myelodysplastic syndrome
Hyperproliferative	
Hemolytic	Hemoglobinopathies Autoimmune Membrane disorder Drug-induced Metabolic abnormalities Glucose-6-phosphate dehydrogenase deficiency Infections

Fig. 13.4 Causes of anemia.

Iron and iron-deficiency anemia

Iron deficiency remains the most common cause of anemia worldwide

Although dietary iron deficiency may occur in infants and adolescence during the rapid growth phase, iron deficiency generally occurs only as a result of chronic bleeding. In women, it is usually due to blood loss from menstruation and pregnancy; in men and postmenopausal women, iron-deficiency anemia is often a clue to pathologic blood loss and warrants a search to discover the source of bleeding.

Two-thirds of body iron is in hemoglobin

Iron is needed to form the complex molecule, heme, which is the oxygen-carrying component of hemoglobin. When aging red cells are destroyed, almost all the iron is salvaged to form new red blood cells. However, a small but critical fraction of red blood cell iron is obtained from the diet. Dietary iron is absorbed mostly in the duodenum and proximal jejunum as part of heme and as in elemental form by the intestinal epithelial cell through cell surface receptors. Heme iron is readily absorbed and released in the cell from the porphyrin ring by heme oxygenase. However, non-heme iron absorption is highly variable. Many types of food such as tea, egg yolk, and bran interfere with iron absorption. Excess iron is stored in the cell as a ferritin complex.

Iron enters and is transported in the plasma by binding to transferrin. Iron–transferrin complexes bind to transferrin receptors which are integral membrane glycoproteins expressed by maturing erythroid cells; this leads to internalization with subsequent release of iron intracellularly. The transferrin and

193

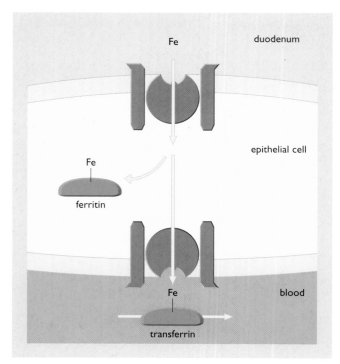

Fig. 13.5 Iron absorption by the gastrointestinal epithelial cell. Iron is absorbed via a cell surface receptor on the epithelial cell. Some of the iron passes through the cell and is carried in the blood by transferrin. Excess iron is stored as ferritin.

transferrin receptor are recycled to the cell membrane (Fig. 13.5).

The amount of physiologic loss of iron is approximately:
- 1 mg/day in men and nonmenstruating women.
- 2–3 mg/day in menstruating women.
- 500–1000 mg with each pregnancy.

The patient's history and physical examination may yield information that suggests the presence of iron-deficiency anemia. The definite diagnosis of iron-deficiency depends essentially on one or more specific laboratory measurements. Serum ferritin levels may be helpful in the assessment of body iron stores. It is associated with iron-deficiency anemia unless there is a concurrent process that abnormally raises the level, such as infection or liver disease. Iron deficiency also results in a low serum iron level and a high total iron binding capacity (TIBC), i.e., a low iron/total iron binding capacity ratio. Microcytosis on the peripheral blood smear is a late finding. The most sensitive and specific test to diagnose iron deficiency is a bone marrow examination of iron stores, the bone marrow iron stain, but this procedure is not usually needed in most clinical situations.

Treatment of iron-deficiency anemia consists of correction of the underlying causes of iron deficiency and iron replacement therapy. Oral administration of ferrous sulfate is the standard treatment for iron-deficiency anemia. Iron is best absorbed when taken on an empty stomach with ascorbic acid, which binds to iron and facilitates iron transport into intestinal cells. At the acidic pH of the stomach, mucin binds to inorganic iron and enhances its absorption, which may otherwise be impaired by antacids or medications that reduce stomach acid production. Commercial preparations of ferrous sulfate usually contain 60 mg of elemental iron, and only 10–20% of the ingested iron is absorbed by iron-deficient patients. In other words, the bioavailability is relatively low. The usual dose is 150–200 mg elemental iron per day, divided into three or four doses. A prompt rise in reticulocyte count confirms that iron deficiency is at least partially responsible for the anemia. The hemoglobin concentration of patients who are optimally treated with 180 mg/day of elemental iron increases by about 1 g/dl/week (mass concentration 10 g/liter/week; substance concentration 0.62 mmol/liter/week), assuming they are otherwise well. Iron supplementation should continue for another 6 months after the hemoglobin level has been normalized to replenish the body's iron stores.

The most common complaint of patients taking iron is gastrointestinal irritation. Sometimes this can be very bothersome. Physicians need to talk carefully with patients in order to foster adherence to this regimen. Lowering the daily doses of iron or taking iron with meals significantly reduces iron-induced adverse effects. Alternatively, a polysaccharide–iron complex preparation is available that may cause less gastrointestinal irritation, but is much more expensive. Parenteral iron preparation is also available and is only indicated for the patients with iron-deficiency anemia unable to tolerate or absorb iron pills, or for those patients who have chronic bleeding disorders or whose needs cannot be met by oral iron therapy alone. The intramuscular route is painful and may cause skin discoloration at the injection site. Alternatively, iron dextran can be slowly infused intravenously, but this must only be carried out with close monitoring, because there is a high incidence of anaphylactoid-like reactions.

Deferoxamine and iron overload

Excessive ingestion of iron may result in acute or chronic iron toxicity (iron overload). Acute iron toxicity is usually seen in young children who ingest an overdose of iron tablets that are used either as a pediatric or prenatal vitamin supplement or for treatment of anemia in a family member or themselves. Iron pills are particularly tempting to young children, as they may appear similar to candies. Acute iron toxicity is the leading cause of death due to toxicological agents in children under 6 years. Chronic iron overload, on the other hand, is commonly seen in patients with inherited hemochromatosis, a disorder characterized by excessive iron absorption, and in patients who have received blood transfusions over a long period of time in the absence of ongoing external blood loss which would lead to iron loss from the body. For example, iron overload is the leading cause of death among thalassemia patients in industrialized nations. This is due to the fact that the body does not have mechanisms to substantially increase elimination of iron.

> **⚠ Warning about oral iron preparations**
>
> - *Taking oral iron leads to black stools that may obscure the diagnosis of gastrointestinal bleeding!*

Iron toxicity can be divided into two categories, corrosive and cellular toxicity. Iron is an extremely corrosive substance in the gastrointestinal system. It acts on the mucosal tissues and its corrosive effects could manifest as hematemesis or diarrhea. Patients may become hypovolemic due to fluid and blood loss. The absorption of excessive quantities of ingested iron will result in systemic iron toxicity. Severe overdose causes impaired oxidative phosphorylation and mitochondrial dysfunction, which can result in cellular death. The most affected organ is the liver. Other organs, including the heart, kidneys, lungs, and the hematologic systems may be impaired as well. With acute ingestion of iron greater than 20 mg/kg body weight, patients will typically show signs of gastrointestinal toxicity. When the ingestion of elemental iron exceeds 40 mg/kg, patients will generally have moderate to severe intoxication. Ingestions exceeding 60 mg/kg may lead to death.

Iron overload may be prevented and treated with a chelating agent capable of complexing with iron and promoting its excretion. The only iron-chelating agent currently available for clinical use is deferoxamine B, a trihydroxamic acid isolated from the bacteria, *Streptomyces pilosus*, with relative specificity for ferric iron. It is used subcutaneously and intravenously to chelate iron in acute and chronic iron overload.

Deferoxamine is given subcutaneously at a dosage of 20–50 mg/kg over 8 to 10 hours, three to five nights per week. Administration of deferoxamine should be continued until the ferritin level is consistently less than 1000 ng/ml. Ascorbic acid (vitamin C), 100 mg, will increase the excretion of iron and is given in combination with the deferoxamine. If there is severe hemosiderosis, deferoxamine is given intravenously at a dose of 100 mg/kg over 12 hours. It is desired to keep the ferritin level below 2000 ng/ml; if the ferritin is above 4000 ng/ml hospital admission should be considered for high dose deferoxamine therapy.

The most common adverse effects of deferoxamine include tinnitus and a reversible transient hearing loss. These effects are not related to the deferoxamine dosage. Decreased night vision is less common. Intravenous infusion exceeding 15 mg/kg/h may induce hypotension and even shock. Allergic reactions including anaphylaxis are not uncommon. Hydrocortisone can be mixed with deferoxamine to decrease this reaction. Diluting the deferoxamine can reduce the irritation at the site of administration. Excessive iron chelation will cause growth disturbance in children and mineral deficiency.

Vitamin B$_{12}$, folate, and other macrocytic anemias

The macrocytic anemias have two subgroups, namely megaloblastic anemia that is caused by a biochemical defect in deoxyribonucleic acid (DNA) synthesis and nonmegaloblastic anemia that is usually associated with a pathological alteration in membrane lipids of the red blood cells. The most common conditions that cause megaloblastic anemia include vitamin B$_{12}$ (cobalamin) deficiency, folate deficiency, myelodysplasia, and medications that inhibit DNA synthesis (see Chapter 27). Both cobalamin and folate are critical cofactors in enzymatic reactions

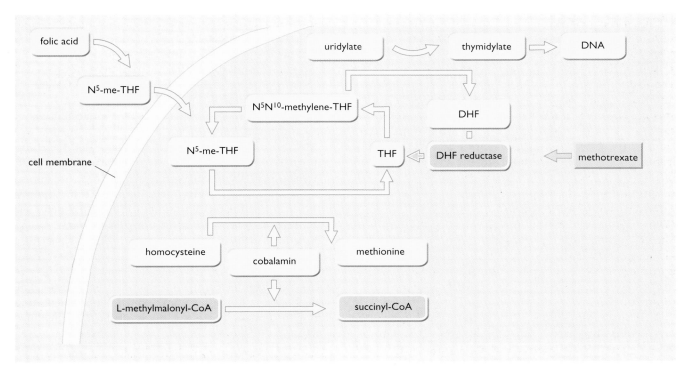

Fig. 13.6 Role of folate and vitamin B$_{12}$ in DNA synthesis. Folate compounds are required as carbon donors in the conversion of deoxyuridine to deoxythymidine. Cobalamin is a cofactor for homocysteine–methionine methyltransferase, which transfers a methyl group from methyltetrahydrofolate to homocysteine to make methionine. Cobalamin is also required for methylmalonyl coenzyme A mutase, which converts methylmalonyl coenzyme A to succinyl coenzyme A. Methotrexate inhibits DNA synthesis by inhibiting DHF reductase which converts DHF to THF. (DHF, dihydrofolate; N^5-me- THF, N^5-methyl-tetrahydrofolate; THF, tetrahydrofolate)

required for DNA synthesis (Fig. 13.6). The interdependency of cobalamin and methylfolate may explain the similar morphologic changes observed when either cobalamin or folate is deficient. Unlike folate deficiency, however, vitamin B_{12} deficiency can also cause neurologic deficits. Paresthesia is the earliest symptom followed by loss of vibratory sense, ataxia, dementia, and coma.

Vitamin B_{12} deficiency

Vitamin B_{12} (cobalamin) is a complex molecule consisting of a central cobalt atom linked to four pyrrole rings and attached to a nucleotide. Humans obtain vitamin B_{12} from dietary animal proteins. The daily requirement for vitamin B_{12} is 0.6–1.2 μg, and the biological half-life of vitamin B_{12} stored in the liver is about 1 year. The total body content of vitamin B_{12} is 3–5 mg, and the normal daily loss is very low; therefore, more than 2 years generally elapse after a complete cessation of vitamin B_{12} intake before clinical manifestations of deficiency become apparent.

■ *The most common cause of B_{12} deficiency is often the disease pernicious anemia*

Vitamin B_{12} is readily absorbed from the gastrointestinal tract with the aid of an intrinsic factor secreted by the parietal cells of the stomach, and the intrinsic factor–cobalamin complex is absorbed via receptors on the ileal cell surface (Fig. 13.7) (see also Chapter 27). As vitamin B_{12} is widely available in animal products, dietary deficiency is an uncommon cause of vitamin

B_{12} deficiency except in the strictest vegetarians. Breast-fed infants of vegans may also develop vitamin B_{12} deficiency. The most common cause of B_{12} deficiency is pernicious anemia, a form of gastric secretory failure with atrophy of gastric parietal cells and a consequent failure to secrete the intrinsic factor. It is strongly suspected that pernicious anemia results from an autoimmune destruction, since antiparietal cell and anti-intrinsic factor antibodies are detected in many patients. In addition, B_{12} deficiency is also seen in patients with partial or total gastrectomy, malabsorption syndrome, inflammatory bowel disease, or small bowel resection.

Diagnosis of vitamin B_{12} deficiency involves measuring serum vitamin B_{12} levels, although a significant minority of deficient patients have levels in the normal range. Vitamin B_{12} deficiency leads to increased serum and urine concentrations of methylmalonic acid. These are sensitive indices of vitamin B_{12} deficiency. A two-stage test, first with radiolabeled vitamin B_{12} alone and then with radiolabeled B_{12} with intrinsic factor (Schilling test), can be performed to determine whether a vitamin B_{12} deficiency is due to pernicious anemia.

Treatment of vitamin B_{12} deficiency should start with parenteral vitamin B_{12}. There are two commercial preparations of vitamin B_{12}, cyanocobalamin and hydroxocobalamin, available for clinical use. The recommended initial dose is 0.1–1 mg of vitamin B_{12} intramuscularly daily for 1–2 weeks. The maintenance dose for treatment of pernicious anemia is monthly injections of 1 mg cyanocobalamin for life. However, oral therapy with 1 mg vitamin B_{12} five times a week has been shown to be equally effective. Despite the lack of intrinsic factor, absorption by passive diffusion still functions and can fulfil the 2–5 μg/day requirement. The application of a vitamin B gel intranasally (ENER-B gel) has been approved by the USA Food and Drug Administration (FDA) for dietary supplementation, but not for the treatment of pernicious anemia, although it does consistently raise serum vitamin B_{12} levels. The serum K^+ concentration may fall after initial treatment with vitamin B_{12} due to an increased need for intracellular K^+ to support new cell synthesis.

Megaloblastic anemia due to vitamin B_{12} deficiency may respond to large doses of folic acid administration. Conversely, supraphysiologic doses of vitamin B_{12} therapy can reverse megaloblastic anemia due to folate deficiency. Importantly, however, the neurologic damage due to vitamin B_{12} deficiency is not reversed by folate. Consequently, an accurate diagnosis is essential in order to select the correct therapy.

Folic acid deficiency

Folates belong to the vitamin B family and are found in a wide variety of fresh foods, but are rapidly destroyed by heating during food preparation (see Chapter 27). Folic acid is widely

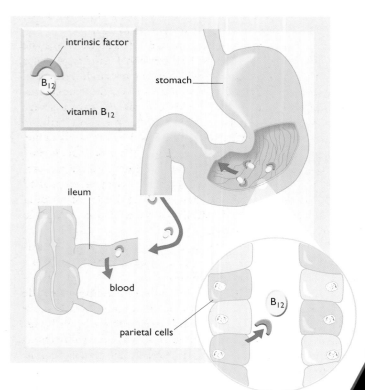

Fig. 13.7 Absorption of vitamin B_{12}. Intestinal absorption of vitamin B_{12} requires intrinsic factor, which is secreted by parietal cells in the stomach, and occurs in the distal ileum via cell surface receptors.

> ⚠ **Warning about using folic acid**
>
> • *Large doses of folic acid can reverse the megaloblastic anemia caused by vitamin B_{12} deficiency, but do not reverse the neurologic damage of vitamin B_{12} deficiency.*

distributed in nature as a conjugate with one or more molecules of glutamic acid. Naturally occurring folates must be reduced to mono- and diglutamates by conjugases in the stomach before they can be efficiently absorbed from the proximal small intestine. Folates are then transported to the liver where they are stored and transformed into 5-methyltetrahydrofolate, which is the form that enters tissue cells. In the cell, 5-methyltetrahydrofolate is converted into the metabolically active tetrahydrofolate by vitamin B_{12}-dependent methyltransferase. The normal daily requirement of folate is about 100 μg, and the tissue storage of folate is estimated at 10 mg. Inadequate dietary folate intake, therefore, will lead to megaloblastic anemia much sooner than those caused by vitamin B_{12} deficiency.

Inadequate intake is the most common cause of folate deficiency

During pregnancy, the need for folates is markedly increased and folate deficiency very early in pregnancy is associated with congenital neural tube defects. Folate supplementation is recommended for all pregnant women or those who are likely to become pregnant, since there is increased requirement for folate even before a woman may realize that she is pregnant. Alcohol abuse is a common cause of folate deficiency anemia as a result of reduced folate intake and diminished folate absorption. As the concentration of folate in bile is several times higher than that in plasma, biliary diversion will reduce the plasma concentration of folate. Patients with prolonged biliary drainage should therefore be given oral folate supplementation. People taking phenytoin and related anticonvulsants tend to have lower serum folate levels due to their reduction in iron absorption, but they rarely have megaloblastic anemia. Antifolates such as methotrexate are widely used to treat hematologic and inflammatory diseases. Methotrexate competes with dihydrofolate for the enzyme dihydrofolate reductase and, even at the relatively low doses used in the treatment of rheumatoid arthritis, there is evidence of red blood cell macrocytosis (see Fig. 13.6 and Chapter 20).

A patient's history, physical examination, and finding of macrocytosis in the peripheral blood smears should alert the clinician to the possibility of folate deficiency. Although folate deficiency and vitamin B_{12} deficiency cause a similar morphologic change in red blood cells, characteristic neurologic changes are only seen in megaloblastic anemia caused by vitamin B_{12} deficiency. Diagnosis of folate deficiency is obtained by measuring serum or red blood cell folate levels; the latter is of greater diagnostic value.

Folate deficiency responds promptly to treatment with 1–5 mg/day of oral folate. An injectable form is available for patients who are unable to take medication orally or have poor enteric absorption. As vitamin B_{12} deficiency may cause concomitant folate deficiency, it is important to make certain that the patient is not vitamin B_{12}-deficient before starting folate treatment. As previously stated, folate may correct the megaloblastic anemia of vitamin B_{12} deficiency, but will not correct the neurologic damage caused by a lack of vitamin B_{12}. Indiscriminate use of folate may therefore mask the symptoms of vitamin B_{12} deficiency and lead to irreversible neurologic deficits.

Folic acid may have a role in preventing arteriosclerosis

Serum homocysteine concentrations are inversely correlated with serum folate levels. There is increasing evidence that an elevated serum homocysteine level is an independent risk factor for arteriosclerosis. As a result, the effect of homocysteine-lowering treatment with folic acid in the prevention of atherothrombotic disease is being evaluated in clinical trials.

Hydroxyurea and sickle cell anemia

Sickle cell anemia is a common hemoglobinopathy, mainly existing in black populations including African-Americans. Fifty years ago, Dr Linus Pauling and his colleagues discovered that sickle cell anemia was caused by the change in a protein molecule due to an allelic change in a single gene. The precise mechanism was later revealed: a point mutation in the β-chain gene of hemoglobin S results in substitution of valine for glutamate at the sixth amino acid position. This alteration markedly reduces the solubility of deoxygenated hemoglobin S, which leads to polymerization of the deoxygenated hemoglobin S, and causes deformity of the red blood cell (sickling) and hemolysis. Patients with sickle cell anemia are homozygous for the sickle gene and have hemoglobin S but no hemoglobin A. In contrast, people with sickle cell trait are heterozygous for the sickle gene and have both kinds of hemoglobin. People with sickle cell trait (occurring in about one out of 10 black people) are usually not symptomatic. However, vigorous physical activity at high altitude, air travel, and anesthesia are potentially dangerous to them.

The majority of clinical manifestations result from episodic sickling leading to microvascular occlusion. Painful crises occur when rigid and deformed sickled cells interact with platelets, endothelium, and coagulation factors to occlude the microcirculation. Patients with sickle cell disease have a severe hemolytic anemia that begins within weeks of birth, as hemoglobin S replaces hemoglobin F, and lasts throughout life. The average red blood cell lifespan in these patients is only 17 days (the norm is 120 days), and thus patients are particularly sensitive to transient bone marrow suppression, caused by a variety of infections, that may lead to the development of aplastic crisis. Repeated episodes of ischemic necrosis lead to progressive organ damage.

Treatment of sickle cell anemia in the past has been primarily supportive, with intravenous fluids, oxygen, analgesics for pain relief, and blood transfusion.

Hydroxyurea (HU) is an inhibitor of the ribonucleotide reductase system that catalyzes the rate-limiting step in the *de novo* biosynthesis of purine and pyrimidine deoxyribonucleotides. It is currently used to treat chronic myelogenous leukemia and polycythemia vera. Recent clinical trials demonstrate that HU raises the population of reticulocytes containing hemoglobin F and stimulates a small rise in the hemoglobin F level. A multicenter clinical trial demonstrated that HU decreased painful crises in severely affected adults and children with sickle cell anemia. However, not all patients benefited from treatment, and crises were not eliminated in most patients. More clinical trials are needed to determine whether HU can prevent chronic organ damage in adults and children with sickle cell anemia. Although HU has been widely used in treatment of a variety of hematologic disorders and is relatively well tolerated, the use of a cytotoxic drug in a nonmalignant condition raises questions about long-term safety regarding carcinogenesis and teratogenesis. A phase I/II clinical trial has recently shown that HU treatment at the maximum tolerated dose for 1-year results in a significant improvement in hematologic changes, including increased hemoglobin concentrations, with mild, transient, and reversible toxicities in pediatric

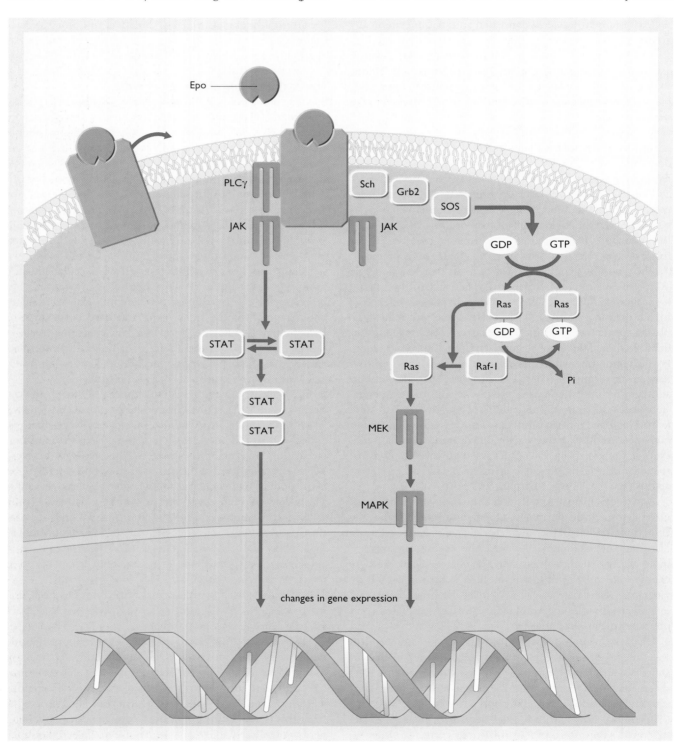

Fig. 13.8 Type I cytokine receptor signal transduction. Stimulation of type I cytokine receptors, in this case erythropoietin receptors (Epo), on hematopoietic progenitor cells induces dimerization of the receptors that trigger activation of JAK/STAT tyrosine kinase signal pathways and the Ras/MAP kinase signal pathway leading to the transcription of genes related to growth and differentiation.

patients with sickle cell anemia. The dosage of HU should be escalated slowly, the aim being to achieve a dose just below that which would produce significant cytopenia. The recommended final dose is about 10–20 mg/kg body weight per day.

Hematopoietic growth factors

Hematopoietic growth factor receptors are members of the type I cytokine receptor family

More than 30 hematopoietic growth factors and cytokines have been well characterized that are involved in regulation of differentiation and proliferation of the blood cells. These include factors regulating specific cell lineage, factors regulating multiple cell lineages, and factors indirectly regulating hematopoiesis by inducing gene expression of hematopoietic growth factors or cytokines. The structure of hematopoietic growth factors and cytokines is variable but the receptors for most of these factors are members of the type I cytokine receptor family. As a group, type I cytokine receptors usually consist of a receptor subunit and an associated transducer subunit. Three transducer subunits shared by the multiple members of this receptor family are glycoprotein 130 (GP 130), common β (βc), and common γ (γc). Unlike the tyrosine kinase receptor family, none of these type I cytokine receptors have an intrinsic tyrosine kinase domain. Instead, the receptors usually form homo- or heterodimers upon binding of their cognate growth factor or cytokines. The ligand-stimulated dimerization of the receptors triggers the activation of JAK/STAT tyrosine kinase signal pathways that mediate differentiation and proliferation of the growth factors or cytokines (Fig. 13.8; also see Chapter 3). Additionally, the Ras/MAP kinase and phosphatidylinositol 3 kinase signal pathways may also be utilized by these receptors to mediate growth stimulation of hematopoietic growth factors.

Preclinical studies and clinical trials have rapidly introduced these factors into the clinic for routine and experimental use. Currently, erythropoietin, G-CSF, GM-CSF, and interleukin-II have been approved for human use by the USA FDA, and many others including thrombopoietin are in the final phases of development.

Erythropoietin (Epo)

Erythropoietin is a physiologic hormone that is the critical hematopoietic growth factor regulating red blood cell proliferation and differentiation in bone marrow. Natural erythropoietin was originally isolated and purified from the urine of patients with anemia. A recombinant form of human erythropoietin is a 165-amino acid glycoprotein with a 34–39 kDa molecular weight. The plasma half-life of intravenously administered erythropoietin is approximately 8 hours. The liver is a major site of erythropoietin degradation.

Erythropoietin is produced in response to tissue hypoxia in the fetal liver and adult kidney. Hemoprotein receptors, sensors in the peritubular cells of the kidneys that are responsive to tissue oxygen content, regulate synthesis and release of erythropoietin (Fig. 13.9). After synthesis, erythropoietin is rapidly released into the blood. In the bone marrow, erythropoietin binds to erythropoietin receptors on erythroid pro-

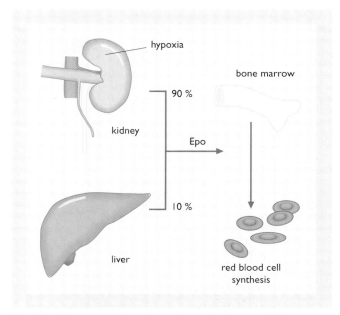

Fig. 13.9 Stimulation of erythropoietin (Epo) synthesis by hypoxia. Low oxygen tension 'sensed' by renal peritubular cells induces these cells to produce Epo, which stimulates the bone marrow to produce red blood cells. The liver also produces a small amount of Epo, which can therefore still be detected in anephric patients.

genitor cells, activates the JAK/STAT and other tyrosine protein kinase signal pathways, and thereby stimulates the cell proliferation and differentiation into red blood cells. (See discussion above, and Fig. 13.8.)

Erythropoietin is an effective treatment of anemia due to renal failure, malignancies, and chronic inflammation. The anemia of chronic renal failure results from a loss of the renal cells that produce erythropoietin. Recombinant human erythropoietin is now a standard treatment for the anemia of chronic renal failure, and subcutaneous or intravenous erythropoietin 150 units/kg three times a week will correct the anemia of 80% of such patients. The reticulocyte response to erythropoietin can develop within 3 days of starting treatment, with a significant rise in hematocrit occurring at 1 week. Maximum effects are achieved after 4–8 weeks. Erythropoietin has also been used for treatment of anemia due to primary bone marrow disorders and secondary anemia associated with inflammation, AIDS, and cancer. Erythropoietin is also an effective treatment of zidovudine-induced anemia in patients with human immunodeficiency virus and in cancer patients receiving chemotherapy.

Complications of erythropoietin treatment include hypertension and thrombosis, which may occur if the hematocrit rises too rapidly. Seizures have been reported in patients with a pre-existing history of seizure disorder. The iron stores of patients with anemia of renal failure are often rapidly depleted during erythropoietin treatment due to active erythropoeisis. Because it may be difficult to supplement with oral iron alone in these patients, because of continuing iron loss associated with blood loss, treatment with parenteral iron may be required.

199

The International Olympic Committee prohibits the use of erythropoietin by athletes who desire to improve performance by utilizing the capability of erythropoietin to increase the red blood cell counts and oxygen delivery. In addition, this practice may be dangerous.

Myeloid growth factors and neutropenia

Neutrophils are the principal defense cells against bacterial and fungal infections. Their continuous turnover and replenishment in the tissues are critical for maintaining an uninfected state. Unlike other blood cells, neutrophils and neutrophil precursor cells spend most of their brief lifespan (15 days) in the bone marrow. Normal granulopoiesis must support a cell population in the blood and tissue compartments that turns over rapidly. The number of neutrophils in the blood and tissue is therefore highly susceptible to rapid depletion when the marrow storage pool is compromised.

Drugs are the most common cause of neutropenia

The most common cause of neutropenia is myelosuppression by cancer chemotherapy, but many commonly prescribed medications can also cause neutropenia. Other causes include congenital, autoimmune, and infectious disorders (Fig. 13.10). The proliferation and maturation of myeloid progenitor cells are regulated in part by specific hematopoietic growth factors called colony-stimulating factors.

Granulocyte colony-stimulating factor (G-CSF) and granulocyte–macrophage colony-stimulating factor (GM-CSF)

Granulocyte colony-stimulating factor (G-CSF) and granulocyte–macrophage colony-stimulating factor (GM-CSF) represent several of the most widely utilized therapeutic proteins in practice today. They were purified from human cell lines and their commercial varieties are produced by recombinant technology. G-CSF and GM-CSF stimulate differentiation and proliferation of various myeloid progenitor cells by activating specific receptors expressed in the cell membrane of these cells. As for erythropoietin receptors, G-CSF and GM-CSF receptors are members of the type I cytokine receptor family, that utilize JAK/STAT and other tyrosine protein kinase signal pathways to mediate cellular responses of G-CSF and GM-CSF.

Drugs and disorders that can cause neutropenia

- Myelosuppressive chemotherapy
- Analgesics and anti-inflammatory drugs
- Antibiotics: sulfonamides, semisynthetic penicillins, chloramphenicol, cephalosporins
- Antipsychotics
- Anticonvulsants
- H$_2$ antagonists
- Autoimmune disorders: systemic lupus erythematosus, rheumatoid arthritis
- Malignancy
- Viruses: human immunodeficiency virus, Epstein–Barr virus
- Tuberculosis

Fig. 13.10 Drugs and disorders that can cause neutropenia.

Although their specific physiologic roles in the normal regulation of myelopoiesis are not clearly defined, both G-CSF and GM-CSF have dramatic stimulatory effects on neutrophil production when administered at pharmacologic dosages. G-CSF and GM-CSF also enhance the functional responsiveness of mature neutrophils to inflammatory signals and may increase neutrophil-dependent host defenses by enhancing the function of neutrophils. G-CSF acts only on hematopoietic cells that are committed to become neutrophils, so it is relatively more lineage-specific than GM-CSF, which also stimulates macrophage development. When recombinant G-CSF or GM-CSF are given intravenously or subcutaneously, the absolute neutrophil count usually rises within 24 hours. When the drug is stopped, the absolute neutrophil count decreases by half within 24 hours and returns to baseline in 1–7 days. The response to these factors is decreased in patients who have been extensively treated with radiation or chemotherapy because they have a reduced number of progenitor cells that can respond to the growth factors.

Treatment with G-CSF is better tolerated than treatment with GM-CSF. Although administration of both may cause bone pain, GM-CSF therapy can also cause a pulmonary capillary leak syndrome with pulmonary edema and heart failure. Treatment with GM-CSF, unlike G-CSF, may also cause constitutional symptoms including fever, headache, and malaise.

Megakaryocyte growth factors and thrombocytopenia

Thrombocytopenia is a condition characterized by a decrease in the number of platelets circulating in the blood to less than 150,000/mm^3. Platelets have a pivotal role in several mechanisms of homeostasis, including blood coagulation, wound healing, and the storage and release of cytokines. Patients with severe thrombocytopenia have a tendency towards bleeding. The etiologies of thrombocytopenia are complex and it may be caused by any one of the following mechanisms:

- Decreased bone marrow production (e.g. in patients with aplastic anemia).
- Increased splenic sequestration of platelets (e.g. in patients with portal hypertension or Gaucher disease).
- Accelerated destruction of platelets in peripheral circulation.
- Dilution in patients undergoing massive red blood cell replacement or exchange transfusions
- The adverse effects of many commonly used drugs.

Oprelvekin (interleukin-II)

Oprelvekin is a recombinant form of interleukin-11 (rIL-11). It is the first growth factor approved by the FDA to be used in the secondary prevention of thrombocytopenia in cancer patients who are receiving cytotoxic chemotherapy. The treatment with oprelvekin prevents severe thrombocytopenia and reduces the need for platelet transfusions following myelosuppressive chemotherapy. Oprelvekin stimulates the production of megakaryocytes and thrombocytes by activation of IL-11 receptors on the progenitor cells of platelets. IL-11 receptors belong to the type I cytokine receptor family (Fig. 13.8) and utilize JAK/STAT tyrosine kinase pathways to produce growth regulation. In addition, oprelvekin possesses nonhematopoietic properties, which include enhancing the healing of gastrointestinal lesions, inducing protein synthesis, inhibiting adipogenesis, inhibiting proinflammatory cytokine production, increasing production of osteoclasts, and stimulating neurogenesis.

Following administration, oprelvekin reaches peak plasma levels in about 3 hours with a terminal half-life of about 7 hours. The bioavailability of oprelvekin for subcutaneous injection is greater than 80%. It has been shown that the clearance of oprelvekin decreases with age. The clearance of oprelvekin in infants and children is 20–60% higher than in adults and adolescents. In animal models, oprelvekin is eliminated via the kidney. However, only a very small amount of intact oprelvekin is recovered in urine suggesting that the drug is metabolized before it is excreted.

The most common adverse effects associated with oprelvekin relate to its tendency to cause sodium retention by the kidneys. The resulting changes in blood volume can lead to cardiovascular consequences (e.g. changes in blood pressure, arrhythmias, edema) and may explain the association between use of this drug and mild decreases in hemoglobin concentrations. These adverse effects may be prevented with the concomitant use of diuretics. Furosemide has been proven successful in eliminating the fall in hematocrit associated with the administration of oprelvekin.

Thrombopoietin (Tpo)

Platelets are formed in the bone marrow from the cytoplasm of large multinucleated cells called megakaryocytes, which, like other hematopoietic cells, are derived from hematopoietic stem cells. Thrombopoietin, a primary growth factor that regulates platelet production, is a 65–85-kDa glycoprotein expressed in a variety of cells with a particular abundance of hepatocytes. Thrombopoietin stimulates platelet production in bone marrow by activation of its c-mpl receptors on the progenitor cells of platelets. The c-mpl utilizes JAK/STAT, Ras/MAP kinase, and phosphatidylinositol 3 kinase signal pathways to promote both the proliferation of megakaryocyte progenitor cells and their maturation into platelet-producing megakaryocytes. Thrombopoietin was originally isolated from human urine and its recombinant form (PEG-rHuMGDF) is produced by expression in human cells. Thrombopoietin is being tested in clinical trials for treatment of patients with either primary or secondary thrombocytopenia, but is awaiting FDA approval.

HEMOSTATIC DISORDERS AND ANTITHROMBOTIC THERAPY

Hemostasis

Normal hemostasis is a delicate balance between procoagulant, anticoagulant, and fibrinolytic processes in the blood vessel. Damage to the blood vessel wall initiates a complex series of events involving platelets, endothelial cells, and coagulation proteins that result in the formation of a platelet–fibrin clot. At the same time, physiologic anticoagulants and the fibrinolytic systems are activated by the products of the coagulation cascade to prevent the formation of unwanted clots (i.e. thrombosis).

▓ Platelets play a critical role in hemostasis

The platelets in the circulation do not normally interact with the vascular endothelium. When endothelial cells are damaged, platelets bind to the damaged site of the vessel wall through the interaction of platelet glycoprotein receptors with

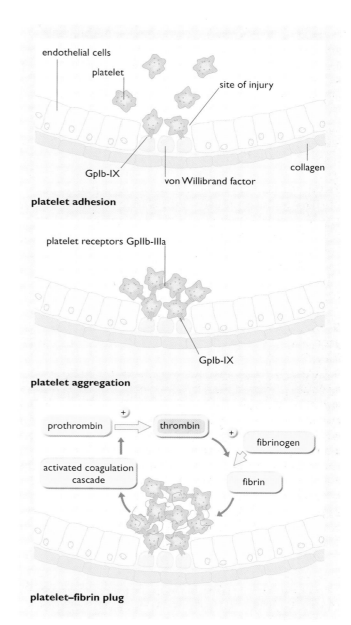

Fig. 13.11 Platelet function in hemostasis. There are three steps in the formation of the platelet–fibrin plug. The first step is platelet adhesion: vascular injury damages the endothelial cells and exposes the underlying collagen matrix. Platelets adhere to the exposed collagen after von Willebrand factors sitting on the collagen have bound to platelet receptors, GPIb-IX. The second step is platelet aggregation: activation of platelets by local factors such as thromboxane A_2, thrombin, and collagen, attracts other platelets, which aggregate through platelet receptors GPIIb-IIIa. The third step is the formation of the platelet–fibrin plug: the platelets provide a phospholipid surface for the activated coagulation cascade to activate thrombin which cleaves fibrinogen to produce fibrin to consolidate the initial platelet plug.

201

subendothelial collagen. The adhesive platelets then undergo activation and degranulation, releasing a number of substances including thromboxane A$_2$ (TXA$_2$), adenosine diphosphate (ADP), epinephrine, and serotonin. These substances activate and recruit additional platelets into the growing platelet-rich thrombus. The activated platelets provide the phospholipid binding surfaces for supporting the assembly of coagulant factor Xase-activating complex (including factor IXa, platelet-bound factor VIIIa, and calcium) and prothrombinase complex (including factor Xa, platelet-bound factor Va, and calcium) thereby markedly increasing thrombin generation. Increased thrombin activates additional platelets and triggers the coagulation cascade (see below).

Activation of platelets by agonists such as ADP and TXA$_2$, particularly thrombin, leads to conformational activation of glycoprotein receptors IIb/IIIa on the cell surface. The activated IIb/IIIa receptors provide functional binding sites for their ligand fibrinogen and other adhesive molecules such as vWF and fibronectin. Binding of bivalent fibrinogen molecules to IIb/IIIa on adjacent platelets forms platelet aggregates. Thus,

activation of the platelet glycoprotein receptor IIb/IIIa is the final pathway of platelet aggregation regardless of agonists that stimulate this process.

■ *The platelet plug is reinforced by fibrin formed from activation of the coagulation cascade: a key role of thrombin*
In addition to thrombin generated from platelet activation and aggregation, the tissue factor–factor VIIa complex plays a key role in initiating coagulation cascade and generating thrombin. Tissue factor (TF) is an intrinsic membrane glycoprotein expressed in many cells that are in contact with blood. It becomes accessible only when proteases are formed or cell injury occurred *in vivo*. After vascular injury, TF functions as cofactor or receptor, in the presence of Ca^{2+}, binding to factor VII and activating factor VII to VIIa. TF/VIIa/Ca^{2+} complex then converts factor X to Xa, which in turn activates prothrombin (factor II) to thrombin (factor IIa). Thrombin then cleaves fibrinogen to fibrin, which stabilizes the primary platelet plug into a permanent plug (Fig. 13.11). The tissue factor–factor VIIa

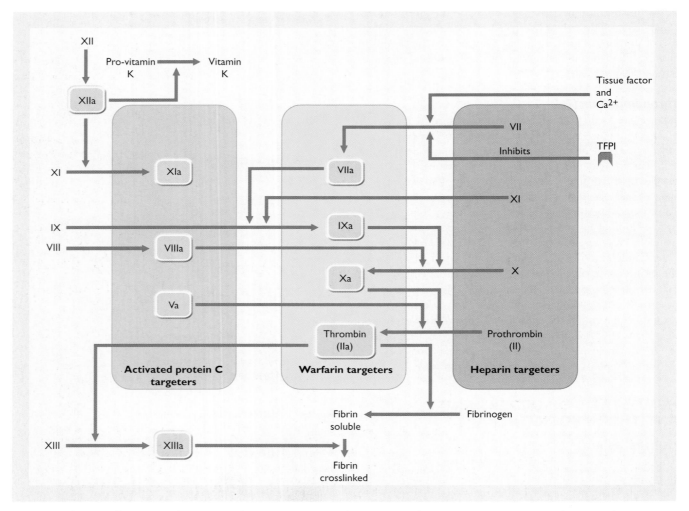

Fig. 13.12 The coagulation cascade. Initiation of coagulation by tissue factor activates factor **VII**, which activates both factor **X** and **IX**. Factor **IX** in turn activates factor **X** to **X**a. Factor **X**a cleaves prothrombin to thrombin, which cleaves fibrinogen to fibrin. By interacting with negatively charged surfaces, factor **XII** is autoactivated into **XII**a that activates its substrates prekallikrein (PK) to K (kallikrein) and factor **XI** results in activation of the intrinsic coagulation pathway. TFPI, tissue factor pathway inhibitors. Factors in the gray rectangle are inhibited by heparin. Factors in the yellow rectangle are inhibited by warfarin. Factors in the green rectangle are negatively regulated by the activated protein C.

complex also activates factor X indirectly by activating factor IX to IXa. Continued activation of factor X requires the factor IXa–factor VIIIa complex (Fig. 13.12). This explains why hemophiliacs with factor VIII or IX deficiency have a bleeding disorder. Another pathway to activate prothrombin to thrombin is the so-called intrinsic system that is triggered by the activation of factor XII, following its contact with highly charged surfaces (Fig. 13.12).

In addition to fibrin conversion, thrombin activates coagulation factor XIII which stabilizes and cross-links the soluble fibrin molecules into an insoluble fibrin clot (Fig. 13.12). Thrombin activates other coagulation factors and cofactors to amplify its own generation, which recruits more platelets and promotes platelet aggregation. Thrombin also causes migration of white cells and regulates vascular tone. Finally, thrombin is a potent activator of vascular smooth muscle cell migration and proliferation. Given thrombin's central role in hemostasis and in thrombogenesis, the goal of many current antithrombotics is to block thrombin activity or prevent its generation (see below).

■ Hemostasis is tightly regulated by specific inhibitors of the activated coagulation factors

There are three groups of physiologic inhibitors in plasma classified according to their mechanism of inhibition, including kinins (pancreatic trypsin inhibitors), serpins (serine protease inhibitors), and α_2-macroglobulins. They limit the extent of hemostasis and protect against thrombus formation.

Tissue factor pathway inhibitor (TFPI) is a member of the kinin family. TFPI first binds to factor Xa and then inactivates tissue factor–factor VIIa complex by forming a quaternary complex. Administration of heparin releases endothelium-associated TFPI into the circulation.

The important members of the serpin family include antithrombin III (ATIII), protein C, and protein S. ATIII is a major inhibitor of thrombin, factor Xa, and factor IXa. Heparin, as a cofactor for ATIII, greatly increases the ATIII inactivation of thrombin and factor Xa. Anticoagulant-activated protein C with its cofactor protein S is the major inhibitor of factor Va and VIIIa. Thrombin activates the protein C pathway by first binding to thrombomodulin, which activates protein C on endothelial cell surfaces. The physiologic relevance of ATIII, protein C and protein S is underscored by the greatly increased risk of venous thrombosis in people who have deficiencies of these natural anticoagulants (Fig. 13.13).

α_2-Macroglobulin functions as a scavenger inhibitor of proteases such as plasmin.

■ The activity of the fibrinolytic system regulates hemostasis

In addition to physiologic anticoagulants, the plasma fibrinolytic

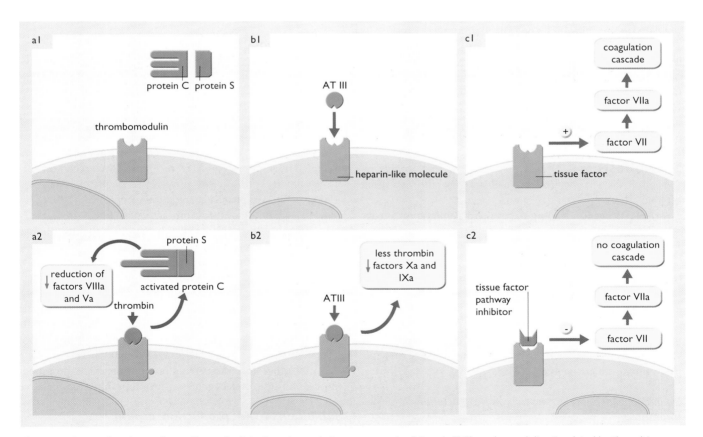

Fig. 13.13 Natural anticoagulants. Three physiologic anticoagulation systems exist. (a1 and a2) Thrombomodulin stimulated by thrombin activates protein C, which with its cofactor protein S, inhibits cofactors Va and VIIIa in the coagulation cascade. (b1 and b2) Antithrombin III (ATIII) stimulated by heparin inhibits thrombin, factor Xa and IXa. (c1 and c2) Tissue factor pathway inhibitor inhibits tissue factor, which is the key activator of the coagulation cascade.

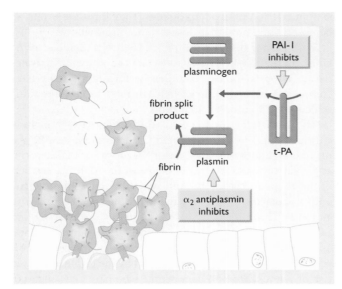

Fig. 13.14 The fibrinolytic system. Fibrin-bound tissue plasminogen activator (t-PA) changes fibrin-bound plasminogen to plasmin, which cleaves fibrin. Physiologic inhibitors are plasminogen activator inhibitor (PAI-1) and α_2 antiplasmin.

system is the major endogenous mechanism that protects against thrombus formation by lysing established fibrin clots. This system consists of plasminogen, plasmin, plasminogen activators, and the respective inhibitors. Fibrinolysis is mainly regulated by the enzyme tissue-type plasminogen activator (t-PA). Circulating t-PA is relatively inactive. Once incorporated into the fibrin clot, it actively converts fibrin-bound plasminogen to plasmin, which degrades the fibrin clot. The plasminogen and plasmin are subject to regulation by various inhibitors, including plasminogen activator inhibitors 1, 2, and 3 (PAI-1, -2, and -3), and α_2 antiplasmin (see Fig. 13.14 and below for more details).

Thrombosis

Thrombosis is a major cause of death and disability as a result of:

- Arterial occlusion leading to myocardial infarction, stroke and peripheral ischemia.
- Venous occlusion causing deep venous thrombosis and pulmonary embolism.

Disabling or fatal thrombotic disease may stem from the formation of thrombi within arteries at the sites of arterial endothelial damage or in veins as a consequence of stasis or increased systemic coagulability. Thrombi may also form within the chambers of the heart, on damaged or prosthetic heart valves, or within the microcirculation as the result of disseminated intravascular coagulation (DIC).

Endothelial injury is the main cause of arterial thrombosis

In the high-flow arterial system, endothelial injury is the dominant influence in thrombogenesis. Arterial thrombi form only at sites with underlying arterial wall pathology (e.g. damage caused by arteriosclerosis, trauma following balloon

angioplasty, or autoimmune vasculitis). Arterial thrombosis due to an increased concentration of plasma homocysteine probably results from its toxic effect on endothelial cells and damage to the arterial wall.

Stasis and hypercoagulability are the main causes of venous thrombosis

In contrast, in venous thrombosis the vessel wall is frequently intact. Stasis plays a more dominant role and permits the build-up of platelet aggregates and nascent fibrin in areas of sluggish flow. Hypercoagulability is also an important contributor. The best-understood and prototypic hypercoagulable states are associated with hereditary deficiencies of the natural anticoagulants antithrombin III, protein C, or protein S. The recent discovery of a relatively common hereditary mutation of factor Va (Leiden), which is much more resistant to inactivation by activated protein C, greatly increases the number of patients with diagnosable hypercoagulable states.

Lifelong anticoagulation

Many patients with an underlying hypercoagulable abnormality require lifelong anticoagulation (see the discussion below for warfarin) once they have had a thrombotic event. In addition, hypercoagulability may also be an important mechanism for the pathogenesis of a thrombotic diathesis in several more common clinical settings such as nephrotic syndrome, following severe trauma or a burn injury, and in disseminated cancer.

Antithrombotic therapy

There are several classes of antithrombotic therapeutics successfully used for arterial and venous thrombotic disorders. As platelets play a critical role in the pathogenesis of arterial thrombotic disorders, these cells are logical targets for antithrombotic therapy. Attenuation of platelet functions can be achieved by inhibition of prostaglandin synthases to reduce TXA_2 production, inhibition of platelet membrane G protein-coupled receptors (e.g. ADP receptor, TXA_2 receptor, and thrombin receptors), and antagonism of platelet adhesion receptor Ib-IX or platelet aggregation receptor GPIIb/IIIa (Fig. 13.15). Given that thrombin-activated fibrin is a major component of thrombi, and that thrombin is the most potent activator of platelets, anticoagulant strategies to inhibit arterial and venous thrombogenesis have focused on inhibiting thrombin activity or preventing thrombin generation. These include the use of indirect inhibitors of thrombin such as oral coumarin derivatives, heparin or low molecular weight heparin (LMWH), and direct inhibitors of thrombin such as hirudin and its derivatives. The third class of antithrombotic therapeutics are thrombolytic agents that actively dissolve thrombi rather than interrupting progression of the thrombotic process by antiplatelet agents or thrombin inhibitors.

Inhibition of TXA_2 production: aspirin

In the hope of helping his father who was suffering from arthritis and the severe adverse effects of the sodium salicylate used to treat it, Felix Hoffman, a German chemist at Farbenfabriken Friedrich Bayer, began working with salicylic

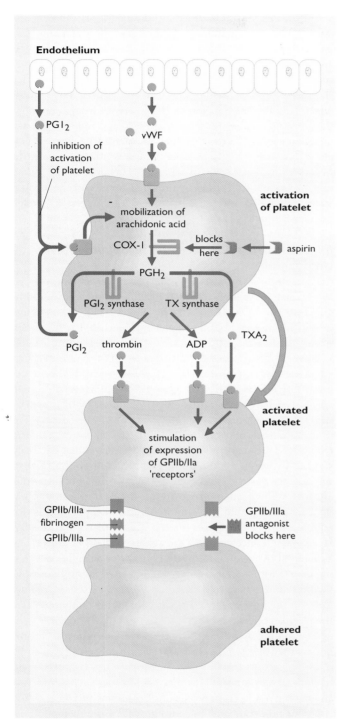

Fig. 13.15 Effects of antiplatelet agents on platelet activation and aggregation. After vascular injury, platelets bind to the vessel wall and undergo activation and degranulation, releasing a number of platelet activators that activate and recruit other platelets. The platelet activators cause the conformation change of platelet GPIIb/IIIa receptors that finally stimulate platelet aggregation. Aspirin, ADP receptor antagonists, and GPIIb/IIIa antagonists block the process at different levels. (PGI$_2$, prostaglandin I$_2$; PGH$_2$, prostaglandin H$_2$; TXA$_2$, thromboxane A$_2$; vWF, von Willebrand factor)

acid in hopes of preserving its anti-inflammatory properties while easing its harsh effects on the stomach. The acetic acid ester of salicylic acid, acetylsalicylic acid was synthesized in 1897. Bayer began marketing it in 1899 under the trade name Aspirin. In the century since, Aspirin has become the most widely consumed drug in the world. Moreover, aspirin is clearly no longer just a pill to pop when your head aches. Instead, it has become the 'gold standard' for antiplatelet agents used in the prevention and treatment of arterial thrombotic disorders such as angina pectoris, myocardial infarction (MI), and ischemic stroke. Clinical trails demonstrate that aspirin has the best benefit/risk and cost/benefit ratios of any of the therapies for acute coronary syndromes.

Aspirin prevents conversion of arachidonic acid to prostaglandin H$_2$ and subsequently reduces production of TXA$_2$ by acetylating the serine residue of enzyme prostaglandin H$_2$ synthase (PGHS, usually referred to as cyclo-oxygenase, COX) and irreversibly inactivating it (Fig. 13.15). There are two COX isoforms, namely COX-1 and COX-2, which are expressed in mammalian cells. COX-1 is constitutively expressed in most cell types and COX-2 is an inducible enzyme that has increased expression in many clinical settings such as inflammation and infection. Human platelets express only COX-1. Aspirin is a relatively selective COX-1 inhibitor, with an approximate 200-fold greater inhibition of COX-1 than COX-2. This is the rationale for the smaller dosage requirements for aspirin as an antithrombotic (involving COX-1) compared with its use as an anti-inflammatory drug (involving COX-2). Inhibition of COX-1 and reduction of TXA$_2$ results in suppression of platelet aggregation for the whole 7–10-day lifespan of the platelet since COX-1 is irreversibly acetylated by aspirin and not resynthesized in platelets which lack nuclei. However, during the treatment of aspirin, substances other than TXA$_2$, such as ADP, epinephrine, and thrombin, can still activate platelets. Aspirin also blocks the synthesis of the platelet inhibitor PGI$_2$ in endothelial cells. However, this effect is limited with low doses of aspirin and short-lived compared with that on TXA$_2$ synthesis in platelets. The effect of aspirin on platelet function is demonstrated by prolonged bleeding times in patients taking aspirin.

Aspirin is rapidly absorbed from the gastrointestinal tract, partially hydrolyzed to salicylate on its first pass through the liver, and widely distributed into most body tissues. Following oral administration, salicylate can be present in the serum within 5–30 minutes and peak serum concentrations are attained within 1 hour. These properties of aspirin are more fully discussed in Chapter 20. However, in order to achieve therapeutic blood levels rapidly for patients with chest pain who might be having an MI, chewed aspirin tablets are recommended, to promote buccal rather than gastric mucosal absorption. Hemostasis returns to normal approximately 36 hours after the last dose of the drug, presumably due to the release of new platelets from the bone marrow.

Aspirin is a cornerstone of therapy for unstable angina or non-Q-wave MI. Several clinical trials have shown that it can reduce the incidence of death or MI by approximately half in these conditions. Also, aspirin serves as the linchpin of therapy for acute MI and the foundation to which other therapies are added, both in the short and long term. It reduces the incidence of reinfarction by one-third and the composite end-point of MI, stroke, or vascular death by one-quarter. Overall, aspirin has been found to be nearly as effective as streptokinase in reducing vascular mortality in acute myocardial infarction. Combining the two agents has an additive effect on mortality in this setting. Doses of aspirin as low as 80 mg/day are effective in the secondary prevention of MI and in reducing mortality in post-myocardial infarction patients. Aspirin is also effective in preventing recurring transient ischemic attacks (TIAs) and in reducing risk of stroke in patients with TIAs. It is also commonly used in settings where there is an increased risk of arterial thrombosis such as coronary catherization, balloon angioplasty, and the postoperative period following vascular surgery. Aspirin is often used in conjunction with the other antiplatelet agents such as ADP antagonists or with anticoagulants such as heparin, or warfarin (see discussion below). Poor response to aspirin may be found in 10–15% of patients, while some develop progressive resistance to aspirin in the course of treatment. Patients with aspirin resistance may be more vulnerable to adverse vascular events.

A loading dose of 325 mg chewable aspirin for acute coronary syndromes is recommended in order to achieve therapeutic blood levels rapidly, followed by 160–325 mg/day during hospitalization. Virtually complete inhibition of COX-1 in platelets can be maintained with a low dose of 80 mg/day with similar efficacy.

Gastrointestinal irritation is the most common adverse effect of aspirin. Tinnitus and central nervous system toxicity do not occur with the low dosages used to achieve antithrombotic effects. Aspirin as with other nonsteroidal anti-inflammatory drugs (NSAIDs) increases the risk of gastric bleeding in a dose-related manner (see Chapter 20). Aspirin may increase the risk of intracerebral hemorrhage; in preventative therapy, it is important to consider the risk/benefit of using aspirin, especially in patients at low risk for cardiovascular events. Some patients may develop severe bronchoconstriction with aspirin (see Chapter 20); in those patients alternative antiplatelet drugs should be considered in the setting of acute myocardial infarction.

Reversible COX inhibitors: Nonsteroidal anti-inflammatory drugs (NSAIDs)

NSAIDs, which are widely used in a variety of inflammatory disorders (see Chapter 20), inhibit platelet COX and result in suppression of TXA_2-dependent platelet aggregation. Unlike aspirin, NSAIDs function as competitive and reversible inhibitors of platelet COX. At typical anti-inflammatory dosages, most NSAIDs produce a 70–85% inhibition of COX activity.

That is insufficient to produce significant antiplatelet benefits. Several NSAIDs, including indobufen, sulfinpyrazone, and triflusal, have been tested in clinical trials for their potential application in a variety of thrombotic conditions. For example, indobufen is a potent inhibitor of COX-1 and has profiles similar to aspirin for biochemical, functional, and clinical effects. At a therapeutic dose of 200 mg twice a day, indobufen inhibits serum TXA_2 by more than 95% and reduces urinary metabolite excretion to an extent comparable to aspirin. Several clinical trials indicate that indobufen is as effective as aspirin in preventing coronary graft occlusion. However, none of these reversible COX inhibitors is indicated for use in the United States in these clinical settings and have no obvious advantage over aspirin in any case.

Inhibition of the ADP receptor: ticlopidine, clopidogrel

ADP receptor antagonists are relatively novel oral antiplatelet agents that block ADP-activated platelet aggregation without affecting the COX-1/2 pathway (Fig. 13.15). These drugs inhibit fibrinogen binding to glycoprotein IIb/IIIa receptors. Additionally, ticlopidine interferes with the binding of von Willebrand factor to platelet membrane gpIB receptors. Platelet adhesion and aggregation are therefore inhibited, and the inhibitory effects on platelet aggregation are irreversible. ADP antagonists have a synergistic effect when used with aspirin or GPIIb/IIIa antagonists.

Ticlopidine hydrochloride and its chemical analog clopidogrel are acidic thienopyridine derivatives that are freely soluble in water. Ticlopidine is rapidly and well absorbed through the gastrointestinal tract. Peak plasma concentrations are achieved within approximately 2 hours after a single oral dose of 250 mg, but the inhibitory effect on platelets is not attained until after approximately 4 days of regular dosing. Steady-state concentrations are achieved in 14–21 days. The half-life of ticlopidine is 24–36 hours after a single dose and up to 96 hours after 14 days of repeated administration. Ticlopidine is extensively metabolized and is excreted mainly through the kidney. Renal impairment significantly increases the plasma concentrations.

Ticlopidine is indicated to prevent a recurrence of thrombotic stroke and TIA. In clinical trials it has been shown to be more efficacious than aspirin. Ticlopidine has also been used in clinical trials for acute coronary syndromes such as unstable angina. The results seem promising. Ticlopidine produces a 46% risk reduction compared to conventional aspirin therapy alone. The combination of ticlopidine and aspirin has been indicated to prevent stent thrombosis in coronary interventions. It is better than aspirin plus oral anticoagulant warfarin in preventing acute stent thrombosis, MI, and repeat interventions. The recommended dose of ticlopidine is 500 mg as an oral loading dose followed by 250 mg twice a day. The loading dose should be given 3 days before the procedure because ticlopidine achieves its maximal effect in 4 days. If the patient receives an intracoronary stent, the dosage of ticlopidine is 250 mg twice a day for 2–4 weeks, along with lifelong aspirin. Ticlopidine may not be useful when a rapid antiplatelet effect is desired because a delayed antithrombotic effect has been found for the first 2 weeks of administration.

The adverse effect of bleeding can be observed with either of these two ADP antagonists. The incidence of gastrointestinal hemorrhage may be slightly lower with ticlopidine or clopidogrel than aspirin. However, if a patient requires elective surgery, ADP antagonists should be stopped about 1 week before operation. Moreover, rare but life-threatening adverse effects such as neutropenia and agranulocytosis have limited ticlopidine use to patients who are intolerant or unresponsive to aspirin.

Clopidogrel, a congener of ticlopidine, has effects, mechanism of action, and clinical indications which are similar to those of ticlopidine but it appears to have minimal bone marrow suppressive effects. For this reason, it is increasingly being used as an alternative to ticlopidine. The recommended dose is 200 mg as an oral loading dose followed by repeated doses of 50–100 mg daily. Using this dose regimen, a steady-state inhibition of platelet aggregation is reached after 4–7 days of treatment. It is interesting to note that the dose for clopidogrel to maintain a maximal inhibition of platelet aggregation (50 mg/day) is only 10% of the dose of ticlopidine (500 mg/day). The most frequent adverse effects of clopidogrel are gastrointestinal upset, bleeding, rash, and diarrhea.

Inhibition of platelet aggregation: antagonists of glycoprotein IIb/IIIa receptors

As described above regardless of the events or modulators that stimulate the aggregation of platelets, the integrin receptor GPIIb/IIIa, functioning as the final common pathway, has a key role in the regulation of platelet–platelet interactions (aggregation) and thrombus formation (Fig. 13.15). The GPIIb/IIIa is a member of the integrin superfamily of receptors, consisting of α and β (e.g. α_{IIb} (gpIIb) and β_3 (gpIIIa)) subunits that form a noncovalently linked heterodimer. The gpIIIa subunit contains a binding site for the tripeptide sequence arginine-glycine-aspartic acid (RGD) found on fibrinogen, vWF, fibronectin, and vitronectin. The gpIIb subunit contains four repeated segments, which are the binding sites for Ca^{2+} and are required for receptor function. Dysfunction of either subunit results in Glanzmann's thrombasthenia, a bleeding disorder in which platelet aggregation does not occur. The GPIIb/IIIa receptor is platelet-specific and the most abundant receptor found on activated platelets.

Antagonists of GPIIb/IIIa receptor interfere with the agonist-induced binding of fibrinogen and other adhesive factors to the platelet membrane receptors. Platelet adhesion and aggregation are therefore inhibited irreversibly. Antagonists of GPIIb/IIIa receptor in clinical use and under development are divided into three categories: (1) monoclonal antibodies against the receptors; (2) naturally occurring RGD-containing peptides isolated from snake venoms or synthetic RGD- or

KGD-containing peptides that compete with fibrinogen for the GPIIb/IIIa receptors; and (3) synthetic small molecule chemicals. Three antagonists of GPIIb/IIIa approved by the FDA for clinical use are monoclonal antibody abciximab, synthetic peptide eptifibatide, and nonpeptide molecule triofiban, each of which is a representative of one of the three categories.

ABCIXIMAB is a mouse/human chimeric monoclonal antibody, which is composed of a Fab fragment of a murine monoclonal antibody against the GPIIb/IIIa complex coupled with the constant regions of human immunoglobulin. Abciximab effectively antagonizes platelet aggregation by blocking of fibrinogen and other adhesive molecules from binding to GPIIb/IIIa. In addition, the potent inhibition of abciximab in thrombus formation leads to a decrease in thrombin generation that may also partially contribute to its antithrombotic effect.

The antiplatelet effect of abciximab is dose-dependent; a definite correlation exists between the percentage of GPIIb/IIIa receptor blocked and inhibition of platelet aggregation. To be effective, more than 90% of the GPIIb/IIIa receptors have to be blocked. Following intravenous bolus administration, free plasma concentrations of abciximab decrease rapidly as a result of rapid binding to platelet GPIIb/IIIa receptors. The half-life of unbound abciximab is approximately 10–30 minutes. However, the bound antibody is cleared only with coated platelets. Optimal duration of treatment based on pharmacokinetic data is unclear.

Current clinical applications of abciximab include its use as an adjunct to percutaneous transluminal coronary angioplasty (PTCA) for the prevention of cardioac ischemic complications and use for acute coronary syndromes. For the latter conditions, abciximab, combined with heparin or aspirin, reduces the occurrence of ischemic events in patients with high- and low-risk unstable angina and non-Q-wave infarction. The recommended dose of abciximab is a bolus of 250 μg/kg followed by an infusion of 10 μg/kg/hour. After cessation of infusion, platelet function gradually returns towards normal, and antiplatelet effect persists for 24–48 hours.

The major adverse effect of abciximab (and also of other GPIIb/IIIa antagonists) is potential for bleeding, in particular in the presence of other antithrombotics. With the currently recommended doses, abciximab may also cause thrombocytopenia, which can be effectively treated with platelet transfusions and is reversible after stopping the treatment. As a chimeric monoclonal antibody, abciximab contains a partial murine peptide segment which can be immunogenic.

EPTIFIBATIDE (INTEGRILIN) was discovered in screening compounds contained in snake venom that inhibit platelet function. The 73-amino acid protein, containing a lysine-glycine-aspartic acid (KGD) sequence rather than the RGD sequence in other GPIIb/IIIa binding compounds, was purified from the southeastern pygmy rattlesnake. Eptifibatide is a synthetic disulfide-linked cyclic heptapeptide using the KGD sequence as the template. The clinical indications for eptifibatide are similar to abciximab. The recommended dose is 0.2–1.5 μg/kg/minute for intravenous infusion. Eptifibatide has a short half-life of about 50–60 minutes. The platelet function returns to normal 2–4 hours after stopping the drug infusion.

TIROFIBAN (MK-383, AGGRASTAT) is a nonpeptide derivative of tyrosine that selectively inhibits the GPIIb/IIIa receptor, with minimal effects on the $\alpha_v\beta_3$ vitronectin receptor. Tirofiban has a short half-life (3 hours versus 3 days for abciximab) and has the potential for oral administration. In high-risk patients undergoing PTCA, tirofiban causes a dose-dependent inhibition of platelet aggregation. The recommended dose of tirofiban is an intravenous bolus 5–10 μg/ml followed by 0.05–0.1 μg/ml/min intravenous infusion for 16–24 hours. The optimal dose for treatment of acute coronary syndromes is still to be established.

ORAL ANTAGONISTS OF GPIIB/IIIA At least a dozen GPIIb/IIIa antagonists have been synthesized and are in various stages of drug development. These drugs have the potential to be given over the long term which is important for patients requiring chronic antithrombotic therapy, although clinical efficacy remains to be established.

DIPYRIDAMOLE Dipyridamole is a coronary vasodilator and the mechanism of action may relate to its ability to increase intracellular levels of cyclic AMP due to inhibition of cyclic nucleotide phosphodiesterase. Dipyridamole is also an antiplatelet agent through inhibition of TXA_2 synthesis or potentiation of the effect of PGI_2 to reduce platelet adhesion to thrombogenic surfaces. The clinical efficacy of dipyridamole, even in conjunction with aspirin, has been a subject of controversy. However, a recent clinical trial reopens this issue. Daily 400 mg of dipyridamole alone or with aspirin reduces stroke risk by 16% or 37% respectively. Additionally, dipyridamole in combination with warfarin is effective in inhibiting embolization from prosthetic heart valves.

ANAGRELIDE High platelet counts due to myeloproliferative diseases such as essential thrombocythemia, unlike the relatively benign reactive thrombocythemia, may have thrombotic consequences. The conventional treatment of these disorders has been with lineage-nonspecific chemotherapeutic agents such as hydroxyurea. Anagrelide, an orally active quinazolin, has a high specificity against megakaryocytes and therefore selectively lowers the platelet count. If long-term trials confirm that anagrelide does not have a leukemogenic potential, this agent may become the treatment of choice for thrombocythemia.

Inhibition of coagulant factor formation: warfarin

The discovery that coumarin has an anticoagulant effect goes back to the 1940s and led to the development of synthetic derivatives such as warfarin. Warfarin is widely used in the clinic as an oral anticoagulant. The synthesis of several coagulation factors (factors II, VII, IX, and X) and cofactors (protein C, and S) in the liver is dependent on vitamin K. The post-translational carboxylation of the glutamic acid residues of these coagulation factors to γ-carboxyglutamic acid requires vitamin K as a cofactor in the enzymatic reaction. In the presence of calcium ions, the γ-carboxyglutamyl residues allow the coagulation factors to undergo a conformational change, which is necessary for their biologic activity. Warfarin inhibits vitamin K epoxide reductase, leading to depletion of reduced vitamin K (KH) and decreased γ-carboxylation (Fig. 13.16), and thereby indirectly impairs the function of coagulation factors. The anticoagulant effects of warfarin have to be effective after disappearance of the existing γ-carboxylated coagulation factors. Prothrombin (factor II) has the longest elimination half-life of 60 hours; therefore 5 days of treatment are required if warfarin is to be fully antithrombotic. This is the rationale for overlapping heparin therapy with warfarin therapy for at least 5 days in the treatment of thrombotic diseases, even if the INR (see below) reaches the therapeutic level before 5 days.

Clinical trials have shown that warfarin is effective for:
- The prevention and treatment of venous thromboembolism and pulmonary embolism (see Chapter 19).
- The prevention of thrombotic and embolic strokes as well as recurrence of infarction in patients with acute myocardial infarction.

Patients with mechanical prosthetic heart valves should be treated with anticoagulants. A combined regimen of warfarin and low-dose aspirin seems to be superior to warfarin alone.

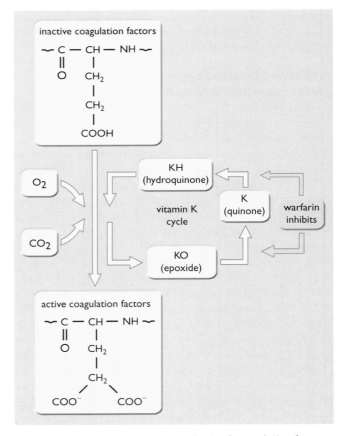

Fig. 13.16 Vitamin K-dependent synthesis of coagulation factors. Warfarin inhibits production of the reduced form of vitamin K (KH), which is required for γ-carboxylation of glutamic acids on factors II, IX, and X, protein C, and protein S.

Indications for oral anticoagulation with warfarin

- Mechanical prosthetic heart valves
- Atrial fibrillation
- Treatment of venous thromboembolism
- Acute myocardial infarction
- Prevention of venous thromboembolism
- Episodic systemic embolism

Fig. 13.17 Indications for oral anticoagulation with warfarin.

There are now convincing data that most patients with atrial fibrillation should be on lifelong anticoagulation treatment with warfarin (Fig. 13.17).

Treatment with warfarin should be initiated with small daily doses 5–10 mg for 1 week to allow an adjustment of the prothrombin time followed by a maintenance dose adjusted to achieve appropriate therapeutic goals. The prothrombin time should be maintained to a level of 20–25% normal activity for long-term warfarin therapy. A standard coagulation assay method for the prothrombin time, the International Normalized Ratio (INR) (test/control), has been used to monitor patients taking warfarin. Currently, two levels of intensity of warfarin therapy are usually recommended: a medium response with an INR of 2.0 to 3.0, and a higher response with an INR of 2.5 to 3.5. Higher INR values greatly increase the risk of bleeding. Recent clinical evidence has shown that a lower INR (2.0–2.5) is effective in the prevention and treatment of most venous and arterial thrombotic disorders.

Warfarin is well absorbed orally and has excellent bio-availability. It is highly bound to plasma proteins (99% albumin) resulting in a small volume of distribution and a long half-life in plasma (36–40 hours), and without urinary excretion of unchanged drug. The drug is metabolized by hepatic microsomes to inactive metabolites excreted in urine and stools.

Many clinical conditions and drug interactions may potentiate or attenuate the anticoagulant effects of warfarin (Fig. 13.18). Fluctuating levels of dietary vitamin K can be an important factor in causing variations in anticoagulation in patients on long-term warfarin therapy.

The major adverse effect of warfarin is bleeding, and this risk is correlated with the intensity of the treatment and the concomitant use of antiplatelet agents such as aspirin. The risk of clinically important bleeding is reduced by lowering the INR therapeutic range from 3.0–4.5 to 2.0–3.0. The most important nonhemorrhagic adverse effect of warfarin therapy is skin necrosis caused by extensive thrombosis of the micro-vasculature within the subcutaneous fat. This phenomenon seems to be associated with protein C and S deficiency.

Drugs and conditions interacting with warfarin

	Activity
Antibiotics	+
Amiodarone	+
Cimetidine	+
Clofibrate	+
Fluconazole	+
Metronidazole	+
Phenytoin	+
Barbiturates	–
Carbamazepine	–
Griseofulvin	–
Nafcillin	–
Rifampin	–
Sucralfate	–
Age	+
Biliary disease	+
Congestive heart failure	+
Hyperthyroidism	+
Hypothyroidism	–
Nephrotic syndrome	–

Fig. 13.18 Drugs and conditions interacting with warfarin.
(+, increased activity; –, decreased activity)

(Proteins C and S are vitamin K-dependent anticoagulants as discussed above.) The thrombotic tendency may be due to a transient procoagulant state during the initial treatment period with warfarin, due to the fact that proteins C and S have much shorter elimination half-lifes than prothrombin. The fall in protein C and S levels, therefore, occurs before there is a reduction in the prothrombin level. Skin necrosis can be avoided by using concurrent therapeutic doses of heparin when starting warfarin therapy.

Warfarin crosses the placenta and is teratogenic, so it must not be given to pregnant women. Women receiving warfarin should be informed of its teratogenic effect and avoid becoming pregnant while taking it. Treatment with heparin and low molecular weight heparins (LMWHs) appears to be safe during pregnancy.

The anticoagulant effects of warfarin can be partially reversed by low doses of vitamin K acting through a warfarin-resistant pathway. Patients also become warfarin-resistant if large doses of vitamin K are given. Fresh frozen plasma or prothrombin complex concentrate can be infused if a rapid reversal of the warfarin effect is needed, as in severe bleeding.

🔑 Warfarin

- Treatment with warfarin requires at least 4–5 days to be fully effective even if the INR of prothrombin activity assay reaches the therapeutic level in 1–2 days

⚠️ *Warning about using warfarin*

- *Warfarin is a teratogen and can produce fetal central nervous system abnormalities or bleeding. Pregnant women with thrombosis should be treated with standard or low molecular weight heparin*

Indirect inhibition of thrombin activity: heparin and low molecular weight heparin

Heparin is a glycosaminoglycan composed of chains of alternating residues of D-glucosamine and an uronic acid. Standard heparin is a heterogeneous preparation with molecular weights ranging from 5000 to 30,000 kDa. The anticoagulant activity of heparin is variable because the chain lengths of the molecules affect the activity and clearance. The higher molecular weight molecules are cleared from the circulation more rapidly than the lower molecular weight species. Furthermore, there are differential activities, with lower molecular weight species being more active against factor Xa than against thrombin.

Heparin primarily exerts its anticoagulant effect through binding to ATIII, thereby greatly altering the conformation of ATIII and accelerating its inhibition of thrombin, factor Xa, and factor IXa. ATIII is an α-globulin that inhibits serine proteases, including several of the clotting factors, by binding at a 1:1 ratio to the serine residue in the reaction center of coagulant factors, leading to the inactivation of these factors. Heparin participates in these reactions as a catalytic agent, catalyzing the inactivation of thrombin by ATIII by acting as a template to which both ATIII and thrombin bind to form a ternary complex. In contrast, ATIII inactivation of factor Xa does not require the formation of a ternary complex. Low molecular weight species of heparin that contain fewer than 18 polysaccharide chains are unable to serve as a template for ATIII inactivation of thrombin, but retain the ability to inactivate factor Xa (Fig. 13.19). However, heparin inhibition of thrombogenesis is incomplete because it is unable to inactivate platelet-bound Xa and fibrin-bound thrombin that remain enzymatically active. This contributes at least partially to the resistance of arterial thrombosis to heparin therapy.

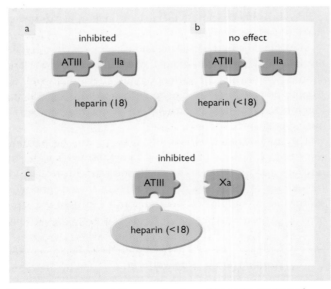

Fig. 13.19 Anticoagulation mechanism of heparin. Binding of heparin with antithrombin III (ATIII) greatly facilitates its inhibition of thrombin (IIa) (a). However, this requires heparin molecules longer than 18 polysaccharide residues (b). Inhibition of factor Xa is not dependent on the size of the heparin molecule (c).

Heparin is poorly absorbed after oral administration and must therefore be given either subcutaneously or intravenously. It is often given intravenously in a bolus dose to achieve rapid anticoagulation and then maintained with a continuous infusion. Alternatively, subcutaneous boluses two or three times a day are equally effective. If immediate anticoagulation is needed, however, the intravenous route is preferred because there is a 1–2-hour delay with subcutaneous heparin. Treatment with heparin requires close laboratory monitoring. Heparin dosages need to be titrated to achieve an activated partial thromboplastin time (aPTT) that is 1.5–2.5 times the normal control.

Heparin is highly negatively charged and binds to endothelial cells and a variety of plasma proteins such as lipoprotein, fibronectin, platelet factor 4, and von Willebrand factor. This property contributes to its reduced bioavailability at low concentrations and limits the amount of heparin available to interact with ATIII. Moreover, the changes in plasma levels of heparin-binding proteins in patients with thrombotic disorders lead to an unpredictable anticoagulant response from heparin and the need for a very high dose of heparin in some (heparin resistance).

The pharmacokinetic properties of heparin are complex. It binds to receptors on macrophages and in the reticulo-endothelial system, where it is rapidly internalized and degraded. Heparin thus has a longer half-life in patients with severe hepatic disease. However, this is a dose-dependent saturable mechanism (zero-order kinetics). Heparin is also cleared more slowly with first-order kinetics, mostly by the kidney. As a result, the biologic half-life of heparin depends on the dose. With an intravenous bolus of heparin at 25 units/kg, the biologic half-life is 30 minutes, but this increases to 60 minutes with 100 units/kg and 150 minutes at 400 units/kg.

Heparin is effective for:
- Preventing venous thrombosis.
- Treating deep venous thromboembolism and pulmonary embolism (see Chapter 19).
- The early treatment of patients with unstable angina and acute myocardial infarction.
- Preventing clotting in catheters used to cannulate blood vessels.
- Anticoagulating extracorporeal devices, as in cardiac bypass surgery and hemodialysis.
- Treating arterial thrombosis, as in acute myocardial infarction, in conjunction with antiplatelet and thrombolytic agents.

The pharmacotherapeutic range of heparin is relatively narrow and bleeding is the major complication. Not surprisingly, bleeding occurs much more frequently when heparin is given in large doses than when it is used in small doses prophylactically. Since heparin preparations are obtained from animal sources and can be antigenic, they can cause hypersensitivity reactions, including chills, fever, urticaria, and even anaphylactic shock. An uncommon but serious complication is heparin-induced thrombocytopenia. The platelet counts of patients receiving heparin should therefore be monitored, and heparin therapy should be stopped if heparin-induced thrombocytopenia is suspected. Paradoxically, thrombocytopenia

Adverse effects of heparin

- Bleeding
- Thrombocytopenia and paradoxical thrombosis
- Osteoporosis
- Hypersensitivity

due to heparin can be a highly prothrombotic disorder. Long-term heparin therapy (usually longer than 3 months) is also associated with bone loss.

Heparin is contraindicated in patients who are hypersensitive to it, in patients with bleeding disorders, in patients with severe hypertension or severe hepatic or renal diseases, in alcoholics, and for patients who have surgery of the brain, spinal cord, or eye.

Heparin-induced bleeding can be rapidly reversed by administration of 100 units heparin/1 mg protamine, a basic peptide and specific antagonist of heparin, which combines with heparin to form a stable complex with loss of anticoagulant activity. Overdose of protamine should be avoided because it is an anticoagulant agent. Neutralization of low molecular weight heparin by protamine is incomplete.

LOW MOLECULAR WEIGHT HEPARIN (LMWH): ENOXAPARIN

Unfractionated heparin is commonly extracted from porcine intestinal mucosa or bovine lung. As a result of the extraction process, the polysaccharides are degraded into a heterogeneous mixture of fragments with molecular weights ranging from 300 to 30,000 kDa. All unfractionated heparin preparations are standardized by the National Institute for Biological Standards and Control.

LMWHs are obtained either by fractionation, chemical hydrolysis, or depolymerization of unfractionated heparin. Commercial preparations have a mean molecular weight of 5000 kDa, ranging from 1000 to 10,000 kDa. It should be noted, however, that the LWMHs produced by different preparative methods should be considered as individual drug agents with different pharmacokinetic and pharmacodynamic properties, rather than being viewed as simply interchangeable. Mechanistically, the anticoagulant effects of LMWHs differ from those of standard heparin because:

- The antithrombin/anti-factor Xa ratio is reduced from 1:1 to 1:4.
- The pharmacokinetic properties have diminished inter-subject variability, at least in part due to decreased protein binding.
- There is decreased interaction with platelets compared to heparin.

LMWHs have a number of advantages over heparin. Maximum plasma levels after subcutaneous injections of LMWHs are reached within 2–3 hours. In comparison, the half-life of LMWHs is about 4 hours (i.e. twice as long as the half-life of standard heparin). In addition, the bioavailability of LMWHs is about 90%, whereas that of standard heparin is only in the range of 20% after subcutaneous injection. LMWHs have a

more predictable anticoagulant response based on a weight-adjusted dose, which means that they can be given subcutaneously once or twice a day without laboratory monitoring. Clinical trials have shown that LMWHs are as effective as standard heparin in the prevention and treatment of venous thrombosis and may be associated with fewer bleeding complications.

Enoxaparin sodium (Lovenox) is the first LMWH approved by the FDA in the USA for prevention of deep-vein thrombosis following hip replacement surgery. Moreover, enoxaparin has been approved for use either in the hospital or at home with once a day dosage. Enoxaparin has been intensively tested in clinical trials for treatment of acute coronary syndromes including unstable angina or acute myocardial infarction to compare its potential effects with standard heparin. Limited data suggest that enoxaparin can be effectively substituted for standard unfractionated heparin either alone or as an adjunct to thrombolytic therapy for the treatment of acute myocardial infarctions. The dosage of enoxaparin for treatment of deep vein thrombophelitis or pulmonary embolism is 30 mg subcutaneous injection twice a day for 6 days or longer depending on clinical requirements. Adverse effects of enoxaparin include bleeding, thrombocytopenia, and local irritation.

Direct inhibition of thrombin activity: hirudin (lepirudin)

While multiple other factors may contribute to the pathogenesis of thrombotic disorders, the thrombogenic effects of thrombin play a central role. Inactivation of this enzyme or prevention of thrombin generation can inhibit thrombin-induced thrombosis.

Hirudin, a 65-amino acid (7 kDa) protein originally purified from the salivary glands of the leech, *Hirudo medicinalis*, is a highly specific antagonist of thrombin. Its recombinant protein, lepirudin (refludan), derived from yeast cells, is now available for clinical application. Lepirudin and other synthetic analogs of hirudin are potent direct inhibitors of thrombin and have shown promise as novel antithrombotic agents. Unlike heparin, which needs ATIII to inhibit thrombin, lepirudin and its derivatives directly inhibit thrombin independently of ATIII. Theoretically, these direct thrombin inhibitors should be safer than heparin because they selectively inhibit thrombin and do not affect platelet function. Furthermore, these agents are not associated with thrombocytopenia.

The FDA has recently approved lepirudin for use in patients with thrombosis complications related to heparin-induced thrombocytopenia (HIT) type II. HIT type II is a rare, allergy-like adverse reaction to heparin, a commonly used anticoagulant. HIT type II is caused by a complex immune mechanism and is characterized by a rapid and serious decline in platelet count, presumably due to sequestration of platelets in the vasculature, leading to an increased risk of severe thromboembolic complications. These complications frequently result in crippling disability, amputation or even death. Lepirudin allows HIT type II patients to maintain antithrombotic therapy and prevents thromboembolic complications. Clinical trials have shown that treatment with lepirudin also produces reductions in death, myocardial infarction and need for invasive cardiac procedures, compared with the current standard treatment in patients with unstable angina. The recommended dosage for HIT type II is 0.4 mg/kg (up to 110 kg) for an intravenous bolus slowly followed by 0.15 mg/kg (up 110 kg)/hour as a continuously intravenous infusion for 2–10 days or longer depending on the clinical situations. The half-life of lepirudin is about 60 minutes; it undergoes rapid hydrolysis. The parent drug and its fragments are eliminated in the urine but will be accumulated in renal insufficiency.

The major adverse effect of lepirudin treatment is bleeding that can be exacerbated by concomitant antithrombotic therapy. Other adverse effects occurring with lepirudin treatment include abnormal liver function and allergic skin reactions. Chronic treatment with lepirudin may lead to development of antibodies against the lepirudin–thrombin complex that may enhance the lepirudin antithrombotic effect.

Thrombolytic agents

Unlike antiplatelet agents and anticoagulant prevention of thrombi formation, thrombolytic agents actively dissolve blood clots by promoting the conversion of plasminogen to plasmin, a serine protease that in turn hydrolyzes fibrin and fibrinogen, leading to dissolution of clots (Fig. 13.20). Consequently, selected acute thromboembolic disorders can be treated by administration of thrombolytic agents. However, thrombolytic agents may increase local thrombin since the clot dissolves, leading to enhanced platelet aggregation and thrombosis. Co-therapy with antiplatelet agents such as aspirin or with anticoagulant heparin may prevent this problem.

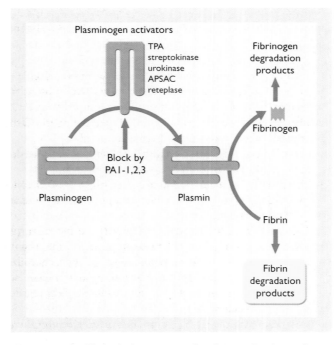

Fig. 13.20 The fibrinolytic system and action mechanisms of thrombolytic agents. The plasminogen activators currently used as thrombolytic agents stimulate conversion of plasminogen to plasmin that degrades fibrin. The action sites of physiologic inhibitors are also illustrated (PAI-1, 2, 3, plasminogen activator inhibitor 1, 2, 3).

The use of thrombolytic agents to dissolve pathologic thrombi has become a standard therapy in acute myocardial infarction. Thrombolytics also appear to be beneficial in the initial treatment of acute peripheral vascular occlusion, deep venous thrombosis, and massive pulmonary embolism. Recently, the FDA has approved rtPA for selected patients with acute ischemic stroke when thrombolytic therapy is initiated within 3 hours of the onset of symptoms.

It is no surprise that hemorrhage is a major adverse effect of administration of thrombolytics, because they do not distinguish the fibrin in unwanted thrombi from that in hemostatic plugs. Thrombolytics are contraindicated in patients with acute pericarditis, active internal bleeding, recent cerebrovascular accident, healing major wounds, or metastatic cancer. In addition, an important complication of thrombolytic therapy for patients with acute myocardial infarction is coronary artery re-occlusion following treatment.

Currently, five thrombolytic agents are commercially available for clinical applications in the USA. Their thrombolytic activities are either directly or indirectly based on the ability to enhance the generation of plasmin from its precursor plasminogen. Pharmacologic and pharmacokinetic properties of these thrombolytic agents are summarized in Fig. 13.21.

- Streptokinase (SK) is derived from group A β-hemolytic streptococci and is highly antigenic. It has no intrinsic enzymatic activity. Following intravenous infusion, it combines with plasminogen to form a 1:1 complex that activates plasminogen to plasmin. The complex hydrolyzes fibrin plugs, fibrinogen, and coagulation factors V and VII.

- Anisoylated plasminogen–streptokinase activator complex (APSAC) is a synthetic SK with the modification that it is pre-bound to a plasminogen molecule. However, it is also without enzymatic activity until its active site is deacylated following administration. It has a fourfold longer half-life than SK and can therefore be given as an intravenous bolus. Like SK, it is also highly antigenic.

- Urokinase (UK) is purified from human fetal kidney cells. UK directly converts plasminogen to plasmin by cleaving the arginine–valine bond in plasminogen. UK directly degrades both fibrin and fibrinogen. As UK is a human protein, it does not induce an antigenic response.

- Alteplase is a recombinant tissue plasminogen activator (rtPA). The enzymatic activity of rtPA depends on the presence of fibrin. Alteplase activates plasminogen bound to fibrin rapidly rather than free plasminogen in the circulation. Theoretically, it should cause less systemic fibrinolytic activation and reduce risk of bleeding. However, at doses sufficient to be clinically effective, rtPA also induces a systemic lytic state and an increased bleeding tendency.

- Reteplase is a modified human tPA constructed by genetic engineering in an attempt to improve the therapeutic properties of tPA without increasing its bleeding potential. The modifications lead to the faster reperfusion rates seen in patients receiving reteplase compared with those receiving alteplase. Several additional second-generation thrombolytic agents produced by recombinant techniques

Pharmacologic and pharmacokinetic properties of thrombolytics

	Streptokinase	Urokinase	APSAC	rtPA	Reteplase
Source	Streptococcal culture	Mammalian cell	Streptococcal culture	Mammalian cell	Mammalian cell
Molecular weight (kDa)	47	32–54	131	70	55
Circulating half-life (min)	12–18	15–20	40–60	2–6	2–4
Systemic fibrinolytic activation	Yes	Yes	Yes	Yes	Yes
Fibrin specificity	1+	2+	1+	3+	3+
Dose (i.v. bolus in minutes)	1.5 MU (30–60)	3 MU (45–90)	30 mg (5)	15 mg bolus, then 50 mg/30 min, then 35 mg/30 min	10 mg bolus, then 10 mg bolus (30)
Duration of infusion (min)	60 or less	5–15	2–5	180 or less	30 or less
Patency at 90 min (%)	53–65	66	55–65	81–88	86–90
Lives saved per 100 treated	2.5	2.5	2.5	3.5	N/A
Early heparin required	No	No	No	Yes	No
Antigenic reactions	Yes	No	Yes	No	No
Intracerebral hemorrhage (%)	0.4	0.4	0.6	0.6	N/A
Hypotension	Yes	No	Yes	No	No
Cost per dose (US$)	300/1.5 MU	2200/MU	1200/30 mg	2300/100 mg	2500/50 mg

Fig. 13.21 **Pharmacologic properties of thrombolytics.** (APSAC, anisoylated plasminogen–streptokinase activator complex; rtPA, recombinant tissue plasminogen activator; MU, million units)

are under development and have shown promise in animal models and in pilot clinical studies.

Novel antithrombotic strategies and agents

The limitations of aspirin and heparin have successfully promoted development of new antithrombotic agents, including inhibitors of TXA_2-independent pathways (e.g. ADP antagonist), platelet adhesive receptor antagonists (e.g. GPIIb/IIIa antagonist), and inhibitors of thrombin generation or activity. New antithrombotic strategies are focusing on the development of more potent and specific inhibitors of platelet function and the chain enzymatic reactions involved in coagulation. Many promising novel antithrombotic agents are currently undergoing clinical trials to determine their role in the management of thrombotic diseases (Fig. 13.22). These include agents to inhibit platelet adhesion, platelet recruitment, and platelet aggregation; agents to block thrombin generation or activity; and agents to enhance natural anticoagulant activity or endogenous fibrinolysis.

BLEEDING DISORDERS

Defects in each of the components of the normal hemostatic mechanisms may cause abnormal bleeding. These defects can be acquired or hereditary and are usually divided into four categories, namely, vascular, platelet, blood coagulation factors, or fibrinolytic defects, according to their place of action in the hemostatic mechanisms (Fig. 13.23).

- Vascular defects include acquired or hereditary structural abnormalities of blood vessel wall.
- Platelet defects include acquired or hereditary abnormalities in platelet quantity (thrombocytopenia) or in platelet quality (thrombocytopathy).
- Von Willebrand's disease (vWD) is the most common inherited coagulopathy. Patients typically present with abnormal bruising and mucosal bleeding such as epistaxis and melena. In contrast, soft tissue bleeding and spontaneous hemarthroses are more characteristic of hemophilias (factor VIII or IX deficiency).
- Acquired defects of coagulant factors include severe liver disease, deficiency of vitamin K, increased fibrinolysis in DIC, and platelet disorders.

Coagulation factor concentrates

Factor VIII concentrates with varying degrees of purity are

Novel antithrombotic strategies and agents

Strategies (mechanisms)	Agents
Inhibit platelet functions	
• Inhibit platelet adhesion	GPIa/IIIb and GPIb/IX antagonists
• Inhibit platelet recruitment	Thromboxane synthase inhibitors
	TXA$_2$ receptor antagonists
	Thrombin receptor antagonists
• Inhibit platelet aggregation	Synthetic GPIIb/IIIa antagonists
Inhibit coagulation	
• Prevent thrombin generation	Factor VII, tissue factor, and VIIa/TF complex inhibitors
	Factor IXa inhibitors
	Factor Xa inhibitors
• Inhibit thrombin activity	Active site inhibitors
Enhance natural anticoagulant activity	
• Modulate protein C pathway	Protein C or activated protein C
	Soluble thrombomodulin
	Thrombin variants
	Allosteric modulators of thrombin
Enhance endogenous fibrinolysis	
• Block type-I plasminogen activator inhibitor	Inhibitors of type-I plasminogen activator inhibitor synthesis
	Inhibitors of type-I plasminogen activator inhibitor activity
• Inhibit procarboxypeptidase B	Inhibitors of procarboxypeptidase B

Fig. 13.22 **Novel antithrombotic strategies and agents.**

Bleeding disorders

Hereditary

Hemophilia A (factor VIII deficiency)
Hemophilia B (factor IX deficiency)
Von Willebrand's disease
Platelet disorders (e.g. Glanzmann's thrombasthenia)

Acquired

Vitamin K deficiency
Liver disease
Disseminated intravascular coagulation
Thrombocytopenia (immune, infection, splenic sequestration)
Platelet disorder (uremia)

Fig. 13.23 **Bleeding disorders.**

Factor VIII concentrates

Product name	Purity
Recombinate	Recombinant
Monoclate-P	High
Koate-HP	Intermediate
Humate-P	Intermediate
Hyate-C	Porcine

Fig. 13.24 **Factor VIII concentrates.**

The development of alloantibodies that inhibit factor VIII or factor IX can be a severe problem in the treatment of hemophilias with factor concentrates. Patients with high levels of factor VIII inhibitor can be treated with porcine factor VIII if the antibodies do not strongly cross-react with the porcine protein. Other options include using factor IX complex concentrates or recombinant factor VIIa concentrates.

Desmopressin

An infusion of desmopressin, 1-deamino-(8-D-arginine)-vasopressin (DDAVP), a synthetic analog of vasopressin, causes the release of von Willebrand factor (vWF) and factor VIII from body storage sites such as Weibel–Palade bodies in endothelial cells.

DDAVP is used in patients with mild factor VIII deficiency (>5%) prophylactically before minor surgical procedures.

commercially available for prophylactic and therapeutic use in patients with hemophilia A. In the past, transmission of viral infections, including human immunodeficiency virus (HIV), has been the major cause of morbidity and mortality in these patients. Since 1985, all factor VIII concentrates have been treated with effective virus attenuation procedures, and the risk of HIV or hepatitis C transmission has essentially been eliminated. Recombinant factor VIII generated from genetically engineered mammalian cells is also now available (Fig. 13.24). The introduction of highly purified factor IX concentrate treated with viral attenuation procedures since 1991 has greatly improved the treatment of hemophilia B patients.

DDAVP cannot be used in patients with severe hemophilia A because they do not have any stored factor VIII. DDAVP is also indicated for the prevention and treatment of bleeding in patients with vWD. vWF is needed to mediate the formation of the platelet plug and also for factor VIII activity by forming a factor VIII–vWF complex. Patients with vWD subtypes that are quantitatively deficient in vWF may respond to DDAVP treatment. Patients with qualitatively defective vWF or a severe deficiency of vWF should be transfused with intermediate-purity factor VIII concentrates which contain functional vWF. Recombinant factor VIII is not an appropriate treatment for these patients. DDAVP has been used for treatment of bleeding in patients with renal failure. Uremia causes complex abnormalities of hemostasis, reflected in part by a prolonged bleeding time. Intravenous infusion of DDAVP can normalize the prolonged bleeding time and ameliorate the tendency toward excessive bleeding.

DDAVP can be given as intranasal spray, or intravenous or subcutaneous injection. The responses to DDAVP treatment vary, and diminish after several doses as a result of depletion of the storage pools. The adverse effects of this medication include flushing, headache, hypertension, and fluid retention.

Vitamin K

Vitamin K is an essential cofactor for the liver synthesis of prothrombin, as well as of factors VII, IX, X, protein C, and protein S. These coagulation factors are synthesized in the liver in a process that requires an adequate dietary intake of vitamin K. Lack of vitamin K or the presence of competitive inhibitors such as warfarin causes the production of non γ-carboxylated prothrombin, which is activated by factor Xa at only 1–2% of the normal level, as discussed on page 208 and in Fig. 13.16.

Vitamin K is used to reverse anticoagulation and bleeding caused by the vitamin K antagonist warfarin. Vitamin K deficiency may also occur in patients with biliary obstruction and liver diseases, and after prolonged treatment with oral anti-biotics, owing to suppression of the intestinal bacteria that synthesize vitamin K.

Natural vitamin K derived from green leafy vegetables is vitamin K_1 (phytomenadione). Vitamin K_2 (menaquinone) is synthesized by intestinal bacteria. Vitamins K_1 and K_2 are fat-soluble vitamins and therefore bile salts are required for their gastrointestinal absorption. Synthesized vitamin K_3 (menadione sodium bisulfite) and vitamin K_4 (menadione diacetate) are water-soluble and can therefore be injected. However, vitamin K_3 and K_4 are rarely used in the clinic because they are thera-peutically ineffective (Fig. 13.25).

A major therapeutic application of vitamin K is to prevent hypoprothrombinemia in the newborn. Vitamin K levels in the newborn may be marginal and exacerbated by inadequate nutritional intake in the first few days of life. The concentrations of factors II, VII, IX, and X in newborn infants are approximately 20–50% of adult plasma levels; premature infants have even lower concentrations. Trace amounts of vitamin K will prevent

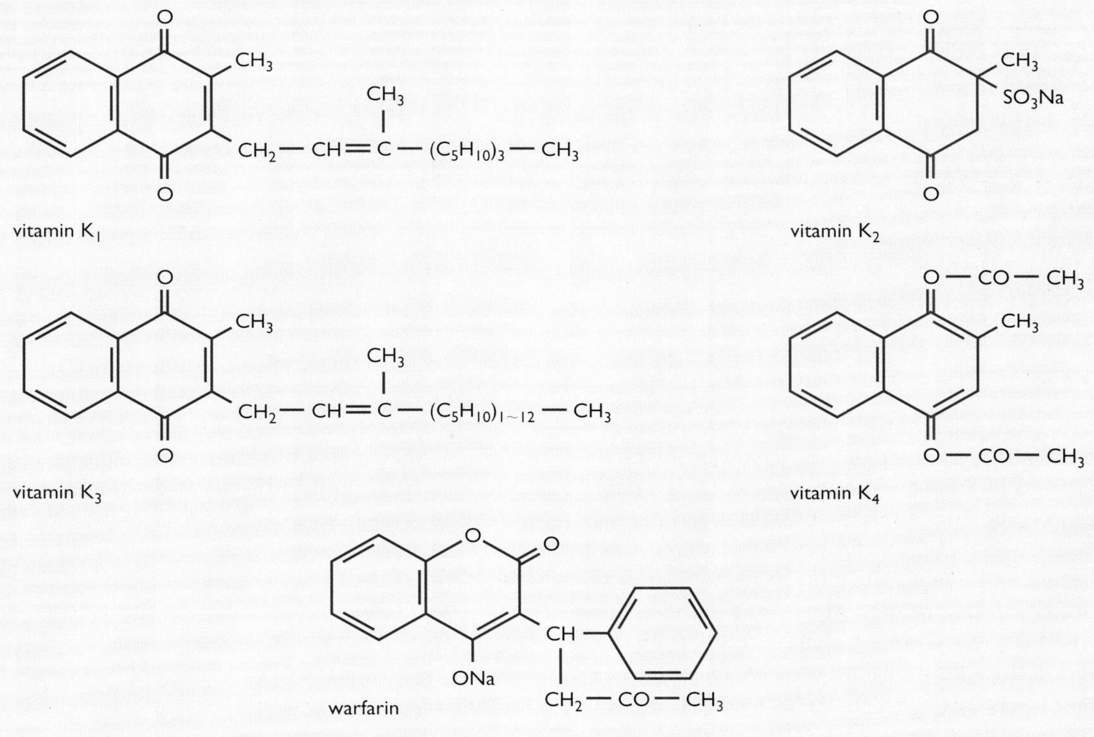

Fig. 13.25 Chemical structures of vitamin K and the antagonist warfarin.

hypoprothrombinemia by attenuating the decline in concentrations of vitamin K-dependent coagulation factors, although this treatment will not raise concentrations of these coagulation factors to adult levels. Prophylactic administration of small doses of vitamin K to newborn infants is routinely recommended and generally considered safe. Excessive dosages can provoke hemolytic anemia, hyperbilirubinemia, and kernicterus in the newborn infant. Premature infants and newborn infants with a congenital deficiency in erythrocyte glucose-6-phosphate dehydrogenase are particularly sensitive to administration of vitamin K. There are several synthetic analogs of vitamin K, including phytonadione (Mephyton), menadione, and menadiol. Phytonadione is the drug of choice for prophylactic treatment in newborn infants since it can be safely administered either orally or parenterally. Although menadione and menadiol do not require the presence of bile for gastrointestinal absorption, they can provoke toxic effects in newborns and are contraindicated in newborn infants and during later pregnancy. An alternative way to give prophylactic phytonadione to newborn infants is to administer it to mothers prior to delivery.

ε *Aminocaproic acid*

ε Aminocaproic acid (EACA) acts as a hemostatic agent by inhibiting the fibrinolytic system. It interferes with lysine-binding sites on plasminogen, blocking plasminogen association with fibrin, and thereby inhibiting the activation of plasminogen to plasmin. It is available in both oral and parenteral formulations, and has been used in the treatment of many bleeding conditions, but most commonly urinary tract bleeding.

The recommended dose of EACA is 6 g four times per day, or a loading dose of 5 g administered by intravenous injection over 30–60 minutes. It is rapidly absorbed orally and eliminated from the body by the kidney. The elimination half-life of EACA is approximately 2 hours.

Adverse effects of EACA include intravascular thrombosis due to inhibition of plasminogen activator, hypotension, myopathy, diarrhea, and nasal stuffiness. Antifibrinolytic agents may exacerbate the thrombotic component of disseminated intravascular coagulation (DIC) and should be avoided in this condition.

Aprotinin

Aprotinin is a 6.5-kDa protein purified from bovine lung. It functions as an inhibitor of several serine proteases including tissue and plasma kallikrein by the formation of reversible enzyme-inhibitor complexes. Aprotinin inhibition of kallikrein results indirectly in decrease in the formation of activated coagulation factor XII (see Fig. 13.12). Consequently, aprotinin inhibits the initiation of both coagulation and fibrinolysis induced by the contact of blood with a foreign surface. Aprotinin is administrated intravenously. The enzymatic activity of the compound is expressed in kallikrein inactivation units (KIU). Plasma concentrations of 125 KIU/ml are necessary to inhibit plasmin, and 300–500 KIU/ml are needed to inhibit kallikrein.

Aprotinin is indicated for reduction of blood loss during cardiac surgery, particularly coronary artery bypass grafting, when the exposure of blood to artificial surfaces in the extracorporeal oxygenator and enzymatic and mechanical injury to platelets and coagulation factors lead to a hyperproteolytic and hyperfibrinolytic state. The use of aprotinin can significantly reduce blood loss by as much as 50% in these surgical procedures.

The major adverse effect of aprotinin is hypersensitivity reactions because it is a herterologous protein. Therefore, a small test dose is necessary before the full therapeutic dose is given. In addition, aprotinin treatment may cause venous or arterial thrombosis. A lower prevalence of stroke among patients treated with aprotinin has been observed in a recent clinical trial.

Topical absorbable hemostatics

The purpose of chemical local hemostatics is to prevent and stop the flow of blood from surgically incised blood vessels or from oozing wound sites. The ideal local hemostatic should have rapid absorption in tissues, no irritation, and hemostatic action independent of the thrombotic mechanisms. The absorbable hemostatics meet most of these requirements and can be put directly on the wound surface to help a blood clot form. The most widely used local absorbable hemostatics include thrombin, micronized collagen, absorbable gelatin sponge, and oxidized cellulose.

THROMBIN (THROMBINAR, THROMBOSTAT) is purified from bovine serum and applied topically to control capillary oozing in surgical procedures and to shorten the duration of bleeding from punctured sites in heparinized patients (e.g. during hemodialysis). One unit of thrombin can make 1 ml of the standard fibrin solution clot in 15 seconds. Thrombin may also be used for localized bleeding in the nose or mouth for patients with vWD. However, thrombin should be never used by systemic injection, because of the high risk of generalized thrombosis.

MICROFIBRILLAR COLLAGEN HEMOSTAT (AVITENE) is purified from bovine corium collagen prepared as the partial hydrochloric acid salt. It acts by attracting and activating platelets to initiate clot formation. It is absorbable and is prepared as a dry, sterile, fibrous, water-insoluble product. Microfibrillar collagen has been found to be as effective as a topical hemostatic agent for large oozing surfaces. It can be used during surgery to control capillary bleeding and as an adjunctive hemostatic method when control of bleeding by ligature or more conventional methods is ineffective or impractical. The product causes a mild, chronic cellular inflammatory response. Additionally, it may interfere with wound healing.

ABSORBABLE GELATIN is a simple protein complex made from animal skin gelatin. It is not antigenic because it has been denatured. There are three forms of preparations of gelatin for different clinical purposes, including absorbable gelatin sponge (Gelfam), absorbable gelatin film (Gelfilm), and absorbable gelatin powder (Gelfoam). Gelatin sponge is produced as a sterile, absorbable, water-insoluble, gelatin-based sponge. It is used for the control of capillary vessel leakage and frank hemorrhage. When implanted in tissue it is absorbed completely in 3–5 weeks without inducing excessive formation of scar tissue. When applied to bleeding areas of skin or to nasal, rectal, and vaginal mucosa, it completely liquefies within 2–5 days. Oral ingestion of 1–10 mg of gelatin powder has been employed to treat gastrointestinal bleeding.

OXIDIZED CELLULOSE (OXYCEL) is a specifically treated form of surgical gauze or cotton that promotes clotting by a physical effect, rather than by any alteration of the normal clotting mechanisms. It is used in surgical procedures to control capillary, venous, and small arterial hemorrhage when ligation or other conventional methods of control are impractical or ineffective. It is also employed in oral surgery and exodontia. Oxidized cellulose should not be used in combination with thrombin because the low pH interferes with the activity of the thrombin. Oxycel is nontoxic and relatively nonirritating but somewhat detrimental to wound healing and requires phagocytosis for removal. Moreover, it should not be employed for permanent packing or implantation in fractures because it interferes with bone regeneration and may result in cyst formation. It is usually made as sterile cotton pledgets, gauze pads, and gauze strips.

FURTHER READING

Dalen JE, Hirsh J (eds) Fifth ACCP consensus conference on antithrombotic therapy. *Chest* 1998; **114**(Suppl): 439S–729S. [An excellent collection of up-to-date reviews on antithrombotic agents.]

Colman RW, Hirsh J, Marder VJ, Salzman EW (eds) *Hemostasis and Thrombosis: Basic Principles and Clinical Practice*, 4th edn. Philadelphia: JB Lippincott; 2000. [An excellent textbook covering all aspects of hemostasis from molecular mechanism to clinical application.]

Gresle P, Fuster V, Page CP, Vermylyn J (eds) The platelet in health and disease. Cambridge: Cambridge University Press; 2002. [A comprehensive overview of platelet biology and antiplatelet drugs.]

Hoffman R, Benz E, Shattil S, Furie B, Cohen H, Silberstein L, McGlave P (eds) *Hematology: Basic Principles and Practice*, 3rd edn. Baltimore: Williams & Wilkins; 2000. [A comprehensive and up-to-date textbook, by authoritative authors, for practicing general hematologists, students of the field, basic scientists involved in hematologic research, as well as practicing internists and pediatricians.]

Smith TW (ed.) *Cardiovascular Therapeutics. A Companion to Braunwald's Heart Disease*. Philadelphia: W. B. Saunders; 1996. [Clinical reference for the therapeutic approaches for cardiovascular diseases.]

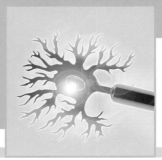

Chapter 14

Drugs and the Nervous System

PHYSIOLOGY OF THE CENTRAL AND PERIPHERAL NERVOUS SYSTEMS

▨ *The nervous system provides for conscious or unconscious control of basic motor and sensory activity, as well as emotional and intellectual functions*

The nervous system is organized as a hierarchy.

- Afferent fibers passing from the peripheral tissues to the spinal cord constitute the part of the peripheral nervous system (PNS) that allows perception of external sensation and body function.
- Efferent neurons from the spinal cord constitute the part of the PNS that regulates the activity of peripheral tissues.
- The central nervous system (CNS) starts at the spinal cord and connects the afferent and efferent neurons of the PNS with the brain, which provides higher processing and executive control.

▨ *The neuron is the basic unit of both the CNS and PNS*

The body contains approximately 10×10^9 neurons (nerve cells) of various types, which differ in length and structure, but are composed of four major areas (Fig. 14.1):

- The cell body, which contains the nucleus and structures concerned with the basic functioning of the cell.
- The axon, which conducts nerve impulses, in the form of an action potential, from the cell body to a distant site, and vice versa.
- Dendrites, which connect neurons with each other and transmit information back to their own cell body.
- Synapses, which are the basis of neurochemical communication.

Axons are either long (as in projection neurons such as peripheral motor and sensory nerves) or short (as in interneurons), and most are covered in myelin. In the PNS this covering (myelin sheath) is provided by Schwann cells, while in the CNS it is provided by neuroglia cells (i.e. oligodendrocytes). At the end of an axon there are usually branches that end in axon terminals or boutons and form synapses with other neurons or tissue cells. Often the connection is with a dendrite from another cell. There are numerous dendrites on most neurons. They have no myelin covering and can be profusely branched. The ends of the axon branches are studded with dendritic spines, which are the points of synaptic connection. The synapse is therefore the point of connection between neurons. Each neuron may have 1000–10,000 synaptic connections with as many as 1000 other neurons.

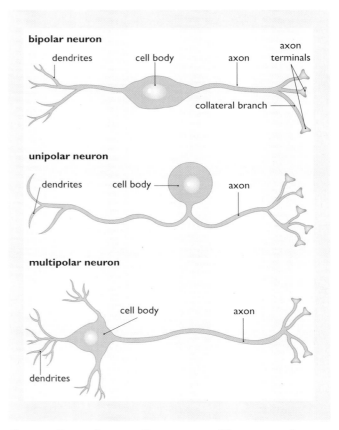

Fig. 14.1 Types of neuron. There are many different types of neuron, which are shaped according to function. Bipolar cells are commonly interneurons, while unipolar cells tend to be sensory neurons and multipolar cells are often motor neurons.

The synapse comprises the axon terminal of the presynaptic neuron, the dendrite of the postsynaptic neuron, and the gap between them, the synaptic cleft (Fig. 14.2). The numerous types of synapses are named according to which two parts of a neuron are connected (i.e. axoaxonic, axodendritic). In addition there are:

- Electrical synapses or gap junctions, which use ions as a transmitter.
- Conjoint synapses which use both ionic and chemical transmitters.

The general actions of drugs at synapses are listed in Fig. 14.3.

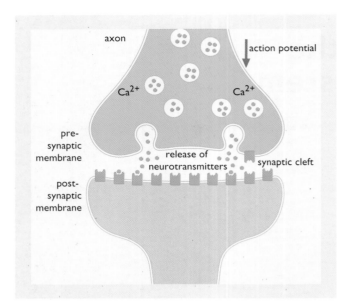

Fig. 14.2 Action potential at the synapse. An action potential passing down an axon to the axon terminal or region with similar function (e.g. axonal varicosities) changes membrane polarization, resulting in Ca^{2+} entry into the cell. This triggers the fusion of neurochemical-containing vesicles and cell membrane and the release of neurochemical (neurotransmitter) into the synaptic cleft. The neurotransmitter diffuses across the cleft and binds to specific receptors on the postsynaptic membrane to initiate a response in the postsynaptic neuron.

Examples of drugs that act at synapses

Mechanism of action	Example
Stimulate synthesis	Levodopa in Parkinson's disease
Stimulate release	Fenfluramine and secondary effect of MAOIs in depression
Release blocker	None in clinical use
Receptor agonist	Bromocriptine in Parkinson's disease
Receptor antagonist	Antipsychotic drugs
Reuptake blocker	Tricyclic antidepressants and SSRIs in depression
Degradative enzyme inhibitor	Vigabatrin in epilepsy

Fig. 14.3 Examples of drugs that act at synapses. (MAOIs, monoamine oxidase inhibitors; SSRIs, selective serotonin reuptake inhibitors)

Neurotransmitter release and neurotransmitter effect depend on the neuronal resting membrane potential and action potential

The resting membrane potential of the cell is negative owing to preferential ion distribution across the cell membrane maintained by the membrane ion pumps and ion channels contained within the neuronal phospholipid membrane. The principal ions are Na^+, K^+, Ca^{2+}, and Cl^- (Fig. 14.4).

An action potential is a brief wave of reversal of membrane potential that moves along the axon away from the cell body (Fig. 14.5). During the action potential Ca^{2+} enters the cell and initiates neurotransmitter release (Fig. 14.6). The action

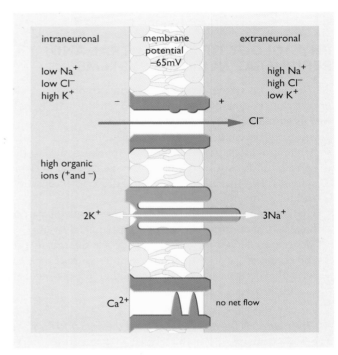

Fig. 14.4 Ion distribution across the neuron membrane at rest. The energy-dependent Na^+/K^+ pump maintains the resting potential by sustaining the Na^+/K^+ concentration gradient across the cell membrane so that the K^+ concentration inside the cell is high. Conversely the Na^+ concentration outside the cell is high.

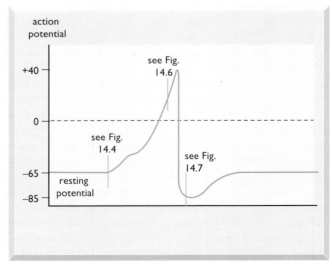

Fig. 14.5 An action potential. This is a brief (0.1–2 msec) wave of reversal of membrane potential (from negative to positive) that moves along the axon away from the cell body.

potential is followed by a period of hyperpolarization when the neuron is more negatively charged than at rest (Fig. 14.7). This prevents further action potentials and the degree of hyperpolarization has implications for nerve cell excitability.

Some neurotransmitters inhibit firing of action potentials by hyperpolarizing the neuron

The classic example of a hyperpolarizing neurotransmitter is γ-aminobutyric acid (GABA), which opens Cl^- channels in the cell membrane, thereby increasing the membrane's negative charge. These Cl^- channels are examples of ligand-gated ion channels (i.e. ion channels that change in response to a specific chemical) (see Chapter 3). The other general type of ion channel is a voltage-gated ion channel (e.g. the Na^+ and Ca^{2+} ion channels involved in the generation of the action potential).

There are receptors for 300-plus endogenous molecules that act in the nervous system

Many drugs used to affect the human nervous system exert their actions by altering the function of the receptors for the endogenous molecules that act in the nervous system. The major classes of receptors and transmitters found in the nervous system are listed in Fig. 14.8.

Receptors can be present in the synapse both pre- and postsynaptically. Many presynaptic receptors inhibit further release of the relevant neurotransmitter, though the effect of activating a presynaptic receptor may depend on:

- The number of receptors activated.
- The affinity of the receptor for the transmitter.
- The efficacy with which the receptor modifies transmitter release.

The two major types of receptor are:

- Those located directly on ion channels such as acetylcholine nicotinic receptors and 5-hydroxytryptamine (5-HT)-3 receptors (both Na^+ and K^+ channels), GABA receptors (Cl^- channels) (Fig. 14.9), and glutamate receptors (N-methyl D-aspartate receptors), which are cation channels.
- G protein-coupled receptors, which can exert their effects via second-messenger systems (e.g. by increasing or decreasing concentrations of cAMP; see Chapter 3). For some G protein-coupled receptors, the activated G protein acts directly on an ion channel without the involvement of a second messenger. Other second messengers include Ca^{2+} and metabolites of the membrane component phosphoinositol (see Chapter 3).

Neurotransmitters are released in response to an action potential

A neurotransmitter is a molecule synthesized in a neuron and released in response to an action potential in physiologically significant amounts. It is then removed or deactivated in the neuron or synaptic cleft. Such a molecule administered as an exogenous drug typically mimics the effects of the endogenous neurotransmitter. A molecule fulfilling some of these criteria is referred to as a putative neurotransmitter.

Neuromodulators are molecules that modulate the response of a neuron to a neurotransmitter, while neurohormones are

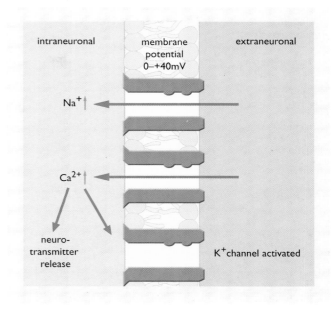

Fig. 14.6 Ion movements during an action potential. An action potential is produced when Na^+ channels open, allowing Na^+ to move along its concentration gradient into the cell. The Ca^{2+} channels then open, allowing Ca^{2+} to enter the cell. Calcium both initiates neurotransmitter release and allows K^+ outflow, which will eventually arrest the action potential.

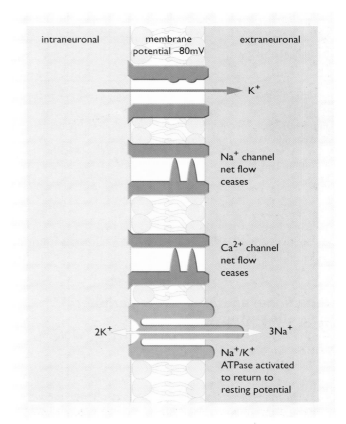

Fig. 14.7 Hyperpolarization. During hyperpolarization, the neuron is more negatively charged than at rest, preventing further action potentials.

Receptor classification for the major CNS neurotransmitters

Transmitter	Receptor
Glutamate	NMDA
	Non NMDA
GABA	GABAa
	GABAb
Glycine	Glycine (strychnine-sensitive)
Acetylcholine	Nicotinic
	Muscarinic
5-HT	5-HT_{1a-d}
	5-HT_2
	5-HT_3
	5-HT_4
	5-HT_5
	5-HT_6
	5-HT_7
Norepinephrine	α_1
	α_2
	β_{1-3}
Dopamine	D_1
	D_2
	D_3
	D_4
	D_5
Cholecystokinin	CCK_A
	CCK_B
Nitric oxide	Activates the enzyme guanylate cyclase

Fig. 14.8 Receptor classification for the major central nervous system (CNS) neurotransmitters. (CCK, cholecystokinin; GABA, γ-aminobutyric acid; 5-HT, 5-hydroxytryptamine; NMDA, N-methyl-D-aspartate)

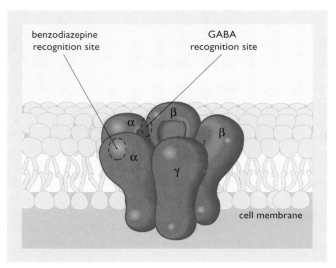

Fig. 14.9 Receptor-operated ionic channels: the γ-aminobutyric acid (GABA) receptor. Each subunit is composed of four protein helical strands. Binding of a benzodiazepine or GABA leads to conformational change. The channel opens and Cl^- passes down its concentration gradient.

Classification of the major central nervous system peptide neurotransmitters

Family	Examples
Opioid	Endorphins, enkephalins, dynorphins
Neurohypophyseal	Vasopressin, oxytocin
Tachykinins	Substance P, neurokinin
Gastrins	Gastrin, cholecystokinin
Others	Neuropeptide Y, substance P, neurotensin, galanin

Fig. 14.10 Classification of the major central nervous system peptide neurotransmitters.

substances that are released into the blood and have effects on neurons (e.g. cortisol and tri-iodothyronine).

The classification for the major CNS neurotransmitters is given in Figs 14.8 and 14.10.

Functional anatomy of the peripheral nervous system

■ *Motor neurons innervate muscle fibers or intrafusal muscle spindles*

Motor neurons send their axons to muscle fibers in the periphery. There are two types of motor neuron:

- α motor neurons are large myelinated fibers and form motor units with the muscle fibers they innervate. The number of muscle fibers innervated by each motor fiber varies with the degree of fine motor control. For fine control only a few fibers are innervated.

- γ motor neurons are much smaller than α motor neurons, have limited myelination, and innervate only intrafusal muscle spindles acting as stretch receptors (Fig. 14.11).

Both α and γ fibers are found in the ventral horn of the spinal cord, and synapse with the descending motor tracts within the spinal cord. Interneuronal connection within the spinal cord integrates the fine motor control provided by the extra-pyramidal system.

Control of skeletal muscle system activity by the motor nervous system is complex and involves intricate CNS regulation. The afferent limb of the system carries information from a variety of sources, including:

- Stretch receptors in the joints and limbs.
- Muscle spindles in the body of skeletal muscles.
- Proprioceptors in joints.
- Labyrinth receptors in the ear.

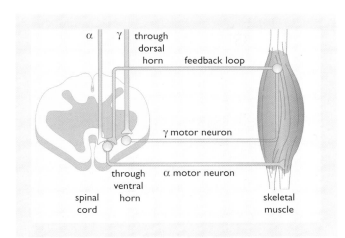

Fig. 14.11 **The motor system of the peripheral nervous system.**
The α and γ neurons provide feedback control of muscle contraction via a loop to the α motor neurons.

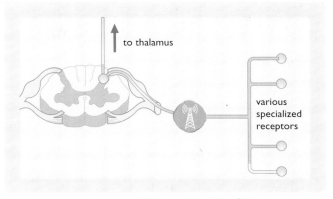

Fig. 14.12 **Sensory system of the peripheral nervous system.**
Sensory neurons originate in peripheral structures and pass into the spinal cord through the dorsal root.

Information arriving at the CNS from these afferent sources is integrated at various levels of the CNS with the cerebellum playing a major role. The voluntary aspects of skeletal muscle control arise in the cerebral cortex. Within the CNS there is a comprehensive interplay between information derived from the cortex (the voluntary component) and that derived from the cerebellum, midbrain nuclei, and spinal cord (the involuntary component).

Efferent motor nerves have myelinated axons and generally one axon supplies one muscle fiber

The focus of this section is the efferent limb of the motor nervous system. Efferent motor nerves arise from the brainstem and at various levels of the spinal cord. Once they leave the CNS there are no ganglia and the motor nerve axons thus conduct impulses rapidly from the CNS to skeletal muscle. These axons are myelinated and so allow rapid propagation of action potentials along them. Each axon normally innervates a single muscle fiber. Multiply innervated muscles are rare and are found in the muscle spindle and the extraocular muscles of the eye.

Once the axon reaches the skeletal muscle fiber it terminates in a highly discrete region. The axon abuts onto the muscle fiber at the neuromuscular junction, and, at this site, the nerve ending sits within the 'cup' of folded end-plate membrane. Here, acetylcholine mediates its molecular action (activation of nicotinic receptors). This, through a cascade of transduction mechanisms, elicits a system response in skeletal muscle (contraction) (see below).

Sensory neurons originate in peripheral structures and transduce stimuli into action potentials

The endings of sensory neurons in peripheral structures comprise a highly specialized network of physiologic receptors, which transduce stimuli into action potentials. The sensory fibers pass into the spinal cord through the dorsal root (Fig. 14.12). Some fibers synapse at the level of entry into the spinal cord, while others pass to the brainstem before synapsing and passing to the thalamus. The special sensory systems such as vision and hearing have a highly individualized arrangement and are discussed in Chapters 24 and 25, respectively.

The autonomic nervous system maintains the internal environment of the body

The autonomic nervous system (ANS) controls visceral functions such as circulation, digestion, and excretion, mostly without voluntary or conscious control. It also modulates the function of the endocrine glands, which regulate metabolism. The ANS has both sensory and motor components, and is divided into sympathetic and parasympathetic systems according to its anatomy and physiology. In general the first neurons of the sympathetic system are located in the intermediate horn of the thoracolumbar region of the spinal cord. These synapse with the second neurons in the para- or prevertebral sympathetic ganglia. In the parasympathetic system the first neurons are located either in the cranial nerve autonomic nuclei or in the intermediate horn of the sacral region of the spinal cord. They synapse with the second neurons either in autonomic ganglia in the case of cranial nerves or in the effecter tissue itself.

The autonomic nervous system is composed of three major elements:
• The afferent limb.
• The central integrated elements.
• The efferent limb.
The afferent limb carries information from sensors (neuronal receptors sited at the ends of afferent nerves) to the spinal cord and the rest of the CNS. Most of this information is then processed within the hypothalamus and other parts of the lower brain. After processing, appropriate signals are passed from the CNS and down the efferent nerves to the effector organs (Fig. 14.13), which are so named because they produce the responses to activity in the CNS.

The efferent part of the autonomic nervous system is divided into three separate types on the basis of its anatomy and neurotransmitters:

223

- The parasympathetic (cholinergic) system.
- The sympathetic (adrenergic) system.
- The nonadrenergic and noncholinergic (NANC) system.

▨ A cholinergic system is one in which the primary neurotransmitter is acetylcholine

Acetylcholine is the neurotransmitter released from presynaptic terminals in the autonomic ganglia and from the prejunctional nerve endings at the effector organ (Fig. 14.14). The receptors of the cholinergic system that bind acetylcholine are cholinoceptors. Cholinoceptors include those classified as muscarinic and nicotinic receptors (see Fig. 14.13).

▨ An adrenergic system is one in which the neurotransmitter is related to certain products of the adrenal medulla (epinephrine and norepinephrine)

The other major limb of the autonomic nervous system is the adrenergic system. The nomenclature is an historical accident,

as when the system was first described, there was no clear separation between two possible transmitters, namely epinephrine and norepinephrine. It is now known that apart from the special case for the adrenal glands, which secrete epinephrine (adrenaline), the neurotransmitter is always norepinephrine.

▨ The sympathetic and parasympathetic systems generally functionally antagonize each other

The sympathetic system prepares the body for action (i.e. the 'fear, fight, or fight response'), while the parasympathetic system is generally concerned with the body at rest (Fig. 14.15). Drugs acting in the CNS often produce their adverse effects by changing the activity of the ANS.

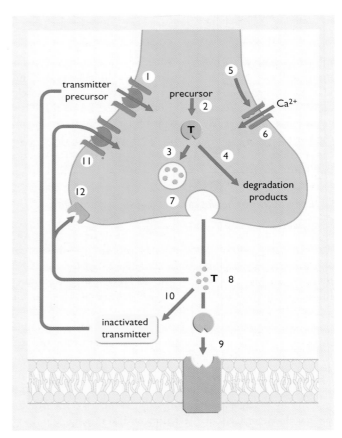

Fig. 14.14 Processes generally involved in the synthesis, storage, and release of neurotransmitters. 1 = uptake of precursors; 2 = synthesis of transmitter; 3 = storage of transmitter in vesicles; 4 = degradation of surplus transmitter; 5 = depolarization by prolonged action potential; 6 = influx of Ca^{2+} through N-type Ca^{2+} channels in reponse to depolarization; 7 = release of transmitter by exocytosis; 8 = diffusion to postsynaptic membrane; 9 = interaction with postsynaptic receptors; 10 = inactivation of transmitter; 11 = reuptake of transmitter or degradation products; 12 = interaction with presynaptic receptors. These processes are well characterized for many transmitters (e.g. acetylcholine, norepinephrine, dopamine, 5-hydroxytryptamine), but may well differ by omission of some of the processes for other transmitters (e.g. amino acids, purines, peptides). (Adapted with permission from *Pharmacology*, 3rd edn, by Rang, Dale, and Ritter, Churchill Livingstone, 1995.)

Fig. 14.13 Acetylcholine (ACh) and norepinephrine (NE) are the major neurotransmitters in the peripheral autonomic nervous system. ACh acts on peripheral tissues via two types of receptor, nicotinic (nic) or muscarinic (mus), depending on the tissue. NE acts on peripheral tissues via at least two types of receptors, α and β, depending on the tissue. (E, epinephrine)

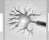

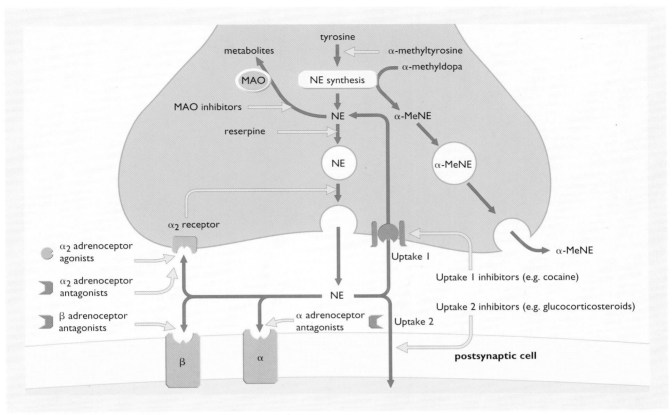

Fig. 14.15 Drug actions on the noradrenergic (sympathetic) nervous system. The molecular actions shown here, at the nerve terminal, affect the noradrenergic system throughout the body. Drugs may affect synthesis, storage, release, uptake, and receptors. (MAO, monoamine oxidase; α-MeNE, α-methylnorepinephrine; NE, norepinephrine) (Adapted with permission from *Pharmacology*, 3rd edn, by Rang, Dale, and Ritter, Churchill Livingstone, 1995.)

The preganglionic transmitter for both the cholinergic and the adrenergic systems is acetylcholine

The efferent nerves for both the cholinergic and the adrenergic systems arise from the appropriate parts of the brainstem and the spinal cord. These efferent nerves then synapse at ganglia situated throughout the body.

- In the adrenergic system, the ganglia lie mainly in a chain close to the spinal cord, known as the paravertebral sympathetic chain.
- In the cholinergic system, the ganglia are usually situated close to or on their effector organ.

Despite this clear anatomical distinction, both types of ganglia use acetylcholine as the principal ganglionic transmitter.

Neurotransmitters can modulate their own release

A further complexity is that neurotransmitters can modulate their own release. Neurotransmitters can act back upon receptors on the nerve ending that originally released them, to inhibit their own release.

The nonadrenergic, noncholinergic system is a third component of the autonomic system

In addition to the cholinergic and adrenergic system, it has been recognized over recent decades that parts of the autonomic nervous system are neither cholinergic nor adrenergic.

This section of the autonomic nervous system is therefore known as the nonadrenergic, noncholinergic (NANC) system. It is not clear which neurotransmitters act in this system, although nitric oxide has recently been suggested to be the major neurotransmitter in NANC nerves in various parts of the body, including the penis and the lung (Fig. 14.16). Nitric oxide is synthesized in nerve endings from the precursor amino acid L-arginine by the enzyme nitric oxide synthase.

An added complication for cholinergic and adrenergic systems is the presence in these nerve endings of chemicals known generically as co-transmitters. These co-transmitters may not serve the primary function of neurotransmission (i.e. passing the neuronal message to effector tissue), but instead have modulator functions. An example is adenosine triphosphate (ATP).

(Co-transmission and NANC transmission will be discussed further below, following a more complete description of the mechanisms by which drugs can affect the functioning of the autonomic nervous system, particularly the cholinergic and adrenergic systems.)

Cholinergic and adrenergic ganglia cannot be differentiated from each other pharmacologically

Both cholinergic and adrenergic ganglia are considered together in the following discussion since they cannot be

225

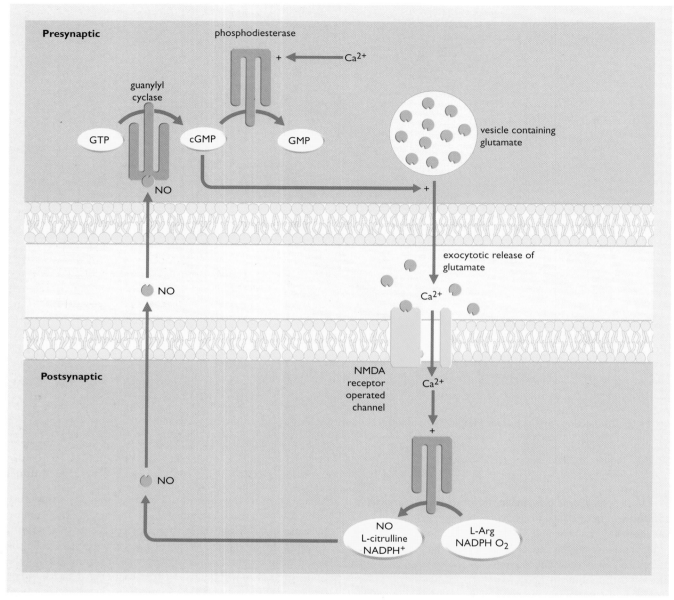

Fig. 14.16 Nitric oxide and glutaminergic neural transmission. In this model, glutamate released from a presynaptic terminal binds to postsynaptic NMDA receptors causing an influx of calcium ions (Ca^{2+}). Alternatively, calcium influx may occur through voltage-gated calcium channels. The increased Ca^{2+} concentration leads to activation of NO synthase, which results in production of nitric oxide (NO). Nitric oxide then diffuses to surrounding tissue, including the presynaptic release terminal, where it binds to and activates guanylate cyclase. This sets into motion a biochemical cascade that results in increased glutamate release from the presynaptic terminal. (Adapted from Holscher C, 1997. Nitric oxide, the enigmatic neuronal messenger: its role in synaptic plasticity. *Trends Neurosci* **20**: 298–303, with permission from Elsevier Science.)

differentiated from each other by pharmacologic means, despite their different anatomic locations.

The term 'preganglionic fibers' refers to neuronal axons that arise in the CNS and terminate on cell bodies in the ganglia; they are primarily cholinergic. Axons arising from the cell bodies in the ganglia and terminating at the effector tissue are known as postganglionic fibers. Some postganglionic adrenergic fibers have been found to innervate cholinergic ganglia, adding further complexity to the two systems.

Drugs and ganglionic transmission

Given that transmission in ganglia is primarily cholinergic, it is possible to understand the mechanisms by which drugs may interfere with ganglionic transmission, either to accentuate or to block transmission.

Drugs can interfere with acetylcholine synthesis and storage

Acetylcholine is synthesized by condensation of the amino alcohol, choline, with acetate to form the chemical ester, acetylcholine. No common pharmacotherapeutic drugs or toxins directly inhibit the enzyme (acetylcholine transferase) responsible for the condensation. However, a variety of cholinomimetics (e.g. analogs of choline) can prevent the formation of acetylcholine and its subsequent storage in vesicles, though such drugs are of experimental interest only.

Drugs and the choline transport system

The release of acetylcholine from nerve terminals requires the opening of N-type Ca^{2+} channels, the entry of Ca^{2+}, the mobilization of vesicles, and vesicle fusion with the neuronal membrane to release their contents into the synaptic gap of the ganglia. Once released, acetylcholine is free to bind to receptors or to be broken down by the enzyme acetylcholinesterase, which splits acetylcholine into its acetate and choline fragments. The released choline is taken back up into the cholinergic neuron ending by a special choline transport system. Experimentally, it is possible to interfere with this choline transport system, but drugs that do this have little clinical importance.

Ganglion blockers can block all transmission in the autonomic nervous system

By blocking all transmission in the autonomic nervous system, ganglion blockers effectively prevent the autonomic nervous system from participating in body responses.

The first antihypertensive drugs were ganglion blockers, and when they were given in effective doses the resulting wide range of signs and symptoms gave a clear insight into the importance of the autonomic nervous system to humans. A full ganglion-blocking dose of the drug produces a variety of signs and symptoms, including the following:

- Inability to accommodate vision for near sight.
- Drying of secretions in the mouth, stomach, and eyes.
- Constipation.
- Difficulty with urination.
- Loss of sexual function in the male.
- Orthostatic hypotension.

These symptoms emphasize the importance of resting tone in the autonomic nervous system. Both parasympathetic and sympathetic ganglia are blocked by ganglion blockers because these drugs are not selective for different ganglia.

The molecular mechanism of action of ganglion blockers is nicotinic antagonism.

Adrenergic nervous system

The adrenergic nervous system innervates many parts of the body, but particularly:

- The gut.
- The heart.
- The lungs.
- Blood vessels.

The adrenergic system innervates some tissues (e.g. the gut and airway smooth muscle) via the cholinergic ganglia. This means that the role of the adrenergic nervous system in the gut and, to a lesser extent, in the lung, is to control activity in the parasympathetic cholinergic ganglia.

The three adrenergic neurotransmitters of interest are norepinephrine, epinephrine, and dopamine

Two of the three adrenergic neurotransmitters are found in the peripheral nervous system and in the CNS, whereas the third, dopamine, is found primarily (although not exclusively) in the CNS.

Norepinephrine, epinephrine, and dopamine are all formed from the same precursor essential amino acid, tyrosine. Tyrosine is exposed to a cascade of enzymes in the adrenergic nerve ending (Fig. 14.15) where synthesis stops at norepinephrine in noradrenergic neurons or dopamine in dopaminergic neurons. Very little of the tyrosine is metabolized to the N-methyl product of norepinephrine (epinephrine) in neurons. However, the adrenal gland, which is a very discrete organ lying above the kidney, is an exception. The outer part (cortex) of the gland is involved in the synthesis of steroid hormones, particularly glucocorticosteroids and mineralocorticoids, whereas epinephrine is synthesized in the center of the gland (medulla). High concentration of cortisol activate expression of phenylethanolamine N-methyl transferase, the enzyme catalyzing the conversion of norepinephrine to epinephrine.

The adrenal medulla is effectively a highly specialized sympathetic ganglion

The adrenal medulla is a ganglion that has a residual post-ganglionic neuron (Fig. 14.13). Stimulation of the adrenal medulla by activation of nicotinic receptors results in the release of epinephrine directly into the adrenal medullary veins and then into the vena cava, from whence it reaches the heart to be distributed around the body. Epinephrine released in this manner can therefore be regarded as a circulating hormone, rather than a neurotransmitter.

The enzymatic cascade producing epinephrine, norepinephrine, and dopamine is the same

Tyrosine is progressively hydroxylated and decarboxylated to produce dopamine. The process can then stop, or can continue with further hydroxylation and methylation to produce norepinephrine, where the process can again stop. Further methylation in the adrenal glands results in the production of epinephrine.

The rate-limiting enzyme or critical control point in the cascade producing dopamine, norepinephrine, or epinephrine is tyrosine hydroxylase. Metyrosine is used in the treatment of some cases of pheochromocytoma; it is an inhibitor of tyrosine hydroxylase.

The release process for norepinephrine, epinephrine, and dopamine from vesicles is similar to that for acetylcholine

Once synthesized, norepinephrine, epinephrine, and dopamine are packaged into vesicles where they are complexed to ATP and a special vesicular protein. Release of the contents of such vesicles is by the same type of process as for acetylcholine. The arrival of an action potential at the postganglionic nerve ending results in the opening of N-type Ca^{2+} channels, which allow the intracellular flow of Ca^{2+}. The elevation of Ca^{2+} in the nerve endings results in the subsequent mobilization of the vesicles, which fuse with the membrane of the nerve ending. As a result the released norepinephrine diffuses across the junctional cleft to bind to adrenoceptors. Postjunctional adrenoceptors, the molecular targets for norepinephrine are discussed in Fig. 14.16. The uses of these drugs are discussed in subsequent chapters.

As with acetylcholine, there is a highly effective system for re-using norephinephrine

Once norepinephrine has acted upon the postjunctional receptor:

- Some diffuses from the junctional cleft.
- Some acts upon prejunctional receptors on postganglionic nerve endings to inhibit the release of more norepinephrine. The receptor here is the α_2 subtype.
- Most is taken back into the nerve terminal. This reuptake requires a special process involving a norepinephrine transporter located in the cell membrane. This transporter carries norepinephrine back into the nerve ending where it is either broken down by the enzyme monoamine oxidase located on mitochondria or it is repackaged into vesicles.

Thus, with acetylcholine and the cholinergic system, there is a highly effective system for reusing the transmitter substance.

Any norepinephrine that escapes from the junctional cleft is exposed to two possible fates.

- The first is metabolism by the enzyme catechol-O-methyl transferase.
- The second is to be taken up by the uptake 2 system.

There are two uptake systems for norepinephrine in tissues. The first, uptake 1, is the physiologically important system since it ensures that the neurotransmitter is used efficiently and that its residence time in the junctional cleft is limited. The second, uptake 2, is of doubtful physiologic relevance.

The major action of a variety of drugs is inhibition of the uptake 1 process. Such drugs are therefore known as uptake 1 inhibitors. Uptake 1 inhibition has complex sympathetic nervous system effects.

Cocaine can produce a hyperadrenergic state

The classic uptake 1 inhibitor is cocaine. If there is sufficient cocaine to block uptake 1, the effects of adrenergic stimulation or injected norepinephrine are markedly increased. The cocaine addict is therefore exposed to some extent to a hyperadrenergic state, and this occurs both centrally and peripherally. Such a hyperadrenergic state may partly account for the sudden death that occurs in some cocaine addicts (see below). Such sudden deaths are believed to be due to fatal arrhythmias.

The adrenergic system can be manipulated at different levels

It is apparent that the adrenergic system can be manipulated at a number of different levels:

- By sympathomimetic drugs, which are agonists.
- By inhibiting uptake 1 or the enzyme monoamine oxidase.
- By interfering with the storage of norepinephrine in vesicles.
- By disrupting the process that results in the release of vesicles.

Drugs that reduce norepinephrine storage and release affect the adrenergic system to reduce the level of activity. Therapeutically, this can be advantageous (e.g. in the treatment of hypertension).

Drugs interfering with the adrenergic system innervating blood vessels may cause postural hypotension

One adverse system effect of adrenergic neuron blockers is postural hypotension (a dramatic fall in blood pressure on rising to a standing position from a previous sitting or supine position). The fall in blood pressure can be profound and cause dizziness or even fainting. This is because normally, on standing up, there is increased activation of the adrenergic system innervating veins and arteries resulting in:

- Vasoconstriction (a squeezing action on capacitance veins), which ensures an adequate venous return to the heart and sufficient cardiac output to maintain blood pressure.
- Vasoconstriction of arteries to maintain the blood pressure.

As a result of these two system mechanisms, blood flow in the cerebral arteries is maintained. Impairment of these mechanisms impairs the ability of patients to stand up.

Cholinergic system

The mechanisms of synthesis and release of acetylcholine in the cholinergic autonomic nervous system are similar to those that occur in the parasympathetic and sympathetic preganglionic neurons of the autonomic nervous system. However, the postsynaptic receptors are muscarinic (not nicotinic) (Fig. 14.17).

The system responses to acetylcholine are diverse, and depend on the type of muscarinic receptor mediating the molecular response (M_1, M_2, or M_3).

The prejunctional or presynaptic neuronal membranes contain autoreceptors of the M_2 subtype, and stimulation of these receptors inhibits the release of acetylcholine and possibly other neurotransmitters. The sites at which parasympathetic transmission may be modulated are shown in Fig. 14.17.

PATHOPHYSIOLOGY AND DISEASES OF THE PERIPHERAL NERVOUS SYSTEM

Major diseases of the peripheral nervous system particularly affect skeletal muscle function. Neural control of skeletal muscles is accomplished mainly through the somatic motor nerves and afferent influence from sensory receptors present in the muscles (e.g. muscle spindles), tendons (e.g. Golgi tendon organs) and joints (proprioceptors). The main controlling influence for somatic nerve activity comes from the motor cortex via the corticospinal tracts (also called pyramidal tracts) to the lower motor neurons (α motor neurons), which is the final neuronal pathway to the muscle.

Skeletal muscle disorders
Myasthenia gravis

Myasthenia gravis is an autoimmune disease affecting the neuromuscular junction (NMJ) (Fig. 14.18). Characteristic symptoms are skeletal muscle weakness and fatigability after a brief period of repeated activity with recovery after a short

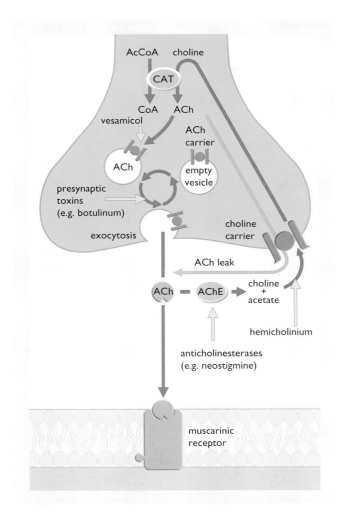

Fig. 14.17 Sites of drug action at a cholinergic nerve terminal.
Drugs can interfere with cholinergic transmission in a variety of ways, including effects on synthesis, storage, release, and uptake, and postjunctional effects. (Adapted with permission from *Pharmacology*, 3rd edn, by Rang, Dale, and Ritter, Churchill Livingstone, 1995.)

period of rest. However, adequate muscle strength may not always return after a period of rest in those patients in whom the disease has progressed to the crisis level. Additionally, about 85% of myasthenic patients experience generalized weakness involving the eyelids, extraocular muscles, limb muscles, diaphragm, and neck extensor muscles. Sometimes the weakness is localized to the eyelids and extraocular muscles, but this occurs in only about 15% of patients and is manifested by the characteristic appearance of drooping eyelids (ptosis).

The prevalence of myasthenia gravis is about 100 cases/ million of the US population and it usually occurs in women under 50 years of age, though it also occurs in a significant number of men over 60 years of age.

The pathophysiologic features of myasthenia gravis result from a deficit in the number of nicotinic cholinergic receptors at the NMJ

The population of nicotinic cholinergic receptors at myasthenic muscle end-plates is only about one-third of that at normal

muscle end-plates. The receptor deficit appears to be linked to an immunologic response involving the thymus gland, since muscle strength usually improves after the thymus has been removed from myasthenic patients. This immunologic link is supported by the finding of cholinergic receptor antibodies in the serum of myasthenic patients. Furthermore, it appears that the antigen may be located in the thymus (Fig. 14.19), since cholinergic receptors have been demonstrated on the surface of muscle-like cells in the thymus. The triggering mechanism for the immune response is uncertain, but it may be due to a defect in the regulation of the immune response in myasthenic patients, as normal individuals also have thymic muscle-like cells with cholinergic receptors.

In myasthenia gravis, neurally induced somatic muscle contraction is inadequate for sustained physical activities

This is because the magnitude of neurally induced contraction depends on the number of interactions between ACh and nicotinic receptors at the NMJ. Normally ACh is released from the nerve terminal and diffuses across the junctional cleft to interact with nicotinic cholinergic receptors on the muscle end-plate (see Fig. 14.18). The transmitter–receptor interactions produce a localized end-plate potential, mainly due to increased Na^+ permeability. If this potential reaches a threshold value, an action potential is produced and invades the muscle fiber, causing contraction. These events are terminated by strategically located acetylcholinesterase enzymes in the synaptic folds; these enzymes metabolize ACh. For sustained muscle contraction, this cycle of events must take place in many muscle fibers, which act together to generate muscle power.

In myasthenia gravis, contraction cannot be sustained because the number of transmitter–receptor interactions is lower than normal, owing to the deficit in nicotinic cholinergic receptors at the muscle end-plate (see Figs 14.18, 14.19). Furthermore, this reduced number of transmitter–receptor interactions means that action potentials can be generated only in a small proportion of the muscle fibers. Contraction is therefore likely to fail after a brief period of muscle activity. However, this failure can be prevented by enhancing the number of cholinergic transmitter–receptor interactions.

Effective drug treatment of myasthenia gravis enhances the number of cholinergic transmitter–receptor interactions

Treatment of myasthenia gravis involves procedures that:
- Increase the junctional synaptic concentration of ACh (e.g. anticholinesterase drugs).
- Suppress the immune response.

Anticholinesterase drugs

ACh is the junctional transmitter that mediates somatic muscle contractions, but it cannot be given effectively as a drug because it is rapidly metabolized by acetylcholinesterase at the NMJ. However, the concentration of ACh at the NMJ can be increased by using anticholinesterase drugs, which inhibit the metabolism of ACh. The peak effects of anticholinesterase drugs are typically obtained promptly during the initial phases of

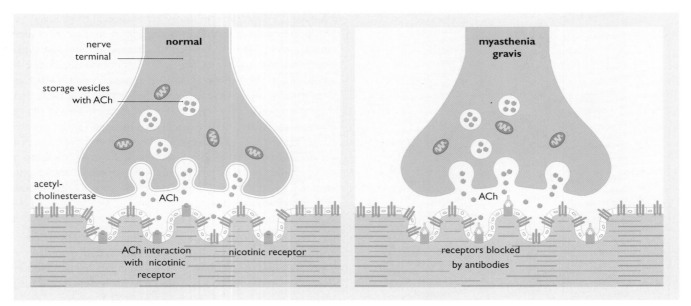

Fig. 14.18 Neurotransmitter release and its interaction with nicotinic receptors at the neuromuscular junction (NMI). In myasthenia gravis the nicotinic receptors are blocked by antibodies, preventing interaction between the neurotransmitter and the receptor. (ACh, acetylcholine)

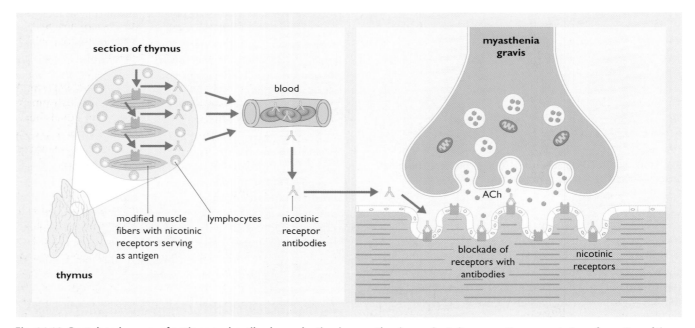

Fig. 14.19 Postulated source of antigen and antibody production in myasthenia gravis. A diagrammatic representation of a section of the thymus gland containing modified muscle cells with nicotinic receptors on the surface. It is suggested that this gland may be the source of the antigen that serves as a template for the production of nicotinic antibodies in myasthenic patients. These antibodies block the nicotinic receptors at the neuromuscular junction and prevent interaction between the neurotransmitter and the nicotinic receptors (see Fig. 14.18). (ACh, acetylcholine)

treatment but, after weeks or months of treatment, the drugs often lose their efficacy. It then becomes necessary to add other drugs to the treatment regimen.

The cholinesterase enzyme, which is inhibited by these drugs, exists in two structurally related forms. One form called acetylcholinesterase (which specifically metabolizes acetylcholine) is found predominantly at the NMJ (and at cholinergic neuroeffector junctions of tissues). The other form is called butyrylcholinesterase (the substrates are non-specific esters) and it is found mainly in the blood plasma. These isoforms of the enzyme have two major binding sites (esteratic and anionic) for which the anticholinesterase drugs compete with acetylcholine to inhibit its metabolism. The drugs that inhibit the acetylcholinesterase enzyme can be grouped into two categories based on the site and stability of the interaction with the enzyme, e.g. reversible and irreversible inhibitors.

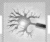

■ *Carbamates represent a major group of reversible anticholinesterases*

The carbamates, particularly neostigmine and pyridostigmine, are among the most widely used anticholinesterase drugs for treatment of myasthenia gravis (Fig. 14.20). Both drugs reversibly inhibit acetylcholinesterase by binding at its anionic and esteratic sites. During the period of inhibition of 3–6 hours, ACh concentration increases at the NMJ and as a result there are repeated interactions with the reduced number of nicotinic cholinergic receptors. This leads to improved muscle contraction in the myasthenic patient. Both drugs are given orally, but pyridostigmine has greater bioavailability and longer duration of action (half-life 4 hours) than neostigmine (half-life 2 hours) which is incompletely absorbed.

■ *Grip strength and lung vital capacity are usually used for monitoring the improvement in muscle strength produced by anticholinesterase drugs*

Another reversible but short acting anticholinesterase such as edrophonium chloride is used for this type of monitoring (and for diagnosis of myasthenia gravis). This monitoring procedure is a precautionary measure to prevent excessive dosing, which may decrease muscle strength by ACh-induced depolarization blockade of nicotinic cholinergic receptors at the NMJ of patients with myasthenia gravis. To produce its effect, edrophonium competes with acetylcholine for reversible binding at the anionic site of acetylcholinesterase. Improvement in muscle strength with edrophonium lasts for about 5 minutes when the drug is given intravenously. However, despite the short duration of action of edrophonium, atropine should be available to counter muscarinic side effects due to accumulation of acetylcholine.

Longer-acting anticholinesterase drugs

Longer-acting (i.e. over 3–8 hours) anticholinesterase drugs such as ambenonium can also be used in the treatment of myasthenia gravis. This drug acts similarly to the carbamates, but it has a longer duration of action. However, the organo-phosphates, which are also long-acting anticholinesterases, are not used because of difficulty in controlling the dose in relation to the patient's need. This difficulty is due to the irreversible binding of this category of drug to the esteratic site of acetylcholinesterase. These drugs are used primarily as insecticides (e.g. parathion, malathion) and as biologic weapons in war (e.g. tabun, sarin). But occasionally, echothiophate is used in treatment of some forms of glaucoma.

ADVERSE EFFECTS OF ANTICHOLINESTERASE DRUGS result from the widespread accumulation of acetylcholine leading to stimulation of muscarinic receptors on many tissues. The effects include abdominal cramps, increased salivation, increased bronchial secretions, miosis, and bradycardia. These effects can be controlled with muscarinic receptor antagonists such as atropine, but this is not usually given as it is preferable not to mask the appearance of the muscarinic effects, which are indicative of excessive anticholinesterase treatment. However, most patients become tolerant to these adverse effects.

DRUG INTERACTIONS WITH ANTICHOLINESTERASES The effectiveness of the anticholinesterases is diminished and the symptoms of myasthenia gravis are worsened if the patient is exposed to either tubocurarine (a nondepolarizing neuromuscular blocker) or an aminoglycoside antibiotic, which interferes with neuromuscular transmission.

DRUGS THAT SUPPRESS THE IMMUNE RESPONSE IN MYASTHENIA GRAVIS Since the effectiveness of anticholinesterase treatment often diminishes within weeks or months, additional therapeutic measures are used. These include the oral use of immunosuppressant drugs such as the glucocorticosteroids which are indicated if muscle strength is inadequate.

Glucocorticosteroids

Glucocorticosteroids are used in the treatment of myasthenia gravis because they can inhibit the synthesis of the antibodies to the nicotinic cholinergic receptors at the NMJ (see Fig. 14.20). Prednisolone or prednisone are typical glucocorticosteroids used for this indication. Their action leads to an increase in the number of free nicotinic cholinergic receptors for interaction with ACh, and as a consequence muscle strength improves in myasthenic patients. It has been suggested that the beneficial effects of prednisolone may be partly due to increased synthesis of ACh receptors, which would also improve neuromuscular transmission in myasthenia gravis.

In the early stages of treatment with prednisolone, muscle weakness may increase, therefore patients should be hospitalized when it is first used. Alternatively, the risk can be minimized by starting therapy with a combination of an anticholinesterase and a small dose of prednisolone of about 20 mg. As the muscle strength improves, the glucocorticosteroid dose can be gradually increased while the anticholinesterase dose is simultaneously reduced until the glucocorticosteroid alone produces a desirable level of muscle strength. However, since glucocorticosteroid treatment of myasthenia gravis is often long term, an alternate-day treatment regimen is preferred to reduce the risk of adverse

Drugs used for the treatment of myasthenia gravis	
Drug	Major effect
Anticholinesterases (e.g. neostigmine, pyridostigmine, ambenonium)	Increase acetylcholine concentration at the neuromuscular junction
Glucocorticosteroids (e.g. prednisolone, prednisone)	Inhibit the synthesis of nicotinic receptor antibody
Azathioprine	Inhibits the synthesis of nicotinic receptor antibody
Cyclosporine	Inhibits the synthesis of nicotinic receptor antibody

Fig. 14.20 **Drugs used for the treatment of myasthenia gravis.**

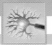

effects. With this regimen, maximum therapeutic benefits are obtained within 6–12 months. The adverse effects of glucocorticosteroids are described in Chapter 15.

Azathioprine

Azathioprine (see also Chapters 12 and 16) is used as an alternative to prednisolone for advanced myasthenia gravis and for other forms of this disease that do not respond adequately to glucocorticosteroid therapy (see Fig. 14.20). Azathioprine is effective because it suppresses nicotinic cholinergic receptor antibody synthesis by inhibiting B-lymphocyte proliferation. Also, its effectiveness may be due to the metabolite, 6-mercaptopurine, which inhibits DNA synthesis (see Chapter 12). However, its therapeutic effectiveness develops slowly, taking up to 1 year to produce satisfactory clinical responses.

MAJOR ADVERSE EFFECTS OF AZATHIOPRINE include a reaction similar to influenza, nausea and vomiting, dermatitis, bone marrow depression and hepatotoxicity. Many of these adverse effects may develop into serious toxicity if azathioprine is used in combination with either 6-mercaptopurine or allopurinol.

Cyclosporine

Cyclosporine is another immunosuppressant drug that can be used in the treatment of myasthenia gravis (see Fig. 14.20). Its effectiveness is due to inhibition of the synthesis of nicotinic cholinergic receptor antibody by blocking the activation of T-helper cells (see Chapter 16) and, as a consequence, the subsequent events that lead to antibody production are suppressed. The therapeutic benefits of cyclosporine are obtained earlier (within 1–2 months) than with azathioprine.

MAJOR ADVERSE EFFECTS OF CYCLOSPORINE include renal toxicity, hepatotoxicity, hypertension, and tremor (see Chapter 12).

Other approaches to the treatment of myasthenia gravis

Surgical removal of the thymus is often recommended when the dose of immunosuppressant drugs needs to be reduced so as to prevent the development of serious adverse effects. The benefits of surgery include removal of the source responsible for the sustained antigenic stimulation that leads to the production of antibodies to the nicotinic cholinergic receptors at the NMJ. This surgical procedure is not recommended for children below the age of puberty because of the need to preserve the role of the thymus in the developing immune system.

PLASMAPHERESIS can be used to remove ACh nicotinic receptor antibodies from the circulation, but it is used as short-term therapy only in patients who are experiencing a myasthenic crisis (i.e. exacerbation of symptoms of the disease). The therapeutic effectiveness of this procedure occurs within days but only lasts for a few weeks.

Spasticity

The major pathophysiologic feature of spasticity is hypertonic skeletal muscle contraction. It often occurs as a symptom of neurologic disorders such as cerebral palsy, multiple sclerosis, and stroke. The causes of hypertonia in muscles are:

- Excessive tendon (stretch) reflexes driven by increased γ neuron activity and triggered by excitation of muscle spindles.
- Flexor muscle spasms, which are due to clonus produced by a volley of discharge from spindle afferents onto several lower motor neurons (α motor neurons).

▇ *Spasticity is treated with drugs that reduce excessive afferent stimulation of the α motor neurons innervating the skeletal muscles*

Drugs that reduce excessive afferent stimulation of the α motor neurons (Fig. 14.21) are preferable to the neuromuscular blockers for treating spasticity because they are more selective. In comparison with these drugs, neuromuscular blockers produce relaxation by disrupting both normal muscle tone and increased tone due to spasm of any etiology.

Baclofen

Baclofen is derived (as a chlorophenyl analog) from the inhibitory neurotransmitter GABA, and it was designed as a source of GABA that could more readily cross the blood–brain barrier.

In the treatment of spasticity, baclofen is most useful for reducing flexor and extensor spasms. These effects are produced at the level of the spinal cord, but they are not associated with any interference with voluntary muscle power or normal tendon reflexes.

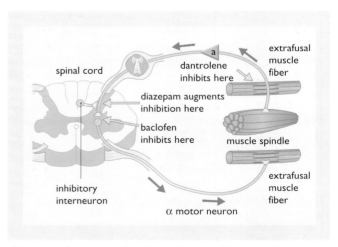

Fig. 14.21 The neuronal pathway that contributes to the development of clonus in spasticity is inhibited by diazepam and baclofen. Stretching the muscle activates the IA afferents from the muscle spindle and sends a flood of impulses to the α motor neuron, triggering contraction of the muscle. This relieves the tension on the spindle and terminates activity in the afferents. However, when the muscle relaxes, the tension on the spindle returns because the sensitivity of the reflex is increased in spasticity and the cycle of events is repeated, giving rise to clonus.

Baclofen produces these effects by inhibiting the afferent input to the α motor neurons via interaction with presynaptic GABA$_B$ receptors on the afferent nerve terminals and associated interneurons. It is believed that the interaction of baclofen with GABA$_B$ receptors (coupled to a G protein) reduces Ca^{2+} influx into the afferent nerve. As a result, less neurotransmitter is released for activating the α motor neurons, which become less active and less susceptible to the cycle of events that sustain spasticity.

▨ *Baclofen is effective for spasticity due to spinal cord lesions and multiple sclerosis, but is ineffective for spasticity due to stroke and other cerebral lesions*
Baclofen is usually given orally and it is rapidly absorbed from the gut. It has a plasma half-life of 3–4 hours and approximately 35% is excreted unchanged by the kidneys and in the feces.

MAJOR ADVERSE EFFECTS OF BACLOFEN include drowsiness (less than with diazepam), motor incoordination, mental confusion, nausea, and hypotension (especially after overdose). An overdose may produce seizures, and it is therefore not recommended for patients with epilepsy. Furthermore, baclofen should be withdrawn gradually at the termination of treatment after prolonged use because sudden withdrawal can cause hallucinations, anxiety, and tachycardia.

Diazepam
▨ *Diazepam is effective for treatment of spasticity associated with spinal cord lesions, but is less effective than baclofen, especially against flexor spasm*
Diazepam is a member of the benzodiazepine group of drugs (see below). It is useful in the treatment of spasticity because it reduces muscle tone by depressing polysynaptic and mono-synaptic reflexes. These reflexes help to maintain muscle spasticity. Although this action of diazepam can be produced at both spinal and supraspinal levels, it appears that the spinal level is the important site of action in reducing spasticity. To produce this effect in the spinal cord, diazepam binds (via benzodiazepine receptors) to GABA$_A$ receptor complexes on afferent nerve terminals that synapse with α motor neurons (see Fig. 14.21). It therefore increases presynaptic inhibition mediated by GABA which increases Cl$^-$ influx following interaction with GABA$_A$ receptors (Fig. 14.22). Diazepam can be given orally or intravenously. Its half-life is about 60 hours to which the active metabolite, nordiazepam, contributes.

▨ *Diazepam causes dose-dependent drowsiness as a side effect*

Dantrolene sodium
Unlike baclofen and diazepam, dantrolene sodium relieves spasticity by a direct action on skeletal muscle (see Fig. 14.22).
Dantrolene sodium is a hydantoin derivative that not only relieves spasticity but also produces muscle weakness, which reduces its clinical usefulness. Its mechanism of action involves interference with skeletal muscle excitation–contraction coupling by decreasing the amount of Ca^{2+} released from the

Drugs used for treatment of spasticity	
Drugs	**Mechanism of action**
Baclofen	Inhibits flexor and extensor muscle spasm via GABA$_B$ receptor-mediated blockade of afferent stimulation of the α motor neuron
Diazepam	GABA$_A$ receptor-mediated presynaptic inhibition of afferent stimulation of the α motor neuron
Dantrolene sodium	Inhibition of skeletal muscle excitation–contraction coupling by decreasing Ca^{2+} released from the sarcoplasmic reticulum

Fig. 14.22 Drugs used for treatment of spasticity. (GABA, γ-aminobutyric acid)

sarcoplasmic reticulum. This reduces the tension generated by the muscle.

▨ *Dantrolene sodium is mainly used to relieve the spasticity of paraplegia and hemiplegia*
Dantrolene sodium is usually given orally, but it is not completely absorbed. It has a half-life of 9 hours and it is metabolized by the liver.

ADVERSE EFFECTS OF DANTROLENE SODIUM include muscle weakness and sedation, and sometimes hepatotoxicity. It is contraindicated in patients with either respiratory muscle weakness or liver disease. Also, it is recommended that regular liver function tests should be done when this drug is used therapeutically.

Movement disorders resulting from defects in muscle excitability
Although many movement disorders are attributed to defects in the basal ganglia, some disorders result from impairment of neuromuscular transmission and skeletal muscle excitability (e.g. Lambert–Eaton syndrome, McCardle syndrome, congenital myotonia, and tetany).

Lambert–Eaton syndrome (myasthenia syndrome)
Lambert–Eaton syndrome is associated with a variety of malignancies, especially lung cancer. This syndrome occurs more frequently in males of age 50–60 years. As the NMJ is the site of the defect, it resembles myasthenia gravis in terms of symptoms of fatigability and depressed limb reflexes. However, it differs from myasthenia gravis because the weakness, which particularly affects the limb muscles, does not respond to treatment with anticholinesterase drugs. This is because, unlike myasthenia gravis, which results from a reduction in the number of nicotinic cholinergic receptors at the NMJ, Lambert–Eaton syndrome results from disrupted coupling between nerve terminal excitation and ACh release at the NMJ (Fig. 14.23). In

233

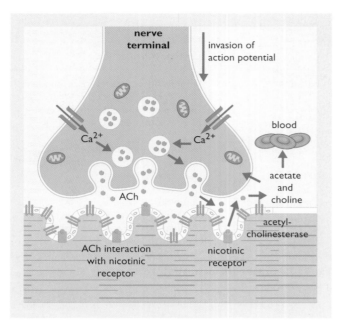

Fig. 14.23 Action potential-induced release of the neurotransmitter acetylcholine (ACh) and its metabolism at the neuromuscular junction.

Treatment of movement disorders due to defects in muscle excitability	
Disorder	Treatment
Lambert–Eaton syndrome	Ca^{2+} salts, physical exercise
McCardle syndrome	Large doses of glucose, injection of epinephrine or glucagon
Congenital myotonia	Membrane stabilizers such as quinine and phenytoin
Tetany	Normalize plasma Ca^{2+}

Fig. 14.24 Treatment of movement disorders due to defects in muscle excitability.

some patients this is associated with autoantibodies directed against neuronal voltage-gated Ca^{2+} channels. It appears that voltage-gated Ca^{2+} channels are present in the tissue of small-cell lung cancer, therefore this malignant tissue represents a source for development of Ca^{2+} channel antibodies which are commonly found in Lambert–Eaton syndrome associated with this malignancy. Approaches to treatment of this syndrome involve procedures that increase the release of transmitter at the NMJ. These include:

- Physical exercise, which improves muscle power.
- Ca^{2+} salts, which seem to be beneficial because Ca^{2+} plays an important role in the release of neurotransmitter from nerve terminals (Figs 14.23, 14.24).
- 3,4-diaminopyridine, which increases neurotransmitter release by blocking K^+ conductance at the nerve terminals. This drug is given orally about 4 to 5 times daily. Its major adverse effect is CNS stimulation.

McCardle syndrome

Characteristically, the main symptoms of this syndrome are disabling weakness, muscle pain, and stiffness after a brief period of exercise. These symptoms are produced because the muscles fail to relax, owing to inadequate production of ATP, which is necessary for Ca^{2+} sequestration in the sarcoplasmic reticulum to terminate contraction. The underlying cause of inadequate ATP production is an inability to liberate glucose from glycogen due to an inherited deficiency of glycogen phosphorylase in the muscles. These patients have only a limited supply of ATP from blood glucose and fatty acids for muscle activity, which is therefore brief. Also, these patients do not show the typical increase in blood lactate and pyruvate after exercise.

Treatment of this syndrome includes the administration of large doses of glucose or the injection of epinephrine or glucagon to increase glucose release from the liver (see Fig. 14.24).

Congenital myotonia

Congenital myotonia is an inherited disorder characterized by violent muscle spasm due to irritability of the muscle fiber membrane. The irritability is due to a structural defect in the muscle fiber membrane that renders the fiber hyperexcitable and therefore easily re-excited by the afterpotential that follows an action potential. It appears that the afterpotential is prolonged by accumulation of extracellular K^+ and decreased Cl^- conductance. Normal Cl^- conductance is required for muscle relaxation.

Membrane stabilizers such as quinine and phenytoin can be used orally to reduce the frequency and severity of the spasm.

Tetany

Tetany is characterized by widespread muscular twitching, together with persistent contraction of muscles in the hands and feet, resulting in painful cramps. The cause of tetany is due to hypocalcemia, which increases excitability of the somatic nerves. It is suggested that low extracellular Ca^{2+} decreases the depolarizing current that is required to open Na^+ channels in somatic nerves and causes repetitive firing, leading to persistent muscle contraction.

Tetany is treated with Ca^{2+} salts (e.g. Ca^{2+} gluconate) to restore extracellular Ca^{2+} concentrations.

Dysautonomias

Dysautonomias are disorders associated with defects in the autonomic nervous system (e.g. familial dysautonomia (Riley–Day syndrome), Shy–Drager syndrome, and Horner syndrome).

Familial dysautonomia

This is an inherited disorder transmitted as an autosomal recessive trait and characterized by a complex mixture of symptoms. It is more common in Ashkenazi Jewish infants than in other ethnic group. Manifestations of the disorder are usually present at birth and the child commonly dies during infancy. The major symptoms include an inability to control body temperature and to produce tears, uncontrollable perspiration, hypertension and sometimes postural hypotension, corneal and pain insensitivity, fever, and frequent episodes of pneumonia. These symptoms are associated with defects in both the parasympathetic and sympathetic divisions of the autonomic nervous system as well as defects in some peripheral sensory nerves (Fig. 14.25). The cutaneous nerves contain a decreased number of unmyelinated fibers, which are the neuronal pathways for pain and temperature sensation. Neurons in the vagus and the glossopharyngeal nerves are typically smaller and reduced in number. Similarly, there appear to be fewer neurons in the cervical and thoracic sympathetic ganglia.

Treatment is symptomatic as there is no cure (Fig. 14.26). Sedatives (e.g. diazepam) and the phenothiazine drugs (e.g. chlorpromazine) are often used for gastrointestinal and behavioral symptoms. In addition, antibiotics are used for pulmonary infection (see Chapter 19), which is quite common.

Shy-Drager syndrome

This syndrome is also due to autonomic nervous system failure. It is characterized by a complex mixture of symptoms, which include severe postural hypotension, urinary incontinence, male erectile dysfunction, akinesia, tremor, muscle rigidity, and the inability to sweat. Pathologic evidence suggests that the autonomic deficiency is due to a loss of preganglionic sympathetic cells from the intermediolateral column of cells in the spinal cord. There also appears to be CNS motor control involvement with the syndrome, as reflected in the symptoms of akinesia and muscle rigidity.

The most troublesome symptom is postural hypotension, which is treated with small doses of fludrocortisone (0.1 mg). This increases Na^+ and water retention and may increase the sensitivity of blood vessels to catecholamines. α Adrenergic agonists are also used, including phenylephrine and ephedrine; however, the disadvantage of these drugs is that they tend to produce hypertension when the patient is supine.

Horner's syndrome

Horner's syndrome results from a loss of cervical sympathetic control to the head. It is characterized by miosis due to the loss of pupillary dilation, slight drooping of the eyelids (ptosis), recession of the eyeball (enophthalmos), facial vasodilation, and loss of the ability to sweat. These symptoms are often unilateral and may result from an injury or tumor involving either the preganglionic or postganglionic cervical sympathetic nerves. Lung cancer is a common cause.

The location of the lesion must be clearly defined for effective treatment, for example:

• If the lesion is confined to preganglionic fibers, both directly and indirectly acting sympathomimetics (phenylephrine, ephedrine, and cocaine) are effective (e.g. restoration of mydriatic response). This is because their effects are mediated via direct action on the tissue receptor and indirectly by the

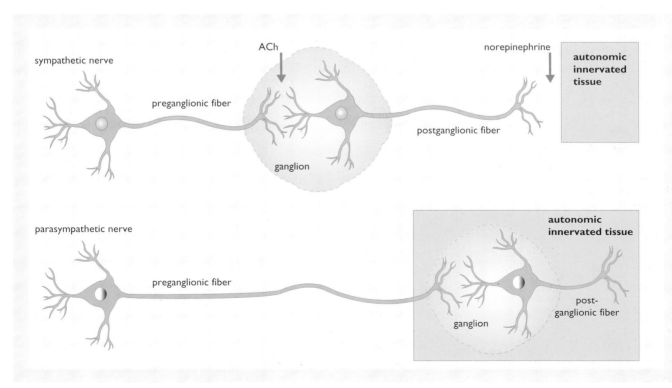

Fig. 14.25 The two major divisions of the autonomic nervous system that may become defective in dysautonomia.

Treatment of dysautonomias

Disorder	Treatment
Familial dysautonomia (Riley–Day syndrome)	Symptomatic (i.e. autonomic drugs, sedatives, phenothiazines, and antibiotics for pulmonary infection)
Shy–Drager syndrome	Fludrocortisone, phenylephrine, and ephedrine to counteract the postural hypotension
Horner's syndrome	Directly and indirectly acting sympathomimetics for preganglionic lesions and directly acting sympathomimetics for postganglionic lesions

Fig. 14.26 Treatment of dysautonomias.

release of stored norepinephrine from the postganglionic nerve terminal, respectively (see Fig. 14.25).

• If the lesion is on the postganglionic fiber, only the directly acting sympathomimetics (e.g. phenylephrine) are therapeutically effective. The indirectly acting agents are ineffective because they act on functioning postganglionic fibers.

FUNCTIONAL ANATOMY OF THE CENTRAL NERVOUS SYSTEM

The spinal cord is part of the CNS and consists of ascending and descending tracts passing information between the brain and the PNS. The tracts are interconnected at various levels by short interneurons, which allow a degree of integration and control of motor function and sensory input at a spinal level (Fig. 14.27).

The medulla oblongata is directly continuous with the spinal cord and is the first part of the brainstem (Fig. 14.28a). It also contains the nuclei for cranial nerves V, IX, X, XI, and XII and is where motor fibers and some sensory fibers cross.

The pons lies between the medulla and midbrain. It can be viewed as a relay station between the cerebellum, the brain, and the PNS. It contains the nuclei for cranial nerves V, VI, VII, and VIII, and motor nuclei in the pontine reticular formation that participate in postural, cardiovascular, and respiratory control (Fig. 14.28b).

The cerebellum lies posterior to the pons (Fig. 14.29), and has incoming and outgoing connections, with sensory and motor tracts ascending and descending the spinal cord. It is the largest motor structure in the brain. Although its function is not entirely clear, the multiplicity of its connections allows the cerebellum to exert fine control over motor functioning and to act as a center for integrating sensory and motor information for performing complex tasks.

Above the pons lies the midbrain (mesencephalon). This is the most primitive part of the human brain and ends in two huge fiber bundles, which form the cerebral peduncles, carrying fibers to and from the thalamus and cerebral hemispheres. It also contains the superior (visual) and inferior (auditory) colliculi (Figs 14.28c, 14.28d), the nuclei for cranial nerves III and IV, two motor nuclei, the red nucleus, and the substantia nigra, which links and acts as a relay between the basal ganglia and the motor system (see Fig. 14.28c).

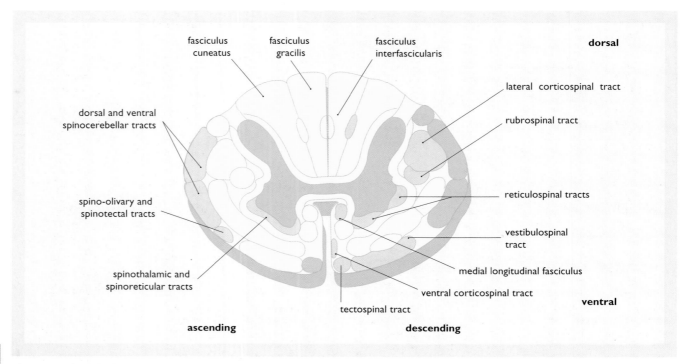

Fig. 14.27 The spinal cord at the midcervical level showing the major tracts of the spinal white matter.

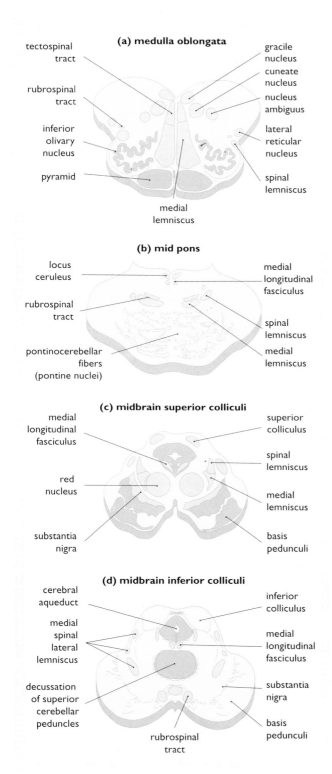

(a) medulla oblongata

tectospinal tract

rubrospinal tract

inferior olivary nucleus

pyramid

gracile nucleus

cuneate nucleus

nucleus ambiguus

lateral reticular nucleus

spinal lemniscus

medial lemniscus

(b) mid pons

locus ceruleus

rubrospinal tract

pontinocerebellar fibers (pontine nuclei)

medial longitudinal fasciculus

spinal lemniscus

medial lemniscus

(c) midbrain superior colliculi

medial longitudinal fasciculus

red nucleus

substantia nigra

superior colliculus

spinal lemniscus

medial lemniscus

basis pedunculi

(d) midbrain inferior colliculi

cerebral aqueduct

medial spinal lateral lemniscus

decussation of superior cerebellar peduncles

rubrospinal tract

inferior colliculus

medial longitudinal fasciculus

substantia nigra

basis pedunculi

Fig. 14.28 The medulla oblongata, pons, and midbrain. (a) The medulla oblongata is the first part of the brainstem and motor fibers and some sensory fibers cross here. (b) The pons lies between the medulla and midbrain. It can be considered as a relay station between the cerebellum, the brain, and the peripheral nervous system. (c) The midbrain superior colliculi allow tracking of visual stimuli. (d) The midbrain inferior colliculi provide selective attention to auditory stimuli.

The diencephalon, the central core of the cerebrum, consists of the hypothalamus, subthalamus, epithalamus, and thalamus (Fig. 14.30).

- The hypothalamus subserves many homeostatic functions such as regulation of the ANS and endocrine function via the pituitary. It also has a role in the control of basic drives such as those involved in hunger, thirst, threat, procreation, and fatigue.
- The subthalamus is involved in motor function and has connections to the basal ganglia, the red nucleus, and the substantia nigra.
- The epithalamus consists of the habenular nuclei and the pineal gland. The habenular nuclei are the center for the integration of olfactory, visceral, and somatic afferent pathways, and are connected to the reticular formation. The function of the pineal gland is unclear, but it contains high

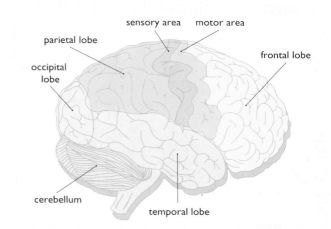

sensory area   motor area

parietal lobe

occipital lobe

frontal lobe

cerebellum

temporal lobe

Fig. 14.29 A lateral view of the brain.

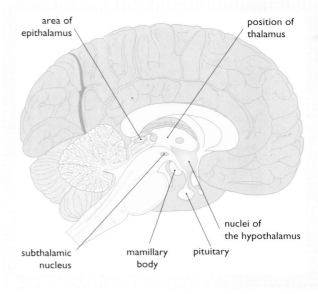

area of epithalamus

position of thalamus

subthalamic nucleus

mamillary body

pituitary

nuclei of the hypothalamus

Fig. 14.30 The diencephalon. This consists of the hypothalamus, subthalamus, epithalamus, and the thalamus.

237

concentrations of melatonin and 5-HT and may have a role in circadian rhythm regulation.

- The thalamus is the largest part of the diencephalon and is closely related both functionally and anatomically to the cerebral cortices. Almost all fibers passing to the cerebral hemispheres pass through and synapse within the thalamus. It has outgoing connections with virtually every part of the cerebrum and its function is most likely to be integration of incoming sensory information via its interconnected nuclei. The information is then passed to the cerebral cortex for interpretation.

Basal ganglia is a collective term given to bilateral masses of deeply sited gray matter (Fig. 14.31). They have afferent and efferent connections with the cerebral cortex, the thalamus, subthalamus, and brainstem, and they are thought to control motor function by an effect on the cerebral hemispheres.

The cerebral hemispheres form the telencephalon. Consciousness and the ability to adapt and react to changing circumstances result from the complexity and size of the right and left hemispheres. The ability to use complex methods of communication is also provided by the telencephalon. These capabilities lead to the capacity for abstract thought and therefore the ability to learn and profit not only from our own experiences but also those of others, and to generate hypotheses. This higher functioning leads to the development of a rich emotional life and therefore the risk of profound mental illness.

Certain functions are associated more with some areas of the cerebral hemispheres than others

The cerebral hemispheres can be divided into the frontal, temporal, parietal, and occipital cortices (see Fig. 14.29). The precise localization of function within the brain is not known,

possibly because no single function resides exclusively in any one particular area. However, as with the lower parts of the CNS, certain functions are associated more with some areas than others:

- Voluntary motor function is subserved by the precentral gyrus of the frontal lobe.
- Sensory function lies in the postcentral gyrus of the parietal lobe.
- Part of the dominant frontal lobe appears to have a primary role in the production of speech.
- Part of the frontal lobes bilaterally appear to be involved in the formation of personality, higher reasoning, and intellectual functioning.
- The temporal lobes provide a large proportion of memory function and integration as well as the auditory centers.
- The parietal lobes appear to have a complex integrating function for sensory and motor and, to a lesser extent, emotional functioning. They also allow planning and initiation of complex actions and have a crucial role in topographic, object and word recognition and their association with emotion.
- The occipital cortices receive and process visual input.

The limbic system has a crucial role in memory and emotion

The limbic system is a collection of connected structures in the cerebrum, including a variety of deep structures such as the amygdala, selected areas of the cerebral cortex such as the cingulate, and segments of other structures such as the hypothalamus (Figs 14.32, 14.33). The basic component of the limbic system is the Papez circuit. In this loop the hippocampus transmits information through the fornices to the mamillary bodies of the hypothalamus, which transmit to the anterior nucleus of the thalamus via the mamillothalamic tracts. Information is then sent via the internal capsule back to the hippocampus. The precise functions of the limbic system remain unclear, but lesions of specific parts that disrupt the various loops lead to:

- Amnesia, which is associated with lesions of the mamillary bodies in Korsakoff's syndrome, or with lesions of the temporal lobes.

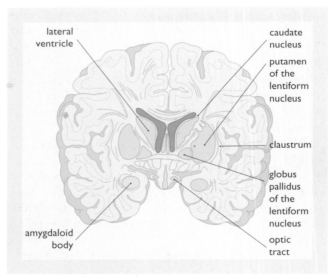

Fig. 14.31 Basal ganglia. The bilaterally represented masses of gray matter form deep structures. The corpus striatum consists of the caudate nucleus and the lentiform nucleus, which are separated by the internal capsule except at the anterior–inferior aspect of the caudate nucleus where the head of the caudate is continuous with the putamen of the lentiform nucleus. The lentiform nucleus consists of the putamen and the globus pallidus.

Labels in figure: lateral ventricle; caudate nucleus; putamen of the lentiform nucleus; claustrum; globus pallidus of the lentiform nucleus; amygdaloid body; optic tract

The major components of the limbic system

- Regions of the limbic cortex (cingulate, parahippocampal gyrus, entorrhinal cortex)
- Hippocampal formation (dentate gyrus, hippocampus)
- Amygdala (basolateral complex, centromedial complex, parts of the stria terminalis and the hypothalamus)
- Nucleus accumbens
- Mamillary bodies
- Anterior and dorsomedial nuclei of the thalamus (some authors also include other cortical regions including the orbitofrontal area, the temporal poles and the insula)

Fig. 14.32 The major components of the limbic system.

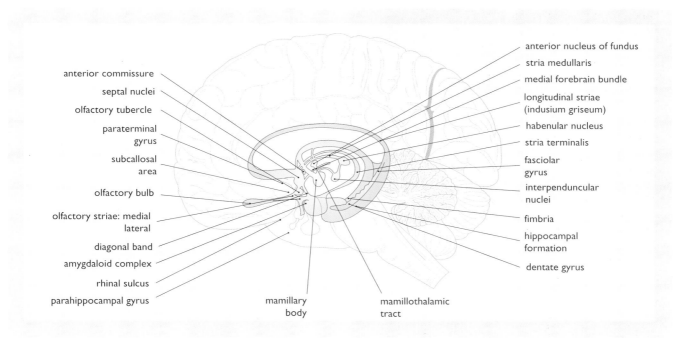

Fig. 14.33 The anatomic relations of the amygdala, the hippocampus, and other components of the limbic system.

- Placidity, which is associated with lesions of the amygdala.
- Rage, which is associated with lesions of the posterior hypothalamus.

The symptoms of hallucinations and delusions in psychiatric patients may result from limbic system dysfunction.

The reticular formation has a nonspecific alerting function and contributes to motor, sensory (pain), and autonomic function

The reticular formation is a network of neurons with diffuse dendritic connections that occupies the midline of the brainstem and extends upwards from the substantia intermedia of the spinal cord to the intralaminar nuclei of the thalamus. It is loosely organized into three longitudinal nuclear columns (i.e. median, medial, and lateral), which are each subdivided into three ventrocaudally (mesencephalic, pontine, and medullary).

The reticular formation has input from ascending sensory neurons, the cerebellum, the basal ganglia, the hypothalamus, and the cerebral cortex. There are outputs to the hypothalamus, the thalamus, and the spinal cord.

The nonspecific alerting function of the reticular formation appears to be related to the ascending reticulothalamocortical pathway (ascending reticular activating system). The reticular formation also makes contributions to motor, sensory (pain), and autonomic function, especially affecting respiration and vasomotor function.

FUNCTIONAL NEUROCHEMISTRY OF THE NERVOUS SYSTEM

The neurotransmitters listed in Figs 14.8 and 14.10 are found within specific regions of the nervous system and together with the complex anatomic arrangement provide for the sophisticated function of the human brain.

Glutamate is the major excitatory neurotransmitter in the CNS

Glutamate is an amino acid and acts on N-methyl-D-aspartate (NMDA) and non-NMDA receptors. It is the primary neurotransmitter in thalamocortical, pyramidal cell, and corticostriatal projections, and is an important transmitter in the hippocampus. It has been suggested that as some drugs that act on the NMDA receptor produce psychotic symptoms, abnormalities of the glutamate system may have a causative role in psychotic illnesses.

GABA is the major inhibitory neurotransmitter in the nervous system

GABA is also an amino acid and acts primarily on $GABA_A$ and $GABA_B$ receptors. $GABA_A$ receptors are the most common and are present on 40% of neurons. The cortical distribution of $GABA_A$ is shown in Fig. 14.34. $GABA_A$ is a receptor-operated Cl^- channel, while $GABA_B$ receptors are coupled to G proteins.

Benzodiazepines and most anticonvulsants have their effects on the GABA receptor:

- Benzodiazepines act on a specific benzodiazepine receptor on a subunit of the GABA receptor and enhance the effects of GABA on the receptor, thereby acting as neuromodulators.
- Some anticonvulsants have similar effects to benzodiazepines, but most act directly on the GABA receptor.

Abnormalities of the GABA system are thought to be associated with anxiety disorders, and recent work has suggested a role for GABA in the etiology of schizophrenia.

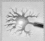

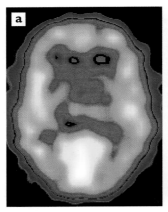 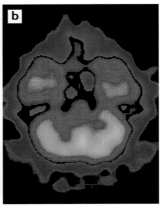

Fig. 14.34 The cortical distribution of γ-aminobutyric acid-A (GABA_A) receptors. This is shown using the radioactively labeled benzodiazepine analog lomazenil and single photon emission tomography (SPET). The brightest areas have the highest density of receptors. (a) The image at the level of the midoccipital cortex. (b) The image at the level of the cerebellum.

■ Glycine is a 'mandatory adjunctive neurotransmitter' for glutamate

Glycine must be present for glutamate to have an effect. It also acts on its own receptor-operated Cl⁻ channel and is inhibitory.

■ Acetylcholine is a central and a peripheral neurotransmitter

ACh can act as a neurotransmitter in the CNS as well as in the periphery (described above).

Centrally, the primary ACh-containing nucleus is the nucleus basalis of Meynert, which is situated in the basal forebrain and has projections to the cerebral cortex and limbic system. Cholinergic fibers in the reticular system project to the cerebral cortex, the limbic system, the hypothalamus, and the thalamus.

■ More than nine distinct 5-HT (serotonin) receptors have been identified

The 5-HT$_{1a}$, 5-HT$_{2a}$, 5-HT$_{2c}$, and 5-HT$_3$ subgroups of 5-HT receptors have been most extensively studied. The major site of serotonergic cell bodies is in the area of the upper pons and midbrain. The classic areas for 5-HT-containing neurons are the median and dorsal raphe nuclei. The neurons from the

raphe nuclei project to the basal ganglia and various parts of the limbic system, and have a wide distribution throughout the cerebral cortices in addition to cerebellar connections (Fig. 14.35).

All the 5-HT receptors identified so far are G protein-coupled receptors except the 5-HT$_3$ receptor, which is a receptor-operated Na⁺/K⁺ channel.

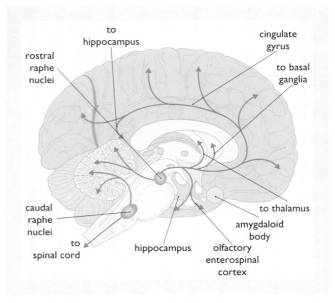

Fig. 14.35 5-Hydroxytryptamine (5-HT) pathways. 5-HT-containing neurons are found in the median and dorsal raphe nuclei, the caudal locus ceruleus, the area postrema, and the interpeduncular area.

Acetylcholine, Parkinson's disease, and Alzheimer's dementia

- The symptoms of Parkinson's disease result from a defect in the balance between acetylcholine and dopamine in the basal ganglia

- Anticholinergic medication is used to treat the parkinsonian adverse effects of antipsychotic medications and idiopathic Parkinson's disease (see page 268)

- Nicotinic and muscarinic agonists or drugs that enhance endogenous acetylcholine function appear to be beneficial in the treatment of Alzheimer's dementia

---

5-Hydroxytryptamine, depression, and anxiety

- Most antidepressant medications inhibit the uptake of 5-HT in the synaptic cleft

- Buspirone is a partial agonist of the presynaptic 5-HT$_{1A}$ receptor and appears to be an effective treatment of anxiety and depression

- 5-HT$_{2A}$ and 5-HT$_{2C}$ receptors appear to play a role in depressive illnesses, the negative symptoms of schizophrenia, and protection against the long-term sequelae of neuroleptics

- There is a relative increase in the number of 5-HT$_{2A}$ receptors in the frontal cortices of suicidal patients

- 5-HT$_{2A}$ receptor antagonists have been used to treat negative schizophrenia with some success

- Antipsychotics with high-affinity antagonistic activity at 5-HT$_{2A}$ receptors (atypical antipsychotics) are a more effective treatment of negative symptom schizophrenia than typical antipsychotics and produce fewer adverse motor effects with a similar level of dopamine blockade

- 5-HT$_3$ receptor antagonists are used in the management of nausea (see page 473)

- Early and current trials of 5-HT$_3$ receptor antagonists in schizophrenia are producing equivocal results

5-HT is synthesized from tryptophan by tryptophan hydroxylase, and the supply of tryptophan is the rate-limiting step in the synthesis of 5-HT. The latter is primarily broken down by monoamine oxidase-a to 5-hydroxyindoleacetic acid (5-HIAA).

Norepinephrine is widely distributed

Norepinephrine can also act as a neurotransmitter in the CNS as well as in the periphery (as described above). Norepinephine can act on several types of adrenoceptor, α_1, α_2, β_{1-3}. The majority of norepinephrine-containing neurons in the CNS are located in the locus ceruleus in the pons/midbrain and their projections to other areas of the brain are shown in Fig. 14.36 (see also Figs 14.28b, 14.28c).

In general it seems that:
- Postsynaptic α_1 receptors are linked to stimulation of phosphoinositol turnover.
- α_2 Receptors inhibit the formation of cAMP.
- β Receptors stimulate the formation of cAMP.

Five types of dopamine receptor (D_1–D_5) have so far been identified in the human nervous system

D_1 and D_5 receptors stimulate the formation of cAMP by activating a stimulatory G protein, while D_2, D_3, and D_4 receptors inhibit the formation of cAMP by activating an inhibitory G protein. D_2 receptors are more ubiquitous than D_3 and D_4 receptors. D_3 receptors are primarily located in the nucleus accumbens (one of the septal nuclei in the limbic system) and D_4 receptors are particularly concentrated in the medial frontal cortex.

🔑 **Norepinephrine and affective and anxiety disorders**

- Norepinephrine is thought to play a crucial role in affective disorders, and to a lesser extent in anxiety disorders
- Abnormalities of norepinephrine-containing neurons are incorporated as part of the monoamine theory of depression (see page 248)
- Most traditional tricyclic antidepressants inhibit the uptake of norepinephrine from the synaptic cleft and thereby increase the availability of synaptic norepinephrine
- Monoamine oxidase inhibitors inhibit the breakdown of norepinephrine
- It is thought that the antidepressant effect of norepinephrine manipulation is mediated by a down-regulation in postsynaptic β receptors

There are a variety of dopaminergic pathways or tracts (Fig. 14.37):
- The nigrostriatal tract projects from the substantia nigra in the midbrain to the corpus striatum, and has a role in motor control.
- The mesolimbic/mesocortical tract has cell bodies in the ventral tegmental area adjacent to the substantia nigra and projects to the limbic system and neocortex in addition to the striatum. It supplies fibers to the medial surface of the frontal lobes and to the parahippocampus and cingulate cortex.
- The third major pathway is the tuberoinfundibular tract. The cell bodies reside in the arcuate nucleus and periventricular

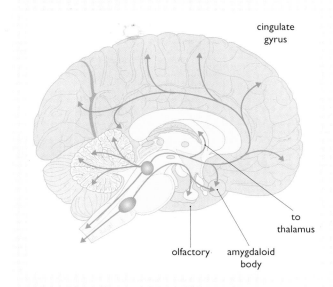

Fig. 14.36 Norepinephrine pathways. Most of the norepinephrine-containing neurons in the central nervous system are located in the locus ceruleus in the pons and midbrain. These neurons project through the medial forebrain bundle to the limbic system, cerebral cortices, the thalamus, and the hypothalamus. A second group of norepinephrine-containing neurons in the ventral tegmental area have projections to the hypothalamus and amygdala.

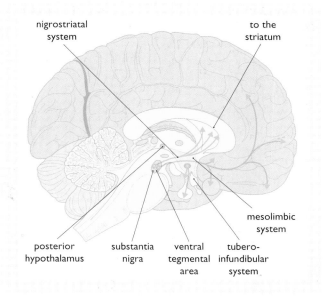

Fig. 14.37 Dopamine pathways. These tracts include the nigrostriatal tract, the mesolimbic/mesocortical tract, and the tuberoinfundibular tract.

241

Dopamine, Parkinson's disease, and psychosis

- Idiopathic Parkinson's disease results from degeneration of cells in the substantia nigra

- Parkinsonian adverse effects of typical antipsychotics (e.g. haloperidol, chlorpromazine) result from blocking of dopamine receptors within the nigrostriatal tract

- Antipsychotic medications are thought to exert beneficial effects on the mesolimbic and mesocortical tract

- The inhibitory drive of prolactin release is removed by dopamine receptor blockade within the tuberoinfundibular tract by antipsychotics and leads to prolactinemia

area of the hypothalamus, and they project to the infundibulum and the anterior pituitary. Dopamine inhibits the release of prolactin within this tract.

Dopamine is synthesized as part of the common pathway for catecholamines (see above), and it is metabolized by two enzymes: MAO-B, which is intraneuronal, and catechol-O-methyl transferase (COMT), which is extraneuronal. The primary metabolite of dopamine is homovanillic acid (HVA).

D_2 receptors were considered to be the most important dopamine receptor in psychosis, as the potency of antipsychotic medications correlated with their affinity for the D_2 receptor. However, the advent of atypical antipsychotics, with equal efficacy but a relatively low potency at the D_2 receptor, raises the possibility that other subtypes of the dopamine receptor may have a more important role in the etiology and treatment of psychosis.

Chronic blockade of dopamine receptors leads to their upregulation and this may contribute to the movement disorders seen with long-term neuroleptic therapy.

There is evidence that the mesolimbic and mesocortical pathways play an important role in the regulation of behaviors governed by positive reinforcers (rewards), and these findings may lead to the development of novel medications for the treatments of addictions.

Peptide neurotransmitters

■ *There may be as many as 300 peptide neurotransmitters in the brain*

A peptide is a short protein consisting of fewer than 100 amino acids. The best-characterized neuropeptides are listed in Fig. 14.10. Often these peptides are synthesized as part of much larger molecules called preprohormones. These are cleaved in the neuronal cytoplasm to prohormones, which are then taken up into vesicles. Within the vesicles the prohormones are further cleaved into the neuroactive peptides. Most peptide neurotransmitters coexist with other neurotransmitters.

■ *Opioids are thought to regulate stress, pain, and mood*

The three endogenous opioid groups listed in Fig. 14.10 (i.e. endorphins, enkephalins, and dynorphins) are synthesized from larger precursor molecules. Enkephalin coexists in noradrenergic and serotonergic neurons. Opioids act on three types of receptors:

- μ, where their action is to decrease production of cAMP and increase K^+ conductance.
- δ, where they have a similar action to that on μ receptors.
- κ, where their action is to decrease K^+ conductance.

■ *The neurohypophysial neuroactive peptides vasopressin and oxytocin are thought to be involved in mood regulation*

The two neurohypophysial hormones vasopressin and oxytocin are synthesized in the hypothalamus and released in the posterior pituitary. There are three receptors for vasopressin and its actions are mediated either by changes in membrane phospholipids or by increasing cAMP.

■ *Tachykinins include substance P and neurokinin*

Substance P is a primary neurotransmitter in most primary afferent sensory neurons and is present in the nigrostriatal tract. It is associated with ACh and 5-HT and has been implicated in Huntington's chorea, Alzheimer's dementia, and affective disorders.

■ *Cholecystokinin may have a role in schizophrenia, panic disorder, eating disorders, and some movement disorders*

Cholecystokinin (CCK) is coexistent in neurons with dopamine and GABA. It acts on two receptor subtypes, CCK-A and CCK-B receptors. The signal transduction mechanisms of the B receptor are not yet understood, but the A subtype acts via an effect on membrane phospholipids.

■ *Neurotensin may have a role in schizophrenia*

Neurotensin is coexistent in neurons with norepinephrine and dopamine. It acts on G protein-coupled high-affinity receptors present in dopamine-rich areas and the enterorhinal cortex implicated in schizophrenia.

PATHOPHYSIOLOGY AND DISEASES OF THE CENTRAL NERVOUS SYSTEM

Psychosis

Psychosis describes a mental state characterized by a loss of touch with reality. The patient may describe a variety of abnormalities of perception, thought, and ideas. Psychosis is not a specific illness and psychotic symptoms may occur in depression and other mood disorders and in medical conditions that interfere with brain function. Psychotic illnesses include schizophrenia, schizoaffective disorder, delusional disorders, and some depressive and manic illnesses. The most prevalent psychotic illness that includes all the cardinal psychotic symptoms is schizophrenia.

Schizophrenia

Schizophrenia is a psychotic illness characterized by multiple symptoms affecting thought, perceptions, emotion, and volition. Its incidence in industrialized countries is approximately 15 new cases/100,000 population/year. Its prevalence is 0.5–1%, rising to 2.8% in some areas (e.g. Northern Sweden).

Schizophrenia characteristically develops in people aged 15–45 years, but it may occur before puberty or be delayed until the seventh or eighth decade. The typical age of onset for males is 23–28 years and for females, 28–32 years. There is an increased rate among people living in inner cities and those from lower social classes, and in immigrant populations. This appears to be because patients 'drift' down the social ladder into inner cities or overseas as part of their illness during the time before their onset of symptoms or admission into hospital.

Florid symptoms of schizophrenia include delusions, hallucinations, abnormal thought processes, and passivity experiences

The premorbid personality is often described as emotionally and socially detached. Such people have few friends, are often cold and aloof, and engage in solitary occupations. Their behavior may be eccentric and they are indifferent to praise or criticism. People with schizophrenia slowly become more withdrawn and introverted, develop new interests, which are sometimes out of character, and drift away from family and friends. They may begin to fail in their occupation or school work. The onset of overt schizophrenia is commonly slow and insidious, taking weeks to years, but eventually, often with an apparently precipitating event, the symptoms of florid illness appear. The florid symptoms are variable, but usually include delusions, hallucinations, abnormal thought processes, and passivity experiences. In addition there may be formal thought disorder, a flat or inappropriate affect, and abnormal motor signs, which are usually called catatonic symptoms.

Delusions are false personal beliefs held with absolute conviction

The beliefs of delusions are outside the person's normal culture or subculture in spite of what everyone else believes and evidence to the contrary. They dominate the individual's viewpoint and behavior. Delusional disorders are disorders in which delusions are prominent and hallucinations and abnormal thought phenomena are vague or absent.

Hallucinations are false perceptions in the absence of a real external stimulus

Hallucinations are perceived as having the same quality as real perceptions and are not subject to conscious manipulation. Hallucinations in schizophrenia are equally varied and may involve any of the sensory modalities. The most common are auditory hallucinations in the form of voices, which occur in 60–70% of patients diagnosed with schizophrenia. Visual hallucinations occur in about 10% of patients, but should raise the suspicion of an organic disorder. Olfactory hallucinations are more common in temporal lobe epilepsy (TLE) than schizophrenia, and tactile hallucinations are probably experienced more frequently than is reported by patients. No one type of hallucination is specific to schizophrenia and the duration and intensity is probably more important diagnostically.

Thought alienation and disordered thought are common in schizophrenia

Disorders of thought possession in schizophrenia are described as thought alienation. The patient has the experience that his thoughts are under the control of an outside agency or that others are participating in his thinking. Disorders of the form of thought are also characteristic, and as a result the speech is difficult to follow or incoherent and follows no logical sequence.

Catatonic symptoms can occur in any form of schizophrenia

Catatonic symptoms form part of a subtype of schizophrenia. However these, mainly motor, symptoms can occur in any form of schizophrenia. They include:

- Ambitendence (alternation between opposite movements).
- Echopraxia (automatic imitation of another person's movements).
- Stereotypies (repeated regular fixed parts of movement, or speech, that are not goal-directed).
- Negativism (motiveless resistance to instructions and attempts to be moved or doing the opposite of what is asked).
- Posturing (adoption of an inappropriate or bizarre bodily posture continuously for a substantial period of time).
- Waxy flexibility (the limbs can be 'moulded' into a position and remain fixed for long periods of time).

The differential diagnosis of acute schizophrenia includes other psychotic illnesses and organic disorders

The differential diagnosis of acute schizophrenia includes other psychotic illnesses such as schizophreniform disorder, schizo-affective disorder, bipolar affective disorder, paranoid psychosis, and psychotic depression. Certain organic causes must be excluded including drug/substance-induced psychosis, early dementia, some forms of epilepsy, endocrine causes, infections, metabolic disorders, systemic lupus erythematosus (SLE), and the long-term sequelae of head injury.

Approximately 50–65% of patients with acute schizophrenia develop chronic schizophrenia

The symptoms seen in acute schizophrenia are generally termed the positive symptoms of schizophrenia and are characteristic of the acute phase of the illness. In chronic schizophrenia some florid (positive) symptoms may remain, but the predominant negative symptoms are:

- Poverty of speech (a restriction in the amount of spontaneous speech and in the information contained in speech; alogia).
- Flattening of affect (a restriction in the experience and expression of emotion).
- Anhedonia–asociality (an inability to experience pleasure, few social contacts, and social withdrawal).
- Avolition–apathy (reduced drive, energy, and interest).
- Attention impairment (an inattentiveness at work and interview).

Some of these symptoms may also occur as part of a florid psychotic episode. Their presence is associated with a poor prognosis, a poor response to neuroleptics, poor premorbid adjustment, cognitive impairment, and atrophic changes seen on computed tomography (CT) scan.

Once schizophrenia has been diagnosed there are four main outcomes

The clinical course of schizophrenia will usually follow one of the following patterns:

- The illness resolves completely, with or without treatment, and never recurs (pattern A, 10–20% of patients).
- The illness recurs repeatedly with full recovery every time (pattern B. 30–35% of patients).
- The illness recurs repeatedly, but recovery is incomplete and a persistent defective state develops, becoming more pronounced with each successive relapse (pattern C, 30–35% of patients).
- The illness pursues a downhill course from the beginning (pattern D, 10–20% of patients).

There is some debate about the impact of effective treatments for acute schizophrenia on the long-term course and prognosis of the illness. Approximately 55% of people with schizophrenia now live and work normally. Factors contributing to a poor prognosis include an early onset, an insidious onset, a lack of a prominent affective component, a lack of clear precipitants, a family history of schizophrenia, poor premorbid personality, confusion or perplexity, a low IQ, a low social class, social isolation, and a previous psychiatric history. The converse of these factors usually points to a better prognosis.

The tendency to develop schizophrenia is genetically transmitted

Although the mode of transmission remains obscure it appears to be polygenic. Twin studies indicate that the genetic contribution to schizophrenia is approximately 50%.

The neurotransmitters dopamine, 5-HT, GABA, and glutamate may have a role in schizophrenia

Many hypotheses have been invoked to explain the manifestations of schizophrenia at the level of neurotransmitters in the brain. The potential pivotal role of excess dopamine in various brain regions has received considerable attention. Although many antipsychotic drugs block dopamine receptors, particularly D_2 and D_2-like receptors, there is little support from current research for a primary receptor-based dopaminergic abnormality in schizophrenia. Recently however it has become increasingly clear that people with schizophrenia may release too much dopamine in response to a stimulus. The precise implications of this are not yet clear. Other neurotransmitters that may have a role in schizophrenia include 5-HT, GABA, and glutamate.

The treatment of schizophrenia and all other psychotic illnesses involves the use of antipsychotic medications (previously called neuroleptics)

Chlorpromazine and other antipsychotics produce a general improvement in all the acute symptoms of schizophrenia, but their efficacy in negative schizophrenia and their ability to affect the course and prognosis of schizophrenia is less clear. The therapeutic effect of these 'typical' antipsychotic drugs was thought purely to be related to their ability to block dopamine (primarily D_2) receptors (Fig. 14.38). However, the development of newer 'atypical' antipsychotic drugs (e.g. clozapine, olanzapine, quetiapine), which have lower affinity for the D_2 receptor, but are still clinically effective, has challenged this simple hypothesis.

Psychotic illness is usually first treated with an oral antipsychotic such as chlorpromazine (sedating), trifluoperazine, or haloperidol

The dose of antipsychotic is titrated against symptoms for a period of 4–6 weeks, which is considered to be necessary for an adequate trial of such a drug. Some authors advocate using the atypical antipsychotics as the first-line drugs because they cause fewer adverse motor side effects at therapeutic doses. If

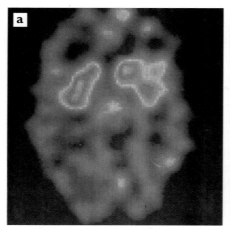
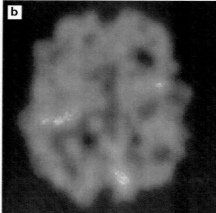
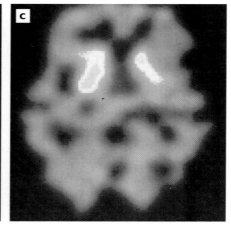

Fig. 14.38 The cerebral distribution of dopamine receptors in treated and untreated schizophrenia. Single photon emission tomography (SPET) scans acquired using the dopamine D_2 ligand I [^{123}I]-iodobenzamine. (a) Striatal dopamine receptors in an untreated schizophrenic patient. (b) Complete blockade of the receptors shown in (a) with a typical antipsychotic. (c) Partial blockade of the receptors shown in (a) with an equally effective dose of clozapine, an atypical antipsychotic. (Courtesy of the Institute of Nuclear Medicine, Middlesex Hospital, London, UK.)

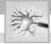

the medication is effective it may then be given as a depot pre-paration if the patient is poorly compliant, or oral treatment can be continued. If the medication is ineffective, an alternative class of typical antipsychotic should be used instead. If the medication is still ineffective, the medication should be changed to an atypical antipsychotic such as clozapine. Approximately 35% of patients do not respond to classic antipsychotics.

The general consensus is that all acute episodes of schizo-phrenia should be treated with an antipsychotic and that the medication should be continued for 1–2 years before being cautiously withdrawn.

Most patients require maintenance therapy after an acute psychotic episode

Generally, the lowest possible dose of antipsychotic should be used for maintenance therapy. In chronic schizophrenia, antipsychotics are used to prevent further acute episodes. Although most studies show a much higher relapse rate for patients whose medication is discontinued, some studies have failed to show a drug/placebo difference. Approximately 16–25% of patients relapse despite the use of medication.

Antipsychotic (neuroleptic) drugs

Antipsychotic drugs are not a homogeneous group, and there are various classes (Fig. 14.39). Typical antipsychotics cause catalepsy in animals via D_2 receptor blockade. Atypical anti-psychotics do not, when administered at therapeutic levels. The phenothiazines include:

- Drugs with aliphatic side chains such as chlorpromazine.
- Drugs with piperidine chains such as thioridazine.
- Drugs with piperazine side chains such as trifluoperazine and fluphenazine.
  Other classes of antipsychotic include
- The thioxanthenes (e.g. flupenthixol and zuclopenthixol).
- The butyrophenones (e.g. haloperidol and droperidol).
- The diphenylbutylpiperidines (e.g. pimozide).
- The substituted benzamides (e.g. sulpiride and amisulpride).

- The dibenzodiazepines (e.g. clozapine).
- The benzixasoles (e.g. risperidone).
- The thienobenzodiazepines (e.g. olanzapine).
- The dibenzothiazepines (e.g. quetiapine).
- The imidazolidinones (e.g. sertindole).

Adverse effects of antipsychotics

ACUTE NEUROLOGIC ADVERSE EFFECTS DUE TO D_2 RECEPTOR BLOCKADE include acute dystonia. This is characterized by fixed muscle postures with spasm and include clenched jaw muscles, protruding tongue, opisthotonos, torticollis, and oculogyric crisis (mouth open, head back, eyes staring up-wards). It appears within hours to days and is most common in young males. It should be treated immediately with anti-cholinergic drugs (procyclidine 5–10 mg or benztropine intra-muscularly or intravenously). The response is dramatic.

MEDIUM-TERM NEUROLOGIC ADVERSE EFFECTS DUE TO D_2 BLOCKADE include akathisia and parkinsonism.

Adverse effects of antipsychotics

- *Acute neurologic effects: acute dystonia, akathisia, parkinsonism*
- *Chronic neurologic effects: tardive dyskinesia, tardive dystonia*
- *Neuroendocrine effects: amenorrhea, galactorrhea, infertility*
- *Idiosyncratic: neuroleptic malignant syndrome*
- *Anticholinergic: dry mouth, blurred vision, constipation, urinary retention, ejaculatory failure*
- *Antihistaminergic: sedation*
- *Antiadrenergic: hypotension, arrhythmia*
- *Miscellaneous: photosensitivity, heat sensitivity, cholestatic jaundice, retinal pigmentation*

The classes of antipsychotic drugs

Type	Class	Examples
Typical antipsychotics	Phenothiazines Butyrophenones Thioxanthenes Diphenylbutylpiperidines	Chlorpromazine, thioridazine, trifluoperazine Haloperidol and droperidol Flupenthixol and zuclopenthixol Pimozide
Atypical antipsychotics	Dibenzodiazepines Benzixasoles Thienobenzodiazepines Dibenzothiazepines Imidazolidinones Benzothiazolylpiperazines Substituted benzamides	Clozapine Risperidone Olanzapine Quetiapine Sertindole Ziprasidone Sulpiride and amisulpride (NB: sulpiride considered by some to be a typical antipsychotic)

Fig. 14.39 The classes of antipsychotic drugs.

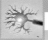
Akathisia is a motor, generally lower limb, restlessness accompanied by an inner feeling of restlessness. It is usually very distressing to the patient. Treatment primarily involves reducing the drug dose.

Parkinsonism is induced by blockade of D_2 receptors in the basal ganglia. The symptoms appear after a few days to weeks and treatment involves anticholinergic drugs (e.g. procyclidine, orphenadrine), reduction of the neuroleptic dose, or switching to an atypical antipsychotic which is less likely to produce such extrapyramidal symptoms (EPS).

CHRONIC NEUROLOGIC ADVERSE EFFECTS DUE TO D_2 BLOCKADE

are tardive dyskinesia and tardive dystonia.

Tardive dyskinesia is usually manifested as orofacial dyskinesia and causes lip smacking and tongue rotating. Tardive dystonia appears as choreoathetoid movements of the head, neck, and trunk. It appears after months to years of drug treatment. There is an increased risk of tardive dyskinesia in older patients, females, the edentulous, and patients with organic brain damage. Approximately 20% of patients who are taking typical antipsychotics over the long term will develop tardive dyskinesia, but there is no relationship to duration, total dose of treatment, or class of antipsychotic used. There is no effective treatment, so prevention by limiting the use of neuroleptics and early recognition of symptoms is important. Increasing the dose may temporarily alleviate the symptoms, while reducing the dose may worsen them. Clozapine has been shown to improve these symptoms. Newer atypical antipsychotics may be less likely to induce tardive dyskinesia.

NEUROENDOCRINE ADVERSE EFFECTS DUE TO D_2 BLOCKADE

include hyperprolactinemia because of the reduction of the negative feedback on the anterior pituitary. High serum concentrations of prolactin can produce galactorrhea, amenorrhea, and infertility in some patients.

NEUROLEPTIC MALIGNANT SYNDROME (NMS)

is the most life-threatening adverse effect of neuroleptic use. It is thought to be due to deranged dopaminergic function, but the precise pathophysiology is unknown. Symptoms include hyperthermia, muscle rigidity, autonomic instability, and fluctuating consciousness. It is an idiosyncratic reaction that appears from a few days to weeks after beginning treatment, but can occur at any time. The mortality is 20% if untreated and immediate medical treatment is required:

- Bromocriptine (a D_1/D_2 agonist) is used to reverse dopamine blockade.
- Dantrolene (a skeletal muscle relaxant) is used for muscular rigidity.
- Dehydration and hyperthermia are managed with supportive treatment.

Renal failure from rhabdomyolysis is the major complication and cause of mortality. NMS can recur on reintroducing antipsychotics. It is therefore recommended to wait at least 2 months before reintroduction and to use a drug of a different class, at the lowest recommended dose.

ANTICHOLINERGIC ADVERSE EFFECTS

Conventional antipsychotics often have anticholinergic adverse effects, which include a dry mouth (hypersalivation with clozapine), difficulty urinating or retention, constipation, and blurred vision. Profound muscarinic blockade may produce a toxic confusional state.

SEDATIVE ADVERSE EFFECTS OF ANTIPSYCHOTICS

may involve the antagonism of histamine-1 (H_1) receptors by these drugs.

ADVERSE EFFECTS DUE TO α ADRENOCEPTOR BLOCKADE

Many neuroleptics have the capacity to block α adrenoceptors, and this may contribute to postural hypotension.

ADVERSE EFFECTS THAT MAY BE DUE TO IMMUNE REACTIONS

include urticaria, dermatitis, rashes, dermal photosensitivity, and a gray/blue/purple skin tinge, which may be autoimmune responses. These are more commonly seen with the phenothiazines, as are the conjunctival, corneolenticular, and retinal pigmentation, which are sometimes reported. Cholestatic jaundice due to a hypersensitivity reaction is a rare adverse effect of chlorpromazine. Weight gain is common.

ADVERSE EFFECTS RELATED TO INDIVIDUAL DRUGS

include neutropenia with clozapine and sudden death secondary to a cardiac arrhythmia with pimozide. It has therefore been recommended that all patients have an ECG before starting pimozide and that it should not be used in patients with a known arrhythmia or a prolonged QT interval. Recently droperidol and thioridazine have been withdrawn from regular clinical use due to fears over their propensity to prolong the QT interval.

Atypical antipsychotics

CLOZAPINE has been used since the 1960s for treatment of schizophrenia, but its use has become restricted (see below) since reports of several associated deaths from neutropenia. Clozapine has a low affinity for the D_2 receptor and a higher affinity for the D_1 and D_4 receptors. The low incidence of extrapyramidal adverse effects associated with its use is thought to be due to its low activity at the D_2 receptor. Clozapine also has antagonistic activity at the $5-HT_{2A}$ receptor and this may possibly underlie its clinical efficacy in improving negative symptoms. Clozapine can be effective at any dose; this is because it has very variable pharmacokinetics. Plasma levels of clozapine above 350 μg/L to 420 μg/L are a better predictor of response.

■ *The use of clozapine is restricted because it can cause a fatal neutropenia*

In the UK and US, clozapine can be used only if a patient:
- Is unresponsive to two other neuroleptics.
- Has tardive dyskinesia or severe extrapyramidal symptoms.

Careful monitoring, especially of the formed elements in blood, is mandatory. Each patient has to be registered and the drug can be dispensed only after the white cell count has been found to be normal. A white cell count is then performed every week for 18 weeks, and then regularly during the treatment period.

The frequency of testing varies by country. Clozapine is contraindicated in patients with a history of neutropenia. The risk of neutropenia is 1–2% and it is usually reversible.

Other adverse effects of clozapine include hypersalivation, sedation, weight gain, tachycardia, and hypotension.

OLANZAPINE, similarly to clozapine also demonstrates antagonistic effects at a wide range of receptors but has a higher affinity for D_2 and 5-HT$_{2A}$ receptors than clozapine and a lower affinity at the D_1 receptor subtype. In acute phase studies olanzapine is definitely efficacious for positive and secondary negative symptoms and may be slightly superior to haloperidol on overall improvement. Olanzapine may also be effective for the primary negative symptoms of schizophrenia. Although olanzapine does not cause neutropenia it shares a similar side-effect profile to clozapine with weight gain and sedation as the most common side effects. EPS are rare at therapeutic doses. The licensed dose range is up to 20 mg, the minimal effective dose recommended is 10 mg. EPS are increasingly seen above doses of 25–30 mg.

QUETIAPINE has a similar receptor binding profile to clozapine. In comparison with clozapine it has relatively lower affinity for all receptors, with very little affinity for muscarinic receptors. Quetiapine is effective in acute phase studies for the treatment of positive and negative symptoms. Its efficacy is similar to 'classical' antipsychotics. The rates of EPS with quetiapine are similar to those seen in placebo-treated groups and significantly lower than in 'classical' antipsychotic comparator groups. The most common side effects demonstrated by quetiapine are somnolence and postural hypotension. Quetiapine demonstrates a lower potential to cause weight gain than clozapine and olanzapine and does not increase serum prolactin. The dose range is from 300 mg to 750 mg. The dose at which quetiapine begins to produce EPS is not known.

RISPERIDONE, in comparison with clozapine, has a very high affinity for 5-HT$_{2A}$ receptors and an affinity for D_2 receptors similar to that of most 'classic' antipsychotics. It appears to be at least as effective as haloperidol for positive symptoms and may be more effective for negative symptoms. At higher doses the adverse effects of risperidone include the extrapyramidal effects of tremor, rigidity, and restlessness, but these occur less frequently than with 'classic' antipsychotics, at doses of less than 6 mg of risperidone. At doses above 8 mg per day EPS are seen with a similar rate to the EPS seen with equivalent doses of haloperidol.

AMISULPRIDE, in contrast to all of the other atypical antipsychotics, only has effects on the dopamine D_2 and D_3 receptors, where it is a potent antagonist. It has a similar efficacy to haloperidol and at low doses (50–300 mg) may have a unique effect in patients with only negative symptoms. The dose range for acute schizophrenia, in contrast, is between 400 and 800 mg per day. Amisulpride has a lower incidence of EPS, at doses below 800 mg per day, than haloperidol. Amisulpride causes less weight gain that other atypical antipsychotics but does increase plasma prolactin.

SERTINDOLE has effects at 5-HT and dopamine receptors similar to those of risperidone, but is also a potent antagonist at adrenoceptor receptors. Sertindole has been withdrawn from routine clinical use due to fears over its propensity to prolong the QT interval.

ZIPRASIDONE is due to be released in the UK in the near future. It has a high affinity for the 5HT$_{2A}$ and the D_2 receptors similar to that of risperidone and sertindole, with a slightly higher 5-HT$_{2a}$/D_2 receptor affinity ratio. It is an agonist at the 5-HT$_{1A}$ receptor. Ziprasidone also has potent affinity for D_3 and moderate affinity for D_4 receptors. It exhibits weak serotonin and noradrenergic reuptake inhibition. Ziprasidone again is as efficacious as haloperidol for acute and chronic schizophrenia. It appears to have relatively low levels of side effects. These may include somnolence, headache and mild weight gain but results of full clinical studies remain to be published.

Affective disorders

The primary affective disorders are major depressive disorder and bipolar affective disorder.

Major depressive disorder

Major depressive disorder has a lifetime prevalence of approximately 9–15%, and perhaps as high as 20% in women. The mean age of onset is 35–40 years, although onset can be at any age. There are no specific correlations with socio-economic status.

The etiology of major depressive disorder is not clear

Life events (e.g. loss of job, moving house) and environmental stress are associated with an increased risk of developing major depressive disorder, but the precise causal relationship is unclear. The effect may be mediated by changes in the neurochemical environment of the CNS in reaction to stress. There is evidence that major depression also has a genetic component. Although the evidence for this is not as strong as for schizophrenia, the concordance rates are similar in twin studies. There appears to be a genetic factor of approximately 50% in the causation of depression.

Putative neurohormonal and neurochemical causes for depression have received considerable attention. The hypothalamic–pituitary–adrenal axis, which controls much of the body's hormonal equilibrium, has been particularly implicated. It has long been noted that depressed patients have a raised baseline cortisol concentration and that cortisol is not suppressed in response to dexamethasone in approximately 50% of depressed subjects. Fast feedback mechanisms have suggested that the cortisol receptors in the hippocampi of depressed subjects are abnormal. Nonspecific abnormalities have also been noted in thyroid hormone and growth hormone responses.

247

The most widely accepted neurochemical etiologic theory involves the biogenic amines, norepinephrine, 5-HT (serotonin), and dopamine

The original hypothesis of depression suggested that depression was due to a functional deficit of a transmitter amine (e.g. norepinephrine, dopamine, 5-HT), partly because tricyclic antidepressants (TCA) and monoamine oxidase inhibitors (MAOI) facilitated neurotransmission in aminergic neuron systems. It was also known that drugs that depleted amine stores (e.g. reserpine) could cause depression. Increased numbers of 5-HT receptors in the brains of people who have committed suicide have been attributed to a low 5-HT concentration as this is a relatively consistent finding in studies of cerebrospinal fluid (CSF) 5-HT metabolites in depressed patients. Subsequent work in animal models has shown that all effective antidepressants decrease the sensitivity of β adrenoceptors and 5-HT_{2A} receptors. The delay in treatment response coincides with the time taken for these receptors to downregulate. It is therefore possible that it is the biogenic amine receptors that are related to depression and not the absolute levels of the transmitters themselves.

The dopaminergic system may also be involved in the etiology, since reducing the central dopamine concentration can lead to depression and drugs that increase the central dopamine concentration improve depression.

Other systems that may be involved in depression include the GABA system and some of the neuropeptide systems, particularly vasopressin and endogenous opiates. Second-messenger systems may also have a crucial role in the efficacy of some treatments.

The cardinal symptoms of depression are usually divided into emotional/cognitive symptoms and biologic symptoms

In order to make a diagnosis of a major depressive disorder, the symptoms must have been present without a return to normality for at least 2 weeks. The emotional/cognitive symptoms include sadness and misery, decreased pleasure in life, hopelessness, guilt and worthlessness, slowed thinking and speech, and suicidal ideation. These symptoms vary throughout the day, but are characteristically worse in the morning. The biologic symptoms include low energy and fatigue, apathy and poor concentration, a change in appetite (usually decreased, with weight loss), a change in sleep pattern, classically with early morning wakening (a change in sleep pattern when the sufferer wakes very early in the morning and cannot return to sleep), low libido, and diurnal variation of mood.

Major depressive disorders can be classified as psychotic depression if they are accompanied by delusions and hallucinations. These are usually consistent with the mood and therefore negative in content.

The differential diagnosis of major depression includes a variety of psychiatric, drug-induced, and medical conditions

The differential diagnosis of major depression includes the depressive phase of bipolar affective disorder, minor depressive disorder, adjustment reaction with depressed mood, anxiety disorders, dementia, and dysthymia. Abuse of various substances (e.g. alcohol, barbiturates, benzodiazepines, cocaine, amphetamines; see below) can produce a depressive syndrome, while certain prescription medications (e.g. some antihypertensives especially reserpine, some antibiotics and analgesics, steroid medications, cimetidine, and some anticonvulsants) can worsen or cause depression. Many medical illnesses are associated with a depressive syndrome, including Parkinson's disease, cerebrovascular disease, Cushing's and Addison's diseases, parathyroid disorders, thyroid disorders, and porphyria.

65% of depressive episodes last 4–6 weeks, provided that the patient is given appropriate treatment

The remaining 35% of depressive episodes have a longer course despite appropriate treatment. Untreated depressive illnesses tend to last 6–13 months. Most depressive illnesses relapse at some time, 65% within 5 years.

Antidepressants

The mechanisms of action of drugs used to treat depression are listed in Fig. 14.40.

Virtually all antidepressants are metabolized by the cytochrome P-450 enzyme system. Some antidepressants, i.e. the selective serotonin reuptake inhibitors (SSRIs), are potent inhibitors of specific P-450 enzymes. These may be associated with pharmacokinetic interactions. A summary of this and other relevant pharmacokinetic data can be seen in Fig. 14.41.

Tricyclic antidepressants (TCAs) and related cyclic drugs

TCAs are an effective therapy for depression, but their adverse effects can reduce patient compliance and acceptability.

All TCAs act by preventing 5-HT and norepinephrine uptake into the presynaptic terminal from the synaptic cleft. The potency of different tricyclic antidepressants for blocking uptake varies, and some have some potency for blocking dopamine uptake. All TCAs also have some affinity for H_1 and muscarinic receptors and for α_1 and α_2 adrenoceptors.

TCAs are relatively dangerous in overdose due to cardiotoxicity.

Evidence for the monoamine hypothesis of depression

- Drugs that deplete monoamines are depressant
- Most antidepressants enhance monoaminergic transmission at some point in the synaptic signaling process
- The concentration of monoamines and their metabolites is reduced in the cerebrospinal fluid of depressed patients
- In various postmortem studies, the most consistent finding is elevation in cortical 5-HT_2 binding

Mechanism of action of drugs used to treat depression

Mechanism of action	Examples
Nonspecific blockers of monoamine uptake	Tricyclic antidepressants (amitriptyline, imipramine, nortriptyline, clomipramine, lofepramine)
Selective serotonin reuptake inhibitors (SSRIs)	Fluoxetine, paroxetine, sertraline, citalopram
Serotonin–norepinephrine reuptake inhibitors (SNRIs)	Venlafaxine
Noradrenergic and specific serotonergic antidepressant (NaSSA)	Mirtazapine
Selective noradrenaline reuptake inhibitor (NARI)	Reboxetine
Noncompetitive, nonselective, irreversible blockers of MAO_A and MAO_B	Monoamine oxidase inhibitors, (MAOIs) (phenelzine, tranylcypromine)
Reversible inhibitors of MAO_A (RIMAs)	Moclobemide, brofaromine

Fig. 14.40 Mechanism of action of drugs used to treat depression.

Pharmocokinetic considerations with antidepressants

Drug	Class	Half-life (hours)	Daily dosing	Cytochrome P-450	Potential interactions	Active metabolites	Route of administration/ formulation
Amitriptyline	TCA	8–24	75–150 mg o.d.		Other sedatives (i.e. alcohol, benzodiazepines (BDZs), antipsychotics), also sympathomimetics, cimetidine	Nortriptyline	Available as liquid
Imipramine	TCA	4–18	75–200 mg o.d.		Other sedatives (i.e. alcohol, benzodiazepines (BDZs), antipsychotics), also sympathomimetics, cimetidine	Desipramine	Available as liquid
Nortriptyline	TCA	18–96	75–150 mg o.d.		Other sedatives (i.e. alcohol, benzodiazepines (BDZs), antipsychotics), also sympathomimetics, cimetidine		
Clomipramine	TCA	17–28	50–250 mg o.d.		Other sedatives (i.e. alcohol, benzodiazepines (BDZs), antipsychotics), also sympathomimetics, cimetidine		Available as liquid and as i.v. forms
Lofepramine	TCA	1.5–6	70–210 mg/day b.d. or t.d.s.		Other sedatives (i.e. alcohol, benzodiazepines (BDZs), antipsychotics), also sympathomimetics, cimetidine	Desipramine	Available as liquid

Pharmocokinetic considerations with antidepressants (Continued)

Drug	Class	Half-life (hours)	Daily dosing	Cytochrome P-450	Potential interactions	Active metabolites	Route of administration/ formulation
Fluoxetine	SSRI	24–140	20–60 mg o.d.	Inhibits: CYP2D6+++ CYPIA2+ CYP3A4+	MAOIs contraindicated Increases plasma levels of TCAs, BDZs, and clozapine No alcohol potentiation	Nor-fluoxetine	Available as liquid
Paroxetine	SSRI	24	20–60 mg o.d.	Inhibits: CYP2D6++	MAOIs contraindicated Increases plasma levels of TCAs, BDZs, and clozapine No alcohol potentiation		Available as liquid
Sertraline	SSRI	24–26	50–150 mg o.d.	Inhibits: CYP2D6+++	MAOIs contraindicated Increases plasma levels of TCAs, BDZs, and clozapine No alcohol potentiation & care with alcohol		
Citalopram	SSRI	33	20–60 mg o.d.	Inhibits: CYP2D6+	MAOIs contraindicated only		
Nefazodone	5-HT$_{2A}$ antagonist & weak SNRI	2–4	200–600 mg/day b.d.	Inhibits: CYP2D6+ CYP3A4+++	MAOIs contraindicated Increases plasma levels of haloperidol, carbamazepine and digoxin		
Venlafaxine	SNRI	5–11	75–375 mg/day o.d. or b.d.	Inhibits: CYP2D6+	MAOIs contraindicated	*O*-desmethyl-venlafaxine	
Mirtazapine	NaSSA	20–40	15–45 mg o.d.	Inhibits: CYP2D6+/– CYP1A2+/– CYP3A4+/–	MAOIs contraindicated, potentiates other sedatives and alcohol		
Reboxetine	NARI	13	8–12 mg/day as b.d.	Inhibits: CYP2D6+/– CYP3A4+/–	MAOIs contraindicated No alcohol potentiation		
Phenelzine	MAOI	1.5	45–90 mg/day as t.d.s.		See text: tyramine reaction common and severe		
Moclobemide	RIMA	1–2	300–600 mg/day as b.d.		See text: tyramine reaction rare, avoid pethidine, sympathomimetics, SSRIs and L-dopa		

Fig. 14.41 Pharmacokinetic considerations with antidepressants. (MAOI, monoamine oxidase inhibitor; NARI, noradrenaline reuptake inhibitor; NaSSA, noradrenergic and specific serotonergic antidepressant; RIMA, reverse inhibitor of MAOI$_A$; SNRI, serotonin and norepinephrine reuptake inhibitor; SSRI, selective serotonin reuptake inhibitor) (+++, strong inhibition; ++ moderate inhibition; +, weak inhibition; +/–, equivocal inhibition not clinically relevant) (Adapted from the South London and Maudsley NHS Trust 2001 Prescribing Guidelines, 6th edn.)

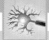

The choice of TCA usually depends on the degree of sedation required:

- Clomipramine is the TCA of choice for obsessive–compulsive disorder.
- Trimipramine is the TCA of choice for agitated states.

Metabolism of TCAs can produce pharmacologically active metabolites (e.g. amitriptyline is metabolized to nortriptyline, imipramine is metabolized to desipramine). Trazodone is a triazolopyridine derivative and is not strictly a tricyclic. It is less anticholinergic and cardiotoxic. Although it is quite sedative it is commonly used in the elderly and may be the antidepressant of choice in epilepsy.

ADVERSE EFFECTS OF TCAs The adverse effects due to muscarinic blockade include dry mouth, constipation, urinary retention, and blurred vision. α_1 Adrenoceptor antagonism may cause postural hypotension, while H_1 receptor antagonism leads to sedation. Alterations in serotonergic function lead to sexual dysfunction, including loss of libido and anorgasmia. Generally, tolerance develops to the anticholinergic adverse effects within 2 weeks. These can be minimized by gradually increasing the dose.

CONTRAINDICATIONS TO TCAs include prostatism, narrow angle glaucoma, recent myocardial infarction, and heart block. Care is needed if the patient has:

- Heart disease (because TCAs increase the risk of conduction abnormalities).
- Epilepsy (because TCAs lower the seizure threshold).

DRUG INTERACTIONS OF TCAs TCAs potentiate the effects of alcohol, other anticholinergic drugs, epinephrine, and norepinephrine. A fatal interaction can occur with lidocaine in local anesthetic preparations.

Selective serotonin (5-hydroxytryptamine) reuptake inhibitors (SSRIs)

SSRI MECHANISM OF ACTION After release from nerve terminals, serotonin activates various subtypes of serotonin receptors on nerve cells. Serotonin is inactivated by several mechanisms. The two primary mechanisms are metabolism by monoamine oxidase (MAO) to the major inactive metabolite 5-HIAA and reuptake of the transmitter into serotonergic nerve endings (Fig. 14.42). This latter important pathway is a very useful target for the development of antidepressant drugs.

Reuptake of serotonin into nerve endings requires a specific transporter expressed on nerve endings. The serotonin transporter is a member of a gene family of neurotransmitter transporters. Transporters for serotonin, as well as for norepinephrine, dopamine, glycine and GABA, have been identified. The overall structure of these transporters involves proteins with 12 putative membrane-spanning domains with N-

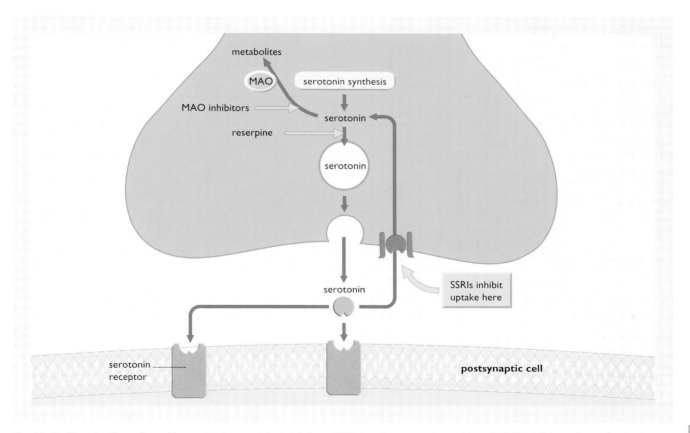

Fig. 14.42 Site of action of specific serotonin reuptake inhibitors (SSRIs) and monoamine oxidase (MAO) inhibitors. Reserpine leads to depletion of serotonin.

glycosylation sites that are likely to be important for transporter function. There is homology between these transporters and transporters for nutrients such as glucose. The expression of the serotonin transporter has been localized primarily to serotonergic nerves. The specificity with which this transporter is expressed in nerve cells and the selectivity with which it moves serotonin across cell membranes is of major importance in the function of serotonergic nerves. It should be emphasized that the serotonin transporter, as well as transporters for dopamine and norepinephrine, are quite distinct from the vesicular monoamine transporters that concentrate transmitters such as norepinephrine into synaptic granules. Those transporters are inhibited by drugs such as reserpine (see Chapter 3).

The serotonin transporters belong to a class of Na^+/Cl^--coupled transporters. Overexpression of this transporter, as well as very extensive experimentation in serotonergic neuronal preparations, has led to the discovery and development of a novel class of therapeutic agents with high specificity for potent inhibition of serotonin reuptake into nerves while having potentially only minimal effects on reuptake of other neurotransmitters or on other targets. These specific serotonin reuptake inhibitors (SSRIs) are efficacious in the treatment of depression. Some of these drugs also inhibit reuptake of norepinephrine. In some animal models SSRIs have been found to change expression of β adrenoceptors and serotonin receptor subtypes in the brain. The potential clinical significance of these differences between SSRIs in terms of specificity and on effects on receptor expression in the brain is not known.

SSRIs have efficacy similar to that of TCAs. In addition they have clinical advantages:

- They have no anticholinergic activity, thus increasing patient acceptability.
- They are not toxic in overdose. This is a major reason for their use.
- They lack cardiotoxic adverse effects and are therefore the drugs of choice in patients also suffering from heart disease.

SSRIs act by inhibiting the uptake of 5-HT from the synaptic cleft and have only a minor effect on noradrenergic uptake. Nefazodone is often classified as an SSRI, but is a weak inhibitor and may in fact have more effect on norepinephrine uptake. Thus it is better thought of as an SNRI. It is also a potent 5-HT_{2A} receptor antagonist and this may underlie its effects in improving sleep and its low level of sexual side effects.

The most potent SSRI is citalopram, followed in descending order by paroxetine, fluoxetine, sertraline, and fluvoxamine. The half-life of fluoxetine (active metabolite 7–9 days) means that it may take longer to reach steady-state concentrations but may be prescribed on alternate days. The half-lifes of the other SSRIs vary from 15 to 24 hours.

ADVERSE EFFECTS OF SSRIs include nausea, diarrhea, insomnia, anxiety, and agitation due to their effect on 5-HT receptors throughout the body. Sexual dysfunction may also occur. The adverse effect profile of nefazodone is similar to that of other SSRIs, but the associated incidence of sexual dysfunction may be lower.

CONTRAINDICATIONS AND INTERACTIONS are few, but SSRIs should not be used with MAOIs as the combination is likely to produce a serotonergic syndrome, which could be fatal. Care should be taken when prescribing SSRIs concurrently with lithium for similar reasons.

Serotonin (5-hydroxytryptamine) and norepinephrine reuptake inhibitors (SNRIs)

The only drug currently in this new class of antidepressants is venlafaxine, a phenethylamine bicyclic derivative. Its half-life is approximately 5 hours and it has an active metabolite with a half-life of 10 hours.

The pharmacologic effects of venlafaxine are similar to those of the TCAs, but it has fewer adverse effects because it has little affinity for cholinergic and histaminergic receptors or a adrenoceptors. Its adverse effects are similar to those of SSRIs, but they occur with a lower frequency. Drug interactions are similar to those of SSRIs, though extra care must be taken with patients with increased blood pressure as venlafaxine increases blood pressure.

Noradrenergic and specific serotonergic antidepressant (NaSSA)

Mirtazapine is the only drug in this class and is pharmacologically unique. Mirtazapine enhances noradrenergic transmission by blocking α_2 autoreceptors, therefore increasing noradrenaline release. It also increases 5-HT neuronal firing by acting on noradrenergic α_2-heteroreceptors on serotonergic neuronal cell bodies thus increasing synaptic serotonin. It is also an antagonist at 5-HT_{2A} and 5-HT_3 receptors. It has weak affinity for muscarinic receptors (but greater than venlafaxine). It also has relatively high affinity for H_1 receptors. Thus mirtazapine causes less nausea, less headache and less anxiety than 'pure' SSRIs as it is blocking the 5-HT receptors which mediate these side effects. However, probably due to the H_1 receptor antagonism, mirtazapine's side effects include increased appetite and weight gain, drowsiness and sedation. These occur in 14–37% of patients treated with mirtazapine and are greater at initiation of therapy.

Selective noradrenaline reuptake inhibitor (NARI)

Reboxetine is currently the only drug in this class, although the TCAs desipramine and nortriptyline are effectively NARIs. These drugs selectively block the reuptake of noradrenaline with little or no effect on serotonergic reuptake. These drugs are said to be better for depression with marked psychomotor retardation. Reboxetine has a better side effect profile than the TCAs with relative selectivity for noradrenaline reuptake. The side effects of reboxetine do include dry mouth, constipation and insomnia. The incidence of impotence and deceased libido increases at higher doses.

Monoamine oxidase inhibitors

MAOIs block the action of MAO-A and MAO-B, which metabolize norepinephrine, dopamine, and 5-HT. MAO-A is primarily located in the gut and preferentially breaks down 5-HT and norepinephrine, while MAO-B is primarily located in the brain. MAO-A inhibitors are used to treat depression.

ADVERSE EFFECTS OF MAOIs Gut MAO-A breaks down tyramine in the diet. Once tyramine enters the circulation it results in the release of norepinephrine, causing a sudden and potentially fatal rise in blood pressure. Patients on MAOIs must therefore avoid foods rich in tyramine, which include:

- Cheese, especially mature varieties.
- Degraded protein such as chicken liver, hung game, pickled herring, and pâté.
- Yeast and protein extract (e.g. Marmite, Bovril, Oxo).
- Beer.
- Chianti wine.
- Broad bean pods.
- Green banana skins.

Drug preparations containing amines to be avoided include:

- Opiates (e.g. meperidine).
- Sympathomimetics, which are often included in cough and cold remedies, nose drops, and laxatives bought over the counter.
- SSRIs.
- Levodopa.
- Some H_1 receptor antagonists.

These restrictions remain for at least 2 weeks after the MAOI is discontinued since MAO blockade is irreversible and requires new protein synthesis to restore function. After ingesting such food or drugs, patients on MAOIs usually experience flushing and a pounding headache, and this may progress to a fatal hypertensive crisis. This so-called 'cheese reaction' is the most important adverse effect of MAOIs.

Other rare adverse effects of MAOIs include hepatotoxicity (especially with phenelzine) and a theoretic risk of precipitating psychosis by increasing the availability of dopamine.

Because of the dietary and drug restrictions, MAOIs are largely reserved for depression resistant to other antidepressants and treatment

Phenelzine has traditionally had a role in treating atypical nonbiologic depression with pronounced anxiety and hypochondriac symptoms. It has also been effectively used in the treatment of phobias and panic disorder.

The three irreversible MAOIs currently available are:

- Phenelzine, which is the most commonly used.
- Tranylcypromine, which has amine uptake and amphetamine-like activity.
- Isocarboxazid, which is now rarely used.

Moclobemide is a newer MAOI that reversibly inhibits MAO-A

Moclobemide carries the risk of an interaction with tyramine resulting in raised blood pressure if high levels of tyramine are consumed (e.g. more than 50 g of mature cheese), but in general no dietary restrictions are required. The likelihood of an interaction with tyramine is reduced if moclobemide is taken after a meal. Although the clinical efficacy of moclobemide is probably similar to that of other anti-depressants (i.e. TCAs and SSRIs), it is not recommended as a first-line treatment.

The adverse effects of moclobemide include insomnia, nausea, agitation, and confusion. Drug interactions include interactions with cimetidine, meperidine, and SSRIs, and moclobemide should be used with caution with TCAs as all these combinations may lead to a 'cheese reaction.'

Depression is usually treated with an antidepressant

The choice of antidepressant depends on:

- The clinical characteristics of the patient's illness.
- The drug's adverse effect profile.
- The danger of overdose.
- Previous treatments.

Generally, if there are no medical contraindications (e.g. heart disorders) and there is no or little risk of suicide, a TCA can be used. The TCA chosen will depend on whether sedation is required. The newer antidepressants (SSRIs, SNRIs, NaSSAs, etc.) are increasingly used as first-line treatments because of better tolerability. If there are medical contraindications, or suicide is a risk, or the patient has previously not tolerated the anticholinergic adverse effects of TCAs, then one of the newer antidepressants should be used.

Bipolar affective disorder

Bipolar affective disorder (BPAD) is characterized by swings in mood from mania (or hypomania) to depression. There is a high concordance rate of BPAD ranging from 33 to 90% in monozygotic twins, and family studies indicate an 18-fold increased risk for BPAD and a tenfold increased risk for major depression in the first-degree relatives of affected probands. The neurochemical basis for BPAD is unclear.

BPAD is characterized by episodes of depression and mania with periods of normality in between

The cycle of depressive and manic episodes in BPAD may take months or years, but may occur over days or weeks. There is no typical sequence of episodes.

Mania and hypomania are distinguished according to their severity and duration:

- A manic episode usually lasts longer than a week, significantly impairs social and occupational functioning, and may

---

> **⚠ Adverse effects of antidepressants**
>
> - *Tricyclics: blurred vision, dry mouth, constipation, urinary retention, mania, hypotension, arrhythmias*
> - *Serotonin and norepinephrine reuptake inhibitors (SNRIs): sedation, mania*
> - *Selective serotonin reuptake inhibitors (SSRIs): nausea, vomiting, dry mouth, agitation*
> - *Monoamine oxidase inhibitors (MAOIs): as for tricyclics plus sympathetic crisis with dietary tyramine*
> - *Reversible inhibitors of monoamine oxidase (RIMAs): mild agitation*

be accompanied by psychotic phenomena such as delusions and hallucinations.

- Hypomania is, by definition, not accompanied by psychotic features.

For ease of explanation, both mania and hypomania are here considered synonymous with the classification manic episode. The signs of a manic episode include an elevated mood, increased motor activity, accelerated thoughts and speech, irritability, decreased sleep, increased or decreased appetite, distractability, grandiose ideas, and delusions and hallucinations, usually of a grandiose nature. Features normally considered to be typical of schizophrenia occur in approximately 10% of patients. Patients with the severest form of manic episode may exhaust themselves, or carry out dangerous plans based on their grandiose ideas.

The depressive episodes in BPAD are clinically identical to depression in the absence of previous manic episodes. The patient may experience several episodes of depression in sequence, or several episodes of mania.

BPAD is treated with a combination of mood stabilizers, antipsychotics, and antidepressants.

Mood stabilizers
Lithium
Lithium is the most widely used mood stabilizer:

- It is used in the prevention of relapse in manic depressive (bipolar) and recurrent unipolar (i.e. no mania) depressive disorders.
- It is an effective treatment in acute mania.
- It can be used in resistant depression to augment anti-depressant activity.

Lithium inhibits the scavenging pathway for recapturing inositol for the resynthesis of polyphosphoinositides. Since the entry of inositol into the brain is relatively poor, this action of lithium may diminish the concentrations of lipids important in signal transduction in the brain (see Chapter 3).

Renal and thyroid function must be checked before starting lithium
Owing to adverse effects and contraindications (see below), before starting therapy, renal (urea, creatinine, electrolytes) and thyroid function must be checked. Once treatment is started, plasma lithium concentration should be monitored every 5 days after an increase in dose until the concentration is between 0.6 and 1 mEq/liter (0.6–1.0 mmol/liter). During maintenance, lithium concentration should measured, with renal function, every 2–3 months. Thyroid function should be measured every 6 months.

ADVERSE EFFECTS AND TOXICITY OF LITHIUM In the early stages of lithium therapy, patients commonly complain of thirst, nausea, loose stools, fine tremor, and polyuria. These often disappear with continued therapy. Other adverse effects include weight gain, edema, and acne. A long-term adverse effect can be diabetes insipidus leading to polydipsia, which occurs because lithium inhibits vasopressin action in the kidney,

leading to obligate water loss, goiter and, less commonly, frank hypothyroidism due to impaired release of thyroid hormone from the thyroid gland.

The first signs of lithium toxicity, which occur at a plasma lithium concentration of 1.5–2 mEq/liter (1.5–2.0 mmol/liter), are anorexia, vomiting, diarrhea, coarse tremor, ataxia, dysarthria, confusion, and sleepiness. Later signs, when the plasma lithium concentration is higher than 2 mEq/liter (2.0 mmol/liter), are impaired consciousness, nystagmus, muscle twitching, hyper-reflexia, and convulsions. Coma and death occur at higher concentrations. At the first signs of toxicity the plasma lithium concentration should be measured urgently. If high, the lithium should be stopped and efforts made to increase lithium elimination, possibly involving hemodialysis.

INTERACTIONS BETWEEN LITHIUM AND OTHER DRUGS often lead to a rise in plasma lithium concentration. Such interacting drugs include:

- Antipsychotics (especially haloperidol), which increase neurotoxicity.
- Nonsteroidal anti-inflammatory drugs (NSAIDs) except aspirin, which increase plasma lithium concentration by decreasing excretion.
- Diuretics (especially thiazides), which increase plasma lithium concentration by decreasing excretion.
- Cardioactive drugs (digoxin, angiotensin-converting enzyme inhibitors), which increase the risk of neurotoxicity possibly secondary to membrane effects.

Carbamazepine
Carbamazepine may be as effective as lithium in preventing relapses in BPAD and in the treatment of acute mania, and is traditionally indicated for rapid cycling bipolar illness.

Carbamazepine shares with lithium a mechanism of action possibly mediated via effects on second-messenger systems. Carbamazepine also inhibits calcium influx through the NMDA and GABA$_B$ receptors. Furthermore carbamezapine treatment also leads to a sodium channel-mediated membrane stabilization and potentiation of α_2 adrenoceptors.

At the start of therapy, carbamazepine induces its own catabolic enzymes in the liver; plasma concentrations therefore should be monitored to establish a maintenance dose.

ADVERSE EFFECTS OF CARBAMAZEPINE include drowsiness, diplopia, nausea, ataxia, rashes, and headache. Hematologic disturbancness include agranulocytosis and leucopenia; patients therefore should be warned about fever and infections as these may indicate agranulocytosis and they should be investigated. It is advised that the plasma carbamazepine concentration is measured and a full blood count is obtained every 2 weeks for the first 2 months.

Acute carbamazepine toxicity is associated with diplopia, ataxia, hyper-reflexia, clonus, tremor, and sedation.

INTERACTIONS BETWEEN CARBAMAZEPINE AND OTHER DRUGS
Carbamazepine interacts with:

- Lithium, potentially resulting in CNS adverse effects of carbamazepine and carbamazepine toxicity despite 'normal' plasma carbamazepine concentrations. It must be noted, however, that the combination of lithium and carbamazepine may be more effective than either drug alone.
- Antipsychotics, resulting in drowsiness and ataxia.
- TCAs, decreasing the plasma TCA concentration as a result of enzyme induction.
- MAOIs, precipitating the cheese reaction.

Carbamazepine is an enzyme inducer (see Chapter 4) and therefore affects the plasma concentrations of many drugs metabolized in the liver.

Valproate sodium and divalproex sodium

Valproate is an effective mood stabilizer and is worth considering as a first-line treatment or as an adjunct in refractory cases. Divalproex sodium is a mixture of valproate sodium and valproic acid; this improves bioavailability and tolerability, and the active moeity remains valproate. The mechanism of action of valproate is not fully understood, but it is known to enhance the synthesis, turnover, and release of GABA. It also inhibits calcium influx through NMDA receptors. Perhaps related to these two actions, valproate leads to an enhancement of serotonergic function and a reduction in dopaminergic function.

ADVERSE EFFECTS OF VALPROATE SODIUM include gastrointestinal effects (nausea, vomiting, diarrhea), CNS effects (sedation, ataxia, dysarthria, tremor), and hepatic effects (persistent elevation of liver transaminases). It may also cause hair loss. A rare adverse effect is hepatotoxicity leading to death.

New anti-epileptics for the treatment of bipolar affective disorder

Although all new anti-epileptics may be potential treatments for bipolar affective disorder, the only drug from this group which seems to have effects superior or equal to existing treatments is lamotrigine. Lamotrigine is thought to inhibit neuronal kindling. It inhibits sodium currents by selectively binding to the inactivated state of the sodium channel and subsequently suppresses the release of the excitatory amino acid, glutamate. Early data suggests that it is well tolerated in bipolar affective disorder and may have a role in treating the depressive phase of the illness.

Anxiety disorders

The sensation of anxiety is common in all humans. The psychologic symptoms include a diffuse, unpleasant, and vague feeling of apprehension, and this is often accompanied by physical symptoms of autonomic arousal such as headache, perspiration, palpitations, 'upset stomach' ('butterflies'), and tightness in the chest, and in some people restlessness. Anxiety warns of impending danger and enables the individual to take measures to deal with a threat that is usually unknown, internal, vague, or conflictual (with stimulatory opposite emotions, e.g. excitement and guilt) in origin. This is in contrast to fear, which is a response to a threat that is known, external, definite, or nonconflictual in origin.

Anxiety is a common symptom in a variety of distinct mental illnesses and is a predominant symptom in phobias, panic disorder, and obsessive–compulsive disorder. Other anxiety disorders include generalized anxiety disorder, post-traumatic stress disorder, and hysterical conversion reactions.

The two neurotransmitters most commonly implicated in the etiology of all anxiety disorders are GABA and 5-HT Norepinephrine also has a role, particularly in panic disorder. There have been no conclusive studies to confirm the role of these neurotransmitters, but functional imaging of benzodiazepine receptors in the brain has shown differences in receptor binding in the temporal lobes between patients with panic disorder and normal subjects. Benzodiazepines act indirectly on GABA receptors.

Anxiety disorders are treated with anxiolytics and antidepressants.

Anxiolytics
Benzodiazepines

Benzodiazepines (Fig. 14.43) act by potentiating the action of GABA, the primary inhibitory neurotransmitter in the CNS. The benzodiazepine receptor lies within the GABA$_A$ receptor complex, and benzodiazepines enhance inhibitory activity (Fig. 14.44). Benzodiazepines reduce anxiety, and the duration of their action will be determined to some extent by their half-lifes.

ADVERSE EFFECTS OF BENZODIAZEPINES include dependence and the potential for abuse. Generally, tolerance develops within 14 days and their efficacy then declines. Sudden cessation after long-term use can result in a withdrawal syndrome characterized by insomnia, anxiety, tremor, loss of appetite, tinnitus, and perceptual disturbances. Controlled benzodiazepine withdrawal is performed by switching to an equivalent dose of a benzodiazepine with a long half-life (e.g. diazepam) and reducing the dose gradually by approximately one-eighth every 2 weeks. This process may take many weeks to 1 year, depending on the severity of tolerance.

The most common adverse effects of benzodiazepines are drowsiness, ataxia, and reduced psychomotor performance, so care should be taken when driving or operating machinery. These effects can become more marked after a few weeks because the long half-life of some benzodiazepines leads to drug accumulation. Disinhibition with aggression may occur, but is rare and more likely to be seen with short-acting benzodiazepines (i.e. midazolam).

Half-lifes of benzodiazepines

Diazepam:	14–70 hours (one metabolite is active for up to 200 hours)
Nitrazepam:	15–30 hours
Lorazepam:	8–24 hours
Temazepam:	3–25 hours
Oxazepam:	3–25 hours

Mechanism of action of drugs used to treat anxiety

Drug	Mechanism of action	Use
Anxiolytics		
Benzodiazepines (diazepam, alprazolam)	Act on GABA receptors	Short-term treatment of anxiety
Buspirone	Acts on 5-HT$_{1A}$ receptor	? Effective in generalized anxiety disorder
Autonomic suppression		
Propranolol	Acts by inhibiting β adrenoceptors	Useful for some social/performance anxiety disorders
Antidepressants		
Imipramine	Tricyclic antidepressant	Most studied biologic treatment in panic disorder
Phenelzine, moclobemide	MAOIs	Useful for social phobia and panic, may also be useful for PTSD
Fluoxetine, sertraline	SSRIs	Proven efficacy in OCD and panic disorder

Fig. 14.43 Mechanism of action of drugs used to treat anxiety. (GABA, γ-aminobutyric acid; 5-HT$_{1A}$, 5-hydroxytryptamine-IA; MAOIs, monoamine oxidase inhibitors; OCD, obsessive–compulsive disorder; PTSD, post-traumatic stress disorder; SSRIs, selective serotonin reuptake inhibitors)

■ *Benzodiazepines are indicated only for short-term relief of severe, disabling, or unacceptably distressing anxiety*

Such severe anxiety may occur alone or in association with insomnia or a short-term psychosomatic, organic, or psychotic illness, and diazepam (5–20 mg/day) is the most commonly prescribed anxiolytic. The use of benzodiazepines to treat short-term 'mild' anxiety is inappropriate as dependence and withdrawal are more problematic with benzodiazepines prescribed as anxiolytics than with those prescribed as hypnotics. Alprazolam is effective for panic attacks.

Azapirones

Buspirone is the first of a new class of agents called azapirones. It is thought to reduce 5-HT neurotransmission by acting as a partial agonist at 5-HT$_{1A}$ receptors. 5-HT$_{1A}$ receptors are inhibitory presynaptic receptors and their activation results in decreased firing of 5-HT neurons. Buspirone has no activity at the GABA-benzodiazepine receptor complex and cannot therefore be used to ameliorate the benzodiazepine withdrawal syndrome. It is not an hypnotic.

ADVERSE EFFECTS OF BUSPIRONE include nervousness, dizziness, headache, and lightheadedness.

■ *Buspirone is indicated for the short-term management of generalized anxiety disorder*

The anxiolytic effect of buspirone gradually evolves over 1–3 weeks. In contrast to benzodiazepines, buspirone does not cause significant sedation or cognitive impairment and carries only a minimal risk of dependence and withdrawal. It does not potentiate the sedative effects of alcohol.

β Adrenoceptor antagonists

β Adrenoceptor antagonists such as propanolol reduce heart rate and other manifestations produced by excess catecholamine. Propranolol:

- May ease the somatic manifestations of an anxiety characterized by marked sympathetic autonomic arousal (e.g. palpitations and tremor).
- Is useful for social phobia and may act by reducing the autonomic arousal, thereby preventing amplification of the sufferer's anxiety.
- Reduces performance anxiety in musicians for whom fine motor control may be critical.

Antidepressants

Certain antidepressants have a specific application in particular anxiety disorders:

- Imipramine has been most studied for use in panic disorder and produces a beneficial effect in 60–70% of patients. Generally, the dose used is higher than that for depression and the therapy must be continued for longer before a response is seen.
- MAOIs have uses in several anxiety disorders including panic disorder, agoraphobia, social phobia, and post-traumatic stress disorder, and some studies have indicated benefits over and above regular TCAs.
- SSRIs, especially fluoxetine and the TCA clomipramine, appear to be most effective in the treatment of obsessive–compulsive disorder. The doses must, however, be higher than those used for depression and the therapeutic effect may take 1–3 months to become fully apparent.

Often patients present with a mixed picture of anxiety and depression (agitated depression). Antidepressants are then indicated, and generally a more sedative one is used.

Eating disorders

The two well-defined eating disorders are anorexia nervosa and bulimia nervosa. There is considerable overlap between the two disorders with patients moving from one to the other. Treatment is almost purely with pyschotherapy, though these

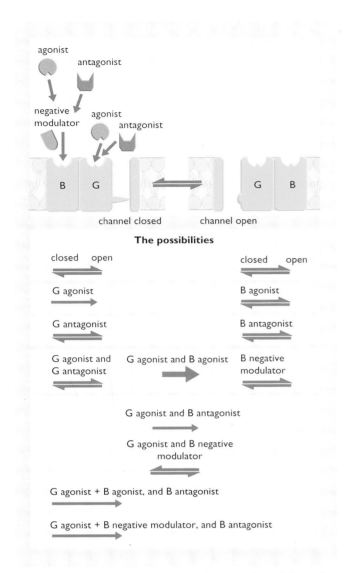

The possibilities

Fig. 14.44 Benzodiazepine agonist and antagonist activity and modulation of γ-aminobutyric acid (GABA) agonist and antagonist activity. A Cl⁻ channel, part of a receptor-operated channel (ROC), exists in an open and a closed state. This ROC has two distinct ligand-recognition sites, a GABA site (G) and a benzodiazepine site (B). Equilibrium between closed and open states of the Cl⁻ channel is altered by GABA agonism. Neither benzodiazepine agonism or antagonism on their own affect channel opening. However, GABA agonist-induced channel opening is facilitated by concomitant benzodiazepine agonism. This potentiation is blocked by benzodiazepine antagonism. In addition, benzodiazepine negative modulators reduce the ability of GABA to open the channel, and benzodiazepine antagonists can block the effect of negative modulators. The G and B ligand-recognition sites presumably interact allosterically, with the B site functioning as a modulator of the G site.

disorders are often accompanied by depression, which may need pharmacologic treatment.

Epilepsy

Epilepsy is characterized by recurrent unprovoked seizures. A seizure is a particular behavior produced by an altered neurologic function resulting from a paroxysmal discharge of neurons in the cerebral cortex. Seizures are sometimes called fits. Approximately 10% of the US population experiences one or more seizures during their lifetime, and epilepsy will develop in approximately 1.5% of the population. Behavior during a seizure varies from immobility and slight twitching of a digit through to violent tonic–clonic movements or even purposeful activity, depending on the type of epilepsy.

The cellular mechanisms of epilepsy are not known, but may involve altered GABA metabolism.

Appropriate drug treatment depends on the nature of the epilepsy

A diagnosis of epilepsy is made from the patient's history, the nature of the seizure (Fig. 14.45), and the electroencephalographic (EEG) pattern.

Partial or focal seizures arise from a restricted region of the cerebral cortex. The resulting effect depends on the involved region of brain and can be sensory (including visual disturbances) or motor in nature. The motor behavior can be quite purposeful. Consciousness is variable and usually there is no memory of the seizure.

Generalized seizures are convulsive or nonconvulsive and range from a blank stare to a generalized tonic–clonic seizure:

- Absence seizures are the most common nonconvulsive seizure. They occur most often in children and can be confused with daydreaming.
- Myoclonic seizures are rapid symmetric arrhythmic jerks of the extremities or body.
- Tonic seizures are characterized by stiffening of body and limbs and can produce fractures.
- Atonic seizures involve loss of muscle tone and can cause a fall.
- A generalized tonic–clonic seizure (grand mal seizure) starts with increased muscle tone (stiffening), which is followed by clonic movements lasting a few minutes. This may be accompanied by vocalization, cyanosis, and incontinence of urine and/or feces. The seizure is followed by confusion and fatigue.

Seizures can be classified into different epileptic syndromes based on:

- Seizure type.
- Other clinical features such as age at onset.
- Anatomic location.
- Etiology (e.g. fever).

Status epilepticus describes a state of continuous seizures.

Drug treatment can control, but not cure, 60–90% of recurrences of seizures and treatment is therefore long term

The aim of pharmacologic treatment is to control seizures without producing adverse drug effects, but this is not always accomplished. Partial seizures are controlled in only approximately 45% of cases despite optimal medical treatment. The appropriate drug depends on the nature of the epilepsy (Fig. 14.46).

Classification of epileptic seizures

Partial (focal, local) seizures

Simple partial seizures (consciousness not impaired) (motor signs, somatosensory or special sensory signs, psychic symptoms)
Complex partial seizures (consciousness impaired) (simple partial onset followed by impaired consciousness, consciousness impaired at onset)
Partial seizures evolving to generalized seizures (tonic, clonic, or tonic–clonic)
  Simple partial seizures evolving to generalized seizures
  Complex partial seizures evolving to generalized seizures
  Simple partial seizures evolving to complex partial seizures evolving to generalized seizures

Generalized seizures (convulsive or nonconvulsive)

Typical absence seizures (brief stare, eye flickering, no motion)
Atypical absence seizures (associated with movement)
Myoclonic seizures
Clonic seizures
Tonic seizures
Tonic–clonic seizures
Atonic seizures

Fig. 14.45 Classification of epileptic seizures. (From the Commission on Classification and Terminology of the International League Against Epilepsy)

Drugs used for epilepsy

Seizure type	Primary drugs	Secondary drugs
Partial and/or generalized tonic–clonic seizures	Carbamazepine, phenytoin	Phenobarbital, primidone, valproate
Absence seizures	Ethosuximide, valproate	Clonazepam
Myoclonic seizures	Valproate	Primidone

Fig. 14.46 Drugs used for epilepsy.

Treatment should always be initiated with a single drug and its use optimized before adding a second drug
Optimization of drug therapy usually involves increasing the dose of a single drug until toxicity appears. The incidence of adverse drug effects has been reported to be 22% in patients on monotherapy, 34% when two anti-epileptic drugs are given, and 44% with three drugs. A single drug is therefore preferable.

The pharmacokinetic properties and adverse effects of any chosen anti-epileptic drug must be known to obtain its maximum therapeutic benefit. Monitoring of blood concentrations is useful with phenytoin in particular because of its zero-order pharmacokinetics and a reasonable relationship between its blood concentration and therapeutic or toxic effects (see Chapter 4).

Adverse effects of anti-epileptic drugs must be considered when starting treatment because of the long duration of their use. Drug interactions (see Chapter 4) are common between other drugs and anti-epileptic drugs, and are particularly important because:

- Anti-epileptic drugs are used long term.
- There are small differences between therapeutic and potentially toxic blood concentrations for several anti-epileptic drugs.

Anti-epileptic drugs
Barbiturates (phenobarbital and primidone)
Phenobarbital was the first effective anti-epileptic drug, and despite the availability of newer agents it can still be useful in reducing the recurrence of tonic–clonic seizures. It is also inexpensive. The anti-epileptic dose is limited because phenobarbital produces sedation, but this tends to lessen with continued use. Sometimes phenobarbital produces excitement instead of sedation in children. Primidone is a structural analog of phenobarbital and is converted to phenobarbital in the body.

The cellular mechanism of action of the barbiturates probably involves synaptic inhibition by enhancing the effects of GABA. Phenobarbital and other barbiturates seem to act at $GABA_A$ receptors.

Not all barbiturates can be used as anti-epileptic drugs because many produce too much sedation at anti-epileptic doses. It is not known why phenobarbital is less sedative.

Phenobarbital is a good inducer of cytochrome P-450 so can be involved in drug interactions (see Chapter 4). Its plasma half-life is 100 hours.

Phenytoin
Phenytoin (diphenylhydantoin) is useful in the treatment of tonic–clonic seizures. At a cellular level it slows the rate of recovery of Na^+ channels from inactivation, thereby reducing neuron excitability, and this may be responsible for its anti-epileptic activity. The use of phenytoin is complicated by its characteristic toxicities and zero-order pharmacokinetics, and the necessity for long-term administration. The zero-order

pharmacokinetics (see Chapter 4) imply that when blood concentrations of phenytoin approach those that will saturate the systems that metabolize phenytoin, a small increase in dose can produce a disproportionately large increase in its plasma concentration with resulting toxicity. This can be partly prevented by measuring plasma phenytoin concentrations.

ADVERSE EFFECTS OF PHENYTOIN may be dose- or nondose-related:

- The dose-related adverse effects of phenytoin affect the cerebellovestibular system leading to blurred vision, ataxia, hyperactivity, and confusion. Gastrointestinal disturbances also occur.
- The nondose-related adverse effects include skin rashes, gingival hyperplasia, lymphadenomas, and hirsutism. Phenytoin is also believed to be teratogenic.

DRUG INTERACTIONS Phenytoin is a good enzyme inducer so is liable to produce drug interactions with drugs such as isoniazid, warfarin, chloramphenicol, erythromycin, and cimetidine (see Chapter 4).

Carbamazepine

Carbamazepine is chemically related to TCAs. Its anti-epileptic activity is similar to that of phenytoin, but it is also useful for pain such as that of trigeminal neuralgia and in the treatment of manic depressive illness. Like phenytoin it acts on Na^+ channels at a cellular level, and this may be involved in its anti-epileptic activity. Serum concentrations of carbamazepine are not clearly related to its therapeutic effects.

Carbamazepine is a powerful inducer of enzymes, including its own metabolizing enzymes. Its plasma half-life is therefore shortened by chronic administration.

ADVERSE EFFECTS OF CARBAMAZEPINE include drowsiness, vertigo, and ataxia. It is probably as teratogenic as phenytoin.

Valproate sodium

Valproate sodium is useful in reducing the frequency of tonic–clonic and particularly absence seizures. Like phenytoin and carbamazepine it interacts with Na^+ channels. It also increases the GABA content of the brain when given long term. The blood concentrations of valproate sodium do not correlate well with its therapeutic effects.

ADVERSE EFFECTS OF VALPROATE SODIUM include gastro-intestinal upset, and more importantly, hepatic failure. Hepatic toxicity appears to be more common when valproate sodium is used with another anti-epileptic drug. Tests of liver function do not predict subsequent liver toxicity.

Ethosuximide

Ethosuximide is the agent of choice for absence seizures. It is believed to act by inhibiting low-threshold Ca^{2+} currents (T-currents) in the thalamus, which is currently thought to be the origin of absence seizures. Plasma ethosuximide concentrations do not correlate well with therapeutic effectiveness.

ADVERSE EFFECTS OF ETHOSUXIMIDE include gastrointestinal upset, drowsiness, lethargy, euphoria, urticarial skin lesions, and most importantly, leukopenia, and rarely bone marrow depression.

Benzodiazepines

Clonazepam is useful for absence and myoclonic seizures while diazepam and lorazepam are effective in the management of status epilepticus. The benzodiazepines enhance GABA-induced increases in Cl^- conductance and this is probably involved in their anti-epileptic activity.

ADVERSE EFFECTS OF THE BENZODIAZEPINES The common adverse effect of the benzodiazepines is sedation. Intravenous diazepam can depress respiration, so resuscitation equipment should be available when treating status epilepticus. Repeated seizures can damage the brain and can be life-threatening so status epilepticus should be controlled.

New anti-epileptic agents

The exact role of the new anti-epileptic agents, gabapentin and lamotrigine, in the treatment of seizures remains to be defined.

GABAPENTIN is a highly lipid-soluble molecule and has been designed to mimic GABA in the CNS. It seems to be a useful add-on therapy for patients with partial seizures and is relatively free from adverse effects other than somnolence, dizziness, and fatigue.

LAMOTRIGINE is intended for use in partial seizures and seems to act through Na^+ channels. Reported adverse effects are dizziness, ataxia, blurred vision, and gastrointestinal upset.

Lamotrigine is metabolized by glucuronidation in the liver, and concomitant administration of phenytoin, carbamazepine, or phenobarbital decreases the serum half-life of lamotrigine from 24 to 15 hours, presumably by inducing increased hepatic glucuronidation of lamotrigine. In contrast, sodium valproate inhibits lamotrigine metabolism and increases the half-life of lamotrigine to 60 hours.

Sleep disorders
Normal sleep

Normal sleep is characterized by patterns of electrical activity that can be recorded on an EEG. On the basis of this record, sleep is separated into five stages. Stages 1–4 are periods of nonrapid eye movement (NREM) sleep, while stage 5 is the period of rapid eye movement (REM) sleep (Fig. 14.47).

- Stage 1 makes up 5% of total sleep and is the lightest sleep.
- Stage 2 makes up 45% of sleep and is characterized on the EEG by 'sleep spindle' waveforms.
- Stages 3 and 4 are the deepest stages of sleep and make up 12% and 13% of total sleep, respectively. These stages are often classified together on the basis of the EEG as slow-wave sleep or δ wave sleep.
- Stage 5 (REM) sleep makes up 25% of sleep and the EEG record shows low-voltage random sawtoothed waves.

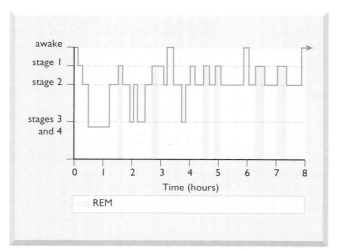

Fig. 14.47 A normal sleep cycle. This shows the normal stages of sleep. (REM, rapid eye movement)

The time between the onset of sleep and the initiation of the first portion of REM sleep is termed REM latency and is usually 90 minutes. NREM is a generally restful state with a regular low blood pressure and heart and respiratory rate; any restless movements are made during these stages and dreaming is lucid and purposeful. Body muscle tone is drastically reduced during REM sleep and the subject is still. However, the blood pressure and heart and respiratory rate are all raised, partial or full penile erections, occur, and dreams are abstract and surreal.

The central control of sleep is complex and involves:
• Serotonergic neurons in the raphe nuclei.
• Noradrenergic neurons in the locus ceruleus.
• ACh-containing neurons within the pontine raphe nuclei, which have a central role in the production of REM sleep.

The sleep–wake pattern may be governed by melatonin secreted by the pineal gland, which is in turn controlled by the hypothalamus. It is hypothesized that the sleep 'on/off switch' is situated in the hypothalamus and is part of a neuronal circuit connecting the hypothalamus with the reticular activating system.

The normal length of sleep required by an adult is 6–9 hours per night. Deprivation of REM sleep causes irritability and lethargy and a subsequent rebound in REM sleep. Prolonged total sleep deprivation can lead to death.

A variety of sleep abnormalities have been noted in psychiatric illness:
• In depression there is a marked decrease in REM latency and an increase in REM sleep.
• Alzheimer's dementia leads to a decrease in REM and slow-wave sleep.

Various drugs alter sleep patterns:
• Benzodiazepines, and to a lesser extent antidepressants, reduce REM sleep.
• Drugs that increase dopamine release (e.g. amphetamine) increase wakefulness.

Insomnia

Insomnia is a common and nonspecific disorder and may be reported by 40–50% of people at any given time. Of these cases:
• 30–35% are due to psychiatric illness.
• 15–20% are psychophysiologic or primary.
• 10–15% are due to alcohol or drugs.
• 10–15% are due to periodic limb movement disorder.
• 5–10% are due to sleep apnea.
• 5–10% are due to medical illness.

Among those seeking treatment, the female:male ratio is 2:1 and there appears to be a preponderance of cases in lower socio-economic groups.

The prognosis, etiology, and treatment of insomnia depend upon the underlying cause

A history should be taken to define the problem (e.g. initial or middle insomnia or early awakening). Is it due to a physical cause (e.g. pain or a cough)? Is it due to environmental factors such as noise?

In many cases, education in 'sleep hygiene' (e.g. reducing caffeine intake, changing sleep habits, or pain relief) might be more appropriate than a sedative medication. Early morning wakening is one of the biologic features of depression, an antidepressant might therefore be appropriate. Generally, treatment should be for the underlying cause. Insomnia without an obvious underlying cause is known as primary or psychophysiologic. Severe psychophysiologic (primary) insomnia is treated with hypnotics.

Hypnotics
Benzodiazepines

Benzodiazepines act by potentiating GABA-ergic neurotransmission and therefore enhance inhibitory activity (see page 257 for adverse effects). The benzodiazepine receptor lies within the $GABA_A$ receptor complex.

Benzodiazepines induce sleep, and their duration of action will be determined to some extent by their half-life.

Benzodiazepines should be used as hypnotics only for severe, disabling, or extremely distressing insomnia, and preferably for only 1 week

Benzodiazepines should never be used as hypnotics for more than 3 weeks and should not be used for chronic insomnia.

Other drugs for insomnia

Chloral hydrate is generally used only in the elderly. Zopiclone and zolpidem are nonbenzodiazepine hypnotics, but bind to particular subtypes of the benzodiazepine receptor. They are rapidly acting, with a short half-life of approximately 2 hours and minimal hangover effects. Long-term use is not recommended and they should not be used for more than 4 weeks.

Narcoleptic syndrome

The narcoleptic syndrome is a relatively rare disorder that occurs in 20–160 per 100,000 adults. It is characterized by excessive daytime sleepiness and cataplexy, which in turn is characterized by a sudden loss of muscle tone in response to emotional stimuli such as laughter, pain, and fear. Cataplexy affects the jaw, neck, legs, or whole body, leading to collapse. Associated symptoms include sleep paralysis, which is an inability to move any muscles on awakening while apparently conscious. It occurs in 40% of narcoleptics and can last several minites. Short-duration sleep paralysis lasting seconds can be a normal phenomenon, as can pre-sleep dreaming (sometimes called hypnagogic hallucinations), which occurs in 30% of people with narcolepsy.

The sleep attacks can occur at any time of the day and cannot be avoided. They usually start in the late teens, and almost invariably before 30 years of age. The attacks may progress in severity and frequency or reach a plateau. Spontaneous re-mission is rare.

The night-time sleep pattern is disrupted, with a markedly reduced REM latency and sleep-onset REM occurring within 10 minutes after the onset of sleep.

Narcolepsy is treated with CNS stimulants
The first management strategy in narcolepsy is to encourage the patient to have regular daytime naps and sometimes this can almost abolish the sleep attacks. However, most patients require medication.

CNS stimulants used to treat narcolepsy
Methylphenidate hydrochloride and amphetamine
Both methylphenidate hydrochloride and amphetamine are indirectly acting sympathomimetics. Their primary effect is to cause the release of catecholamines from presynaptic neurons. They also inhibit catecholamine reuptake. These actions lead to stimulation of many brain regions, including the ascending reticular activating system and the striatum.

ADVERSE EFFECTS OF METHYLPHENIDATE AND AMPHETAMINE include anxiety, irritability, insomnia, dysphoria, and an increased blood pressure and heart rate. Long-term effects include a delusional disorder similar to schizophrenia. Over-dose leads to psychosis, cardiovascular symptoms, and seizures.

Modafinil
Modafinil is a centrally acting stimulant. It is an effective treatment of excessive daytime sleepiness (EDS). It may reduce attacks and improve performance in narcolepsy, and is thought to have a better adverse effect profile and less addictive potential than the sympathomimetics. Its mechanism of action is not clear, but it may act as an agonist at α_1 adrenoceptors.

Other drugs used in the treatment of narcolepsy
These include:
- The MAO_B inhibitor selegiline.
- Anticholinergic medications to treat cataplexy.
- SSRIs (e.g. fluoxetine) and SNRIs (e.g. venlafaxine) to improve cataplexy.

Sleep apnea
This disorder has been recently recognized and is characterized by disturbed sleep at night and excessive daytime sleepiness. Its prevalence is not yet known, but it appears to be relatively common, particularly in the obese and the elderly, and the apnea is lengthened and made more likely to occur by alcohol.

There is little pharmacologic treatment at this time although modafinil may help EDS in patients who do not respond to continuous positive airway pressure therapy.

Periodic limb movement disorder
Like sleep apnea, periodic limb movement disorder is characterized by disturbed night-time sleep and daytime sleepiness. It is, however, less well understood than sleep apnea or narcolepsy. Possibly up to 30% of patients over 60 years of age and as many as 10% of people with insomnia have this disorder.

The night-time symptoms typically involve a stereotypic extension of the big toes with flexion of the ankle and knee, leading to partial awakening. If they occur more than 30 times during the night they usually lead to daytime somnolence.

The prognosis and etiology are unknown, but the disorder occurs in other sleep disorders and in parkinsonism and is worsened by TCAs and MAOIs.

The most effective treatments to date have been clobazam, clonazepam, selegiline (a MAO_B inhibitor, see above) and levodopa (the dopamine precursor used in Parkinson's disease).

Circadian rhythm disorders
These are an important group of sleep disorders that affect most people at some time or another. The sufferer has by definition a sleep–wake cycle that is out of step with his or her environment, resulting in impaired social or occupational functioning.

The most common reasons for this disorder include:
- Shift working, and particularly changing shifts to opposite sides of the day/night.
- Jet lag, in which the sufferer has travelled east or west across more than one time zone.
- Delayed sleep phase syndrome, which affects adolescents, particularly males. In this syndrome the sleep onset and awakening times steadily advance by 1–2 hours/day until the sufferer is out of synchrony with his or her environment.

Circadian rhythm disorders are usually self-limiting; however, re-establishment of a normal sleep–wake pattern with a hypnotic and with bright light exposure may be helpful. Melatonin is a hormone secreted by the pineal gland and is involved in the sleep–wake cycle experimentally. It is available over the counter and may have some uses in re-establishing a normal sleep–wake cycle in delayed sleep phase syndrome and jet lag.

Dementia
Dementia is defined as a global impairment of higher cortical functions, including memory, the capacity to solve the problems of day-to-day living, the performance of learned perceptual–motor skills (e.g. playing an instrument), the correct use of social skills, and control of emotional reactions, in the absence of gross clouding of consciousness. The condition is

261

Common causes of dementia

- Alzheimer's disease
- Vascular (multi-infarct dementia)
- Pick's disease
- Dementia of parkinsonism
- Huntington's disease
- Creutzfeldt–Jacob disease

often irreversible and progressive. A shorter definition is 'Dementia is an acquired global impairment of intellect, memory, and personality, but without an impairment consciousness.'

Senile dementia of Alzheimer's type (Alzheimer's disease)

Alzheimer's disease (AD) is the most common cause of dementia, accounting for 50–60% of all cases. It is senile and presenile (i.e. onset before 65 years of age) dementia and women are affected twice as often as men after the age of 70 years, but equally at younger ages. The average duration of the disease is 5–10 years and is increasing as general health improves.

Signs of AD are progressive global memory loss, parietal lobe function abnormalities of spatial orientation, deteriorating social skills, loss of drive, initiative, and intellect, depression, anxiety, aggression, emotional lability, unconcern, agitation, and disruption of the sleep–wake cycle.

Pharmacologic treatments for Alzheimer's dementia target the cholinergic system

Pharmacologic treatments for AD are still being developed and three approaches (Fig. 14.48) are in use:

- An ACh precursor such as lecithin choline, but while this has been shown to increase CNS ACh concentrations in the rat, there has been no demonstrable improvement in cognition in patients with AD.

Treatment strategies for Alzheimer's dementia

Strategy	Drug
To increase the concentration of acetylcholine or to stimulate brain cholinergic receptors directly using a precursor	Lecithin
Release enhancers	Hydergine
Cholinesterase inhibition	Tacrine, velnacrine, donepezil, rivastigmine, galantamine

(Not all of these are currently licensed in the US or UK)

Fig. 14.48 Treatment strategies for Alzheimer's dementia.

- Medications that enhance the release of ACh, such as Hydergine (ergoloid mesylates), which increase ACh release from rat cortical slices. However, there have not yet been any trials of these drugs in humans.
- Cholinesterase inhibitors such as tacrine, donepezil, rivastigmine, galantamine and velnacrine, which are significantly better than placebo at increasing short-term memory, selective attention, language abilities, and praxis functions in AD. However, the clinical benefits are generally quite modest with only about a 10% improvement.

ADVERSE EFFECTS OF TACRINE AND VELNACRINE include abdominal cramps, nausea, polyuria, and diarrhea. Serious adverse effects have been noted with tacrine, including a persistent rise in liver transaminases in 15–30% of patients, as well as severe liver toxicity. This is thought to be due to a mild drug-induced dose-dependent hepatic inflammation. The more recently introduced anticholinesterase inhibitors donepezil, rivastigmine and galantamine are better tolerated than tacrine and velnacrine but still exhibit side effects such as nausea, vomiting and diarrhea. These are worse at higher doses and during a rapid titration.

Vascular dementia (multi-infarct dementia)

Multi-infarct dementia (MID) is traditionally thought to be the second most common dementia, and accounts for 15–30% of all cases of dementia. However, some experts believe that diffuse Lewy body disease is more common, but this remains to be confirmed. MID can coexist with other degenerative dementias and this accounts for 15% of all dementias.

MID is more common in men and in people with a high risk of cardiovascular problems. The onset is usually relatively acute and the progression is typically stepwise as each infarct occurs. The site and extent of the infarcts determines the cognitive deficits. Neurologic signs are generally more common than in AD.

The typical clinical features of MID include an abrupt onset, emotional incontinence, stepwise deterioration, a history of hypertension, a fluctuating course, a history of strokes, nocturnal confusion, atherosclerosis, relative preservation of personality, depression, focal neurologic symptoms and signs, somatic complaints, and patchy cognitive deficits.

Pharmacologic treatments for MID are based on attempting to reduce the risk of further cerebral infarction

Hypertension should be treated with appropriate antihypertensives (see Chapter 18), and any coexisting conditions that predispose to emboli formation (e.g. cardiac arrhythmias, cardiac valve disease) should be treated appropriately. Daily enteric-coated aspirin is indicated for any patient suspected of suffering from MID, because of its antithrombotic activity (see Chapter 13). If there are coexistent features of AD, a therapeutic trial of cholinergic medication (see above) may be prescribed.

Parkinson's disease

Parkinson's disease is a neurologic disorder characterized by impaired voluntary movements. Voluntary movements are controlled centrally by neuronal pathways that travel in the pyramidal (corticospinal) tracts from the motor cortex and down the spinal cord to the lower motor neurons (α motor neurons). The lower motor neurons directly control the activity of voluntary muscles. Although these are the main neuronal pathways, neuronal inputs from other sources also exert some influence on the pyramidal pathways. These subsidiary pathways provide the extrapyramidal influence, which smoothes voluntary movements. One major extrapyramidal source is the basal ganglia (caudate nucleus, putamen, and pallidum), and disease of these structures (e.g. Parkinson's disease) affects the smooth execution of voluntary movements.

Parkinson's disease is characterized by the major symptoms of:
- Bradykinesia (i.e. slow initiation of movements).
- Tremor at rest involving the hands in 'pill-rolling' movements.
- Muscle rigidity, reflected as resistance to passive limb movements.
- Abnormal posture (Fig. 14.49).

The signs displayed by parkinsonian patients include:
- A characteristic shuffling gait.
- A blank facial expression.
- Speech impairment.
- An inability to perform skilled tasks.

The disease occurs more frequently in the elderly and gets progressively worse with time unless it is treated.

Parkinsonism is usually idiopathic, but it can be induced by neuroleptics

Although there is usually no identifiable underlying cause of Parkinson's disease, it is associated with loss of dopaminergic neurons in the basal ganglia and it has been suggested that it may be caused by an environmental toxin. For example, in primates, 1-methyl-4-phenyl-1,2,3,6-tetrahydropyridine (MPTP), which is a chemical contaminant produced in the synthesis of a heroin substitute, causes irreversible damage to the nigrostriatal dopaminergic pathway that can lead to the development of symptoms similar to idiopathic Parkinson's disease seen in humans. It appears that a metabolite (MPP^+) produced from MPTP by MAO_B is actually responsible, and MAO_B inhibitors (e.g. selegiline) can prevent the damage produced by MPTP.

Parkinsonism can be induced by drugs that block striatal dopaminergic receptors (e.g. neuroleptics such as chlorpromazine). Indeed, when such drugs are used in the treatment of schizophrenia, a parkinsonian-like syndrome can occur as an adverse effect. Similarly, drugs such as reserpine, which deplete the nigrostriatal nerves of their dopamine content, also produce a parkinsonian-like syndrome.

At postmortem, the brains of parkinsonian patients contain a substantially reduced concentration of dopamine (less than 10% of normal) in the corpus striatum and substantia nigra.

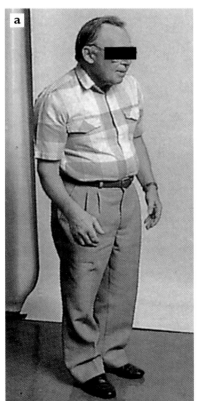
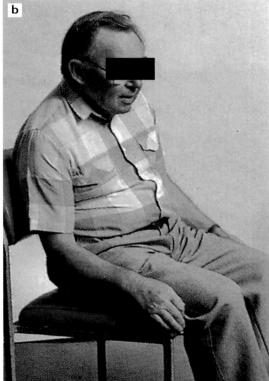
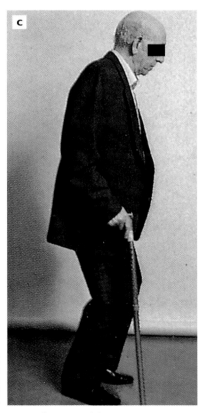

Fig. 14.49 Parkinson's disease. Posture and gait can give important clues to neurologic diagnosis. (Courtesy of Dr R. Capildeo)

Striatal cholinergic hyperactivity is also associated with the development of Parkinson's disease. Usually, the activity of this neuronal pathway is opposed by the dopaminergic pathway that projects from the substantia nigra (Fig. 14.50).

■ *Treatment of Parkinson's disease involves enhancing striatal dopaminergic activity and inhibiting striatal cholinergic activity*

The approach to treating Parkinson's disease is based on correcting the imbalance at the basal ganglia between the dopaminergic and cholinergic systems, and two major groups of drugs are used:

- Drugs that increase dopaminergic activity between the substantia nigra and the corpus striatum.
- Drugs that inhibit striatal cholinergic activity.

Tissues rich in dopamine (e.g. chromaffin cells from the adrenal medulla) have been surgically implanted into the corpus striatum to improve dopaminergic activity, but the clinical effectiveness of such procedures is uncertain. Gene therapy to increase striatal dopamine content by transfecting the tyrosine

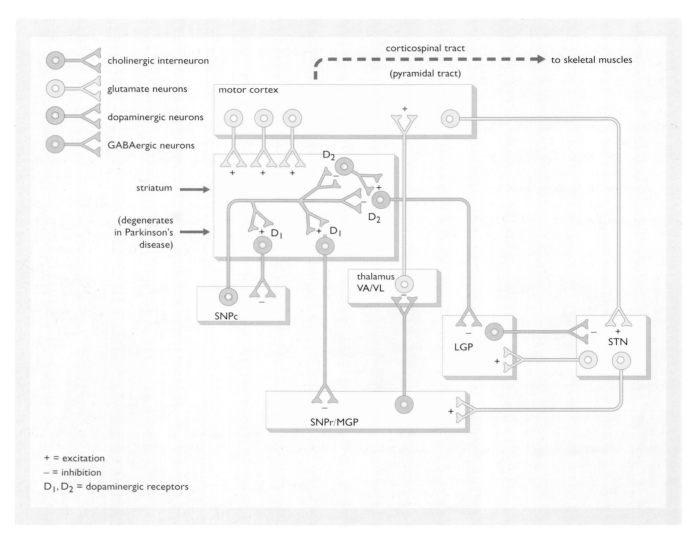

Fig. 14.50 Schematic diagram of the basal ganglia systems involved in Parkinson's disease. In Parkinson's disease, inhibitory dopaminergic activity of the extrapyramidal pathway from the substantia nigra pars compacta (SNPc) to striatal GABAergic neurons is considerably depleted (20–40%), usually through neurodegeneration. This results in unopposed cholinergic excitation of the striatal GABAergic neurons leading to the pathologic features of Parkinson's disease. Normally, two neuronal pathways from the basal ganglia regulate thalamic feedback input to the motor cortex for smooth execution of movement. Both pathways are activated by glutamate neurons from the motor cortex. The direct pathway consists of striatal GABAergic neurons which send inhibitory activity to the substantia nigra pars reticulata (SNPr) and the medial globus pallidus (MGP) leading to disinhibition of the output from these sites to the thalamus and thus allowing thalamic feedback input to the motor cortex. The indirect pathway also consists of another group of striatal GABAergic neurons which send inhibitory activity to the lateral globus pallidus (LGP), to prevent it from inhibiting excitatory neuronal output from the subthalamic nucleus (STN) to the SNPr and MGP. Excitation of the latter sites leads to inhibition of the thalamic feedback input to the motor cortex and interferes with the smooth execution of movement. The relative activity of these two pathways is regulated by dopaminergic neuronal activity from the SNPc to the striatum. ACh is found in interneurons that exist in the indirect pathway. VA and VL are ventroanterior and ventrolateral thalamic nuclei.

hydroxylase gene to the corpus striatum to enhance the rate of synthesis of dopamine has also been considered.

Drugs that increase dopaminergic activity
Levodopa (L-dopa)

Levodopa is used instead of dopamine, which does not cross the blood–brain barrier, to replenish the dopamine content of the striatum. It is a precursor from which dopamine is produced by decarboxylation (Fig. 14.51). Levodopa crosses the blood–brain barrier, undergoes decarboxylation, and increases the content of releasable dopamine which opposes the excessive striatal cholinergic activity and restores balance between the two systems.

Levodopa is rapidly absorbed from the small intestine by an active transport system for aromatic amino acids. Its absorption can be impaired by dietary aromatic amino acids, and by gastric juice hyperacidity, delayed gastric emptying, and the presence of food. Peak plasma concentrations are reached 1–2 hours after an oral dose. The plasma half-life is only 1–3 hours, owing to extensive metabolism in the wall of the intestine (Fig. 14.52). Levodopa is also metabolized in the blood and peripheral tissues and only about 1% of the administered dose is left to enter the brain and produce therapeutic effects. Dopamine is the major peripheral product of levodopa metabolism and it is responsible for most of the peripheral adverse effects. Other metabolic products derived from levodopa include HVA and 3,4-dihydroxyphenylacetic acid (see Fig. 14.51). The extensive peripheral metabolism of levodopa means that large doses have to be given to produce therapeutic effects in the brain, but such doses produce many adverse effects (see below).

■ *The peripheral adverse effects of levodopa can be reduced by combining it with a peripheral dopa decarboxylase inhibitor or by co-administering domperidone or selegiline*

These effects can be reduced by combining levodopa with a peripheral dopa decarboxylase inhibitor such as carbidopa or benserazide, which reduce the peripheral metabolism of levodopa so that it can be used at lower doses. Neither carbidopa nor benserazide cross the blood–brain barrier; consequently, they interfere with levodopa metabolism only in the periphery. However, this drug combination not only maximizes the therapeutic effectiveness of levodopa but also increases the unwanted central effects of dopamine. Additionally, pyridoxine (vitamin B_6), which usually exacerbates peripheral metabolism of levodopa, does not interfere with the therapeutic effectiveness of the drug combination.

Some of the peripheral adverse effects of levodopa can also be decreased by co-administration of the dopaminergic D_2 antagonist, domperidone, which does not cross the blood–brain barrier. Alternatively, selegiline, an MAOI that selectively blocks MAO_B, can be used to inhibit dopamine metabolism selectively in the brain. MAO_B is the predominant MAO isoform responsible for metabolizing dopamine in the brain (MAO_A predominates in the periphery). Unlike the nonselective MAOIs, selegiline does not inhibit the peripheral metabolism of tyramine to produce the 'cheese reaction' (see above).

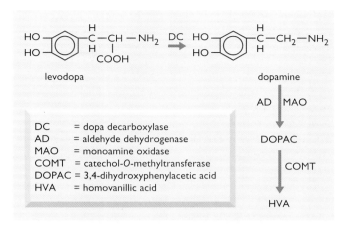

Fig. 14.51 Conversion of levadopa to dopamine and other metabolites.

DC   = dopa decarboxylase
AD   = aldehyde dehydrogenase
MAO   = monoamine oxidase
COMT = catechol-O-methyltransferase
DOPAC = 3,4-dihydroxyphenylacetic acid
HVA   = homovanillic acid

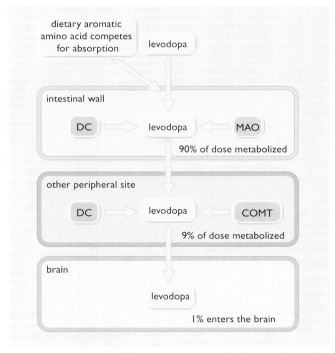

Fig. 14.52 Percentage of levodopa entering the brain after oral administration. There is extensive metabolism in the wall of the intestine by dopa decarboxylase (DC) and to a lesser extent by monoamine oxidase (MAO). Levodopa is also metabolized in the blood and peripheral tissues by catechol-O-methyltransferase (COMT) and DC. The extent of peripheral metabolism is of the order of 99%, leaving only about 1% of the administered dose of levodopa to enter the brain to produce therapeutic effects.

Although selegiline is used mainly with levodopa to prolong and increase central dopaminergic effects, it has been proposed that this drug can be used alone in the early stages of Parkinsonism to slow the progressive loss of dopaminergic neurons in the basal ganglia.

Other therapeutic approaches to increase central levodopa concentration include the use of catechol-O-methyl transferase (COMT) inhibitors (e.g. entacapone, tolcapone). These drugs

265

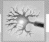

prevent the metabolism of levodopa to 3-o-methyldopa. This effect is produced peripherally by both drugs and centrally by tolcapone, which crosses the blood–brain barrier.

EFFECTS OF LEVODOPA DURING TREATMENT When levodopa is first used, the parkinsonian symptoms of rigidity, bradykinesia, and motor functions, as well as facial expression, speech, and handwriting, usually improve. However, the effectiveness of levodopa decreases after several years of treatment, possibly owing to a progressive loss of dopaminergic neurons in the nigrostriatal pathway.

The beneficial effects of levodopa can fluctuate during effective therapy, leading to a worsening of symptoms (e.g. rigidity and bradykinesia). This phenomenon, termed the 'on–off effect' (see below), results in difficulty initiating movement, even while walking or attempting to rise from a chair. The mechanism of this phenomenon is not understood, but it occurs when the plasma levodopa concentration is falling. More frequent but lower doses of levodopa may therefore reduce its occurrence, as may the addition of bromocriptine with lower doses of levodopa.

▨ *The beneficial effects of levodopa are produced mainly through the actions of dopamine on D_2 receptors*

The D_2 receptors are distributed postsynaptically on striatal GABAergic neurons that form part of the basal ganglia indirect pathway which regulates thalamic feedback input to the motor cortex (see Fig. 14.50). At the cellular level, activation of D_2 receptors inhibits adenylyl cyclase and as a consequence decreases production of the second messenger, cAMP. This reduction in cAMP opposes the excitatory effect of the cholinergic interneurons on the GABAergic neurons (of the indirect pathway). Consequently, these GABAergic neurons are inhibited and thus prevented from activating the indirect pathway, which opposes thalamic feedback input to the motor cortex. There is also evidence that D_1 receptors are distributed postsynaptically on another group of striatal GABAergic neurons that form part of the basal ganglia direct pathway which facilitates thalamic feedback input to the motor cortex. Activation of these D_1 receptors leads to stimulation of adenylyl cyclase and increased production of cAMP. This second messenger activates the basal ganglia direct pathway and as a consequence facilitates thalamic feedback input to the motor cortex (see Fig. 14.50).

As a result of these actions, dopamine re-establishes regulatory control on the neuronal output from the basal ganglia to the thalamus (see Fig. 14.51), which sends appropriate feedback nerve impulses to the motor cortex for smooth execution of movement and alleviation of the symptoms of Parkinson's disease.

ADVERSE EFFECTS OF LEVODOPA These include:
- Nausea, vomiting, and anorexia.
- Hypotension and cardiac arrhythmias.
- Abnormal involuntary movements (dyskinesias).
- The 'on–off' effect.
- Behavioral changes.

Nausea, vomiting, and anorexia result from stimulation of dopaminergic receptors in the chemoreceptor trigger zone of the area postrema. They can be minimized by giving levodopa with either domperidone or a dopa decarboxylase inhibitor (e.g. carbidopa).

The cardiac effects are usually tachycardia or extrasystoles, both of which are due to increased catecholamine stimulation following the excessive peripheral metabolism of levodopa. Although the explanation for the hypotension is uncertain, there is evidence that central interference with sympathetic activity may be involved. However, the hypotension diminishes with continued levodopa treatment in many patients.

Dyskinesias develop after long-term treatment with levodopa and involve mainly the face and limbs. They are more common when levodopa is used in combination with a dopa decarboxylase inhibitor or when other measures are taken to produce a substantial increase in central dopamine concentration. The abnormal movements can be improved by reducing the doses of levodopa and thereby reducing the central dopamine concentration, but rigidity may reappear.

The 'on–off' effect is manifested as rapid fluctuations in clinical features, varying from increased mobility and general improvement, to increased rigidity and a general deterioration in the patient's ability to perform voluntary movements. This effect occurs suddenly and for short periods lasting from a few minutes to a few hours. At present, there is no clear explanation for the effect, but similar worsening can occur when the plasma levodopa concentration falls (see above).

Behavioral changes include insomnia, confusion, and other effects that are commonly seen in schizophrenia. Schizophrenia is attributed to increased dopaminergic activity in the mesolimbic area of the brain and can be controlled with a neuroleptic such as clozapine.

Bromocriptine

Bromocriptine is a member of a group of drugs (including pergolide and lisuride maleate) derived from ergot alkaloids.

It is used in the treatment of Parkinson's disease because it is a dopamine agonist at D_2 receptors in the corpus striatum. However, it also activates other central D_2 receptor sites (e.g. in the anterior pituitary gland) and D_1 receptors. Members of the ergot alkaloid group can also be used in the treatment of hyperprolactinemia and to suppress growth hormone release in acromegaly (see Chapter 15).

Bromocriptine is often added to levodopa in the treatment of Parkinson's disease when levodopa alone does not adequately

---

⚠ **Adverse effects of levodopa**

- *Involuntary movements*
- *'On–off' effect*
- *Nausea*
- *Hypotension*
- *Some cardiac arrhythmias*

control the symptoms or when patients experience severe 'on–off'. Usually, the combination consists of submaximal doses of levodopa and bromocriptine, but occasionally full doses of bromocriptine are given alone. Good therapeutic results are obtained with both regimens and the incidence of involuntary movements is reduced. However, it has not been clearly established that bromocriptine is effective in patients who have become refractory to levodopa. The plasma half-life of bromocriptine (6–8 hours) is longer than that of levodopa, although peak plasma concentration of both drugs are reached over the same period (1–3 hours) following oral administration.

ADVERSE EFFECTS OF BROMOCRIPTINE are similar to those of levodopa, except that in some patients hypotension can be severe enough to cause fainting after the first dose of bromocriptine. It is therefore recommended that, before starting full treatment with bromocriptine, patients should be tested for susceptibility to the hypotensive effect by using a 1-mg test dose of the drug after a meal and with the patient lying in bed. Other unwanted effects include visual and auditory hallucinations and erythromelalgia involving the feet and hands. Dyskinesia occurs much less frequently than with levodopa, perhaps because the agonist effect at the D_2 receptor in the striatum is greater than the partial agonist effect at the D_1 receptor at this site.

Pergolide relieves the symptoms of Parkinson's disease as effectively as bromocriptine

Both pergolide and lisuride are agonists at D_2 receptors, and pergolide relieves the symptoms of Parkinson's disease as effectively as bromocriptine.

Pergolide is also an agonist at D_1 receptors and it produces less nausea, vomiting, and hypotension, but this drug is still undergoing clinical evaluation.

Other recently introduced D_2 agonists include cabergoline (an ergot derivative), ropinirole and pramipexole. These drugs are recommended for use in combination with levodopa to reduce 'on–off' effects, and motor fluctuations, and to allow the use of lower maintenance doses of levodopa. Clinical experience with these drugs suggests that they are as effective as bromocriptine; however, they are still being evaluated.

Amantadine

Amantadine is useful in the treatment of Parkinson's disease because it increases central dopamine release. However, it is less effective than the dopaminergic agonists, possibly because of its mechanism of action, which is thought to be facilitation of neuronal dopamine release and inhibition of its uptake into nerves. A modest anticholinergic effect may also contribute to its therapeutic effectiveness. However, based on its dopaminergic mechanism of action, it is expected that the effectiveness of amantadine would be brief, since there is progressive degeneration of the nigrostriatal dopaminergic neurons through which amantadine produces its therapeutic effects in Parkinson's disease. Amantadine is therefore only of short-term benefit, since most of its effectiveness is lost within 6 months of initiating treatment. Nevertheless, addition of amantadine

to the levodopa regimen leads to synergistic effects and an improvement in the therapeutic benefits.

Amantadine is usually given orally and is quickly absorbed from the gastrointestinal tract. Its plasma half-life is 2–4 hours, but it can accumulate in the body during renal impairment because it is excreted unchanged in the urine.

ADVERSE EFFECTS OF AMANTADINE are similar to, but less severe than, those of levodopa. They include hallucinations, confusion, nightmares, and anorexia. Prolonged use of amantadine may lead to development of livedo reticularis owing to catecholamine-induced vasoconstriction in the lower extremities.

Drugs that inhibit striatal cholinergic activity

Inhibition of striatal cholinergic activity is also a therapeutic strategy used for treating Parkinson's disease. The drugs most commonly used are antagonists at the muscarinic receptors that mediate striatal cholinergic excitation in opposition to dopaminergic inhibition of striatal GABAergic nerve activity (see Fig. 14.50). Their major function in the treatment of Parkinson's disease is to reduce the excessive striatal cholinergic activity that characterizes the disease.

The prototype of this group of drugs is trihexyphenidyl hydrochloride; other members of the group are benztropine mesylate, biperiden, orphenadrine hydrochloride (which has H_1 receptor antagonist properties) and procyclidine hydrochloride. As a group, their therapeutic effectiveness is less than that of levodopa and the tremor is reduced more than the

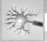

rigidity and bradykinesia. They also reduce the excessive salivation associated with Parkinson's disease. These drugs are given orally. There is no major difference in the therapeutic effectiveness among members of the group.

ADVERSE EFFECTS OF MUSCARINIC ANTAGONISTS USED IN PARKINSON'S DISEASE The typical peripheral anticholinergic adverse effects (i.e. dry mouth, blurred vision, urinary retention, and constipation) are common. More often, patients experience a variety of CNS adverse effects, including mental confusion, delusions, hallucinations, drowsiness, and mood changes. As parkinsonism can worsen when these drugs are discontinued, any termination of treatment should be gradual.

Huntington's disease

Like Parkinson's disease, Huntington's disease is a movement disorder associated with defects in the basal ganglia and related structures. But, unlike Parkinson's disease, it is a hyperkinetic disorder characterized by excessive and abnormal movements. The movements are involuntary, irregular and jerky; different groups of muscles of the face, trunk, and neck are involved. The disorder is also characterized by progressive dementia.

Huntington's disease is hereditary and often appears during adult life. The symptoms are associated with biochemical defects in the basal ganglia that in many ways are the mirror image of the defects that produce the symptoms of Parkinson's disease. For example, increased concentrations of dopamine are found in the putamen of patients with Huntington's disease at postmortem. Reduced glutamic acid decarboxylase (an enzyme that synthesizes GABA) and choline acetyltransferase activities have also been demonstrated and correlate with the production of deficient levels of GABA and ACh in the basal ganglia. It is thought that these deficiencies reduce the inhibitory influence (via striatal GABA neurons) on the nigrostriatal dopaminergic neurons (see Fig. 14.50) and lead to the dopaminergic hyperactivity associated with Huntington's disease. Further evidence for this pathophysiologic process is provided by the observations that the symptoms of Huntington's disease are suppressed by drugs that block dopaminergic receptors and worsened by drugs that increase basal ganglia dopaminergic activity.

■ *Treatment of Huntington's disease involves the use of drugs to reduce basal ganglia dopaminergic activity*
DRUGS THAT DEPLETE CENTRAL DOPAMINE STORES by blocking entry into the neuronal storage vesicles include reserpine (given in small doses of 0.25 mg daily; no longer used in the UK) and tetrabenazine. The adverse effects of these drugs include hypotension, depression, sedation, and gastrointestinal disturbances. These effects occur less frequently with tetrabenazine than with reserpine.

DRUGS THAT REDUCE DOPAMINERGIC ACTIVITY BY BLOCKING THE RECEPTORS include the phenothiazines (e.g. perphenazine) and the butyrophenones (e.g. haloperidol), which are neuroleptics. The major adverse effects associated with their use include restlessness and parkinsonism.

Migraine and headache

Migraine is a common condition affecting 5% of men and 15% of women. It is a familial disorder in which two major syndromes have been identified, firstly classic migraine, or migraine with aura; secondly common migraine or migraine without aura. Migraine is characterized by periodic, often unilateral pounding pulsatile headaches, that often begin in childhood. It is exacerbated by physical activities and/or emotional stress. Accompanying symptoms include phonophobia, photophobia, nausea and vomiting. The classic view of the mechanism of migraine is that it is the result of complex vascular factors, and in particular the distension and excessive pulsation of branches of the external carotid artery.

The treatment of migraine consists of two parts: treatment of acute attacks, and prophylaxis of future attacks.

Treatment of an acute attack should be initiated during the neurologic (visual) prodrome, or if this is absent, at the very start of the headache. Treatment of mild to moderate headaches is with an NSAID, acetaminophen or propoxyphene. Codeine or oxycodone can be combined with aspirin or acetaminophen, caffeine and butalbital, but only for short periods as this combination can cause dependence. For more severe attacks, the ergot alkaloids, ergotamine tartrate or dihydroergotamine (DHE) are used. Ergotamine is an α adrenergic agonist that has strong affinity for 5-HT_1, receptors, stimulation of which leads to vasoconstriction. These drugs can be administered subcutaneously or intramuscularly and can be re-administered 30–60 minutes later if necessary. Ergotamine is contraindicated in patients with coronary artery or peripheral vascular disease. A single dose of the H_1 receptor antagonist promethazine or the dopamine agonist metoclopramide, helps relax the patient and reduce the nausea and vomiting. Recent evidence suggests that a single dose of sumatriptan, a highly selective agonist of the 5-HT_{1D} receptor is effective in the treatment of migraine. It is well tolerated and administered orally (100 mg), although it is not as effective as when administered subcutaneously. Sumatriptan is not used for prophylaxis.

In patients with frequent migraine attacks, efforts at prophylactic prevention are important and considerable success has been obtained with the β adrenoceptor antagonists, propranolol or altenolol. In patients who do not tolerate these drugs, a calcium channel blocker such as verapamil or nifedipine can be used. The monoamine oxidise inhibitor phenelzine can sometimes be useful. Methysergide can also be used to prevent migraine attacks, as can the NSAIDs ketoprofen and tolfenamic acid.

CLUSTER HEADACHES are another type of headache having a characteristic 'cluster pattern' which occur predominantly in young adult men. Cluster headache is usually treated with a single dose of ergotamine. Subcutaneous DHE or sumatriptan can also be used.

STROKE

Stroke is one of the leading causes of death in the Western world and may be the most important disease causing long-term disability. The management of strokes has changed considerably as it is now possible to intervene and ameliorate neurologic deficits in many patients if treatment is initiated quickly after symptoms develop. In view of these developments, stroke needs to be viewed in the same context as acute myocardial infarction where public education has influenced people to go quickly to emergency medical departments.

The initial diagnosis of stroke is primarily clinical and will not be discussed here. The major distinction between ischemic and hemorrhagic stroke must be made quickly as the early treatment, and therapies aimed at secondary prevention are quite different for these two disorders. Computerized tomography (CT) of the brain, or possibly magnetic resonance imaging (MRI) in some cases, may be the most useful way to make this demarcation even if the clinical presentation seems straightforward. Ischemic stroke is usually caused by occlusion of an cerebral artery. The clinical deficits found in the early stage of ischemic stroke are due to the local death of neuronal cell function; at this stage, the loss of function may be reversible if cerebral blood flow can be restored. The time window for this opportunity is not clear. Once this is exceeded, the damage will progress to an irreversible stage associated with neuronal cell death. Thrombolytic therapy is appropriate in many patients with ischemic stroke whereas it is contraindicated in patients with hemorrhages.

Thrombolytic therapy for acute strokes

Systematic reviews of multiple controlled trials have demonstrated benefit from thrombolytic therapy, especially in decreasing neurologic deficits and dependent living when evaluated after 3–6 months. Although thrombolytic therapy with tissue plasminogen activator (TPA), streptokinase, or urokinase can cause intracranial bleeding, the efficacy more than outweighs this risk. Moreover, for patients with an ischemic stroke treated within 3 hours of onset, the risk of intracranial bleeding is less and the benefits are greater. These results of clinical trials highlight the importance of emergency treatment of ischemic stroke. While further information is necessary in order to characterize the use of TPA in patients with concomitant diseases such as diabetes and hypertension, current evidence favors implementing TPA therapy at an early time. This therapy is generally contraindicated in patients taking anticoagulants or having clotting disorders or low platelet counts. The use of TPA in thrombotic states is described in Chapter 13.

There may be a small benefit in using aspirin in the early phases of acute stroke. The potential benefits of anticoagulants during acute stroke are not established; unfortunately, no experimentally attractive neuroprotective agents have been shown to be effective in clinical trials.

Stroke prophylaxis

Aspirin has a well-established benefit in preventing stroke, especially in patients who have had a transient ischemic attack (TIA) or have carotid atherosclerosis. Aspirin and other antiplatelet drugs are discussed in Chapter 13.

Anticoagulation with warfarin has established benefit in preventing stroke in patients with atrial fibrillation. The use and therapeutic monitoring of warfarin is discussed in Chapter 13.

DRUGS AND INFECTIONS OF THE CENTRAL NERVOUS SYSTEM

Infections can occur in every part of the CNS and include:
- Meningitis (inflammation of the meninges).
- Radiculitis (inflammation of the spinal nerve roots).
- Myelitis (inflammation of the spinal cord).
- Encephalitis (inflammation of the brain).
- Brain abscess (a localized collection of pus).

In addition, new imaging techniques such as MRI have revealed that many regions of the CNS show dynamic fluctuating inflammatory processes in unnamed syndromes involving the CNS. The cause of these lesions is unknown, but could be a virus or similar microbiologic agent.

The CNS is protected by the skull, spinal column, and meningeal membranes, but infectious agents can gain access:
- Through any breach in the CNS protection (e.g. a skull fracture).
- Via the blood (e.g. septicemia with subsequent abscess formation).
- Via the nerves (e.g. rabies virus).
- By uncertain means (e.g. herpes simplex virus (HSV)).

The local immune response of the CNS varies with the site and the infecting organism, and the degree and nature of the tissue response to different microbial agents is therefore quite diverse.

The biologic agents that infect the CNS range from helminthic parasites (e.g. *Trichinella spiralis*, a nematode), to fungi and bacteria (e.g. *Coccidioides immitis* and *Mycobacterium tuberculosis*) through to viruses (e.g. HSV) and subviral proteins (e.g. prions in Creutzfeldt–Jacob disease).

■ *Diagnosis of a CNS infection is based on findings from the patient's history, physical examination, and laboratory tests*

The signs and symptoms vary and depend on the site affected. They include fever, irritability to the extent of convulsions, altered mentation, altered motor function, and lassitude, drowsiness, or coma. As abscesses and parasitic cysts are space-occupying lesions they can produce symptoms and signs resulting from pressure on or destruction of adjacent structures (e.g. visual field defects due to pressure on or destruction of the optic nerve).

Examination of the CSF can be helpful:
- An increased initial pressure and an increased concentration of CSF protein suggest that there is an infection.
- Microscopy may reveal increased leukocytes (bacterial infection), increased lymphocytes (viral infection), or increased eosinophils (parasitic infection).
- A Gram stain may demonstrate meningococcus (*Neisseria meningitidis*) or *Streptococcus pneumoniae* as the infective agent, while India-ink staining may reveal a fungal infection.

269

- Biochemical examination may reveal the presence of viruses or parasites or their corresponding antibodies.
- Special CNS scanning techniques such as computerized axial tomography (CAT) or MRI also help in the diagnosis, especially of an abscess or other space-occupying lesion.

Whenever bacteria enter the blood stream (septicemia) there is a possibility that a cerebral abscess will develop. Although rare, this can occur after staphylococcal skin infections, for example.

Encephalitis can occur without inflammation of the meninges and vice versa, but they often occur together. Meningeal irritation is due to either an infection or the presence of an inflammation-inducing substance in the CSF (e.g. blood). The particular symptoms and signs of meningeal irritation are:

- A stiff neck.
- Pain on neck flexion.
- Pain accompanying limitation of passive straight leg raising. These physical findings should always lead to further investigations.

◼ The primary use of drugs for CNS infections is to control or eliminate the causative organism

The organism must be identified and the drug most likely to be selectively toxic is chosen. This drug must be able to reach the site of infection in adequate concentration. It must therefore cross the blood–brain barrier at an adequate rate and there must be adequate access of the drug to the infected site (i.e. abscesses must be surgically treated in addition to any pharmacologic treatment).

◼ A secondary use of drugs for CNS infections is to control responses to the infection

Such responses include seizures, which are treated with antiepileptic drugs (see page 257), and allergic and other immunologic tissue responses, which are treated with glucocorticosteroids (see Chapter 15).

◼ Antibiotics and antiviral agents do not readily penetrate into the CNS, presumably because of the blood–brain barrier

The relative concentration of penicillin G in the CSF compared with that in the serum is 5%, while that for ampicillin is 15%, nafcillin 5%, vancomycin 10%, chloramphenicol 30%, gentamicin 20%, cefotaxime 15%, ceftriaxone 5% and ceftazidime 20%. The tissue distribution of antibiotics and antivirals is discussed in Chapters 8 and 9.

The question of whether antibiotics should be given directly into the CSF has not been satisfactorily answered, but the mortality rate of children with meningitis due to Gram-negative bacilli increases when gentamicin is injected into the cerebral ventricles. This suggests that injecting antibiotics into the CSF carries considerable risk.

Viral meningitis and encephalitis

Almost any virus can cause encephalitis accompanied by varying degrees of meningeal inflammation, including rubeola or mumps virus, a variety of herpes viruses, HSV types 1 and 2,

Epstein–Barr virus (EBV), cytomegalovirus (CMV), varicella zoster virus (VZV), coxsackie virus, and human immuno-deficiency virus (HIV) (see Chapter 8).

Treatment involves the use of the appropriate antiviral drug, if such a drug exists, and intravenous administration of drug is almost always required:

- Acyclovir is the drug of choice for treating encephalitis due to HSV-1 and its use has reduced the mortality rate due to this infection from 80% to 20%.
- Ara-A or foscarnet are used for acyclovir-resistant HSV-1 encephalitis.
- Sorivudine is selective for VZV infections.
- Ganciclovir is useful for CMV encephalitis, but must be used with caution because of bone marrow toxicity and, since it is excreted primarily by the kidneys, renal function should be monitored.

The treatment of cerebral disease in patients with HIV is evolving and involves decisions as to whether HIV or some other agent is causing the problem (see fungal and parasitic infections below).

Several viruses that cause encephalitis (e.g. the virus causing eastern equine encephalitis) are not susceptible to antiviral drugs.

Bacterial meningitis and encephalitis

The bacterium most likely to produce meningitis varies with the age of the patient. The commonest bacteria causing meningitis are:

- Gram-negative bacilli and group B streptococci in neonates less than 1 month old.
- *Haemophilus influenzae*, *N. meningitidis*, and *S. pneumoniae* in children aged 1 month to 15 years.
- *N. meningitidis*, *S. pneumoniae* and staphylococci in adults (i.e. those over 15 years of age).

A bacterial cause of a CNS infection must be diagnosed as soon as possible so that specific antibiotic therapy can be instituted. The CSF should be cultured to identify which bacteria are present and appropriate sensitivity tests are indicated to guide the choice of antibiotic.

If the etiology of the CNS infection is unknown but believed to be bacterial, the initial antibiotic therapy listed in Fig. 14.53 is used. If the bacterial etiology is known, the currently recommended antibiotics of choice for beginning therapy, as shown in Fig. 14.54, are used.

CNS tuberculosis and syphilis

Mycobacterium tuberculosis and *Treponema pallidum*, the cause of tuberculosis and syphilis, respectively, are important causes of CNS infections.

M. tuberculosis can infect the CNS and cause meningitis, tuberculous abscesses, or widespread miliary tuberculosis in the brain and spinal cord. All these are serious diseases and require appropriate therapy with antibiotics (see Chapter 19).

Syphilitic meningitis and neurosyphilis are manifestations of infection with *T. pallidum* during secondary and tertiary syphilis. Neurosyphilis is often accompanied by changes in

Initial antibiotic therapy for meningitis or encephalitis if the etiology is unknown but believed to be bacterial

Patient group	Antibiotics
Neonates less than 1 month old	Ampicillin plus either gentamicin or ceftriaxone or cefotaxime
Children aged 1 month to 15 years	Ampicillin plus either chloramphenicol or ceftriaxone or cefotaxime
Adults (i.e. those over 15 years of age)	Ampicillin or penicillin G
Immunocompromised adults	Ampicillin plus ceftriaxone or cefotaxime plus gentamicin
Postcraniotomy patients	Nafcillin plus ceftriaxone or cefotaxime plus gentamicin

Fig. 14.53 Initial antibiotic therapy for meningitis or encephalitis if the etiology is unknown but believed to be bacterial.

Currently recommended initial antibiotic therapy for bacterial meningitis or encephalitis if the bacterial etiology is known

Bacterial cause	Antibiotic
S. pneumoniae, streptococcus A and B, *Listeria monocytogenes*, *N. meningitidis*	Penicillin G
H. influenzae (β lactamase negative)	Ampicillin
Methicillin-sensitive *Staphylococcus aureus*	Nafcillin
Methicillin-resistant *Staph. aureus*	Vancomycin
H. influenzae (β lactamase positive)	Cefotaxime or ceftriaxone
Escherichia coli, *Klebsiella*, and *Proteus*	Cefotaxime or ceftriaxone with gentamicin
Pseudomonas aeruginosa	Gentamicin plus ceftazidime

Fig. 14.54 Currently recommended initial antibiotic therapy for bacterial meningitis or encephalitis if the bacterial etiology is known.

mental status and can be mistaken for other forms of mental illness. During tertiary syphilis, syphilitic gummas (areas of focal degeneration of brain tissue similar to abscesses) may form in the CNS. All stages of syphilis should be treated with penicillin as soon as they are diagnosed; even gummas are reduced by penicillin treatment.

Fungal CNS infections

Several fungi can cause meningitis and/or focal lesions in the brain and spinal cord, particularly in immunocompromised patients (e.g. in people with AIDS or those who have been treated with anticancer or immunosuppressant drugs). Such fungi include *C. immitis* and *Histoplasma capsulatum* (see Chapter 10). The behavior of these organisms resembles that of *M. tuberculosis* in that they are inhaled, and the resulting disease usually involves the lungs, but may involve the CNS, presumably because the organism is transported to the CNS in the blood. The CSF contains complement-fixing antibody in 95% of cases of coccidioidomycosis, and the demonstration of such antibodies justifies starting antifungal therapy. In approximately 50% of cases *C. immitis* can be found on microscopic examination of CSF. Complement-fixing antibodies are less common in histoplasmosis and its diagnosis depends on isolating *H. capsulatum* in culture.

Treatment of both coccidioimycosis and histoplasmosis is difficult, but centers on amphotericin B.

Protozoal CNS infections

MALARIA Worldwide, cerebral malaria resulting from infection by *Plasmodium falciparum* (see Chapter 11) is probably the most serious and common CNS infection. There are approximately two million deaths due to malaria each year. African children with cerebral malaria account for about half a million of these deaths. The death rate of cerebral malaria is approximately 20% despite the best current treatment, which involves intravenous quinine (or quinidine) or *Artemisia* derivatives such as artemether.

TOXOPLASMOSIS CNS infections with *Toxoplasma gondii* can occur in immunosuppressed patients. If the immunosuppression has a cause other than AIDS, 2–5% of CNS infections are due to this agent, but in patients with AIDS, the incidence rises to 25–80%. In these conditions, there are often cerebral lesions, which are best detected by MRI. Motor weakness, hemiparesis, and convulsions can occur, depending on the location of the lesions.

The drugs of choice in treating toxoplasmosis are pyrimethamine plus a sulfonamide, but bone marrow depression due to the antifolate activity of pyrimethamine can be a problem. Another antifolate, trimethoprim, is of little value in this disease. The macrolide antibiotic clarithromycin may be of use.

Helminthic CNS infections

Three helminths can infect the CNS: *Trichinella spiralis*, *Taenia solium*, and *Echinococcus granulosis*. The first two are ingested in infected inadequately cooked pork or game (e.g. bear). *E. granulosis* is harbored by dogs and the eggs are excreted in the feces; they can then be ingested by humans. Once in the intestine, all three parasites can be transported in the blood to the brain where they produce space-occupying cerebral lesions that can be seen on CAT or MRI scans. The neurologic signs they produce will depend on the location of the lesions.

271

TRICHINOSIS INVOLVING THE CNS is definitively diagnosed by identifying the larvae in the CSF. It is usually treated with prednisone to suppress the CNS immune response to the nematode, which is often accompanied by marked eosinophilia in the CSF. Mebendazole is given to suppress the parasite.

T. SOLIUM cysticerci (larvae) develop in the brain. The definitive diagnosis is obtained by biopsy of one of the cystic lesions. Drug treatment involves glucocorticosteroids to suppress immune responses, plus albendazole or praziquantel.

ECHINOCOCCAL CYSTS usually develop in the liver or lungs but, if they rupture, eggs can then be carried to the brain, where new cystic lesions develop. Such cysts are often detected by CAT or MRI scan. Surgical removal of the cyst is the definitive therapy, but the cyst must not be ruptured otherwise eggs will be spread elsewhere by the blood. Giving albendazole during the surgery may reduce this risk of spreading the infection.

PAIN

Pain is a normal manifestation of everyday life and serves a vital defensive function. However, uncontrolled pain can dramatically diminish quality of life. Pain is often associated with a range of other psychologic and central disturbances (e.g. anxiety, depression, insomnia, anorexia) and profound changes in autonomic function (e.g. heart rate, blood pressure, micturition).

Pain can be subdivided into acute and chronic forms.

- Acute pain is short term, generally persisting only for the duration of the tissue damage, and represents a natural, physiologic defense reaction of the body.
- Chronic pain is evident even when the normal healing mechanisms have been completed, and in diseases such as rheumatoid arthritis may persist for weeks, months, or even years.

It is not known what physiologic function, if any, can be ascribed to chronic pain. However, it is clear that pain is an important component of the response to trauma (e.g. accidents, burn damage), surgery (e.g. postoperative pain), and disease (e.g. arthritis, cancer, cardiac pain, sickle cell crisis, herpes zoster, myofascial pain).

▇ *Pain perception is best viewed as a three-stage process*
A full understanding of the processes that control pain perception in both damaged tissues and the spinal cord and higher brain centers is useful when trying to provide effective therapy for pain. Although possibly an oversimplification, the three stages of pain perception can be seen as:

- Pain 'appreciation' in peripheral tissues following activation of specialized pain sensors (nociceptors).
- Transmission of pain information from the periphery to the dorsal horn of the spinal cord where it is inhibited or amplified by a combination of local (spinal) neuronal circuits and descending tracts from higher brain centers.
- Onward passage of pain information to higher brain centers, from which any appropriate action can be initiated.

Each of these stages is controlled by a variety of local hormones at peripheral sites, and neurotransmitters at central sites. The interactions between the various neurotransmitters are highly complex and have not yet been clearly defined.

▇ *The first step in the perception of pain appears to be activation of pain-specific receptors called nociceptors in the peripheral tissues*
Unlike other sensory receptors that detect, for example, mechanical pressure or temperature changes, nociceptors (Fig. 14.55) are poorly defined anatomically. It seems likely that they are simply bare nerve endings in the skin, muscle, and deeper viscera. Exactly how they are activated following, for example, tissue damage, remains a mystery, although a number of chemical mediators known to be present at the site of tissue disease or decay can stimulate nociceptors and therefore promote pain (see Fig. 14.55). Inflammatory mediators included in this group include histamine (also causes itching) and bradykinin (BK). When applied in low doses to an exposed blister base in human volunteers, both histamine and BK are able to trigger a painful response (Fig. 14.56). BK acts via G protein-linked receptors (B_1 and B_2) to produce a range of proinflammatory effects including vasodilation and edema. BK receptor stimulation also activates membrane-bound phospholipase A_2 enzyme activity, which in turn causes membrane de-esterification, leading to the release of free arachidonic acid (eicosatetraenoic acid) and the subsequent

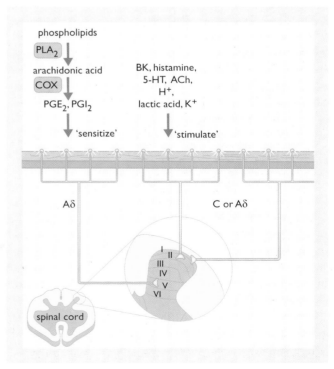

Fig. 14.55 Perception of pain. (ACh, acetylcholine; BK, bradykinin; COX, cyclo-oxygenase; 5-HT, 5-hydroxytryptamine; PG, prostaglandin; PLA, phospholipase A)

Pain

 Pain-related definitions

- Pain is an unpleasant sensory and emotional experience associated with actual or potential tissue damage

- Acute pain is pain of recent onset and limited duration. It usually has an identifiable cause relating to injury or disease

- Chronic pain is pain that persists for long periods, usually beyond the time of tissue healing, and for which the cause may not necessarily be easily identifiable

- Hyperalgesia is tenderness and/or pain arising from relatively innocuous stimulation

- A noxious stimulus is a stimulus that damages or is potentially damaging to the tissue

- Nociception is the process of detecting and signaling the presence of a noxious stimulus. This term is frequently reserved to describe the process in experimental animals

- Pain behavior is behavior that leads an informed observer to conclude that a human or an experimental animal is experiencing pain

- An algogen is a chemical mediator that promotes pain behavior and is usually generated within diseased or damaged tissue

- An analgesic drug is a drug or therapy that effectively removes or at least curtails pain sensation in humans

- An antinociceptive drug is a drug or therapy that effectively removes or at least curtails pain behavior

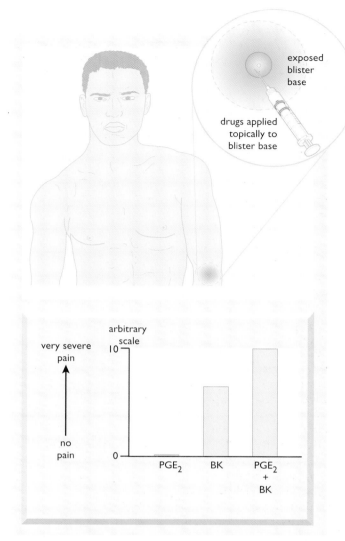

Fig. 14.56 The role of bradykinin (BK) and prostaglandin (PG) in pain. In low doses BK is algesic (i.e. causes pain), whereas PGE$_2$ is hyperalgesic (i.e. not painful by itself, but potentiates BK-induced algesia).

biosynthesis of prostaglandins (e.g. PGE$_2$ and prostacyclin, PGI$_2$) by cyclo-oxygenase (COX) (see Chapters 16 and 20 for further details). It is therefore not surprising that there are prostaglandins (PGs) at the site of the inflammatory response (e.g. PGs are found in synovial fluid aspirated from the joints of patients with rheumatoid arthritis or osteoarthritis). PGs cause hyperalgesia but not algesia. Physiologic concentrations of PGs (PGE$_2$, PGI$_2$) do not cause pain when applied to exposed blister bases in human volunteers or following intradermal injection in animals. However, such concentrations of PGs powerfully accentuate the pain-producing effect of mechanical or chemical stimulation, as well as that resulting from the application of chemical agents such as histamine and BK (see Figs 14.55, 14.56). 5-HT is another local hormone that triggers pain responses from peripheral nociceptors. It is released from degranulating mast cells at the site of tissue damage and triggers a powerful pain response, which is probably greater than that elicited by either BK or histamine. A variety of metabolic substances released from damaged cells (e.g. ATP, lactic acid, K$^+$) also exhibit algesic activity.

The second step in pain perception is the transfer of information from stimulated nociceptors in the periphery to the spinal cord.

Information is transferred from stimulated nociceptors in the periphery to the spinal cord by:

- Myelinated Aδ fibers, which transmit information rapidly at a rate of approximately 15 m/second and appear to produce a sharp and intense pain sensation.
- Unmyelinated C fibers, which transmit information more slowly at a rate of approximately 1 m/second and appear to produce a less well-localized pain that may be described as a dull and throbbing ache.

The cell bodies of both Aδ and C fibers lie within the dorsal root ganglion, from which fibers enter the dorsal spinal cord through the dorsal root to synapse with so-called 'nocirespkonsive' neurons located in the superficial laminae I and II and to a lesser extent lamina V (Aδ fibers only) (see Fig. 14.55, and Fig. 14.57). Excitatory amino acids (EAA) such as glutamate, and neurokinins such as substance P and neurokinin A, act as neurotransmitters at the junction between primary afferent nerve terminals and spinal cord nocirespkonsive neurons.

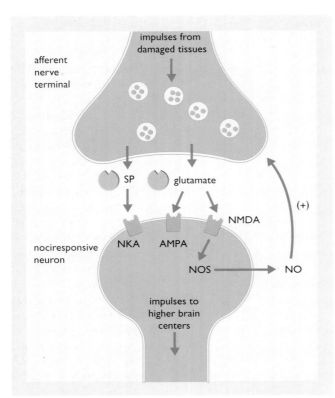

Fig. 14.57 Mechanism of pain perception. Activation of nociceptors in damaged, diseased, or inflamed tissues by a range of algesic and hyperalgesic chemical mediators stimulates Aδ and C sensory afferent nerves, which terminate in the superficial laminae (I and II) and lamina V of the spinal cord. Nitric oxide (NO) is the retrograde transmitter, increasing substance P (SP) and glutamate release to cause 'wind-up.' (AMPA, 2-amino-3, 3-hydroxy-5-methylisooxazol-4-yl propionic acid; NKA, neurokinin A; NMDA, N-methyl-D-aspartate receptors; NOS, nitric oxide synthase)

■ *Electrophysiologic analysis of membrane potentials from dorsal horn nociresponsive cells in response to peripheral noxious stimuli reveals a complex pattern of electrical activity*

An early rapid membrane depolarization takes place and has been ascribed to activation of AMPA (2-amino-3, 3-hydroxy 5-methlisooxazol-4-yl propionic acid) receptors by glutamate released from primary afferent nerves. This initial response is followed by a more slowly developing secondary depolarization. Glutamate acting on N-methyl-D-aspartate (NMDA) receptors and substance P are generally considered to be the major neurotransmitters at this site, but other neuropeptides such as vasoactive intestinal polypeptide, somatostatin, and cholecystokinin may also regulate this process.

An additional important role for glutamate acting on NMDA receptors located on the spinal nociresponsive neurons is the induction of a process called spinal 'wind up.' This electrophysiologic phenomenon is analogous to 'long-term potentiation' in other brain areas and can be defined as the increase in amplitude of membrane depolarization in spinal nociresponsive neurons, following repetitive stimulation of their C fiber input by a painful stimulus applied to a peripheral tissue. In this way, pain (e.g. inadvertently hitting a thumb with a hammer) may not only provoke instantaneous pain (carried by Aδ fibers) but also cause a dull and throbbing painful sensation in the damaged region several minutes or even hours later. This secondary pain reaction is triggered by the formation of proinflammatory algesic mediators such as BK and histamine in the damaged tissue, in this case the thumb. As inflammation proceeds, the resulting activation of nociceptors sets up a barrage of impulses along sensory C fibers, gradually 'winding up' nociresponsive neurons in the spinal cord. Ultimately, a situation is reached where usually nontroublesome stimuli, such as lightly brushing the thumb or applying an adhesive plaster, can cause tenderness and pain (i.e. hyperalgesia). Spinal 'wind up' may explain why acute pain sometimes converts into chronic pain spontaneously and for no good physiologic reason. The cellular mechanism of this phenomenon is now believed to involve the following steps:

- Activation of NMDA receptors by glutamate, either on the nociresponsive neuron itself or on adjacent neurons.
- Opening of NMDA-linked Ca^{2+} channels in these neurons.
- Activation of Ca^{2+}–calmodulin-dependent nitric oxide synthase (NOS) to yield nitric oxide (NO).

NO is a freely diffusible and highly lipid-soluble mediator and rapidly passes retrogradely to the primary afferent nerve terminal to increase efflux of glutamate (and perhaps also substance P). In this way, the initial release of even a very small amount of glutamate from sensory C fiber terminals is able to trigger the efflux of larger and larger quantities of glutamate, enhancing depolarization of the nociresponsive neuron and ultimately completing the 'wind up' process. It might therefore be predicted that breaking this 'circle' by administering NOS inhibitors such as L -N^{G}-nitro-arginine methyl ester (L-NAME) in experimental animals will relieve pain. Whether such drugs will be effective for chronic pain awaits the identification of novel NOS inhibitors, with fewer adverse effects, that can be studied in humans.

■ *Electric activity of spinal nociresponsive neurons is 'fine tuned' by neurotransmitters released from spinal neurons and major supraspinal descending nerve bundles*

Perhaps the greatest local control over spinal cord pain sensitivity is provided by opioid peptides, particularly Met-enkephalin and β-endorphin, and perhaps to a lesser extent Leu-enkephalin and dynorphin. Each of these peptides is located within neurons of laminae I and II of the dorsal spinal cord and each provokes analgesia by interacting with specific opioid receptors (i.e. μ, δ, and κ).

Since intrathecally applied opioids such as morphine are analgesic, their site of action must be spinal, but systemically administered opioids may also influence pain perception by an effect on higher brain centers. The mechanism of action of opioids at the spinal level involves inhibiting the release of substance P and glutamate from C fiber terminals, but the cellular mechanism of action is not clear.

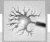

■ *Opioid receptors have been cloned. The μ, δ, κ₁, and κ₂ receptors belong to the G protein-coupled family of receptor proteins*

Activation of opioid receptors has a number of cellular consequences, including inhibition of adenylyl cyclase activity leading to a reduction in intracellular cAMP concentration. This fall in neuronal cAMP was believed to account entirely for the analgesic effect of opioids. However, more recent studies indicate that other cellular results of opioid receptor activation are also important including:

- Opening of K^+ channels to cause hyperpolarization of the nociresponsive neuron, thereby reducing excitability.
- Blocking the opening of voltage-gated Ca^{2+} channels to inhibit glutamate and substance P release from primary afferent terminals.

Other neurotransmitters that play a part in controlling the function of nociresponsive neurons include GABA, which has also been detected by mapping the synthetic enzyme glutamic acid decarboxylase (GAD) in the dorsal spinal cord. Like opioids, GABA acting on GABA_B receptors located presynaptically on primary afferent nerve fibers is believed to reduce the release of glutamate and substance P. In this way, baclofen, which is a GABA_B agonist, produces behavioral antinociception in experimental animals.

■ *The third step in the perception of pain is the onward passage of pain information to higher brain centers*

The plethora of excitatory and inhibitory neuronal inputs acting on nociresponsive neurons in the dorsal spinal cord highlights the major importance of these neurons in transferring information from nocireceptors in the tissues to the brain. This function underlies the 'gate control' theory of pain put forward by Melzack and Wall in the mid-1960s, according to which nociresponsive neurons of laminae I and II act as intelligent 'gatekeepers' between damaged tissues and the brain. The information they receive is modified by both spinal and supraspinal influences before being transmitted as a 'package' of knowledge about the painful stimulus to higher centers. The ascending nociceptive pathways involved in this final stage of the process travel in the ventrolateral and dorsolateral funiculi of the spinal cord and terminate mainly in the thalamus and reticular formation. Further ascending tracts terminate in the cerebral cortex and limbic systems where the cognitive and emotional aspects of pain are coordinated.

Testing analgesic drugs

A wide variety of procedures are available to assess analgesic drugs. Tests used in human volunteers include:

- Application of a tourniquet to the upper arm, measuring the length of time the volunteer can bear the resulting ischemia-induced discomfort. This is probably the best-characterized human model of pain.
- Application of radiant heat or pressure to the skin.
- Electric shock stimulation of the skin or tooth pulp.
- Cold pressor tests in which the arm or hand is placed in ice-cold water and the time to removal recorded.

■ *Experimental subjects use a variety of techniques to quantify their perception of the level of pain*

Objective measurement of pain is not usually possible. Experimental subjects (volunteers or patients) are therefore required to express an opinion on their perception of the level of pain. This is commonly obtained using a sliding scale, which can either be verbal (e.g. 0 for no pain to 10 for worst possible pain) or visual (e.g. placing a mark on a 10-cm line graded from no pain to the worst possible pain). Occasionally such a system cannot be used. For example, assessing pain in young children is difficult, using such scales. The children can then be asked to draw a face that can be graded between a happy face to indicate no pain and a sad face to indicate intense pain. Clearly, all these measurements are highly subjective, and properly trained personnel and rigorous statistical evaluation of the results are needed, to avoid misleading or biased conclusions. Furthermore, the personality of the individual and other factors, such as the nature of the environment in which testing takes place and the general attitude of the investigator, can markedly affect the response of individuals to pain. There is therefore a need for randomization, allocating subjects to control and test groups. Despite these problems, however, each of the tests described above has been used with varying degrees of success to demonstrate drug-induced analgesia.

Drug therapy of pain
Nonsteroidal anti-inflammatory drugs (NSAIDs)

The NSAIDs inhibit the biosynthesis of hyperalgesic and proinflammatory PGs and form a chemically disparate group of drugs. Pharmacologically, NSAIDs exhibit anti-inflammatory, antipyretic, and mild analgesic activity. Tissue damage (associated with, for example, inflammation) and the accompanying plasma membrane distortion activate phospholipase A_2 enzyme activity, which cleaves free arachidonic acid from its binding sites in membrane phospholipids and renders it susceptible to attack by cyclo-oxygenase (COX or PGH synthase). All NSAIDs inhibit the COX enzymes and this effect underlies their analgesic activity. Two separate isoforms of COX have been identified:

- COX-1 is a constitutive (constantly present) enzyme found in a wide variety of cells throughout the body; it maintains the formation of PGs involved in 'housekeeping' (i.e. control of vascular flow through individual organs, regulation of platelet aggregator, etc.).
- COX-2 is synthesized *de novo* in inflammatory cells, such as neutrophils and mast cells, following exposure to stimuli such as bacterial endotoxins and/or cytokines (e.g. tumor necrosis factor (TNF) and interleukin-1β). It is responsible for generating PGs at the site of inflammation and/or tissue damage.

The majority of available NSAIDs show little or no selectivity as inhibitors of the two COX isoforms. Some compounds such as meloxicam and nimesulide have been reported to exhibit some preference for inhibiting the COX-2 enzyme although the selectivity of these compounds vis-à-vis COX-1 is not great. More recently, two highly selective COX-2 inhibitors (celecoxib and rofecoxib) have become available. Both of these compounds

275

are several orders of magnitude more potent as COX-2 versus COX-1 inhibitors, and exhibit potent anti-inflammatory and analgesic activity both in experimental animals and man. An added advantage is that these compounds appear to be associated with markedly reduced gastrointestinal side effects (a consequence of COX-1 inhibition) than do the classical NSAIDs.

Aspirin is the archetypal NSAID and was first used clinically in 1899. It acts by covalently modifying serine residues in both COX-1 (serine 530) and COX-2 (serine 516), effectively preventing further prostanoid biosynthesis. Over the last three decades numerous other NSAIDs have been developed. These are probably best classified according to their chemical structure. On this basis they can be divided into, (i) salicylic acids (e.g. aspirin along with diflunisal, olsalazine and sodium salicylate); (ii) p-aminophenol derivatives notably acetaminophen; (iii) indole acids such as indomethacin and sulindac; (iv) arylacetic acids such as tolmetin and ketorolac, and arylpropionic acids such as the widely used ibuprofen, as well as flurbiprofen, naproxen and ketoprofen; (v) anthranolic acids including mefanamic acid; and finally (vi) enolic acids such as piroxicam and tenoxicam. Unlike aspirin, most of these newer compounds bind reversibly to COX-1 and COX-2 isoforms. For the treatment of pain, NSAIDs are generally given orally and the analgesic activity is likely to persist for approximately 6–8 hours, although the effect of some NSAIDs such as piroxicam and phenylbutazone (withdrawn several years ago) can last much longer (i.e. 12 hours to several days).

All NSAIDs exhibit the same profile of biologic activity (notably anti-inflammatory, antipyretic and analgesic). However, it should be noted that NSAIDs are generally not effective against severe pain (particularly that of visceral origin) for which opioids are much better. Also, the maximal degree of pain relief available with NSAIDs is less than that provided by opioids. NSAIDs provide an effective pain-relieving strategy for mild to moderate pain as follows:

- Pain associated with an inflammatory component (e.g. gout, rheumatoid arthritis, osteoarthritis, toothache, ultraviolet light-induced sunburn).
- The pain of cancer metastases, injury (e.g. bone fractures, surgical produceres), and some types of headache, which are also associated with an inflammatory reaction.
- Dysmenorrhea, which results from increased uterine PG formation.

In this respect, the most commonly used analgesic NSAIDs are aspirin and the various salicylates. In the clinical setting there is usually very little to choose between the various NSAID classes. However, some NSAIDs (e.g. acetaminophen and ketorolac) are good analgesics but have relatively weak anti-inflammatory activity. Acetaminophen is a relatively weak inhibitor of COX enzymes and its precise mechanism of action in controlling pain remains something of a mystery.

ADVERSE EFFECTS OF NSAIDS (with the possible exception of selective COX-2 inhibitors such as celecoxib) include the ability to cause gastric blood loss and ulceration, particularly with aspirin. This may be less prevalent with other NSAIDs such as

> ⚠️ **Adverse effects of nonsteroidal anti-inflammatory drugs**
>
> - *Gastric bleeding and ulceration*
> - *Reduced platelet aggregation*

ibuprofen. Inhibited gastric formation of PGE_2 and PGI_2, which are vasodilating and cytoprotective, is important in the development of this adverse effect. Replacement therapy with synthetic PG (e.g. 15-methyl PGE_2) is available if gastric damage presents a major problem. NSAIDs also inhibit platelet aggregation and accelerate bleeding time as a result of inhibiting platelet formation of thromboxane A_2 (TxA_2), which is vasoconstricting and pro-aggregatory. Other adverse effects include dizziness, headache, and water and sodium chloride retention (all adverse effects of piroxicam). Finally, large doses of aspirin (1000–1500 mg/day) and other NSAIDs can cause auditory and visual disturbances accompanied by fever and changes in blood pH, and sometimes coma.

Opioids

All opioid drugs, whether naturally occurring such as morphine, or chemically synthesized, interact with specific opioid receptors to produce their pharmacologic effects. The three major classes of opioid receptors are μ, δ, and κ. A fourth opioid receptor (σ) was suggested, but a variety of other nonopioid drugs also appear to act as ligands at this site so it is doubtful whether this receptor should now be considered a true opioid receptor. Further subclassification of some opioid receptors (e.g. into μ_1 and μ_2) has been suggested on the basis of ligand binding and other experiments, but the pharmacologic and clinical significance of individual subtypes remains largely unclear. Drugs interact with opioid receptors as either full agonists (e.g. morphine and methadone), partial agonists, quite commonly as mixed agonists (full agonist on one opioid receptor, but partial agonist on another, e.g. pentazocine and butorphanol); or antagonists, such as naloxone and naltrexone (see Chapter 3 for definitions). Presently available opioids (with major opioid receptor target shown in brackets) include morphine ($\mu > \kappa$), methadone (μ), etorphine and bremazocine (μ, δ, and κ), levorphanol (μ and κ), fentanyl (μ) and sufentanil (mainly μ).

■ *Opioids are useful for most moderate to severe pain, and particularly for postoperative or cancer-related pain.*

Opioids have less effect against nerve pain (neuropathic pain) such as trigeminal neuralgia or phantom limb pain. In addition to their analgesic effect, opioid drugs have a variety of other actions within the CNS, but not all are beneficial. For example, opioids cause euphoria accompanied by a general sense of peace and contentment, which accounts for the illicit use of such drugs by addicts (see below). This calming activity undoubtedly contributes to their analgesic efficacy by helping relieve the anxiety and distress associated with pain, and this can be important in the treatment of acute myocardial infarction, for example. Morphine-induced euphoria appears to be mediated by activation of μ and/or κ receptors, which are presumably located within the limbic system.

Opioid analgesics are administered systemically (orally, intramuscularly, or subcutaneously) or directly into the spinal cord (intrathecally). Usually a loading dose is given, followed by maintenance dosing to ensure steady-state plasma concentrations.

TOLERANCE AND DEPENDENCE   Tolerance to the analgesic effect of opioids develops rapidly and can often be detected within 12–24 hours of administration. As a result, larger and larger doses of the drug are needed to achieve the same clinical effect, leading to an increased severity and incidence of adverse effects. Physical dependence may develop and is characterized by a definite abstinence syndrome following drug withdrawal. This syndrome comprises a complex mixture of irritable and sometimes aggressive behavior coupled with extremely unpleasant autonomic symptoms such as fever, sweating, yawning, and papillary dilation (see below).

ADVERSE EFFECTS OF OPIOIDS   limit the dose that can be given and the analgesia that can be maintained. They are all direct consequences of opioid receptor activation and relate largely to the preponderance of opioid receptors in the medulla and peripheral nervous system. They can therefore be inhibited by opioid receptor antagonists such as naloxone. The most serious adverse effect is probably respiratory depression, which results from reduced sensitivity of the medullary respiratory centers to carbon dioxide. Respiratory depression is the most common cause of death from opioid overdose. Another common adverse effect is constipation due to changes in lower gastrointestinal smooth muscle tone resulting in decreased propulsion. Other adverse effects include pupillary constriction (miosis) and vomiting via an action on the CTZ in the medulla (see page 474). The antitussive activity of opioids is an adverse effect that has been exploited clinically and as a result codeine and dextromethorphan are frequently included in proprietary cold medicines (see Chapter 19).

Pharmacologic adjuncts to analgesia

BENZODIAZEPINES   Severe pain can lead to intense emotional distress and therefore drug therapy of the associated anxiety is frequently considered to be helpful. The benzodiazepines (see pages 255) are often used for this purpose. Diazepam and lorazepam are usually the drugs of choice, providing effective anxiolytic cover over a long period, coupled with a mild amnesic effect which, although beneficial in some patients, can cause distress and confusion, particularly in older patients.

NITROUS OXIDE (N₂O)   (see Chapter 20) is another adjunct to analgesia. It is a useful analgesic in its own right for acutely painful procedures of short duration (e.g. dental procedures, childbirth) and the analgesia it provides when inhaled (sometimes as a 50% mixture in air, i.e. entonox) is rapid in both onset and offset.

KETAMINE   (see Chapter 20) was originally introduced as a dissociative anesthetic, but can also provide useful short-term analgesia, although unpleasant adverse effects such as delirium and bizarre hallucinations limit its widespread use.

■ *Opioids and NSAIDs are the mainstay of pain relief, but cannot be considered to be 'ideal' analgesics*

Both opioids and NSAIDs are relatively effective against different types of pain, but the relatively high incidence of adverse effects and other problems associated with their clinical use means that neither group can be considered to be the 'ideal' analgesic. It is hoped that the continually improving understanding of the physiologic basis of pain will ultimately be translated into the development of more powerful and safer analgesic drugs.

DRUGS OF ABUSE

Since drugs that act on the CNS can have profound effects on emotions, mood and behavior it is not surprising that such drugs are used for such actions in a nontherapeutic setting. This nontherapeutic use of drugs is generally categorized as being abuse of those drugs. Such a term is widely understood and can be used effectively, despite the fact that a more precise term might be 'substance abuse,' since common substances such as gasoline and solvents are sometimes inhaled for their pharmacologic effect. Furthermore, substances such as ethanol, caffeine and nicotine, in all their forms, are not generally commonly regarded by the public as being drugs in the therapeutic use of that term. Since such substances are taken for the effect that they produce in the human brain there is no need, pharmacologically speaking, to separate such substances from drugs of abuse. It could be even speculated that the excessive intake of food in general or of particular types of foods, is abuse in much the same way as drug abuse. The common theme of such use, or overuse, is an attempt of the taker to achieve some form of psychological reward.

Each of the drugs of abuse is used for its own particular purpose, and whatever that is, it appears to involve mechanisms that are common to other mammals. Thus drugs of abuse will, with the use of the appropriate experimental paradigm, produce an analogous pattern of abuse in other species.

All of the drugs and substances that are taken for nonthera-peutic reasons have their own profile with respect to various

> ⚠️ **Adverse effects of opioid drugs**
>
> - *Respiratory depression (μ, δ, and κ receptors)*
> - *Constipation (variable, μ, and κ receptors)*
> - *Nausea and vomiting*
> - *Pupillary constriction (μ/δ receptors)*
> - *Rapid development of tolerance*
> - *Physical dependence and abstinence syndrome*

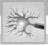

properties. The most important of these properties is the pharmacologic action of the drug in question. Drugs that are abused have a wide variety of pharmacologic actions that can be very loosely divided into at least four categories: depressant, stimulant (excitant), opioid, and hallucinogenic. Drugs in the first category are recognized to reduce activity in the CNS to the point, in the case of drugs such as barbiturates and general anesthetics, of coma and death. The term depressant is of course not exact or very descriptive. Stimulant drugs on the other hand induce alertness, excitement and euphoria and presumably are taken for such reasons. Opioid drugs are agonists at the opioid receptors and produce a mix of actions in that, in addition to producing euphoria, they also have depressant actions. Hallucinogenic drugs produce altered perception especially with respect to time and space and related to this is their ability to produce hallucinations. Dissociative anesthetics, besides producing anesthesia, also produce hallucinations.

The extent, onset and duration of the above effects are very dependent upon the route of administration and pharmacokinetic properties. Thus in order to achieve the greatest effect most rapidly, use is made of the intravenous route. An alternative to this is nasal administration (especially cocaine and nicotine) where absorption into arteries and veins is very rapid and avoids first-pass exposure in the liver. An analogous route is by inhalation into the lungs in the form of smoke and this is used especially for the opiates. The oral route, while being the easiest, is often not the favorite one since it involves an unavoidable delay between ingestion and effect.

There are many classes of drugs that are used as drugs of abuse. Many of these affect the CNS and can induce tolerance and dependence. This is best illustrated by the opioids.

Opioids

Opioids are well known as drugs of dependence and have been and are commonly abused in many societies with economic and social consequences. In many countries an extensive illegal economy exists for producing and marketing drugs of abuse and this is particularly the case for opioids, as well as for cocaine, marihuana and recreational drugs such as 'ecstasy.' In the case of the opioids the starting point is opium produced organically from the poppy *Papaver somniferum*. The opiate latex is collected from the seed pod and then variously treated for local use or export. A relatively simple chemical process converts the main alkaloid, morphine, to heroin. The latter is the choice for those whose preferred route of administration is intravenous injection.

Abusers of opioids can show tolerance and psychological dependence to opiate effects and in addition show withdrawal when opioids are discontinued after regular use. Tolerance, or more correctly, physiologic dependence is when the same dose shows lesser effects upon repeated administration or, alternatively, larger and larger doses are needed to produce the same physiologic effect. The mechanisms underlying tolerance to opiates appear to involve some form of adaptation to the continued presence of the drug. This adaptation is neuroadaptive in the sense that up- and down-regulation of receptors and neurotransmission occurs in an attempt to maintain normal function. In animal experiments, physiologic dependence or tolerance can be seen to develop within hours.

Psychological dependence is seen when a drug is used repeatedly because it provides a psychological reward of some kind, whether of pleasure or freedom from pain and anxiety. This rewarding effect relates to the main pharmacologic actions of the drug. There are elements of habit formation with any psychological dependence and there may be very little difference between an ingrained habit and psychological dependence on a drug.

The signs and symptoms of withdrawal are often opposite in nature to the acute effects of the drug. With stimulants the withdrawal syndrome is often depression, while for depressants the withdrawal syndrome is marked by excitation. In addition some of the changes seen upon withdrawal are compounded by autonomic responses to the accompanying stress.

Depending upon the particular opiate considered, as a result of its pharmacologic actions and pharmacokinetics, tolerance, psychological dependence and withdrawal can be pronounced or limited. For such reasons both morphine and heroin produce marked physiologic and psychological dependence and withdrawal whereas methadone produces much less. Much of these differences can be attributed to pharmacokinetic factors, namely the slower excretion of methadone. Drugs that are slowly eliminated from the body generally show limited withdrawal effects.

When considering drugs of abuse there is a need to consider the dangers to society associated with abuse of that drug, as well as dangers to the individual abuser. The opiate abuser generally does not constitute an immediate problem to society since the acute pharmacologic effects of opiates lead to social withdrawal and inactivity. In the longer term, the abuser incurs a social cost in terms of criminal activity related to obtaining illegal drugs and in terms of interpersonal relationships. The pharmacologic and toxicological harmful effects of opiates include confusion and, in severe cases, respiratory depression. More importantly, the mode of taking the drug carries a great risk when dirty needles and solutions are used to inject heroin (or other drugs). The risk of AIDS is very high in addicts who inject drugs.

TREATMENT The primary treatment for heroin and morphine abuse is substitution with methadone. It is administered orally, which is a benefit, and withdrawal symptoms are limited since it is eliminated slowly from the body. Methadone, is of course an opiate receptor agonist. Supportive and symptomatic therapy is an important component in treating opiate abuse.

A summary of opioid abuse is provided below:
- Analogs: morphine, heroin, fentanyl, methadone.
- Routes: oral, smoked, parenteral, particularly intravenous.
- Type of action: opiate depressant.
- Desired psychological actions: euphoria, analgesia, relaxation.
- Pharmacologic actions/effects of overdose: confusion, respiratory depression.
- Psychological dependence: marked and develops rapidly if intravenous route used.
- Tolerance: very marked.

- Withdrawal symptoms: can be severe but generally not fatal, includes shaking, tremors, diarrhea, dysphoria, sleep disturbance.
- Note: methadone has slower metabolism and produces less marked effects; therefore it is used as morphine and heroin opiate replacement.

The properties of other classes of drugs of abuse are summarized below.

Cocaine ('coke')
- Analogs: none.
- Route: oral (South America), nasal, smoked, intravenous.
- Type of action: stimulant.
- Desired psychological actions: highly rewarding for euphoria and arousal.
- Pharmacologic actions/effects of overdose: psychosis, cardiovascular death (arrhythmias and hypertensive crisis), tissue damage at site of application or injection. Fetal damage.
- Psychological dependence: strong particularly for intravenous form.
- Tolerance: limited.
- Withdrawal symptoms: depression, dysphoria, sleep disturbance.

Amphetamines
- Analogs: methamphetamine (ecstasy).
- Routes: oral, or sometimes parenteral.
- Type of action: stimulant.
- Desired psychological actions: euphoria, arousal and increased state of wakefulness.
- Pharmacologic actions/effects of overdose: psychosis, cardiovascular death (arrhythmias and hypertensive crisis), hyperthermia.
- Psychological dependence: strong but 'rush' not so apparent as with cocaine.
- Tolerance: limited.
- Withdrawal symptoms: depression, dysphoria, sleep disturbance.

Nicotine
- Analogs: none.
- Forms of use: smoked tobacco in cigarettes, cigars, pipe; intranasally as snuff; chewing tobacco (buccal cavity); transdermal patches; and chewing gum for treating nicotine addiction.
- Type of action: stimulant.
- Desired psychological actions: some euphoria, relaxation and increased concentration.
- Pharmacologic actions/effects of overdose: due to stimulation of nicotinic receptors. Overdose occurs with accidental poisoning since nicotine insecticides are absorbed through the skin and cause death from cardiovascular accidents and neuromuscular blockade. Smoking, snuff and oral administration associated with cancer (principally in lungs and oral cavity), while smoking specifically results in emphysema, bronchitis and cough.
- Psychological dependence: can be surprisingly strong.

- Tolerance: limited.
- Withdrawal symptoms: irritability, weight gain with increased appetite, headache.

Caffeine
- Analogs: none for abuse but theophylline used therapeutically.
- Forms of use: chiefly, orally ingested as drinks (coffee, tea, cocoa, chocolate, cola and some other soft drinks).
- Type of action: stimulant.
- Desired psychological actions: increased alertness and concentration.
- Pharmacologic actions/effects of overdose: anxiety, tremors, arrhythmias and convulsions in children.
- Psychological dependence: very limited.
- Tolerance: limited.
- Withdrawal symptoms: limited.

Barbiturates
- Analogs: large number exist but relatively few abused.
- Route: usually oral.
- Type of action: depressant.
- Desired psychologic actions: sedation.
- Pharmacologic actions/effects of overdose: sedation, confusion, coma, respiratory depression resulting in death.

Benzodiazepines
- Analogs: large number.
- Pharmacologic actions/effects of overdose: coma and death due to respiratory depression.
- Withdrawal symptoms: potentially the most lethal of all drugs: convulsions, tremors, shakes.

Ethanol ('alcohols')
- Analogs: by far the most important is ethanol but other low molecular weight alcohols are also abused, especially methanol.
- Route: oral.
- Type of action: depressant.
- Desired psychological actions: euphoria, release of inhibitions, increased sociability.
- Pharmacologic actions/effects of overdose: excitement, confusion, ataxia, and coma and death with acute overdose. Chronic abuse leads to hypertension, and cardiac, brain and liver pathology. Damaging to the fetus (fetal alcohol syndrome).
- Psychological dependence: moderate to severe.
- Tolerance: limited.
- Withdrawal symptoms: can be fatal, convulsions, seizures, hallucinations (pink elephants).

Phencyclidine ('dissociative anesthetics')
- Analogs: ketamine.

Solvents
- Analogs: gasoline, glue and other solvents.
- Route: inhalation.
- Type of action: depressant.

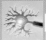

LSD ('Hallucinogens')

- Analogs: LSD principally, also mescaline, cohabe, peyote.
- Route: oral or snuff for some analogs.
- Type of action: hallucinogen.
- Desired psychological actions: hallucinations and disturbances of perception of space and time.
- Pharmacologic actions/effects of overdose: psychosis and 'flashbacks.'
- Psychologic dependence: limited.
- Tolerance: limited.
- Withdrawal symptoms: very rare probably reflecting infrequent pattern of use.

Cannabinoids

- Analogs: cannabinoid alkaloids from *Cannabis sativa*, principally delta-9-tetrahydrocannabinoid (Δ9THC).
- Route: oral (cookies) or smoked.
- Type of action: weak hallucinogen.
- Desired psychological actions: relaxation, euphoria, disturbance of perception of time and space, pleasurable effects are to some extent learned.

- Effect of overdose: not conspicuous.
- Psychological dependence: moderate.
- Tolerance: moderate or weak.
- Withdrawal symptoms: limited, sleep disturbance, anxiety.

FURTHER READING

Kaplan HI, Sadock BJ, Grebb JA. *Synopsis of Psychiatry: Behavioral Sciences, Clinical Psychiatry*, 8th edn. Baltimore: Williams & Wilkins; 1997. [An excellent general psychiatry text with comprehensive coverage of biology and psychopharmacology.]

Kopin IJ. The pharmacology of Parkinson's disease therapy: an update. *Annu Rev Pharmacol Toxicol* 1993; **32**: 467–495. [Recommended for a better understanding of the basis for the therapeutic regimens used in the treatment of Parkinson's disease.]

Pleuvry BJ, Lauretti GR. Biochemical aspects of chronic pain and its relationship to treatment. *Pharmacol Ther* 1996; **71**: 313–324. [A good general overview of the role of neurotransmitters in acute and chronic pain and of analgesic drugs.]

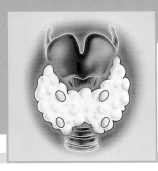

Chapter 15

Drugs and the Endocrine and Metabolic Systems

GENERAL PHYSIOLOGY OF THE ENDOCRINE AND METABOLIC SYSTEMS

The endocrine and metabolic system consists of a variety of organs (glands) that secrete substances (hormones) into the blood which affect the function of target tissues elsewhere in the body. Glands include the hypothalamus, pituitary, thyroid, adrenals, gonads, pancreatic islets of Langerhans, and the parathyroids. The endocrine system regulates seven major physiologic functions (Fig. 15.1). A cardinal feature of the drug therapy of endocrine diseases is the interaction between exogenously administered drugs and the 'endogenous pharmacology' of hormones.

The endocrine regulation of Ca^{2+} homeostasis is discussed in Chapter 20 and disorders of circulatory volume in Chapter 18. Additional information on disorders of the genitourinary function is presented in Chapter 22.

Functional anatomy of the endocrine and metabolic systems

Endocrine function	Regulatory factors	Endocrine organ/hormone	Target tissues
Availability of fuel	Serum glucose, amino acids, enteric hormones (somatostatin, cholecystokinin, gastrin, secretin), vagal reflex, sympathetic nervous system	Pancreatic islets of Langerhans/insulin, glucagon	All tissues, especially liver, skeletal muscle, adipose tissue, indirect effects on brain and red blood cells
Metabolic rate	Hypothalamic thyrotropin releasing hormone (TRH), pituitary thyrotropin (TSH)	Thyroid gland/ triiodothyronine (T_3)	All tissues
Circulatory volume	Renin, angiotensin II, hypothalamic osmoreceptor	Adrenals/aldosterone Pituitary/vasopressin	Kidney, blood vessels, CNS
Somatic growth	Hypothalamic growth hormone releasing hormone (GHRH), somatostatin, sleep, exercise, stress, hypoglycemia	Pituitary/growth hormone Liver/insulin-like growth factors (IGFs)	All tissues
Calcium homeostasis	Serum Ca^{2+} and Mg^{2+} concentration	Parathyroid glands/parathyroid hormone, calcitonin, vitamin D	Kidney, intestines, bone
Reproductive function	Hypothalamic gonadotropin releasing hormone (GnRH), pituitary follicle stimulating hormone (FSH) and luteinizing hormone (LH), inhibins	Gonads/sex steroids Adrenals/androgens	Reproductive organs, CNS, various tissues
Adaptation to stress	Hypothalamic corticotropin releasing hormone (CRH), pituitary adrenocorticotropic hormone (ACTH), hypoglycemia, stress	Adrenals/glucocorticosteroids, epinephrine	Many tissues: CNS, liver, skeletal muscle, adipose tissue, lymphocytes, fibroblasts, cardiovascular system

Fig. 15.1 Functional anatomy of the endocrine and metabolic systems. The endocrine and metabolic systems regulate seven major bodily functions. For each target tissue effect, endocrine glands release hormones in response to regulating factors, which include physiologic (e.g. sleep and stress), biochemical (e.g. glucose and Ca^{2+}), and hormonal (e.g. hypothalamic and enteric hormones) stimuli.

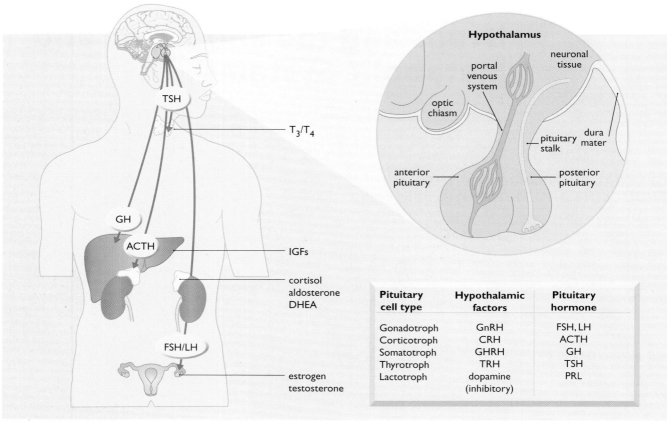

Pituitary cell type	Hypothalamic factors	Pituitary hormone
Gonadotroph	GnRH	FSH, LH
Corticotroph	CRH	ACTH
Somatotroph	GHRH	GH
Thyrotroph	TRH	TSH
Lactotroph	dopamine (inhibitory)	PRL

Fig. 15.2 The hypothalamic–pituitary axis. The cells of the anterior pituitary are regulated by hypothalamic hormones, which are released into the portal veins leading from the hypothalamus to the anterior pituitary via the pituitary stalk. Anterior pituitary hormones are released into the inferior petrosal veins for delivery to endocrine organs elsewhere in the body. The posterior pituitary consists of specialized neurons that synthesize the peptide hormones, vasopressin and oxytocin, for release into the systemic circulation. (ACTH, adrenocorticotropic hormone; CRH, corticotropin-releasing hormone; DHEA, dehydroepiandrosterone; FSH, follicle-stimulating hormone; GH, growth hormone; GHRH, growth hormone-releasing hormone; GnRH, gonadotropin-releasing hormone; IGFs, insulin-like growth factors; LH, luteinizing hormone; PRL, prolactin; T_3, triiodothyronine; T_4, tetraiodothyronine; TRH, thyrotropin-releasing hormone; TSH, thyroid-stimulating hormone.)

The hypothalamic–pituitary axis

The hypothalamus and pituitary glands integrate physiologic signals and release hormones that regulate the function of other glands

With the exception of energy metabolism and electrolyte homeostasis, pituitary hormones regulate most endocrine systems. The pituitary regulates thyroid, glucocorticosteroid, sex steroids, and growth factor secretion by synthesizing and secreting specific hormones which regulate these glands. The pituitary also secretes two hormones (prolactin and vasopressin) that act directly on target tissues. It consists of anterior and posterior divisions (Fig. 15.2). The anterior pituitary (adeno-hypophysis) develops from Rathke's pouch in the embryonic oropharynx whereas the posterior pituitary (neurohypophysis) is an extracranial extension of neuronal tissue from the diencephalon. The blood supply to the anterior pituitary is first delivered to a capillary bed in the hypothalamus, then by conduit veins to the capillary bed of the pituitary. This portal venous system provides a pathway for delivery of hypothalamic hormones which regulate anterior pituitary function. As a result of low perfusion pressures in the portal venous system the anterior pituitary is vulnerable to ischemic damage, particularly

during postpartum hemorrhage (Sheehan's syndrome). The cells of the anterior pituitary are a mixed population of cell types that secrete different peptide hormones.

Regulation of thyroid hormone secretion is a typical example of a hypothalamic–pituitary–endocrine axis control loop (Fig. 15.3). If a low concentration of circulating thyroid hormone is detected by hypothalamic receptors sensitive to thyroid hormones there is a resulting release of thyrotropin-releasing hormone (TRH) from the hypothalamus (tertiary level of regulation) into portal veins supplying the anterior pituitary. Stimulation of TRH receptors on pituitary thyrotroph cells leads to the release of thyroid-stimulating hormone (TSH, thyrotropin) into the systemic venous system (secondary level of regulation). TSH stimulates thyroid hormone release from the thyroid gland (primary level of hormone production). Thyroid hormone acts directly on target tissues and also has negative feedback effects on the hypothalamus and pituitary. The endocrine systems regulating the sex steroids and the adrenal response to physiologic stress share this four-tiered pattern of hypothalamic, pituitary, primary endocrine gland, and target tissue response.

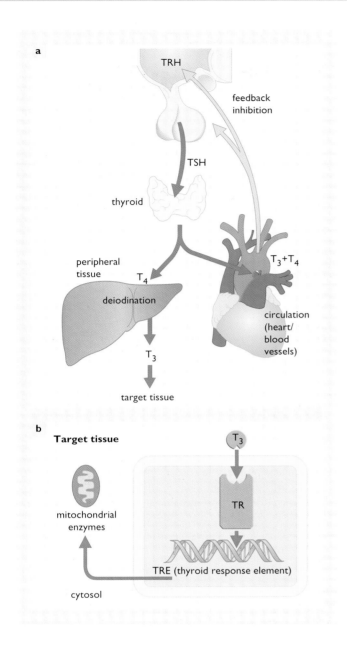

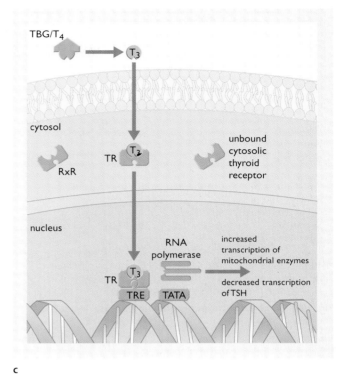

c

Fig. 15.3 The hypothalamic–pituitary–thyroid axis. (a) Thyroid hormone regulation illustrates the features of endocrine systems regulated by the hypothalamus and pituitary. Hypothalamic thyrotropin-releasing hormone (TRH) is released into the portal circulation and stimulates pituitary thyroid-stimulating hormone (TSH) release. Circulating TSH stimulates the thyroid gland to release thyroxine (tetraiodothyronine or T_4) and triiodothyronine (T_3) from stores in the thyroid follicles. (b) Thyroid hormones are largely bound to the proteins thyroid-binding globulin (TBG) and prealbumin in the circulation. The major circulating hormone, T_4, is metabolized in the peripheral tissues to the more active hormone T_3, which enters cells and binds thyroid hormone receptors. (c) The ligand-bound thyroid receptor may dimerize with itself or with the retinoic acid receptor (RxR) before translocation to the nucleus. Bound thyroid hormone receptors (TR) interact with specific thyroid response elements (TREs) of thyroid hormone-responsive genes. The hypothalamus and pituitary also contain thyroid hormone receptors, which mediate feedback inhibition by circulating thyroid hormone. Thyroid hormone is stored in the follicles of the thyroid gland. TSH stimulates endocytosis of thyroglobulin stores and release of thyroid hormone into the circulation. The scalloped margins of the thyroglobulin stores result from resorption by the cells lining the thyroid follicle.

▸ *Many endocrine systems share a common pattern of diseases*

Endocrine systems regulating metabolic rate (thyroid hormone), reproductive function (sex steroids), adaptation to physiologic stress (glucocorticosteroids) and somatic growth (growth hormone–IGF axis) share a common pattern of diseases affecting each level of endocrine regulation. While disease at any level in the regulatory system may produce a similar effect (i.e. hypo- or hyperstimulation of end-organ effects), different approaches to drug therapy may be preferred depending on the site of pathology. For example, hypogonadism due to failure of pituitary gonadotrophs may respond to therapy with exogenous gonadotropins, but gonadal failure will not. Diagnostic strategies in endocrine disease attempt to identify the site of

pathology by identifying the pattern of hormonal responses, which is characteristic for different diseases (Fig. 15.4). The primary alterations and compensatory responses of regulatory hormones accompanying the different patterns of endocrine disease must be understood to allow both diagnosis and treatment.

PATHOPHYSIOLOGY AND DISEASES OF THE ENDOCRINE AND METABOLIC SYSTEMS

Pharmacologic principles

Drugs affecting the endocrine and metabolic systems act at a variety of steps in the process of hormonal signaling where

Common patterns of endocrine disease

	Primary hormone	Regulatory hormones	Target tissue effects
Primary hormone deficiency	Decreased	Increased	Decreased
Secondary hormone deficiency	Decreased	Decreased	Decreased
Primary hormone excess	Increased	Decreased	Increased
Secondary hormone excess	Increased	Increased	Increased
Target tissue resistance	Increased	Increased	Decreased

Fig. 15.4 Common patterns of endocrine disease. Hyperfunction and hypofunction of an endocrine system may result from disease of the primary endocrine organ, at the secondary regulatory level, or at the target tissues. Diagnosis and treatment must consider patterns of adaptation to disease at these different levels. For example, symptoms of adrenal insufficiency associated with a low cortisol and high adrenocorticotropic hormone (ACTH) concentrations suggest a diagnosis of primary adrenal failure (Addison's disease), whereas similar symptoms associated with a low ACTH concentration suggest pituitary disease.

they promote or inhibit target tissue effects. This allows for different pharmacotherapeutic approaches to achieve the same pharmacologic effect by either modifying hormone action or altering hormone production. Pharmacologic intervention comprises two forms: replacement therapy (to restore depleted levels of hormones to normal), and drug therapy (administration of hormone antagonists, or other drugs, that affect an endocrine system). Replacement therapy sometimes utilizes a synthetic analog of an endogenous hormone.

In endocrine systems that are regulated by hormonal feedback to the hypothalamus and pituitary, drugs which reduce hormonal stimulation of target tissues may lead to increased hormone secretion. The cortisol synthesis inhibitor metyrapone, for instance, reduces glucocorticosteroid inhibition of adrenocorticotropic hormone (ACTH) release. Its use leads to increased ACTH stimulation of the adrenal gland which may overcome the effect of metyrapone therapy.

Diseases of the pituitary

Hypothalamic and pituitary diseases affect either single or multiple hormonal systems and lead to symptoms which resemble those of diseases of the primary endocrine glands. Owing to the critical role of the pituitary in the regulation of many endocrine functions, pituitary disease affects many body functions.

Pituitary hypofunction (hypopituitarism)

Pituitary hypofunction is caused by destructive neoplasms,

Causes of hypopituitarism

Mass lesions	Pituitary tumors Craniopharyngioma Meningioma
Infarction	Postpartum pituitary necrosis (Sheehan's syndrome)
Inflammatory/infiltrative diseases	Sarcoidosis Histiocytosis X Hemochromatosis Lymphocytic hypophysitis
Infectious diseases	Tuberculosis Syphilis
Physical insults	Trauma Surgery Radiation
Isolated hypothalamic/pituitary hormone deficiencies	

Fig. 15.5 Causes of hypopituitarism.

trauma, vascular infarction, inflammatory diseases or granulomatous infection of the pituitary (Fig. 15.5). The cardinal features of hypopituitarism are: (1) hypofunction of several endocrine-responsive target tissues; (2) low concentrations of the primary hormones affecting these tissues; and (3) concentrations of pituitary hormones that are below the level of normal compensatory response during hormone deficiency. In some cases, pituitary hormone concentrations may be increased, but not sufficient to fully correct the hormonal deficit. Pituitary hypofunction is treated by pharmacologic replacement of thyroid hormone, sex steroids, glucocorticosteroids, and vasopressin, and in some cases growth hormone.

Prolactin excess (hyperprolactinemia)

Excess prolactin secretion by the pituitary is a common condition with multiple causes. Prolactin secretion is tonically inhibited by dopamine from the hypothalamus which acts via D_2 receptors to reduce intracellular cAMP in the lactotrophs cells of the anterior pituitary. Excess prolactin usually results from either a secretory lactotroph adenoma or a variety of hypothalamic–pituitary conditions that reduce the tonic inhibition by dopamine (Fig. 15.6). Excess prolactin is a common cause of infertility and galactorrhea, and may be associated with symptoms and signs due to the physical size of a pituitary tumor, such as headaches and compression of the optic nerves.

Prolactin secretion, even from pituitary adenomas, is suppressible by dopaminergic agonists

Dopaminergic agonists with D_2 receptor activity suppress prolactin secretion (Fig. 15.7). The first drug in this class, the ergot-derivative bromocriptine, is effective in lowering prolactin concentrations but is poorly tolerated due to nausea, fatigue and other side effects. Rare but dangerous adverse effects such as seizures, cardiac arrythmia and cerebrovascular accident have been reported. Recently, the long-acting D$_2$ agonist, cabergoline, has demonstrated improved tolerability profile compared with bromocriptine. In addition to prolactin-lowering effects, D$_2$ agonist therapy also leads to shrinkage of pituitary lactotroph adenomas by suppressing DNA synthesis and cell division. In many cases, shrinkage of the prolactinoma occurs within several days of initiating therapy. Normalization of prolactin concentration is achieved in 70–80% of patients treated with dopaminergic agonists, whereas, surgical cure is achieved in approximately 50–60% of microadenomas. For this reason, these agents have now replaced surgery as the primary treatment for this type of pituitary tumor. Therapeutic benefits also include reversal of amenorrhea and infertility, and prevention of hypogonadism-related bone loss.

Causes of hyperprolactinemia	
Compression of pituitary stalk by mass lesions	
Pituitary lactotroph adenoma	
Physiologic stimuli	Suckling Chest wall trauma
Hormonal effects	Pregnancy Estrogen therapy Hypothyroidism
Drugs	Antipsychotic drugs (dopamine antagonists) Cimetidine Verapamil Opiates
Renal failure and hepatic cirrhosis	

Fig. 15.6 Causes of hyperprolactinemia.

Prolactin-lowering dopaminergic agents

- *Nausea and vomiting*
- *Orthostatic hypertension*
- *Nasal congestion*
- *Exacerbation of psychosis*
- *Digital vasospasm*

Dopaminergic agonists for hyperprolactinemia

Agent	Pharmacology	Dose	Efficacy	Pharmacokinetics	Adverse events
Bromocriptine	D$_2$-selective agonist Ergot derivative	1.25–5 mg b.i.d.	70–80%, normalize prolactin levels	Limited absorption (30%) Extensive first-pass metabolism Rapid initial plasma clearance (t$_{1/2}$ = 2 hours) Distributes to tissues Slow terminal elimination	Nausea Fatigue Postural hypotension Nasal congestion Exacerbation of psychosis Seizures Cerebrovascular accident
Pergolide	D$_1$ and D$_2$ receptor agonist Ergot derivative	0.025–0.5 mg q.d.	Similar to other agents (limited data available)	Extensive hepatic metabolism t$_{1/2}$ = 27 hours after steady-state dosing	Nausea Postural hypotension Syncope Palpitation Arrhythmia Edema
Cabergoline	D$_2$-selective agonist Ergot derivative	0.25–1 mg twice weekly	77% normalize prolactin concentrations ~70% experience shrinkage (>25%) of prolactinoma 0.05 mg is more effective than 2.5 mg b.i.d. of bromocriptine	t$_{1/2}$ = 60 hours Tissue distribution to pituitary, biliary excretion No CYP metabolism	Nausea, less than bromocriptine
Quinagolide	D$_2$-selective agonist Nonergot derivative	0.025–0.3 mg q.d.	60–80% normalize prolactin concentrations	t$_{1/2}$ = 17 hours Renal and hepatic excretion	Nausea Fatigue Postural hypotension

Fig. 15.7 Dopaminergic agonists for hyperprolactinemia.

Abnormalities of the growth hormone–insulin-like growth factor axis
Growth hormone excess (acromegaly)

The growth hormone–insulin-like growth factor (IGF) axis is another endocrine system for which the pathology lies largely within the pituitary and hypothalamus. Growth hormone is a 191-amino acid peptide which promotes protein synthesis and tissue growth. Many of the effects of growth hormones are mediated by the release of insulin-like growth factors (IGF) from the liver. These IGFs are peptide hormones which produce anabolic effects by stimulating receptors linked to tyrosine kinases. Excess production of growth hormone is rare and is usually due to an adenoma of pituitary somatotrophs. Growth hormone excess in adulthood after closure of the epiphyseal plates (i.e. acromegaly) does not usually increase stature. The main signs of adult growth hormone excess are coarse facial features (Figs 15.8 and 15.9), enlargement of hands and feet, thickening of soft tissues, and enlargement of organs such as the heart (cardiomegaly). In children, growth hormone excess may lead to giantism.

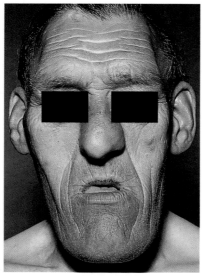

Fig. 15.8 Characteristic facial features of acromegaly. (Courtesy of Dr CD Forbes and Dr WF Jackson.)

Symptoms and signs of acromegaly

- Coarse facial features
- Enlargement of hands and feet
- Thickening of soft tissues
- Dental misalignment
- Arthralgias
- Excessive sweating
- Glucose intolerance
- Enlargement of organs (e.g. heart)
- Hypertension
- Skin tags

Fig. 15.9 Signs and symptoms of acromegaly.

Treatment of growth hormone-secreting tumors with a dopaminergic agonist or octreotide is sometimes indicated

Treatment of growth hormone-secreting tumors usually involves surgery and radiation therapy. If appropriate, two types of drug can be used:

- Dopaminergic D_2 receptor agonists which suppresses growth hormone secretion in a small percentage of cases.
- Somatostatin analogs such as octreotide or lanreotide.

Somatostatin is a 14-amino acid peptide hormone produced at many sites in the body, including the central nervous system (CNS), the digestive tract, and pancreatic δ cells, that inhibits the release of a variety of hormones (Fig. 15.10). Somatostatin receptors are G protein-coupled receptors (GPCR) that inhibit hormone release by reducing cAMP formation. Somatostatin has not been developed as a therapeutic agent, but the synthetic octapeptide analog octreotide is used clinically for the treatment of acromegaly, carcinoid tumors and bowel dysfunction.

In the treatment of acromegaly, octreotide is titrated from 50 µg t.i.d. s.c. to a maximum dose of 500 µg s.c. t.i.d. according to symptomatic and hormonal response. After maximum therapeutic response is achieved, patients may be switched to the more convenient depot preparation (octreotide-SAR 20 mg i.m.) for once-monthly injections. Octreotide therapy normalizes growth hormone and IGF-1 concentrations in approximately 50–80% of acromegalic patients. Recently, the long-acting somatostatin analog, lanreotide, has demonstrated 60–75% efficacy in normalizing hormone concentrations. Therapeutic response to these agents includes reduction in arthralgia, hyperhidrosis, headache, sleep apnea and improvement in cardiac function. Adverse effects include injection site pain, alterations in bowel function, and increased risk of cholelithiasis.

Growth hormone deficiency

Short stature is a common clinical complaint which is only rarely caused by deficiency in growth hormone (Figs 15.11, 15.12). Growth hormone deficiency may result from panhypopituitarism, selective impairment of pituitary somatotrophs, or deficient hypothalamic GHRH release.

Growth hormone (hGH) derived from cadaveric pituitary extracts have been used in the past, but resulted in some cases of Creutzfeldt–Jacob disease. Currently, recombinant human growth hormone, somatropin, and a closely related hGH analog, somatrem, are marketed for the treatment of pediatric growth hormone deficiency, short stature related to Turner syndrome, and adult-onset growth hormone deficiency. Somatrem contains the 191 amino acids of native hGH and an additional terminal methionine residue. Growth hormone binds to GH receptors in many tissues which act by intracellular tyrosine kinase pathways. In the liver, GH receptor activation leads to secretion of insulin-like growth factors (IGF-I and IGF-II) which are monomeric proteins with high homology to insulin. IGFs bind to IGF receptors in many tissues and stimulate tyrosine kinase signaling pathways (see Chapter 3, Fig. 3.9).

Administration of recombinant hGH accelerates linear skeletal growth, exerts an anabolic effect on organs and soft

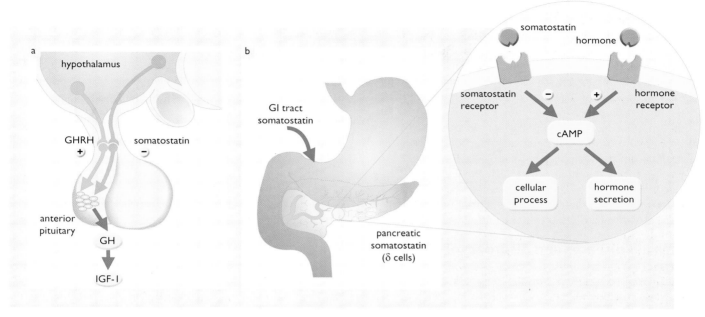

Fig. 15.10 Somatostatin physiology. Somatostatin is synthesized and released locally in the hypothalamus, pancreatic δ cells (a) and gastrointestinal (GI) tract (b). Somatostatin inhibits cellular processes related to growth hormone (GH), insulin, glucagon, and enteric hormone secretion by reducing cAMP accumulation and inhibiting cellular depolarization (inset). Octreotide is a synthetic peptide analog of somatostatin used in the treatment of GI carcinoid tumors, hormone-mediated bowel disease, and occasionally, acromegaly. (GHRH, growth hormone releasing hormone; IGF-I, insulin-like growth factor-I)

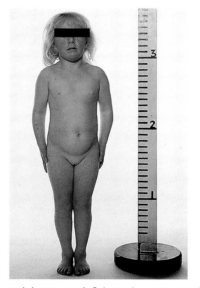

Fig. 15.11 Growth hormone deficiency in a 10-year-old girl.
(Courtesy of Dr WF Jackson.)

Causes of short stature	
Constitutional short stature	
Familial (genetic) short stature	
Chronic illness	
Intrauterine growth retardation	
Psychosocial dwarfism	
Endocrine conditions	Hypopituitarism Growth hormone (GH) deficiency GH resistance (dwarfism) Hypothyroidism Glucocorticosteroid excess Vitamin D disorders
Genetic syndromes	Achondroplasia Turner's syndrome Noonan's syndrome Genetic obesity syndromes

Fig. 15.12 Causes of short stature.

tissues, promotes electrolyte retention and enhances glucose and fatty acid mobilization. Since the endogenous release of endogenous growth hormone is intermittent and pulsatile, continuous plasma levels of exogenous growth hormone are not necessary for therapeutic efficacy. Intermittent hGH administration results in sustained increases in plasma concentration of IGF-I. Recombinant growth hormone has a plasma elimination half-life of approximately 4 hours after subcutaneous administration, and is effective in a daily dosing regimen in pediatric patients (0.18–0.3 mg/kg/week divided in 6 daily doses). Somatropin is cleared from plasma with a half-life of 20 minutes, but apparent plasma clearance after subcutaneous injection is prolonged due to delayed absorption.

Growth treatment of growth hormone-deficient children results in mean final adult height that is within 0.5–0.7 standard deviations of the normal population mean. Treatment of patients with Turner syndrome results in increases of 6–7 cm in final adult height. In children, hGH therapy produces few side effects, and has not been associated with an increased risk of diabetes or cancer to date. Pediatric hGH therapy is discontinued at the time of epiphysial closure. Treatment of growth hormone-deficient adults results in mild improvements in exercise ability, subjective symptoms and lean body mass, but long-term health outcomes have not been fully assessed. Growth hormone therapy may exacerbate glucose intolerance in adults. Administration of growth hormone to critically ill adults in an attempt to reverse tissue catabolism resulted in an unexpected increase in mortality. Illicit use of growth hormone has become popular among performance athletes, due to anabolic effects on muscle. As a recombinant human hormone, illicit use of somatropin is difficult to diagnose by drug assay.

Thyroid diseases and disorders of metabolic rate

■ *Thyroid hormone controls the metabolic activity of all tissues by regulating genes whose protein products are critical for cellular respiration*

Many tissues respond to hormonal and paracrine stimuli by increasing cellular metabolism. Skeletal muscle, for example, responds to continuous stimulation with activation myosin–ATPase and subsequent increased glycolysis to sustain muscle contraction. Independent of this type of tissue- and function-specific regulation of cell metabolism, thyroid hormone exerts a broad regulation of cell metabolism and protein synthesis, loosely referred to as 'metabolic rate.' Thyroid hormone has multiple effects (Fig. 15.13). They are best understood in terms of regulating the body's overall level of cellular metabolic activity and energy expenditure.

Conditions such as starvation or severe illness reduce thyroid hormone activity and conserve energy expenditure by many tissues. Conversely, the hypothalamic–pituitary–thyroid axis is stimulated under conditions of CNS arousal such as fear and anxiety. Although thyroid hormone is not considered to be part of the hormonal 'fight or flight' response, because of its slow time course of effect, it has a complementary function in modulating the body's response to more prolonged periods of stress.

Physiologic effects of thyroid hormone
• Fetal development (physical and cognitive)
• Metabolic rate
• Body temperature
• Cardiac rate and contractility
• Peripheral vasodilation
• Red cell mass and circulatory volume
• Respiratory drive
• Peripheral nerves (reflexes)
• Hepatic metabolic enzymes
• Bone turnover
• Skin and soft tissue effects

Fig. 15.13 Physiologic effects of thyroid hormone.

■ *The synthesis, release and target-organ effects of thyroid hormones involve numerous steps, several of which are sites of drug action*

Active thyroid hormone (triiodothyronine or T_3) and its precursor (thyroxine, tetraiodothyronine, or T_4) are formed by the addition of I^- anions to two sites on the aromatic rings of tyrosine residues on a large peptide (thyroglobulin) stored in the thyroid gland. The iodination of tyrosine molecules, and the linkage of two iodotyrosine molecules together to form thyronine requires three key functions in thyroid epithelial cells:

- The ability to accumulate high intracellular concentrations of I^- by active transport from the blood (I^- transport).
- The action of an oxidizing enzyme, thyroid peroxidase, to catalyze the binding of hypoiodate (IO^-) to the tyrosine ring and the coupling of two iodinated molecules of tyrosine.
- The large polypeptide, thyroglobulin, with numerous tyrosine residues suitable for iodination and coupling (Fig. 15.14).

Thyroglobulin in the extracellular thyroid follicles stores iodinated thyronine, which is released as thyroid hormone into the blood after endocytosis and cleavage by thyroid follicular cells. The thyroid follicles store preformed thyroid hormone, usually in sufficient amounts to sustain T_4 release for approximately 6 weeks. T_3 has a tenfold greater binding affinity for the thyroid receptor than T_4, and is therefore considered to be the active form of the hormone. Although some T_3 is released from the thyroid gland, most is formed by deiodination of T_4 by deiodinase enzymes distributed throughout the body (peripheral conversion). The deiodinase enzyme isoforms in the pituitary (type II) and the periphery (type I) are differentially regulated. During systemic illness or starvation, the activity of the type I isozyme is reduced, while that of the type II isozyme is maintained. This mechanism appears to reduce peripheral metabolic demands, while preventing a compensatory increase in TSH release.

Hypothyroidism

Thyroid hormone deficiency is a common disorder that is usually caused by autoimmune destruction of the thyroid gland. Its symptoms include lethargy, weight gain, cold intolerance, dry skin, and mental sluggishness. In its most severe form (myxedema), it may cause coma. In neonates hypothyroidism is an important cause of lifelong cognitive impairment and abnormal skeletal development (cretinism).

Primary failure of the thyroid gland, due to autoimmune disease (Hashimoto's thyroiditis), is the most common cause of hypothyroidism, although other inflammatory conditions and physical damage may also impair thyroid gland activity (Fig. 15.15). Autoimmune thyroid disease, like many autoimmune diseases is more prevalent in women, and in rare cases may be associated with other autoimmune endocrine deficiencies, such as adrenal failure, insulin-dependent diabetes mellitus, or hypogonadism. Impaired thyroid hormone action may also be due to reduced pituitary TSH secretion (secondary hypothyroidism) or the rare condition of cellular resistance (thyroid hormone resistance).

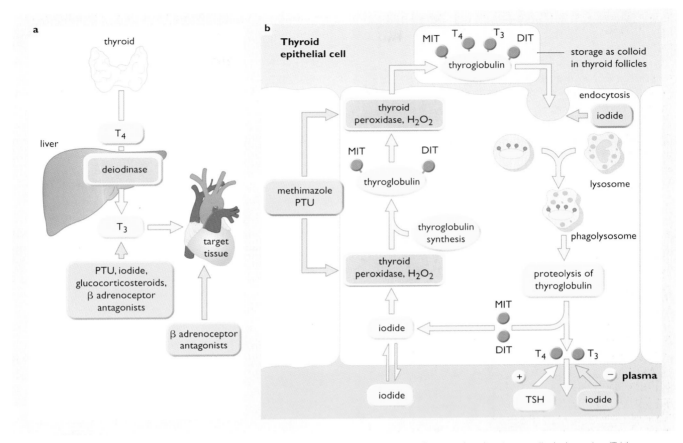

Fig. 15.14 Thyroid hormone pharmacology. (a) Thyroxine (tetraiodothyronine or T$_4$) undergoes deiodination to triiodothyronine (T$_3$) by diodinase at peripheral sites such as the liver. The sites of action of antithyroid drugs are also shown. (b) Iodide is actively transported into thyroid epithelial cells. Thyroid peroxidase, a microsomal enzyme, catalyzes the iodination of the aromatic rings of tyrosine at the 3 and 5 positions, creating monoiodotyrosine (MIT) and diiodotyrosine (DIT). Thyroid peroxidase also couples iodotyrosines to form thyronine residues in thyroglobulin. Thyroglobulin is secreted and stored in the thyroid follicles. Thyroid-stimulating hormone (TSH) causes stored thyroglobulin to undergo endocytosis and lysosomal proteolysis to release thyroid hormone. (PTU, propylthiouracil)

Causes of hypothyroidism	
Primary	Chronic lymphocytic thyroiditis (Hashimoto's disease)
	Subacute thyroiditis
	Painless thyroiditis (postpartum thyroiditis)
	Radioactive iodine ingestion
	Iodine deficiency or excess
	Inborn errors of thyroid hormone synthesis
Secondary	Pituitary disease
Target tissues	Thyroid hormone resistance

Fig. 15.15 Causes of hypothyroidism.

▋ Synthetic thyroid hormones are widely used to treat hypothyroidism

Synthetic levothyroxine (1-T$_4$) is a convenient to use, orally active, hormone replacement therapy. Although it requires metabolic activation to form active T$_3$, it is commonly used because of its long elimination half-life of 6 days. This prolonged action is largely due to extensive binding to plasma thyroid-binding globulin, and to prealbumin, resulting in reduced clearance and a large store of circulating drug. Drugs with long elimination half-lifes are generally useful in the treatment of chronic diseases as the impact of a single missed dose on the steady-state plasma concentration is small. The disadvantage of levothyroxine therapy is its slow rate of achieving steady-state effects: dose adjustments can be evaluated only after treatment for 5 weeks. Liothyronine (1-triiodothyronine sodium) is bound less avidly by thyroid binding globulin; hence, the un-bound fraction of this agent is higher than 1-T$_4$. Liothyronine achieves biologic effects more rapidly than levothyroxine, but is also cleared more rapidly and requires twice daily administration to avoid wide fluctuations in plasma concentrations between doses.

The dose of levothyroxine in most adults is 75–150 μg/day (1.7 μg/kg/day) and symptomatic improvement is seen within 4 weeks. In elderly patients, a starting dose of 1 μg/kg/day is recommended. Overdosage of thyroxine may increase the risk of atrial fibrillation. Treatment-related increases metabolic rate may also worsen angina pectoris, although normal thyroid replacement therapy does not contribute to thrombosis of

289

Causes of hyperthyroidism

- Thyroid hormone ingestion
- Diffuse toxic goiter (Graves' disease)
- Hyperfunctioning adenoma (toxic nodule)
- Toxic multinodular goiter
- Painless thyroiditis
- Subacute thyroiditis
- Thyroid stimulating hormone (TSH)-secreting adenoma
- Human chorionic gonadotropin (HCG)-secreting tumors

Fig. 15.16 Causes of hyperthyroidism.

coronary arteries. For these reasons, hypothyroidism in the frail elderly should be treated initially with 25 μg/day of 1-T$_4$, and doses should be increased by 25 μg/day at 4-week intervals with appropriate monitoring. Doses should be adjusted to maintain TSH concentrations within the normal range.

Hyperthyroidism

Hyperthyroidism is a syndrome of excessive tissue metabolism due to excessive thyroid hormone action resulting from either:

- Overproduction of endogenous hormone.
- Ingestion of exogenous hormone.

Thyroid hormone excess is usually due to immunologically stimulated thyroid hormone release, or a hormone-producing thyroid adenoma (Fig. 15.16). Autoimmune disease (Graves' disease) is the most common cause. In Graves' disease, antibodies activate TSH receptors, leading to diffuse enlargement of the thyroid gland, excess hormone release, and the classic stigmata of hyperthyroidism (i.e. nervousness, weight loss, tremor, eyelid retraction, sweating, and heat intolerance (see Fig. 15.17)). Other forms of hyperthyroidism share these features, but Graves' disease is the only form of hyperthyroidism in which there is an immunologic attack on the extraocular muscles, which causes protrusion of the globe (proptosis, exophthalmos). Other immunologic forms of thyroiditis may also result in excess thyroid hormone production by allowing preformed thyroid hormone to leak from an inflamed thyroid gland.

The major causes of nonimmunologically mediated hyperthyroidism are adenomas, either single (hyperfunctioning adenoma) or multiple (multinodular goiter). Multinodular goiter is common in the elderly and is usually clinically insignificant. Occasionally, thyroid hormone production and release by a thyroid adenoma exceeds daily requirements and leads to hyperthyroidism.

Antithyroid drugs inhibit thyroid hormone synthesis, release, peripheral conversion, and target tissue effects

The different drugs used to treat hyperthyoidism act at almost every step of thyroid hormone synthesis and release (see Fig. 15.14).

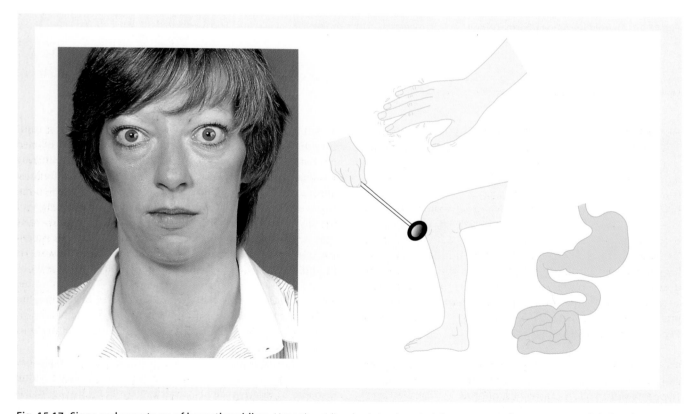

Fig. 15.17 Signs and symptoms of hyperthyroidism. Hyperthyroidism leads to characteristic symptoms of nervousness, weight loss, heat intolerance, and fatigue. Signs such as tachycardia, tremor, accelerated reflexes, smooth skin, hyperhidrosis, and ocular stare are common to hyperthyroidism of any cause. Proptosis, diplopia, and corneal inflammation are specific findings in Graves' disease. (Photograph courtesy of Dr CD Forbes and Dr WF Jackson.)

Antithyroid therapy for hyperthyroidism

Agent	Major mechanism	Typical dose	Efficacy	Adverse effects	Pharmacokinetics	Drug interactions
Common features of thioureas	Inhibit iodine coupling to thyroglobulin by TPO. Inhibit T_4 to T_3 conversion		90% achieve remission with initial therapy	Common, dose-dependent: skin rash fever, arthralgia. Uncommon: granulocytopenia		Discontinue prior to ^{131}I ablation therapy
Methimazole		10–30 mg b.i.d., maintenance dose: 5–10 mg/day		Neonatal scalp aplasia (contraindicated in pregnancy and breastfeeding) Cholestatic hepatic disease (rare)	$t_{1/2}$ = 6 hours (range 3–12 hours) Distributes to thyroid tissue Hepatic metabolism	
Carbimazole	Prodrug form of methimazole	10–30 mg b.i.d. maintenance dose: 5–10 mg/day		Same as methimazole	Same as methimazole	
Propylthiouracil		100–200 mg t.i.d.–q.i.d. Maintenance dose: 50–150 mg q.d.		Hepatocellular hepatitis Aplastic anemia (rare)	$t_{1/2}$ = 1–2 hours Distributes to thyroid tissue High protein binding Less transplacental passage than methimazole, Renal excretion of conjugates (dose reduction in renal failure)	

Fig. 15.18 Antithyroid therapy for hyperthyroidism.

METHIMAZOLE AND PROPYLTHIOURACIL (Fig. 15.18) bind TPO, the thyroid peroxidase enzyme (molecular action) leading to reduced thyroid hormone formation and storage in the thyroid follicles (cellular action). However, the tissue action (decreased thyroxine secretion) may not be detectable for several weeks if there are stores of previously synthesized hormone. Propylthiouracil also inhibits the deiodination reaction that produces active T_3 from T_4. This may be desirable if the hyperthyroidism is life-threatening. Methimazole, however, has a longer elimination half-life allowing once- or twice-daily doses and so improving compliance. Both drugs can cause allergic reactions and rarely are hepatotoxic and cause bone marrow suppression. Their use therefore requires careful clinical monitoring.

IODIDE found in dietary supplements, radiocontrast agents, and some cough syrups can reduce thyroid hormone release. In addition, I^- reduces conversion of T_4 to T_3. In acute thyrotoxicosis due to Graves' disease, iodide administration (e.g. supersaturated potassium iodide solution (SSKI), Lugols's solution, or oral radiographic contrast agents) is the most rapidly acting suppressive treatment available.

β_1 ADRENOCEPTOR ANTAGONISTS (e.g. propranolol and esmolol) are commonly used to counteract the effects of excess thyroid hormone. This form of 'functional' (uncompetitive) antagonism (see Chapter 3) occurs because many of the effects of thyroid hormone and β adrenoceptor agonism are the same (e.g. tachycardia, increased metabolic rate, nervousness, and tremor). Thus the actions of thyroid hormone and epinephrine/norepinephrine can be additive or even synergistic. Thyroid hormone also upregulates the number of adrenoceptors in many tissues thereby exacerbating the interaction.

 Antithyroid drug therapy

- Propylthiouracil and methimazole inhibit thyroid hormone synthesis
- I^- blocks the release of stored thyroid hormone
- I^-, propylthiouracil, and β adrenoceptor antagonists inhibit conversion of thyroxine (tetraiodothyronine or T_4) to triiodothyronine (T_3)
- β Adrenoceptor antagonists functionally antagonize the target organ effects of thyroid hormone

Disorders of carbohydrate metabolism

Although thyroid hormone regulates the basal metabolic rate of tissues, its effect on the delivery of fuel precursors to cells is minor. Instead this critical endocrine function is performed mainly by the endocrine pancreas. Unlike most other endocrine systems, regulation of the endocrine pancreas does not occur through a hypothalamic–pituitary axis. Instead, carbohydrate and lipid metabolism is regulated by:

- Signals from the gut (gastric distension and food content).
- Signals from the blood stream (circulating glucose levels).
- Intracellular signals (intracellular energy stores).

The overall homeostatic function of carbohydrate (and lipid) metabolism is to deliver energy substrates for use, and storage, after eating, and to mobilize energy stores during the fasting (postabsorptive) state.

The regulation of carbohydrate (and fatty acid) metabolism is the key function of insulin and the associated counter-regulatory hormones. The maintenance of adequate levels of circulating glucose is essential for brain tissue and red blood cell intermediary metabolism since these tissues lack insulin-dependent glucose transporters and depend on circulating glucose concentration for their energy supply.

■ Insulin receptor stimulation activates glucose transporters on the plasma membranes of insulin-sensitive tissues

The intracellular mechanism of insulin action is not completely understood. The insulin receptor is a membrane-bound receptor linked to tyrosine kinase (Fig. 15.19). As with other intracellular kinases, phosphorylation of intracellular proteins alters their enzymatic activity resulting in sequential phosphorylating and dephosphorylating steps in an intracellular signaling cascade. Insulin receptor stimulation leads to translocation of glucose transporters from an endosomal storage site to the plasma membrane, leading to increased glucose uptake. The regulation of glucose transporters on peripheral tissues is essential to fuel delivery, while on pancreatic β cells it is essential to the glucose-sensing mechanism, which regulates insulin release.

Insulin release occurs in response to food-related stimuli such as glucose, amino acids and gut-derived hormones, which reflect increasing fuel availability. These signals lead to depolarization of β cells in the pancreatic islets of Langerhans and Ca^{2+}-mediated exocytosis of insulin into the portal vein (Fig. 15.20). The resting membrane potential of the β cells is regulated by an ATP-sensitive potassium channel (iK_{ATP}) which is a molecular target for drugs of the sulfonylurea class. Insulin concentrations are high in the portal circulation, leading to substantial effects on the liver, before being diluted in the general circulation. Although insulin has numerous effects on fuel metabolism in these tissues (Fig. 15.21), the overall effect is coordinated glucose disposal, glycogen storage, fatty acid storage, and protein synthesis. These different metabolic effects of insulin can occur at different doses. Inhibition of ketone body formation in the liver occurs at lower doses of insulin than those required to stimulate glucose uptake in skeletal muscle.

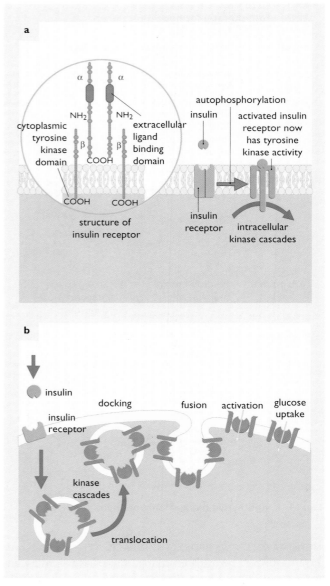

Fig. 15.19 Insulin action. (a) The insulin receptor is a heterodimeric transmembrane receptor consisting of two α and two β subunits. The intracellular portions of the β subunits contain tyrosine kinase activity (see Chapter 3). Insulin receptor stimulation leads to phosphorylation of multiple intracellular signaling molecules. Phosphorylation of tyrosine kinase residues on intracellular kinases leads to activation of serine/threonine kinase cascades. (b) Intracellular kinase cascades cause translocation of glucose transporters from an endosomal compartment to the plasma membrane where they increase glucose uptake.

■ Counter-regulatory hormones from the pancreas, pituitary, adrenal cortex, and adrenal medulla protect against hypoglycemia

In the fasting state, as glucose concentrations decline insulin release is suppressed. Multiple neurohormonal responses occur

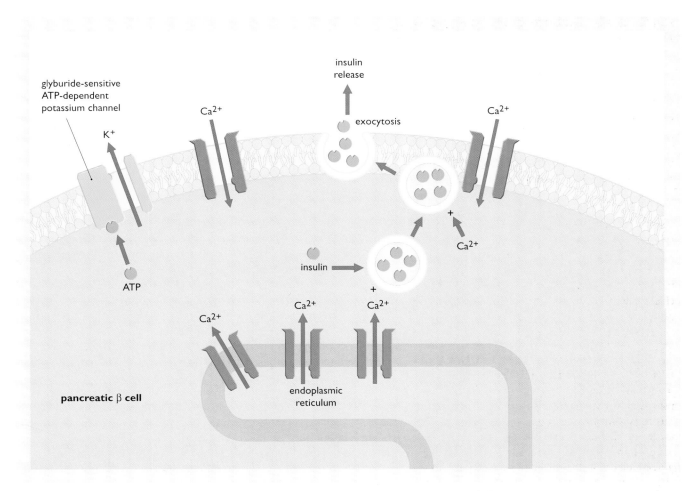

Fig. 15.20 Insulin secretion. Insulin release from pancreatic β cells is stimulated by the release of Ca^{2+} from the endoplasmic compartment by voltage-sensitive channels, and by influx of extracellular Ca^{2+}. The ATP-dependent K^+ channel on the plasma membrane maintains the intracellular resting potential. Inhibition of this K^+ channel by sulfonylurea or meglitinide agents results in depolarization and activation of Ca^{2+} channels, resulting in enhanced insulin secretion.

Effects of insulin on fuel homeostasis

Carbohydrates	Increases glucose transport
	Increases glycogen synthesis
	Increases glycolysis
	Inhibits gluconeogenesis
Fats	Increases lipoprotein lipase activity
	Increases fat storage in adipocytes
	Inhibits lipolysis (hormone sensitive lipase)
	Increases hepatic lipoprotein synthesis
	Inhibits fatty acid oxidation
Proteins	Increases protein synthesis
	Increases amino acid transport

Fig. 15.21 Effects of insulin on fuel homeostasis.

if the plasma glucose falls below a critical concentration. These include:

- Pancreatic glucagon release.
- Sympathetic nervous system activation.

- Hypothalamic–pituitary–adrenal release of growth hormone, cortisol, and epinephrine.

These counter-regulatory hormones increase glycogenolysis and inhibit insulin release. The prodromal symptoms of hypoglycemia (nervousness, tachycardia, tremor, sweating) result from sympathetic nervous system activity. Failure of the counter-regulatory response, as seen in extreme insulin excess and panhypopituitarism, leads to an insufficient supply of glucose to the brain and coma. Somatostatin, which is synthesized in pancreatic δ cells and elsewhere, inhibits the release of both insulin and counter-regulatory hormones, providing a mechanism to dampen the escalating insulin and counter-regulatory hormone release.

Diabetes mellitus

Diabetes mellitus was originally diagnosed if urine tasted sweet due to the presence of glucose.

Two types of diabetes mellitus share the features of hyperglycemia and vascular pathology. They differ in their pathogenesis and in the ability of residual insulin to suppress ketone formation from fatty acids (Fig. 15.22).

Features of insulin-dependent (IDDM) and noninsulin-dependent (NIDDM) diabetes mellitus

	IDDM	NIDDM
Age at onset	<30 yrs	>30 yrs
Family history of diabetes mellitus	Uncommon	Common
Body weight	Not obese	Obese
Ketoacidosis	Common	Rare
Insulin treatment	All patients	Some patients
Other autoimmune endocrine deficiencies	Yes (rare)	No
Prevalence in adult population	0.5%	5%
HLA association	Yes	No

Fig. 15.22 Features of insulin-dependent (type 1) and noninsulin-dependent (type 2) diabetes mellitus.

TYPE 1 DIABETES MELLITUS (INSULIN-REQUIRING, KETOSIS-PRONE DIABETES MELLITUS) results from autoimmune destruction of pancreatic β cells. The autoimmune attack begins years before insulin secretion fails. By the time diabetes mellitus is diagnosed the β cells are irreversibly damaged. Since this usually occurs before age 30 the description 'juvenile-onset' diabetes mellitus has been used. The cardinal finding in type 1 diabetes mellitus is an inability to secrete even the modest amounts of insulin needed to suppress ketone formation, resulting in recurrent episodes of diabetic ketoacidosis.

TYPE 2 DIABETES MELLITUS is the other major form of diabetes mellitus. Insulin is secreted, but is ineffective in normalizing plasma glucose. However, the circulating insulin concentrations are sufficient to suppress ketone formation under most circumstances, so patients with this condition do not have repeated bouts of diabetic ketoacidosis. Although insulin may be used therapeutically, type 2 patients are not usually dependent on insulin therapy to prevent ketoacidosis. β-Cell function in type 2 patients declines over time, to the extent that some type 2 patients develop insulin deficiency and may be prone to ketoacidosis in the setting of infection or serious illness. Early in the course of type 2 diabetes, the cardinal feature of this disorder is inadequate lowering of blood glucose in response to insulin administration. This phenomenon is termed 'insulin resistance,' but is not due to a receptor mutation that impairs the response to insulin. Insulin resistance and type 2 diabetes mellitus define a syndrome that may include several different disease processes including:
- Glucose transporter defects.
- Desensitization of insulin receptors.
- Toxic effects of hyperglycemia.

- The metabolic demands of obesity.
- Conditions associated with excessive counter-regulatory hormones (e.g. pheochromocytoma, Cushing's syndrome, and acromegaly).
- Conditions associated with a loss of pancreatic function (e.g. pancreatic cancer surgery and pancreatitis).

Type 1 and type 2 diabetes share the clinical features of hyperglycemia

Insufficient insulin action, whether due to insulin deficiency (type 1) or insulin resistance (type 2) results in hyperglycemia. Although impaired glucose delivery into target tissues following food ingestion results in postprandial hyperglycemia, deficient insulin-mediated suppression of hepatic gluconeogenesis is the primary cause of diabetic hyperglycemia. Ingestion of dietary sugar accounts for a small portion of the hyperglycemic state in most diabetics. Fasting plasma glucose concentrations >7 mmol/L (126 mg/dl) are associated with increased risk of long-term diabetic complications (see below). Symptomatic hyperglycemia (polyuria, polydipsia, unexplained weight loss) usually occurs at higher levels of hyperglycemia. Glucosuria occurs only when the concentration of glucose in the renal tubules exceeds the threshold of maximum absorption (Tm) at approximately 9 mmol/L (160 mg/dl). For this reason monitoring of urinary glucose is not an effective method for monitoring diabetic therapy. Elevated plasma glucose concentrations increase the rate of glycation (nonenzymatic covalent bonding of glucose) of many proteins in the body. Elevated glycated hemoglobin (HbA_{1c}) reflects prolonged hyperglycemia and is a useful test for monitoring glycemic control in diabetes.

Insulin resistance can occur in the absence of hyperglycemia

Severe insulin resistance leads to impaired glucose regulation and the development of clinical diabetes mellitus, but many patients with hypertension and hypercholesterolemia demonstrate insulin resistance without abnormal glucose regulation. This observation has led to the term 'syndrome X' to describe patients with hypertension, hypercholesterolemia, and insulin resistance. Such patients constitute a large fraction of the population at risk of premature arteriosclerosis. The pathogenetic mechanism underlying this syndrome is not known, but impaired insulin action is associated with increased hepatic very low density lipoprotein (VLDL) production and lower circulating high density lipoprotein (HDL) concentrations (see below), which increase the risk of arteriosclerosis.

Both types of diabetes mellitus lead to microvascular and neuronal dysfunction which contribute to 'end-organ complications'

Although type 1 and type 2 diabetes mellitus differ in disease etiology, the occurrence and prevalence of ketoacidosis, and the role of insulin resistance, they both produce the same pathologic sequelae. The so-called 'end-organ complications' include retinal disease, renal failure, peripheral nerve dysfunction, peripheral vascular disease, and arteriosclerosis. Owing to the prevalence of obesity in affluent societies, type

2 diabetes mellitus is nine times more common in adults from such societies than type 1. Diabetes is a leading cause of blindness and renal failure, and a major cause of morbidity and mortality, due to arteriosclerosis resulting in cerebrovascular thrombosis, myocardial infarction, and amputations of the extremities.

Insulin and the treatment of diabetes mellitus

Different insulin preparations with different patterns of absorption are used to match insulin delivery to caloric intake

Before the discovery and therapeutic use of insulin in the 1930s, type 1 diabetes was lethal in childhood. A variety of insulin preparations have since been developed to provide a 'physiologic' pattern of insulin replacement (Fig. 15.23). An insulin pump attached to a small subcutaneous needle, delivering a basal rate of insulin and small boluses on demand at mealtimes, is the most successful way of creating a physiologic pattern of insulin administration. However, this method does not achieve better glucose control than that achieved in compliant patients using multiple insulin injections daily. The success of such multiple injection regimens depends upon the availability of insulins with different pharmacokinetic patterns of absorption. Estimates of the duration of action of different insulins (see below) are, however, imprecise. The hypoglycemic response to each type of insulin varies widely between patients, and requires close therapeutic monitoring.

SHORT-ACTING INSULINS (REGULAR, SEMILENTE) are insulin preparations intended for prompt, meal-related insulin delivery. Most regular insulin is human insulin produced by recombinant DNA technology, although semisynthetic regular insulin, produced by modification of porcine insulin, is also available. Regular insulin consists of an insulin/Zn^{2+} suspension, but has no additives or formulations to delay absorption. Short-acting insulins spontaneously form dimeric or hexameric aggregates which retard absorption. Since subcutaneous absorption is slower than pancreatic release, such preparations are injected 30–45 minutes before a meal and exert their action for approximately 6 hours afterwards.

Insulin preparations

Insulin preparation	Action	Peak activity (h)	Duration (h)
Regular	Rapid	1–3	5–7
Semilente	Rapid	3–4	10–16
Neutral protamine Hagedorn (NPH)	Intermediate	6–14	18–28
Lente	Intermediate	6–14	18–28
Ultralente	Prolonged	18–24	30–40

Fig. 15.23 Insulin preparations.

INTERMEDIATE- AND LONG-ACTING INSULINS have a more gradual onset and offset. This is due either to using a buffer which alters solubility (Lente), or to addition of the cationic protein, protamine (neutral protamine Hagedorn or NPH), to regular insulin Zn^{2+} suspensions. Depending on the formulation, and the species origin (human, pig or beef) of the insulin, intermediate insulins have an onset of action within 2 hours, a peak effect at 10 hours, and are usually inactive after 20 hours. Long-acting insulin (Ultralente) contains Zn^{2+} and an acetate buffer to delay absorption further. It begins to act within 4 hours and lasts up to 36 hours. Insulin glarginine is a recently-introduced insulin analog which is absorbed over 24 hours without a discernible peak in the absorption versus time profile. Insulin glarginine differs from recombinant human insulin by the replacement of arginine by glycine at amino acid 21, and addition of two arginine residues to the C terminus of the B chain. Unlike Ultralente, insulin glarginine begins to act within 1 hour of injection. It may provide adequate basal insulin concentrations in a single daily injection.

INSULIN LISPRO AND INSULIN ASPART are genetically engineered recombinant insulin analogs which do not undergo spontaneous dimerization. These monomeric insulins are absorbed more rapidly than regular insulin. These analogs have an onset and duration of action shorter than that of regular insulin and are therefore given immediately before meals. Due to a shorter time course of action, monomeric insulin analogs produce less hypoglycemia than regular insulin.

INSULIN REGIMENS generally include combinations of short or rapid-acting insulin with intermediate- or long-acting insulin to provide a maximal effect during hepatic neogenesis in the morning and during daytime meal ingestion, but a minimal effect during fasting periods. Treatment of type 1 diabetes requires a close matching of insulin administration with caloric intake and therefore a combination of regular and intermediate insulin is usually necessary. Many type 2 patients, who have residual cell function, only need intermediate or long-acting insulin to improve glycemic control. Insulin administration is guided by the timing and pattern of food intake, but the early morning increase in activity of the hypothalamic–pituitary–adrenal (HPA) hormones such as cortisol, growth hormone and epinephrine may increase blood sugar even without food intake. The slow rate of absorption of intermediate insulin and the 'dawn phenomenon' of the HPA axis allows intermediate insulin to be taken at bedtime with minimal nocturnal hypoglycemia.

The goal of insulin therapy in type 1 diabetes is physiologic replacement

To reproduce the pattern of normal pancreatic function, type 1 diabetics require low levels of insulin from bedtime until early morning, higher levels of insulin from early morning until bedtime, and significant increases in short-acting insulin at the time of meal ingestion (Fig. 15.24). The first two objectives can be achieved by administration of intermediate (NPH, Lente) or long-acting insulin (Ultralente) twice per day,

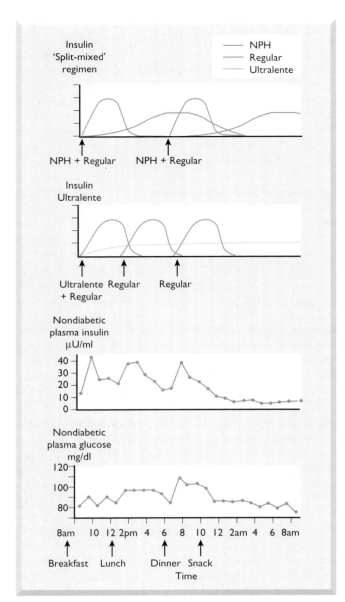

Fig. 15.24 Insulin therapy. Exogenously administered insulin does not mirror the rapid meal-related increases of pancreatic insulin secretion owing to delayed absorption from the site of injection. The goal of insulin dosing regimens is to coordinate peaks in insulin delivery with the times of caloric ingestion. Systemic insulin levels are higher during insulin therapy of type 1 diabetes mellitus than with endogenous pancreatic regulation. Pancreatic insulin release into the portal venous system may suppress hepatic gluconeogenesis at lower doses than those needed with systemic insulin administration.

ideally at bedtime and in the morning. The evening dose of long-acting insulin is adjusted to achieve euglycemia before breakfast, without nocturnal hypoglycemia. When fasting morning euglycemia is achieved, then the morning dose of long-acting insulin is adjusted to achieve euglycemia before the evening meal. Insulin glarginine may permit basal insulin requirements to be met with a single dose of this long-acting insulin analog. Short-acting (regular or monomeric insulin analogs) should be administered with each meal to achieve 2-hour postprandial blood glucose levels of <160 mg/dl

(9 mmol/L). Due to variation in activity and caloric intake, the dose of short-acting insulin should be adjusted according to the blood glucose prior to the meal. Difficulty in administering insulin around midday may be accommodated by the use of intermediate-acting insulin (instead of long-acting) insulin in the morning, and adjustment of the size of the midday meal. Blood glucose at bedtime should be between 100 and 140 mg/dl (5.5–7.7 mmol/L) and subjects should check blood glucose at 2 a.m. on several occasions after any change in the insulin regimen.

Oral hypoglycemic drugs for diabetes

Oral hypoglycemic drugs act to increase insulin secretion, or the sensitivity of tissues to endogenous insulin. Oral hypoglycemic agents are used to treat patients with diabetes mellitus who do not require insulin to prevent ketoacidosis. These drugs can be categorized according to whether they increase insulin release, increase sensitivity to insulin, or block glucose uptake (Fig. 15.25).

SULFONYLUREA DRUGS and meglitinides enhance β-cell function by:

- Blocking ATP-dependent K^+ current (iK_{ATP}) in pancreatic cells, and as a result,
- Causing depolarization which activates voltage-sensitive Ca^{2+} channels,
- Increasing intracellular Ca^{2+} which increases insulin exocytosis.

Sulfonylurea agents were discovered after it was observed that sulfonamide antibiotic administration occasionally produced hypoglycemia. The second-generation sulfonylurea hypoglycemic agents share a similar efficacy and safety profile, although they differ slightly in dose and frequency of administration (Fig. 15.25). Earlier (first-generation) sulfonylureas such as tolbutamide, chlorpropamide, acetohexamide and tolazamide have lower molar potency but demonstrate intrinsic efficacy similar to that of the more commonly used second-generation agents. Second-generation agents are metabolized in the liver to inactive forms; hence, they may pose less risk of hypoglycemia in patients with reduced renal function than renally excreted agents such as chlorpropamide. Although glipizide and glyburide differ in plasma elimination half-life (3 hours versus 10 hours respectively) both agents may be effective in single daily doses, and plasma drug levels do not closely correlate with glucose-lowering efficacy. Repaglinide is

 Oral antagonists for non-insulin-dependent diabetes mellitus

- Sulfonylureas stimulate insulin release by inhibiting K^+ channels on pancreatic β cells
- Biguanides and troglidazole enhance the insulin sensitivity of target tissues
- All hypoglycemic therapies improve insulin release and action by reducing hyperglycemic β cell dysfunction (glucose toxicity)

Oral hypoglycemic agents

	Major mechanism	Typical dose	Efficacy	Adverse effects
Biguanides	Inhibit hepatic gluconeogenesis Increases glucose transporters Increases tissue insulin sensitivity		1.5–2% reduction in HbA1c Mild triglyceride lowering Mild LDL lowering No weight gain Reduced coronary mortality in obese type 2 diabetes mellitus	Abdominal bloating, diarrhea Potential metabolic acidosis Contraindicated in renal insufficiency
Metformin		0.5–0.85 g t.i.d. 1 g b.i.d.		
Sulfonylureas	Stimulate insulin release from pancreas		1.5–2% HbA1c reduction Mild triglyceride-lowering	Hypoglycemia Weight gain
Glyburide		5–10 mg q.d.-b.i.d.		
Glipizide		5–10 mg q.d.-b.i.d.		
Glipizide extended-release		5–20 mg q.d.		
Glimepiride		1–8 mg q.d.-b.i.d.		
Repaglinide	Stimulates insulin release from pancreas	0.5–4 mg ac (t.i.d.–q.i.d.)	1.7% decrease HbA1c	Hypoglycemia
Thiazolidinediones	Increase tissue insulin sensitivity Inhibit hepatic gluconeogenesis		1–1.5% HbA1c reduction 10–15% HDL increase 10–20% triglyceride reduction	Mild LDL increases Weight gain Worsens congestive heart failure Possible hepatotoxicity
Rosiglitazone		4–8 mg q.d. (or 2–4 mg b.i.d.)		
Pioglitazone		15–30 mg q.d.		
α-Glucosidase inhibitors	Inhibit hydrolysis of disaccharides Reduce glucose absorption		0.7–1% HbA1c reduction mild triglyceride lowering	Abdominal bloating, diarrhea, flatulence Titration of dose q. 2 weeks recommended Hepatotoxicity (rare)
Acarbose		25–100 mg b.i.d.–t.i.d. with meals		
Miglitol		25–100 mg t.i.d. with meals		

Fig. 15.25 Oral hypoglycemic agents.

a recently introduced non-sulfonylurea agent that blocks iK_{ATP} and possibly other molecular targets on pancreatic β cells. Repaglinide is rapidly absorbed and has a plasma elimination half-life of approximately 1 hour. It is metabolized by CYP 3A4 and eliminated in the feces. Repaglinide (0.5–4 mg) is administered 15–30 minutes before each meal, and its glucose-lowering efficacy is similar to that of the sulfonylurea drugs.

METFORMIN is the most commonly used agent in another class of hypoglycemic agents, the biguanides. The biguanides are synthetic analogs of agents found in herbal diabetic therapies indigenous to southern Europe. The first biguanide, phenformin, was found to cause severe lactic acidosis and is no longer used clinically. This adverse effect is rarely reported with metformin. Metformin acts to increase tissue sensitivity to insulin, especially in the liver where it significantly reduces hepatic gluconeogenesis by a mechanism that is not well understood. Metformin has a short plasma elimination half-life (6 hours) and is eliminated exclusively by the kidneys. Due to the risk of metabolic acidosis, it is contraindicated in patients with renal insufficiency, hepatic dysfunction, congestive heart failure, and during radiographic contrast procedures. Metformin has a low therapeutic index. The minimally effective dose for most patients is 1500 mg/day and the maximal dose is 1 g b.i.d. or 850 mg t.i.d. Due to abdominal bloating and altered bowel function, doses should be administered with food and titrated every 2 weeks from a low starting dose (e.g. 500 mg p.o. b.i.d.). Metformin has three therapeutic advantages over other oral agents: it does not cause weight gain; it does not produce hypoglycemia; it reduces both microvascular (renal, retinal, neuronal) and macrovascular (death from myocardial infarction) end-points. For these reasons, it should be considered the preferred treatment for obese type 2 diabetics. The glucose-lowering effects of metformin are similar to those of sulfonylureas, and combined use of biguanides with sulfonylureas produces additive efficacy.

THIAZOLIDINEDIONES, OR TZDs are a class of newly synthesized organic molecules that act as agonists for the gamma subclass of peroxisomal-proliferator activator receptors (PPAR-γ). PPARs are ligand-activated transcription factors, similar to the thyroid/steroid receptor family. Since the endogenous ligand for these receptors is unknown, they are termed 'orphan' receptors. TZDs in current clinical use (rosiglitazone, pioglitazone) induce genes which enhance insulin action in skeletal muscle, adipose tissue and the liver. This results in increased insulin-mediated glucose delivery into tissues and reduced hepatic gluconeogenesis. Although plasma elimination half-lifes of rosiglitazone (3–4 hours) and pioglitazone (3–7 hours) are relatively short, administration once or twice per day appears to be equally effective. Several weeks are required to achieve steady-state pharmacodynamic effects. As glucose-lowering agents, TZDs are less efficacious than metformin or sulfonylureas. Their advantages include the ease of once-daily dosing, low potential for hypoglycemia, and the ability to increase HDL cholesterol concentrations. While long-term cardiovascular outcomes have not yet been reported, low HDL cholesterol is a common feature of dyslipidemia and coronary artery disease in type 2 diabetes. TZDs may cause weight gain and expansion of blood volume which may exacerbate congestive heart failure. The first drug in this class, troglitazone, was discontinued due to hepatic toxicity, but the agents in current clinical use do not appear to share this feature.

INHIBITORS OF INTESTINAL α-GLUCOSIDASE (ACARBOSE, MIGLITOL) provide an alternative strategy in type 2 diabetes by reducing glucose absorption. The α-glucosidase inhibitors are less efficacious than other oral agents, but may be useful for patients with predominantly postprandial hyperglycemia. They are administered immediately prior to meals and are eliminated by the gut without significant systemic absorption. Due to impaired glucose absorption and increased glucose delivery to the colon, they frequently cause flatulence and abdominal cramping.

Control of type 2 diabetes usually requires multiple agents

Only a small proportion of patients with type 2 diabetes achieve satisfactory glucose control (fasting blood glucose <140 mg/dl) using metformin or a sulfonylurea alone, and glycemic control worsens over time, regardless of which agent is used. For this reason combination therapy may be required to achieve the maximum reduction of microvascular diabetic complications that results from maintenance of normoglycemia. A practical approach to combination therapy involves addition of a second oral agent or insulin to the existing maximum dose of the initial therapy. Agents that do not cause hypoglycemia when used alone (e.g. metformin, TZD), may do so when combined with sulfonylureas or insulin. Unlike oral agents, insulin may

be continually titrated upward as hyperglycemia progresses over time; hence, most type 2 diabetic patients will eventually need insulin therapy. The simplest approach to initiating insulin therapy is with a single dose of bedtime long-acting insulin (e.g. 20 units), combined with daytime use of an oral agent. This approach produces very little insulin-related weight gain, and is well accepted by patients. If hyperglycemia persists in spite of >50 units of bedtime insulin, daytime insulin injections should be added. Diabetic subjects with minimal insulin resistance require 0.5–1.0 μg/kg of insulin per day, most of which is administered as intermediate- or long-acting insulin. In most type 2 patients, however, the insulin dose cannot be predicted due to variable degrees of insulin resistance.

Agents that target the pathophysiology of end-organ complications may reduce the morbidity of diabetes mellitus

The large-scale prospective Diabetes Control and Complications Trial (DCCT) has demonstrated that maintenance of near normoglycemia using fastidious dietary control and multiple daily injections of insulin reduces the rate of development of retinal disease, nephropathy, and peripheral neuropathy in type 1 diabetes. The United Kingdom Prospective Diabetes Study (UKPDS) has demonstrated similar benefits of glycemic control on these end-points in type 2 diabetes. Despite this, maintenance of normoglycemia is difficult to achieve clinically and therefore other therapies that can reduce the severity of diabetic complications are needed. Based on the high rate of coronary artery and cerebrovascular disease in diabetes, careful management of hypertension and dyslipidemia appear to deliver significant clinical benefit. In type 2 diabetics with hypertension, antihypertensive agents of the ACE-inhibitor and β-blocker classes appear to be equally efficacious in reducing death from myocardial infarction, cerebrovascular accident, and progression to renal failure. ACE inhibitors have been demonstrated to reduce renal failure in type 1 diabetes, and the rate of progression of proteinuria in type 2 diabetes, regardless of the presence of hypertension. The ACE inhibitor, ramipril, has also demonstrated efficacy in the primary prevention of coronary artery disease in diabetic patients, regardless of the presence of hypertension. While a specific study of the prevention of coronary artery disease in patients with diabetes has not yet been published, gemfibrozil has demonstrated significant reduction in recurrent myocardial infarction in men with the low HDL dyslipidemia that is typical of diabetic patients. HMG CoA reductase inhibitors ('statins') are also efficacious in the prevention of recurrent myocardial infarction in diabetic patients.

Hypoglycemia

Pathologic hypoglycemia is treated surgically if the cause is an insulinoma

Hypoglycemia is a confusing term used to describe either a pathologically low blood sugar, or a set of symptoms similar to those produced by glucose counter-regulatory hormones. Pathologic hypoglycemia is best defined as deprivation of adequate glucose in glucose-dependent tissues (particularly the brain). This leads to impaired mental function (neuroglycopenia) and symptoms of the counter-regulatory responses such as nervousness, tachycardia, tremor, hunger, and sweating. Pathologic hypoglycemia is rare and usually results from administration of hypoglycemic agents and less commonly from tumors that either secrete insulin or consume glucose, or rare disorders of alimentary function.

In the past, hypoglycemia was frequently diagnosed by the occurrence of blood sugars below the normal fasting range 3 hours after a dose of oral glucose. It is now understood that such 'postabsorptive' glucose concentrations may be low without impairing energy supply to glucose-sensitive tissues. A variety of neuropsychiatric complaints have been attributed to 'hypoglycemia' as a result of inappropriate use of the oral glucose tolerance test.

Pathologic hypoglycemia may occur in a variety of conditions, but the classic hypoglycemic syndrome is that due to an insulin-secreting tumor of the pancreas (insulinoma). Surgery is the main therapy for this condition, although nonresectable tumors are occasionally treated pharmacologically with octreotide or diazoxide. Diazoxide is a drug that reduces insulin secretion by activating IK_{ATP} channels and hyperpolarizing pancreatic β cells. This contrasts with the inhibitory effects of sulfonylurea agents on this channel.

GLUCAGON The natural counter-regulatory hormone, glucagon, is available as a therapeutic agent for parenteral administration, but its short half-life limits its use to the short-term correction of severe hypoglycemia resulting from the treatment of diabetes mellitus. In conscious patients, however, oral glucose administration is the primary treatment for hypoglycemia.

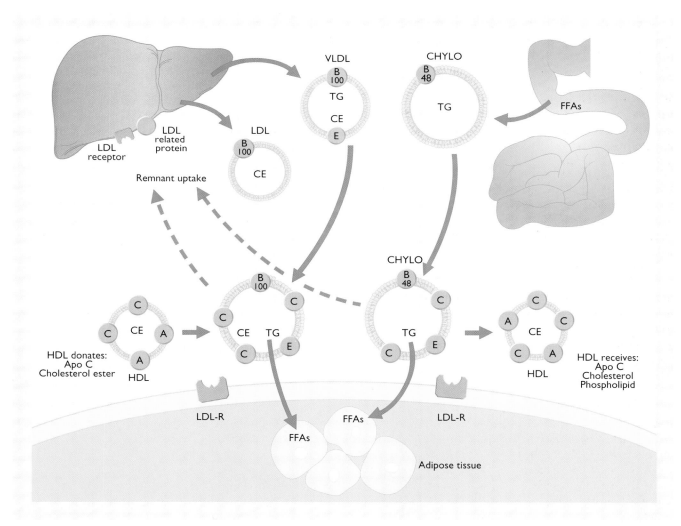

Fig. 15.26 Lipoprotein metabolism. Ingested fatty acids (FFAs) are converted to triglycerides (TG), combined with apoprotein (Apo) B-48, and covered by a phospholipid monolayer to form chylomicrons (CHYLO) in the intestinal lymph. Similarly, triglycerides synthesized in the liver are combined with Apo B-100 to form very low density lipoprotein (VLDL) in the liver. These triglyceride-rich lipoproteins acquire Apo C proteins from high-density lipoprotein (HDL). Apo C is a cofactor for lipoprotein lipase (LPL) in the vascular endothelium, which delivers fatty acids to target tissues. As triglyceride-rich particles are metabolized, HDL recovers Apo C and phospholipids for reuse by other nascent particles. Remnant particles are taken up by the liver and secreted by the liver in LDL particles, which contain cholesterol ester (CE) as their predominant core constituent.

299

Disorders of lipid metabolism

Ingested fats and those that are synthesized endogenously, form a variety of functionally important compounds such as cell membrane components, bile, steroid hormones, and intercellular signaling molecules (e.g. prostaglandins and leukotrienes). The processes of dietary fat intake, hepatic synthesis of fat molecules, and delivery to target tissues is known collectively as lipoprotein metabolism (Fig. 15.26).

■ The lipoprotein system shuttles triglycerides to peripheral tissues and orchestrates the movement of cholesterol

At the point of origin, the lipoprotein aggregate (either intestinal chylomicron or hepatic VLDL particle) has its highest triglyceride content and therefore its lowest density. While circulating through peripheral vascular beds, lipoprotein lipase removes triglycerides for uptake by the tissues. Apoproteins of the C class act as cofactors for lipase activity and are exchanged between triglyceride-rich particles and circulating high-density lipoprotein (HDL). As the triglyceride content is progressively lost and the density increases, intermediate-density lipoprotein (IDL) particles and chylomicron remnants are eventually taken up by a hepatic uptake mechanism that recognizes B and E class apolipoproteins.

In addition to shuttling triglycerides to peripheral tissues, the lipoprotein system also orchestrates the movement of cholesterol. The liver synthesizes cholesterol and produces LDL particles for cholesterol delivery to peripheral tissues. Cholesterol is taken up by cholesterol-requiring tissues via the LDL receptor, the LDL receptor-related protein, and nonreceptor-mediated pathways. Defects of the LDL receptor lead to familial hypercholesterolemia, a lipoprotein disorder characterized by very high cholesterol levels and premature arteriosclerosis.

The liver also synthesizes components of the HDL particle that contain apolipoproteins which facilitate cholesterol esterification and transfer to triglyceride-rich particles. HDL also recovers nonesterified cholesterol and Apo C components from chylomicrons and VLDL remnants for reuse by new triglyceride-rich particles. This 'centripetal' cholesterol transport is one mechanism for removing cholesterol from the peripheral circulation and distributing it in triglyceride-rich lipoprotein particles. Although HDL particles contain considerable amounts of cholesterol, they do not contain the B and E class lipoproteins needed for receptor-mediated uptake of LDL and IDL particles. Cholesterol in HDL and triglyceride-rich VLDL particles is less atherogenic than the cholesterol contained in LDL and IDL particles.

■ Lipid-lowering drugs act at many of the multiple steps in the lipoprotein metabolic pathway

Hyperlipidemia is common in many countries and is associated with cardiovascular diseases such as arteriosclerosis and its complications. The most commonly encountered manifestations are elevations of LDL, VLDL, or both lipoproteins, and are due to a combination of familial tendencies and dietary excess. Several hyperlipidemic syndromes have very specific patho-

genetic mechanisms, but these account for a minority of hypercholesterolemic patients. The specific mechanisms include:

- Defective LDL receptors (familial hypercholesterolemia).
- Overproduction of apolipoprotein B (familial combined hyperlipidemia).
- Deficiency of lipoprotein lipase (type I hyperlipidemia, primary hypertriglyceridemia).
- Deficient remnant particle clearance (type III hyperlipidemia, familial dysbetalipoproteinemia).

The Fredrickson classification of hyperlipidemias is commonly used for these disorders (Figs 15.27, 15.28).

Drug treatment of hyperlipidemia includes a variety of agents that affect cholesterol synthesis, cholesterol losses in bile, and LDL and VLDL metabolism. The steps involved in cholesterol and lipoprotein metabolism affected by such drugs are shown in Fig. 15.29.

HMG CoA reductase inhibitors

Studies of cholesterol biosynthesis in the 1950s led to the discovery of nonsterol compounds that inhibited various steps in the metabolic pathway. Inhibition of the rate-limiting enzymatic step, the enzyme hydroxymethylglutaryl (HMG) CoA reductase, by fungally derived compounds resulted in cholesterol reduction without build-up of toxic sterol intermediates. HMG CoA reductase releases the cholesterol precursor mevalonic acid from coenzyme A. Competitive inhibition by HMG CoA reductase inhibitors ('statins') leads to compensatory cellular responses such as increased expression of HMG CoA reductase enzyme and LDL receptors. Owing to the compensatory increase in HMG CoA reductase, cellular cholesterol synthesis is only slightly reduced, but clearance of cholesterol via the LDL receptor mechanism is markedly enhanced.

The Fredrickson classification of hyperlipidemias

Type	Serum cholesterol and TG concentrations	Specific lipoproteins
I	TG very elevated Cholesterol mildly elevated	Chylomicrons increased VLDL normal
IIa	Cholesterol increased TG normal	LDL increased
IIb	Cholesterol increased TG increased	LDL and VLDL increased
III	Cholesterol increased TG increased	Excess IDL remnant particles
IV	TG increased Cholesterol normal	VLDL increased LDL normal
V	TG very elevated Cholesterol mildly elevated	Chylomicrons increased VLDL increased

Fig. 15.27 The Fredrickson classification of hyperlipidemias. (IDL, intermediate density lipoprotein; LDL, low density lipoprotein; VLDL, very low density lipoprotein; TG, triglyceride)

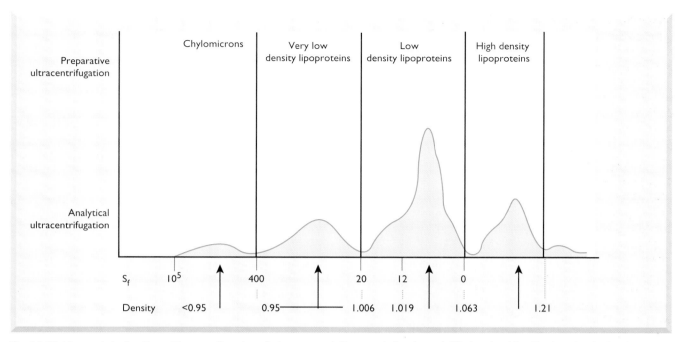

Fig. 15.28 Lipoprotein fractions. Ultracentrifugation of plasma reveals lipoprotein fractions of differing densities. The low density fraction contains both low (LDL) and intermediate-density lipoproteins (very low density lipoprotein remnants). The most commonly used cholesterol assays do not use ultracentrifugation, but instead estimate the concentration of LDL after measuring triglycerides and high-density lipoproteins.

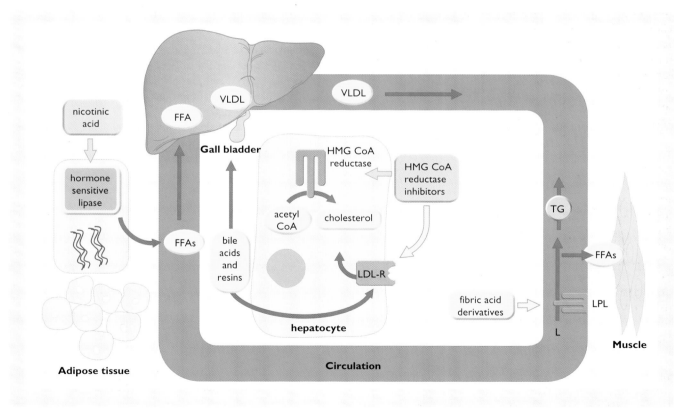

Fig. 15.29 Sites of action of hypolipidemic agents. HMG CoA reductase inhibitors lead to increased expression of low density lipoprotein receptor (LDL-R) expression on hepatocytes and improved clearance of LDL from the plasma. Bile acid resins similarly lead to an increased LDL clearance as well as increased cholesterol losses in bile. Fibric acid derivatives enhance lipoprotein lipase (LPL) action in peripheral tissues, which leads to improved clearance of triglyceride-rich particles. Nicotinic acid limits the flux of free fatty acids (FFAs) from adipose tissue, which reduces the stimulus for hepatic very low density lipoprotein (VLDL) production. By the reduction of VLDL production, fewer remnant particles are available for LDL synthesis.

The statins have limited systemic bioavailability after oral administration. Most are subject to extensive (50–80%) first-pass hepatic metabolism and drug concentrations in the systemic circulation are low. Plasma elimination half-life varies from approximately 2 hours (pravastatin, fluvastatin, cerivastatin) to 14 hours (atorvastatin). Simvastatin and lovastatin are pro-drugs which require oxidative cleavage of a lactone ring to become pharmacologically active. Most statins (except pravastatin and fluvastatin) are metabolized by CYP 3A4, and subject to adverse drug interactions. Although not a CYP 3A4 substrate, pravastatin plasma concentrations are increased by cyclosporine, possibly by interaction with the P-glycoprotein drug transport system.

HMG CoA reductase inhibitors produce the greatest reductions in LDL cholesterol of any single class of hypolipidemic agents (Fig. 15.30). The most pronounced effect of the 'statins' is reduction of LDL cholesterol, but there is also a reduction in the cholesterol content of VLDL particles, while HDL cholesterol may increase slightly. Their modest efficacy at lowering VLDL and raising HDL cholesterol limits their use as a monotherapy for combined hyperlipidemias. Other mechanisms of action such as direct inhibition of atherogenic processes in vascular tissue have been proposed but not clearly confirmed in clinical studies.

Bile acid sequestrant resins

Lower plasma cholesterol concentrations can be achieved by combining a reduced dietary intake of cholesterol with the use of bile acid sequestrants to eliminate cholesterol. The bile acid-binding resins cholestyramine, colestipol, and colesevelam inhibit bile acid reabsorption. Hepatic uptake of cholesterol from blood is increased to meet the body's ongoing needs for bile synthesis, and this leads to more rapid clearance of circulating LDL and IDL particles. Maximal doses of resin lead to reductions of LDL cholesterol of approximately 20%, with little effect on HDL cholesterol concentrations. VLDL concentrations usually increase during the initial period of therapy; hence these agents may exacerbate hypertriglyceridemia. Bile acid sequestrant resins are not systemically absorbed and therefore have no direct systemic pharmacologic activity. They do, however, bind other lipid-soluble factors such as vitamins

A and D as well as some drugs. These interactions may lead to symptoms related to malabsorption of drugs and nutrients. Bile acid sequestrants cause mild gastrointestinal adverse effects such as bloating and constipation.

Fibric acid derivatives

In contrast to the predominantly LDL-lowering effects of HMG CoA inhibitors, fibric acid derivatives (fibrates) such as gemfibrozil, fenofibrate, bezafibrate and clofibrate enhance the clearance of VLDL particles. The first compound in this class (clofibrate) was discovered in the early 1960s by screening novel organic compounds for cholesterol-lowering activity in rats. More recently, fibrates have been found to be agonists for the α class of peroxisomal-proliferator-activator receptors (PPAR-α) nuclear transcription factors. Fibrates increase the activity of peripheral lipoprotein lipase (LPL) by decreasing the transcription of apoprotein CIII, an inhibitory cofactor for LPL. Enhanced LPL function facilitates the entry of triglycerides from VLDLs and chylomicrons into target tissues. Fibrates also increase the transcription of apolipoproteins AI and AII which facilitate transfer of cholesterol esters from VLDL to HDL, thereby reducing the cholesterol content of remnant particles and increasing that of HDL particles. With maximal doses of gemfibrozil, HDL cholesterol increases by approximately 20% while circulating triglyceride concentrations are reduced by approximately 50%. Through poorly understood mechanisms, LDL cholesterol is reduced by approximately 10%.

GEMFIBROZIL has a plasma elimination half-life of approximately 1.5 hours, and is administered twice daily. Another commonly used fibrate, fenofibrate, demonstrates a plasma elimination half-life of approximately 20 hours in a sustained-release formulation which may be administered once daily. Despite these pharmacokinetic differences, all fibrates in current clinical use demonstrate comparable maximal efficacy. Fibric acid derivatives are most appropriate for the clinical disorders associated with increased circulating triglycerides (type IIb and type IV hyperlipidemias), and are particularly effective for familial dysbetalipoproteinemia (type III hyperlipidemia), which results from impaired remnant clearance due to Apo E abnormalities. A genetic deficiency of lipoprotein lipase (type I hyperlipidemia) is characterized by markedly elevated triglycerides, but is not responsive to fibric acid derivatives. Gemfibrozil reduces the risk of initial myocardial infarction in middle aged men with non-HDL cholesterol concentrations >200 mg/dl (Helsinki Heart Study), and reduces the risk of recurrent myocardial infarction in men with HDL cholesterol concentrations <40 mg/dl (VA-HIT Study). Fibrates are well-suited for the treatment of dyslipidemia in diabetic patients who often demonstrate hypertriglyceridemia and low levels of HDL.

Niacin (nicotinic acid)

Niacin is a vitamin precursor of the nicotine adenine dinucleotides (NAD and NADP). At pharmacologic doses, niacin's effects on lipoprotein metabolism are independent of its role as a precursor for nicotinamide. Although niacin has

---

> ⚠ **Lipid-lowering agents**
>
> - *HMG CoA reductase inhibitors: elevation of liver enzymes and creatine phosphokinase (myositis)*
> - *Bile acid sequestrant resins: gastrointestinal bloating, constipation, impaired drug absorption*
> - *Fibric acid derivatives: cholelithiasis, elevation of creatine phosphokinase (myositis)*
> - *Niacin: vasomotor flushing, pruritus, hyperuricemia, glucose intolerance, peptic ulcer, cholestatic jaundice, hyperpigmentation*
> - *Sustained-release niacin preparations and combined use of HMG CoA reductase inhibitors and fibric acid derivatives lead to an increased risk of myositis*

Lipid-lowering agents

	Major mechanism	Typical dose	Efficacy	Adverse effects
HMG CoA reductase inhibitors ('statins')	Competitive inhibition of cholesterol biosynthetic enzyme induces LDL receptor expression and enhanced LDL clearance		Significant LDL lowering (see individual agents) 10–20% triglyceride reduction 5–10% HDL increase	Myopathy Hepatic transaminase elevation Potentiation of myopathy with fibrates
Lovastatin		10–80 mg/day	20–40% LDL reduction	CYP 3A4 interactions (cyclosporine, erythromycin, diltiazem)
Atorvastatin		10–80 mg/day	40–60% LDL reduction	CYP 3A4 interactions
Pravastatin		10–40 mg/day	20–35% LDL reduction	
Simvastatin		10–80 mg/day	30–50% LDL reduction	CYP 3A4 interactions
Fluvastatin		20–80 mg/day	20–30% LDL reduction	
Cerivastatin		0.2–0.3 mg/day	25–30% LDL reduction	
Fibric acid derivatives ('fibrates')	Enhanced VLDL catabolism (Apo C) Increases HDL cholesterol content (Apo AI/II)		40–60% triglyceride reduction 10–20% HDL elevation Mild LDL lowering	Dyspepsia Possible increased risk of cholelithiasis Potentiation of myopathy with statins
Gemfibrozil		600 mg b.i.d.		
Fenofibrate (micronized)		200 mg q.d.		
Niacin (nicotinic acid)	Decreases fatty acid flux from adipose tissue Decreases VLDL production		30–80% triglyceride reduction 10–30% HDL elevation 10–20% LDL reduction	Cutaneous flushing, pruritis, rash Hepatotoxicity Impaired glucose tolerance Hyperuricemia Exacerbation of peptic ulcer Acanthosis nigricans
Immediate release (crystal) niacin		0.5–2 g t.i.d.		
Sustained release niacin (Niaspan)		1–2 g p.o. q.d.		
Bile acid resins	Increase intestinal clearance of cholesterol		10–25% LDL reduction	Abdominal bloating, constipation Mild triglyceride elevation Drug interactions (if administered 1 h before or up to 4 h after resin dosing) Fat malabsorption (rare)
Cholestyramine		4–8 g b.i.d.–t.i.d. (1 g/tablet, 4 g/packet, or 4 g/scoop of granules		
Colestipol		5–15 g b.i.d. (1 g/tablet, 5 g/packet, or 5 gm/scoop of granules)		
Colesevelam		625 mg b.i.d.		No drug interaction with concurrently administered digoxin, warfarin, metoprolol or quinidine

Fig. 15.30 Lipid-lowering agents.

303

been used to treat hyperlipidemia for many years, its mechanism of action is poorly understood. Its major effect is to decrease production of VLDLs by reducing the flux of fatty acids from adipose tissue to the liver. Lower VLDL concentrations lead to a reduced exchange of cholesterol with HDL (and therefore higher HDL cholesterol concentrations) as well as reduced delivery of IDL to the liver for LDL formation. Because of these compensatory changes in lipoprotein metabolism, niacin therapy produces the optimal therapeutic effect of increasing HDL while lowering LDL cholesterol and triglycerides. For these reasons, it is useful in the treatment of combined hyperlipidemias.

The adverse effects of niacin include acute dose-related effects such as flushing and pruritus, which are the most common. These are prostaglandin-mediated and may be prevented by concurrent aspirin administration. Patients become tolerant to such adverse effects, but not to the therapeutic effect on lipoproteins with gradual increases in dose and prolonged exposure. Other adverse effects, such as an aggravation of peptic ulcer disease, hyperuricemia, glucose intolerance, and hepatic and skeletal muscle toxicities may, however, limit the use of this inexpensive and effective agent. Niacin is also used as a sustained-release preparation, which is well tolerated by most patients. Sustained-release niacin demonstrates greater potency in LDL reduction compared with immediate-release niacin, although maximal efficacy is similar for the two formulations. Doses of 1.5–2 g/day of sustained-resease niacin are comparable to 3 g/day of the immediate-release (crystalline) formulation. Although previous sustained-release niacin preparations were associated with dose-dependent hepatotoxicity, this was largely due to administration of >2 g/day.

Other hypolipidemic agents

PROBUCOL is a hypolipidemic agent with minimal cholesterol-lowering effects, but may act by reducing the oxidation of LDL. Oxidized LDL is taken up more avidly by macrophages to produce foam cells and atherosclerotic plaques. However, probucol is not commonly used because it reduces HDL to a greater degree than LDL cholesterol and has been associated with ventricular arrhythmias.

FISH OILS contain ω_3 fatty acids such as eicosapentaenoic acid, which is an essential fatty acid constituent of biologic membranes. Ingestion of fish oils results in decreased VLDL synthesis and improved clearance of remnant particles. These ω_3 fatty acids reduce the production of arachidonic acid metabolites, and may thereby reduce platelet aggregation. The usual dose for reduction of hypertriglyceridemia is 5 g b.i.d. Nausea and malodorous eructation are the most common adverse effects. The hypolipidemic effect of this dietary constituent is thought to contribute to the low prevalence of coronary artery disease in many maritime cultures.

Secondary causes and combined therapy of hyperlipidemia

Dietary reduction of cholesterol intake and treatment of cholesterol-elevating conditions such as diabetes mellitus, renal disease, cholestatic disorders, hypothyroidism, and hypogonadism are recommended before starting drug therapy for hyperlipidemia. Weight loss is associated with the combined health benefits of improved lipoprotein metabolism, reduced blood pressure, and improved insulin sensitivity. If lifestyle modification is inadequate, and complicating medical conditions have been appropriately managed, cholesterol-lowering therapy can be initiated according to the predominantly elevated component, for example:

- Nicotinic acid or fibric acid derivatives for triglycerides.
- Bile acid sequestrants or HMG CoA reductase inhibitors for LDL cholesterol.

Combined therapy with bile acid sequestrants and other agents is safe and usually produces additive cholesterol-lowering effects. Combinations of nicotinic acid, HMG CoA reductase inhibitors, and fibric acid derivatives are effective, but may cause either hepatic or skeletal muscle toxicity.

Disorders of glucocorticosteroids and the stress response hormones

The hypothalamic–pituitary–adrenal (HPA) axis releases adrenal hormones such as glucocorticosteroids and epinephrine. These mediate a complex set of physiologic effects best characterized by the term 'general adaptation syndrome.' In the 1940s Hans Selye coined this term to describe the adrenal response to 'fight or flight' situations. This concept of hormonally regulated adaptation to conditions of acute physiologic stress such as trauma, hypovolemia, systemic infection, or environmental exposure, provides a general framework for understanding the varied actions of glucocorticosteroids and catecholamines (Fig. 15.31).

Under conditions of stress, the hypothalamic hormone, corticotropin-releasing hormone (CRH), causes pituitary ACTH release, resulting in increased production of cortisol in the zona fasciculata of the adrenals. The sympathetic nervous system, activated under similar conditions, releases neuronal norepinephrine and secretes epinephrine from the adrenal medulla. Among its varied effects, cortisol enhances epinephrine synthesis and sensitizes the peripheral tissues to the effects of catecholamines. The net effect of glucocorticosteroid and catecholamine action is to prepare the body for short periods of high physical or stressful activity. In this light, the varied effects of glucocorticosteroids, i.e. increasing gluconeogenesis and lipolysis, mobilizing fuel substrates from muscle, increasing CNS arousal, increasing blood pressure, suppressing inflammation, and delaying wound healing, seem to serve a common purpose. The sympathetic nervous system reinforces these effects by increasing blood pressure, cardiac output, blood glucose, lipolysis, CNS arousal, skeletal muscle blood flow, and platelet coagulability.

Sustained increases of 'stress' hormones lead to widespread physiologic disturbances

While short-term activation of 'stress' hormones may have been useful during evolution, major disorders can result from prolonged excess of the hormones that mediate the general adaptation syndrome:

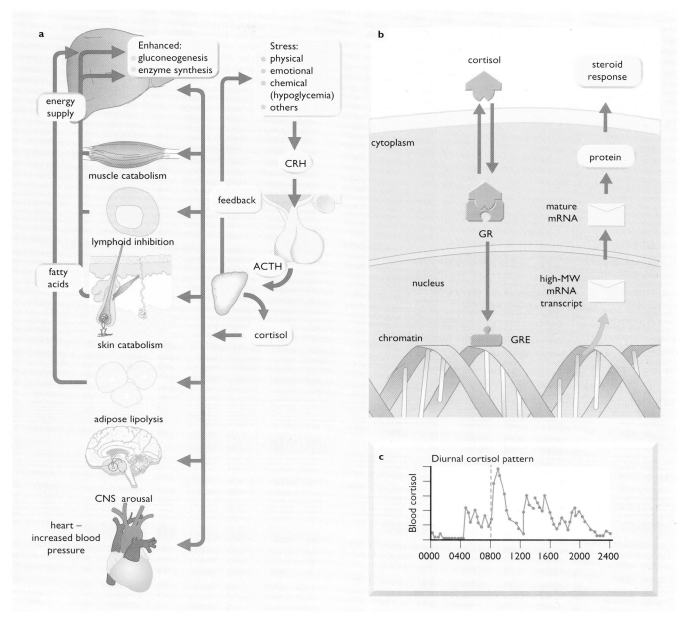

Fig. 15.31 Glucocorticosteroids and adaptation to stress. (a) A variety of sensorineural inputs regulate the pattern of corticotropin-releasing hormone (CRH) release in the hypothalamus. CRH releases adrenocorticotropic hormone (ACTH). ACTH leads to cortisol production in the adrenal zona fasciculata. Cortisol circulates to peripheral tissues where it binds cytosolic glucocorticosteroid receptors (GR) (b). After hormone binding, these receptors are translocated to the nucleus where they lead to transcription of glucocorticosteroid-responsive genes. The products of these genes lead to diverse target tissue effects such as enhanced gluconeogenesis, lipolysis, tissue catabolism, inhibition of lymphocyte function, pressor effects in the vasculature, and CNS behavioral effects. (c) The diurnal cortisol pattern reflects peak activity of the hypothalamic–pituitary–adrenal axis in the early morning.

- Chronic suppression of lymphocyte function by glucocorticosteroids predisposes to a variety of infections, including opportunistic parasitic and fungal diseases.
- Similarly, chronic glucose counter-regulation may lead to diabetes mellitus.
- Chronic cardiovascular activation may result in hypertension.

Glucocorticosteroids also have other poorly understood effects. These include:
- Stimulation of bone resorption.
- Inhibition of intestinal Ca^{2+} absorption.

- Inhibition of gonadotropin release.
- An increase in abdominal adipose tissue.
- Permissive effects on the action of vasopressin in the kidney.

As sex steroids are important anabolic agents for bone, the combined effects of glucocorticosteroid therapy on gonadotropins, Ca^{2+} balance, and bone physiology mean that it is an important risk factor for osteoporosis in both men and women.

Glucocorticosteroid deficiency

Glucocorticosteroid deficiency leads to profound symptoms

305

even under nonstressful conditions. Glucocorticosteroid deficiency results from either:

- Hypothalamic–pituitary disease leading to reduced ACTH secretion.
- Destruction of the adrenal cortex by autoimmunity (Addison's disease), destructive tumors, infarction, or infection.
- Suppression of hypothalamic–pituitary axis (HPA) function following treatment with exogenous glucocorticosteroids for inflammatory, autoimmune, or allergic diseases (iatrogenic adrenal insufficiency).

All these syndromes share the hallmark clinical features of glucocorticosteroid deficiency such as poor appetite, weight loss, fatigue, myalgia, arthralgia, and reduced cardiovascular reserve.

Patients with glucocorticosteroid deficiency due to deficient pituitary function do not demonstrate:

- Deficiency of the adrenal salt-retaining hormone aldosterone, since this is maintained by the renin–angiotensin system.
- Compensatory rises in ACTH and the related pituitary hormone melanocyte-stimulating hormone (MSH), which leads to increased skin pigmentation.

Patients with primary adrenal deficiency (Addison's disease) demonstrate the additional features of low blood pressure and hyperkalemia, owing to loss of aldosterone.

Synthetic glucocorticosteroids differ in their potency, duration and concurrent mineralocorticosteroid actions

Glucocorticosteroids are used to correct for the following:

- Adrenal insufficiency.
- Suppression of an overactive HPA axis.
- Suppression of autoimmune diseases.
- Prevention of rejection in organ transplants.
- Treatment of lymphocyte-derived tumors.
- Treatment of allergic disorders such as asthma and skin disorders.

As a result of these uses, glucocorticosteroids are among the most commonly prescribed drugs in clinical use. In the treatment of adrenal insufficiency, the goal is to mimic the physiologic patterns of cortisol action. In the treatment of other diseases, glucocorticosteroids are given in supraphysiologic doses where the therapeutic goal is to maximize therapeutic benefit while minimizing dose-related adverse effects such as iatrogenic adrenal insufficiency, osteoporosis, arteriosclerosis, infections, and neuropsychiatric disorders.

Glucocorticosteroid therapy

- Osteoporosis
- Glucose intolerance
- Increased risk of atherosclerotic disease
- Myopathy
- Immune suppression
- Cataracts
- Avascular necrosis of bones (e.g. hip)
- Neuropsychiatric disorders

Dosing and drug-delivery strategies are used to reduce the adverse effects of glucocorticosteroid therapy

One strategy aimed at minimizing adverse effects of glucocorticosteroid therapy is intermittent dosing, for example alternate-day therapy for allergic diseases. This strategy exploits the differences in pharmacodynamic half-lifes seen with different glucocorticosteroid effects. It has been demonstrated that glucocorticosteroids may suppress allergic phenomena when given every 48 hours, whereas pituitary suppression is shorter-lived. Even with the same average dose, glucocorticosteroid administration every 2 days may achieve the desired therapeutic effect with less iatrogenic adrenal insufficiency than more frequent dosing.

Another strategy for optimizing therapy is local administration. Topical glucocorticosteroids used for psoriasis and contact dermatitis (see Chapter 23) and inhaled glucocorticosteroids used for asthma and chronic lung disease achieve high local concentrations, but produce only modest elevations of systemic glucocorticosteroid (see Chapter 19). Such relative localization depends on dose, however, since topical glucocorticosteroids can be systemically absorbed in quantities sufficient to suppress pituitary function. Therapy is further enhanced with topical glucocorticosteroids whose high rates of drug metabolism lead to rapid elimination of systemic drug (e.g. triamcinolone acetonide).

Potency and duration of effect must be compared before substituting glucocorticosteroids for one another

The therapeutic effect of glucocorticosteroid therapy is determined by four factors:

- Drug concentration in effector tissue.
- Potency.
- Elimination half-life.
- Half-life of biologic responses.

Potency comparisons between glucocorticosteroids provide a general guideline for therapeutic substitution (Fig. 15.32). However, estimates of potency are imprecise because they do not fully reflect the duration of effect. For example, dexamethasone has sevenfold greater binding affinity for the glucocorticosteroid receptor than hydrocortisone but is 150-fold more potent in suppressing adrenal function 1 day after a single dose. In general, long-acting synthetic glucocorticosteroids such as dexamethasone and betamethasone are more likely to produce pituitary suppression than are the short-acting ones.

When hydrocortisone therapy is used for adrenal insufficiency, in an attempt to mimic physiologic release of cortisol, unequally divided doses are given in the early morning and afternoon to try to mimic the physiologic condition (Fig. 15.33). Endogenous cortisol production is approximately 10 mg/day (28 mmol/day), and although hydrocortisone is highly bioavailable, greater daily exposure to glucocorticosteroid is often needed in replacement therapy.

Although synthetic glucocorticosteroids also have mineralocorticosteroid activity to varying degrees, a synthetic mineralocorticoid (e.g. fludrocortisone) is also administered in the treatment of adrenal insufficiency.

Some characteristics of synthetic glucocorticosteroids

	Equipotent dose (mg)	Relative glucocorticosteroid potency	Relative mineralocorticosteroid potency	Elimination half-life (h)	Duration of effect (h)
Hydrocortisone (cortisol)	20	1	1	1.5–2	8–12
Prednisone	5	4	0.8	3.5	18–36
Prednisolone	5	4	0.8	3.5	18–36
Methylprednisolone	4	5	0.5	2–3	18–36
Triamcinolone	4	5	0	3	18–36
Dexamethasone	0.75	20–50	0	3.5	18–36
Betamethasone	0.6	20–50	0	4.0	18–36

Fig. 15.32 Some characteristics of synthetic glucocorticosteroids.

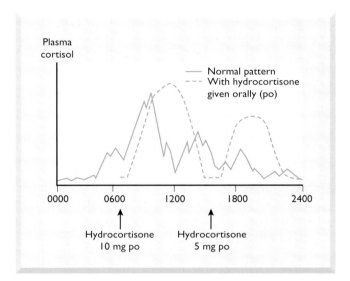

Fig. 15.33 Glucocorticosteroid replacement therapy. An average adult produces approximately 10 mg/day of cortisol. Cortisol production shows marked diurnal variation, with an initial elevation in the pre-waking hours. Physiologic replacement with oral hydrocortisone attempts to mimic this endogenous pattern.

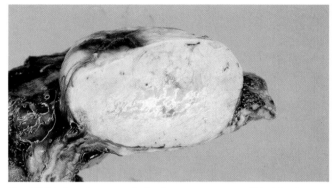

Fig. 15.34 An adrenocortical adenoma, a cause of Cushing's syndrome. (Courtesy of Dr Thomas Ulbright.)

Glucocorticosteroid excess

The physiologic role of glucocorticosteroids is best expressed during conditions of acute stress, but cortisol is secreted in biologically active amounts under normal conditions. Cortisol synthesis and release follows a diurnal pattern, with increased activity in the pre-dawn hours due to the activation of the HPA axis. Thus cortisol secretion is highest in the early morning, and may wane to very low levels at night.

Excess glucocorticosteroid action leads to Cushing's syndrome. This syndrome is characterized by muscle weakness, central fat deposition, 'moon' facies, purple abdominal striae, atrophic skin, capillary fragility, hypertension, glucose intolerance, and neuropsychiatric disorders. Cushing's syndrome results from a variety of causes (Fig. 15.34, 15.35), but is usually due to an ACTH-secreting pituitary adenoma (Cushing's disease), a cortisol-secreting adrenal tumor, or ectopic ACTH production from other neoplasms (e.g. neuroendocrine tumors of the lung and gut).

Inhibitors of cytochrome P-450 steroidogenic enzymes have different effects on glucocorticosteroid, mineralocorticosteroid, and androgen production

The mainstay of treatment for Cushing's syndrome is surgical removal of the hormone-secreting tumor from the pituitary, adrenal gland, or anywhere it occurs. When surgery is not successful, pharmacologic therapy is used to counteract glucocorticosteroid excess. The most useful drugs are inhibitors of adrenal glucocorticosteroid synthesis such as ketoconazole, metyrapone, aminoglutethimide, and mitotane. There are no drugs that reduce ACTH secretion from pituitary adenomas, and the glucocorticosteroid receptor antagonist mifepristone (RU-486) has not proved practical for treating chronic hypercortisolism. Inhibitors of steroid biosynthesis have characteristic activity at different steps in cortisol synthesis, and lead to predictable effects on other adrenal steroids (Fig. 15.36).

METYRAPONE predominantly inhibits the terminal step in cortisol synthesis, 11-hydroxylation, leading to an increase in the precursor 11-deoxycortisol. An accumulation of precursors such as 17-hydroxyprogesterone may lead to increased adrenal androgen formation and hirsutism in women. Although metyrapone has no effect on aldosterone synthesis, the precursor, 11-deoxycortisol, has mineralocorticosteroid activity, which may result in salt retention and hypertension.

Signs and symptoms of Cushing's syndrome

- Myopathy
- Peripheral muscle wasting
- Central obesity
- 'Moon' facies
- Supraclavicular and dorsocervical fat pads
- Pigmented abdominal striae
- Acne
- Hirsutism
- Plethora
- Bruising and capillary fragility
- Hypertension
- Glucose intolerance
- Hypokalemia
- Arteriosclerosis
- Infections
- Neuropsychiatric disorders
- Osteoporosis
- Hypogonadism

Fig. 15.35 Signs and symptoms of Cushing's syndrome. Causes of pathologic hypercortisolism are adrenocorticotropic hormone (ACTH)-secreting pituitary adenomas (Cushing's disease), ectopic ACTH production from other neoplasms (ectopic ACTH syndrome), and adrenocortical adenomas. Cushing's syndrome, unlike mild hypercortisolism seen in obesity, acute psychiatric disease, and alcoholism, leads to progressive physiologic derangements.

KETOCONAZOLE AND AMINOGLUTETHIMIDE Ketoconazole, an imidazole antifungal agent, and aminoglutethimide, an anti-epileptic drug (see Chapter 14), inhibit multiple sites in steroidogenesis, including the entry point of cholesterol side-chain cleavage as well as important steps in androgen and cortisol biosynthesis. Ketoconazole's effectiveness as an antifungal agent is due to inhibition of a cytochrome P-450 enzyme involved in fungal ergosterol biosynthesis (see Chapter 10).

ADVERSE EFFECTS OF KETOCONAZOLE, AMINOGLUTETHIMIDE AND METYRAPONE All the steroidogenic enzymes inhibited by ketoconazole, aminoglutethimide, and metyrapone are part of the large family of cytochrome P-450 enzymes, which catalyze mono-oxygenation reactions. Cytochrome P-450 enzymes are involved in many biosynthetic and drug metabolism reactions, which may be the basis of the adverse drug interactions that occur with these types of agents. Since input into the steroidogenic pathway is reduced and multiple enzyme sites are inhibited, biologically active steroid precursor molecules do not accumulate. However, these drugs do inhibit sex steroid production and this may lead to hypogonadism in men.

MITOTANE inhibits steroidogenesis at the ACTH-regulated step of cholesterol side-chain cleavage and also causes atrophy of the adrenal cortex. Its only use is in the treatment of adrenal cancer because of its gastrointestinal toxicity.

Pheochromocytoma and catecholamine excess

In most cases of hypertension, a reversible cause cannot be identified. In a small percentage of patients, hypertension is caused by excess production of mineralocorticosteroids, glucocorticosteroids, or catecholamines (pheochromocytoma). In the latter condition, norepinephrine or epinephrine is secreted from neoplasms of the adrenal medulla or ectopic medullary tissue. High plasma concentrations of catecholamines elevate blood pressure via α_1 adrenoceptors on the vasculature and β_1 adrenoceptors on the heart. Potential blood pressure-lowering effects such as β_2 adrenoceptor-mediated vasodilation or reduced sympathetic neuronal discharge due to presynaptic α_2 adrenoceptors are not sufficient to normalize blood pressure. Common symptoms of pheochromocytoma include headache, palpitation, diaphoresis, and weight loss. The nonselective α adrenergic antagonist, phenozybenzamine, is the mainstay of medical therapy, prior to surgical resection.

Phenoxybenzamine is a competitive but irreversible antagonist of both α_1 and α_2 adrenoceptors. It exerts long-acting antagonist effects due to its long plasma elimination half-life (approximately 24 hours) and to the irreversible nature of receptor binding. Dosing is initiated at 10 mg p.o. twice daily and titrated upward, according to blood pressure response, at intervals of 3–5 days.

Phentolamine, a competitive reversible α_1 and α_2 adrenoceptor antagonist with a short half-life (20 minutes) is used for intraoperative management of transient hypertensive episodes, but is infrequently used in the ambulatory management of pheochromocytoma. Adverse effects include postural hypotension, nasal congestion and sexual dysfunction. Selective α_1 adrenergic antagonists such as terazosin and doxazosin have not been studied for use in pheochromocytoma.

In cases of refractory or malignant pheochromocytoma, the catecholamine biosynthesis inhibitor α-methyltyrosine may be used. Methyltyrosine is a competitive inhibitor of tyrosine hydroxylase, the rate-limiting step in catecholamine synthesis. Methyltyrosine has a relatively short plasma elimination half-life (4–7 hours) and is titrated from a starting dose of 250 mg to 1 g p.o. q.i.d. Adverse effects such as sedation, fatigue and extrapyramidal effects (rigidity, tremor) are frequent.

Mineralocorticosteroids, vasopressin, and disorders of circulatory volume

The hypothalamus, pituitary, and the adrenal glands are also involved in the hormonal regulation of extracellular fluid volume (Fig. 15.37). The pituitary and adrenal glands regulate circulatory volume by two interdependent mechanisms which regulate: (i) Na^+ balance (adrenal mineralocorticosteroids), and (ii) free water balance (pituitary vasopressin).

Since Na^+ and its accompanying anions (Cl^- and HCO_3^-) are the main osmotic constituents of extracellular fluid, regulation of Na^+ loss through the kidney, gut, and skin (sweat glands) is critical in determining extracellular fluid volume. Extracellular

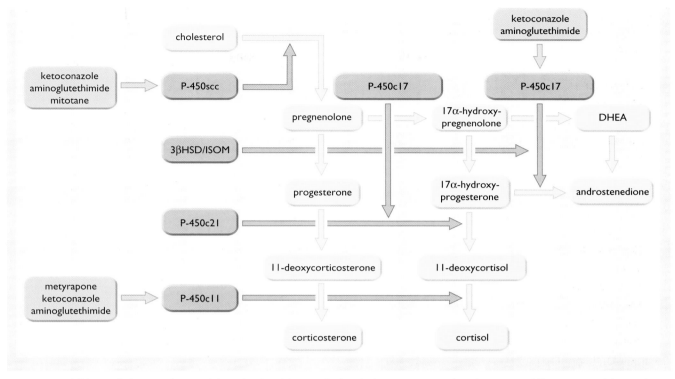

Fig. 15.36 Inhibitors of glucocorticosteroid synthesis. Inhibitors of adrenal glucocorticosteroid synthesis act at different steps of the synthetic pathway. Ketoconazole, aminoglutethimide, and mitotane act at the initial step of cholesterol side-chain cleavage (P-450scc), which delivers steroidogenic substrate into the pathway. Ketoconazole and aminoglutethimide are competitive inhibitors of cytochrome P-450 enzymes, and have other sites of action in the synthetic pathway. These agents reduce the production of adrenal androgen (DHEA and androstenedione) by inhibition of 17α-hydroxylase (P-450c17) and may lead to androgen deficiency in males. Metyrapone inhibits the terminal step in cortisol synthesis, 11β -hydroxylase (P-450c11), leading to a build-up of precursors with androgenic and mineralocorticosteroid potency. (DHEA, dehydroepiandrosterone; 3βHSD/ISOM, 3β-hydroxysteroid isomerase, P-450c21, 21α-hydroxylase)

fluid is partitioned between the vascular and interstitial compartments and therefore extracellular volume is a major determinant of circulatory blood volume and blood pressure homeostasis. The osmotic content of extracellular water drives free water from the large intracellular reservoir to the extracellular fluid compartments.

▓ *Sodium retention in the distal renal tubule is modulated by aldosterone via genes responsible for the synthesis of Na⁺/K⁺ ATPase and the Na⁺/H⁺ exchanger*

Body Na^+ is regulated in the kidney through the mineralocorticosteroid hormone aldosterone, angiotensin II, the sympathetic nervous system, atrial natriuretic peptides, and intrinsic renal mechanisms.

The renal sensing mechanism for circulatory volume as well as its effector limb, the renin–angiotensin–aldosterone (RAA) axis, are also discussed in Chapter 17. Afferent inputs such as renal afferent arteriole baroreceptors, the renal tubular Na^+ sensor, and volume receptors in the central veins, stimulate renin release in response to decreased blood volume or reduced renal perfusion. The actions of renin lead to the synthesis of the peptides angiotensin II and angiotensin III, which act on the adrenal zona glomerulosa to increase the synthesis of aldosterone (Fig. 15.38). The synthetic pathways for aldosterone

are similar to those for cortisol synthesis except for the two-step formation of the 18-aldehyde group by the angiotensin II-sensitive enzyme, corticosterone methyloxidase I and II. This enzyme is present only in the zona glomerulosa.

Like other steroid hormones, aldosterone induces genes in tissues expressing the mineralocorticosteroid receptor (i.e. kidney, brain, vasculature). Although the mineralocorticosteroid receptor can bind both aldosterone and cortisol, it is protected from glucocorticosteroid stimulation as a result of a unique enzyme, 11β-hydroxysteroid dehydrogenase. This enzyme, which is expressed in mineralocorticosteroid target tissues, selectively inactivates any cortisol in the proximity of mineralocorticosteroid receptors.

The classic target tissue for mineralocorticosteroids is the renal distal convoluted tubule epithelial cell where mineralocorticosteroid stimulation induces genes for Na^+/K^+ ATPase, ion channels, and mitochondrial enzymes critical to Na^+ recovery and K^+ or H^+ excretion. Outside the kidney, mineralocorticosteroids conserve Na^+ in the gastrointestinal tract and sweat glands, and increase blood pressure by effects on the brain and the vasculature. Mineralocorticoid receptors also influence collagen synthesis by fibroblasts, and may thereby play an important role in remodeling of vascular tissues damaged by ischemia or hemodynamic stress. Aldosterone

309

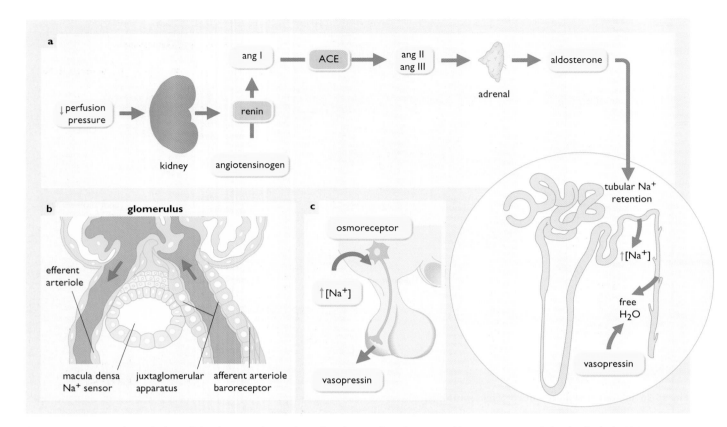

Fig. 15.37 Hormonal regulation of circulatory volume. Central cardiovascular reflexes, renal baroreceptors, and the distal tubular Na^+ sensor provide physiologic input about circulatory volume (a, b). In response to decreased renal perfusion, the juxtaglomerular cells of the afferent glomerular arteriole release renin. Renin converts circulating angiotensinogen to angiotensin (ang) I, which is then converted to ang II by the converting enzyme (ACE) in the vascular endothelium (a). Ang II and ang III stimulate aldosterone production, which leads to Na^+ reabsorption in the distal convoluted tubule. Na^+ reabsorption increases the osmolality of extracellular fluids. This stimulates the hypothalamic osmoreceptor to release vasopressin from the posterior pituitary. Vasopressin leads to enhanced free water reabsorption in the collecting duct, which expands extracellular volume and reduces plasma osmolality (c).

secretion is stimulated by high serum K^+. This stimulation is the major mechanism in the body for protection against life-threatening hyperkalemia. Excess mineralocorticosteroid action leads to a renal loss of K^+ and H^+ (i.e. hypokalemia and alkalosis) and increased extracellular fluid volume, while a lack of mineralocorticosteroid leads to hyperkalemia and volume depletion.

■ *Free water balance is coupled to Na^+ balance via hypothalamic osmoreceptor stimulation and release of vasopressin from the posterior pituitary*
While the RAA system and the sympathetic nervous system regulate the Na^+ content of extracellular water, such control extends to extracellular volume only if the free water balance is also regulated so as to maintain osmotic equilibrium. Marked Na^+ retention by aldosterone leads to both an increased Na^+ content and increased osmolality in extracellular water. As a result, water shifts from the intracellular to the extracellular space, and a hyperosmotic stimulus acts on osmoreceptor cells in the hypothalamus. The osmotic sensing mechanism in the brain causes vasopressin (antidiuretic hormone, ADH) release from the posterior pituitary (Fig. 15.39).

Vasopressin is a 9-amino acid peptide hormone. Circulating vasopressin stimulates V_2 GPCR receptors, which increase the permeability of the renal collecting tubules by a cAMP-mediated mechanism. This allows water in the tubule to move into the extracellular space of the renal interstitium. As a result, free water returns to the circulatory compartment, and then provides negative feedback to the osmoreceptor in the brain. Thirst is also activated and suppressed by similar circumstances. In addition to free water regulation, vasopressin stimulates V_1 receptors on the vasculature to cause vasoconstriction via a Ca^{2+}-dependent intracellular signaling pathway.

Vasopressin release is suppressed by reduced osmolality, resulting in increased free water losses in response to excess fluid intake. If there is a severe reduction in blood pressure (shock), vasopressin is released regardless of osmolality in an attempt to maintain circulatory volume at the expense of osmolality.

Mineralocorticosteroid deficiency
Mineralocorticosteroid deficiency is usually due to destruction of the adrenal cortices (Addison's disease), in which case there are the expected symptoms of mineralocorticosteroid deficiency

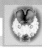

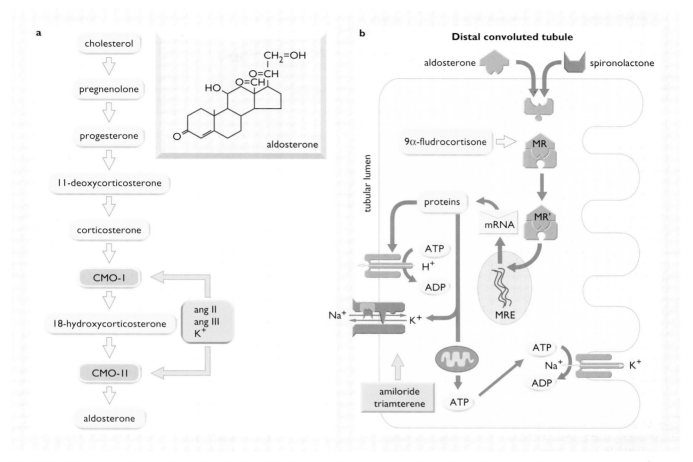

Fig. 15.38 Mineralocorticosteroids and regulation of Na⁺ balance. Angiotensins (ang II and III) regulate the corticosterone methyloxidase (CMO) I and II enzymes, which catalyze the hydroxylation and aldehyde formation at 18-C of corticosterone (a). Circulating aldosterone binds to cytosolic mineralocorticosteroid receptors (MR), which then translocate to the nucleus to regulate the expression of genes containing a mineralocorticosteroid response element (MRE). Renal tubular epithelial cells express Na⁺/K⁺ ATPase, the luminal Na⁺ permease, luminal proton pumps, and mitochondrial enzymes necessary for the production of ATP. The net effect of aldosterone stimulation in the distal convoluted tubule is to reabsorb Na⁺ while excreting K⁺ and H⁺ (b). Spironolactone is a competitive antagonist at mineralocorticosteroid receptors, while diuretics such as amiloride and triamterene functionally antagonize Na⁺/K⁺ ATPase.

(hyperkalemia, acidosis, hypovolemia), as well as symptoms of glucocorticosteroid deficiency (anorexia, weakness, weight loss). The hallmark of mineralocorticosteroid deficiency is reduced extracellular volume and resulting postural hypotension, poor skin turgor, and reduced urine output. Since intracellular water passively follows its osmotic gradient, serum Na⁺ concentration may be normal despite reductions in total body Na⁺. Mineralocorticosteroid deficiency may also result from secondary deficiency of renin and/or angiotensin release in chronic renal disease (hyporeninemic hypoaldosteronism).

SODIUM SUPPLEMENTS AND MINERALOCORTICOSTEROID REPLACEMENT are used to treat mineralocorticosteroid deficiency whatever the cause. Synthetic mineralocorticosteroids include 9α-fludrocortisone, which is a potent mineralocorticosteroid agonist with minimal glucocorticosteroid activity (see Fig. 15.38b).

Vasopressin deficiency (diabetes insipidus)

Some of the consequences of vasopressin deficiency, and the receptors responsible for vasopressin actions, are described in Chapter 17.

A deficiency of action of vasopressin results from either impaired release or impaired action on the kidney:

- Impaired vasopressin release is usually due to destructive lesions (neoplasms, granulomatous inflammation or trauma) of the posterior pituitary.
- An impaired renal response to vasopressin is caused by renal disease and certain drugs (Fig. 15.40).

Vasopressin deficiency is diagnosed by an inability to concentrate urine when the extracellular fluid osmolality increases (hypernatremia). In contrast to the normal serum Na⁺ concentration found with mineralocorticosteroid deficiency, serum Na⁺ concentration is increased in free-water deficiency states.

▣ Treatment of diabetes insipidus requires differentiation between pituitary and renal causes

Nephrogenic diabetes insipidus is treated by removal of any causative drugs and treatment of the intrinsic renal disease.

Pituitary disease leading to vasopressin deficiency is not

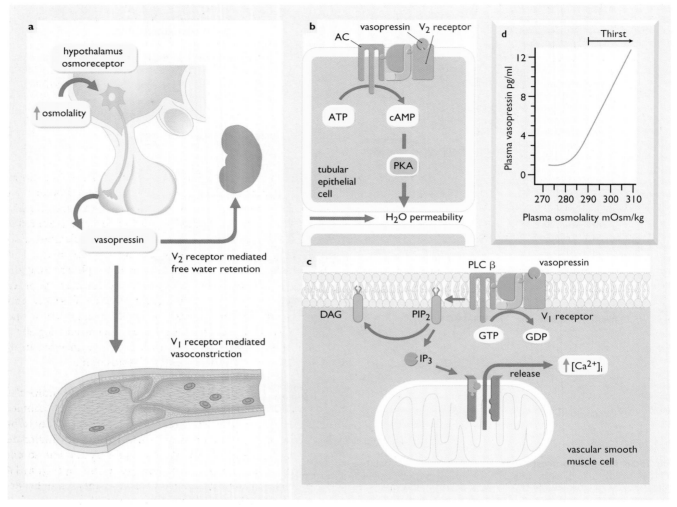

Fig. 15.39 Vasopressin and regulation of free water balance. Osmotic stimulation leads to vasopressin release from the posterior pituitary (a), and vasopressin then stimulates V_2 receptors on distal tubular epithelial cells. V_2 receptors are G protein-coupled receptors that stimulate adenylyl cyclase (AC) to increase intracellular cAMP and activate protein kinase A (PKA). This leads to enhanced permeability of the tubular epithelium (b). Increase in permeability of the collecting duct results in free water movement into the hypertonic renal medullary interstitium. PKA control of a water pore is shown in Fig. 17.14. Vasopressin also acts on other tissues: in the vasculature, via V_1 receptors that are linked to a phospholipase C (PLC β) signaling pathway. Release of inositol-1,4,5-triphosphate (IP_3) and diacylglycerol (DAG) from phosphoinositol (PIP_2) increases intracellular Ca^{2+} and potentiates vasopressor responses (c). As plasma osmolality increases with an increase in plasma vasopressin levels, so thirst mechanisms are activated (d).

usually reversed by treatment of the underlying tumor or inflammation.

VASOPRESSIN REPLACEMENT THERAPY involves administration of synthetic vasopressin analogs (desmopressin or lypressin). These compounds differ from native vasopressin by either a lysine substitution at the eighth amino acid position (lypressin) or deamination of the first-position cysteine residue (desmopressin). They can be administered by nasal spray (currently the preferred route of administration) or subcutaneous or intramuscular injection. Twice-daily treatment is usually required, with at least one dose in the evening to allow uninterrupted sleep. Desmopressin is also used intravenously in the management of hemophilia owing to its unexplained ability to increase the activity of von Willebrand's factor.

Mineralocorticosteroid excess

Mineralocorticosteroid excess is an important, but uncommon, cause of hypertension. Like other hormonal excess syndromes, it is caused by either:

- A primary excess of adrenal mineralocorticosteroid production.
- A secondary excess of the mineralocorticosteroid-regulating hormone angiotensin II.

Secondary mineralocorticosteroid excess due to excessive production of renin and angiotensin is usually caused by renal diseases such as renal artery stenosis, which impair the kidney's ability to respond appropriately to systemic arterial pressure. The mineralocorticosteroid excess is mild and the pressor effects of angiotensin II dominate.

Primary mineralocorticosteroidism usually results from

Causes of diabetes insipidus
Neurogenic (vasopressin deficiency)
Hypothalamic and pituitary tumors Lymphocytic hypophysitis Sarcoidosis Infections (tuberculosis, syphilis) Histiocytosis X
Nephrogenic (renal vasopressin resistance)
Chronic renal disease Hypokalemia Drugs (lithium, demeclocycline, anesthetics)

Fig. 15.40 Causes of diabetes insipidus.

either an aldosterone-producing adenoma, or angiotensin II hypersensitivity leading to bilateral hypertrophy of the zona glomerulosa (idiopathic hyperaldosteronism). Surgical resection of an aldosterone-producing adenoma often reverses the hypertension, but bilateral adrenalectomy will not correct the hypertension in idiopathic hyperaldosteronism.

Mineralocorticosteroid excess increases extracellular Na+

As a result of the increased extracellular Na^+ and indirect stimulation of vasopressin release produced by mineralocorticosteroid excess, water moves from the intracellular space and extracellular fluid volume increases. As circulatory volume and renal perfusion increase a pressure–natriuresis response occurs in the kidney and Na^+ excretion increases. The effects of mineralocorticosteroid-related Na^+ retention and pressure–natriuresis reach equilibrium at a modest level of volume expansion, but do not progress to overt volume excess (edema). Serum Na^+ concentrations remain normal, but K^+ is progressively lost, leading to hypokalemia.

Diseases that reduce renal perfusion by reducing circulatory volume as a result of hypoalbuminemia or reduced cardiac output lead to progressive Na^+ and volume retention, which is not corrected by the pressure–natriuresis response. This accounts for the edema seen in conditions such as congestive heart failure, cirrhosis, and the nephrotic syndrome. Although mineralocorticosteroid levels are high in such conditions, they are elevated by an appropriate physiologic response to reduced renal perfusion.

The major therapy for an aldosterone-producing adenoma is surgery, but many cases of mineralocorticosteroid excess require medical therapy.

SPIRONOLACTONE (see Chapter 17 for full details) is a steroidal mineralocorticosteroid and androgen receptor antagonist. As an antagonist of mineralocorticoid receptors in the distal tubule and collecting duct, its potassium-sparing diuretic effect is useful in states of secondary mineralocorticoid excess such as congestive heart failure and hepatic cirrhosis. Low doses of spironolactone in patients with congestive heart failure demonstrate greater mortality reduction than would be

Clinical and laboratory diagnosis of volume disorders

- Clinical findings of hypervolemia (edema) reflect Na^+ excess, while signs of hypovolemia (orthostatic hypotension, dehydration, oliguria) reflect Na^+ deficiency
- The laboratory finding of hypernatremia reflects free water deficiency, while hyponatremia usually reflects free water excess

expected on the basis of its diuretic effect. This observation suggests that mineralocorticoid effects on tissues other than the kidney may be important in cardiovascular health. Spironolactone is metabolized to at least two active metabolites that have long elimination half-lifes. Spironolactone also antagonizes androgen receptors, leading to gynecomastia and hypogonadism in some males. It is used in the pharmacological treatment of hirsutism, in women. In contrast to other androgen antagonists that interrupt pituitary feedback and result in compensatory increases of testosterone, spironolactone also reduces androgen synthesis. The androgen-reducing effect of spironolactone is likely due to competitive antagonism of enzymes involved in biosynthesis of testosterone.

DIURETICS (see Chapter 17) that functionally antagonize the mineralocorticosteroid effects on renal tubules provide another common pharmacologic strategem for treating mineralocorticosteroidism. The potassium-sparing diuretics amiloride and triamterene reduce tubular Na^+ reabsorption but do not interact with androgen receptors to cause hypogonadal symptoms in male patients. However, they may cause hyperkalemia and their use requires close monitoring.

Vasopressin excess

Vasopressin excess is a common cause of hyponatremia and has numerous etiologies, including vasopressin-secreting tumors, drug effects, pulmonary disease, and neurologic disease. Through poorly understood mechanisms, these conditions lead to a vasopressin release which is not inhibited by low serum osmolality, a condition termed 'syndrome of inappropriate ADH secretion.' Excess vasopressin secretion leads to renal free water retention. Since Na^+ regulation is not similarly affected, the excess water retention leads to a dilutional hyponatremia. Most of the excess free water diffuses into the intracellular space, and therefore increases in circulatory volume (hypertension) and extracellular water (edema) do not occur. The mild expansion of extracellular water is sufficient, however, to increase renal perfusion and lead to increased tubular Na^+ excretion. Increased Na^+ excretion is an inappropriate response to hyponatremia, but is an appropriate physiologic response to increased circulatory volume.

Treatment of elevated vasopressin release is usually directed toward correcting its underlying cause. In some cases, vasopressin secretion by tumors or neurologic disease requires medical therapy, including restriction of free water intake. Antibiotic tetracyclines such as demeclocycline antagonize the

313

action of vasopressin on the kidney, but can cause renal toxicity. Paradoxically, diuretics improve the hyponatremia, probably by reducing the renal medullary osmotic gradient for free water reabsorption.

DRUGS AND THE ENDOCRINOLOGY OF THE REPRODUCTIVE SYSTEM

The following section concentrates on the endocrinology of the reproductive tract. The genitourinary aspects of this topic are covered in greater detail in Chapter 22. Unlike other endocrine systems, which regulate important physiologic functions on a short-term basis, the hypothalamic–pituitary–gonadal (HPG) axis regulates the differential expression of secondary sexual characteristics that take place over a lifetime. Functions such as sustaining spermatogenesis, follicular development, and the menstrual cycle require short-term regulation, while others such as puberty and menopause take place over long periods. Hypothalamic gonadotropin hormone-releasing hormone (GnRH) and pituitary gonadotropin release are coordinated by complex neuroendocrine mechanisms. The major regulator of sex steroid production is luteinizing hormone (LH), while that for gamete development is follicle-stimulating hormone (FSH). These hormones are secreted in an episodic or 'spiking' pattern with lower basal levels during much of the day. Androgens and estrogens exert feedback inhibition on gonadotropin secretion, but these effects vary during the menstrual cycle.

■ *Androgens are produced in the gonads and adrenals, while estrogens are produced from androgen precursors in the gonads and adipose tissue*

LH and FSH stimulate gonadal steroidogenesis and conversion of adrenal androgens to testosterone and estrogens, as shown in Fig. 15.41. The syntheses of estrogens and androgens share biosynthetic steps with other adrenocortical steroids, but glucocorticosteroids and mineralocorticosteroids are not synthesized because gonadal tissues do not express the appropriate enzymes. Under normal conditions, most sex steroids are produced in the gonads. With adrenal disease, however, production of the steroid dehydroepiandrosterone in large quantities in the zona reticularis can lead to the production of substantial amounts of sex steroids. Dehydroepiandrosterone (DHEA) has only slight androgenic activity but is readily converted to other sex steroids in the gonads, leading to the production of potent androgens. DHEA, when administered orally, is extensively conjugated by the liver, and produces small increases in concentrations of active androgens. Estrogens are also produced as a result of aromatase activity in the gonads and adipocytes. The aromatase enzyme converts androgens to estrogens and is expressed in adipose tissue where it is responsible for most postmenopausal estrogen production and higher estrogen levels in obese men and women.

Physiology of the female reproductive tract

■ *The ovary provides the gametes for fertilization and synthesizes hormones for reproductive tissues and to maintain the secondary female sex characteristics*

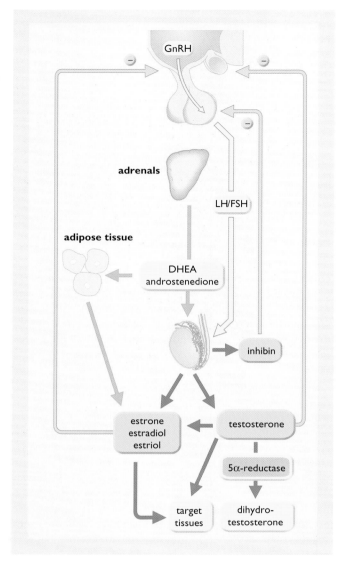

Fig. 15.41 Regulation of sex steroids. Hypothalamic gonadotropin-releasing hormone (GnRH) stimulates the release of luteinizing hormone (LH) and follicle-stimulating hormone (FSH) from the gonadotrophs of the anterior pituitary. LH and FSH stimulate sex steroid production in the gonads. Adrenal androgens are further metabolized to more potent androgens in the gonads. The aromatase enzyme in both the gonads and adipose tissue converts androgens to estrogens. In certain target tissues, the enzyme 5α-reductase converts testosterone to the more potent androgen dihydrotestosterone. In postpubertal males, sex steroid production is constant. In females, gonadotropins and sex steroids are released in a complex pattern during the menstrual cycle (see Fig. 15.45). (ACTH, adrenocorticotropic hormone; DHEA, dehydroepiandrosterone)

The ovary consists of spherical follicles embedded in a stroma, surrounded by a membrane, the tunica albuginea (Fig. 15.42). Each follicle contains a gamete (oocyte, ovum, egg). There are originally about 7 million ova, but a large proportion die before birth and during childhood, leaving some 400,000 at puberty; of these about 0.1% (i.e. 400) will ovulate. The most important hormones from the ovary are the sex steroids estrogen (mainly estradiol, but also estrone and estriol) and progesterone. Their

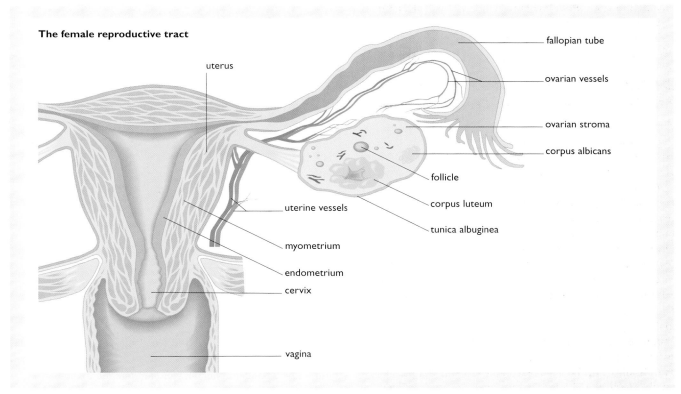

The female reproductive tract

Fig. 15.42 Structure of the female reproductive tract. This consists of two ovaries, each surrounded by a fallopian tube that is approximately 10 cm long and joins a short muscular organ, the uterus. The lower end of the uterus narrows to form the cervix, which is a muscular structure containing many secretory glands and protruding into the vagina. The cervix produces mucus to act as a barrier to infection between the vagina and uterus. The vagina is a thick-walled muscular tube lined by stratified nonkeratinized squamous epithelium. The outer layers of epithelium are constantly shed and these cells form the bulk of the cells seen in vaginal smears, which are taken to determine whether the vaginal mucosa is atrophic or being stimulated by estrogen, and to reveal the presence of infection.

production is controlled by the hypothalamic–pituitary axis (Fig. 15.43).

The menstrual cycle, the period between two ovulations, lasts 24–32 days

Day 1 of menstruation begins with shedding of the uterine endometrium which takes 3–5 days. This is followed by the follicular or proliferative phase of the cycle until day 14 (or midcycle) when ovulation occurs (Fig. 15.44). In the follicular phase, the developing follicles produce estradiol, which causes the uterine endometrium to proliferate. If the ovum is not fertilized, there is a luteal or secretory phase lasting 14 days until the endometrium is shed at menstruation. During the luteal phase, the ruptured follicle becomes a corpus luteum which produces progesterone and causes the endometrium to become secretory.

Luteinizing hormone (LH) increases androgen and progesterone production, while follicle-stimulating hormone (FSH) increases estrogen production from androgens

The production of estrogen and progesterone is controlled by the hypothalamic–pituitary axis (see Fig. 15.43):
- LH increases production of androstenedione and testosterone via receptors on the follicular thecal wall.

- FSH induces aromatization of the androgens to estrogens via receptors on granulosa cells.
- In the late follicular phase, some granulosa cells differentiate so that they express LH receptors and respond to LH by secreting progesterone. This is the first step in the conversion of the granulosa cells to luteal cells. Only the follicle possessing this second set of receptors will respond to the LH surge and ovulate.

An LH surge induces ovulation, reduces androgen and estrogen synthesis, and increases progesterone production

Estrogen concentrations rise as the follicles mature. Normally the sex steroids control the rate of their own secretion by negative feedback on the hypothalamus and pituitary to reduce LH and FSH secretion. Through a poorly understood mechanism this feedback effect is reversed at midcycle when high estradiol concentrations (>200 pg/ml) promote LH secretion for a 2-day period (the LH surge; Fig. 15.45).

The LH surge:
- Appears to desensitize the LH receptors on the theca, thereby terminating androgen/estrogen synthesis.
- Stimulates LH receptors on the differentiated granulosa cells to start secretion of progesterone.
- Stimulates resumption of meiosis in the ovum. The second

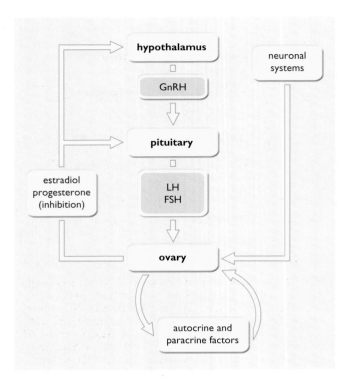

Fig. 15.43 The hypothalamic–pituitary–ovarian axis. Endocrine control of ovarian function is exerted by hormones, the most important being estrogen and progesterone. Their production is controlled by the hypothalamic–pituitary axis. Neurons within the preoptic area of the hypothalamus secrete pulses of a decapeptide called gonadotropin-releasing hormone (GnRH), which enters the hypophysial portal system and reaches the pituitary. It acts on specific receptors on the gonadotropin-secreting pituitary cells, and stimulates the pulsatile release of both follicle-stimulating hormone (FSH) and luteinizing hormone (LH). These two gonadotropins then act on specific receptors in the ovary and stimulate the production of steroid and peptide hormones and ovulation.

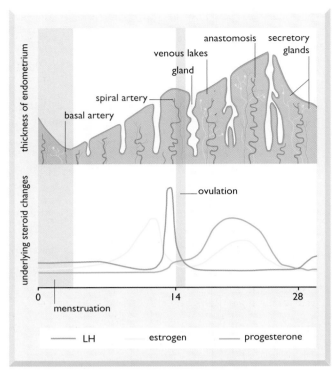

Fig. 15.44 Changes in human endometrium during human menstrual cycle. Underlying steroid changes are indicated (LH, luteinizing hormone).

meiotic division then starts, but is arrested in the metaphase and is completed only at fertilization.

- Induces the release of ovarian cytokines, plasminogen activators, prostaglandins, and histamine, causing the first dissolution of the thecal wall and then contraction of the weakening structure resulting in its rupture (ovulation). This occurs approximately 36 hours after the surge.

■ *The corpus luteum forms after ovulation and produces large quantities of progesterone, which maintains the uterine endometrium*

Under LH stimulation the granulosa cells of the ruptured ovarian follicle differentiate to form the corpus luteum (see Fig. 15.46). The corpus luteum produces large amounts of 17-hydroxyprogesterone and progesterone as well as estrogen. Progesterone primes the uterine endometrium for implantation. If fertilization does not take place the corpus luteum becomes senescent and starts to regress in the midluteal phase (day 21 onward of the cycle). In the later luteal phase, declining progesterone concentrations cause the endometrium to be shed at menstruation.

In response to fertilization, progesterone secretion is maintained by rising concentrations of human chorionic gonadotropin. Progesterone has several physiologic effects to inhibit menstrual cycling and sustain pregnancy:

- Maintenance of secretory endometrium for embyro and placental development.
- Feedback inhibition of gonadotropin secretion.
- Antiestrogenic effects on cervical mucus to reduce fertility.
- Promotion of mammary duct development.

Diseases treated by estrogens and estrogen antagonists
Estrogen-responsive diseases
In women, many disorders are influenced by estrogens, but few are directly caused by altered estrogen production. Common conditions such as menstrual abnormalities, uterine neoplasms, breast cancer, and the predisposition to autoimmune diseases are influenced by estrogen levels, but are not caused by an estrogen excess or deficit. Excess estrogen production in women, like excess testosterone production in men, does not produce readily noticeable signs or symptoms.

Estrogen therapy is used:
- To replace normal hormone production in deficiency states.
- To suppress endogenous hormone production (contraceptives).
- To treat other hormone-responsive conditions.

ESTROGENS AND ESTROGEN AGONISTS Daily output of estrogen (largely estradiol and estrone) in premenopausal women varies

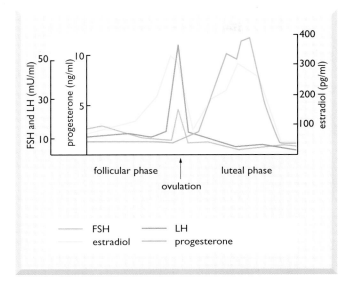

Fig. 15.45 Changes in the concentrations of circulating hormones during the menstrual cycle. Note that the hormone concentrations are drawn to different scales. During menstruation and in the early follicular phase, the steroid concentrations are low, and as there is little steroid negative feedback gonadotropin secretion (especially FSH) is slightly elevated. FSH stimulates the follicles in the ovary to grow, mature, and secrete estrogen. The increasing estrogen concentration then exerts negative feedback, reducing gonadotropin concentrations. However, when the estrogen concentration reaches a critical concentration (>200 pg/ml) for a critical length of time (2 days), the negative feedback switches to a positive feedback, stimulating a dramatic transient release of LH (the LH surge) and to a lesser extent FSH from the pituitary. The increased concentration of LH appears to desensitize the LH receptors on the theca, thereby terminating androgen and therefore estrogen synthesis, resulting in a rapid decline of the circulating estrogen concentration. However, LH receptors on the differentiated granulosa cells continue to respond to LH and start to secrete progesterone.

during the menstrual cycle from 20 to 100 mg/day. Estrogens are readily conjugated in the liver by sulfation and subsequently excreted in bile and urine. This first-pass hepatic metabolism limits oral estrogen therapy and daily doses of 1–2 mg synthetic estradiol are needed to achieve adequate hormone replacement. Most estrogen therapies use drugs that are less susceptible to first-pass hepatic metabolism:

- Conjugated estrogens, either isolated from the urine of pregnant mares or synthetic, contain predominantly estrone sulfates, which are subsequently hydrolyzed and converted to more active estrogens in the peripheral tissues.
- Transdermal estrogen patches deliver estradiol to the systemic circulation and increase exposure of the peripheral tissues before eventual hepatic metabolism.
- Ethinylestradiol is used in a variety of oral contraceptive pills. It contains a substitution at the C-17 of estradiol, which reduces metabolism. It therefore has potent estrogenic effects at doses of 20–50 mg/day.

One of the oldest synthetic estrogens, diethylstilbestrol (DES), is a nonsteroidal synthetic estrogen. Its use in pregnant women to prevent miscarriage in the 1970s was found to cause reproductive tract abnormalities in the daughters of these

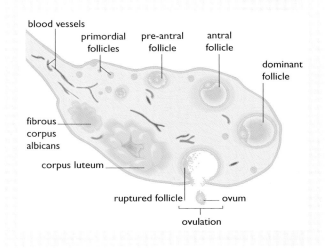

Fig. 15.46 The life cycle of the follicle. The follicles formed in fetal life consist of the ovum surrounded by two or three layers of granulosa cells and are called primordial follicles. Each day, some of these primordial follicles start maturation and begin to form a wall (theca) which becomes vascularized. This is the pre-antral stage and any further maturation is under the control of follicle-stimulating hormone (FSH) and luteinizing hormone (LH). If the FSH levels are below a critical concentration, the pre-antral follicles die (hence the huge losses over a lifetime). In the early follicular phase, FSH levels are above a critical concentration (see Fig. 15.45) and so the pre-antral follicles mature and pass into the antral stage. Only one follicle reaches complete maturity and is ready to ovulate, i.e. the dominant or Graafian follicle (selection phase). This is the source of 90% of the ovarian estrogen hormones. The remaining antral follicles die.

women and has led to a greater recognition of the long-term developmental effects of sex steroid exposure in *utero*. Use of any estrogen or antiestrogen during pregnancy is therefore contraindicated.

The adverse effects of estrogens include abnormal menstrual bleeding, water retention, nausea, increased hepatic synthesis of hormone-binding globulins, an elevation of triglyceride levels, increased blood clotting, and an increased risk of breast and uterine cancer. The increased risk of uterine cancer is eliminated by concurrent progesterone therapy.

SELECTIVE ESTROGEN RECEPTOR MODULATORS (SERMs, ANTIESTROGENS) The role of estrogen in promoting the growth of breast and uterine neoplasms has led to the use of nonsteroidal estrogen receptor antagonists for these conditions and other indications. Previously termed 'antiestrogens,' it is now appreciated that this class of drugs is tissue-selective in displaying estrogen agonist (bone, lipid, endometrium, coagulation) and estrogen antagonist (e.g. breast, pituitary) effects. In addition to tissue-selectivity of agonist versus antagonist effects, these agents display varying degrees of partial agonist activity on estrogen agonist end-points. The tissue-selective pattern of effects appears to be due to differential binding to tissue-specific transcription factors affecting both estrogen receptor- and nonestrogen receptor-mediated gene transcription.

Tamoxifen is an estrogen antagonist in breast tissue but has partial agonist effects on the endometrium, the genitourinary

317

epithelium, bone remodeling, and cholesterol metabolism. Not all responses are equally sensitive to tamoxifen's partial agonist actions. Much of tamoxifen's antagonist activity results from its metabolism to 4-hydroxy-tamoxifen, an active metabolite with greater antagonist potency. Tamoxifen and its active metabolites have long elimination half-lifes (5–14 days). Tamoxifen undergoes extensive oxidative metabolism. Tamoxifen has been used for fertility induction in some countries, but its primary indication is for the adjuvant treatment of breast cancer. Tamoxifen therapy reduces the risk of breast cancer recurrence after primary treatment for up to 5 years. Some cases of recurrent breast cancer reveal an agonistic effect of tamoxifen on the growth of some breast cancer cells. Some patients with breast cancer respond to the weak agonist effects of tamoxifen with an initial increase in tumor mass, a phenomenon termed 'tamoxifen flare,' but this is usually short-lived and antagonist effects soon predominate. Clomiphene is an SERM used for fertility induction that is chemically similar to tamoxifen (see below).

Raloxifene is a nonsteroidal SERM of a different chemical class than tamoxifen and clomiphene. Raloxifene has an elimination half-life of approximately 26 hours and is metabolized by glucuronide conjugation and biliary excretion. Raloxifene was initially developed as a breast cancer therapy, but subsequently found to have antiresorptive effects on bone in postmenopausal women, leading to its use in osteoporosis therapy. Raloxifene shares estrogen agonist effects on bone resorption, LDL-lowering, and coagulation parameters with other SERMs. It differs from tamoxifen in its lack of stimulation of the uterine endometrium. Its estrogen antagonist in the breast and hypothalamus contribute to reduced incidence of breast cancer and exacerbation of postmenopausal vasodilatation (hot flush).

Progesterone pharmacology

Progesterone is produced in large quantities (10–20 mg/day) by the ovary during the luteal phase of the menstrual cycle, and by both ovaries and the placenta during pregnancy. Progestational agents are used therapeutically for:
* Contraception.
* Menstrual irregularities.
* Endometriosis.
* Postpartum suppression of lactation.

Progestins share binding affinity for the androgen receptor, and many progestational agents show androgenic adverse effects. Progestins also have limited binding affinity for mineralocorticosteroid and glucocorticosteroid receptors. Many synthetic progestins are in clinical use. The progesterone receptor antagonist mifepristone (RU-486) is a potent antagonist at both progesterone and glucocorticosteroid receptors. It is used as an abortifacient.

Contraception and menstruation

Drugs can be used to:
* Inhibit normal female reproductive function and thereby prevent fertility (i.e. contraception).
* Replace missing hormones or correct patterns of hormone

secretion so as to facilitate fertility or prevent amenorrhea (absence of menstruation) without inducing fertility.

Steroid contraceptives

There are a variety of orally active natural and semisynthetic estrogens and progestogens (analogs of progesterone). The major estrogen is ethinyl estradiol, an acetylene derivative of estradiol. Progestogens have been developed from two structures, 19-nortestosterone or 17-hydroxyprogesterone.

19-NORTESTOSTERONE DERIVATIVES The first generation of progestogens lacked potency and had androgenic activity. Levonorgestrel (the d-isomer of norethisterone) is a second-generation analog and is more potent. The androgen receptor affinity of first and second generations of progestins contribute to acne and reduced HDL cholesterol concentrations. The effects of progestogen–estrogen combination therapy on hepatically mediated parameters such as lipoproteins, binding globulins and coagulation factors appears to represent a summation of estrogen agonist and androgen-mediated estrogen antagonist effects. Third-generation progestogens (desogestrel, gestodene, and norgestimate) have minimal androgenic activity, and thus permit greater expression of estrogen agonist effects on HDL cholesterol and clotting factors when combined with estrogens.

17-HYDROXYPROGESTERONE ACETATE DERIVATIVES These analogs have no androgenic or estrogenic activity. They are used in intramuscular or depot preparations for dysfunctional uterine bleeding and contraception in premenopausal women. The most common is medroxyprogesterone (brand name Depo-Provera). Medroxyprogesterone acetate is an oral preparation that is commonly used in combined hormone replacement therapy.

Combined oral contraceptives

Combined oral contraceptives (COCs) include second- and third-generation progestogens combined with ethinyl estradiol (EE) (Fig. 15.47). The combination of estrogen and progestogen displays additive and synergistic pharmacologic activity that makes these agents uniquely effective:
* Progestogens suppress menstrual cycling by hypothalamic and pituitary effects.
* Progestogens render cervical mucus inhospitable to sperm.
* Estrogens upregulate progesterone receptors and enhance sensitivity to the progestogen.
* Estrogens counteract the androgenic effects of synthetic progestogens.
* Estrogens contribute to negative feedback on the hypothalamus and pituitary.

The combination is usually taken for 21 days before stopping for 7 days to allow withdrawal bleeding (monophasic preparation). It is possible to take the monophasic preparation daily for 12 weeks (i.e. four packets) before having a 7-day break, particularly if there are adverse effects during the pill-free week. Triphasic preparations have a three stepwise changes in estrogen/progestogen ratio, in an attempt to mimic the natural pattern of cyclic steroid release. In order to further minimize

Combined oral contraceptives (COCs; all doses in μg except where noted)

Agent	Estrogen	Progestogen	Pharmacological features
Monophasic			Continuous administration may be extended up to 12 weeks to minimize inconvenience/symptoms of breakthrough Available in 21- or 28-day dose packs
	ME 50	NE 1 mg	
	EE 50	NE 1 mg	
	EE 50	NG 500	
	EE 35	NE 1 mg	
	EE 35	NE 500	
	EE 35	NE 400	
	EE 35	LNG 150	
	EE 35	LNG 100	
	EE 30	DEG 150	Less androgenic effects
	EE 30	NG 300	Less androgenic effects
	EE 30	LNG 150	
	EE 20	LNG 100	Less nausea and bloating Increased breakthrough bleeding
Multiphasic			Reduced overall progestogen dose minimizes weight gain, fluid retention, dysmenorrhea
	EE 30, 40, 30	LNG 50, 75, 125	
	EE 35	NGM 180, 215, 250	Less androgenic effects
	EE 35	NE 50, 100, 50	
	EE 35	NE 0.5, 0.75, 1 mg	
	EE 35	NE 0.5, 1 mg	
Low dose COC			Minimizes headache, menorrhagia
	EE 20	NE 1 mg	
	EE 20, 0, 10	DEG 150	Less androgenic effects
Antiandrogenic	EE 50	CYP 2 mg	Reduces androgenic effects in polycystic ovary syndrome (not registered in US)

Fig. 15.47 Combined oral contraceptives (COCs). (EE, ethinyl estradiol; ME, mestranol; NE, norethindrone; NG, norgestrel; LNG, levonorgestrel; DEG, desogestrel; NGM, norgestimate. All doses in μg except where noted)

side effects, low-dose estrogen pills (20 μg EE), and combinations with antiandrogenic progestogens (cyproterone acetate) have been developed. Side effects of all COCs include breakthrough bleeding, nausea, migraine headache, breast discomfort, and increased risk of deep vein thrombosis. Early COC preparations containing >50 μg of ethinyl estradiol resulted in excessive cerebrovascular and cardiovascular morbidity. The currently recommended dose of 20–35 μg of ethinyl estradiol does not increase cardiovascular risk in the absence of other risks such as smoking, advanced age and diabetes.

ADVANTAGES OF COMBINED STEROID CONTRACEPTIVES result from suppression of the menstrual cycle and establishment of an endocrine condition similar to that of pregnancy or lactation and include:

- Highly effective contraception (i.e. 0.5 pregnancies/100 woman-years).
- A reduction in the incidence and/or severity of premenstrual tension, dysmenorrhea, and menstrual loss, and therefore a lower incidence of anemia.
- Improved acne (some preparations).
- Suppression of benign breast disease.
- Suppression of ovarian cysts.
- Reduced lifelong risk of ovarian cancer.
- Possible suppression of endometriosis.

> **Fertility and pregnancy in ex-pill and pill users**
>
> - The incidence of spontaneous abortion and abnormalities among ex-pill users is not increased, and there is a decreased incidence of stillbirths
> - Most women experience a rapid return to fertility on stopping 'the pill' and conception can occur after only a 1- or 2-day delay in starting a new packet

- Suppression of uterine fibroids.
- Reduced risk of pelvic inflammatory disease, possibly by thickening the cervical mucus so that bacteria cannot penetrate into the reproductive tract.

Disadvantages of combined steroid contraceptives

Figure 15.48 shows that the relative risk of taking steroid contraceptives compared with other everyday risks is small, and less than the risk of childbirth. Adverse effects are related to the following:

- Estrogen doses over 50 mg, especially in smokers, may be associated with an increased risk of cardiovascular disease. Most preparations now contain 35 mg or less. Estrogen is primarily the cause of thrombotic disorders since it affects clotting factors.

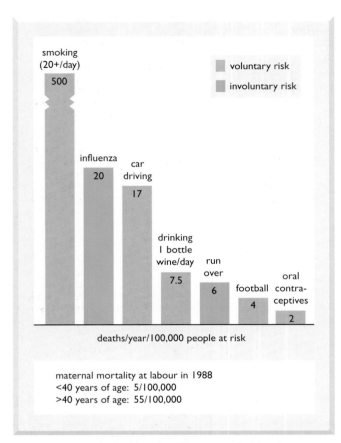

smoking (20+/day)
500

voluntary risk
involuntary risk

influenza
20

car driving
17

drinking 1 bottle wine/day
7.5

run over
6

football
4

oral contraceptives
2

deaths/year/100,000 people at risk

maternal mortality at labour in 1988
<40 years of age: 5/100,000
>40 years of age: 55/100,000

Fig. 15.48 The risk of taking the pill compared with other voluntary and involuntary risks.

- Oral contraceptives reduce the incidence of ovarian and endometrial cancer, but some data suggest an increased risk of breast cancer.
- Oral contraceptives impair glucose tolerance, especially in those predisposed to diabetes mellitus. Changes usually return to normal within 6 months of ceasing treatment. Those at risk are usually given the progestogen-only pill to avoid estrogen treatment.

Progestogen-only pill (minipill)

The progestogen-only pill (POP) is taken continuously and, since ovulation still takes place in many women, menstruation is normal, although its timing can be irregular. Contraceptive efficacy is primarily mediated by fertility-reducing effects on cervical mucus and endometrium. A higher dose of progestogen is used in the POP compared with COC, due to the lack of synergy with estrogen.

Depot progestogen preparations

These include depot medroxyprogesterone acetate i.m. (12-week cover), norethindrone given i.m. every 8 weeks, subdermal implants of ethinyl estradiol combined with a progestogen, or of progestogen alone. Levonorgestrel implants last for 5 years. The two main areas of action are cervical mucus, which is thickened and therefore prevents sperm penetration, and ovulation, which is suppressed in 50% of cycles.

The effects of these depot preparations are reversible and they provide extremely reliable contraception (as effective as sterilization) as a result of the stable blood levonorgestrel concentration. Such depot preparations can cause erratic menstrual bleeding, and a delayed return to fertility with some types. They can worsen depression and premenstrual tension/syndrome in vulnerable women, and increase appetite and weight.

The postcoital pill (emergency contraception)

High dose estrogen–progestogen combinations administered within 72 hours of insemination are approximately 75% effective in preventing pregnancy. A number of mechanisms contribute to the efficacy of this approach:
- If ovulation has not occurred, the LH surge may be diminished, resulting in an anovulatory cycle.
- Progesterone effects on the cervix and endometrium reduce sperm viability.
- Estrogen impairs passage of the ovum through the fallopian tube.

The usual postcoital contraceptive regimen includes four COC tablets (30–35 μg EE with at least 300 μg norgestrel or 125 μg levonorgestrel) taken twice within 72 hours of intercourse. Nausea is commonly encountered. Specifically labelled emergency contraceptive products containing four tablets of 50 μg of EE and 25 μg of levonorgestrel each, and two tablets of 75 μg of levonorgestrel only have also been registered for clinical use. Nausea and vomiting may be less with the progestogen-only regimen.

Hormone replacement therapy

Hormone replacement therapy (HRT) is used to treat symptoms of estrogen deficiency (hot flushes, urogenital atrophy) and maintain bone strength after menopause. Urogenital menopausal symptoms include vaginal dryness, dyspareunia (painful intercourse), recurrent urinary tract infections, urinary incontinence, and atrophy of the urethral mucosa. Vasomotor menopausal symptoms include hot flushes, sweats, and palpitations. These latter symptoms cease spontaneously after some time (months or years), but can recur. The mechanisms underlying menopausal vasomotor problems are not clearly understood. Estrogen deficiency also results in progressive loss of bone mineral mass and collagen over several years, leading to osteoporosis (characterized by a low bone mass and deterioration of the bone microarchitecture, associated with an increased susceptibility to fracture, see Chapter 20).

Drug treatment of menopausal symptoms

HORMONAL TREATMENTS Estrogen replacement therapy relieves symptoms and reduces the risk of osteoporosis and cardiovascular disease. Postmenopausal hormone replacement is usually with natural estrogens. These include special formulations of estradiol or conjugated estrogens extracted from either plant sources, or pregnant mare's urine (Premarin). Conjugated estrogen preparations contain multiple estrogenic substances including 17β-estradiol, estrone sulfate, and equilin (an estrogen not produced in the human). Tibolone, a synthetic steroid with estrogen and progestogenic effects, has been

> **Estrogen and progesterone replacement in the menopause**
>
> - Benefits are lower overall mortality rates, decreased risk of arteriosclerotic disease, prevention of osteoporosis, atrophic vaginitis, and neuropsychiatric effects
> - Risks are menstrual bleeding, venous thromboembolism, cholestatic disease, breast tenderness, fluid retention, migraine headaches, and a slightly increased risk of breast cancer

reported to ameliorate estrogen deficiency symptoms. Phytoestrogen-containing dietary supplements containing isoflavones from soybean, black cohosh or red clover also reduce climacteric (menopausal) symptoms.

When estrogen replacement is administered alone it:
- Induces endometrial hyperplasia, which may become neoplastic.
- Stimulates uterine fibroids to grow, which may lead to heavy irregular breakthrough bleeding.

As a result, estrogens are therefore usually given with a progestogen to inhibit endometrial growth. If progestogen is given over the last 10 days of a 28-day cycle, it induces a withdrawal breakthrough bleeding. If this is unacceptable, the two steroids can be given together continuously. Progestogen does not reduce the benefits due to estrogens. The steroids are usually given orally but can be applied as transdermal patches, gels or subcutaneous implants which can reduce the minor adverse effects (nausea, vomiting, migraine and weight gain). Androgens have beneficial effects on mood and libido in menopausal women, but are not effective in antagonizing estogenic effects in the uterus. Combination therapy with estrogen and testosterone is most appropriate for symptomatic women who have undergone hysterectomy.

NONHORMONAL TREATMENTS provide a second-line treatment for menopausal symptoms, but do not relieve urogenital symptoms, or prevent the increased cardiovascular risk. Clonidine (an α_2 adrenoceptor agonist) and veralipride (a dopamine antagonist) can prevent hot flushes. Propranolol (a β adrenoceptor antagonist) is useful for palpitations. The treatment of osteoporosis is discussed in Chapter 20.

Disorders of sex steroids in premenopausal women

The common disorders of the female reproductive tract are shown in Fig. 15.49.

Hypogonadism and infertility

Isolated gonadotropin deficiency is a congenital deficiency of gonadotropin-releasing hormone (GnRH) leading to hypogonadotropic hypogonadism, characterized by eunuchoid features, incomplete development of secondary sex characteristics, and absence of menarche (onset of menstrual cycles). Hypothalamic function is closely controlled by steroid feedback, but body composition and diet are also controlling influences. For instance, the onset of puberty (menarche) occurs at a critical

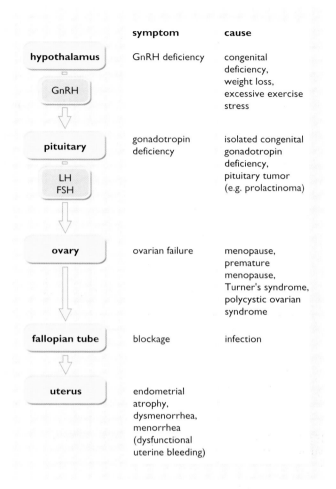

Fig. 15.49 Causes and symptoms of common reproductive disorders. (FSH, follicle-stimulating hormone; GnRH, gonadotropin-releasing hormone; LH, luteinizing hormone)

body weight, and a certain fat:lean ratio. More than a 20% loss in body weight, or strenuous physical exercise, specifically reduces fat and can cause both amenorrhea and oligomenorrhea (infrequent menstrual cycles). It is associated with low female steroid levels and anovulation (infertility). These changes may lead in turn to a diminished bone mass.

GONADOTROPIN THERAPY Exogenous gonadotropins are indicated for infertility secondary to congenital or acquired gonadotropin deficiency. Clomiphene is the first line of therapy (see below). If clomiphene fails to produce ovulation, preparations containing FSH and LH may be administered sequentially.

Gonadotropin preparations include:
- Human menopausal gonadotropin (HMG), extracted from postmenopausal urine, has equal FSH and LH bioactivity. HMG is a biologic extract that is difficult to standardize.
- Metrodin, a purified preparation, also from postmenopausal urine, contains 94% FSH and no LH activity.
- Recombinant FSH and LH are currently under clinical development.

321

- Human chorionic gonadotropin (HCG) is produced by the blastocyst in very early pregnancy and later by the syncytiotrophoblast of the placenta. Structurally it is similar to LH and acts on LH receptors. It therefore has similar biologic actions, but a much longer half-life (20 hours compared with 12 minutes).

To avoid multiple pregnancies, low doses of an FSH preparation are injected for 14 days and daily ultrasound is used to observe follicular growth. The dose is increased only if maturation fails. Alternatively, a high dose of FSH is given at the start of treatment followed by stepwise decrements to mimic the natural cyclic pattern of FSH secretion. Another regime is to obliterate all endogenous gonadotropin secretion by suppressing GnRH release with a GnRH analog. This allows for more precise monitoring of the gonadotropin dosage and timing, and it has been reported that this method reduces miscarriage rates.

GONADOTROPIN-RELEASING HORMONE (GnRH) AND ITS AGONIST ANALOGS GnRH is a decapeptide. Analogs are substituted at amino acids 6 and 10 to increase potency and the duration of action. Currently used preparations are gonadorelin (GnRH itself), buserelin, goserelin, and leuprorelin. Chronic administration of GnRH agonists can ultimately inhibit the release of pituitary gonadotropins after a period of the expected stimulation. The continuous high levels desensitize the GnRH receptors on the gonadotrophs, resulting in a hypogonadal hypopituitary state. Attempts have been made to use this effect for contraception by administering the analogs as a nasal spray. However, they can induce marked estrogenic deficiency, leading to menopausal symptoms.

▨ Administration of the recombinant GnRH decapeptide, gonadorelin, in a pulsatile manner, is used in patients with hypothalamic dysfunction

Administering exogenous GnRH in a similar manner stimulates endogenous gonadotropin release and preserves the feedback mechanisms that avoid the development of multiple pregnancies. GnRH is administered by intravenous or subcutaneous cannula according to a programmed regimen which can give good ovulation rates (i.e. >90%). If the patient is not interested in fertility, replacement therapy can be given with the COC pill, which will provide the steroids necessary for the maintenance of bone density and healthy vasculature. Potent agonist analogs of GnRH are used to induce desensitization and down-regulation of pituitary gondadotropin release in conditions of sex steroid excess (see below).

Ovarian disease

POLYCYSTIC OVARIAN SYNDROME Polycystic ovarian syndrome (PCOS) is one of the most common causes of infertility. It is associated with infertility, obesity, insulin resistance, and hirsutism and the following hormone profile:

- A high LH concentration (i.e. a low FSH:LH ratio).
- Chronically high estrogen and androgen levels.
- Low progesterone levels.

The unopposed estrogen increase the risk of endometrial carcinoma while the high levels of androgens can lead to hirsutism and acne. Treatment varies according to symptoms, and can involve:

- Prevention of amenorrhea or oligomenorrhea and unopposed estrogen effects.
- Induction of ovulation and fertility.
- Prevention and removal of the virilizing effects of the androgens.

Amenorrhea, oligomenorrhea, and dysfunctional uterine bleeding are treated with progestogens, which overcome the unopposed estrogen, while ovulation is induced with clomiphene or other antiestrogens (see below). If clomiphene fails to induce ovulation, gonadotropin preparations or pulsatile administration of GnRH analogs can be tried (see above).

▨ Clomiphene is used to treat infertility in patients with polycystic ovarian syndrome.

Clomiphene, an antiestrogen, antagonizes the normal negative feedback of endogenous estrogen on the hypothalamus and the pituitary resulting in increased FSH release, which induces follicular growth. Although the frequency of ovulation after clomiphene is 70%, the pregnancy rate is only 30%. Clomiphene has a long plasma elimination half-life, and may produce antiestrogenic effects on the uterus after successful stimulation of ovulation. It has not been used as an antiestrogen in breast cancer. Clomiphene is well tolerated. Adverse effects are seen only with higher doses or after prolonged treatment; they include ovarian enlargement and vasomotor symptoms (i.e. flushing and palpitations).

▨ Danazol and GnRH agonists modulate the gonadotropin axis

A variety of disorders in women respond to a reduction in estrogen action. These include breast and uterine neoplasms, endometriosis, dysfunctional uterine bleeding, and estrogen-responsive immunologic syndromes. Estrogen receptor antagonism is one therapeutic option, but modulators of pituitary FSH and LH secretion also reduce estrogen production (Fig. 15.50).

Danazol is a weak androgen that inhibits gonadotropin secretion resulting in a subsequent reduction in estrogen synthesis. More recently, leuprolide, nafarelin, and histrelin, which are GnRH agonists, have proven useful. These agents have greater potency for the GnRH receptor on the pituitary than the endogenous agonist GnRH. After a brief period of stimulation they desensitize the GnRH receptor and so reduce gonadotropin secretion. However, these agents require parenteral administration and lead to menopausal adverse effects such as vasomotor symptoms, bone loss, and genitourinary atrophy.

Androgen excess in women

Hirsutism and acne are common conditions in women, and only occasionally are related to androgen excess. Hirsutism is a common symptom of PCOS. Androgenic action on the

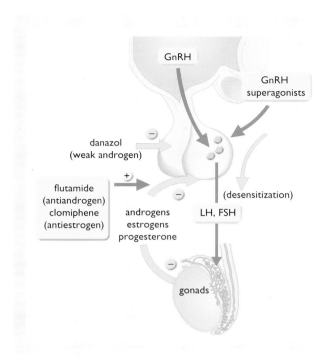

Fig. 15.50 Modulators of the gonadotropin axis. Several commonly used drugs act by altering the function of the hypothalamic–pituitary–gonadal axis. Agonists of the gonadotropin receptor (leuprolide, nafarelin, histrelin) produce desensitization of gonadotroph responses, leading to reduced concentrations of luteinizing hormone (LH) and follicle-stimulating hormone (FSH). The weak synthetic androgen, danazol, mimics the feedback inhibition of endogenous androgens and reduces gonadotropin secretion without marked peripheral androgenic adverse effects. Androgen and estrogen receptor antagonists interrupt feedback inhibition of gonadotropin secretion by sex steroids. The resultant rise in gonadotropins that occurs with the estrogen antagonist, clomiphene, promotes ovarian folliculogenesis in the treatment of infertility, whereas the reflex LH increase that occurs with the androgen receptor antagonist, flutamide, may stimulate testosterone synthesis and lead to failure of the antiandrogen effect. Flutamide may therefore be combined with a gonadotropin releasing hormone (GnRH) agonist in the treatment of prostatic cancer.

pilosebaceous unit (sebaceous gland and hair follicle) induce conversion of vellus to terminal hair and increasing growth rate. Removal of androgenic stimulation does not reverse the process but prevents further growth.

STEROIDAL ANTIANDROGENS include:

- Spironolactone, an aldosterone antagonist and potent antiandrogen, which has higher potency for androgen receptors than cyproterone. It also inhibits cytochrome P-450 mono-oxygenases and alters steroidogenesis, reducing testosterone synthesis and increasing its metabolism. Potassium retention requires periodic monitoring.
- Cyproterone, which also has progestogen actions which require periodic interruption of therapy to allow break-through menstrual bleeding. Alternatively, it can be given with ethinyl estradiol and so provide contraceptive protection. It is not registered in the US.

■ *Combined oral contraception is widely used in the treatment of PCOS-related androgen excess, when infertility is not an immediate issue.*

NONSTEROIDAL ANTIANDROGENS including flutamide and nilutamide, and the 5α-reductase inhibitor, finasteride, have shown no greater efficacy than the steroidal antiandrogens in the treatment of female androgen excess.

Small clinical trials using thiazolidenedione or biguanide (metformin) insulin-sensitizing agents have demonstrated reduction in androgen excess in PCOS. GnRH agonists reduce ovarian steroidogenesis, but are poorly tolerated due to menopausal symptoms.

Androgen excess and deficiency in men

The adrenals and the testes produce a variety of compounds capable of stimulating androgen receptors. Dihydrotestosterone and testosterone are the most potent, but androgenic precursors such as dehydroepiandrosterone and androstenedione also exert androgenic effects. 17-Carbon androgenic precursors from either the adrenals or the gonads can be converted to testosterone by 17-hydroxysteroid dehydrogenase in the testis or in the ovary. The enzyme 5α-reductase produces the more potent androgen dihydrotestosterone in tissues such as the prostate, skin, sebaceous glands and brain. Due to tissue-specific expression of 5α-reductase, androgenic effects on prostate growth and male pattern baldness are largely mediated by dihydrotestosterone. Testosterone, dihydrotestosterone and other androgens act via the androgen receptor, a DNA-linked ligand-activated transcription factor with homology to mineralocorticoid and progesterone steroid receptors.

■ *Androgens are important therapeutic factors in the treatment of disorders of puberty, prostatic disease, and hirsutism*

Androgen excess in prepubertal boys due to unregulated testicular testosterone production ('testotoxicosis') leads to premature puberty, short adult stature, and behavioral problems. Conversely, constitutional pubertal delay can be treated with short courses of androgen therapy that stimulate the HPG axis in adolescent boys. After puberty, androgen excess is clinically silent in men, but leads to androgenic responses ranging from hirsutism to virilization in women. Androgen deficiency in adult males is an important cause of male osteoporosis.

ANDROGEN REPLACEMENT Like the estrogens, testosterone has poor bioavailability owing to hepatic metabolism, and as a result synthetic analogs, transdermal delivery systems, and intramuscular formulations are used clinically (Fig. 15.51). Commonly used intramuscular testosterone preparations (testosterone enanthate, testosterone cypionate, testosterone propionate) use an oil-based vehicle to slow absorption from the site of injection. This leads to dosing intervals of 2–4 weeks, in contrast to the 3-day dosing interval with aqueous testosterone injections. Transdermal testosterone delivery systems or topical gels provide another mechanism of bypassing first-pass hepatic metabolism of exogenous testosterone.

323

Androgen agonists

	Indication and dose	Typical dose	Pharmacokinetics	Adverse effects
Testosterone	Male hypogonadism		Elimination half-life 0.3–1.5 hours Hepatic metabolism	Testosterone class effects: Erythrocytosis, priapism, HDL lowering
Transdermal		Truncal 4–6 mg q.d. Scrotal 5 mg q.d. Topical gel (1%) 5–10 g q.d.		Testosterone class effects
Intramuscular (enanthate, cypionate or propionate esters)		200–400 mg i.m. q. 2–4 weeks		Testosterone class effects
Nandrolone decanoate		Anemia of bone marrow failure (50–200 mg i.m. q. week)	Prolonged absorption, elimination half-life 4 hours, hepatic metabolism	Testosterone class effects
Oral synthetic androgens				
Methyltestosterone	Male hypogonadism Delayed puberty Cryptorchidism Breast cancer palliation Breast engorgement	10–50 mg q.d. p.o. 75 mg q.d. × 5 days for postpartum breast engorgement	45% Hepatic first-pass metabolism, $t_{1/2}$ = 0.2–2 hours 90% renally excreted as testosterone sulfates and glucuronides Extensive protein binding	Oral androgen class effects: fluid retention, erythrocytosis, priapism, acne, reduced HDL cholesterol, prostate hypertrophy, oligospermia, gynecomastia, peliosis hepatis, hepatic adenoma (rare)
Fluoxymesterone	Delayed puberty Breast cancer palliation	50–200 mg q.d. p.o.	$t_{1/2}$ = 9 hours	Class effects
Oxymetholone	Aplastic anemia	50–150 mg p.o. q.d.		Class effects
Oxandrolone	Delayed puberty Cachexia	5–10 mg q.d. – b.i.d. p.o.	$t_{1/2}$ = 5–13 hours Less hepatic first-pass metabolism 30% renal excretion High protein binding (95%)	Class effects
Stanozolol	Hereditary angioedema	2 mg q.d.–t.i.d. p.o.		Class effects

Fig. 15.51 Androgen agonists.

Testosterone replacement therapy is indicated for hypogonal men who demonstrate clinical (reduced shaving frequency, exercise endurance, libido and testicular size) and laboratory findings (reduced free or free plus albumin-bound testosterone concentrations). After appropriate evaluation for possible pituitary or testicular disease, initiation of testosterone replacement therapy improves physical performance, sexual function, mood, and lipid profiles within 4 weeks in most cases. In healthy men, the use of high-dose testosterone or synthetic androgens produces small increases in muscle mass and exercise performance, while posing the risks of aggressive mood disorder, priapism, erythrocytosis, oligospermia and worsened lipid profile. Adverse hepatic effects such as blood-filled hepatic cysts (peliosis hepatis), hepatic adenomas and cholestatic hepatic injury have been reported primarily with oral synthetic androgens. In elderly men, androgen supplementation increases serum concentrations of prostate-specific antigen and may worsen prostate hypertrophy.

The orally active androgens, methyltestosterone and fluoxymesterone, are not commonly used for androgen replacement, but are commonly abused by body builders. Other orally active androgenic steroids (testolactone, oxandrolone,

The effects of androgen therapy

Central nervous system	Gonadotropin suppression Behavioral effects
Body habitus	Hirsutism Virilization Acne Baldness Gynecomastia
Hematologic	Erythrocytosis
Metabolic	Dyslipidemia
Hepatic	Cholestatic jaundice Peliosis hepatis Hepatocellular carcinoma
Genitourinary	Priapism Prostatic hypertrophy Prostatic cancer

Fig. 15.52 The effects of androgen therapy.

Androgen replacement therapy

- Intramuscular preparations (testosterone enanthate, or cypionate) are inexpensive and can be given at 2–4-week intervals
- Transdermal testosterone delivery systems are effective, but more expensive
- Oral androgens are associated with a high risk of hepatic disease

stanozolol, oxymetholone) and intramuscular preparations (nandrolone) have androgenic effects and are used clinically for their anabolic actions in cancer and refractory anemia. Close monitoring for hepatic dysfunction is needed during oral androgen therapy, and for a variety of androgen-related adverse effects during all androgen therapies (Fig. 15.52).

ANTIANDROGENIC THERAPIES (Fig. 15.53) are used to treat prostatic disease in men:
- Nonsteroidal androgen antagonists (flutamide, nilutamide) are devoid of effects on other steroid receptors. Their use

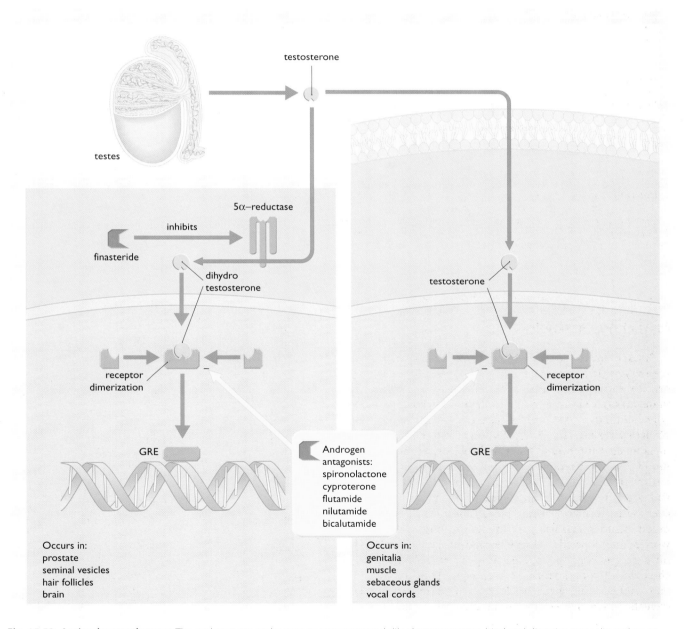

Fig. 15.53 Antiandrogen therapy. The endogenous androgens, testosterone and dihydrotestosterone, bind and dimerize cytosolic androgen receptors (AR), translocate to the nucleus and regulate gene transcription through the glucucorticoid response element (GRE). Dihydrotestosterone is produced from testosterone in selective target tissues that express the enzyme 5α-reductase. Androgen antagonists competitively inhibit androgen binding to the AR. The steroidal antiandrogen, spironolactone, may also inhibit testosterone synthesis. 5α-Reductase inhibitors selectively reduce dihydrotestosterone synthesis in target tissues such as the prostate gland.

325

leads to increased LH secretion and testosterone synthesis, which may result in therapeutic failure.

- A gonadotropin-suppressing progestagen, megestrol acetate, is used to lower androgen concentrations in metastatic prostate cancer, but has no direct androgen receptor antagonist activity. Orchidectomy is also used to lower endogenous androgens.
- Spironolactone, the mineralocorticosteroid antagonist, is also an androgen agonist and is a commonly used drug for female hirsutism, but has not proved efficacious in prostate cancer treatment.

In men, the observation that androgen effects such as prostatic growth and male pattern baldness depend on androgen receptor stimulation by dihydrotestosterone has led to the therapeutic use of the 5α-reductase inhibitor finasteride. Testosterone is converted to the more potent dihydrotestosterone by the enzyme 5α-reductase, which is expressed in the skin, liver, and genital tissues. Finasteride is mildly effective in improving the symptoms of prostatic hypertrophy, but less so than α adrenoceptor antagonists.

FURTHER READING

DeFronzo RA. Pharmacologic therapy for Type 2 diabetes mellitus. *Ann Int Med* 1999; **131**: 281–303. [Comprehensive review of oral agents including guidelines for multi-drug therapy and clinical decision making.]

Ginsberg J (ed.) *Drug Therapy in Reproductive Endocrinology*. London: Arnold, and New York: Oxford University Press; 1996. [Up-to-date and comprehensive series of reviews.]

Klibanski A, Zervas NT. Diagnosis and management of hormone-secreting pituitary adenomas. *N Engl J Med* 1991; **324**: 822–831. [A review of diagnostic and treatment issues in acromegaly, hyperprolactinemia, Cushing's disease, and other pituitary tumors.]

Oppenheimer JH, Braverman LE, Toft A, Jackson IM, Ladenson PW. A therapeutic controversy. Thyroid hormone treatment: when and what. *J Clin Endocrinol Metab* 1995; **80**: 2873–2883. [A discussion of clinical controversies in thyroid hormone therapy for treatment of hypothyroidism and thyroid cancer.]

Pollard I. *A Guide to Reproduction*. Cambridge: Cambridge University Press; 1994. [Provides details of the physiology and endocrinology of the female reproductive system.]

Strobl JS, Thomas MJ. Human growth hormone. *Pharmacol Rev* 1994; **46**: 1–34. [A thorough review of the pharmacology and clinical use of growth hormone in the treatment of short stature.]

Summary of the second report of the National Cholesterol Education Program (NCEP) expert panel on detection, evaluation, and treatment of high blood cholesterol in adults. *JAMA* 1993; **269**: 3015–3023. [Current recommendations from an expert panel on the evaluation of arteriosclerotic risk factors and the integration of pharmacologic and nonpharmacologic approaches to hyperlipidemia.]

Tyrrell JB. Glucocorticoid therapy. In: *Endocrinology and Metabolism*, 3rd edn. New York: McGraw-Hill; 1995. [A thorough review of pharmacologic issues in the use of glucocorticosteroids.]

Zinman B. The physiologic replacement of insulin. An elusive goal. *N Engl J Med* 1989; **321**: 363–370. [A detailed review of therapeutic issues in the treatment of diabetes mellitus with insulin.]

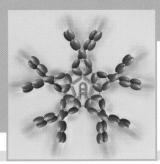

Chapter 16

Drugs and the Inflammatory and Immune Response

PHYSIOLOGY OF THE IMMUNE SYSTEM AND INFLAMMATORY RESPONSE

The immune system and the inflammatory response are involved in the defense against invading organisms. However, inappropriate activation of these systems results in a wide range of inflammatory disorders. Inflammation is characterized by a number of features:

1. Vasodilation leading to redness
2. Increased vascular permeability leading to swelling of tissues
3. Recruitment of leukocytes into tissues
4. If 1–3 occur chronically, this can lead to alterations in tissue function.

A key feature of the immune response is the ability of lymphocytes to recognize foreign proteins (antigens) which can be surface proteins on pathogens or, in some people, otherwise innocuous proteins (such as grass pollen or animal dander) which are responsible for inducing allergic responses (see below). Lymphocytes are derived from bone marrow stem cells. T lymphocytes then develop in the thymus, while B lymphocytes develop in the bone marrow (Fig. 16.1).

T cells have T-cell antigen receptors (TCRs) on their cell surfaces

T cells specifically recognize antigens in association with the major histocompatibility complexes (MHC) (HLA antigens) on antigen-presenting cells (APCs) such as macrophages and dendritic cells. When T cells are activated by an antigen through a TCR (Fig. 16.2) they produce soluble proteins, called cytokines, which signal to T cells, B cells, monocytes/macrophages, and other cells (Fig. 16.3).

T cells are classified into two subsets:

- CD4-positive (CD4+) T cells, which interact with B cells and help them to proliferate, differentiate, and produce antibody. They are therefore called helper T (T_H) cells. T_H cells can be subdivided further into T_{H_1} and T_{H_2}, based on the profile of cytokines which they release (Fig. 16.4).
- CD8-positive (CD8+) T cells, which destroy host cells that have become infected by viruses or other intracellular pathogens. This kind of action is called cytotoxicity and these T cells are therefore called cytotoxic T (T_C) cells.

B cells use surface immunoglobulins as their antigen receptors

B cells specifically recognize a particular antigen and when stimulated by an interaction between surface immunoglobulin and specific antigen, they proliferate and differentiate into plasma cells, which produce large amounts of the receptor immunoglobulin in a soluble form. This is known as an

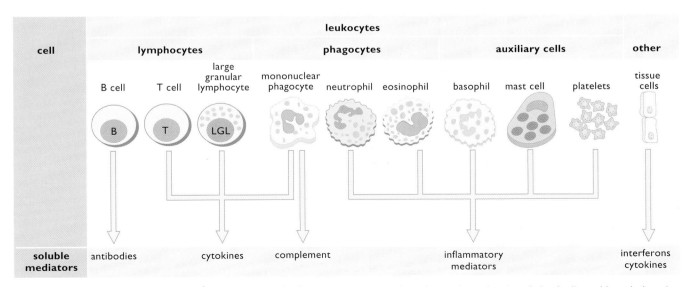

Fig. 16.1 **The principal components of the immune and inflammatory system.** Complement is made primarily by the liver, although there is some synthesis by mononuclear phagocytes. Each cell produces and secretes only a particular set of cytokines or inflammatory mediators.

327

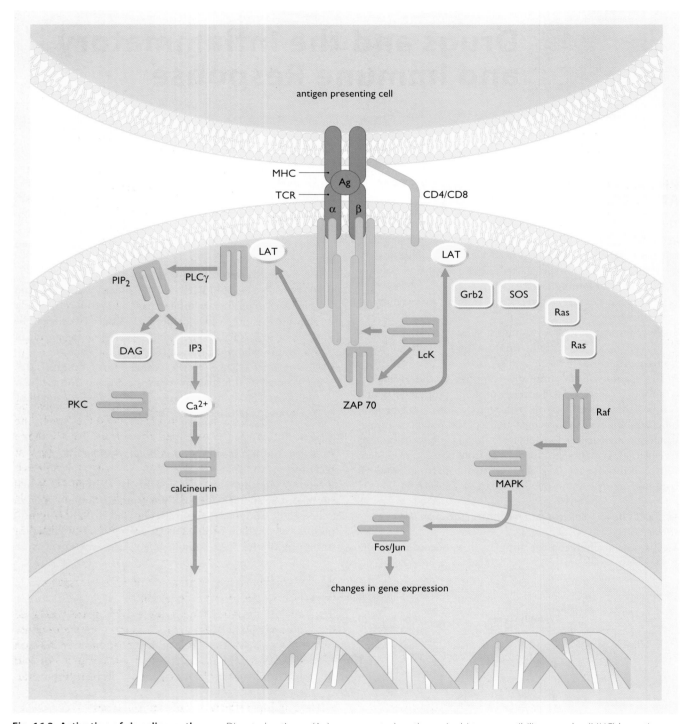

Fig. 16.2 Activation of signaling pathways. Digested antigens (Ag) are presented on the major histocompatibility complex (MHC) by antigen-presenting cells (APCs). Once these presented antigens are recognized by the T-cell receptor (TCR) complex, tyrosine kinases such as LCK and ZAP70 are activated and in turn activate sequential molecules such as the ras-MAPK pathway. At the same time, PLCγ triggers activation of the PKC and Ca–calcineurin pathways. These signals are finally transmitted into the nucleus, and generate synthesis of proteins such as cytokines.

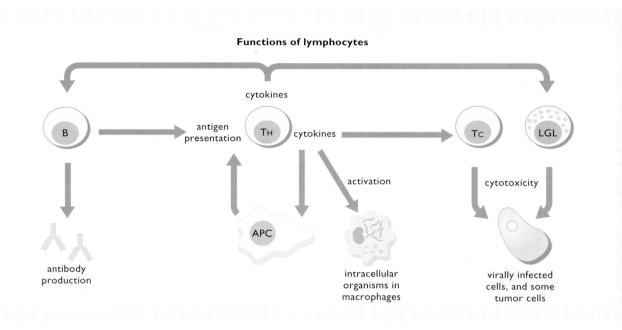

Functions of lymphocytes

cytokines

B — antigen presentation — TH — cytokines — Tc   LGL

activation

cytotoxicity

APC

antibody production

intracellular organisms in macrophages

virally infected cells, and some tumor cells

Fig. 16.3 Functions of B cells and T cells. B cells produce antibodies, while T-helper (TH) cells are stimulated by antigen-presenting cells (APCs) and B cells to produce cytokines, which control immune responses. Macrophages are activated to kill intracellular micro-organisms. Cytotoxic T (Tc) cells and large granular lymphocytes (LGL) recognize and kill target host cells.

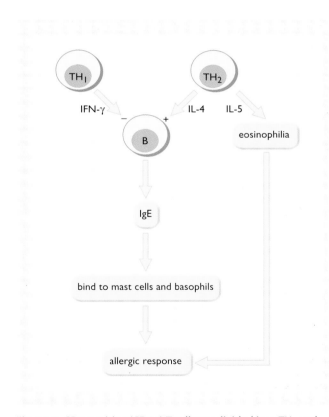

Fig. 16.4 CD4-positive (CD4+) T cells are divided into TH₁ and TH₂ based on the profile of cytokines they release. TH₁ cells release IFN-γ which can inhibit the ability of B cells to make immunoglobulin E, the antibody that is central to the induction of allergic responses. Meanwhile TH₂ lymphocytes release both interleukin-4, which is a necessary co-factor for the induction of IgE synthesis by B cells, and interleukin-5 (IL-5), which is a powerful chemoattractant for eosinophils that characterize the allergic responses.

antibody, which is present in the blood and tissue fluids and can bind to the antigen that initially activated the B cells. The presence of antibodies activates other parts of the immune system, which then eliminate the pathogen carrying that antigen. TH₁ cells normally direct B cells to make IgG. However, when TH₂ cells make IL-4, this signals B cells to make IgE, the antibody thought to be important in allergic conditions. People with atopy have an inherited disposition to develop IgE to inhaled and/or ingested allergens that are not usually allergenic in non-atopic subjects.

Cytokines are a large group of molecules that signal between cells during immune responses

A variety of cytokines and growth factors are produced by various cell populations involved in the immune response (Fig. 16.5) and have a vital role in the initiation and regulation of these immune responses. All are proteins or peptides, and some contain sugar molecules (glycopeptides). In general, cytokines:

- Have multiple effects on different cell types.
- Often share similar or synergistic effects.
- Presumably act in the immune response as an array of molecular messages that orchestrate the interplay and control of individual component cells.

INTERLEUKINS are a large group of cytokines (IL-1 to IL-18) produced mainly by T cells, but some are also produced by macrophages and other cells. Those produced by lymphocytes (T cells) are also called lymphokines. They have a variety of functions but most are involved in directing other cells to divide and differentiate. Each interleukin acts on a specific

329

Cytokine effects in the immune response

Cytokines	Cell sources	Target cells and functions
IL-1	Macrophages	T and B cell activation
IL-2	T cells	T cell activation and proliferation
IL-3	T cells	Stem cell proliferation and differentiation
IL-4	T cells	B cell differentiation and IgE class switch TH_2 cell differentiation
IL-5	T cells	Eosinophil differentiation and activation
IL-6	T cells	B cell differentiation
IL-7	Stromal cells	B cell proliferation and differentiation
IL-8	Macrophages	Neutrophil chemotaxis
IL-10	T cells	Inhibition of TH_1 cells
IL-12	Macrophages	TH_1 cell differentiation
GM-CSF	T cells	Eosinophil activation
IFN-γ	T cells, NK cells	Inhibition of TH_2 cells, macrophage activation MHC class I and II induction
IFN-α	Macrophages	NK cell activation, MHC class I induction
TNF-α	Macrophages	Activation of macrophages, granulocytes, and TC cells

Fig. 16.5 Cytokine effects in the immune response. (GM-CSF, granulocyte–monocyte colony-stimulating factor; IFN, interferon; IL, interleukin; MHC, major histocompatibility complex; NK cells, natural killer cells; Tc cells, cytotoxic T cells; TH cells, helper-T cells; TNF, tumor necrosis factor)

limited group of cells, which express the specific receptors for the corresponding interleukin. For instance, IL-2 is a key cytokine for inducing T-cell proliferation and activation to initiate immune responses. IL-4 stimulates B cells to produce IgE, and IL-5 specifically activates eosinophils.

INTERFERONS (IFNs) are produced early in viral infections and are particularly important in limiting their spread. IFN-α and IFN-β are produced by virally infected macrophages; IFN-γ is produced by certain activated T cells. They induce their antiviral effects by MHC class I and class II induction, macrophage activation, natural killer (NK) cell activation, and activation of CD8+ and some CD4+ T cells (TH_1 cells) which are involved in cell-mediated immunity.

COLONY-STIMULATING FACTORS (CSFs) are involved in directing the division and differentiation of the bone marrow stem cells and the precursors of the blood leukocytes. Some CSFs also activate mature leukocytes.

Other cytokines include tumor necrosis factors (TNF-α and TNF-β) and transforming growth factor-β (TGF-β), which have a variety of functions, but are particularly important in mediating inflammation and cytotoxic reactions.

Neutralizing antibodies for cytokines and soluble forms of cytokine receptors block the binding of cytokine to the receptor and prevent cytokine-mediated cellular responses. Anti-TNF-α antibody and a soluble TNF-α receptor protein have been introduced into therapy for rheumatoid arthritis to inhibit the effects of TNF-α, and are quite effective in reducing inflammation of joints. Such anticytokine therapeutic trials are now in progress for a variety of immunologic and inflammatory diseases.

PATHOPHYSIOLOGY AND DISEASES OF THE IMMUNE SYSTEM

Hypersensitivity reactions and immunologic diseases

Hypersensitivity reactions

Hypersensitivity reactions are pathologic processes resulting from specific interactions between antigens (exogenous or endogenous) and either humoral antibodies or sensitized lymphocytes. They are classified into four types according to their pathogenetic mechanisms.

TYPE I (ANAPHYLACTIC OR IMMEDIATE) reactions result from the binding of antigens (allergens) to specific IgE antibodies bound to high-affinity IgE receptors (FcεRI) on the cell surface of tissue mast cells and blood basophils, and the subsequent release of potent vasoactive and inflammatory mediators such as histamine, prostaglandins and leukotrienes (Fig. 16.6). These mediators then produce vasodilation, increased vascular permeability, smooth muscle contraction, mucosal edema, glandular hypersecretion, and tissue infiltration with eosinophils and other inflammatory cells. Examples of allergic diseases are

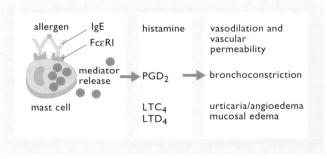

Fig. 16.6 Mechanism of type I hypersensitivity reaction. The binding of allergens to specific IgE antibodies bound to the cell surface IgE receptors (FcεRI) induces degranulation and release of mediators such as histamine and leukotrienes (LT) from mast cells and basophils. (PG, prostaglandin)

rhinitis (hay fever), bronchial asthma (see Chapter 19), atopic dermatitis (see Chapter 23), conjunctivitis (see Chapter 24) and systemic anaphylaxis.

TYPE II (CYTOTOXIC) reactions occur when antibody reacts with antigenic components of a cell or tissue. This leads to cell lysis or tissue damage as a result of antibody-dependent cell-mediated cytotoxicity (ADCC) by NK cells and macrophages through Fc receptors or by activation of the full complement system (Fig. 16.7). Such reactions often form the basis of adverse reactions to drugs, particularly when the drug binds to red blood cells. Ingestion of the offending drug leads to a type II cytotoxic reaction on the surface of red blood cells, leading to lysis of red blood cells and hemolytic anemia.

TYPE III (IMMUNE COMPLEX-MEDIATED) reactions result from deposition of soluble antigen–antibody complexes in vessels or other tissues. The immune complexes activate complement components and thereby initiate a sequence of events that results in polymorphonuclear leukocyte chemotaxis, tissue injury, and vasculitis (Fig. 16.8).

TYPE IV (CELL-MEDIATED OR DELAYED) reactions are mediated by sensitized CD4+ T cells following contact with antigen. Circulating antibodies are not involved and are not needed to produce tissue injury. The activation of sensitized CD4+ T cells

results in their proliferation and the release of cytokines, which activate macrophages, granulocytes, and NK cells (see Fig. 16.5). Type III and IV hypersensitivity reactions are involved in hypersensitivity pneumonitis, allergic bronchopulmonary aspergillosis, and eosinophilic pneumonias (discussed in Chapter 19).

Drug therapy for allergic diseases
H₁ receptor antagonists

Histamine is released from the granules of mast cells activated by cross-linking of two IgE molecules by specific allergen. Histamine is an important mediator of allergic responses in the skin, eye and nose. Histamine causes vasodilation, increased vascular permeability (edema) and smooth muscle contraction (bronchial and gastrointestinal) via activation of H_1 receptors. A number of different chemical classes of H_1 receptor antagonists have been described (Fig. 16.9) which are widely used in the symptomatic treatment of allergic diseases.

All the H_1 receptor antagonists are orally active and many of them cross the blood–brain barrier leading to sedation. However, some of the newer derivatives do not as readily cross the blood–brain barrier and are therefore now used as drugs of choice as they induce less sedation. Nonetheless, even these drugs may interfere with complex motor tasks in some individuals. These new derivatives have longer duration of action and have lesser anticholinergic effects, such as dry

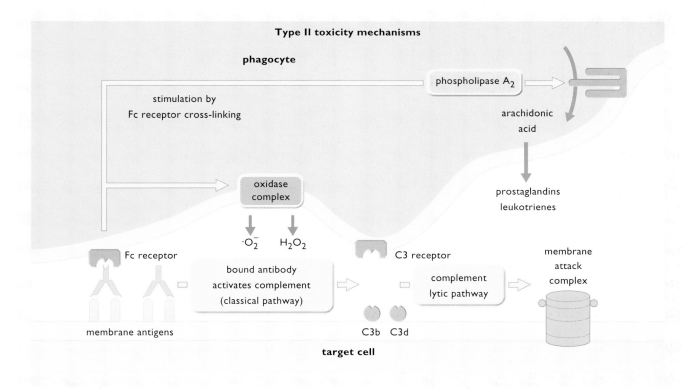

Fig. 16.7 Mechanism of type II hypersensitivity reaction. Antibody bound to membrane antigens on target cells opsonizes them for phagocytes. Cross-linking of the Fc receptors on the phagocyte activates a membrane oxidase complex to secrete oxygen radicals and increases arachidonic acid release from membrane phospholipids (effected by phospholipase A₂). Immune complexes induce complement C3b deposition, and this can also interact with receptors on phagocytes. Activation of the lytic pathway results in the assembly of the membrane attack complex by components C5–C9 of the complement cascade.

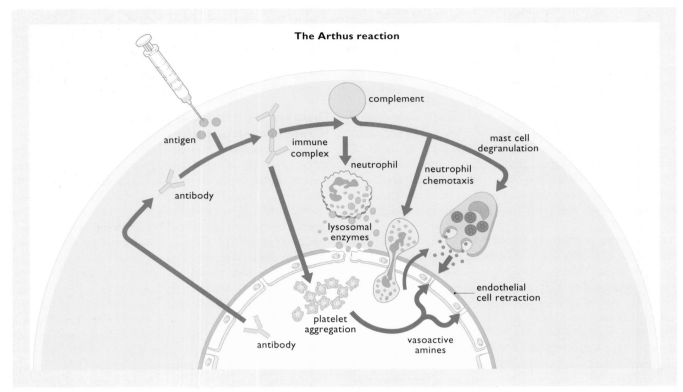

The Arthus reaction

antigen

antibody

immune complex

complement

neutrophil

lysosomal enzymes

mast cell degranulation

neutrophil chemotaxis

endothelial cell retraction

platelet aggregation

vasoactive amines

antibody

Fig. 16.8 Mechanism of type III hypersensitivity reactions. Antigen injected intradermally combines with specific antibody from the blood to form immune complexes. The complexes activate complement and act on platelets, which release vasoactive amines. Immune complexes also induce macrophages to release tumor necrosis factor (TNF) and interleukin-1 (IL-1) (not shown). Complement C3a and C5a fragments cause mast cell degranulation and attract neutrophils into the tissue. Mast cell products, including histamine and leukotrienes, increase blood flow and capillary permeability. The inflammatory reaction is potentiated by lysosomal enzymes released from the polymorphs. Furthermore, C3b deposited on the complexes opsonizes them for phagocytosis. The Arthus reaction can be seen in patients with precipitating antibodies (e.g. those with extrinsic allergic alveolitis associated with farmer's lung disease).

mouth, tachycardia, dilated pupils, and urinary retention, compared with classical H_1 receptor antagonists. However, some of these drugs cause dangerous arrhythmias such as prolongation of the QT interval and *torsade de pointes*, especially in combination with macrolide antibiotics, ketoconazole, and itraconazole.

Cysteinyl-leukotriene receptor antagonists and 5-lipoxygenase inhibitors

Cysteinyl-leukotrienes (LTC_4 and LTD_4) are synthesized *de novo* by a number of inflammatory cells from arachidonic acid released from membrane phospholipids (see Fig. 16.10). Cysteinyl-leukotrienes mimic many of the inflammatory responses induced by histamine, but are often more potent. In humans, the potency of LTC_4 and LTD_4 is 3000 times that of histamine in terms of producing airway smooth muscle contraction. Montelukast, zafirlukast and pranlukast are examples of orally active leukotriene receptor antagonists. The synthesis of leukotrienes involves the enzyme 5-lipoxygenase (see Fig. 16.10) and this can be inhibited by the orally active drug zileuton, which can also be used to treat allergic diseases such as rhinitis and asthma (see Chapter 19).

Anti-allergy drugs

Cromolyn sodium and nedocromil sodium are active topically and are delivered by use of inhalers. Only 1% of orally administered cromolyn is absorbed from the gastrointestinal tract and the maximum plasma concentration appears within 15 minutes. These drugs are used prophylactically to prevent allergic responses. The mechanism of action responsible for this prophylactic activity is not fully understood, but all are known to 'stabilize' mast cells, preventing the release of histamine and other inflammatory mediators, although it is clear that this is not the only activity of these drugs. They are capable of affecting many inflammatory cell types including macrophages and preventing the recruitment of inflammatory cells into tissues. Side effects of cromolyn and nedocromil are rare and mild, including bronchospasm, cough, and pharyngeal edema. In addition, ketotifen is an orally active anti-allergic drug which also has pronounced H_1 receptor antagonism. This drug has a duration of action of 12 hours, possessing anticholinergic effects, as well as sedation.

Epinephrine

Epinephrine is a potent α and β adrenoceptor agonist (see Chapter 14) which can functionally antagonize the effects of inflammatory mediators on smooth muscle, blood vessels and other tissues. In addition, epinephrine inhibits the antigen-induced release of inflammatory mediators from mast cells via the activation of β_2 receptors. Epinephrine is part of the treatment of anaphylaxis and anaphylactoid reactions (see below).

H_1 receptor antagonists

Class	Drugs	Duration of action (hours)	Side-effects
Ethylenediamines	Pyrilamine	4–6	Gastrointestinal symptoms and weak CNS effects
	Tripelennamine	4–6	
Ethanolamines	Diphenhydramine	4–6	Strong anticholinergic and sedative effects
	Dimenhydrinate	4–6	
	Clemastine	12–24	
Alkylamines	Chlorpheniramine	4–6	Relatively weak sedative effects and CNS excitement
	Dexchlorpheniramine	4–6	
	Triprolidine	4–6	
Piperazines	Meclizine	12–24	Weak sedative effects
	Cyclizine	4–6	
	Hydroxyzine	6–24	
Phenothiazines	Promethazine	4–6	Anticholinergic effects
	Trimeprazine	4–6	
New derivatives	Cyproheptadine	6–8	† QT prolongation and *torsade de pointes*
	Terfenadine*†	12–24	
	Astemizole*†	24	
	Loratadine*	24	
	Cetirizine*	12–24	

*Crosses the blood–brain barrier relatively less readily, and therefore induces less sedation. †Causes dangerous arrhythmias, especially in combination with macrolide antibiotics, ketoconazole and itraconazole.

Fig. 16.9 H_1 receptor antagonists.

Glucocorticoids

Glucocortocoids are used widely to treat allergic diseases, as they inhibit inflammatory cell infiltration and reduce edema formation by acting on the vascular endothelium. The mechanism of action of glucocorticoids as anti-inflammatory drugs is complex:

- They induce synthesis of the polypeptide lipocortin-1, which inhibits phospholipase A_2, a key enzyme in the production of inflammatory mediators, including prostaglandins, leukotrienes and platelet-activating factor (PAF) (Fig. 16.10).
- They interact with 'glucorticosteroid response elements' in inflammatory cells, which are believed to neutralize the transcription factors for the synthesis of cytokines such as interleukin (IL)-5 and tumor necrosis factor (TNF)-α (Fig. 16.11).
- They are unique in having the ability to resolve established inflammatory responses in the airways, though the mechanism responsible for this is not clear.

These drugs can be used topically in the treatment of allergic rhinitis, allergic asthma, and atopic skin diseases (see Chapters 19, 23 and 24, respectively), and can also be used orally and intravenously. However, oral glucocorticosteroids have systemic adverse effects and can cause suppression of the hypothalamic–pituitary axis. Chronic use can lead to a variety of serious adverse effects, including stunting of growth in children (see Chapter 15).

Anaphylaxis

Anaphylaxis is a systemic, life-threatening, IgE-mediated type I hypersensitivity reaction that occurs in a previously sensitized person exposed to the sensitizing antigen. It occurs when the antigen reaches the circulation, and the most common causative antigens are foreign serum, parenteral hormones and enzymes, blood products, penicillin, cephalosporins, allergen extracts and insect stings. Histamine, leukotrienes and other mediators released from IgE-activated mast cells and basophils induce the features of anaphylaxis: smooth muscle contraction (bronchial and gastrointestinal), vasodilation and increased vascular permeability (Fig. 16.6).

Anaphylaxis is associated with airway obstruction associated with laryngeal edema and bronchospasm which leads to asphyxia and hypoxia. Vasodilation and plasma extravasation into tissues causes hypovolemic shock with marked hypotension, urticaria and angioedema. The latter features are thought to be caused by histamine acting on H_1 receptors. The vascular collapse is also thought to be caused mainly by histamine acting on H_1 receptors on blood vessels although H_2 receptors, for example in veins, may also play a role. Airways obstruction may be mainly caused by leukotrienes. Typically, within 1–15 minutes after exposure to the antigen, the patient feels uneasy and complains of nausea, abdominal distress, palpitation, pruritis, urticaria, and difficulty in breathing due to laryngeal edema and bronchospasm. The manifestations of shock may develop within another

333

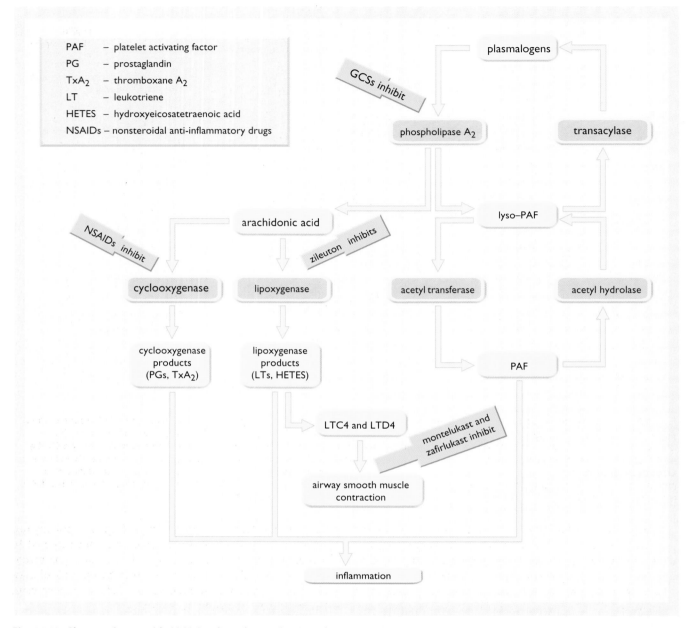

PAF   – platelet activating factor
PG   – prostaglandin
TxA$_2$ – thromboxane A$_2$
LT   – leukotriene
HETES – hydroxyeicosatetraenoic acid
NSAIDs – nonsteroidal anti-inflammatory drugs

Fig. 16.10 Glucocorticosteroids (GCSs) reduce the production of a variety of lipid inflammatory mediators.

1–2 minutes and primary cardiovascular collapse can occur with respiratory systems.

The primary treatment of anaphylaxis is epinephrine, and the earlier it is administered, the more likely is the achievement of a therapeutic response. Additionally, use of H$_1$ histamine receptor antagonists (possibly in combination with H$_2$ receptor antagonists) and a glucocorticosteroid may be of benefit.

Early recognition of an anaphylactic reaction is essential, as death may occur minutes to hours after the first symptoms. Epinephrine, the initial drug of choice should be given immediately. It is likely that a intramuscular injection is appropriate in all but the more mild reactions where a subcutaneous injection of epinephrine may be adequate. In hypotensive patients with anaphylaxis, subcutaneous injections may lead to erratic and delayed drug absorption due to changes in blood flow to the skin. Absorption from muscle is generally more reliable. However, on occasion, it may be necessary to administer epinephrine intravenously (very cautiously with a dilute solution of drug) in severely ill patients; however, this route of administration is more likely to cause adverse effects such as cardiac arrhythmias. An intravenous infusion of fluids is needed to maintain intravascular volume and allow additional medication.

When the above measures have been instituted, an H$_1$ histamine receptor antagonist should be given intravenously to forestall laryngeal edema and block the effect of further histamine release. The additional use of an H$_2$ histamine receptor antagonist may provide additional benefit.

334

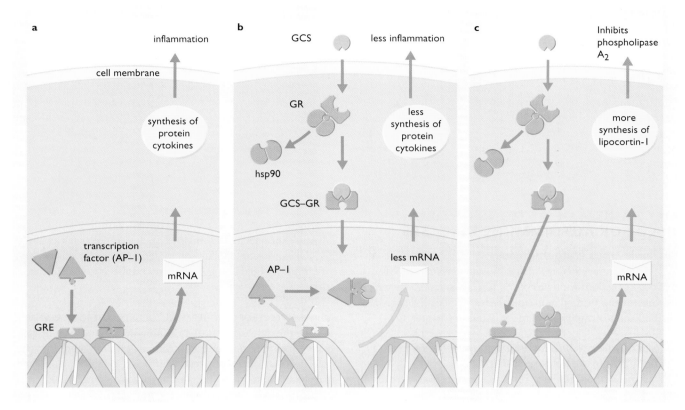

Fig. 16.11 Effect of glucocorticosteroids on gene transcription. (a) Transcription factors (e.g. AP-1) bind to receptors on DNA to bring about mRNA synthesis. This then leads to the synthesis of new proteins (e.g. cytokines) which are released by the cell to cause inflammation. (b) Glucocorticosteroids (GCSs) bind to cytosolic glucocorticosteroid receptors (GR), which are normally associated with two molecules of a 90-kDa heat shock protein (hsp90). The GCS–GR complex translocates to the nucleus and binds to glucocorticosteroid response elements (GRE) in the promoter sequences of target genes. (c) This leads to increased transcription of new proteins (e.g. lipocortin-1), or decreased transcription of proteins via binding to transcription factors (e.g. AP-1), resulting in reduced synthesis of inflammatory products (i.e. cytokines, neurokinin 1 (NK1) receptors, inducible nitric oxide synthase (NOS), cyclo-oxgenase-2, endothelin-1, phospholipase A_2 (PLA_2)).

Glucocorticosteroids (40 mg methylprednisolone or equivalent) have no effect on the acute event, but should be given intravenously to suppress slow-onset urticaria, angioedema, bronchospasm, laryngeal edema, or hypotension.

Inhalation therapy with a β_2 agonist, or other measures may be indicated for bronchospasm that does not respond to the epinephrine.

ANAPHYLACTOID REACTIONS are clinically similar to anaphylaxis, but the mechanism is quite different. They occur after

> **Causes of anaphylaxis and anaphylactoid reactions**
>
> - Anaphylaxis is an IgE-mediated hypersensitivity that occurs in a previously sensitized person; penicillins, cephalosporins, many other drugs, and insect stings are the most common causes
> - Anaphylactoid reactions are due to a dose-related pharmacologically induced mediator release; aspirin, other nonsteroidal anti-inflammatory drugs, and radiographic contrast media are the most common causes

the first injection of certain drugs (aspirin, polymyxin, pentamidine, opioids, and radiographic contrast agents) in susceptible patients, and are due to a dose-related, pharmacologically induced mediator release from basophils and mast cells rather than an immunologically mediated mechanism. Treatment is as for anaphylactic reactions.

Allergic rhinitis

Allergic rhinitis is an IgE-mediated disorder and results from the deposition of airborne allergens (e.g. pollens, molds, animal danders, and house dust mite feces) on the nasal mucosa. The mechanisms and treatment of allergic rhinitis are discussed in detail in Chapter 19.

Urticaria

Urticaria and angioedema are essentially anaphylaxis limited to the skin and are characterized by wheals and erythema in the dermis and a diffuse swelling of subcutaneous tissues, respectively. Causes of urticaria include drug allergy, insect stings or bites, injections of allergen extracts, or ingestion of certain foods (particularly eggs, shellfish, nuts, or fruits).

ACUTE URTICARIA is a self-limiting condition that generally subsides within one to a few days. The symptoms are usually relieved with oral H$_1$ antagonists (e.g. doxepin, diphenhydramine, chlorpheniramine, or terfenadine). Parenteral administration of an H$_1$ antagonist (e.g. diphenhydramine) and/or a glucocorticosteroid (e.g. prednisone) may be necessary for more severe reactions, particularly when associated with angioedema. Topical glucocorticosteroids are of no value. Epinephrine is the first treatment to use for acute pharyngeal or laryngeal angioedema.

Hypersensitivity pneumonitis and allergic bronchopulmonary aspergilosis are examples of types III and IV hypersensitivity reactions. The pathogenesis and treatment of these conditions is discussed in detail in Chapter 19.

MECHANISM OF ACTIONS OF DRUGS USED FOR AUTOIMMUNE DISEASES

Systemic lupus erythematosus

Systemic lupus erythematosus (SLE) is an autoimmune disease that occurs predominantly in young women and is characterized by the production of autoantibodies, especially anti-DNA antibodies. It is discussed in more detail in Chapter 17.

■ *Glucocorticosteroids have a profound inhibitory effect on many cells in the immune system*

The immunosuppressive effects of glucocorticosteroids in relation to the treatment of autoimmune diseases such as SLE are summarized in Fig. 16.12. They suppress the proliferative responses of T cells to antigens and mitogens by inhibiting the synthesis of IL-2; *in vivo*, delayed-type hypersensitivity reactions with antigens are suppressed after 2 weeks of glucocorticosteroid therapy. Glucocorticosteroids also suppress the early stages of B-cell activation and proliferation but, once activation and proliferation have occurred, B cells are resistant to glucocorticosteroid-mediated suppression of immunoglobulin (antibody) production. After several weeks of glucocorticosteroid therapy, the serum levels of IgG and IgA, and to a lesser degree IgM, are lowered, probably as a result of decreased production.

Glucocorticosteroids also modulate monocyte activity. They reduce the production of monocyte-derived cytokines such as IL-1, markedly inhibit the expression of Fc and C3 receptors and monocyte chemotaxis *in vitro* and *in vivo*, and suppress the bactericidal capacity of monocytes.

Glucocorticosteroids also diminish pathophysiologically adverse endothelial cell functions, such as vascular permeability and the expression of adhesion molecules, which probably have an inhibitory effect on leukocyte migration into inflammatory sites.

ADVERSE EFFECTS OF LONG-TERM GLUCOCORTICOSTEROID TREATMENT include the development of a Cushingoid habitus, weight gain, hypertension, opportunistic infections, capillary fragility, acne, osteoporosis, ischemic necrosis of bone, cataracts, glaucoma, diabetes mellitus, hyperlipidemia, myopathy, ulcers, hypokalemia, irregular menses, irritability, insomnia, and psychosis.

■ *Cytotoxic drugs such as cyclophosphamide are used in combination with glucocorticosteroids in the treatment of SLE*

Cyclophosphamide, a derivative of nitrogen mustards, acts as a cytotoxic agent by alkylating DNA and thereby interfering with DNA synthesis and cell division. Cyclophosphamide is activated by the cytochrome P-450 system of the liver, and the active nucleophilic metabolites bind to DNA, interfering with the DNA replication. It is active during all phases of the cell cycle including the resting (G0) stage, but is most active during the S phase of DNA synthesis. Cyclophosphamide is thus used for the chemotherapy of leukemias, lymphomas, and other neoplasms.

Cyclophosphamide exerts a strong immunosuppressive activity that prevents the clonal expansion of both B and T cells and induces lymphocytopenia by depleting these cells. B cells are more sensitive than T cells. Cyclophosphamide:

- Inhibits B-cell antibody production and serum immunoglobulin levels *in vitro*.
- Suppresses the antigen-induced proliferative response and cytokine production of T cells.
- Inhibits T cell-mediated activities such as delayed-type hypersensitivity reactions.
- Inhibits many of the inflammatory and immune activities of monocytes.

Intravenous cyclophosphamide (10 to 15 mg/kg, once every 4 weeks) is used for diffuse proliferative lupus nephritis, which saves lupus patients more efficiently from renal failure than glucocorticosteroid alone. In addition, cyclophosphamide can also be used in daily oral doses (50 to 150 mg/day).

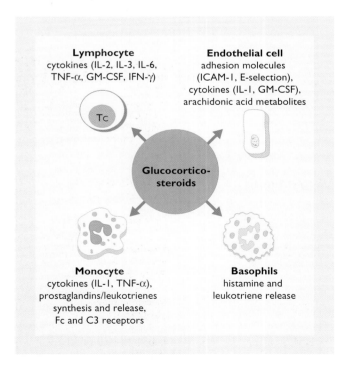

Fig. 16.12 Suppressive effects of glucocorticosteroids on immune and inflammatory responses. (GM-CSF, granulocyte–monocyte colony stimulating factor; ICAM, intercellular adhesion molecule; IFN, interferon; IL, interleukin; TNF, tumor necrosis factor)

ADVERSE EFFECTS OF CYCLOPHOSPHAMIDE include bone marrow suppression, hemorrhagic cystitis, permanent amenorrhea and azoospermia, and an increased risk of malignancy. The bone marrow suppression is dose-dependent and leukopenia is usually self-limiting and reversible once the drug therapy has ceased.

▨ *Nonsteroidal anti-inflammatory drugs (NSAIDs) (see below), including salicylates inhibit cyclo-oxygenase which is an enzyme involved in the synthesis of prostaglandins* (Fig. 16.10)
In particular PGE_2 can induce vasodilation and can induce hyperalgesia contributing to the symptoms of arthralgia.

Although NSAIDs can improve arthralgia in SLE, some adverse effects of NSAIDs such as hepatitis, aseptic meningitis, and renal impairment are particularly common in patients with SLE. The clinical use of NSAIDs is described in more detail in Chapter 20.

▨ *The skin rashes may respond to hydroxychloroquine*
Hydroxychloroquine is used to treat the skin rashes of patients with SLE, but its adverse effects include retinal toxicity, rash, myopathy, and neuropathy.

Rheumatoid arthritis
Rheumatoid arthritis (RA) is a chronic inflammatory synovitis that usually involves the peripheral joints in a symmetric distribution; it is discussed in more detail in Chapter 17. The pathophysiology of rheumatoid synovitis is characterized by the infiltration of CD4+ T cells and monocytes, proliferation of synovial lining cells and fibroblasts, and neovascularization. It is thought to be mediated by proinflammatory cytokines such as IL-1 and TNF-α produced by these cells (Fig. 16.13).

▨ *Nonsteroidal anti-inflammatory drugs are used for symptomatic relief*
A detailed comparison of various NSAIDs is given in Chapter 20. Aspirin and other NSAIDs are widely used to relieve the symptoms of the local inflammatory process. Many chemical classes of NSAID are listed in Fig. 16.14. NSAIDs can inhibit COX_1 enzymes, which are involved in the generation of prostaglandins and thromboxanes, mediators involved in the inflammatory response. Recently it has been shown that a second set of COX enzymes, COX_2 is regulated in certain inflammatory conditions, and this has led to the development of COX_2-selective inhibitors for the treatment of inflammatory pain. These drugs include celicoxib and rofecoxib and are thought to be safer than nonselective NSAIDs as they do not interfere with the synthesis of prostaglandins by COX involved in physiologic processes.

▨ *Disease-modifying antirheumatic drugs (DMARDs) may alter the course of rheumatoid arthritis*
A heterogeneous group of agents has been classified as disease-modifying drugs and may have the capacity to alter the course of RA (Fig. 16.15). They include:
• Gold salts.
• D-Penicillamine.

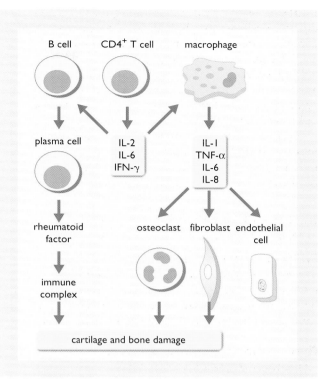

Fig. 16.13 Cytokine network in the pathogenesis of rheumatoid arthritis. Activation of CD4+ T cells, B cells, and macrophages is involved in the initiation of rheumatoid synovitis. These cells release proinflammatory cytokines such as interleukin-1 (IL-1) and tumor necrosis factor (TNF)-α, resulting in proliferation of synovial lining cells and fibroblasts, neovascularization, and cartilage and bone injury.

Classes of NSAIDs	
Propionic acids	Fenoprofen Ibuprofen Ketoprofen Naproxen Oxaprozin
Acetic acids	Indomethacin Sulindac Tolmetin Diclofenac
Oxicoms	Piroxicam Pyroxolone Phenylbutazone
Fenamates	Meclofenamate Mefenamic acid
Salicylates	Aspirin Diflunisal Magnesium salicylate Salsalate

Fig. 16.14 Classes of nonsteroidal anti-inflammatory drugs (NSAIDs).

Disease-modifying antirheumatic drugs used in treatment of rheumatoid arthritis					
Drug	Usual dose	Plasma half-life	Elimination	Time to benefits	Side-effects
Injectable gold salts	25–50 mg i.m., every 2–4 weeks	25 days	70% renal	3–6 months	Rash, stomatitis, myelosuppression thrombopenia, proteinuria, interstitial pneumonia
Oral gold	3 mg oral daily, or twice daily	17–25 days	60% renal	4–6 months	Same as injectable gold but less frequent, plus frequent diarrhea
D-penicillamine	250–750 mg oral daily	2 hours	Liver	3–6 months	Rash, stomatitis, dysgeusia, proteinuria, myelosuppression, autoimmune diseases
Hydroxychloroquine	200 mg oral twice daily	40 days	60% renal	2–4 months	Rash, diarrhea, retinal toxicity
Sulfasalazine	1000 mg oral twice or 3 times daily	4 hours	Liver	1–2 months	Rash, myelosuppression, gastrointestinal intolerance
Methotrexate	7.5–15 mg oral per week	8–10 hours	80% renal	1–2 months	Gastrointestinal symptoms, stomatitis, rash, alopecia, myelosuppression, interstitial pneumonia
Azathioprine	50–150 mg oral daily	0.2 hours	Metabolized in the liver, the metabolites secreted to urine	2–3 months	Myelosuppression, hepatotoxicity, infections, gastrointestinal symptoms
Leflunomide	20 mg oral daily after 100 mg oral for 3 days	11–18 days	43% renal 48% feces	1–2 months	Diarrhea, alopecia, liver dysfunction, rash, fetal death, teratogenic effect

Fig. 16.15 Disease-modifying antirheumatic drugs used in treatment of rheumatoid arthritis. (i.m., intramuscular)

- The antimalarials.
- Sulfasalazine.

These agents have minimal direct nonspecific anti-inflammatory or analgesic effects, usually have a slow onset of efficacy, reduce clinical symptoms over 1–3 months, and induce remissions in a few patients. As many as two-thirds of patients show some clinical improvement as a result of therapy with any of these agents, but the induction of true remissions is unusual. In addition to clinical improvement, there is frequently an improvement in the serologic parameters of disease activity such as C-reactive protein concentration, titers of rheumatoid factor, and the erythrocyte sedimentation rate. Despite this, there is minimal evidence that disease-modifying drugs actually retard the development of bone erosions in the joints.

GOLD SALTS are used in the treatment of RA, but have limited efficacy as single agents. Approximately 20–35% of patients treated with the intramuscular preparation show a significant response, which is maximal at 6–12 months. This remission is sustained in about 50% of the responders. A 5-year follow up revealed no difference between treated and untreated patients when gold salt therapy was used alone.

Gold salts act mainly on monocytes and macrophages, inhibiting their functions. They reduce the migration, phagocytosis, and expression of Fc and CR3 receptors of macrophages as well as accessory cell function, as indicated by the suppression of lymphocyte blastogenesis. They may also inhibit aggregation of γ globulin and induce complement C1 inactivation.

The adverse effects of gold salts include rashes, leukocytopenias, and proteinuria (Fig. 16.15). Oral gold salt therapy is less effective when used as a single agent, but is easier to administer than the parenteral courses of gold salt therapy and has fewer adverse effects.

D-PENICILLAMINE has been used in the treatment of RA. Although its mechanism of action remains unknown, it has immunomodulatory effects *in vitro*, the most important of which may be inhibition of TH cell function. Its adverse effects include gastrointestinal intolerance, skin rash, nephrotoxicity, and elicitation of autoantibodies with associated autoimmune diseases.

HYDROXYCHLOROQUINE can also control the symptoms of RA, but its mechanism of action in the therapy of RA is unknown. It may inhibit the release of prostaglandins or lysosomal enzymes, inhibit lymphocyte proliferation and immunoglobulin production by interfering with IL-1 production by macrophages, or alter the processing and presentation of peptide antigen in the macrophage. Hydroxychloroquine is principally used as the basal agent for attenuating a mild inflammatory process or stabilizing a remission. It should be discontinued if the patient fails to show any improvement after 6 months.

The adverse effects of hydroxychloroquine include dermatitis, myopathy, and corneal opacity, which is usually reversible. Irreversible retinal degeneration can occur and is a cause for concern, but is not common at the doses currently used. Ophthalmologic examination is required every 6 months during treatment.

SULFASALAZINE may reduce the rate of progression of erosions in RA. Its adverse effects include gastric symptoms, neutropenia, hemolysis, hepatitis, and rash.

METHOTREXATE is another immunosuppressive drug that is useful in the treatment of RA. It is a folic acid antagonist and is given in a single oral low dose (7.5–15 mg) once a week. This treatment of RA is discussed in more detail in Chapter 17. Methotrexate inhibits cell division by competitively binding dihydrofolate reductase, resulting in decreased thymidine and purine nucleotide synthesis. Its action is therefore cell-cycle specific, destroying cells during the S phase of DNA synthesis but having little to no effect on resting cells. Methotrexate suppresses primary and secondary antibody responses *in vivo*, but few effects have been observed on pre-existing delayed-type hypersensitivity reactions.

The effect of weekly low-dose methotrexate may be anti-inflammatory and not immunosuppressive. Methotrexate significantly reduces the generation of the 5-lipoxygenase pathway products by leukocytes, and may also decrease IL-1 production by macrophages.

The major adverse effects of methotrexate include bone marrow suppression (leukopenia and thrombocytopenia), opportunistic infections, and hepatotoxicity with fibrosis. Liver fibrosis is most common in those who have a cumulative dosage of 1.5 g, in those receiving the drug daily, and in those with pre-existing liver disease, alcoholism, or diabetes mellitus. Other adverse effects include interstitial pneumonitis, gastrointestinal upset, stomatitis with oral ulcerations, dermatitis, osteoporotic fractures, and fetal malformation. Unlike other cytotoxic drugs, methotrexate is not associated with an increased risk of malignancy.

AZATHIOPRINE is another immunosuppressive drug used for RA. Azathioprine is pro-drug of 6-mercaptopurine (6-MP) and

transformed to 6-MP in the liver. The metabolites of 6-MP block purine synthesis, cause DNA damage, and have cytotoxic actions. Azathioprine suppresses T cell-mediated immune responses including delayed-type hypersensitivities to greater degree than antibody production. Adverse effects of azathioprine include bone marrow suppression and an increased risk of malignancy. The immunosuppressive effects and adverse effects of azathioprine are milder than those of cyclophosphamide. (A detailed discussion of these drugs is found in Chapter 12.) The effects of azathioprine are amplified by allopurinol, an inhibitor of xanthine oxidase that also inactivates 6-MP.

LEFLUNOMIDE is a newly developed selective inhibitor of *de novo* pyrimidine synthesis. Unlike other proliferating cell types, lymphocytes cannot undergo cell division when the pathway for the *de novo* synthesis of pyrimidines is blocked. Thus, leflunomide selectively suppresses lymphocyte proliferation. Leflunomide is similar to both sulfasalazine and methotrexate in efficacy for RA. Adverse effects of leflunomide include diarrhea, liver dysfunction, alopecia, and rash. This drug is contraindicated in pregnant women because of teratogenicity.

Glucocorticosteroids can be used in the treatment of RA

This is discussed in more detail in Chapter 20.

CYCLOSPORINE AND T-CELL SUPPRESSION Cyclosporine has a selective inhibitory effect on T cells by inhibiting the TCR-mediated signal transduction pathway. It specifically binds to its cytoplasmic binding protein, cyclophilin, and this complex then binds to calcineurin, inhibiting phosphatase activity and therefore the nuclear translocation of the nuclear factor of activated T cells (NF-AT) (Fig. 16.16). Cyclosporine inhibits IL-2 production, T-cell proliferation, TH-cell activity for antibody production, and Tc cell generation, and so could have a beneficial effect on autoantibody production and immune complex-mediated diseases. Cyclosporine has therefore been used to treat autoimmune diseases, though most available data are for RA. A clinical improvement is generally observed, but the adverse effects of cyclosporine, as well as the flares that occur after cyclosporine is discontinued may limit its use. Cyclosporine is also an effective therapy for ocular Behçet's disease, psoriasis, atopic dermatitis, aplastic anemia, transplant rejection and nephrotic syndrome, and may have therapeutic activity in polymyositis, dermatomyositis, and severe glucocorticosteroid-dependent asthma.

The major adverse effect of cyclosporine is renal toxicity (primarily proximal renal tubular changes), which is usually dose-related and reversible. Other adverse effects include hypertension, hepatotoxicity, tremor, hirsutism, and gingival hyperplasia. Bone marrow suppression is unusual. Lymphomas have been reported in some cyclosporine-treated renal transplant recipients. Cyclosporine interacts with a variety of drugs. Phenobarbital, phenytoin, and rifampin decrease plasma cyclosporine levels through the induction of the hepatic P-450 system. On the other hand, macrorides, ketoconazole, itraconazole, and grapefruit juice increase plasma levels of this drug. Therefore, monitoring of plasma cyclosporine levels is

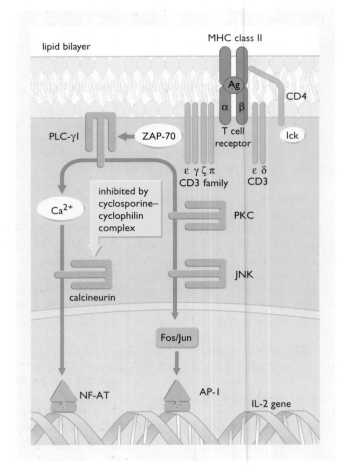

Fig. 16.16 Cyclosporine and T-cell suppression. Stimulation of T cells through the T-cell receptor (TCR) phosphorylates the CD3ζ chain of the TCR–CD3 complex. Phosphorylated CD3ζ then binds and activates ZAP-70, a tyrosine kinase. Subsequently, phospholipase C (PLC)-γ1 is activated by tyrosine phosphorylation and cleaves phosphatidylinositol bisphosphate to the second messengers inositol 1,4,5-triphosphate and diacylglycerol. The former produces a sustained rise in intracellular calcium ($[Ca^{2+}]_i$), while the latter activates protein kinase C (PKC). These two signals then synergize to induce and activate transcription factors required for interleukin-2 (IL-2) gene transcription. The rise in $[Ca^{2+}]_i$ activates the calmodulin-dependent phosphatase calcineurin, which leads to alteration of the preformed cytoplasmic component of the nuclear factor of activated T cells (NF-AT), allowing it to move into the nucleus. There it combines with newly formed Fos and Jun proteins induced by the PKC pathway to create NF-AT, which binds to a response element in the IL-2 enhancer. Fos and Jun also bind as an AP-1 complex to a separate enhancer site (TRE; TPA-responsive element). Other transcription factors NF-κB and NF-IL-2A are also involved in IL-2 gene transcription. Cyclosporine specifically binds to its cytoplasmic binding protein (cyclophilin) and thereby inhibits IL-2 production by T cells. (lck, a tyrosine kinase)

necessary in order to obtain adequate immunosuppressive effects and minimize adverse effects.

Polymyositis and dermatomyositis

Polymositis and dermatomyositis are immunologically mediated inflammatory muscle diseases characterized by lymphocyte infiltration in the skeletal muscle. Patients with polymyositis have symmetric proximal muscle weakness, elevated serum

---

> ### ⚠ Immunosuppressive drugs
>
> - *The major adverse effects of cytotoxic drugs are bone marrow suppression and opportunistic infections*
> - *Cyclophosphamide causes hemorrhagic cystitis, amenorrhea and azoospermia, and an increased risk of malignancies*
> - *Methotrexate causes hepatotoxicity and interstitial pneumonitis*
> - *Cyclosporine causes renal toxicity*

levels of muscle-associated enzymes such as creatine kinase (CK), electromyographic abnormalities characteristic of inflammatory myopathy, and histologic evidence of muscle damage and lymphocyte infiltration in a muscle biopsy. These features are also seen in patients with dermatomyositis in addition to a characteristic heliotrope skin rash and Gottron's erythema.

The pathogenetic mechanisms of polymyositis and dermatomyositis may differ. Interstitial infiltration of CD8$^+$ T cells surrounding and invading otherwise normal-appearing myocytes is a prominent feature in polymyositis. In contrast, perivascular infiltration of CD4$^+$ T cells and B cells and perifascicular muscle fiber atrophy are prominent in dermatomyositis. The myositis-specific autoantibodies may also play a pathogenetic role: for example, anti-Jo-1 autoantibody is directed against histidyl-tRNA synthetase and is found in 20–30% of patients with myositis.

■ Glucocorticosteroids are the mainstay of therapy for polymyositis and dermatomyositis

Polymyositis and dermatomyositis are treated with high doses of glucocorticosteroids (prednisone or prednisolone 1–2 mg/kg/day). The glucocorticosteroid is continued in a high dose until the serum CK level returns to normal. The dose is then tapered very slowly. The condition may improve within 1–4 weeks, but in some patients treatment may be needed for 3 months before there is an improvement. Muscle strength may not improve for weeks to months after the serum concentrations of muscle-derived enzymes have normalized. Patients who have a poor prognosis (i.e. patients with acute severe myositis who have bedridden muscle weakness, dysphagia or respiratory muscle weakness, and patients with interstitial pneumonitis) are treated with intravenous 'pulses' of 1000 mg methylprednisolone for 3 days, followed by maintenance with daily glucocorticosteroids. Sometimes it is difficult to distinguish glucocorticosteroid-induced myopathy (increasing muscle weakness during glucocorticosteroid therapy) from a relapse of the myositis.

■ Other immunosuppressive drugs are sometimes used

Immunosuppressive drugs are used:
- For severe polymyositis or dermatomyositis.
- If the response to glucocorticosteroids is inadequate after 1–3 months of treatment.
- If there are frequent relapses.

Oral methotrexate is a major therapeutic option for glucocorticosteroid-resistant patients. Cyclosporine may be beneficial for conditions such as interstitial pneumonitis.

Systemic sclerosis

Systemic sclerosis (SSc) is a multisystem disorder of unknown etiology, characterized by fibrosis of the skin, lungs, and gastro-intestinal tract, Raynaud's phenomenon, and microvascular abnormalities of the skin and visceral organs. Its characteristic immunologic and microvascular abnormalities include:

- Antinuclear antibodies, particularly anti-Scl-70 autoantibody found in 30–70% of patients and directed against the nuclear enzyme DNA topoisomerase I.
- Hypergammaglobulinemia.
- Perivascular infiltration of CD4+ T cells and macrophages in the dermis.
- Intimal thickening with narrowing of the vascular lumen in the skin and kidneys.

MANAGEMENT D-Penicillamine has been used to reduce fibrosis and prevent the development of skin thickening and significant organ involvement. This drug interferes with inter- and intra-molecular cross-linking of collagen and is also immuno-suppressive, including the inhibitory effect on Tн-cell function. Its immunosuppressive activity may also lead to decreased collagen production.

Glucocorticosteroids are indicated for inflammatory myositis in SSc. They also reduce edema associated with the edematous phase of early skin involvement, but are not indicated in the long-term treatment of SSc. High doses of glucocorticosteroids may cause acute renal failure.

Polyarteritis nodosa

Polyarteritis nodosa (PN) is an immune complex-mediated necrotizing vasculitis that characteristically affects small- and medium-sized muscular arteries, especially at their bifurcations. Most lesions occur in the kidney, heart, liver, gastrointestinal tract, musculoskeletal system, testes, peripheral nervous system, and skin. The symptoms and signs depend on the severity and location of vessel involvement and the resulting ischemic changes. Nonspecific features include fever, weight loss, malaise, neutrophilia, increased C-reactive protein, and increased erythrocyte sedimentation rate. Circulating immune complexes have also been detected. The lesions contain immunoglobulins and complement components, and in some cases hepatitis B

Characteristic features of autoimmune diseases

- Autoimmune diseases are characterized by the presence of autoantibodies and autoreactive T cells against self-antigens
- Disease-specific autoantibodies are frequently detected: anti-DNA antibody in systemic lupus erythematosus; rheumatoid factor (autoantibody to IgG) in rheumatoid arthritis; anti-Jo-1 antibody in polymyositis; and anti-Scl-70 antibody in systemic sclerosis
- Glucocorticosteroids and immunosuppressive drugs are effective treatments

antigen is detected. The deposited immune complexes produce lesions by activating complement components and attracting and activating inflammatory cells.

MANAGEMENT Glucocorticosteroids are the mainstay of therapy, but the addition of cyclophosphamide nearly doubles the 5-year survival rate to 90%.

Transplantation rejection

Antilymphocyte globulin is used as an immunosuppressive agent for the treatment of transplantation rejection and certain types of aplastic anemia.

Many polyclonal antibodies have been prepared, but more recently a mouse ant-CD3 monoclonal antibody, Muromonab, has been introduced for immunosuppression in an attempt to minimize the xenogeneic antibody response in the patient.

FURTHER READING

Frank MM, Austen KF, Calman HN, Unanue ER (eds) *Samter's Immunologic Diseases*, 6th edn. Boston: Little, Brown; 2001. [This book describes, in depth, the mechanism and therapy of immunologic diseases, including hypersensitivity and autoimmune diseases.]

Holgate ST, Church MK (eds) *Allergy*, 2nd edn. London: Mosby; 2000.

Roitt IM, Brostoff J, Male DK (eds) *Immunology*, 6th edn. London: Mosby; 2001. [These two books are updated standard textbooks, with well-drawn illustrations, for understanding the basics of clinical allergy and immunology.]

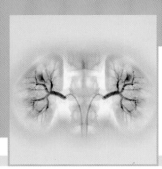

Chapter 17

Drugs and the Renal System

PHYSIOLOGY OF THE KIDNEY

The essential functions of the kidney include:
- Excretion of nitrogenous waste products of metabolism such as urea and creatinine.
- Regulation of the volume of extracellular fluid.
- Regulation of the concentration of various ions in the body.
- Regulation of the pH of body fluids.

The renal system includes the bladder where urine is temporarily stored before final excretion through the urethra (see Chapter 22).

▓ The kidney has two distinct regions: cortex and medulla

Two distinct regions can be macroscopically identified in the kidney: a dark outer region, the cortex, and a paler inner region, the medulla. The medulla is further divided into a number of conical areas, the renal pyramids (Fig. 17.1).

The individual functional unit of the kidney is the nephron with each kidney containing approximately one million nephrons. The nephron is a blind-ended tube with the blind end forming a capsule, the Bowman's capsule, which surrounds a knot of capillaries, the glomerulus. Glomerular capillaries receive their blood from the afferent arteriole, a resistance blood vessel. Blood leaves the glomerulus not in a vein (capacitance vessel) but in a second resistance vessel, the efferent arteriole. This arrangement of afferent and efferent vessels permits generation of a hydrostatic force that drives ultrafiltration (see below). The other parts of the nephron are the proximal tubule, loop of Henle, distal tubule, and the collecting duct (see Fig. 17.6). Many distal tubules join a collecting duct which merges into larger ducts before draining into a renal calyx and, finally, into the renal pelvis.

▓ There are two distinct populations of nephron: cortical and juxtamedullary nephrons

- Cortical nephrons have glomeruli in the outer two-thirds of the cortex with short loops of Henle, which either extend a short distance into the medulla or do not reach the medulla. This type of nephron accounts for 85% of all nephrons. The efferent arteriole of cortical nephrons forms a network of peritubular capillaries that encircle all parts of the nephron.
- Juxtamedullary nephrons (15% of all nephrons) have glomeruli in the inner third of the cortex with long loops of Henle extending deep into the medulla (see Fig. 17.6) and are responsible for generating hypertonic fluid in the

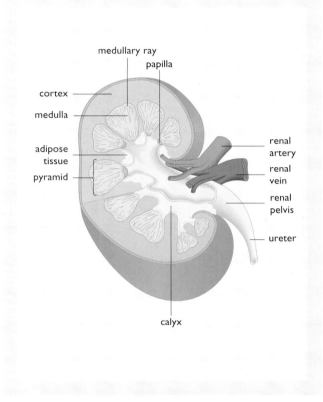

Fig. 17.1 Structure of the kidney. The kidney consists of two visible regions, the cortex and medulla, with the latter being divided into the renal pyramids.

medullary interstitium. The efferent arteriole of juxtamedullary nephrons gives rise to some peritubular capillaries, but also forms a series of vascular loops (the vasa recta) which descend into the medulla and surround the loop of Henle.

▓ Urine is a modified ultrafiltrate of plasma produced by three filtration barriers

The force that drives ultrafiltration (i.e. filtration of small molecules only) is glomerular capillary hydrostatic pressure. This pressure is dependent on the ratio of the resistance in the afferent arteriole to that of the efferent arteriole. In contrast to other vascular beds, the presence of a second arteriole, the efferent arteriole, ensures that the hydrostatic pressure in glomerular capillaries declines very little along their length.

343

Ultrafiltration occurs from the glomerular capillaries into Bowman's capsule through the following three filtration barriers:

- The endothelial cells of glomerular capillaries which contain numerous fenestrations (pores 60 nm in diameter) that act as a filtration barrier only to the cellular elements of the blood (Fig. 17.2).
- The basement membrane, which lies immediately beneath the endothelial cells, and consists of collagen and other glycoproteins. It is the main filtration barrier that allows passage of molecules according to their size and charge.
- Podocytes, which are specialized cells of Bowman's capsule with numerous projections (foot processes or pedicels) that cover the basement membrane. The main function of the podocytes is to lay down and maintain the basement membrane. In addition, the gaps between the interlocking pedicels of adjacent podocytes present a further filtration barrier to negatively charged macromolecules (see Fig. 17.2).

Ultrafiltration prevents molecules with a molecular mass of 70 kDa or more from passing into the proximal tubule. They remain within the glomerular capillaries and pass into the efferent vessels. In contrast, molecules less than 7 kDa (such as glucose, amino acids, Na^+ and K^+) are freely filtered and enter the proximal tubule at a concentration similar to that found in the blood entering the glomerulus. Molecules of 7–70 kDa are retarded by filtration to an extent which is proportional to their molecular mass. The charge on a molecule may also influence the degree of filtration because the basement membrane and podocytes have negative charges which repel anionic macromolecules. This is relevant to the filtration of albumin (69 kDa), which is filtered to a much smaller extent than would be anticipated on the basis of molecular mass alone because it has a net negative charge at physiologic pH.

Ultrafiltrate is modified in the tubules

Ultrafiltrate produced at the glomerulus enters the proximal tubule and is modified by a series of reabsorptive and secretory processes occurring along the length of the nephron (Fig. 17.3). These processes involve the following transport mechanisms:

- Active transport directly coupled to adenosine triphosphate (ATP) hydrolysis.

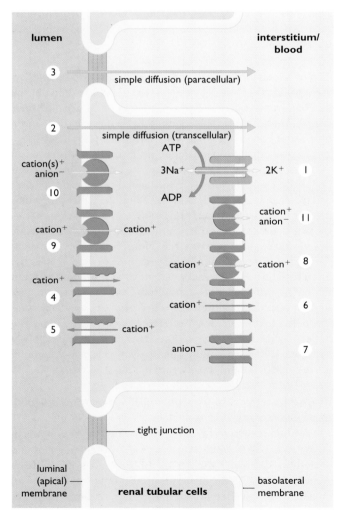

Fig. 17.3 Transport mechanisms in renal tubule cells. Solutes are translocated across renal tubular cells by active transport (a process involving hydrolysis of ATP) (1); by diffusion (2, 3); through ion channels (4–7); by countertransport (transport of solutes in opposite directions across a membrane) (8,9); and by cotransport (transport of solutes in the same direction across the membrane) (10, 11).

Fig. 17.2 Structure of the glomerular filter. The barriers to ultrafiltration in the glomerulus are the capillary endothelium, the basement membrane, and the gaps between the foot processes of the podocytes.

- Simple diffusion using transcellular (across cells) or paracellular (across the tight junctions between cells) routes.
- Movement through ion channels.
- Cotransport (symport), which is carrier-mediated transport with substances conveyed in the same direction.
- Countertransport (antiport), which is carrier-mediated transport with substances moved in opposite directions.

Ion channel proteins form pores in membranes that allow the passage of specific ions such as Na^+ or K^+. Transporter proteins also span the membrane and bind a few substrate ions or molecules at a time. After binding, the transporter undergoes a conformational change to transfer the substrate across the membrane. Since movement of the substrate molecules/ions requires a conformational change, transporters move substrates across cell membranes at a rate about 1000-fold slower than channels.

Many transport mechanisms are not directly linked to ATP hydrolysis, but indirectly depend on electrochemical gradients established by active transport of Na^+ and K^+ across the basolateral membrane. This is mediated by Na^+/K^+ ATPase, which moves three Na^+ ions out of the cell while transporting two K^+ ions into the cell (see Chapter 18). The activity of Na^+/K^+ ATPase drives Na^+ reabsorption and cotransport of solutes such as glucose across the apical membrane. The details of transport mechanisms of particular sections of the nephron are described in relation to the mechanism of action of different diuretic drugs (see below).

PATHOPHYSIOLOGY AND DISEASES OF THE RENAL SYSTEM

Edema

▓ *Edema is an increase in the volume of interstitial fluid resulting in tissue swelling*

Edema results from an imbalance between the rate of interstitial fluid formation and its reabsorption. Formation of interstitial fluid depends upon capillary hydrostatic pressure and oncotic pressure (protein osmotic pressure) of interstitial fluid, while reabsorption of interstitial fluid depends upon hydrostatic pressure of interstitial fluid and capillary oncotic pressure (Fig. 17.4).

▓ *Nephrotic syndrome is the most common kidney disorder that can cause edema*

Edema in nephrotic syndrome results from increased permeability of the glomerular basement membrane to proteins, particularly albumin. This leads to marked proteinuria (protein in the urine) and a reduced plasma protein oncotic pressure resulting in edema. In addition, the increase in interstitial fluid volume decreases the effective circulating volume and therefore activates the renin–angiotensin system (see Chapter 18) that in turn stimulates secretion of aldosterone. Enhanced secretion of aldosterone promotes Na^+ and water retention, thereby increasing blood volume and venous and capillary pressures, which lead subsequently to further edema formation. An expansion of blood volume also reduces the concentration of plasma proteins and therefore plasma oncotic pressure (see Fig. 17.4).

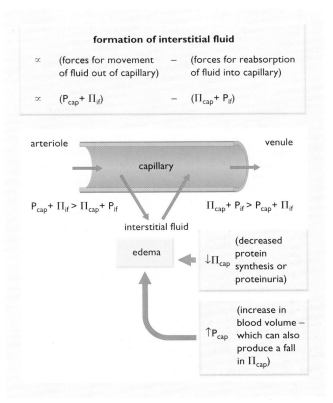

Fig. 17.4 Factors that govern the formation of interstitial fluid. Edema (an increase in the volume of interstitial fluid that results in tissue swelling) occurs as a result of either a fall in capillary oncotic pressure, or an increase in capillary hydrostatic pressure. (P_{cap}, capillary hydrostatic pressure; P_{if}, interstitial fluid hydrostatic pressure; Π_{cap}, capillary oncotic pressure; Π_{if}, interstitial fluid oncotic pressure)

Edema

- Edema is an increase in the volume of interstitial fluid resulting in tissue swelling
- A decrease in plasma protein concentration and an increase in venous pressure reduce the reabsorption of interstitial fluid back into the capillaries, thereby increasing the volume of interstitial fluid
- Activation of the renin–angiotensin system plays an important role in the development of edema by increasing the blood volume, which in turn increases venous pressure and reduces the concentration of plasma proteins
- Edema develops in patients with the nephrotic syndrome, liver disease, and congestive heart failure

Nephrotic syndrome is seen mainly in children and it is usually attributable to 'minimal change nephropathy.' This condition is a glomerulopathy in which glomeruli appear normal, but the negative charges on the basement membrane are diminished. In adults, a multitude of glomerular lesions may cause nephrotic syndrome. Treatment of nephrotic syndrome may be symptomatic or involve treating the renal lesion.

345

There are two approaches to treating nephrotic syndrome:
- Symptomatic, which aims to correct the syndrome, in particular to reversing the edematous state with diuretic drugs.
- Treatment of the underlying renal lesion, which may reverse or delay progression of nephrotic syndrome. Glucocorticosteroids and immunosuppressant drugs, such as cyclophosphamide, are frequently required (see Chapter 16 for details of immunosupressive drugs).

Congestive heart failure and liver disease are other causes of edema

The nephrotic syndrome is an example of a disorder of the kidney that directly results in edema, but edema can also be secondary to disorders of other systems, such as heart failure and liver disease. The mechanism by which congestive heart failure causes edema and the use of drugs to treat this condition are described in Chapter 18. Liver disease may also cause edema, particularly in the peritoneal cavity, where it is called ascites. Ascites results from increased hydrostatic pressure in the hepatic portal vein together with decreased albumin synthesis. Loss of fluid from the capillaries into the peritoneal cavity decreases circulating blood volume, which activates the renin–angiotensin system. This leads, as outlined previously, to increased Na^+ and water absorption in the kidney, which further contributes to the edema.

Diuretics will relieve edema

Edema is relieved by appropriate use of diuretic drugs, which promote loss of extracellular fluid via urine such that extracellular volume is returned toward normal. However, excessive use of diuretics can decrease effective circulating volume and reduce organ perfusion.

Diuretics

Diuresis means an increase in urine volume. Diuretics increase renal excretion of Na^+ and water. The cellular action of most

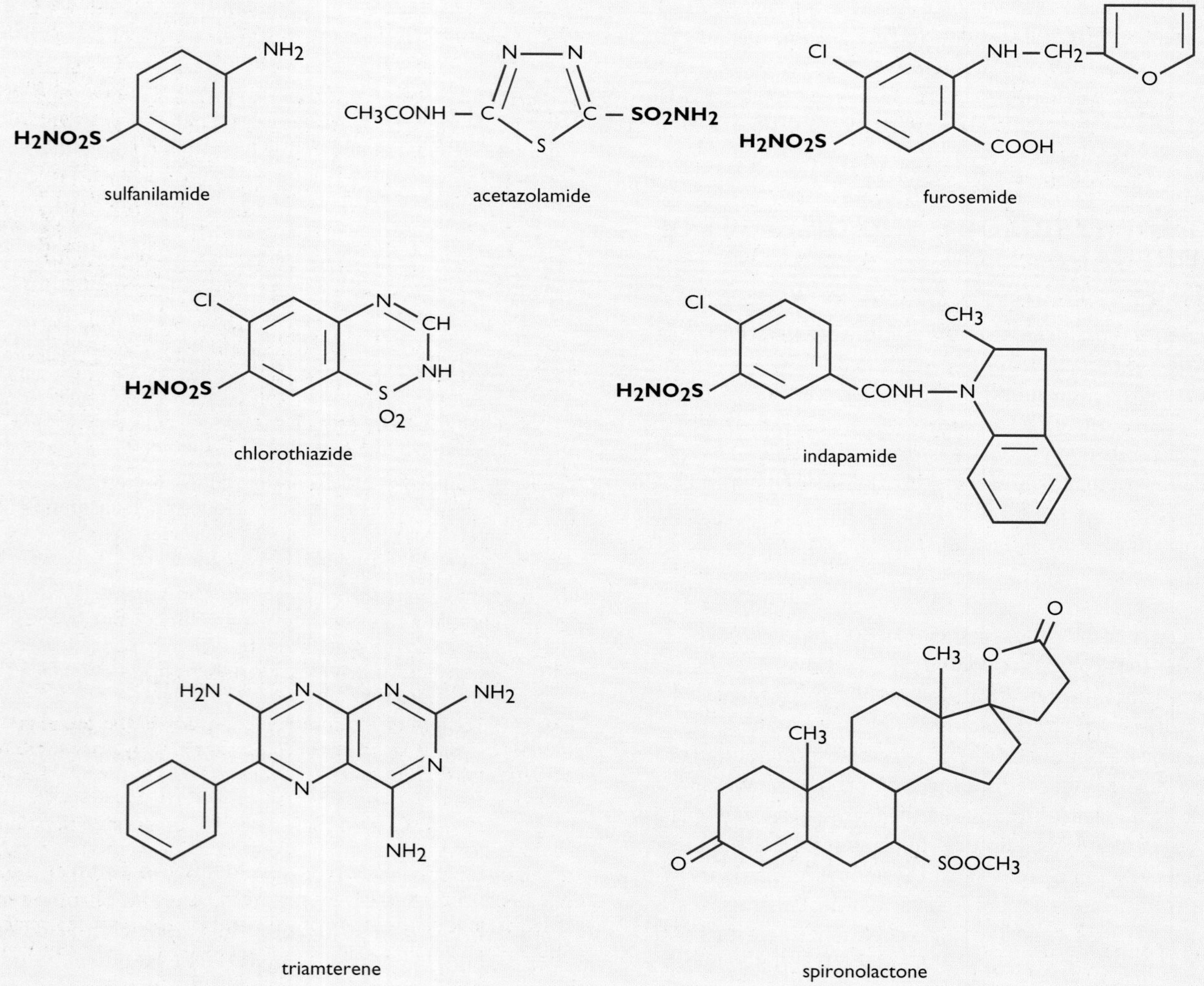

Fig. 17.5 Structures of representative drugs from each diuretic class. The sulfonamide moiety is shown in bold.

diuretic drugs is to reduce the reabsorption of Na⁺, with increased water loss occurring as a secondary consequence. Many diuretic drugs have been developed from modifications of the structure of the sulfonamide drug sulphanilamide and as a result retain the sulfonamide moiety (Fig. 17.5).

All diuretic drugs, other than osmotic diuretics, act directly on renal tubule cells at distinct regions within the nephron (Fig. 17.6). Generally the molecular sites of action for such diuretics are located on the apical membrane following filtration of the drug at the glomerulus and secretion into the proximal tubule. By contrast, aldosterone antagonists act on an intracellular target subsequent to diffusion across the basolateral membrane.

Carbonic anhydrase inhibitors
The development of these drugs arose from the observation that sulfanilamide produced mild diuresis associated with a

metabolic acidosis. The prototype of this class of diuretics is acetazolamide. The primary site of action of acetazolamide is the proximal tubule, although a secondary site is the collecting duct where carbonic anhydrase is involved in acid secretion (see below, Fig. 17.13).

Carbonic anhydrase is located in the cytoplasm of proximal tubule cells and in the apical cell membrane. Activity of the enzyme at both sites plays a role in the reabsorption of sodium and bicarbonate as shown in Fig. 17.7. Normally 1% or less of Na⁺ filtered at the glomerulus is excreted on a typical diet

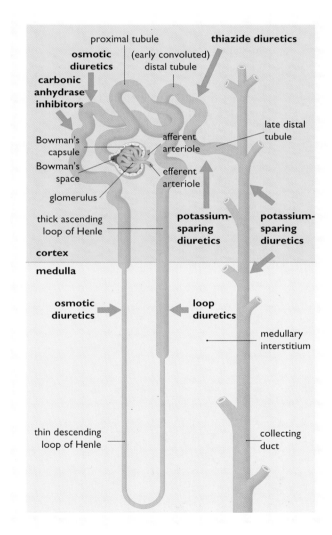

Fig. 17.6 The nephron and collecting ducts showing sites of action of diuretic drugs. The basic functional unit of the kidney is the nephron, which filters blood at the glomerulus. The resulting ultrafiltrate is modified by a series of reabsorptive and secretory processes as it passes along the nephron, before draining into collecting ducts and then into the renal pelvis.

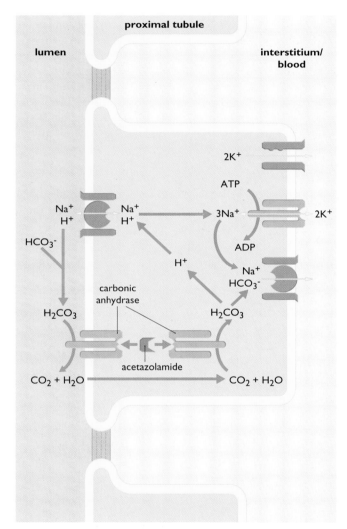

Fig. 17.7 Sodium bicarbonate reabsorption in the proximal tubule and mode of action of the carbonic anhydrase inhibitor acetazolamide. Countertransport of Na⁺ and H⁺ across the apical membrane moves Na⁺ into the cell and H⁺ into the lumen. The latter reacts with tubule fluid bicarbonate (HCO_3^-), producing carbonic acid (H_2CO_3) that dissociates to form CO_2 and H_2O, a reaction catalyzed by carbonic anhydrase bound to the apical membrane. Both CO_2 and H_2O readily enter the cell where carbonic acid is formed by the action of cytoplasmic carbonic anhydrase. Carbonic acid dissociates into HCO_3^-, which is transported across the basolateral membrane with Na⁺, and H⁺. The latter moves into the lumen via the Na⁺/H⁺ countertransporter to begin the cycle again. Inhibition of both membrane-bound and cytoplasmic forms of the enzyme by acetazolamide inhibits Na⁺ and HCO_3^- reabsorption.

whilst the action of acetazolamide results in the excretion of up to 5% of filtered Na^+. The increased urinary loss of bicarbonate, which results in alkalinization of the urine, can produce metabolic acidosis. However, metabolic acidosis is self-limiting since, as it develops, the filtered load of bicarbonate decreases to the extent that the uncatalyzed reaction between water and carbon dioxide is sufficient to allow bicarbonate reabsorption. Moreover, the diuresis produced by acetazolamide is transient since a reduction in bicarbonate filtered at the glomerulus reduces the ability of the drug to inhibit sodium reabsorption. As with other diuretics that result in an increased Na^+ load being delivered to the collecting duct, acetazolamide increases K^+ excretion which can lead to hypokalemia (see Figs 17.8 and 17.9 for adverse effects and drug interactions).

The pharmacokinetics of acetazolamide are outlined in Fig. 17.10.

Acetazolamide can be used to relieve edema resulting from congestive heart failure but such use is rare. Acetazolamide is mainly used for its nonrenal actions; for example, glaucoma where carbonic anhydrase inhibition reduces aqueous humor formation (see Chapter 24).

Loop diuretics

Modifications of the sulfonamide structure have resulted in a group of diuretics with an action on the loop of Henle. These loop diuretics include furosemide (Fig. 17.5), bumetanide and torsemide whilst ethacrynic acid, a phenoxyacetic acid derivative, also produces diuresis through an action on the loop of Henle. These drugs inhibit the cotransport of Na^+, K^+ and $2Cl^-$ ions across the apical membrane of the thick ascending limb of the loop of Henle, by binding to and inhibiting a particular transporter protein (bumetanide-sensitive cotransporter-1, BSC-1) (Fig 17.11). Loop diuretics, sometimes referred to as high ceiling diuretics, are the most powerful of all diuretic agents, resulting in the excretion of 15–25% of sodium filtered at the glomerulus.

The thick ascending limb of the loop of Henle is impermeable to water and therefore movement of Na^+ and Cl^- ions into the medullary interstitium (see Fig. 17.6), without accompanying water, increases the osmotic pressure in this region. The high osmotic pressure of the medullary interstitium drives reabsorption of water from the collecting duct in the presence of vasopressin (see below). Loop diuretics reduce the ion concentration in the medullary interstitium and so inhibit water reabsorption from the collecting duct.

Reabsorption of Ca^{2+} and Mg^{2+} is also inhibited by loop diuretics since absorption of these ions is driven by a lumen-positive potential produced by recycling of K^+ across the apical membrane via a K^+-selective channel (Fig. 17.11). Loop diuretics increase the delivery of Na^+ to the collecting duct,

Adverse effects of diuretic drugs				
	Carbonic anhydrase inhibitors	**Loop diuretics**	**Thiazide and thiazide-like diuretics**	**Potassium-sparing diuretics**
Effects directly attributable to diuretic property	Metabolic acidosis Hypokalemia Abnormal taste, lethargy, decreased libido (reduced by administration of $NaHCO_3$)	Hypokalemia (corrected by K^+ supplements or combination with potassium sparing diuretics) Metabolic alkalosis Hypovolemia and hypotension Hypocalcemia Hypomagnesemia	Hypokalemia (corrected as for loop diuretics) Metabolic alkalosis Hyponatremia Hypovolemia and hypotension Hypomagnesemia Hypercalcemia	Hyperkalemia Metabolic acidosis
Effects not directly related to diuretic property	Occasionally hepatitis and blood dyscrasias as a result of immunological hypersensitivity reactions	Hyperuricemia which may precipitate gout (enhanced uric acid absorption in proximal tubule as a result of volume depletion or decreased secretion due to competition at organic acid secretory mechanism) Ototoxicity (hearing loss, tinnitus; more likely with ethacrynic acid)	Hyperuricemia (mechanism as loop diuretics) Hyperglycemia which may reveal latent diabetes mellitus (due to reduced insulin secretion and alterations in glucose metabolism) An increase in plasma levels of low density lipoproteins (LDL) and cholesterol Impotence	Nausea and vomiting (amiloride and triamterene) Diarrhea and peptic ulcer (spironolactone) Spironolactone binds to other steroid receptors which can result in: Gynecomastia Menstrual disorders Impotence Hirsutism Loss of libido

Fig. 17.8 Adverse effects of diuretic drugs.

Notable interactions between diuretics and other drugs

Diuretic drug(s)	Drug(s) interacting	Consequence	Comment
Acetazolamide	Phenytoin Phenobarbital Primidone	Osteomalacia and rickets	Uncertain mechanism
Acetazolamide	Aspirin or salicylates	Lethargy, confusion and coma	Acetazolamide-induced acidosis results in more salicylate entering the central nervous system, which can lead to salicylate intoxication
Thiazide, thiazide-like and loop diuretics	Cardiac glycosides	Increased cardiac glycoside-induced arrhythmias	Hypokalemia potentiates action of cardiac glycosides
Thiazide, thiazide-like and loop diuretics	Sulfonylureas (oral hypoglycemic drugs) and insulin	Hyperglycemia	Thiazides and to a lesser extent loop diuretics decrease insulin secretion
Thiazide, thiazide-like and loop diuretics	Lithium	Increased plasma levels of lithium with risk of toxic effects	Increased tubular reabsorption of lithium
Thiazide, thiazide-like and loop diuretics	Uricosuric agents	Reduced effect of uricosuric agents	Decreased tubular secretion of uricosuric agents
Thiazide, thiazide-like and loop diuretics	Nonsteroidal anti-inflammatory drugs	Reduced diuretic response	Interaction a result of inhibition of prostaglandin synthesis
Loop diuretics	Aminoglycosides Cisplatin	Increased risk of ototoxicity	Synergism of ototoxicity
Potassium-sparing diuretics	ACE inhibitors and K supplements	Increased risk of hyperkalemia	Additive hyperkalemic effects

Fig. 17.9 Notable interactions between diuretics and other drugs.

which increases K^+ and H^+ secretion, leading to a hypokalemic alkalosis (see below).

Loop diuretics are water-soluble weak acids that are highly bound to plasma albumin (>90%) at therapeutic concentrations. The greater part of a dose of furosemide is excreted by the kidneys as a result of secretion in the proximal tubule (Fig. 17.10). Bumetanide and torsemide are largely cleared by metabolism in the liver and, as a result, accumulate less in renal failure than furosemide. Hence bumetanide and torsemide have a lower potential to produce toxic effects in renal failure.

Loop diuretics also have an indirect venodilator action

In addition to their diuretic properties, loop diuretics have an indirect venodilator action as a result of the release of a substance from the kidney (most probably a prostaglandin). This action leads to a fall in left ventricular filling pressure and helps relieve pulmonary edema before the onset of the diuretic effect.

Furosemide acts within an hour of oral administration (20–80 mg) and diuresis is complete within 6 hours. Consequently, furosemide can be given twice daily without diuresis interfering with sleep. Once-daily dosing can result in 18 hours when the kidney avidly reabsorbs sodium, resulting in 'rebound

Na^+ retention,' which may be of sufficient magnitude to negate the prior diuresis. Such problems do not arise when the drug is given by continuous intravenous infusion.

CLINICAL INDICATIONS for loop diuretics include:
- Acute pulmonary edema for which they are administered intravenously to ensure a rapid onset of action (this is a major use).
- Other edematous states such as the nephrotic syndrome, ascites of liver cirrhosis, and chronic renal failure when drug would be administered orally.
- Hypertension in patients who have not responded to other diuretics or antihypertensive drugs, usually in the presence of renal insufficiency (see Chapter 18).
- Acute renal failure, when they are given to increase urine production (see below).
- Hyponatremia; this can produce swelling of brain cells that results in neurological dysfunction characterized by lethargy, confusion and even coma. (Loop diuretics dissipate the high solute concentration in the medullary interstitium. This promotes additional water loss in relation to sodium ex-

349

Pharmacokinetic parameters for some diuretic drugs

Drug	Routes of administration	Oral absorption (%)	Half-life (h)	Volume of distribution (L/kg)	Elimination	Comments
Acetazolamide	p.o., i.v., i.m.	100	8 (6–9)	0.2	Unchanged in urine	Decrease dose in elderly and other patients with diminished renal function. Alkalinization of urine may decrease urinary excretion of weak bases (e.g. quinidine) and increase their pharmacological effect
Furosemide	p.o., i.v., i.m.	52 (27–80)	1.5 (0.5–2.0)	0.2–0.3	About 75% of dose is excreted unchanged in urine	Food intake reduces absorption
Chlorothiazide	p.o., i.v.	7–33	15–27	0.3	Unchanged in urine	Oral absorption decreases with dose
Indapamide	p.o.	High	17 (10–22)	60 L	Extensive metabolism	
Triamterene	p.o.	30–83	1.5–2.5	2.2–3.7	Rapid metabolism	
Spironolactone	p.o.	60–70	1.3 ± 0.3 (SD)	Not known	Extensive metabolism	Absorption is variable because of poor solubility in water but is improved after food. Canrenone is an active metabolite

Fig. 17.10 Pharmacokinetic parameters for some diuretic drugs. (p.o., oral administration; i.v., intravenous; i.m., intramuscular)

cretion and accounts for the use of loop diuretics, combined with hypertonic saline, in the treatment of hyopnatremia). The main adverse effects and principal drug interactions that occur with loop diuretics, compared with other diuretics, are shown in Figs 17.8 and 17.9.

Thiazide and thiazide-like diuretics

The original members of this class of drugs were benzothiadiazine compounds and, as a result, they were termed thiazide diuretics. This group includes bendroflumethiazide, chlorothiazide, polythiazide and hydrochlorothiazide (Fig. 17.5). More recently discovered diuretics with a similar mode of action, but not of a thiazide structure, are called thiazide-like diuretics. This group includes indapamide, chlorthalidone and metolazone, all of which retain the sulfonamide moiety (Fig. 17.5).

■ Thiazide diuretics inhibit the Na⁺/Cl⁻ cotransporter in the distal convoluted tubule

The molecular mechanism of action of thiazide diuretics is inhibition of the Na^+/Cl^- cotransporter (TSC, thiazide-sensitive cotransporter) in the distal convoluted tubule (Fig. 17.12). Compared with loop diuretics, thiazides produce a moderate diuresis. One reason for this is that by the time the filtrate has

reached the distal tubule, 90% of the sodium originally filtered at the glomerulus has already been reabsorbed. The action of thiazides results in the urinary excretion of up to half the sodium that passes to the distal nephron; that is 5% of sodium filtered at the glomerulus. However, in contrast with loop diuretics, which are used to treat hyponatremia, thiazides are prone to produce this potentially fatal problem. Thiazides may precipitate hyponatremia since they increase sodium excretion without affecting the kidney's ability to concentrate urine.

Differences amongst thiazide and thiazide-like diuretics

Thiazide and thiazide-like drugs are well absorbed following oral administration and are eliminated by the kidney via secretion in the proximal tubule (Fig. 17.10). However, a significant fraction of doses of bendroflumethiazide, polythiazide and indapamide is also eliminated by metabolism. Chlorthalidone has a particularly prolonged action, such that it can be given on alternate days in the control of edema. Indapamide differs from other drugs in this class in that it lowers blood pressure at doses below those required to elicit a diuresis; an effect attributed to L-type calcium channel blockade. In addition, indapamide has less effect on uric acid secretion and glucose metabolism than other members of this group of diuretics (see Fig. 17.8).

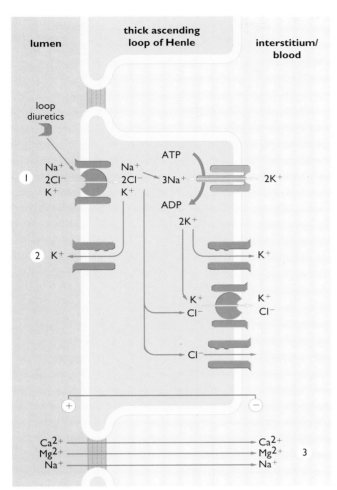

Fig. 17.11 Transport mechanism in the thick ascending loop of Henle. Loop diuretics block the Na$^+$/K$^+$/2Cl$^-$ cotransporter (1), thereby preventing the absorption and hence increasing tubular excretion of Na$^+$ and Cl$^-$. These drugs also decrease the potential difference across the tubule cell which is generated by the recycling of K$^+$ (2). As a result, increased excretion of Ca^{2+} and Mg^{2+} occurs because of inhibition of paracellular diffusion (3).

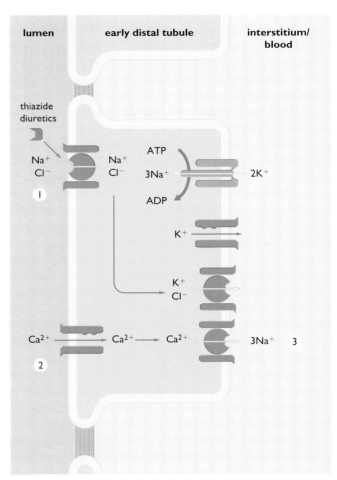

Fig. 17.12 Transport mechanisms in the early distal tubule. Thiazide diuretics increase the excretion of Na$^+$ and Cl$^-$ by inhibiting the Na$^+$/Cl$^-$ cotransporter (1). The reabsorption of Ca^{2+} (2) is increased by these drugs through a mechanism that may involve stimulation of Na$^+$/Ca^{2+} countertransport (3) due to an increase in the concentration gradient for Na$^+$ across the basolateral membrane.

Thiazides decrease Ca^{2+} excretion

In contrast with loop diuretics, thiazides decrease the excretion of Ca^{2+}, although the exact mechanism underlying this effect is uncertain. In the distal tubule, Ca^{2+} is reabsorbed from the lumen via an epithelial calcium channel (ECaC) that is distinct in structure and function from the L-type voltage-dependent calcium channel found in the heart and blood vessels. Entry of calcium is followed by exchange across the basolateral membrane via a Na$^+$/Ca^{2+} exchange countertransporter (Fig. 17.12). Since the intracellular concentration of Na$^+$ is reduced as a consequence of the primary molecular action of thiazide, the increase in the Na$^+$ concentration gradient across the basolateral membrane may be sufficient to enhance the removal of Ca^{2+} across the basolateral membrane via the Na$^+$/Ca^{2+} exchanger. There is a parallel here with the cellular mechanism by which digitalis affects intracellular Ca^{2+} in the heart in the treatment of heart failure (see Chapter 18), which also involves an indirect effect on the Na$^+$/Ca^{2+} exchanger secondary to a change in Na$^+$ homeostasis.

PHARMACOTHERAPEUTIC INDICATIONS FOR THIAZIDE DIURETICS include:

- Edema associated with congestive heart failure, hepatic cirrhosis, and nephrotic syndrome.
- Hypertension (see Chapter 18), where they are used either alone or in combination with other antihypertensive drugs. Clinical studies have shown that, when used alone to treat hypertension, the maximal daily dose of a thiazide diuretic should not exceed 25 mg of hydrochlorothiazide or equivalent for other thiazide or thiazide-like drugs. Higher doses produce a greater diuresis but with no proportional decrease in blood pressure, and have a greater risk of hypokalemia, which predisposes to cardiac arrhythmias such as *torsades de pointe* and ventricular fibrillation (see Chapter 18).
- Renal stone disease (nephrolithiasis) (see below).

351

Thiazide and loop diuretics cause metabolic alkalosis and hypokalemia

These effects are due to increased K^+ and H^+ secretion in the late distal tubule (connecting tubule) and collecting duct. There are two types of cells in the late distal tubule and collecting duct:

- Principal cells, which are sites for Na^+, K^+, and water transport.
- Intercalated cells, which are sites for H^+ secretion into the lumen (Fig. 17.13 and Fig. 17.14).

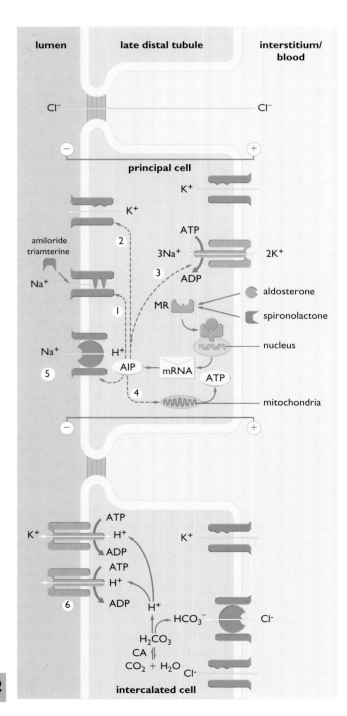

Fig. 17.13 Transport mechanisms in the late distal tubule and collecting duct, and mode of action of potassium-sparing diuretics. Amiloride and triamterene block apical Na^+ channels resulting in a diminished potential difference across the principal cell (lumen negative with respect to interstitium). The loss of potential results in a decreased driving force for K^+ secretion from the principal cell and H^+ secretion from the intercalated cell. The net effect is increased Na^+ excretion and decreased K^+ and H^+ excretion. Aldosterone binds to a cytoplasmic mineralocorticosteroid receptor (MR) resulting in stimulation of the synthesis of aldosterone-induced proteins (AIP), which (1) activate silent (nonfunctional) Na^+ channels; (2) increase the synthesis of K^+ channels; (3) increase the synthesis of Na^+/K^+ ATPase; (4) increase mitochondrial production of ATP; (5) increase the synthesis of the Na^+/H^+ countertransporter; and (6) increase the synthesis of H^+ ATPase. The overall effect of these changes is a decrease in Na^+ excretion and an increase in K^+ and H^+ excretion. Spironolactone, an aldosterone antagonist, has opposite effects. CA, carbonic anhydrase; this enzyme also catalyzes the formation of carbonic acid in principal cells which provide H^+ for Na^+/H^+ countertransport.

Na^+ reabsorption across the apical membrane of principal cells occurs mostly via Na^+ channels as opposed to transporters. This amiloride-sensitive epithelial sodium channel (ENaC) differs in structure and function from the voltage-regulated Na^+ channel in nerves and cardiac muscle. The epithelial Na^+ channels provide a high conductance pathway for Na^+ to move across the apical membrane and down the electrochemical gradient generated by Na^+/K^+ ATPase in the basolateral membrane (Fig. 17.13). The high permeability of the apical membrane to Na^+ results in depolarization of this membrane but not the basolateral membrane. This creates a potential difference across the cell with the lumen negative with respect to the interstitium. This potential difference provides a driving force for the secretion of K^+ into the tubular lumen. K^+ is transported into the cell by Na^+/K^+ ATPase and moves across the apical membrane via ROMK-1, an inwardly rectifying channel of the ROMK (rat outer medullary K^+ channel) family of K^+ channels. A proportion of K^+ that enters via Na^+/K^+ ATPase moves back across the basolateral membrane via K^+ channels.

The action of thiazides and loop diuretics result in an increase in apical Na^+ concentration in the late distal tubule and collecting duct. This increases K^+ secretion because:

- Increased Na^+ delivery results in enhanced Na^+ reabsorption that increases the lumen-negative potential, which is the driving force for K^+ secretion.
- Increased intracellular Na^+ concentration in the principal cell increases the activity of Na^+/K^+ ATPase; this increases uptake of K^+, which is then available for secretion.
- Increased flow in the distal parts of the nephron generated by the diuretics flushes away secreted K^+, thus maintaining the concentration gradient for further secretion.

In addition, thiazides and loop diuretics can cause contraction of extracellular fluid and a fall in blood pressure which activate the renin–angiotensin system (see Chapter 18). This system is the primary stimulus for the secretion of aldosterone a hormone that promotes the secretion of K^+ (see below).

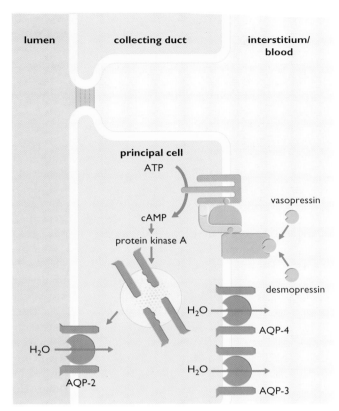

Fig. 17.14 The mechanism for controlling water permeability of the collecting duct. Vasopressin or its analog (e.g. desmopressin) bind to G protein-coupled V_2 receptors on the basolateral membrane of principal cells in the collecting duct. This, via activation of adenylyl cyclase and protein kinase A, leads to the migration of vesicles containing pre-formed water channels (aquaporin-2; AQP-2) to the apical membrane. AQP-2 channels are released from the vesicle and inserted into the membrane, thereby increasing water permeability. Water channels of the aquaporin 3 and 4 type (AQP-3, AQP-4) are present in the basolateral membrane to allow passage of water into the interstitium.

Intercalated cells are the site of H^+ secretion either via H^+ ATPase or a H^+/K^+ ATPase. The H^+ ions for these transport enzymes are generated by carbonic anhydrase (Fig. 17.13). In addition, there is an Na^+/H^+ countertransporter in principal cells that reabsorbs Na^+ in exchange for H^+. With regard to overall Na^+ reabsorption, Na^+/H^+ transport in the late distal tubule and collecting ducts is of minor importance compared with this transport system in the proximal tubule (see above). Secreted H^+ is buffered in the lumen by HCO_3^- and other ions such as HPO_4^{2-}.

Thiazide and loop diuretics produce a metabolic acidosis because of increased urinary loss of H^+ with a corresponding greater reabsorption of HCO_3^-. This occurs because:

- Increased Na^+ delivery to the distal tubule stimulates Na^+/H^+ exchange.
- The increased lumen-negative potential produced by increased Na^+ reabsorption enhances H^+ secretion by H^+ ATPase.
- Enhanced secretion of K^+, due to increased Na^+ reabsorption, increases the activity of H^+/K^+ ATPase.

- Elevated aldosterone secretion, due to extracellular volume reduction, produces increased expression of the transporters and enzymes involved in H^+ secretion (see Fig. 17.13).

Potassium-sparing diuretics

Potassium-sparing diuretics act on the late distal tubule and collecting duct

These drugs are divided into two groups:

- ENaC channel blockers, of which there are two, triamterene and amiloride. (These compounds are organic bases that do not contain the sulphonamide group; Fig. 17.5.)
- The aldosterone antagonists (e.g. spironolactone and its metabolite, potassium canrenoate) that block mineralocorticosteroid receptors, which are DNA-linked receptors (see Chapter 3). Spironolactone has a 4-ring structure that is characteristic of steroids (Fig. 17.5).

Both types of potassium-sparing diuretic drug have limited diuretic actions resulting in the loss of 2–3% of Na^+ filtered at the glomerulus, although the magnitude of the diuresis produced by aldosterone antagonists depends on the levels of aldosterone.

Blockade of apical Na^+ channels in principal cells by amiloride or triamterene reduces Na^+ movement across the apical membrane (Fig. 17.13). Amiloride also inhibits Na^+/H^+ exchange, although this occurs at concentrations much higher than are likely to be achieved during therapeutic use. The resultant lowering of intracellular Na^+ concentration by amiloride and triamterene reduces activity of basolateral Na^+/K^+ ATPase activity such that less Na^+ is pumped out and less K^+ moves in to the cells. The reduction in Na^+ movement across the apical membrane reduces the lumen-negative potential difference and consequently decreases the driving force for K^+ secretion. The net effect of these drugs is therefore to reduce Na^+ reabsorption and decrease K^+ secretion, hence the term potassium-sparing diuretics. The latter effect can, however, result in the development of hyperkalemia.

Amiloride and triamterene can cause metabolic acidosis

The diuretic action of amiloride and triamterene indirectly decreases H^+ secretion, which can cause metabolic acidosis. The reduction in the lumen-negative potential difference produced by these ENaC blockers decreases H^+ secretion via H^+ ATPase whilst the reduction in K^+ secretion decreases H^+ secretion via K^+/H^+ ATPase.

Aldosterone increases Na^+ reabsorption and K^+ and H^+ secretion

The cells of the late distal tubule and collecting duct contain cytoplasmic receptors for mineralocorticosteroids which, when bound to aldosterone, migrate to the nucleus and initiate DNA transcription, translation, and production of specific proteins (aldosterone-induced proteins). These proteins:

- Activate silent Na^+ channels (cause inactive channels present in the membrane to become functional conducting channels, although the exact mechanism for this effect is unclear).
- Increase the synthesis of K^+ channels.
- Increase the synthesis of Na^+/K^+ ATPase.

353

- Increase mitochondrial production of ATP.
- Increase the synthesis of the Na^+/H^+ antiporter (exchanger).
- Increase the synthesis of H^+ ATPase (see Fig. 17.13).

As a result of these actions, the net effect of aldosterone is to increase Na^+ reabsorption, and K^+ and H^+ secretion.

Spironolactone indirectly reduces Na^+ reabsorption and K^+ and H^+ secretion

Spironolactone competitively inhibits the binding of aldosterone to its receptor (Fig. 17.13), thus blocking stimulation of the synthesis of proteins that modify the transport functions of the late distal tubule and collecting duct. The effects of spironolactone are therefore to reduce Na^+ reabsorption and K^+ and H^+ secretion. The latter actions can lead to hyperkalemia and metabolic acidosis.

Mineralocorticoid receptors are expressed not only in epithelial cells but also in tissues such as brain, heart and blood vessels. Chronic stimulation of these receptors in heart and blood vessels by aldosterone has been shown to induce harmful effects such as fibrosis and hypertrophy. Spironolactone improves survival of patients with severe heart failure when added to conventional treatment, such as angiotensin-converting enzyme inhibitors. Such beneficial effects may owe more to blockade of nonepithelial receptors than blockade of epithelial receptors in the kidney.

Both amiloride and triamterene are effective when given orally and, whilst amiloride is eliminated predominately unchanged in the urine, triamterene is extensively metabolized to the active metabolite 4-hydroxytriamterene. Spironolactone is well absorbed following oral administration and is extensively metabolized in the liver (Fig. 17.10). It has a short half-life of 1.3 hours but is metabolized to the longer-acting active metabolite canrenone (half-life 17 hours), which prolongs the diuretic effect.

CLINICAL INDICATIONS Triamterene, amiloride, and spironolactone are used in combination with potassium-losing diuretics (thiazides and loop diuretics) to preserve K^+ balance. The inclusion of potassium-sparing diuretics in diuretic treatment is an alternative to the use of K^+ supplements with potassium-losing diuretics. Amiloride and triamterene are used in combination with thiazide and loop diuretics to treat edema associated with congestive heart failure and liver disease. One example of such a diuretic combination is 50 mg of triamterene plus 40 mg furosemide contained in one tablet with 0.5 to 2 tablets taken once daily. These drugs are also used in combination with thiazides for the treatment of hypertension (see Chapter 18) but only when hypokalaemia develops.

Aldosterone antagonists are useful in the treatment of:

- Primary aldosteronism (Conn's syndrome): a tumor of the adrenal gland that secretes large amounts of aldosterone which results in hypertension, hypokalemia and an increase in extracellular fluid. This condition can be managed by dietary Na^+ restriction and spironolactone (100–200 mg daily) although adverse effects limit long-term use of spironolactone (see Fig. 17.8). Surgical excision of the tumor is the usual treatment.

- Secondary aldosteronism: increased production of aldosterone in response to activation of the renin–angiotensin system that occurs in an accelerated phase of hypertension due to overproduction of renin or as a consequence of edema (see above).
- Chronic heart failure: primarily for extrarenal effects as discussed above.

Osmotic diuretics

Osmotic diuretics such as mannitol (given intravenously) and isosorbide (given orally) are freely filtered at the glomerulus and undergo little, if any, reabsorption. These are rare examples of drugs whose action does not involve a particular molecular target but is a general function of their physicochemical properties. Osmotic diuretics increase the osmotic pressure of tubular fluid, thereby reducing the reabsorption of water and lowering luminal Na^+ concentration, with a subsequent decrease in Na^+ reabsorption in the proximal tubule and descending loop of Henle. Osmotic diuretics increase the extracellular fluid volume by increasing water loss from intracellular compartments, and this increase inhibits renin release and decreases blood viscosity, which in turn increase renal blood flow. In addition, renal vasodilation and the subsequent increase in medullary blood flow produced by osmotic diuretics may involve the release of prostaglandins. The increase in medullary blood flow contributes to the overall diuretic effect by reducing medullary hypertonicity.

CLINICAL INDICATIONS Osmotic diuretics are rarely used because of the greater therapeutic effectiveness of other diuretics. However, they are sometimes used in the treatment of oliguria (see below), but not in the treatment of edema. If given to patients with heart failure, they may cause pulmonary edema

---

 Mechanisms of action of diuretic drugs

- Loop diuretics block the $Na^+/K^+/2Cl^-$ cotransporter in the thick ascending loop of Henle, resulting in the excretion of 15–25% of filtered Na^+
- Thiazide diuretics block the Na^+/Cl^- cotransporter in the distal convoluted tubule, resulting in the excretion of 5% of filtered Na^+
- Potassium-sparing diuretics increase the Na^+ excretion by 2–3% and decrease K^+ excretion by acting on the late distal tubule and collecting duct
- Potassium-sparing diuresis is produced by blockade of luminal Na^+ channels (e.g. with amiloride or triamterene) or by blockade of cytoplasmic mineralocorticosteroid receptors (e.g. with spironolactone)
- Osmotic diuretics reduce water reabsorption resulting in a subsequent decrease of Na^+ reabsorption in the proximal tubule and descending limb of the loop of Henle
- Carbonic anhydrase inhibitors indirectly block Na^+/H^+ exchange in the proximal tubule, which results in the excretion of up to 5% of Na^+ filtered at the glomerulus

as a result of extracting water from intracellular compartments and expanding the extracellular fluid volume. As a result of increasing the osmotic pressure of plasma, osmotic diuretics induce the movement of water out of the eye and brain. Such effects are used in the treatment of acute attacks of glaucoma and in the reduction of a raised intracranial pressure due to cerebral edema. These uses are unrelated to the renal actions of osmotic diuretics, with their useful effects disappearing following filtration in the kidney.

Polyuria

Polyuria is excessive production of a dilute urine and is usually accompanied by polydipsia (increased drinking). The main causes of polyuria are:

- Diabetes mellitus (see Chapter 15).
- Diabetes insipidus, which is caused either by a failure to produce sufficient vasopressin (central diabetes insipidus) or because the collecting ducts fail to respond to vasopressin (nephrogenic diabetes insipidus).

Vasopressin receptors and agonists

Vasopressin, also known as 8-arginine vasopressin (AVP) or antidiuretic hormone (ADH), is a nonapeptide released from the posterior pituitary in response to an increase in plasma osmolality or reductions in blood volume and/or arterial blood pressure (see Chapter 15). There are two subtypes of receptor for vasopressin, V_1 and V_2, and both are G-protein-linked. Stimulation of V_1 receptors produces smooth muscle contraction, particularly vascular smooth muscle. V_2 receptors mediate the effects of vasopressin on water permeability of the collecting duct. The affinity of V_2 receptors for vasopressin is greater than that of V_1 receptors and therefore cardiovascular effects are seen only at higher doses than those that affect renal function.

In addition to arginine vasopressin itself, other vasopressin agonists used to treat diabetes insipidus include:

- Lypressin (8 lysine vasopressin): a nonselective agonist with similar potency and duration of action to vasopressin, but administered as a nasal spray.
- Desmopressin (dDVAP, 1-deamino-8-D-arginine-vasopressin) which is approximately 3000 times more selective for V_2 receptors and has a longer duration of action (half-life 75 minutes) than vasopressin (half-life 10 minutes).

◼ Vasopressin increases the number of water channels (aquaporins) in the apical membrane of the collecting duct

Vasopressin increases the permeability of collecting ducts to water; whereas in its absence the collecting ducts are impermeable to water. Vasopressin binds to V_2 receptors on the basolateral membrane of principal cells of the collecting ducts (Fig. 17.14). These receptors are positively coupled to adenylyl cyclase and the resultant increase in cAMP activates protein kinase A. By ill-defined mechanisms, protein kinase A-induced protein phosphorylation triggers a shuttling of vesicles, which contain preformed water channels, to the apical membrane where there is exocytosis of the vesicles and insertion of the channels into the membrane. A further effect of activation of

protein kinase A is a decreased rate of removal of water channels from the membrane. The overall effect of V_2 receptor activation is increased numbers of water channels in the apical membrane, which results in elevated water permeability. As mentioned above, water channel proteins are called aquaporins and the protein inserted in the apical membrane of the collecting duct is a particular type designated aquaporin-2 (AQP-2). The basolateral membrane also contains water channels to allow movement of water into the interstitium; these channels are of the aquaporin-3 and -4 type (AQP-3 and AQP-4) (Fig. 17.14).

◼ Desmopressin is the drug of choice for central diabetes insipidus

Administration of desmopressin can distinguish central from nephrogenic diabetes insipidus, since the drug will increase urine osmolality in a patient with central diabetes insipidus but will have little or no effect in patients with the nephrogenic form of the disorder. Desmopressin administered via a nasal spray is the drug of choice for treating central diabetes insipidus and, for most patients, therapy is lifelong. The duration of effect from a single nasal dose (10–40 μg) is 6–20 hours and it has no vasoconstrictor effects, unlike arginine vasopressin and lypressin, due to its low affinity for V_1 receptors. In some patients nasal administration is not possible; for example, in patients with chronic allergic rhinitis. In such cases desmopressin can be given by oral or subcutaneous routes.

Lypressin is also administered as a nasal spray but has a short duration of action of 4–6 hours. Since it is a nonselective vasopressin agonist, lypressin can produce V_1 receptor-mediated effects, such as cutaneous vasoconstriction and increased intestinal activity manifest as belching and abdominal cramps. However, for patients who do not respond to desmopressin, lypressin is a viable alternative.

Arginine vasopressin is not used in long-term treatment of diabetes insipidus due to a short duration of action and to V_1 receptor-mediated effects. It is used as an alternative to desmopressin for evaluation of patients with suspected diabetes insipidus and for treatment of transient polyuria, when it is administered by intravenous infusion, or subcutaneous or intramuscular injection.

Some patients with polyuria are capable of releasing vasopressin but in inadequate amounts. Such patients are described as suffering from partial central diabetes insipidus, and can be treated with nonhormonal drugs such as chlorpropamide or carbamazepine. Both drugs potentiate the antidiuretic effect of residual vasopressin, but the molecular and cellular mechanisms responsible for this action are unclear.

◼ Nephrogenic (renal) diabetes insipidus is treated with a long-acting thiazide and indomethacin

In some patients, nephrogenic diabetes insipidus has been attributed to mutations in the V_2 receptor or aquaporin-2. The polyuria of nephrogenic diabetes insipidus can be controlled by long-acting thiazide diuretics (e.g. chlorothiazide) alone or in combination with amiloride. Addition of amiloride prevents the development of hypokalemia and is particularly useful in

355

the treatment of lithium-induced nephrogenic diabetes insipidus (see below). The cyclo-oxygenase inhibitor indomethacin also reduces the polyuria of diabetes insipidus and is used together with thiazide diuretics.

The paradoxical antidiuretic action of thiazides and that of indomethacin in nephrogenic diabetes insipidus are poorly understood:

- The response to thiazides begins with a reduction in effective circulating fluid volume and this may increase the oncotic pressure of plasma proteins and reduce the hydrostatic pressure in the peritubular capillaries of the proximal tubule. This would favor Na^+ and water reabsorption in this region of the nephron, with decreased fluid delivery to collecting ducts with reduction in polyuria.
- Indomethacin has been reported to decrease glomerular filtration rate and enhance fluid reabsorption from the proximal and distal tubules. In addition, it potentiates the effect of vasopressin on the principal cells of the collecting duct (prostaglandins attentuate the effect of vasopressin in patients with a partially effective V_2 receptor system). These effects of indomethacin are a consequence of inhibition of cyclo-oxygenase-1 (COX-1).

Syndrome of inappropriate vasopressin secretion

The syndrome of inappropriate (excess) vasopressin secretion consists of water retention, hyponatremia, and reduced plasma osmolality. The urine osmolality often exceeds that of the plasma. Although plasma Na^+ concentrations are diminished, Na^+ excretion in urine may be normal, and the patient is neither edematous, nor dehydrated. The causes of inappropriate (excess) vasopressin secretion include:

- Some tumors; for instance carcinomas of the bladder, prostate and pancreas.
- Pulmonary infections such as tuberculosis.
- Head injuries.

◼ *Treatment is with demeclocycline*

Treatment is with the tetracycline demeclocycline, which blunts the action of vasopressin on the collecting ducts. This action has been attributed to inhibition of adenylyl cyclase. The resulting fall in cAMP reduces aquaporin-2 insertion in the apical membrane with a decrease in water permeability and an increase in urine flow.

Diabetes insipidus

- This condition is characterized by polyuria
- It is due to either decreased production of vasopressin (central diabetes insipidus) or insensitivity to the renal effects of vasopressin (nephrogenic diabetes insipidus)
- Central diabetes insipidus is controlled by desmopressin (desamino vasopressin)
- Nephrogenic diabetes insipidus can be treated with thiazide diuretics

---

Renal stones (nephrolithiasis)

Renal stones develop when poorly soluble substances crystallize in the urine and the crystals aggregate to form particles large enough to lodge within the urinary system. Large stones in the upper urinary tract (renal pelvis and ureter) increase resistance to urine flow, resulting in back pressure that opposes glomerular filtration. Accordingly prolonged or severe obstruction results in functional impairment of the affected kidney.

◼ *Thiazide diuretics prevent Ca^{2+} stone formation*

Most renal stones are composed of calcium oxalate and/or calcium phosphate. Management of renal stones consists of removing the stones (by means of surgery or ultrasound) and by preventing further stone formation. Thiazide diuretics can be used to prevent stone formation because in the long term they diminish urinary excretion of Ca^{2+} (see above).

◼ *Allopurinol prevents uric acid stone formation*

Renal stone disease also results from precipitation of uric acid. In this case treatment with allopurinol, an inhibitor of xanthine oxidase, is beneficial because this drug reduces urinary uric acid levels and the incidence of stone formation (see also treatment of gout in Chapter 20). Oxalic acid stones can be caused by excess dietary oxalate, pyridoxine (vitamin B_6) deficiency, polyethylene glycol (antifreeze) intoxication, or may arise secondarily to gastrointestinal diseases such as inflammatory bowel disease.

◼ *D-penicillamine prevents cystine stone formation*

There are some rare inherited disorders associated with stone formation. Cystinuria is an autosomal recessive condition that impairs cystine, ornithine, arginine, and lysine transport in the proximal renal tubules. Cystine is much less soluble than the other dibasic amino acids whose transport is affected, and renal stones develop in homozygous individuals. These can be prevented by D-penicillamine, which by thiol exchange reacts with cystine to form a soluble penicillamine–cysteine product. (See Chapter 20 for more details on penicillamine.)

Uricosuric drugs

Gout is characterized by elevated plasma levels of uric acid that lead to precipitation of sodium urate crystals in tissues (see Chapter 20). This condition can be treated by drugs that facilitate urinary excretion of uric acid (uricosuric drugs). Uric acid is cleared from the blood mainly by glomerular filtration with some secretion into the proximal tubule. However, the bulk of uric acid in tubule fluid is reabsorbed by counter-transport systems in both the apical and basolateral membranes of tubule cells. These exchange urate for either organic or inorganic anions. Uricosuric drugs inhibit the transport of urate across the apical membrane.

The principal uricosuric drugs are probenecid and sulfinpyrazone, and these are useful in patients who have a low urine clearance of uric acid. To prevent urates from crystallizing in the early stage of uricosuric therapy, patients need to maintain a high fluid intake (2 liters/day) and to take sodium bicarbonate or potassium citrate to produce an alkaline urine (pH $\geq$ 6.0).

ADVERSE EFFECTS Uricosuric drugs should be avoided in patients who overproduce uric acid. Paradoxically, uricosuric drugs can cause gout in some patients and they should not be given during an acute attack.

Probenecid and sulfinpyrazone cause gastrointestinal disturbances and are contraindicated in patients with peptic ulceration. Probenecid blocks the renal tubule secretion of organic acid drugs, such as benzylpenicillin, which may prolong their effects and increase the risk of toxicity.

Oliguria

Oliguria describes a reduced urine volume. In normal adults, urine output is about 1.5 liters/24 h, but in oliguric patients urine volume is inappropriately low, generally less than 400 ml/24 h. When urine production falls to less than 50 ml/24 h, the patient is said to be anuric.

■ Oliguria is a clinical feature of acute renal failure

Severe hypoperfusion of the kidneys, acute damage to the tubules, or blockage of the urinary tract can each individually cause acute renal failure. Hypoperfusion of the kidney can be corrected by restoring the effective circulating volume, and obstruction of the urinary tract is rectified by surgery. In both situations, renal function usually returns to normal. If the tubule cells have been damaged, oliguria persists for 2–4 weeks before there is a recovery phase and a gradual return to normal renal function, which occurs in most patients.

■ No drugs prevent or treat acute renal failure, but mannitol or furosemide may be useful

At present, there are no satisfactory drugs for prevention or treatment of acute renal failure. However, diuretic therapy with either mannitol or furosemide may be of value if intratubular obstruction plays a role in the pathogenesis of renal dysfunction. These drugs increase renal blood flow and the diuresis they evoke helps to maintain tubule patency by eliminating debris from the tubule lumen. In order to produce diuresis in acute renal failure, doses of furosemide may need to be as high as 250 mg daily compared with doses of 20–80 mg that are used to relieve edema.

Many organs or body systems are adversely affected by acute renal failure and drugs may be used in the management of such secondary effects. For example:
- Antihypertensive drugs are used for hypertension (see Chapter 18).
- Anticonvulsant drugs are given to patients who develop seizures (see Chapter 14).
- H_2-antagonists have proved beneficial in preventing gastric ulceration (see Chapter 21).
- Antibacterial drugs may be used, as infections develop in many cases and are a major cause of morbidity and mortality.

Chronic renal failure

Chronic renal failure describes deteriorating renal function due to a loss of functional nephrons and is common to the later stages of all chronic renal disease. Common causes include:

- Severe hypertension.
- Diabetes mellitus.
- Glomerulonephritis.
- Obstruction of the urinary tract.

■ Drugs are used to treat the symptoms of chronic renal failure

The only effective treatments for chronic renal failure are chronic dialysis or renal transplants. However, drugs can be used to aid patient management and these include:
- Loop diuretics, used in an attempt to increase urine volume and Na^+ excretion.
- Acetazolamide, used to correct metabolic alkalosis associated with vomiting in renal failure.
- Antihypertensive drugs (see Chapter 18) to control the hypertension associated with chronic renal failure since they have been shown to reduce the rate of decline in renal function; angiotensin-converting enzyme inhibitors are particularly effective. Most patients with chronic renal failure have hypertension, which can damage the kidney, leading to proteinuria and hyperfiltration with subsequent loss of glomeruli.
- Antiemetics (see Chapter 14) to control the symptoms of nausea and vomiting experienced by many patients with late renal failure.
- Recombinant human erythropoietin to treat the anemia that develops following the loss of the major source of erythropoietin from the peritubular cells in the renal cortex. Erythropoietin stimulates the production of red blood cell precursors in the bone marrow (see Chapter 13).
- Hydroxylated derivatives of vitamin D (1α-hydroxycholecalciferol and 1,25-dihydroxycholecalciferol) to maintain plasma Ca^{2+} and prevent hyperparathyroidism. In chronic renal failure, vitamin D metabolism (see Chapter 15) is abnormal because there is impaired hydroxylation of 25-hydroxycholecalciferol to 1,25-dihydroxycholecalciferol within the kidney. As a result, absorption of dietary Ca^{2+} is reduced and plasma Ca^{2+} is low. Secondary hyperparathyroidism (see Chapter 15) then develops, which can lead to bone disease.

Drugs contraindicated in renal failure

Drugs should be prescribed with care in patients with impaired renal function because:
- There can be diminished excretion of drugs that are primarily excreted by the kidney. As a result, plasma drug concentrations may increase to dangerous levels.
- Some drugs are not effective when renal function deteriorates.
- The impairment of health resulting from renal failure may lower the threshold for adverse effects to drugs.

Examples of drugs that fall into these categories are given in Fig. 17.15. Nephrotoxic drugs should not be used in patients with renal disease, if possible, because the consequences of nephrotoxicity are likely to be more severe if the functional capacity of the kidney is already limited.

Key classes of drugs to be avoided or used with caution in renal failure		
	Drug	**Comment**
Sensitivity increases	Opioid analgesics	Morphine and its analogs may produce prolonged central nervous system (CNS) depression and unusual neurologic effects
	Anxiolytics/sedatives	Dosage should be reduced because of increased CNS sensitivity in severe renal failure
Reduced activity	Uricosuric agents	Probenecid and sulfinpyrazone are ineffective
	Antibacterial drugs	Nitrofurantoin and nalidixic acid fail to achieve effective concentrations in urine
Increased risk of toxicity	Cardiac glycosides	Reduced renal excretion of digoxin and increased risk of arrhythmias
	Potassium-sparing diuretics	Such drugs will aggravate the hyperkalemia of acute renal failure Potassium supplements are also contraindicated
	Antibacterial drugs	Increased risk of peripheral neuropathy with isoniazid and nitrofurantoin
Adverse effects poorly tolerated	Biguanide antihypoglycemics	Metformin increases the risk of lactic acidosis
	Tetracyclines	Tetracyclines, except doxycycline and minocycline, inhibit protein synthesis and induce a catabolic effect that results from increased metabolism of amino acids. This may aggravate renal failure

Fig. 17.15 Key classes of drugs to be avoided or used with caution in renal failure.

Glomerulonephritis

The term 'glomerulonephritis' is used to describe a range of kidney diseases characterised by inflammatory changes to the glomerulus. Typically, patients with glomerulonephritis exhibit both hematuria (blood in urine) and proteinuria, as well as diminished renal function, which is often associated with fluid retention, hypertension and edema. Glomerulonephritis occurs as a primary renal disease or may result from secondary involvement in a systemic disease such as systemic lupus erythematosis (Chapter 20). The causes of primary glomerulonephritis are unclear but many cases occur subsequent to bacterial or viral infection.

■ Drug therapy attempts to slow the progression of glomerulonephritis

Drug treatment of glomerulonephritis is similar to that used in management of the nephrotic syndrome (see above). There are no drug therapies that are effective in every form of glomerulonephritis, but in some patients, preservation of, or an improvement in, renal function may be achieved by:

- Antihypertensive drugs to control blood pressure. ACE inhibitors such as captopril are the drugs of choice because they decrease intraglomerular pressure and proteinuria.
- Thiazides or loop diuretics to reduce fluid retention.
- Immunosuppression with either glucocorticosteroids alone or in combination with cytotoxic drugs such as cyclophosphamide.

Dialysis and drug therapy

■ Dialysis may complicate drug therapy

Dialysis is the separation of diffusible from less diffusible solutes by use of a semipermeable membrane. This technique is used for patients with end-stage renal disease to remove waste products and excess water from the body. Furthermore, dialysis may be a useful adjunct to the management of drug overdose and poisoning.

There are two types of dialysis:

- Hemodialysis involves passage of blood through a system containing a dialysis solution separated from blood by an artificial semipermeable membrane.
- Peritoneal dialysis is performed by introducing the dialysis solution into the peritoneal cavity. In this case, the tissues within the peritoneal cavity act as the semipermeable membrane.

In both techniques, solutes diffuse from blood into the dialysis fluid.

Dialysis complicates drug therapy because drug is cleared from blood not only by the body's own elimination mechanisms but also by the process of dialysis. If clearance by dialysis makes a significant contribution to the overall elimination of drug from the body, it may be necessary to give supplementary doses of drug to replace the amount lost during dialysis.

The clearance of drugs by dialysis is dependent on the nature of the dialysis technique, the fraction of drug unbound in blood and its molecular size. Hemodialysis clears drugs more efficiently than peritoneal dialysis. Accordingly, it is the method of choice for therapy in drug overdose or poisoning. Only unbound drug contributes to the concentration gradient that drives diffusion from blood into the dialysis fluid; hence a high degree of plasma protein binding is a major constraint on clearance by dialysis. Most drugs used clinically are small enough to diffuse readily across either artificial or endogenous tissue membranes.

Nephrotoxic drugs

The kidney has a central role in the removal of drugs and/or their metabolites from the body. As a consequence, the kidney is susceptible to adverse drug effects because renal tissue is exposed to drug in blood and in the renal tubule. The concentration in the renal tubule can be much higher than in the blood and consequently more toxic. Many nephrotoxic drugs have their primary effects on discrete parts of the nephron. This results from factors such as regional differences in transport characteristics, cellular energetics, repair mechanisms, and capacity to bioactivate or detoxify potential toxins. The reasons for the selective renal toxicity of some drugs are still to be elucidated. The sites of action of some nephrotoxic drugs are shown in Fig. 17.16.

Antimicrobial drugs

Aminoglycosides, amphotericin B, and some of the first-generation cephalosporins are nephrotoxic.

Aminoglycosides play an important role in the treatment of severe Gram-negative infections, but 10–15% of patients who receive these drugs develop acute renal failure. The primary site of injury is the proximal tubule. The order of these drugs, in terms of toxicity, with the most toxic first, is gentamicin, tobramycin, amikacin, and netilmicin.

The systemic antifungal drug amphotericin B is also nephrotoxic. It has been estimated that about 80% of patients given amphotericin B develop impaired renal function. This drug causes renal vasoconstriction, and although several regions of the nephron are damaged by amphotericin B, the primary site of toxicity is the distal tubule.

Some first-generation cephalosporins (cephaloridine and cephalothin) are potential nephrotoxins, but they are not as toxic to the kidney as aminoglycosides and amphotericin B.

Antineoplastic drugs

Alkylating agents, platinum derivatives, and increased urate excretion due to cell destruction following cytotoxic therapy, can cause renal damage

Nephrotoxicity is a prominent feature of many alkylating agents. Cyclophosphamide and ifosfamide are metabolized to products that release acrolein, a nephrotoxic compound that induces hemorrhagic cystitis. This adverse effect can be prevented by the simultaneous administration of mesna (2-mercaptoethane sulfonate), which reacts with acrolein to render it nontoxic in the urinary tract.

The platinum derivatives, cisplatin and to a lesser degree carboplatin, are also nephrotoxic. Cisplatin-induced injury mainly affects the straight portion of the proximal tubule. To minimize renal damage due to these drugs, it is routine to hydrate the patient with an infusion of 1–2 liters of saline before the drug is administered.

The destruction of cells by antineoplastic drugs results in the release of large amounts of purines as a result of the breakdown of nucleic acids. Further catabolism of purines leads to excessive urate formation and excretion. Increased uric acid secretion leads to an increased risk of renal stone formation.

Immunosuppressant drugs

Cyclosporine and tacrolimus are markedly nephrotoxic

The structural basis for the nephropathy caused by cyclosporine and tacrolimus is unique, as both drugs adversely affect the renal vasculature. Most patients who receive cyclosporine develop an acute reversible impairment of renal function during early treatment. This is associated with afferent arteriolar vasoconstriction, which can be reversed by dopamine and

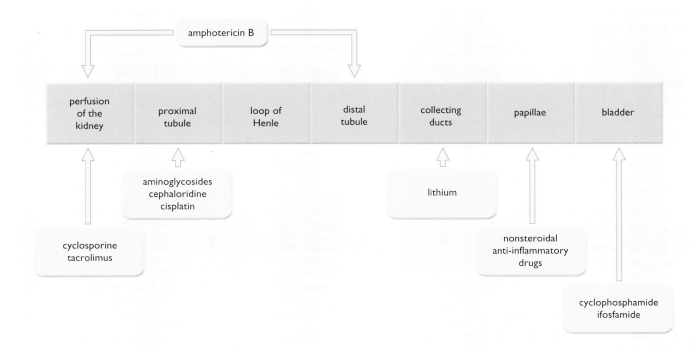

Fig. 17.16 Primary renal sites of action of some nephrotoxic drugs.

nifedipine. Chronic nephrotoxicity is also common among patients given cyclosporine and may result from damage to the afferent arteriole with sclerosis of downstream glomeruli.

Analgesics

Acetaminophen and nonsteroidal anti-inflammatory drugs can damage the kidney

Acute renal failure develops as a result of acute tubular necrosis in about 2% of patients who have taken an overdose of acetaminophen (paracetamol). Renal dysfunction is usually accompanied by severe hepatic failure, but in a few cases there is acute renal failure in the absence of hepatic damage. Acute renal failure arises several days after ingestion and is mainly oliguric in type.

Chronic nonsteroidal anti-inflammatory drug (NSAID)-induced nephropathy is characterized by interstitial nephritis and renal papillary necrosis. Renal damage results from long-term ingestion of NSAIDs and is unusual in patients under 30 years of age. It occurs mainly in women aged 40–60 years. The loss of papillary tissue may lead to secondary nephron damage and eventually to impaired renal function.

Lithium

A minority of patients who are treated with lithium for affective disorders develop nephrogenic diabetes insipidus, which is usually reversible on stopping the drug. The mechanism for this effect is a reduction in V_2 receptor-mediated stimulation of adenylyl cyclase by vasopressin. Amiloride can be used to reverse lithium-induced diabetes insipidus by inhibiting reabsorption of lithium through Na^+ channels in the collecting ducts.

Some drugs can cause acute interstitial nephritis

Many drugs can lead to an acute deterioration of renal function by causing inflammation of the renal interstitium (acute interstitial nephritis), which may be due to a hypersensitivity reaction. These drugs include:

- Penicillins.
- Sulfonamides (including co-trimoxazole).
- NSAIDs.
- Diuretics (thiazides and furosemide).
- Allopurinol.
- Cimetidine.

Patients often have a fever, skin rash, and hematuria.

FURTHER READING

Brenner BM (ed.) *Brenner and Rector's The Kidney, vols 1 and 2*, 6th edn. Philadelphia: WB Saunders; 2000. [A comprehensive reference text on renal physiology, pathophysiology, and the treatment of renal diseases.]

Couser, WG. Glomerulonephritis. *Lancet* 1999; **353**: 1509–1515. [An excellent review of the pathogenesis and treatment of glomerulonephritis.]

Greger RF, Knauf H, Mutschler E (eds) *Diuretics: Handbook of Experimental Pharmacology*, vol 117. Berlin: Springer-Verlag; 1995. [A review of renal physiology coupled with a detailed analysis of the development, pharmacodynamics, pharmacokinetics, and clinical use of each class of diuretic agent.]

Hook JB, Goldstein RS (eds) *Toxicology of the Kidney*, 2nd edn. New York: Raven Press; 1993. [A detailed review of the adverse effects of chemicals on the kidney.]

Klahr S, Miller SB. Acute oliguria. *N Engl J Med* **338**: 1998; 671–675. [A succinct review of the causes of oliguria, its prevention and management.]

Lote CJ. *Principles of Renal Physiology*, 4th edn. Dordrecht, The Netherlands: Kluwer Academic; 2000. [A clear and concise introduction to renal physiology.]

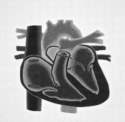

Chapter 18

Drugs and the Cardiovascular System

PHYSIOLOGY OF THE CARDIOVASCULAR SYSTEM

■ *The cardiovascular system is composed of the heart and the blood vessels*

The heart is a pump that supplies the body with blood, which is distributed throughout the body by blood vessels. The cardiovascular system provides a blood supply that maintains an optimal environment for the body tissues by supplying oxygen and nutrients and removing waste products. The normal partial pressures of oxygen and carbon dioxide in oxygenated arterial blood are:

- pO_2 100 mmHg.
- pCO_2 40 mmHg.

The human heart contracts about 70 times every minute and pumps approximately 7000 liters (5 liters/min) of blood every day. In adults, the heart weighs approximately 300 g. It has four chambers: two smaller ones, located towards the base called the atria, and two larger ones, located towards the apex, called ventricles (Fig. 18.1). The wall of the heart chambers is made up of three layers: the epicardium (outer layer), the mid-myocardium (the middle layer), and the endocardium (the inner layer).

■ *A series of valves ensures that blood flows only in one direction*

The right atrium and ventricle receive deoxygenated blood from the body, and pump it into the pulmonary artery to the lungs. The left atrium and ventricle receive the re-oxygenated blood via the pulmonary veins and pump it out through the aorta to the rest of the body. The location and names of the valves are shown in Fig. 18.1.

Heart valves

- Valves prevent the backward flow of blood through the heart
- Atrioventricular valves are sited between the atria and the ventricles
- Backflow into arteries is prevented by semilunar valves
- Artificial valves can replace valves damaged by diseases such as rheumatic fever

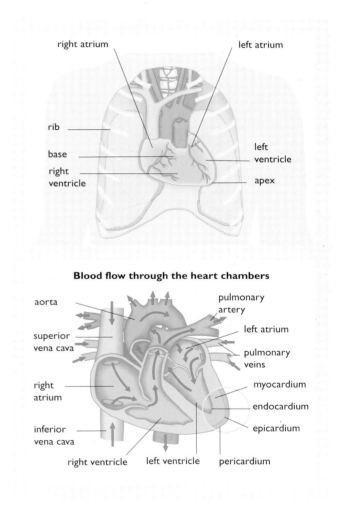

Blood flow through the heart chambers

Fig. 18.1 The heart consists of four chambers and is located in the chest cavity. The direction of blood flow through the heart is shown.

Vascular tree

The body's vascular system is often referred to as a vascular tree. There are two main types of blood vessel, namely arteries and veins, each with a lining of endothelial cells which are in contact with the blood. The endothelium is more than a simple barrier between the blood and the surrounding vessel, as it releases many important vasoactive substances (e.g. nitric oxide) that affect vessel diameter and blood clotting, thereby locally regulating blood flow (Fig. 18.2).

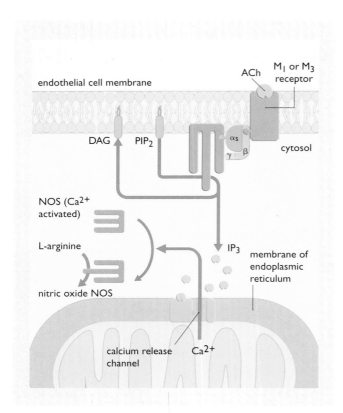

Fig. 18.2 Example of release of vasoactive substance (here, nitric oxide) from endothelium. Acetylcholine (ACh), bradykinin, thrombin, serotonin, shear stress, and other substances can release nitric oxide. ACh utilizes numerous intermediates in the cellular response that ultimately facilitates nitric oxide release. (DAG, diacylglycerol; NOS, nitric oxide synthase; IP$_3$, inositol-1,4,5-triphosphate; PIP$_2$, phosphatidylinositol)

Normal resting systolic/diastolic blood pressure is approximately 120/80 mmHg

Blood pressure in a vessel is generated by, and is proportional to, the output of the heart (cardiac output) and the resistance to flow in the arterioles. Resistance depends on factors such as vessel caliber, elasticity, geometry, and blood viscosity. Arterial blood pressure is expressed as systolic pressure/diastolic pressure and the usual normal value is 120/80 mmHg. Peak blood pressure occurs during systole which is when the left ventricle contracts and pumps blood into the aorta. The trough occurs during diastole when the left ventricle relaxes and fills with blood returning to the heart (Fig. 18.3). As blood flows through the body's circulatory system the mean blood pressure falls from approximately 90 mmHg, to about 5 mm Hg in the major central veins. Blood pressure is intermediate in the capillaries, which are small vessels that connect arterioles and venules. Nutrients and metabolites leave and enter the vasculature through capillary membranes.

Cardiac electrophysiology

The unequal distribution of K$^+$, Na$^+$, Cl$^-$ and Ca^{2+} across ventricular and atrial cell membranes results in a resting (diastolic) membrane potential of approximately −85 to −90 mV. In sinoatrial (SA) and atrioventricular (AV) nodal tissue, the membrane potential value is unstable and during diastole the minimum value it attains is more positive than that in other atrial or ventricular cells. Resting membrane potential stays at these levels because of the K$^+$ gradient, there being a high concentration of K$^+$ inside the cell relative to outside. This gradient is maintained by the Na$^+$/K$^+$ pump (also known as Na$^+$/K$^+$ ATPase, see Chapter 3) and because during diastole the membrane is more permeable to K$^+$ than to other ions.

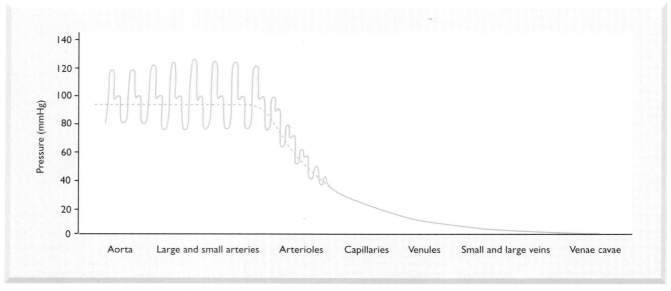

Fig. 18.3 Blood pressure in various blood vessel types. Systolic and diastolic blood pressures are shown, as well as mean arterial pressure. (Adapted from *Principles of Anatomy and Physiology*, 8th edn, by Tortora and Grabowski. This material is used by permission of John Wiley & Sons, Inc.)

The Na$^+$/K$^+$ pump moves three Na$^+$ ions outward in exchange for two K$^+$ ions inward (i.e. it is an electrogenic pump, Fig. 18.4).

■ An action potential is generated when an atrial or ventricular cell is depolarized sufficiently quickly to approximately –70 mV

The upstroke of the action potential (Fig. 18.5) is due to opening of Na$^+$ channels with voltage-dependent gates, with channel opening being triggered by depolarization (see Chapter 3). Activation of these Na$^+$ channels is transient and, if the membrane remains depolarized for more than a few milliseconds, the channel inactivates and the inward current terminates. Such inactivation results in a period during which a second action potential cannot be triggered. This is known as the effective refractory period.

The characteristic plateau phase of the cardiac ventricular action potential results from an influx of Ca^{2+} through L-type Ca^{2+} channels leading to an inward current balanced by an outward current. These channels, like the Na$^+$ channels, are voltage-dependent, but the resulting current has a much slower time course. The currents that arise from the opening of Na$^+$ and Ca^{2+} channels are therefore often referred to as:

- The fast inward Na$^+$ current (I_{Na}).
- The slow inward Ca^{2+} current (I_{Ca} or I_{si}).

During the depolarization phase of the action potential, other voltage-dependent channels are activated, particularly a variety of different types of K$^+$ channel. These carry K$^+$ ions in the out-

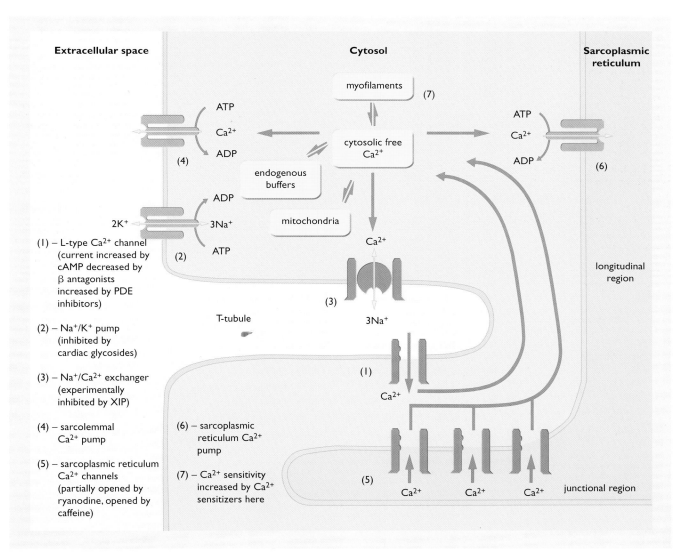

Fig. 18.4 Ion transport pathways in the heart, focusing on Ca^{2+} movements during the cardiac cycle. Membrane depolarization at the start of the action potential is the trigger for the opening of Ca^{2+} channels which span the surface membrane (sarcolemma). The local increase in Ca^{2+} concentration in the interior of the cell (cytosol) causes further release of Ca^{2+} from the intracellular stores (sarcoplasmic reticulum). Some Ca^{2+} may also enter the cell via the Na$^+$/Ca^{2+} exchanger. Once inside the cytosol, Ca^{2+} is bound to endogenous buffers, which include the inner surface of the sarcolemma and the contractile machinery (myofilaments; not shown functioning in this mode), which are activated by the presence of Ca^{2+}, leading to contraction. At the end of the action potential, Ca^{2+} leaves the cell by the Na$^+$/Ca^{2+} exchanger, and is also taken up again into the sarcoplasmic reticulum by ATP-driven Ca^{2+} pumps. (PDE, phosphodiesterase; XIP, exchanger inhibitory peptide)

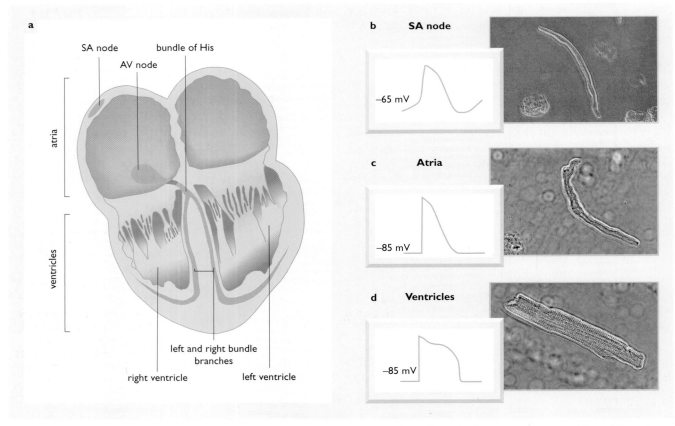

Fig. 18.5 Regional variation in cell structure and action potential configuration throughout the heart. Action potential from different heart regions are quite different due to differences in the ion channels that underlie action potentials in these regions. (a) Location of the sinoatrial (SA) node, the atrioventricular (AV) node, and the bundle of His. (b) An action potential from the SA node and an SA node cell. (Courtesy of Dr Hilary F. Brown.) (c) An action potential from the atria and an atrial cell. (d) An action potential from the ventricles and a ventricular cell.

Cardiac K⁺ currents

- Delayed rectifier current (I_K), which is activated by depolarization and has two components (r and s)
- Transient outward current (I_{to}) which causes the initial repolarization phase, referred to as the 'notch' of the action potential, which is important in some, but not all, regions of the heart
- Inward rectifier current (I_{K1}), with a main role of stabilizing the resting membrane potential
- ATP-sensitive current ($I_{K(ATP)}$), which is blocked by basal levels of ATP, and is therefore important when ATP is reduced (e.g. in disease conditions such as ischemia)

ward direction, which causes repolarization of the membrane potential.

The heart's normal beating starts as a result of spontaneous depolarization (pacemaker activity) in specialized cells in the sinoatrial (SA) node

The SA node in humans (Fig. 18.5) rhythmically fires impulses approximately 70–80 times/min, a rate that is faster than that for any other region of the heart. The node is innervated by autonomic nerves; release of acetylcholine from the vagus nerve decreases the rate of firing while norepinephrine increases it. The SA node action potential is conducted rapidly through the atria, and then delayed at the AV node for about 70 milliseconds (msec) because of the small diameter of the fibers and the dependence of conduction on I_{si} at this location. The AV node is the only electrical connection between the atria and the ventricles; it controls the movement of action potentials from the atria to the ventricles. Once in the ventricle, the action potential is then rapidly conducted through the left and right branches of the bundle of His (described by His in 1893; see Fig. 18.5), from where it spreads throughout the ventricular mass through a conduction network known as the Purkinje fibers (described by Purkinje in 1845) to finally reach all the ventricular muscle.

Ventricular and SA node action potentials are quite different in shape (height and width) because the currents that cause them (produced by the opening and closing of ion channels) are not exactly the same (Figs 18.6, 18.7).

Excitation is coupled to contraction in atria and ventricles

One of the most important events in the cardiac action potential is the voltage-dependent opening of L-type Ca^{2+} channels (see

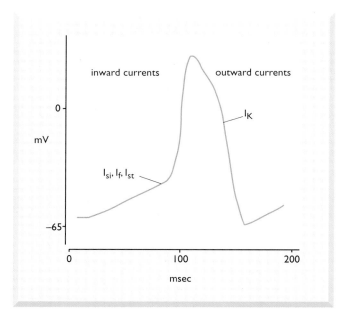

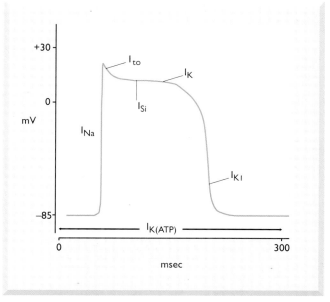

Fig. 18.6 Ion channels and currents (I) underlying the sinoatrial node action potential. (I_{si}, an inward current carried by Ca^{2+} ions; I_f, 'funny' or hyperpolarization-activated cation current that may have a role in pacemaking and is carried by Na^+ and Ca^{2+} ions; I_{st}, the sustained inward Na^+ current that may be important in pacemaker activity; I_K, the delayed rectifier current which is an outward K^+ current; note that there is no I_{Na}, the inward Na^+ current, or I_{K1}, the inward rectifier K^+ current)

Fig. 18.7 Configuration of a typical ventricular action potential showing the activation of the most important ionic currents. (I_{Na}, fast inward Na^+ current; I_{si}, slow inward Ca^{2+} current; I_{to}, transient outward K^+ current; I_K, delayed rectifier K^+ current; I_{K1}, inward rectifier K^+ current; $I_{K(ATP)}$, ATP-sensitive K^+ current; note, the last of these is activated only during ischemia or hypoxia)

Chapter 3). This leads to a relatively small inward movement of Ca^{2+} ions across the sarcolemmal membrane, which in turn activates a process known as Ca^{2+}-induced Ca^{2+} release, whereby a small increase in intracellular Ca^{2+} triggers a much larger amount of Ca^{2+} to be released from intracellular stores (i.e. sarcoplasmic reticulum). As a result, intracellular Ca^{2+} rises from 100 nM at rest (diastole) to 10 μM during contraction. As the cytosolic Ca^{2+} concentration rises, Ca^{2+} binds to troponin C, which regulates the position of actin and myosin filaments, causing them to slide past one another, leading to contraction.

After contraction, Ca^{2+} is re-sequestered into the stores by an adenosine triphosphate (ATP)-dependent Ca^{2+} pump, whereupon it is ready to take part in the next cycle. In addition, Ca^{2+} is extruded from the cell during diastole via the electrogenic Na^+/Ca^{2+} exchanger. This exchanges one Ca^{2+} ion out of the cell for the inward movement of three Na^+ ions, thereby generating an inward current (note, however, that the direction of exchange can change during the action potential and may be affected in disease states by changes in intracellular concentration of Na^+). Figure 18.4 shows schematically how cell Ca^{2+} is controlled, as well as how drugs may modulate the processes involved.

The sequence of events during one heart beat, also known as the cardiac cycle, takes place in the following order:
- Depolarization of the atria.
- Right atrial contraction and generation of pressure which ejects blood through the open tricuspid valve into the right ventricle.

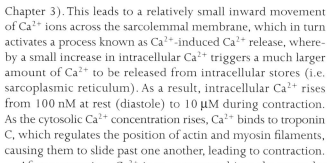

Pharmacologic tools used to block ion channels experimentally

- Tetrodotoxin to block I_{Na}
- Nicardipine to block I_{st}
- 4-Aminopyridine to block I_{to}
- Tetraethylammonium to block I_K
- Barium to block I_{K1}
- Glyburide to block $I_{K(ATP)}$

- Left atrial contraction and generation of pressure which ejects blood through the open mitral valve into the left ventricle.
- After a short interval, ventricular depolarization and contraction, with left ventricular contraction preceding right ventricular contraction.
- When the pressure in the right and left ventricles increases, this opens the pulmonary valve and the aortic valve, respectively, allowing ejection of blood into the pulmonary artery and aorta.

■ *The electrocardiogram is a recording from the surface of the body of the electrical changes that result from the heart's electrical activity*

The electrocardiogram (ECG or EKG) records the average signal of the depolarizations and repolarizations occurring in all the cardiac myocytes. It can be recorded on the surface of the body using electrodes.

An understanding of the normal EKG (see Fig. 18.9a) is essential before considering treatment of cardiac arrhythmias. The sequence of events in the normal EKG is the following:

- The P wave corresponds with atrial contraction.
- The PR interval is the time from the beginning of the P wave to the beginning of the QRS complex. It is equivalent to the time taken for electrical activity to propagate through the AV node.
- The QRS complex represents ventricular depolarization; atrial repolarization is hidden beneath this large complex.
- The T wave corresponds with ventricular repolarization.
- The ST segment is the interval between the QRS complex and the T wave, and its position above or below the baseline is characteristically changed during ischemia (so-called elevation or depression of the ST segment).
- The QT interval is the time from the start of the QRS complex to the end of the T wave and represents the ventricular depolarization to repolarization interval.

PATHOPHYSIOLOGY AND DISEASES OF THE HEART

Arrhythmias

Arrhythmia literally means no rhythm, whereas dysrhythmia means an abnormal heart rhythm. In practice, both terms are used interchangeably to mean an abnormal or irregular heart beat. There are many underlying causes of arrhythmias, such as acute myocardial infarction (see page 383 and Chapter 15) and adverse effects of therapeutic drugs (paradoxically this includes many antiarrhythmic drugs).

Arrhythmias may be classified according to their anatomic origin:

- Supraventricular (originating in the SA node, atria or AV node).
- Ventricular (originating in the ventricles).

Arrhythmias range from asymptomatic (some supraventricular arrhythmias) to life-threatening, (i.e., asystole and some fast ventricular arrhythmias). Lethal ventricular arrhythmias are the most common cause of death in the USA and in other economically developed countries, with around 350,000 such deaths every year in the USA alone. Sudden cardiac death, that is, without prior symptoms, or symptoms of less than 30 minutes, duration, is primarily a euphemism for lethal ventricular arrhythmias; ventricular fibrillation (most commonly) or asystole (in a minority of cases) occur without warning, and usually out of hospital.

■ *Myocardial ischemia is an important cause of serious ventricular arrhythmias*

Myocardial ischemia means lack of blood flow in a region of the heart and occurs clinically when, for example, a coronary artery becomes obstructed by a clot arising as a result of thrombosis in the setting of arteriosclerosis. As a result, insufficient blood reaches the myocardium to meet the tissues' needs for oxygen and nutrients, and removal of metabolic waste. If the region of myocardium (especially within the ventricles) rendered ischemic is sufficiently large, arrhythmias may occur, with the time course after onset of ischemia shown in Fig. 18.8. The molecular and cellular causes of an ischemia-induced arrhythmia are not clear. Possibilities include accumulation of extracellular K^+ (which contributes to diastolic depolarization and abnormal repolarization) and activation of cyclic adenosine monophosphate (cAMP) production which may trigger spontaneous action potentials. Perhaps surprisingly, there are no therapeutic drugs that specifically target these changes to suppress arrhythmias.

Reperfusion, which means removal of obstruction of coronary flow to the previously ischemic region, is essential if the tissue is to recover and cell death (infarction) is to be avoided. However, early reperfusion, especially after a brief (less than 30 minutes) period of ischemia can itself cause arrhythmias.

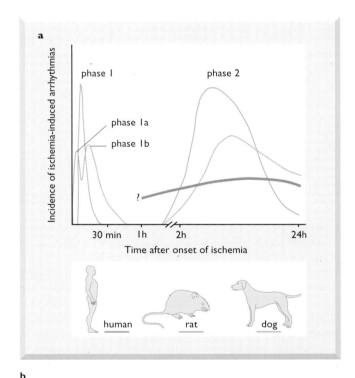

Possible mediators of ischemia-induced arrhythmogenesis

Angiotensin II	Opioids
Endothelin	Palmitoyl carnitine
Histamine	Platelet activating factor
5-Hydroxytryptamine	Extracellular K^+
Leukotrienes	Prostaglandins
Lysophosphatidyl choline	Protons
Norepinephrine	Thromboxane A_2

Fig. 18.8 Time course of ventricular arrhythmias due to ischemia in mammalian hearts. (a) There are two main phases of arrhythmias, phase 1 and phase 2. In the dog, phase 1 arrhythmias may be further subcategorized into phase 1a and 1b arrhythmias. Very little is known about phase 1 arrhythmias in the human, but they are thought to exist. (b) Possible mediators of ischemia-induced arrhythmogenesis.

Ischemia

- Ischemia resulting from a reduced blood flow is associated with contractile failure, EKG abnormalities, and chest pain
- Silent ischemia is characterized by contractile failure and EKG abnormalities without chest pain
- Myocardial infarction occurs if sustained ischemia results in cell death
- Stunning is a reversible impairment of cardiac or vascular function that is detectable during the first few hours or days after the start of reperfusion
- Hibernation myocardium occurs if the myocardial function is depressed during relative ischemia. It preserves energy substrates, thereby aiding recovery when reperfusion occurs
- Preconditioning is caused by a short period of ischemia and describes the resulting protection (from arrhythmias and contractile dysfunction) afforded to the heart against the effects of a longer period of ischemia

Arrhythmias are defined according to their EKG configuration

Diagnosis of arrhythmias (Fig. 18.8) depends on the appearance of the EKG:

- A flat-line EKG is indicative of asystole.
- SA nodal re-entry is associated with a normal EKG configuration, but an abnormally rapid rate.
- Atrial premature beats appear on the EKG as abnormal P waves and are often asymptomatic.
- Atrial flutter is a condition, common in the elderly, in which the atria beat rapidly (>300 beats/min) and is often complicated by AV block (resulting from the ability of the normal AV node to filter incoming high frequency impulses) so that not every atrial beat is conducted to the ventricles. In the EKG, the P waves are repetitive and tend to vary in frequency.
- Atrial fibrillation, also common in the elderly and in people with mitral valve disease, occurs when the atria beat asynchronously so that the active pumping function of the atria is impaired. In the EKG, the P waves are generally not recognizable.
- Paroxysmal supraventricular tachycardia is a rhythm disorder originating from a region of injury and slow conduction in the AV node. It can result in retrograde conduction through the node and tachycardia in the atria. In itself this is not life-threatening but it can become so if it sustains a dangerously rapid ventricular rate.
- Ventricular premature beats (VPBs, Fig. 18.9b) are sometimes referred to as ventricular ectopic beats, and are defined as discrete and identifiable premature QRS complexes (usually of an abnormal shape).
- Ventricular tachycardia (Fig. 18.9c) is defined as a run of consecutive VPBs (an arbitrary number, usually a minimum of four, but note that some cardiologists chose any number between two and more than 10 when defining and diagnosing this arrhythmia). Sustained ventricular tachycardia

may cause marked hemodynamic effects in some patients, such as hypotension, yet have relatively little effect in others.
- Ventricular fibrillation (Fig. 18.9d) is a lethal arrhythmia if it lasts for more than a few minutes since the heart stops pumping blood with this arrhythmia. Ventricular fibrillation may be defined as a signal from which individual EKG deflections vary in size and frequency on a cycle-to-cycle basis (although cardiologists tend to use a variety of different definitions).
- *Torsades de pointes*, (a French term meaning 'twisting of peaks' because of its characteristic EKG appearance), is a syndrome characterized by a clinically serious ventricular arrhythmia similar to fibrillation, with rapid asynchronous complexes and an undulating baseline on the EKG, which is spontaneously reversible (unlike ventricular fibrillation which usually is not). A risk of *torsades de pointes* is usually associated with a prolonged QT interval in the EKG, which may be

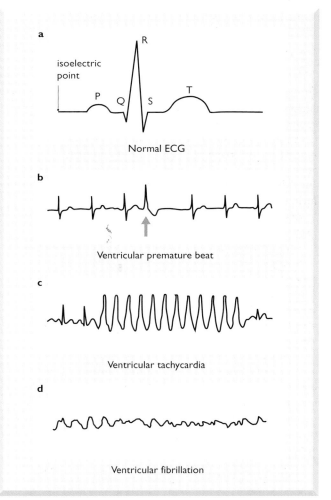
Fig. 18.9 Electrocardiograms (EKGs or ECGs). (a) The normal EKG. (b) Ventricular premature beats. (c) Ventricular tachycardia. (d) Ventricular fibrillation. Note that in (a), the P wave represents depolarization of the atria, the QRS complex reflects depolarization of the ventricles, and the T wave, repolarization of the ventricles. Arrhythmias are manifest as abnormalities in the configuration of the EKG. Arrhythmias are defined according to the Lambeth Conventions.

congenital (in congenital long QT syndrome) or drug induced (e.g. by class Ia and class III antiarrhythmics, see Fig. 18.13). Induction of *torsades de pointes* is facilitated by several predisposing factors: hypokalemia, bradycardia, and the administration of numerous drugs.

- Wolff–Parkinson–White syndrome is due to a congenital, accessory connection between the atrium and the ventricle known as the bundle of Kent. This connection allows impulses to be conducted quickly from the atria to the ventricles and bypass the AV node. It is diagnosed from the EKG as a short PR interval followed by a 'delta wave' on the wide QRS complex, and it may give rise to atrial fibrillation.

Mechanisms for arrhythmias

At the cardiac electrophysiologic system level, most arrhythmias are initiated by abnormal impulse (action potential) generation and the rest are initiated by abnormal impulse conduction. Abnormal impulse generation can be spontaneous, or triggered by a normal beat (Fig. 18.10). All arrhythmias are maintained by abnormal impulse conduction, and all arrhythmias except parasystole are maintained by re-entry (Fig. 18.11). Abnormal impulse initiation and conduction are the system targets for antiarrhythmic drugs.

AUTOMATIC ABNORMAL IMPULSE GENERATION Automaticity describes the development of an ectopic (out of place) focus of arrhythmia generation and there are two types:

- That occurring in tissues capable of automatic impulse generation under normal conditions (enhanced normal automaticity).
- That occurring in atrial or ventricular tissue—not normally automatic (abnormal automaticity).

Mechanisms of arrhythmogenesis
Abnormal impulse generation
Automatic rhythms Enhanced normal automaticity Abnormal automaticity
Triggered rhythms Early after-depolarizations Delayed after-depolarizations
Abnormal impulse conduction
Conduction block First-, second- or third-degree block
Re-entry Circus movement Reflection

Fig. 18.10 **Mechanisms of arrhythmogenesis.**

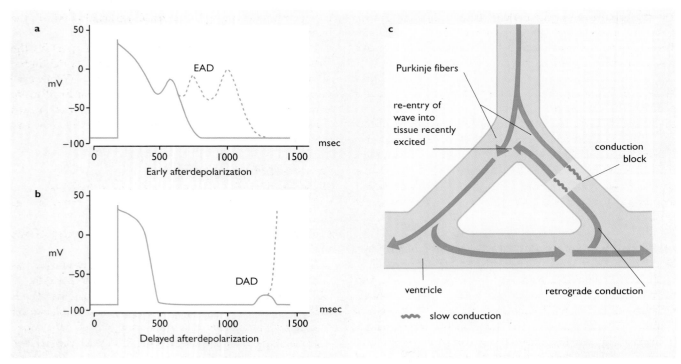

Fig. 18.11 **Main mechanisms of arrhythmogenesis.** (a) Early after-depolarizations (EADs) occur during the repolarization phase of the action potential. The dotted line indicates repetitive EADs. (b) Delayed after-depolarizations (DADs) occur after repolarization of the action potential, during diastole. The dotted line shows an action potential generated from a DAD. (c) Unidirectional block. The impulse moves from the sinoatrial node to the atrioventricular node and then into the Purkinje fibers, from where it passes into the mass of ventricular tissue. However, conduction is blocked in an area of ischemia in a unidirectional fashion; this allows retrograde conduction of an impulse from the ventricle back into the Purkinje fibers, hence re-exciting tissue that has passed through its refractory period and is excitable once more.

Under normal conditions the subsidiary (slow) pacemakers (the AV node, the His bundles, and Purkinje fibers) are suppressed by the faster rate of the SA node ('overdrive suppression'). This normally prevents potential ectopic foci from becoming dominant. During pathologic processes such as ischemia, however, abnormal automaticity often arises in the Purkinje fibers, which may become partially depolarized, giving rise to a faster rate of automaticity. Local release of catecholamines, as occurs during ischemia, can enhance this automaticity. Examples of arrhythmias likely to be caused by automaticity are:

- Nodal tachycardias.
- VPBs associated with developing myocardial infarction.

TRIGGERED ABNORMAL IMPULSE GENERATION Triggered activity is a form of abnormal automaticity and can also be of two types:

- Early after-depolarizations (EADs).
- Delayed after-depolarizations (DADs, Fig. 18.11).

Impulses are triggered by the previous 'normal' impulse. EADs occur during the repolarization phase of the action potential (i.e. during phase 2 or 3), whereas DADs occur after the action potential has ended (i.e. during phase 4).

Early after-depolarizations are associated with an abnormally prolonged action potential

EADs are facilitated by bradycardia and drugs that prolong the action potential duration (for example, this includes pro-arrhythmic effects of class III antiarrhythmics; see page 374). The mechanism underlying EADs is not known. It may involve a decrease in the repolarizing delayed rectifier K⁺ (I_K) current. There is experimental evidence that EADs may initiate *torsades de pointes* and reperfusion-induced arrhythmias.

Delayed after-depolarizations typically occur as a result of cellular Ca²⁺ overload

DADs typically occur as a result of cellular Ca^{2+} overload, as may occur during ischemia, reperfusion, or digitalis intoxication. It is believed that this leads to an oscillatory release of Ca^{2+} from the sarcoplasmic reticulum. This then leads to the production of an inward current (resulting in the DAD), which may be carried by the Na^+/Ca^{2+} exchanger (the transient inward current, I_{TI}).

ABNORMAL IMPULSE CONDUCTION Conduction block (heart block) and re-entry are examples of abnormal conduction.

The most common site of heart block is the AV node, and the block is called first-, second-, or third-degree, as follows:

- In first-degree AV block conduction through the AV node is slowed. This is manifested on the EKG as a prolonged PR interval.
- In second-degree AV block some of the impulses generated in the SA node are not conducted to the ventricles (i.e. a beat is missed) and, on the EKG, no QRS complex follows those P waves.
- In third-degree AV block, which is clinically the most serious type, there is a complete block of conduction through the AV node, with no impulses being conducted to the ventricles. This generally leads to a slow ventricular escape rhythm that may not maintain adequate cardiac output. Abnormal conduction of this type can lead to premature beats (VPBs) via automatic or re-entry mechanisms.

Re-entry maintains (and may initiate) ventricular tachycardia and ventricular fibrillation. In 1914, Mines established the criterion for re-entry, in excised rings of cardiac tissue, as an area of unidirectional block of the impulse that can allow reverse (retrograde) conduction, which then re-excites the tissue beyond the block; this is known as circus movement re-entry. The following criteria must be fulfilled to provide definitive evidence of a circus movement mechanism:

- The path for circus movement must have adequate boundaries to prevent short circuiting.
- The length of the path must be greater than the wavelength (ω) determined by the effective refractoriness of the path (ERP) and conduction velocity (CV), and described by the equation, $\omega = ERP \times CV$.
- Unidirectional conduction block must be present.

The area of unidirectional conduction block may be anatomic (as in the tachycardia resulting from Wolff–Parkinson–White syndrome), or functional (e.g. prolonged refractoriness resulting from ischemia or from the arrhythmia itself), or both. Re-entry can be terminated by interrupting the circuit by premature activation, by overdrive pacing, and by administration of certain drugs (see Treatment of arrhythmias below).

A second type of re-entry is known as reflection. It occurs in nonbranching bundles in which an impulse can return over the same bundle owing to electrical dissociation within the bundle.

Re-entry is involved in the maintenance and possibly the initiation of atrial tachycardia, atrial fibrillation, atrial flutter, AV nodal re-entrant tachycardia, Wolff–Parkinson–White syndrome, ventricular tachycardia, and ventricular fibrillation. There are many other putative arrhythmogenic mechanisms and details may be found in the Further Reading list at the end of this chapter.

Treatment of arrhythmias

There may be several objectives in treating arrhythmias:

- To restore the cardiac rhythm to normal—the first objective.
- To prevent arrhythmia recurrence.
- To ameliorate the hemodynamic consequences of the arrhythmia.
- To reduce the risk of a more severe arrhythmia such as ventricular fibrillation, a cause of sudden cardiac death.

Cardiac arrhythmias are treated by nonpharmacologic methods such as electrical defibrillation, surgery, and implantation of artificial pacemakers, as well as by drugs. The non-pharmacologic methods are growing in importance, and are believed by some cardiologists to have the potential to outmode much of the present pharmacologic therapy (which has relatively poor efficacy, especially for treating life-threatening arrhythmias). The first objective of drug treatment, to restore sinus rhythm without production of adverse effects, is not well achieved for many available drugs. The specific dose needed

369

may depend on the individual patient and, in particular, on their particular arrhythmia profile; nonetheless, typical dosages for most of the compounds in use in the US are shown in Fig. 18.12. Monitoring of plasma drug concentrations is required for many of these drugs (for general description of therapeutic drug monitoring, see Chapter 6).

The Vaughan Williams classification of antiarrhythmic drugs

Antiarrhythmic drugs may, in theory, be classified according to their mechanism of action at the molecular, cellular, or tissue level. Since the first antiarrhythmic drug, quinidine, was discovered in 1914 by Wenckebach, the list of antiarrhythmic drugs has grown, but a fully coherent system of classification has not grown with it. The first classification system, devised by Vaughan Williams in 1970, was later modified by Harrison (Fig. 18.13). This classification is of somewhat limited value, however, owing to the difficulty of determining arrhythmia mechanisms in individual patients, and uncertainty concerning precisely how antiarrhythmics actually achieve their effects.

Classification of antiarrhythmic drugs might be expected to assist selection of appropriate treatments. However, there are few arrhythmias for which a single class of drug is the only available choice. This is partly because the available agents are not effective in every patient. In the case of supraventricular arrhythmias this is not necessarily a major problem since if one agent is ineffective, another can be administered. However, the need to select a drug that is likely to work is more critical in the case of ventricular arrhythmias (some of which are rapidly lethal). Because lethal ventricular arrhythmias are particularly unresponsive to antiarrhythmic drugs, drug selection is often based on sequential testing of drugs' abilities to suppress arrhythmias induced by programmed electrical stimulation of the left ventricle in individual patients in the hospital. However, evidence-based studies demonstrate that this method does not very well predict improvement in survival in the long term. Nevertheless it continues to be used as a guide to selecting therapy targeted to the individual. Drugs of a different class are often used in combination (e.g. mexiletine plus β adrenoceptor antagonist) in prophylaxis against ventricular arrhythmias. However, in view of these considerations, the most important emerging treatment for life-threatening ventricular arrhythmias is nonpharmacologic: the automatic implantable cardiac defibrillator (AICD).

The Vaughan Williams classification does not help drug selection on the basis of the tissue mechanism of the arrhythmia. EADs and re-entry can represent tissue targets for protective drugs yet also represent tissue mechanisms of arrhythmia facilitation (pro-arrhythmia) by drugs (including some

Mean dosage and route of administration of the main antiarrhythmic drugs used in the US

Drug	Mean effective plasma concentration (μg/ml)	Route of administration
Disopyramide	3	i.v./p.o.
Lidocaine	3	i.v.
Procainamide	7	i.v./p.o.
Quinidine	4	i.v./p.o.
Mexiletine	1	i.v./p.o.
Tocainide	7	i.v./p.o.
Phenytoin	15	i.v./p.o.
Flecainide	0.7	i.v./p.o.
Encainide	0.75	i.v./p.o.
Propafenone	1.5	i.v./p.o.
Bretylium	1	i.v./p.o.
Amiodarone	1.5	i.v./p.o.
Verapamil	0.1	i.v./p.o.

Fig. 18.12 Mean dosage and route of administration of antiarrhythmic drugs used in the US. Note that the dosage given is only a guide and will vary enormously from patient to patient. (i.v., intravenous; p.o., oral)

Vaughan Williams classification of antiarrhythmic drugs

Class	Type of drug	Electrophysiologic actions	Examples
Ia	Na⁺ channel blocker	Blocks conduction, increases ERP	Quinidine Disopyramide
Ib	Na⁺ channel blocker	Blocks conduction, decreases ERP	Lidocaine Mexiletine
Ic	Na⁺ channel blocker	Blocks conduction, no effect on ERP, or an increase	Flecainide Encainide
II	β Adrenoceptor antagonist	Decreases sinus node automaticity, sympatholytic activity	Propranolol Sotalol
III	A drug that prolongs the action potential duration	No effects on conduction, delays repolarization	Bretylium Amiodarone Sotalol
IV	Ca²⁺ antagonist	Slows conduction velocity in the atrioventricular node	Verapamil Diltiazem

Fig. 18.13 Vaughan Williams classification of antiarrhythmic drugs. (ERP, effective refractory period)

antiarrhythmics). The prevalent effect (pro- or antiarrhythmic) of a drug will depend on the underlying condition and drug dosage. In animal experiments it is possible to evoke EADs with class III antiarrhythmic drugs, yet prevent re-entry with the same drugs. Class I drugs can facilitate re-entry by slowing conduction velocity, and block re-entry by converting unidirectional block of conduction to bidirectional block. Thus it is not easy to predict whether the overall effect of a antiarrhythmic drug will be beneficial or detrimental to cardiac rhythm unless the underlying tissue mechanism is known (and in man this is rarely the case).

The characteristic molecular action of class I antiarrhythmic drugs is blockade of cardiac Na⁺ channels

The molecular mechanism of action of class I drugs (inhibition of opening of Na^+ channels) was confirmed by showing that tetrodotoxin, a highly selective Na^+ channel-blocking toxin (that is more selective than any available drug), is antiarrhythmic in animal arrhythmia models (note that tetrodotoxin is never used as an antiarrhythmic in man because it blocks Na^+ channels in nerves at doses below those affecting the heart). The cellular mechanism of action of class I antiarrhythmics is blockade of the inward (depolarizing) Na^+ current. The resultant tissue and system mechanisms of action are less clear, but animal experiments suggest that conversion of unidirectional block to bidirectional block may prevent the occurrence of re-entry. Some class I drugs (class Ia, see below) also have an additional molecular and cellular action, i.e. block of K^+ channels, and therefore block of repolarizing K^+ currents. This prolongs the effective refractory period and may contribute to the drugs' effects on re-entry (see class III drugs for explanation; page 374).

QUINIDINE, the first antiarrhythmic drug to be used, is a Na^+ and K^+ channel blocker. It was pharmacologically identified by Frey in 1918 to be the most active cinchona alkaloid among quinine, quinidine, and cinchonine in patients with atrial fibrillation.

Class I antiarrhythmics were subclassified in the late 1970s by Harrison because, although all class I drugs shared the property of blocking conduction (manifested as a widening of the QRS complex), they fell into three groups depending on their effect on ventricular effective refractory period (see Fig. 18.13). Quinidine is a class Ia drug, meaning that it widens QT interval, as well as slowing conduction at therapeutic doses. The molecular selectivity of quinidine (and other class Ia drugs) for Na^+ versus K^+ channels is poor. As a result, some investigators now attribute quinidine's antiarrhythmic effects not to Na^+ channel blockade but to its ability to widen QT interval via block of cardiac K^+ channels (illustrating a degree of overlap between the molecular, cellular and tissue actions of class Ia and class III agents). This serves to illustrate that classifying a drug according to the Vaughan Williams system does not really provide a clear description of even the molecular mechanism of action.

The oral dose of quinidine may vary widely (200–300 mg every 3 to 4 hours) because of interindividual variations in

> **Adverse effects of quinidine**
>
> - Nausea
> - Fever
> - Syncope
> - Blood dyscrasia
> - Torsades de pointes

pharmacokinetics. Quinidine may be used to treat atrial fibrillation and flutter (restoring sinus rhythm), Wolff–Parkinson–White syndrome, and ventricular tachycardia. Like other class Ia drugs, quinidine does not reduce the incidence of sudden cardiac death (i.e., ventricular fibrillation) following acute myocardial infarction. A vagolytic action may elicit adverse sinus tachycardia. Another less common adverse effect, 'quinidine syncope' is now thought to result from quinidine-induced *torsades de pointes*, especially if hypokalemia is present. This may relate to the QT widening effect of the drug. Meta-analyses (see Chapter 6 for explanation) suggest that quinidine when used to treat atrial arrhythmias may increase the chance of sudden cardiac death. With long-term use of quinidine, gastrointestinal irritation is common, and the more rare 'cinchonism' syndrome (deafness, tinnitus, blurred vision, flushing and tremor) may also occur. Quinidine may elevate blood concentrations of digoxin potentially leading to an adverse drug interaction. Quinidine, along with other class Ia drugs, is contraindicated in patients with AV block or a history of long QT/*torsades de pointes*.

PROCAINAMIDE has similar properties to quinidine. Its differences include a more rapid absorption by mouth, and the availability of intravenous and intramuscular formulations. It has an active metabolite, N-acetylprocainamide (NAPA), which possesses relatively selective class III antiarrhythmic properties. Unlike quinidine, procainamide has approval in the USA only for treatment of ventricular arrhythmias (not supraventricular). It is a first-line drug for suppression and prophylaxis of ventricular tachycardia, especially when given intravenously in acute care and emergency settings. Nevertheless, there is no evidence that procainamide reduces the prevalence of mortality from ventricular fibrillation and death following acute myocardial infarction. A requirement for frequent dosing, resulting from rapid metabolism, limits patient compliance and hence may jeopardize therapeutic effectiveness. Gastrointestinal side effects are common (as for quinidine). Procainamide can cause leukopenia and (sometimes lethal) agranulocytosis. Complete blood counts are recommended during the first 12 weeks of therapy. Thrombocytopenia and positive Coomb's tests are rare. Long-term use (>6 months) is associated with an increasing susceptibility to development of a 'lupus-like-syndrome', which differs from systemic lupus erythematosus only in terms of its lack of renal involvement and its milder severity and greater reversibility.

DISOPYRAMIDE, another class Ia drug, has similar indications and properties to quinidine. It has particularly pronounced vagolytic effects, and the anticholinergic adverse profile extends to additional atropine-like actions including blurred vision, and dry mouth and urinary retention in elderly males. It has an advantage over quinidine in that there is no adverse drug interaction with digoxin.

LIDOCAINE is the proptotypical class Ib antiarrhythmic but is distinct from other Ib agents in that it is administered exclusively by the intravenous route for arrhythmia suppression, which results in a high concentration of drug reaching the heart. Lidocaine is otherwise metabolized in the liver (metabolism here is avid) and so oral administration is unfeasible. Characteristically for class Ib drugs, lidocaine has few effects on the normal EKG, and electrophysiologic actions occur selectively in the ischemic myocardium and during ventricular tachycardia (wherein, curiously, an ability to delay repolarization renders the drug quinidine-like, meaning that the Ib classification may not be appropriate in ischemia). It has been used for many years in the early phase of acute myocardial infarction (see page 383) to reduce the incidence of ventricular fibrillation. However, despite its ability to reduce the frequency of VPBs in this setting, lidocaine has no beneficial influence on long-term survival, suggesting that its therapeutic role has been overestimated. Overdose results in actions on nervous tissue, leading to paresthesias, and convulsions. This is particularly a risk in patients with hypotension, who may have diminished liver blood flow, decreasing elimination of lidocaine. Therapy monitoring is important in the safe use of this drug. Its mode of administration means that it is used only in emergency settings, and not for maintenance therapy. Lidocaine's other use as a local anesthetic is discussed in Chapter 26.

MEXILETINE is an orally active class Ib antiarrhythmic. It is no longer used for its original indication as an anticonvulsant. It is now exclusively used for suppression of VPBs and ventricular tachycardia but, following acute myocardial infarction, mexiletine has little or no effect on survival (typical of class Ib drugs). Adverse effects, while not as severe as those of dysopyramide, can nevertheless necessitate discontinuation. Neurologic adverse effects, which are not closely dose-related, are the most common (dizziness, paresthesias, ataxia and tremor). Pharmacokinetic-based drug interactions occur with antacids (which increase mexiletine's gastric absorption), but low plasma protein binding means that displacement of highly plasma protein-bound drugs is not a concern. The combination of mexiletine with a β_1 adrenoceptor antagonist is more effective than either drug alone, and allows a dosage reduction of each in suppression of ventricular arrhythmias.

TOCAINIDE is an orally active class Ib agent, which is used less often than mexiletine.

PHENYTOIN is an orally active anticonvulsant with class Ib antiarrhythmic properties similar to those of lidocaine. Its general and anticonvulsant properties are discussed in detail in Chapter 14. As an antiarrhythmic, phenytoin has been used to treat ventricular arrhythmias, digitalis overdose-induced arrhythmias, and *torsades de pointes*.

FLECAINIDE is the prototypical class Ic antiarrhythmic. The characteristics of class Ic agents are high potency and selectivity for cardiac Na^+ channels, with slow dissociation of the drug from the Na^+ channels. This causes detectable EKG effects (QRS widening) associated with slowed ventricular conduction in healthy cardiac tissue at normal heart rates (this is potentially hazardous; see below). Flecainide is used exclusively orally to treat supraventricular arrhythmias (paroxysmal supraventricular tachycardia, atrial flutter and fibrillation), and is contraindicated in patients with structural heart disease. This is because it was shown in the notorious Cardiac Arrhythmia Suppression Trial (CAST study) that flecainide may double the likelihood of death in patients with myocardial infarction (Fig. 18.14). This adverse effect is assumed to result primarily from a seemingly paradoxical pro-arrhythmic effect: nonlethal VPBs are suppressed but lethal arrhythmias (especially ventricular fibrillation) are facilitated. This is now presumed to be due to slowed conduction in healthy parts of the ventricle. Aside from this, the adverse effects of flecainide are minor.

ENCAINIDE is a class Ic drug with similar properties to flecainide, and a similar risk of pro-arrhythmia.

PROPAFENONE is another class Ic agent, used since the 1970s in Germany, and in the USA more recently. Although it appears to share a qualitatively similar pharmacologic and pro-arrhythmic profile with flecainide and encainide, it was not evaluated in the CAST study and therefore there is less of a perception that it is strongly contraindicated in patients with structural heart disease and myocardial infarction. Furthermore, propafenone possesses weak β_1 adrenoceptor antagonist activity which may offset any pro-arrhythmic adverse effects.

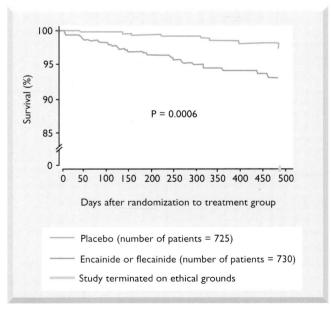

Fig. 18.14 Survival of patients in the Cardiac Arrhythmia Suppression Trial. Note that patients were allocated to groups in a randomized blinded fashion and that the cause of death in each case was cardiac-related.

Overall, class I drugs have been widely used but have limited effectiveness. It is generally regarded that mexiletine, quinidine, disopyramide and procainamide are equally effective in suppressing ventricular arrhythmias. No class I drug reduces the likelihood of death following acute myocardial infarction, and many are pro-arrhythmic.

Class II antiarrhythmics act by reducing sympathetic activity

An increase in sympathetic tone can stimulate myocardial β_1, β_2, or α_1 adrenoceptors and precipitate or aggravate arrhythmias in animal models, and it is believed that inappro-priate cardiac adrenoceptor activation (especially β_1) may contribute to arrhythmogenesis in man, although this is probably the case only during exercise or mental stress (where sympathetic tone is high). The prototype class II drug is propranolol, which is a nonselective β_1 and β_2 antagonist (Fig. 18.15). Conventionally, β_1 antagonism has been regarded as the molecular mechanism of action of class II antiarrhythmics, although recent animal studies suggest that β_2 antagonism may also contribute to the action of some class II drugs. Metoprolol and esmolol are 'cardioselective' class II agents, meaning that they are selective β_1 antagonists. The cellular and tissue mechanisms of the antiarrhythmic action of class II agents are not clear.

β Adrenoceptor antagonists used in cardiovascular disease

Drug	Selectivity	Main uses	Usual dose (mg/day)	Plasma half-life (h)	Elimination	Adverse effects
Propranolol	β_1/β_2	Essential and renal hypertension Angina pectoris Myocardial infarction Atrial arrhythmias Hypertrophic obstructive cardiomyopathy	40–320 p.o. 120–240 p.o. 160 p.o. 30–160 p.o. 30–160 p.o.	3–6	Hepatic metabolism and renal excretion	Generally mild/rare: Bronchospasm Hypoglycemia Bradycardia Fatigue Lassitude
Metoprolol	β_1	Hypertension Myocardial infarction	100–200 p.o.	3–4	Hepatic	Similar to propranolol (less hypoglycemia)
Atenolol	β_1	Hypertension Angina Atrial arrhythmias Acute myocardial infarct	50 p.o. 100 p.o. 50–100 p.o. Up to 10 i.v.	3–6	Mainly renal	Similar to propranolol (less hypoglycemia)
Acebutolol	β_1 partial agonist	Hypertension Angina pectoris Atrial arrhythmias	400 p.o. 400–1200 p.o. 400–1200 p.o.	3–6	Mainly renal	Similar to propranolol (less hypoglycemia)
Carvedilol	β_1	Hypertension Angina	12.5–50 p.o. 12.5–25 p.o.	7	Hepatic metabolism and renal excretion	Similar to propranolol + postural hypotension
Betaxolol	β_1	Hypertension	20–40 p.o.	3–6	Mainly renal	Similar to propranolol (less hypoglycemia)
Bisoprolol	β_1	Hypertension Angina	5–20 p.o. 5–20 p.o.	10–12	Hepatic metabolism (50%) and renal (50%)	Similar to propranolol (less hypoglycemia)
Nadolol	β_1	Hypertension Angina Arrhythmias	80–240 p.o. 40–160 p.o. 40–160 p.o.	14–17	Mainly fecal + hepatic metabolism and renal excretion	Similar to propranolol (less hypoglycemia)
Pindolol	β_1 partial agonist	Hypertension Angina	5–45 p.o. 5–15 p.o.	2.5–4	Hepatic (50%) and renal (50%)	Similar to propranolol (less hypoglycemia)
Labetalol	β_1/α_1	Hypertension	100–2400 p.o.	6	Hepatic metabolism and renal excretion (60%) + fecal (40%)	GI disturbance Male sexual dysfunction Liver damage (overall mild)

Fig. 18.15 β Adrenoceptor antagonists used in cardiovascular disease. (p.o., orally; i.v., intravenously)

β Adrenoceptor antagonists should be avoided in patients with:

- Asthma
- Diabetes mellitus with hypoglycemic reactions
- Severe intermittent claudication

Adverse effects of propranolol

- Bradycardia
- Depression
- Fatigue
- Cold extremities

Class II agents, especially propranolol, are particularly useful in suppression of atrial fibrillation and flutter associated with exercise or mental stress. Several adrenergic receptor antagonists have been shown to reduce mortality in patients with myocardial infarction, a benefit that has not been reproducibly demonstrated for any other antiarrhythmic drug class. This favorable effect may be due to other therapeutic actions (unrelated to arrhythmia suppression) of this class of drugs for this indication. Metoprolol, timolol, propranolol and atenolol have been shown to reduce the risk of a subsequent myocardial infarction in patients treated promptly after a first myocardial infarction (secondary prevention). The adverse effects of β_1 adrenoceptor antagonists are described in detail in the section on treatment of angina (page 377).

Class III antiarrhythmics act by prolonging the action potential duration

Prolongation of the cardiac action potential by class III antiarrhythmics is manifest on the EKG as an increase in QT interval. This leads to suppression of re-entry, although as noted earlier, it may exacerbate EADs. Thus anti- and pro-arrhythmic effects are possible, depending on the underlying tissue mechanism of the arrhythmia (EAD versus re-entry). Bretylium, amiodarone, sotalol, d-sotalol and dofetilide are all class III drugs.

Bretylium is the oldest, but least effective class III agent, and its adrenergic neuron-blocking effects (see Chapter 14) represent a lack of molecular selectivity and account for adverse effects such as hypotension.

Amiodarone was developed as a coronary vasodilator, and its antiarrhythmic effects were found by chance. Although amiodarone is generally referred to as a class III antiarrhythmic, it also blocks Na$^+$ and Ca^{2+} channels and (weakly) α adrenoceptors. Amiodarone may also decrease expression of β_1 adrenoceptors in cardiac myocytes but does not interact directly with these receptors. This nonselectivity means that its molecular mechanism of action is unclear, and its classification as a class III agent is questionable. Its onset of action is quite

fast (within 60 minutes) when given intravenously, but by the oral route the drug must be administered for up to 3 weeks before a pharmacotherapeutic effect is achieved. Amiodarone has a very long half-life of over 50 days, which means that it is not possible to achieve rapid modification of effects (beneficial or adverse) by altering the dosage. It has been shown to be effective against both atrial and ventricular arrhythmias. Amiodarone is much more effective than quinidine, class II agents, verapamil and digitalis in suppressing paroxysmal supraventricular tachycardia related to Wolff–Parkinson–White syndrome. Its effectiveness against supraventricular tachycardia is enhanced when used in combination with digoxin, although care must be taken as serum digoxin concentrations are commonly increased via a drug–drug interaction. Combination with class IV antiarrhythmics (described on page 375) may provide benefit against severe supraventricular tachycardia, although care must be taken to avoid AV block. Prevention of sudden cardiac death by suppression of ventricular fibrillation following myocardial infarction may be achieved with amiodarone, but serious side effects jeopardize the success of long-term therapy, limiting effectiveness (see Adverse effects box). One advantage of amiodarone over many β blockers, however, is that it is not contraindicated in patients with common disorders such as asthma, diabetes, coronary artery disease, or renal failure.

Until recently, all the class III drugs used clinically were believed to share a common molecular action, i.e. the ability to block cardiac K$^+$ channels. However, other molecular actions can lead to the tissue response characteristic of class III drugs (i.e. action potential prolongation). These include α_1 adrenoceptor agonism and inhibition of Na$^+$ channel inactivation. The latter is believed to contribute to the molecular mechanism of action of ibutilide, a class III agent approved in the USA for the treatment of supraventricular tachycardia.

The broad-spectrum antiarrhythmic dl-sotalol (commonly referred to simply as sotalol) is a mixed class II/class III agent. It is less effective than amiodarone for suppressing uncomplicated atrial flutter and fibrillation, and as effective as amiodarone in Wolff–Parkinson–White syndrome. Its effectiveness in preventing ventricular fibrillation following myocardial infarction is not proven, although benefit through the combined molecular effects of β_1 adrenoceptor blockade and K$^+$ channel blockade is likely. This lack of demonstrated benefit is a result of an absence of data due to the shift of focus onto more selective ('pure') class III agents that began in the 1980s; the trend in perception was that greater selectivity would lead to greater efficacy (a perception now no longer held).

Adverse effects of amiodarone

- Thyroid abnormalities
- Corneal deposits
- Pulmonary disorders
- Skin pigmentation

A new generation of class III agents began with the introduction of d-sotalol, the sotalol enantiomer that possesses class III effects on K$^+$ channels with little or no class II effects on β$_1$ adrenergic receptors. It was the first 'pure' class III agent. It is less effective than dl-sotalol for supraventricular arrhythmias. However, early studies reported promising effects against serious ventricular arrhythmias. Most of the new class III agents (dofetilide, almokalant, clofilium) selectively block the channel responsible for the rapid form of the delayed repolarizing potassium current, I$_{Kr}$ (an important repolarizing K$^+$ current in atria and ventricles). Other drugs that act on other K$^+$ channels are less selective and target I$_{Kr}$ plus the channels responsible for the transient outward K$^+$ current, I$_{to}$ (tedisamil), the inward rectifying K$^+$ current, I$_{K1}$ (terikalant) or the ATP-dependent K$^+$ current I$_{K(ATP)}$ (glyburide). None are used clinically as antiarrhythmics owing to adverse effects. Of the new generation of class III agents, only dofetilide remains in widespread clinical use (for supraventricular tachycardia). It is notable that, in the SWORD clinical trial (Survival with Oral d-Sotalol), the highly selective I$_{Kr}$ blocker, d-sotalol, was found paradoxically to increase mortality following myocardial infarction, by an unknown mechanism, possibly pro-arrhythmic effects on EADs leading to *torsades de pointes*. Subsequently, a fear that *torsades de pointes* may be a class effect has meant that most of the new generation of I$_{Kr}$-selective class III agents (as well as most of the nonselective K$^+$ channel blockers) have been withdrawn from development. One exception is dofetilide, for which clinical development had progressed substantially at the time the SWORD trial findings were published. Today, dofetilide at low doses is an alternative therapy for supraventricular tachycardia, particularly that involving re-entry through the AV node. Low dosage avoids K$^+$ channel-blocking effects in the ventricles, reducing the risk of *torsades de pointes*. However low dosages also precludes the possibility of benefit against serious ventricular arrhythmias and death following myocardial infarction. Dofetilide is virtually free of adverse drug interactions and side effects, with the exception of an ability to evoke *torsades de pointes* in susceptible patients. The risk of this is low.

Class IV antiarrhythmics are Ca²⁺ antagonists

VERAPAMIL (a papaverine derivative) is the prototype of class IV antiarrhythmics (Fig. 18.16). It:

- Decreases SA nodal rate.
- Decreases AV nodal conduction.
- Causes negative inotropy.
- Causes coronary and peripheral vasodilation.

The main calcium antagonists used in cardiovascular disease

Drug	Main uses	Usual doses (mg/day)	Plasma half-life (h)	Metabolism and elimination	Adverse effects
Verapamil	Essential hypertension Hypertensive emergency Angina pectoris Acute myocardial infarction secondary prevention Supraventricular tachycardia	160–480 p.o. 5 i.v. 160–480 p.o. 360 p.o. 2.5 i.v. repeated	2–7	Hepatic metabolism by CYP3A/CYPIA2 Urinary excretion	Constipation (most common) Hypotension
Diltiazem	Angina pectoris Myocardial infarction Variant angina Hypertension Supraventricular tachycardia Raynaud phenomenon	180 p.o. up to 360 p.o. 360 p.o. 180–360 p.o. 20 i.v. over 2 min	2–6, prolonged in elderly	Hepatic metabolism High first-pass + urinary excretion of metabolites	Hypotension Edema Headache (all rare)
Nifedipine	Hypertension (all forms) Ischemic heart disease (all forms) Raynaud phenomenon Heart failure	15–30 or 40 sublingual 0.2 intracoronary or 10–60 p.o.	5	Hepatic metabolism by CYP3A4 High first pass + urinary excretion of metabolites	Hypotension
Nicardipine	Angina pectoris Hypertension	30–120 p.o. 60–120 p.o. (30–60 sustained release)	1–2	Similar to nifedipine	Hypotension
Felodipine	Arterial hypertension	10–20 p.o.	24	Similar to nifedipine (but slower)	Similar to diltiazem
Amlodipine	Essential hypertension	10 in single daily dose	30–60	Hepatic metabolism (slow, no first pass)	Hypotension Bradycardia

Fig. 18.16 The main calcium antagonists used in cardiovascular disease. (p.o., orally; i.v., intravenously)

⚠	**Adverse effects of verapamil**
	• Bradycardia
	• Nausea and vomiting
	• Constipation

⚠	**Adverse effects of adenosine**
	• Acceleration of tachycardia in Wolff–Parkinson–White syndrome
	• Atrial fibrillation in Wolff–Parkinson–White syndrome
	• Bronchospasm and hypotension

DILTIAZEM has a similar pharmacologic profile to verapamil. The antiarrhythmic application of these drugs is mainly for the treatment of supraventricular arrhythmias (both have other applications unrelated to arrhythmia suppression; see pages 380 and 398). In studies in rats and dogs it appears that, during acute ischemia, ventricular arrhythmias may be suppressed by verapamil. However, clinical trials of Ca^{2+} antagonists in patients with coronary artery disease have rarely demonstrated any useful suppression of ventricular arrhythmias. One reason for this may be that, as a result of the vasoselective nature of these drugs, the maximum safe doses used are insufficient to act in the ventricles to inhibit arrhythmias.

Adenosine is an antiarrhythmic that falls outside the Vaughan Williams classification

ADENOSINE is not orally active but can be very effective when used intravenously as a treatment for paroxysmal supra-ventricular tachycardia. It has a short half-life, and its effects are blocked by commonly used drugs (theophylline) and by caffeine. Its molecular mechanism of action is agonism at A_1 adenosine receptors in the SA node, AV node and atria. Its cellular mechanism of action following receptor stimulation is a cascade beginning with activation of an inhibitory G-protein (Gi), which leads to inhibition of adenylyl cyclase activity and other actions mediated by Gi. Activation of A_1 receptors leads to opening of the same K^+ channels as those affected via this transduction cascade by acetylcholine. Because these channels are absent in the ventricles, adenosine has no effect on ventricular arrhythmias by this mechanism. The tissue action is hyperpolarization and a decrease in action potential duration leading to termination of re-entry. These actions account for a range of therapeutic effects: slowing of ventricular rate during atrial fibrillation (as a result of AV block, an action similar to that produced by digitalis), termination of sinoatrial re-entrant tachycardia (a rare condition of re-entry within the SA node), termination of paroxysmal supraventricular tachycardia involving re-entry through the AV node, and termination of Wolff–Parkinson–White syndrome involving retrograde conduction through the AV node. (However, in the latter, class Ia and Ic agents are preferred since adenosine may accelerate the tachycardia as a result of its ability to shorten the atrial refractory period.) In addition, through mechanisms that are less well-established, A_1 activation by adenosine activates K_{ATP} channels, and this may account for the anti-ischemic effects of adenosine in ventricles reported in preclinical studies. Adenosine's ability to evoke bronchospasm as a consequence of bronchial A_1 agonism means that it is contraindicated in asthma.

CVT-510 is a selective A_1 agonist currently in clinical development as an antiarrhythmic. It has greater selectivity for the AV node than adenosine.

There are four types of adenosine receptor (A_1, A_{2A}, A_{2B} and A_3). Coronary vascular A_{2A} receptor activation leads to coronary vasodilation, although this has not been exploited clinically (in angina, for example).

Digitalis cardiac glycosides are used primarily to treat heart failure, but have additional antiarrhythmic actions

Digitalis can be used to treat supraventricular tachycardia. Its mechanism of action is unusual. Supraventricular tachycardia may have a rate in excess of 300 beats/min and can be dangerous if the ventricles 'follow' the atria, as they will do over a wide range of supraventricular rate. The resultant rate may be too fast for effective diastolic filling so cardiac output falls. Digitalis converts supraventricular tachycardia to fibrillation by shortening the atrial refractory period, but its effects on the AV node mean that ventricular rate actually slows (Fig. 18.17).

Once the ventricular rate has stabilized, the atrial fibrillation can be terminated by electroshock. However, it may be necess-

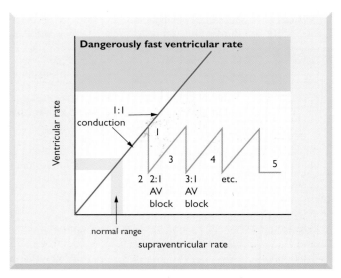

Fig. 18.17 The unusual mechanism by which digitalis ameliorates supraventricular tachycardia. 1 Digitalis prolongs AV refractory period by releasing acetylcholine from vagus. **2** This causes 2:1 AV block. **3** However, digitalis also shortens atrial refractory period increasing supraventricular tachycardia rate. **4** This exacerbates the AV block (since the AV recovery time is reduced). **5** Eventually AV dissociation occurs leading to a safer ventricular rate.

ary to pretreat patients with heparin or warfarin depending on the suspected duration of the atrial fibrillation. This is because in atrial fibrillation (especially chronic fibrillation) a stasis thrombus may form in the atrial cavity, and restoration of sinus rhythm may dislodge the thrombus which, after passing into the circulation, may lodge in cerebral arterioles causing stroke. Digitalis must not be used for supraventricular tachycardia caused by Wolf–Parkinson–White syndrome, as the accessory pathway would allow the ventricles to 'follow' the atria and fibrillate. Digoxin is the antiarrhythmic cardiac glycoside of choice.

THE 'SICILIAN GAMBIT' (Task Force of the Working Group on Arrhythmias of the European Society of Cardiology, 1991) is an alternative approach to the Vaughan Williams classification of antiarhythmic drugs (Fig. 18.18).

In this scheme, an approach to classification is proposed, which encourages consideration of a drug's action at the molecular and cellular level, and its action at the tissue level on certain 'vulnerable parameters.' This reappraisal of antiarrhythmic drugs is primarily intended as an open-ended guide to drug selection, based on the opinion that the Vaughan Williams classification oversimplifies the properties and mechanisms of action of 'groups' of drugs. The Vaughan Williams classification:

- Is a hybrid, with class I and class IV representing a molecular mechanism (ion channel blockade), class II representing a molecular mechanism (blockade of receptors), and class III representing a tissue mechanism (prolongation of action potential).
- Does not take into account the fact that drugs may act differently in normal and diseased tissue.
- May oversimplify the situation, so that it is assumed that all members of one class are the same (although, for example, different class III antiarrhythmics act via blockade of different K^+ channel subtypes).
- Fails to acknowledge that antiarrhythmic drugs may act on pumps, carriers, exchangers, and second-messenger systems, as well as on receptors and ion channels, and so it is difficult to use this system to classify new compounds.

However, the Vaughan Williams classification does have the advantages of being physiologically based, and easily learnt and recalled. The Sicilian Gambit approach to classification has not been generally adopted.

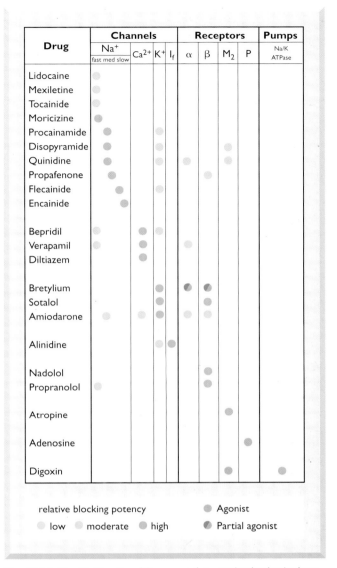

Fig. 18.18 The Sicilian Gambit approach to antiarrhythmic drug classification. This is an alternative approach to antiarrhythmic drug classification introduced by the Task Force of the Working Group on Antiarrhythmias of the European Society of Cardiology. This scheme summarizes the actions of a variety of antiarrhythmic drugs on ion channels, drug receptors, and ion pumps. I_f, hyperpolarization activated current; M_2, muscarinic subtype 2 receptors; P, purinergic receptors; Na/K ATPase, Na^+/K^+ pump. (Reproduced with permission from *Circulation* 1994; **84**: 1848. Copyright 1994 American Heart Association.)

Angina pectoris

There are a number of disease conditions where insufficient blood flow can occur in one or more coronary arteries. The resultant regional (localized) myocardial ischaemia can produce characteristic pain in the chest (angina pectoris, see below) but pain may not necessarily occur (silent angina). Angina is a word derived from the Latin *ango*, to choke, but is today understood and misunderstood to denote chest pain. In medicine there are many types of angina but the most important, in terms of prevalence, is angina associated with myocardial ischemia. Myocardial ischemia can be partial or complete; it can be temporary, lasting for a few minutes, or permanent leading to the death of tissue.

Myocardial ischemia can result from:
- Fixed partial obstruction of an artery or arteries due to atheroma or other pathologic processes.
- Inappropriate arterial vasospasm.
- A thrombus.

If myocardial ischemia is sufficiently severe, and maintained for a sufficient period of time, death of tissue occurs (infarction).

■ *Angina pectoris results from an imbalance between coronary blood supply and myocardial oxygen demand*

Angina pectoris (actually a symptom, not a disease) is a condition in which episodes of ischemia in the ventricular myocardium generates paroxysmal pain in the chest (especially the pectoral region). It is often precipitated or worsened by exercise, emotion, meals and cold and is characteristically alleviated by rest. The triggering stimuli result in an increase demand for cardiac work and hence coronary flow. If the coronary flow cannot increase enough to meet demand, ischemia is the result. Thus angina pectoris may be regarded as an expression of a coronary blood supply–demand mismatch. The various possible reasons for this are listed in Fig. 18.19.

Unstable angina is commonly associated with pathologic changes in atherosclerotic plaques lining coronary arteries.

Unstable (also known as crescendo) angina occurs suddenly at rest or with limited physical activity and increases in frequency and severity and often occurs prior to a myocardial infarction. Very often unstable angina reflects pathologic changes in a coronary artery associated with platelet aggregation and atherosclerotic plaque anatomy; therapy is aimed at relieving pain and halting progression of the coronary lesion.

■ *Variant angina and Syndrome X are rare forms of angina*

A rare form of angina is variant angina pectoris (Prinzmetal's angina). It is associated with coronary arteries that are usually free of a fixed obstruction. It occurs at rest (it is not specifically provoked by exercise) and is associated with coronary artery spasm. The clinical features of variant angina differ from those of typical angina (Fig. 18.20). Syndrome X refers to angina in the setting of apparently normal coronary arteries, although its clinical importance is uncertain.

Diseases that cause unstable angina

- Coronary arteriosclerosis
- Transient platelet aggregation and coronary thrombosis
- Coronary artery spasm
- Coronary vasoconstriction following adrenergic stimulation
- Accumulation of potent vasoconstrictors at sites of endothelial injury

Fig. 18.19 Diseases that cause unstable angina.

Clinical features of variant angina pectoris

- Chest pain at rest
- Pain at the same time of day (early morning)
- ST segment elevation during chest pain
- Chest pain accompanied by ventricular arrhythmias
- Nitroglycerin relieves chest pain and ST segment elevation

Fig. 18.20 Clinical features of variant angina pectoris.

 Types of angina

- Angina pectoris presents as a radiating chest pain, is due to insufficient oxygen supply to the myocardium, and can occur during exercise and stress
- Chronic stable angina is caused by a fixed coronary stenosis (narrowing)
- Unstable angina occurs at rest or with physical activity and has a crescendo pattern
- Variant angina or Prinzmetal's angina occurs at rest and is caused by coronary vasospasm

---

Treatment of angina

The approaches to treatment depend on the type of angina:
- For acute attacks of angina, sublingual nitrates provide rapid relief by reducing preload and afterload. Nitrates can be used for preventing an attack if given just before the precipitating activity.
- For anginal attacks that occur in a predictable manner, several different classes of drug may be used on a prophylactic basis to prevent attacks. Such drugs include long-acting nitrates, nonselective or β_1-selective adrenoceptor antagonists, and Ca^{2+} antagonists. Each of these differ in their molecular, cellular, and tissue mechanisms of action, but all affect one or more of preload, afterload, myocardial oxygen consumption, and heart rate. The general pharmacology of beta blockers is shown in Fig. 18.15.
- For unstable angina, therapy is aimed at relieving pain and preventing progression to an acute myocardial infarction. It is common to use aspirin to reduce the likelihood of platelet aggregation to reduce risk of a myocardial infarction.
- Maintained acute anginal pain, especially when caused by coronary thrombosis (heart attack), may be treated with morphine.
- There are no specific therapies for Syndrome X.

■ *Nitrates dilate the systemic veins and arterioles and large and medium-sized coronary arteries*

Nitrates when administered sublingually (to achieve rapid absorption) may relieve angina within a few minutes. The main tissue mechanism of action in angina is dilation of the systemic veins. This reduces preload which in turn reduces myocardial wall tension and oxygen demand. The molecular mechanism of action for this effect is associated with an increase in vascular guanylyl cyclase activity, which increases cyclic guanosine monophosphate (cGMP) levels (Fig. 18.21). cGMP is an important transduction component (see Chapter 3). Most nitrates are pro-drugs, and decompose to form nitric oxide (NO), which then activates guanylyl cyclase (Fig. 18.21). By the same molecular and cellular mechanism, nitrates also cause vasodilation of large and medium-sized coronary arteries, thereby increasing coronary blood flow and oxygen delivery to the subendocardial region of the myocardium. However, this is clinically relevant only if vasospasm is present. Indeed, if there is a fixed coronary obstruction (arteriosclerosis) dilation

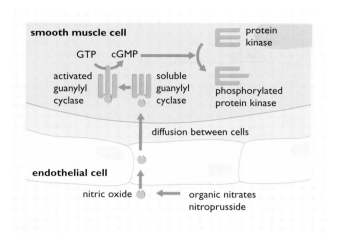

Fig. 18.21 Molecular and cellular mechanisms of action of nitrate and nitrite vasodilators. The product, phosphorylated protein kinase, causes vascular smooth muscle relaxation by phosphorylating (and inactivating) myosin light chain kinase.

of adjacent healthy coronary arteries can shunt blood away from the ischemic region (coronary 'steal'). Peripheral arteriolar dilation may also occur, but this is short-lived and its clinical significance is unclear. Sympathetic reflexes may overcome the short-lived ability of nitrates to reduce afterload. Several preparations are available, including:

- Nitroglycerin.
- Erythrityl tetranitrate.
- Isosorbide dinitrate.
- Nitroglycerin.
- Pentaerythritol tetranitrate.

Only sublingual nitroglycerin is used to treat an acute attack, although the other nitrates are used to prevent attacks.

▨ Nitrate tolerance is associated with continuous nitrate administration

Long-acting nitrates such as isosorbide dinitrate are usually given at 6–8-hour intervals during the day, whereas the shorter-acting drug, nitroglycerin, may be applied as a patch preparation on the chest at any time, although it is generally not applied overnight. These treatment regimens minimize the effect of nitrate tolerance, which can occur over time with repeated nitrate administration. As a general principle, tolerance is avoided by careful planning of dosing in relation to the drug's pharmacokinetics to ensure that a steady-state plasma concentration is not sustained over a 24-hour period. The patient must be free of nitrate for at least 8 hours of the day to prevent development of tolerance.

▨ β_1 Adrenoceptor antagonists reduce myocardial oxygen demand

β_1 Adrenoceptor antagonists (also known as β blockers) block activation of the β_1 adrenoceptors by the peripheral autonomic nervous system and by epinephrine released from the adrenal medulla. These drugs:

- Decrease exertionally-induced increases in heart rate.

- Decrease systolic blood pressure, particularly if hypertension is present.
- Decrease cardiac contractile activity.

As a result β_1 adrenoceptor antagonists reduce myocardial oxygen demand by means of blunting the heart's response to sympathetic tachycardic stimuli. The details of their molecular mechanisms of action are shown in Fig. 18.22. Drugs in this class include those listed in Fig. 18.23.

At relatively low doses, β_1-selective agents such as metoprolol, atenolol and acebutolol tend to reduce heart rate responses and myocardial contractile activity without affecting bronchial smooth muscle (in which circulating epinephrine effects a physiologically important bronchodilation, in some patients, due to β_2 agonism). However, at higher doses, any selectivity is lost and the effects resemble those of nonselective β (β_1 and β_2) adrenoceptor antagonists, such as propranolol, which may exacerbate bronchospasm in some asthmatics as a result of β_2 antagonism in the respiratory tract.

▨ β Adrenoceptor antagonists cause a variety of adverse effects including fatigue, insomnia, dizziness, male sexual dysfunction, bronchospasm, bradycardia and heart block

β Adrenoceptor antagonists should be used cautiously, or may be contraindicated, in patients with bradycardia (heart rate less than 55 beats/min), bronchospasm, hypotension (systolic

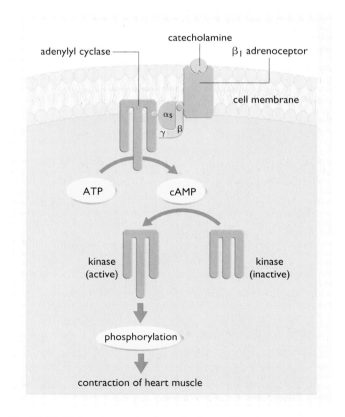

Fig. 18.22 Molecular mechanism of action of β_1 adrenoceptor antagonists. Stimulation of β_1 adrenoceptors by catecholamines leads to activation of adenylyl cyclase and an elevation of cAMP. This process is inhibited by β_1 adrenoceptor antagonists.

β Adrenoceptor antagonists used in patients with angina		
Drug	**Selectivity**	**Classification**
Acebutolol	β_1 Selective	Partial agonist
Alprenolol	β_1 Selective	Partial agonist
Atenolol	β_1 Selective	Antagonist
Metoprolol	β_1 (low doses)	Antagonist
Oxprenolol	β_1, β_2 Nonselective	Partial agonist
Pindolol	β_1, β_2 Nonselective	Partial agonist
Propranolol	β_1, β_2 Nonselective	Antagonist
Sotalol	β_1, β_2 Nonselective	Antagonist
Timolol	β_1, β_2 Nonselective	Antagonist

Fig. 18.23 β Adrenoceptor antagonists used in patients with angina.

pressure less than 90 mmHg) or any degree of heart block. β Adrenoceptor antagonists can promote acute pulmonary edema in patients with compensated heart failure or severe congestive heart failure (although, apparently paradoxically, these drugs are used to treat heart failure under carefully controlled circumstances, see page 389).

Calcium antagonists block L-type Ca²⁺ channels to alleviate angina pectoris

Calcium antagonists block L-type Ca^{2+} channels to alleviate angina pectoris

Calcium antagonists are effective in angina because of the following three tissue mechanisms of action:

- They reduce venous pressure (preload).
- They reduce arteriolar pressure (afterload).
- They reduce myocardial oxygen consumption.

Each of these effects occurs as a result of the same molecular mechanism of action, which is block of L-type Ca^{2+} channels. This decreases Ca^{2+} current and Ca^{2+} entry into vascular and cardiac cells, and so reduces the concentration of intracellular Ca^{2+} concentration (the cellular mechanism of action), resulting in reduced contractile activity in vascular and cardiac muscle.

Calcium antagonists include verapamil, bepridil (phenethylalkylamines), diltiazem (a dibenzazepine), nifedipine, nicardipine, felodipine and amlodipine (1,4-dihydropyridines). These drugs possess slightly different tissue and system mechanisms of action, despite having similar molecular and identical cellular mechanisms of action.

Phenethylalkylamines and dibenzazepines affect cardiac tissue (reducing cardiac contractility and in high doses slowing atrioventricular conduction) and blood vessels (causing vasodilation). They reduce myocardial oxygen consumption at rest and during exercise by reducing heart rate and cardiac contractile activity, increasing coronary blood flow, and reducing

preload and afterload. Although verapamil and diltiazem may have favorable effects on ventricular response rates in patients with uncontrolled atrial fibrillation, these drugs may adversely slow conduction through the AV node, leading to AV block (see section on antiarrhythmic drugs, page 375).

The 1,4-dihydropyridines are very vascular-selective, causing vasodilation without slowing AV conduction or heart rate or reducing cardiac contractility. Indeed, immediate-action formulations of nifedipine (e.g., sublingual chewable capsules) may indirectly increase heart rate as a reflex response to hypotension due to the associated systemic arterial vasodilation, although this appears to be a less common adverse effect of slow-release formulations of nifedipine (which are now the predominant formulations used), and for amlodipine, felodipine and nicardipine. The basis for this vascular selectivity is a marked voltage dependence such that the ability to block L channels is minimal at membrane potentials encountered in (the relatively hyperpolarized) working myocardium and cardiac nodal tissue during diastole, compared with effects in (the relatively depolarized) blood vessels. Verapamil and diltiazem also show voltage dependence, but this is not as marked as that seen with dihydropyridines, so AV conduction slowing is possible with therapeutic doses (see section on antiarrhythmic effects of calcium antagonists, page 375). The beneficial actions of 1,4-dihydropyridines in angina are attributed to increases in coronary blood flow to the epicardial regions of the myocardium, and peripheral vasodilation (a reduction in afterload).

Calcium antagonists are effective in preventing chest pain in patients with stable angina following exercise or stress, either alone or in combination with nitrates and/or β_1 adrenoceptor antagonists. If nifedipine, nicardipine, felodipine or amlodipine is combined with a β_1 adrenoceptor antagonist there is only a low risk of AV block and of impairing cardiac output as a result of reduced ventricular contractility (effects that would be particularly hazardous if the patient has congestive heart failure or AV conduction abnormalities). Nifedipine, nicardipine, felodipine and amlodipine can therefore be used in patients with these conditions. However, there is a greater risk for this type of adverse drug interaction if verapamil, diltiazem or bepridil are combined with a β_1 adrenoceptor antagonist. Since verapamil, diltiazem and bepridil have negative inotropic effects they should not be given to patients with severe heart failure. Bepridil is less selective at the molecular level for L-type Ca^{2+} channels than verapamil or diltiazem, because it blocks cardiac Na^+ and K^+ channels at high doses, possibly sufficiently to slow cardiac conduction and delay repolarization. This has been associated with the adverse effect of *torsades de pointes*. Because of this, bepridil is recommended only for severe stable angina that is not fully responsive to other interventions.

Calcium antagonists have several adverse effects, with nifedipine being the least well tolerated. The systemic vasodilating effects of nifedipine (primarily the rapid-onset formulations) may cause dizziness and palpitations. Nifedipine also causes venodilation, which may explain the peripheral edema that occurs in some patients. Amlodipine and nicardipine are generally better tolerated than nifedipine, causing little or

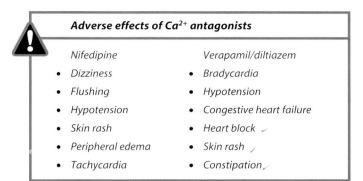

Adverse effects of Ca²⁺ antagonists

Nifedipine	Verapamil/diltiazem
• Dizziness	• Bradycardia
• Flushing	• Hypotension
• Hypotension	• Congestive heart failure
• Skin rash	• Heart block
• Peripheral edema	• Skin rash
• Tachycardia	• Constipation

no peripheral edema, and have no adverse interactions with β_1 adrenoceptor antagonists (owing to their lack of direct effect on the myocardium). Moreover, amlodipine and nicardipine do not cause reflex tachycardia at therapeutic doses. The main adverse effect of verapamil is constipation, but bradycardia, hypotension, and heart failure may also occur. Verapamil in combination with a β_1 adrenoceptor antagonist results in a marked bradycardia and should not be used in patients with heart failure, bradycardia, hypotension, or AV block (if at all). Diltiazem is also associated with bradycardia.

Aspirin is used in the treatment of patients with coronary artery disease to decrease cardiac risk

Although aspirin is considered primarily as a treatment for unstable angina (see below) it is also recommended in stable angina at a moderate dose (80–325 mg/day). The aim is to reduce the chance of coronary thrombosis rather than specifically to treat the stable angina. Aspirin is a potent inhibitor of cyclo-oxygenase, which is an enzyme with a pivotal role in the biosynthesis of thromboxanes in platelets and prostacyclin in vascular endothelium (Fig. 18.24, and see Chapters 13 and 16):

• Platelet-derived thromboxane is a potent vasoconstrictor, so aspirin may reduce coronary occlusion by inhibiting its synthesis.
• Endothelium-derived prostacyclin is a potent vasodilator and inhibits platelet aggregation, so inhibition of its synthesis is potentially hazardous.

Aspirin's molecular mechanism of action is acetylation of the α amino group of the terminal serine residue of the cyclo-oxygenase enzyme. This irreversibly inhibits the activity of the enzyme.

Adverse effects related to aspirin use include:
• Gastrointestinal bleeding, which is common.
• Possible gastric ulceration, especially with overdosage.
• Reduced renal function as a result of a reduction in renal blood flow with inappropriately high doses.
• Occasional bronchospasm with inappropriately high doses.

Treatment of unstable angina

The main use of aspirin in angina pectoris is to prevent unstable angina leading to myocardial infarction

Aspirin may reduce the platelet aggregation that is initiated by coronary endothelial injury and can participate in the etiology

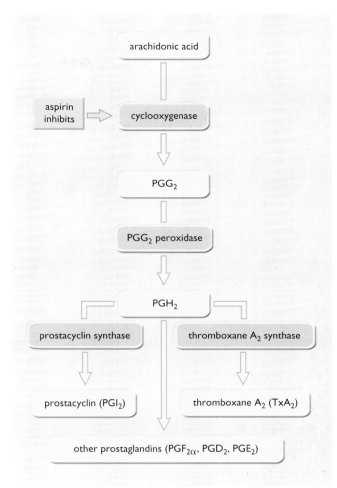

Fig. 18.24 Mechanism of action of aspirin. Aspirin blocks the activity of cyclo-oxygenase and reduces the formation of prostacyclin and thromboxane A_2. PGG_2 and PGH_2 are both prostaglandin cyclic endoperoxides and are unstable intermediates.

of unstable angina. If platelets aggregate they can occlude severely narrowed coronary arteries and release potent vasoconstrictors, which worsen the angina. These vasoconstrictors include thromboxane A_2, serotonin (5-HT), adenosine diphosphate (ADP), thrombin, and platelet-activating factor.

The molecular mechanism of action of aspirin is a selective inhibition of thromboxane synthesis. This is achieved because platelets do not possess a cell nucleus and are therefore unable to resynthesize cyclo-oxygenase, whereas endothelial cells can resynthesize cyclo-oxygenase within a few hours. Low-dose aspirin (30 mg/day) is insufficient to block the activity of cyclo-oxygenase completely, so its use can achieve a maintained suppression of thromboxane synthesis, with only a transient inhibition of prostacyclin synthesis, and an overall effect of reduced platelet aggregation. These actions contribute to the benefit achieved by prophylactic use of aspirin against acute myocardial infarction (see below and Fig. 18.25). There is emerging evidence that adding clopidogrel to aspirin reduces mortality.

HEPARIN FOR UNSTABLE ANGINA Intravenous heparin has been shown to reduce the occurrence of chest pain in unstable angina (Fig. 18.26). Heparin inhibits blood clotting by preventing fibrin formation and platelet aggregation, probably as a result of its thrombin-inhibitory effects since thrombin is a potent platelet aggregator. Heparin's molecular mechanism of action involves binding to the lysine site on antithrombin III, which accelerates the rate of reaction of antithrombin III, the endogenous inhibitor of thrombin. Antithrombin III also inhibits the other serine proteases in the coagulation cascade: factors XIIa, XIa, IXa, and Xa. The arginine site on antithrombin III interacts with the serine site on thrombin, thereby rendering it inactive. Heparin increases the risk of bleeding disorders so its risk/benefit ratio requires careful consideration if there is a history of a pre-existing bleeding disorder (e.g. peptic ulceration). Heparin is discussed in more detail in Chapter 13.

GPIIB/IIIA RECEPTOR ANTAGONISTS GPIIb/IIIa receptor antagonists inhibit the final steps of platelet aggregation. These drugs may have efficacy in some patients with unstable angina and are particularly useful in patients undergoing urgent or elective coronary angioplasty. The drugs may be particularly useful in patients with unstable angina with elevations of troponin T or I which might be surrogate markers for thrombosis formation. These drugs are described in detail in Chapter 13. Abciximab is a monoclonal antibody that can be administered only intravenously, and consequently is not appropriate for long-term use. Interestingly, infused abciximab is largely platelet-bound; consequently, if necessary, its effects can be reversed by a platelet transfusion. For longer term therapy, especially following coronary angioplasty, several orally active GPIIb/IIIa antagonists are available; these drugs are also described in Chapter 13.

NITRATES, CALCIUM ANTAGONISTS, β BLOCKERS AND OTHER TREATMENTS FOR UNSTABLE ANGINA Nitrate therapy relieves pain in patients with unstable angina. It is given orally or transdermally, but patients who still have unstable angina are given intravenous nitrates. Intravenous nitroglycerin is given at a dose that does not cause hypotension or tachycardia. Calcium antagonists or β adrenoceptor antagonists can be given if unstable angina persists. β Adrenoceptor antagonists may be preferred for patients with angina at rest and ST segment elevation during the pain without an elevated heart rate or

> **Drug therapy for angina**
>
> - Nitrates are effective because they decrease oxygen demand. The principal tissue mechanism of action is a reduction in preload
> - β Adrenoceptor antagonists decrease heart rate, systolic blood pressure, and cardiac contractile activity
> - Calcium antagonists reduce preload and afterload and may increase coronary flow
> - Aspirin inhibits platelet and endothelial cyclo-oxgenase and reduces the incidence of coronary thrombosis

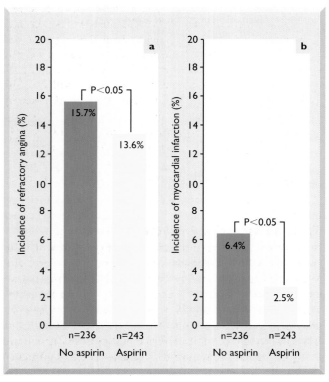

Fig. 18.25 Effect of aspirin (325 mg twice daily) on incidence of (a) angina and (b) myocardial infarction.

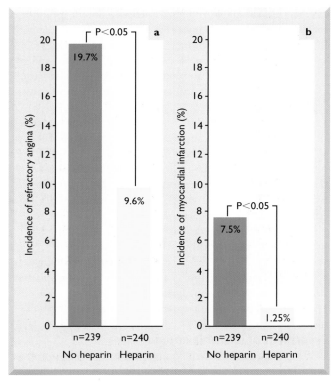

Fig. 18.26 Effect of heparin (1000 units/hour) on the incidence of (a) angina and (b) myocardial infarction.

blood pressure. Thrombin modulators are given to patients with persistent angina despite drug therapy (i.e. nitrates, Ca^{2+} antagonists, or β adrenoceptor antagonists) to reduce the risk of myocardial infarction by reducing the likelihood of coronary thrombosis.

SURGICAL INTERVENTION IN UNSTABLE ANGINA Cardiac catheterization or coronary artery revascularization is necessary for patients with unstable angina that persists despite pharmacologic intervention.

Coronary arteriography is:

- Recommended for patients with unstable angina and no other severe medical conditions, following successful control of their angina by drug intervention.
- Essential for patients with recurring unstable angina, even after drug treatment.

Coronary artery bypass graft surgery (CABG) or percutaneous transluminal coronary artery angioplasty (PTCA), often followed by the insertion of a stent, are advised for this second group of patients. Coronary artery revascularization extends life for patients with left main coronary stenoses, or with three-vessel coronary stenoses and depressed left ventricular function.

Variant angina and its treatment with drugs that dilate the coronary arteries

Variant angina is caused by coronary vasospasm and is also known as Prinzmetal's angina (after the physician who first characterized it). Variant angina is the only form of angina in which dilation of coronary arteries is the principal tissue mechanism of action of the drugs used to treat it. It should initially be treated with nitrates, either alone or with a Ca^{2+} antagonist:

- Nifedipine (40–160 mg/day) alone may be sufficient to prevent variant angina in up to 75% of patients. Its effectiveness is not modified by the presence of concurrent partially obstructive coronary arteriosclerosis.
- Verapamil (Fig. 18.27) and diltiazem may also be used, as well as the newer agents, nicardipine, israpidine, and amlodipine.

Despite differences in tissue selectivity (vasculature versus AV node), all these Ca^{2+} antagonists appear to be equally effective, although individual patients may respond better to one drug than to another. For unknown reasons, the combination of diltiazem and nifedipine may be beneficial if the agents are less than completely effective when used alone. β Adrenoceptor antagonists are not recommended in these patients because they are often ineffective and may increase the frequency and severity of spasm.

Emerging drugs

Several studies are currently examining the following drugs for use in the treatment of different forms of angina:

- **Ranolazine.** This agent has a complex molecular and cellular action, but has the potential advantage over many other antianginal agents of having no effect on heart rate or blood pressure, and little or no adverse effects. It acts on mito-

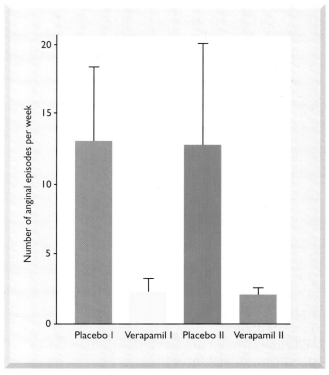

Fig. 18.27 Effect of verapamil in patients with variant angina. I and II refer to two different patient populations.

chondria to inhibit fatty acid oxidation, stimulating glucose oxidation and improving oxygen metabolism.

- **Lovastatin.** This HMG-CoA-reductase inhibitor, used primarily for hyperlipidemia (see Chapter 15), is presently under investigation for prevention of unstable angina as well as myocardial infarction when administered to healthy people with average to moderately elevated levels of HDL cholesterol. It is speculated that this action will slow the development of, and possibly reverse atherosclerosis, by preserving endothelial function.
- **Dalteparin** and **enoxaparin**. These low molecular weight heparin fragments are presently under investigation for use in short-term aggressive treatment of unstable angina. Dalteparin is already approved for this use in many countries.

Acute myocardial infarction

The pathological processes underlying angina can worsen to the point at which potentially irreversible occlusion and maintained ischemia occurs and myocardial infarction begins. Patients who suddenly and unexpectedly experience maintained symptoms of angina pectoris may be undergoing an acute myocardial infarction (AMI). This is a syndrome that elicits a well established pattern of clinical signs and symptoms. The word infarction describes dead (scarred) tissue, and animal studies have proven that myocardial tissue has to undergo severe ischemia for more than 60 minutes before cell death occurs, but the term AMI is used clinically for the syndrome associated with severe irreversible regional myocardial ischemia. Although the syndrome of AMI comprises events (e.g., angina and ventricular arrhythmias) which have been previously discussed in this chapter, its treatment *en bloc* requires special consideration.

Early palliative treatment of acute myocardial infarction

Early palliative intervention is begun immediately the patient is admitted to hospital, or sooner if possible. Thus, intravenous morphine can be given for chest pain.

Morphine has two beneficial system effects:

- Its analgesic properties, discussed in Chapter 14, relieve chest pain.
- It has a relatively selective ability to reduce preload (venous tone) and afterload (arterial tone) in the agitated patient with raised sympathetic tone.

This second effect results from the suppression of excess sympathetic nervous system activity. This reduces myocardial oxygen demand and this contributes to the relief of chest pain and, possibly, the progression of ischemic damage.

Limitation of death of heart cells in patients with acute myocardial infarction

A major objective of treatment of acute myocardial infarction is to target the underlying system pathology (the blocked artery) and limit myocardial ischemia and resultant myocyte cell death. This is achieved by drugs (in most cases their mechanism of action has already been described in this chapter), or by mechanical intervention involving cardiac catheterization. The first therapeutic objective is to reperfuse the ischemic myocardium so as to limit the eventual extent of cell death (infarction). This is achievable if effected early; if infarction is established, reperfusion is of limited value. A Q wave in the ECG is indicative of infarction.

Thrombolytics are used to facilitate reperfusion. Although vasospasm in the absence of thrombosis is uncommon as a sole cause of AMI, nitrates are additionally useful in patients with thrombotic occlusion because they reduce preload and chest pain (see section on treatment of angina), especially if blood pressure is elevated, although their contribution to improved long-term survival as a consequence of their ability to facilitate reperfusion is not substantial. Thrombolytics, administered as soon as possible after the onset of symptoms, include intravenous tissue plasminogen activator, streptokinase and heparin. These are by far the most important drugs for reperfusion in AMI, as thrombosis is the most common cause of coronary occlusion in AMI. Their cellular and molecular actions are described in Chapter 13. Aspirin (325 mg twice a day) has een shown to reduce the risk of secondary coronary thrombosis and death if treatment is begun immediately and continued long term (Fig. 18.25). Likewise, intravenous heparin infusion has been shown to reduce the incidence of myocardial infarction and subsequent death (Fig. 18.26), as has streptokinase (given as an intracoronary infusion over 1 hour). The combination of streptokinase and aspirin is optimal, whereas heparin (given subcutaneously or intra-

venously) confers no additional benefit either as adjunct, or as a substitute for streptokinase. Subcutaneous heparin, which is absorbed unpredictably, has been documented to cause death by cerebral haemorrhage in AMI patients. In addition to causing bleeding disorders, streptokinase is antigenic and can elicit allergy reactions in some patients.

Tissue-type plasminogen activator (tPA) is somewhat more effective as a thrombolytic than streptokinase in the treatment of patients with acute myocardial infarction, and the recombinant form (r-tPA, also known as alteplase) is non-allergenic. In the USA, tPA is first-line therapy but in other countries it has not completely replaced streptokinase, since streptokinase compared with tPA is inexpensive and almost equally efficacious. However, the occurrence of streptokinase antibodies (from previous infection with *Streptococcus* sp. or previous treatment with this agent) can limit its use. tPA is an endogenous enzyme that initiates a cascade of extracellular events (see Chapter 13). tPA activates plasminogen (a pro-enzyme) to form plasmin (an enzyme). Plasmin can hydrolyze fibrin, an integral component of the architecture of a thrombus. Both streptokinase and tPA must be infused into a blood vessel to have benefit. In the case of streptokinase, intracoronary infusion is more effective than intravenous infusion of this agent, whereas intravenous infusion of tPA is sufficiently effective.

There is a form of streptokinase which has a fourfold longer plasma half-life compared with the native preparation. This is anisolylated plasminogen-streptokinase activator complex (known as APSAC or anistreplase). One advantage that APSAC has over streptokinase and tPA is its ease of use; owing to its longer half-life, a single intravenous bolus is as effective in achieving reperfusion as intracoronary or intravenous infusions of streptokinase or tPA.

Other drugs used in AMI

A variety of interventions used in AMI do not treat the underlying myocardial ischaemia itself, but target the effects of ischemia. Their molecular and cellular mechanisms of action have been discussed elsewhere in this chapter. The interventions include the routine use of β adrenoceptor antagonists, aspirin, antiarrhythmic agents, and (in specific circumstances) sympathomimetics.

- Antiarrhythmic agents may produce immediate beneficial effects (suppression of arrhythmias) without improving long-term survival, whereas β adrenoceptor antagonists and aspirin may have little immediate effect but can improve long-term survival.
- Once the patient has stabilized, continued administration of aspirin and β adrenoceptor antagonists is strongly recommended.
- Prophylactic use of antiarrhythmics (to prevent recurrence of life-threatening arrhythmias) is now not recommended (likewise, in the acute phase, antiarrhythmics are useful only if arrhythmias are already present, and not as prophylaxis).
- Sympathomimetics are used only for emergency treatment of cardiogenic shock, and are discussed first.

Sympathomimetic drugs are used for cardiogenic shock in AMI

Cardiogenic shock can complicate AMI. This occurs if cardiac output is severely impaired, typically due to a large loss in cardiac muscle. Animal studies suggest that involvement of more than 40% of the left ventricle may generate cardiogenic shock in the absence of other complications. Prognosis in man is very poor with a high death rate. Emergency treatment (prior to surgical intervention; see below) has been with intravenous adrenoceptor agonists which activate β_1 receptors in the heart (norepinephrine, dopamine or dobutamine). The aim is to infuse the lowest dose sufficient to achieve improvement of CNS and coronary blood flow without increasing afterload or preload. The tissue mechanism of action is a combination of positive inotropy (in uninvolved healthy myocardium) and vasoconstriction (in splanchnic perfusion beds) thereby re-distributing cardiac output to the CNS and coronary perfusion beds. The therapeutic dose window is narrow, and pulmonary edema and exacerbation of heart failure are common. Supportive surgical intervention by intra-aortic balloon (which is inflated and deflated in time with the cardiac cycle so as to direct more of the cardiac output to the coronary and carotid arteries) is instigated as soon as possible.

Antiarrhythmics are used for suppressing arrhythmias in the acute phase of AMI

If non-life-threatening ventricular arrhythmias occur, these may be suppressed by intravenous lidocaine. Procainamide (intravenous) may be used if ventricular tachycardia is present on hospital admission. If ventricular fibrillation occurs, electrical cardioversion is necessary. Accelerated idioventricular rhythm resulting from abnormal automaticity in infarcting Purkinje fibers (2 hours or more after the acute event) can be overdrive-suppressed by administering atropine which, by blocking M_2 muscarinic receptors in the sinoatrial node, allows sinus rate to increase, recapturing cardiac rhythm.

The use of antiarrhythmics for improving survival once the patient has stabilized is controversial

Surprisingly, intravenous lidocaine, which has been shown by meta-analysis to have no effect on death rate in 1-year follow up, is still routinely administered immediately following AMI (even if ventricular arrhythmias are minimal or absent), in many parts of the world. Although lidocaine may immediately suppress non-life-threatening arrhythmias, it has no beneficial effect on long-term survival, and may disturb the patient by eliciting adverse effects in the CNS (particularly paresthesias) and cardiovascular system (asystole). The maintained use of class I antiarrhythmics (procainamide, quinidine) or class III antiarrhythmics (sotalol, amiodarone) in the days and weeks after the acute events is questionable owing to lack of effectiveness against ventricular fibrillation and possible adverse effects (including pro-arrhythmia), as discussed earlier in this chapter. Other class I and III antiarrhythmics have been, and may continue to be used, but their effects on survival are dubious at best (see the CAST and SWORD studies mentioned earlier).

Class II agents (β_1 adrenoceptor antagonists) are the only antiarrhythmics proven to reduce death rate in the year following hospital discharge after AMI, although the mechanism of action is unclear (it may not even be the result of suppression of arrhythmias).

Drug treatment versus nonpharmacologic interventions in AMI

- Drug treatment in AMI is most critical for establishing reperfusion of the ischemic myocardium and prevention of re-occlusion.
- Once it occurs, ventricular fibrillation is best treated by electrical cardioversion, and its occurrence in hospital has no bearing on survival in the long term.
- Percutaneous transluminal coronary angioplasty (PTCA), bypass graft surgery or stenting are key nonpharmacologic interventions designed to restore and maintain coronary perfusion. PCTA is the most common procedure, but it damages coronary endothelium, exposing Von Willebrand factor in underlying smooth muscle, which can initiate platelet aggregation, thrombosis and re-occlusion.
- Coronary artery bypass grafts, using a vein from the patient's lower limb, has been the most common surgical procedure. Unfortunately these are particularly thrombogenic owing to the size and shape of the vein used in the graft. It is hoped that artificial grafts (stents) will be less problematic.
- Dipyridamole (plus warfarin), ticlopidine and aspirin all have a role to play before and after surgical reperfusion, preventing acute coronary thrombosis or maintaining graft patency.
- Aspirin reduces death post-AMI and is the only drug proven to reduce the risk of new AMI.
- β Blockers reduce the chance of death in the months following AMI, but the mechanism by which they achieve this is uncertain.
- Following the acute phase of AMI, survivors may develop heart failure if a sizeable infarct develops. The treatment strategies for this are discussed earlier in this chapter.

Treatment of syndromes related to AMI

In animal experiments, a variety of syndromes and conditions, such as reperfusion injury (cardiac and vascular) myocardial stunning, preconditioning, hibernation and ventricular re-modeling have been characterized following permanent ischemia, or temporary ischemia followed by reperfusion. Their clinical counterparts probably exist, but these syndromes and conditions are difficult to characterize well in man, so it is uncertain whether any of the many interventions used in AMI have any beneficial effects upon them.

One exception is ventricular remodeling. This has been characterized in animals, with experimental coronary artery ligation, as the combination of ventricular hypertrophy, wall thickening (and possibly wall thinning) that occurs in uninvolved myocardium during the days and weeks after ischemic tissue becomes infarcted, and which is associated with progressive increases in preload and a reduced cardiac output, each of which contribute to the symptoms of congestive heart failure (the treatment of which is discussed later in this chapter). Because certain treatments for heart failure such as ramipril and captopril have well-documented beneficial effects on remodeling in animals with experimental infarction, it is suspected that their overall benefit in man is achieved, at least in part, through amelioration of adverse remodeling.

Another possible exception is myocardial reperfusion injury. Adenosine (whose molecular and cellular actions are described on page 376) is under investigation as an adjunct to reperfusion (by thrombolysis or PTCA) because an initial clinical trial (AMISTAD-I) found that myocardial infarct size appeared to be reduced when intravenous adenosine was given as an adjunct to reperfusion.

Finally, although treatments for the various aspects of AMI are used, overall success (in terms of survival) is poor. The reduction in 1-year mortality with optimal use of all available interventions is probably no better than 20%. Moreover, in many AMI victims, the first symptom is ventricular fibrillation, and 35–50% die outside of hospital from their first AMI before medical attention can be received. Thus, those patients most at risk of death are not included in most statistics on effectiveness of interventions. In the long term, prevention of coronary artery disease by diet and avoidance of risk factors such as cigarette smoking, combined with AICDs for those identified as being at risk of acute coronary obstruction, will probably be more effective than pharmacologic intervention after the acute event.

Congestive heart failure

Congestive heart failure (CHF) is the most common reason for hospitalization of people over 65 years of age in the US, where over 400,000 new cases are reported each year. Diagnosis is made on the basis of impaired cardiac function and reduced tolerance to exercise. The major causes of congestive heart failure are ischemic heart disease, and hypertensive and valvular heart disease, as well as various forms of cardiomyopathy. The specific cause of the congestive heart failure may have an impact on therapeutic strategies.

Heart failure refers to the chronic failure of the heart to provide a sufficient cardiac output for the body's physiologic needs. Congestive describes abnormal accumulation of venous blood and edema. The heart can fail to provide sufficient cardiac output for various underlying reasons which include:

- Loss of viable myocytes (cardiomyopathy) due to infarction, infection or exposure to chemicals/drugs (e.g. cobalt/adriamycin).
- Excessive afterload (leading to cardiac hypertrophy) due to arterial hypertension or aortic stenosis.
- Valvular defects (e.g., mitral regurgitation) and tachycardia (e.g. in thyrotoxicosis) that reduce stroke volume.

CHF is most amenable to drug treatment if it is the result of cardiomyopathy or arterial hypertension. Classification of cardiomyopathies is based upon physiologic and anatomic considerations (Figs 18.28, 18.29). Myocarditis resulting from bacterial infection is discussed on page 410. Regardless of the type of cardiomyopathy, the common end-point is a gradual

 Common diseases that contribute to the development of congestive heart failure

- Cardiomyopathy
- Myocardial ischemia and infarction
- Hypertension
- Cardiac valve disease
- Congenital heart disease
- Coronary artery disease

 Clinical features of congestive heart failure

- Reduced force of cardiac contraction
- Reduced cardiac output
- Reduced tissue perfusion
- Increased peripheral vascular resistance
- Edema

reduction in heart function and precipitation of CHF. The failure may be acute or chronic and usually involves both ventricles. CHF becomes symptomatic if insufficient oxygenated blood is supplied to the organs of the body or if central venous pressure rises sufficiently to cause edema.

CHF may involve a failure in the cardiac excitation–contraction coupling processes. In CHF there is progressive systolic and diastolic ventricular dysfunction, which is characterized by structural and metabolic changes to cardiac muscle that can be acute or chronic, with a spectrum of symptoms depending upon the severity of the dysfunction (Fig. 18.30):

- Acute CHF can result from exposure of cardiac muscle to toxic levels of drugs or as a result of coronary artery occlusion, usually due to thrombosis.
- Chronic CHF occurs when the heart is damaged by conditions such as primary hypertension or myocardial ischemia and infarction, adriamycin or cobalt exposure, and surviving myocytes often become hypertrophic.

▨ *Left ventricular heart failure (the most common form) is characterized by reduced cardiac output and blood pressure, and pulmonary congestion*

Left ventricular heart failure produces 'forward failure,' with reduced cardiac output and blood pressure, and 'backward failure' due to pulmonary congestion. Blood pressure may not necessarily fall as fluid retention may compensate for the impaired cardiac output but, if so, edema is a likely occurrence.

▨ *Right ventricular heart failure is characterized by dyspnea, edema, and fatigue*

The characteristics of right ventricular heart failure (dyspnea, edema, and fatigue) result from 'backward failure.' In this condition central venous and right atrial pressures are both

Classification of cardiomyopathies

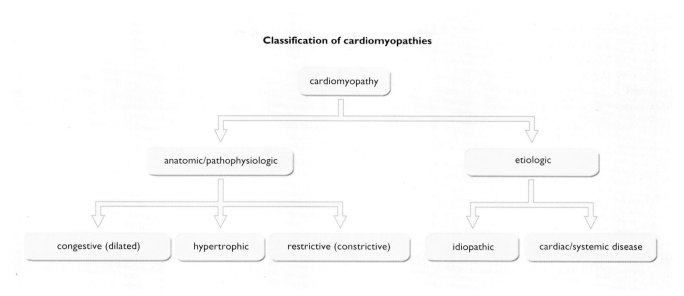

Fig. 18.28 Classification of cardiomyopathies based upon anatomic, pathophysiologic, and etiologic considerations.

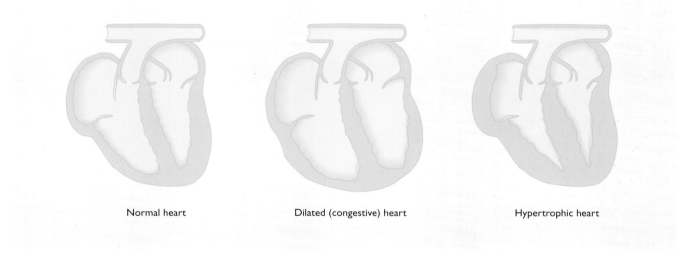

Normal heart　　　　Dilated (congestive) heart　　　　Hypertrophic heart

Fig. 18.29 Types of cardiomyopathies involving both the right and the left ventricle.

high, producing general venous congestion. Any obstruction to right ventricular inflow or excessive load imposed on the right ventricle can precipitate this condition. It ultimately leads to left ventricular failure since the left ventricle's demand for oxygenated pulmonary venous blood cannot be met.

◼ *Compensatory reflexes initially alleviate, then exacerbate the symptoms of heart failure*

Regardless of the type of heart failure, both cardiac output and (often, though not always) blood pressure are reduced. The cardiovascular system compensates for these decreases, initially maintaining adequate organ and tissue perfusion. Two processes usually occur:

- Activation of extrinsic neurohumoral reflexes.
- Intrinsic cardiac compensation.

Both work in conjunction, improving cardiac function. However, in the long term the symptoms of heart failure are made worse.

◼ *Extrinsic neurohumoral reflexes initially help to maintain cardiac output and blood pressure*

Hypotension activates baroreceptors, which increase the activity of the sympathetic nervous system, leading to an increased heart rate and vasoconstriction. Cardiac contractility and arteriolar resistance therefore increase. The latter increases cardiac 'afterload.' Cardiac afterload is defined as the resistance against which the cardiac muscle must pump to expel blood from the ventricles. When it increases, the ejection fraction (the amount of blood ejected from the ventricles with each heart beat) and perfusion to organs such as the liver and kidneys are

387

reduced. A reduction in renal perfusion activates the renin–angiotensin system, leading to renin secretion which increases plasma angiotensin II formation. Angiotensin II subsequently releases aldosterone from the adrenal cortex.

Symptoms associated with congestive heart failure	
Acute	**Chronic**
Tachycardia	Various arrhythmias
Shortness of breath	Hypertension
Edema (peripheral/pulmonary)	Cardiomegaly
Decreased exercise tolerance	Edema (peripheral/pulmonary)

Fig. 18.30 Symptoms associated with congestive heart failure. The severity of the symptoms depends upon the degree of heart failure.

Angiotensin II causes peripheral vasoconstriction while aldosterone increases Na^+ retention leading to the following sequence of events:
- Increased water retention.
- Increased venous and arterial blood pressures.
- Increased vascular and interstitial fluid volume.
- Congestion and edema both systemically and in the lungs.
- Increased cardiac preload (Fig. 18.31).

■ *Intrinsic cardiac compensatory mechanisms are activated by an increase in cardiac preload*
The cardiac changes that occur include:
- Ventricular dilation.
- An increase in the volume and pressures generated by the ventricles.

As preload increases, there is incomplete emptying of the ventricles and a resulting increase in end-diastolic pressure, which initially maintains cardiac output by increasing the muscle tension. In cardiac muscle the tension depends on the

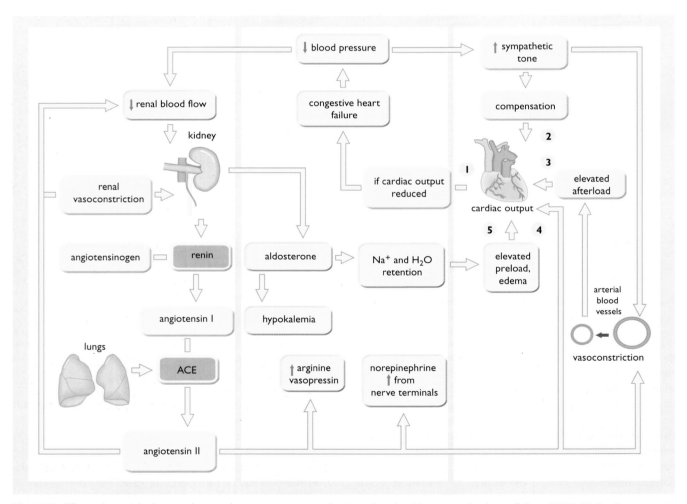

Fig. 18.31 The major extrinsic neurohumoral compensatory mechanisms involved in congestive heart failure (CHF). (1) Cardiac output is reduced in CHF. (2) Reflex sympathetic compensation can increase cardiac output, but (3) an associated increase in afterload can reduce cardiac output. The cascade of other events can lead to hypertrophy (4) owing to actions of angiotensin II on the heart, which increases cardiac output and Na^+ retention. This may increase cardiac output (5) by raising preload and left ventricular end-diastolic pressure, but this may cause death by initiating pulmonary edema.

degree of stretch of the muscle fiber (i.e. preload at the onset of contraction). This relationship is described by the behavior of cardiac muscle length–tension curves, which parallel the output–volume relationship of the heart (Frank–Starling ventricular function curve, see below, Fig. 18.35).

The hypertrophy and dilation that develop as a consequence of CHF increase cardiac muscle mass, which facilitates ventricular systole and increases the efficiency of blood ejection from the ventricles. It is also an adaptive mechanism which reduces ventricular wall stress.

The relationship between heart wall tension and ventricular chamber pressure is known as Laplace's law: $T = (P \times r)/w$, (where T is the tension developed in the heart muscle wall, P is the transmural pressure, r is the radius of the ventricle, and w is wall thickness). If ventricular wall stress were not relieved, severe damage would result. From Laplace's law, however, ventricular wall tension varies inversely with wall thickness, and the ventricular hypertrophy may reduce the developing wall stress as preload increases. However, this adaptive process cannot compensate for CHF indefinitely and, with time, the ventricles usually become much less compliant than normal, and cardiac output falls.

Compensatory mechanisms activated during CHF result in positive inotropism

An increase in the rate of contractility ($(+dP/dt)_{max}$) is defined as positive inotropism. This is achieved as a consequence of increased sympathetic drive to the heart, and activation of β_1 adrenergic receptors. This leads to increased efficiency in systolic emptying. However, the benefit of this compensatory mechanism is not well maintained. Failure results from ventricular overload due to increased ventricular filling pressures, systolic wall stress, and increased myocardial energy requirements.

Treatment of congestive heart failure

There are two phases of treatment of CHF: acute and chronic. Drug treatment should not only provide relief from symptoms but also reduce mortality. The immediate objectives are to:
- Reduce congestion (edema).
- Improve cardiac systolic and diastolic function (contraction and relaxation, Fig. 18.32). Many drugs can be used to achieve this purpose (Fig. 18.33).

Cardiac glycosides have been used for heart failure for more than 200 years

Digoxin is the prototype cardiac glycoside and is extracted from the leaves of the purple (*Digitalis purpurea*) and white (*D. lanata*) foxglove, a common flower. These natural occurring compounds are known collectively as cardiac glycosides. Although there are several other cardiac glycosides, digoxin has the most widespread clinical use.

All cardiac glycosides share a similar chemical structure. Digoxin, digitalis, and ouabain all possess an aglycone steroid nucleus that is essential for pharmacological activity. An unsaturated (C17-linked) lactone ring is present, which confers the cardiotonic actions, and C3-linked sugar moieties which influence potency and pharmacokinetic characteristics.

Pharmacotherapeutic approach to congestive heart failure	
Problem	**Approach**
Fatigue	Rest, positive inotropes
Edema	Diet (salt restriction), diuretics, digitalis
Poor cardiac contractility	Positive inotropes
Dyspnea	Diuretics (thiazides/loop)
Congestion	Nitrovasodilators
Increased cardiac preload and afterload	Angiotensin-converting enzyme inhibitors, venodilators, vasodilators
Irreversible heart failure	Heart transplantation

Fig. 18.32 Pharmacotherapeutic approach to congestive heart failure. The most important approach is to reduce congestion (edema) and improve cardiac contractility.

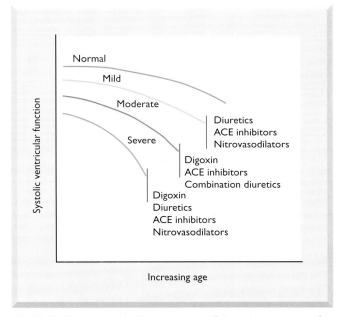

Fig. 18.33 Drugs used in the treatment of the various stages of congestive heart failure. The slow decline in ventricular function with age is exacerbated by disease. (ACE, angiotensin-converting enzyme)

Cardiac glycosides inhibit membrane-bound Na⁺/K⁺ ATPase

Cardiac glycosides achieve their effects at the molecular level by inhibiting membrane-bound Na^+/K^+ ATPase (Fig. 18.34). This enzyme is involved in establishing the resting membrane potential of most excitable cells by virtue of its ability to pump three Na^+ ions out of the cell in exchange for two K^+ ions into

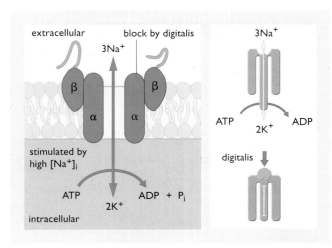

Fig. 18.34 Mechanism of action of digitalis glycosides. The binding site for digitalis is on the extracellular aspect of the α–β heterodimer structure of the Na⁺/K⁺ ATPase enzyme. Inhibition of this enzyme raises intracellular Na⁺ concentration, which raises intracellular Ca²⁺, and mediates the positive inotropic actions of cardiac glycosides.

the cell against their concentration gradients, thereby establishing intracellular concentrations which are high (140 mM) for K^+ and low (25 mM) for Na^+. The pump's energy is derived from the hydrolysis of ATP. Inhibition of the pump results in an increased intracellular cytoplasmic Na^+ concentration.

The increase in Na^+ concentration leads to inhibition of a membrane-bound ion exchanger (Na^+/Ca^{2+} exchanger), and as a consequence there is a marked increase in cytoplasmic Ca^{2+} concentration. The exchanger is an ATP-independent antiporter (see Chapter 3) that normally causes a net extrusion of Ca^{2+} from cells. The increased cytoplasmic Na^+ concentration passively reduces the exchange function so that less Ca^{2+} is extruded. The raised cytoplasmic Ca^{2+} concentration is then actively pumped into the sarcoplasmic reticulum and becomes available for release during subsequent cellular depolarizations, thereby enhancing excitation–contraction coupling. The resultant tissue mechanism of action is a greater force of contractility, known as positive inotropism (Fig. 18.35).

In the failing heart, the positive inotropic actions of the cardiac glycosides produce changes in the Frank–Starling ventricular function curve. Figure 18.35 outlines the actions of positive inotropic agents on cardiac output.

Despite widespread use, there is no convincing evidence that digitalis, the most commonly used cardiac glycoside, has a

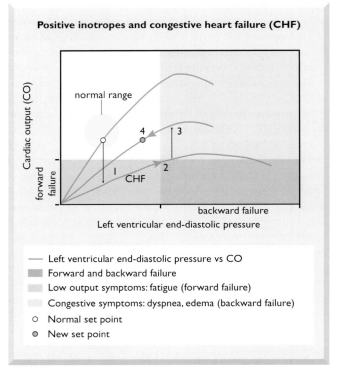

Fig. 18.35 The Frank–Starling curve, positive inotropes, and congestive heart failure (CHF). Normal cardiac output is determined by the pressure in the left ventricle at end-diastole. In CHF, the set point for cardiac output is reduced and cardiac output falls (1). Compensatory neurohumoral responses become activated which increase end-diastolic pressure and improve cardiac output; however, this can give rise to backward failure (2). Positive inotropic agents increase cardiac output (3). The improved cardiac output reduces the drive for a high end-diastolic pressure, and decompensation occurs to a new set point (4).

beneficial effect on the long-term prognosis of patients with CHF. The symptoms are improved in many patients but digitalis does not reduce mortality due to CHF.

■ *Cardiac glycosides additionally alter the electrical activity in the heart*

In addition to improving the force of contraction, cardiac glycosides alter the electrical activity in the heart, both directly and indirectly.

At pharmacotherapeutic doses, cardiac glycosides indirectly alter the heart rate by increasing activity in the vagus nerve (cranial nerve X) as a result of the stimulation of afferent elements in the paravertebral (nodose) ganglion and a reflex increased in activity in the vagus nerve arcs. Increased vagal firing activity predominates in the supraventricular regions and causes:

- Slowing of the SA node firing rate.
- Slowing of AV node conduction velocity (widening the PR interval of the EKG).
- Shortening of the atrial action potential.

At toxic doses, cardiac glycosides also increase efferent cardiac sympathetic tone. However, the rate of neural discharge is not

---

🔑 **Positive inotropes that improve cardiac contractility**

- Cardiac glycosides (e.g. digoxin)
- Phosphodiesterase inhibitors (e.g. inamrinone)
- β₁ Agonists (e.g. dobutamide)

uniform for all sympathetic nerves and this can result in nonuniform myocardial excitability and arrhythmias, including AV node block, AV junctional tachycardia, and ventricular premature beats.

The direct effects of cardiac glycosides on cardiac tissue are most marked at high doses and relate to the loss of cytoplasmic K^+ due to inhibition of Na^+/K^+ ATPase. The continued loss of cytoplasmic K^+ to the extracellular space reduces the resting membrane potential of the cell, resulting in:

- Enhanced automaticity.
- Decreased cardiac conduction velocity.
- Increased AV node refractory period.

Owing to the increase in cytosolic Ca^{2+} concentration, eventually the Ca^{2+} binding capacity of the sarcoplasmic reticulum (SR) may become saturated. With increasing cardiac glycoside concentrations, the free Ca^{2+} concentration reaches toxic levels. These high cytoplasmic Ca^{2+} concentrations saturate the SR sequestration mechanism, resulting in oscillations in Ca^{2+} due to Ca^{2+}-induced Ca^{2+} release and resultant oscillations in membrane potential (oscillatory afterpotentials). Arrhythmias resulting from oscillatory afterpotentials include single and multiple ventricular premature beats and tachyarrhythmias.

Cardiac glycosides can increase peripheral vascular resistance by a direct α_1 adrenoceptor-mediated vasoconstriction in peripheral vessels and a centrally mediated increase in sympathetic tone. In CHF, the elevated peripheral resistance that is present falls as treatment is maintained. The improvement in hemodynamics occurring as a result of the increased cardiac output results in diuresis (as a consequence of an increase in renal blood flow).

All cardiac glycosides have a low therapeutic ratio because the pharmacotherapeutic and toxic actions both result from increased cytoplasmic Ca^{2+} concentrations. The most important adverse effects are cardiac arrhythmias.

In addition to the heart, other organ system toxicities are common with cardiac glycosides, but usually only during prolonged therapy. The most frequent noncardiac adverse effects of cardiac glycosides involve:

- Actions on the gastrointestinal tract (gastric irritation).
- Central nervous system (CNS) effects due to stimulation of the vagal afferents and the chemoreceptor trigger zone, resulting in nausea, vomiting, diarrhea, and anorexia.
- Other CNS effects, including visual disturbances, headaches, dizziness, fatigue, and hallucinations, which are especially common in the elderly.
- Rare adverse effects, including eosinophilia and a skin rash, and gynecomastia may occur in men (thought to be due either to hypothalamic stimulation or peripheral estrogenic actions of cardiac glycosides).

Plasma monitoring of cardiac glycoside concentrations is important since the pharmacotherapeutic window is so narrow. The pharmacokinetics of individual cardiac glycosides varies according to the lipophilicity of the compound.

Cardiac glycoside toxicity can be treated

Cardiac glycoside toxicity may be worsened by hypokalemia (which may be associated with the use of diuretics or second-

> **Adverse effects of cardiac glycosides**
>
> - Toxicity because the therapeutic dose ratios are narrow
> - May promote cardiac K^+ loss and hypokalemia which precipitate life-threatening arrhythmias when used with diuretics
> - Abdominal discomfort, emesis, and anorexia
> - Arrhythmias with cardioversion, which should therefore be used with extreme caution

ary aldosteronism). Cardiac glycosides and K^+ ions compete for a common binding site on Na^+/K^+ ATPase. Hypokalemia facilitates cardiac glycoside binding to the enzyme, thereby enhancing pharmacologic activity and toxic effects in equal measure.

Treatment of cardiac glycosides toxicity is achieved by:
- Oral administration of K^+ supplements to raise serum K^+ concentration.
- Antiarrhythmic drugs such as procainamide and phenytoin to reverse cardiac glycoside-induced arrhythmias.
- Monoclonal antibodies specific to cardiac glycosides if the arrhythmias are unresponsive to antiarrhythmic drugs.
- Intravenous digoxin-immune fragment for antigen binding (Fab), derived from specific antibodies to digoxin, for patients with life-threatening intoxication. The high affinity of cardiac glycosides for the antibody prevents binding to Na^+/K^+ ATPase and the drug can be cleared from the circulatory system.

Although cardiac glycoside toxicity may be reversed by these treatments, it should be minimized or prevented by careful monitoring of serum electrolytes and cardiac glycoside blood levels. A very important factor in the risk of developing digoxin toxicity is renal function. Since digoxin is primarily excreted unchanged by the kidneys, maintenance doses of digoxin must be adjusted in patients with renal insufficiency.

PHOSPHODIESTERASE (PDE) INHIBITORS These are agents used in patients with CHF unresponsive to other treatment. Their molecular mechanism of action is inhibition of the F-III isoform of the enzyme (PDE3) found in myocardial and vascular smooth muscle. Their cellular mechanism of action is a cascade that begins with inhibition of cAMP degradation and ends with an elevation of cytosolic Ca^{2+} content.

There are many tissue-specific PDE isoforms. Inhibitors such as inamrinone (known as amrinone in the UK), milrinone and recently vesnarinone, are bipyridines that increase cAMP levels by inhibiting PDE3. This inhibition results in a more prolonged influx of Ca^{2+} during the cardiac action potential and increases contractility. cAMP breakdown is also inhibited in arterial and venous smooth muscle, resulting in marked vasodilation.

This group of drugs increase cardiac output, decrease pulmonary capillary wedge pressure, and reduce total peripheral resistance, without producing any significant changes in heart rate or arterial blood pressure.

Inamrinone is a PDE inhibitor useful for short-term (acute) treatment of CHF

Inamrinone is used clinically for the short-term treatment of patients with CHF that is unresponsive to digitalis and diuretic therapy. It can be used alone or in conjunction with β_1 agonists to:

- Improve cardiac output.
- Increase stroke volume.
- Reduce right atrial and pulmonary capillary wedge pressures.

Prolonged intravenous use does not result in a loss of response, i.e. tachyphylaxis does not occur, but such use can cause adverse effects. There is a high incidence of nausea and vomiting in patients treated with inamrinone, but liver function abnormalities and thrombocytopenia are the adverse effects that cause most concern. These adverse effects disappear on discontinuation of treatment. Inamrinone can also cause supraventricular and ventricular arrhythmias and can therefore only be used clinically if the EKG is frequently monitored.

Milrinone is a potent PDE3 inhibitor that must not be used in long-term therapy

Milrinone is an inamrinone analog, but is a more potent inhibitor of PDE3. It has a similar spectrum of dose-limiting toxicities to that of inamrinone, but is rarely associated with thrombocytopenia. There is less gastrointestinal upset if it is used orally. Its use is limited, however, because it can precipitate lethal arrhythmias; therefore it is not used for chronic therapy. Similar findings have limited the use of a similar agent, enoximone.

Vesnarinone is a PDE inhibitor with additional potentially useful molecular actions

Studies suggest that vesnarinone may increase cardiac contractility by additional mechanisms such as activation of the Na^+/Ca^{2+} exchange antiporter, which will lead to an increase in cytosolic Ca^{2+} during systole. This may be a direct effect or indirect (secondary to the drug's ability to widen the cardiac action potential duration by an unknown mechanism). In addition, vesnarinone may stimulate the L-type Ca^{2+} current (I_{si}). The major limiting adverse effect is agranulocytosis, which occurs in 1–3% of patients. However, this is reversible when the drug is stopped. Its effectiveness in the long-term therapy of heart failure is unknown.

β_1 Adrenoceptor agonists are cardioselective sympathomimetics

The β_1 adrenoceptor is found predominantly in cardiac tissue, and agonism (the molecular action of the β_1 adrenoceptor agonist) results in elevated intracellular Ca^{2+} concentrations (cellular action), which elicits a positive inotropic response (tissue action). Selective β_1 agonists are preferable to non-selective sympathomimetics which possess undesirable α_1 adrenoceptor agonist activity (peripheral vasconstriction will occur).

Dobutamine and dopamine are the two most widely used β_1 agonists, but their use is limited to emergency intravenous therapy for reasons explained below.

Dobutamine (a racemate) is a relatively selective cardiac β_1 adrenoceptor agonist at intravenous doses less than 5 mg/kg/min. Less peripheral vasoconstriction is therefore produced than if epinephrine, for example were administered. Higher doses result in actions on β_2 and (to a lesser extent) α_1 adrenoceptors. Dobutamine acutely improves many indices of cardiac function that are impaired in CHF:

- Cardiac output is increased.
- Mean arterial pressure is decreased.
- Systemic vascular resistance is decreased.
- Ventricular filling pressure is reduced.

Dobutamine is used in the emergency treatment of severe left ventricular dysfunction associated with pulmonary edema or shock that is unresponsive to more conventional drugs. A short half-life means that it is unsuitable for oral or chronic use. It does not increase renal blood flow. Sustained β_1 agonist activity is detrimental to the heart in the long term. Dobutamine can be used acutely to assess heart function as part of 'stress' echocardiography.

Dopamine is a widely used β_1 agonist that also possesses dopamine receptor agonist activity. It is actually an endogenous neurotransmitter and has actions in the peripheral nervous system (it is not fully selective for β_1 adrenoceptors, but it does not cross the blood–brain barrier so has no central effects when administered). When given as an intravenous infusion it has a positive inotropic effect on cardiac muscle as a result of:

- β_1 Agonism (direct effect).
- Release of endogenous norepinephrine (indirect effect, of little therapeutic relevance).

Dopamine produces renal arteriolar vasodilation and therefore increases urinary output and relieves edema. It is useful in emergency due to cardiogenic, traumatic, and hypovolemic shock, where blood pressure is low and renal blood flow is poor.

Other β_1 agonists such as isoproterenol, norepinephrine, and epinephrine are never used in CHF, owing to excessive positive chronotropic effects (all three agents), or peripheral vasoconstriction via α_1 agonism (norepinephrine and epinephrine only).

The use of β_1 agonists in CHF must be considered in terms of the pharmacodynamic events that occur at the receptor level. In CHF, the high cardiac sympathetic tone produces β_1 adrenergic receptor down-regulation. Therefore, repeated exposure of cardiac muscle to β_1 agonists may result in tachyphylaxis or a loss of β_1 function in the failing heart, which may be a result of receptor uncoupling to the transduction cascade. So, paradoxically, the long-term use of selective β_1 agonists may enhance receptor down-regulation and worsen myocardial function in CHF. For this reason, and because of their ability to 'waste' myocardial oxygen (ATP production during β_1 agonism requires more oxygen than in the absence of β_1 agonism), to evoke cardiac arrhythmias, and even to cause myocardial necrosis, β_1 agonists are never used in long-term treatment of CHF, and are only used in an emergency (e.g., in the acute phase of a massive myocardial infarction, see page 383). In fact, β_1 antagonists are emerging as agents for long-term treatment of CHF (see below).

β₁ Adrenoceptor antagonists have paradoxical benefit in CHF

These agents are a surprising addition to the range of drugs for CHF, given that β adrenoceptor agonists are used in emergency treatment. Although difficult to prove, it is suspected that the system mechanism of action of β₁ adrenoceptor antagonists is antagonism of the adverse effects of a raised sympathetic tone (commonly seen in heart failure). At the cellular level, it is suspected that β₁ adrenoceptor antagonists reduce down-regulation of β₁ adrenoceptor expression that occurs in response to the high level of sympathetic tone. Consequently there may be a resetting of β₁ adrenoceptor expression which is more consistent with a healthy cardiovascular status. However, even though the cellular, tissue and system mechanisms of action are not clear, two β₁-selective antagonists, metoprolol and bisoprolol, have been shown to reduce death rate during long-term treatment, suggesting that at the molecular level, β₁ antagonism is the mechanism of action. Therapeutically, both cardiac output failure and sudden cardiac death (exact cause of death uncertain) are reduced. Another β₁ antagonist, carvedilol has also been shown to reduce death rate in CHF patients. However, this drug, in addition to blocking β₁ adrenoceptors, also blocks β₂ adrenoceptors and α₁ adrenoceptors and possesses antioxidant actions, so its exact molecular mechanism of action is not clear. All of these agents may reduce heart rate and cardiac output when treatment is begun, and this may make the patient feel worse. However, if the initial dosage is low this is not a problem. As treatment is maintained, cardiac output increases and CHF symptoms diminish. The effectiveness of the above β₁ blockers has been established in all classes of CHF except the most severe (New York Heart Association class IV).

Diuretics are routinely used with digitalis glycosides to treat congestive heart failure

Diuretics reduce cardiac preload by reducing vascular volume as a result of enhancing Na⁺ excretion by the kidney. Cardiac pump efficiency increases with the resulting reduction in venous pressure, and so the signs and symptoms of edema decrease (Fig. 18.36). Thiazide (e.g. hydrochlorothiazide) and loop diuretic (e.g. furosemide) therapy reduce intravascular and extravascular fluid accumulation in CHF and have beneficial effects in both acute and chronic CHF (albeit proof of this is difficult to establish, since diuretics are commonly included in both the treatment and control arms of present clinical trials, as a consequence of a perception of established benefit and a resultant ethical necessity to give these drugs to all patients).

 Additional drugs used in congestive heart failure to reduce edema and cardiac preload and afterload

- Diuretics (e.g. thiazides, furosemide)
- Angiotensin-converting enzyme (ACE) inhibitors (e.g. captopril)
- Nitrovasodilators (e.g. intravenous nitroprusside oral hydralazine, topical nitroglycerin)

Oral thiazides and loop diuretics are used chronically, whereas furosemide is also used intravenously, for acute CHF.

The detailed pharmacology of diuretics is discussed in Chapter 17. They are also considered later again in this chapter in the section on hypertension (see page 395).

Adverse effects resulting from diuretic therapy are usually seen only with long-term use. They include:

- Activation of hormone pathways.
- Changes in electrolyte balance.
- Changes in metabolic processes.

Electrolyte imbalances occur for serum Na⁺, Mg²⁺, Ca²⁺, and K⁺ ions. The loss of K⁺ ions from serum (hypokalemia) is especially serious and may precipitate ventricular arrhythmias. Potassium-sparing diuretics such as spironolactone or triamterene can be used to preclude K⁺ loss.

The main metabolic changes that can occur include increased concentrations of glucose and uric acid in some patients. Diuretic use should be carefully monitored in the elderly, in whom reduced renal function is common and in whom azotemia, urinary incontinence, hypovolemia, and dizziness may occur with diuretic therapy.

Drug interactions with diuretics are rare. However, the diuretic action of loop diuretics such as furosemide may be

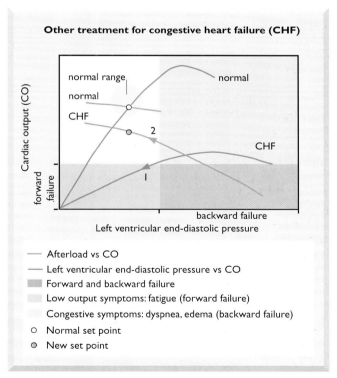

Fig. 18.36 The mechanism of action of other drugs used to treat congestive heart failure (CHF). Venodilation, diuretic therapy, and angiotensin-converting enzyme (ACE) inhibitors reduce backward failure and the symptoms of edema and congestion by reducing end-diastolic pressure. However, when used alone they may precipitate forward failure by this mechanism (1). Vasodilators and ACE inhibitors improve cardiac output by reducing cardiac afterload resulting from increased peripheral vasoconstriction and pulmonary congestion, thus providing a new set point out of the forward and backward failure domains (2).

reduced when used concomitantly with aspirin-like non-steroidal anti-inflammatory agents (NSAIDs). The mechanism probably involves NSAID inhibition of renal prostaglandin (PG) synthesis, especially PGI_2 and PGE_2, which are endogenous vasodilators.

Ototoxicity and nephrotoxicity can result when loop diuretics are used with aminoglycoside antibiotics.

Angiotensin-converting enzyme inhibitors are first-line therapy for congestive heart failure

Angiotensin-converting enzyme (ACE) inhibitors (Fig. 18.37) were first used in CHF after it was found that neurohumoral systems are activated during periods of reduced organ perfusion and increased ventricular volume. The renin–angiotensin cascade decreases cardiac performance by producing angiotensin II, which increases systemic vascular resistance (cardiac afterload) and releases aldosterone, which causes Na^+ and water retention (and edema). Inhibition of this cascade by ACE inhibitors such as captopril, enalapril, and lisinopril therefore reduces circulating angiotensin II levels. This in turn reduces peripheral vascular resistance (cardiac afterload) and prevents aldosterone-mediated Na^+ retention and blood volume expansion (i.e. reduces cardiac preload) (see Fig. 18.36). The increase in sympathetic tone is also reduced, allowing for a reduction in circulating epinephrine levels and an increased efficiency in systolic emptying (increase in cardiac output). Sustained use of ACE inhibitors may also reduce angiotensin II-induced cardiac hypertrophy and ventricular remodeling.

ACE inhibitors are the only agents that have been shown in a number of clinical trials to prolong life in CHF patients, and are therefore major therapeutic agents in this syndrome.

The ACE inhibitors are generally well tolerated. Hypotension is common as a result of the reduced arterial pressure and may cause dizziness and lightheadedness. Renal dysfunction and hyperkalemia occur, but are reversible if the drug is stopped. Approximately 10% of patients develop an irritating and even debilitating cough. Less frequent adverse effects include skin rashes, gastrointestinal upset, altered taste, and angioneurotic edema, which may occur as a result of accumulation of bradykinin and other kinins (see later, Fig. 18.52).

Adverse effects occur when ACE inhibitors are used with NSAIDs. Concomitant use of these agents prevents the auto-regulatory mechanism of PG-mediated efferent arteriolar vasodilation and results in renal hypertension.

Nitrovasodilators achieve benefit in heart failure without directly acting on the heart

Nitrovasodilators are chemically diverse agents that mediate a

Angiotensin-converting enzyme inhibitors

Drug	Main uses	Usual doses (mg/day)	Elimination plasma half-life (h)	Elimination	Adverse effects
Captopril	Congestive heart failure Hypertension	50–100	4	Renal + hepatic	Hypotension (aggravated by NSAIDs), cough
Enalapril	Congestive heart failure Hypertension	2.5–30	30–35	Renal + hepatic	Similar to captopril + GI cancer (low risk)
Benazepril	Hypertension	10–40	24	Renal + hepatic	Similar to captopril
Lisinopril	Congestive heart failure Hypertension	2.5–10	> 30	Exclusively renal	Similar to captopril
Cilazapril	Congestive heart failure Hypertension	1.25–20	30–50	Renal	Similar to captopril
Ramipril	Congestive heart failure Hypertension	2.5–10 (1.25 in renal impairment)	85–190	Renal + hepatic	Similar to captopril
Quinapril	Congestive heart failure Hypertension	10–20	30–50	Renal + hepatic	Similar to captopril
Fosinopril	Essential hypertension	20–40	12	Renal + hepatic	Milder than captopril
Moexipril	Hypertension	7.5–30	12	Renal + fecal	Similar to captopril
Trandolapril	Hypertension Left ventricular hypertrophy	2–8	Up to 8 days	Renal	Similar to captopril

Fig. 18.37 Angiotensin-converting enzyme inhibitors.

potent vasodilating action on both arterial and venous smooth muscle. The molecular mechanism of action remains poorly characterized. However, these agents:

- Are thought to produce vascular relaxation at the cellular level by nitrosothiol intermediate enhancement of cGMP activity.
- May regulate intracellular Ca^{2+} release from the sarcoplasmic reticulum, alter sympathetic tone, and produce smooth muscle-relaxing autacoids such as PGI_2 and PGE_2.
- Reduce diastolic pressure and improve diastolic function in the heart (see Fig. 18.36).

Nitroprusside is a standard first-choice nitrovasodilator in the treatment of acute CHF, especially in patients with elevated arterial blood pressure because it reduces both cardiac preload and afterload. It reduces left ventricular filling pressures by reducing venous tone, and by doing so increases venous capacitance and produces a shift in blood volume distribution.

Since nitroprusside has no important direct effect on ventricular contractility, the increase in cardiac output and stroke volume occur as a result of a reduction in cardiac afterload. The increase in cardiac output is not accompanied by a reflex increase in blood pressure or heart rate, and nitroprusside lowers myocardial oxygen consumption.

Nitroprusside must be given intravenously at 0.10–0.20 mg/kg/min with dose titration, and is used as an acute short-term treatment of CHF.

Liver metabolism of nitroprusside produces cyanide, which is then cleared by the kidney. Cyanide can accumulate in patients with renal insufficiency, resulting in nausea, confusion, and convulsions. Nitroprusside can also be metabolized to prussic acid, which avidly binds hemoglobin.

The major adverse effect of nitroprusside is hypotension, which may be severe.

Nitroglycerin (glyceryl trinitrate) and isosorbide dinitrate predominantly decrease cardiac preload, but produce a slight reduction in cardiac afterload. Tolerance develops rapidly and so administration has to be intermittent. A high first-pass metabolism can be avoided by sublingual administration or topical application. Hypotension is the most common adverse effect.

Hydralazine used in combination with nitrates has been shown to increase the life expectancy of patients with CHF. This combination is therefore an alternative first-line therapy to ACE inhibitors, especially for patients who are unable to tolerate the latter.

In addition to reducing cardiac afterload, hydralazine has an indirect positive inotropic effect on cardiac muscle action, resulting from enhanced sympathetic nervous system activity due to arterial vasodilation. It is therefore useful when withdrawing dobutamine or β_1 agonist treatment. Hydralazine also increases renal blood flow. Hydralazine alone is insufficient to reduce vascular congestion adequately, and is therefore used with topical nitroglycerin or oral isosorbide dinitrate to induce venodilation.

The adverse effects of hydralazine include:

- Reflex activation of the sympathetic nervous system.
- Drug-induced systemic lupus erythematous, which is rare with doses of hydralazine less than 200 mg/day.

> **Adverse effects of drugs used in the treatment of congestive heart failure**
>
> - Cardiac glycosides have a narrow therapeutic index and may precipitate arrhythmias
> - Short-term treatment with phosphodiesterase inhibitors can cause thrombocytopenia and arrhythmias
> - β_1 Agonists may precipitate tachyarrhythmias, and long-term use may worsen myocardial function
> - Diuretics produce serious electrolyte imbalances such as hypokalemia, which may produce ventricular arrhythmias
> - Angiotensin-converting enzyme (ACE) inhibitors produce few adverse effects, and generally only hypotension
> - Nitrovasodilators have few adverse effects

Since myocardial oxygen consumption increases with hydralazine, this drug is contraindicated in patients with CHF who have ischemic coronary artery disease unless nitrates are used at the same time.

EMERGING DRUGS Several studies are currently examining the following drugs for use in the treatment of moderate to severe CHF:

- Novel phosphodiesterase inhibitors (OPC-18790).
- Potent angiotensin-II receptor antagonists (losartan).
- Selective adenosine A_1 antagonists (CVT-124).

Although there are many drugs that relieve the signs and symptoms of CHF, they do not prevent the underlying deterioration of cardiac function. Valve surgery (if valve insufficiency is the cause) or heart transplantation (if a major myocardial infarction or viral myocarditis are the cause) may be required if drugs fail to relieve the symptoms.

Hypertension

Hypertension is a condition of an elevated blood pressure relative to a perceived 'normal' level. Hypertension is defined arbitrarily as sustained increases in systemic blood pressure, typically either systolic or diastolic blood pressure, greater than 140/90 mmHg respectively. Isolated systolic hypertension refers to an elevated systolic blood pressure (typically greater than 140–160 mmHg) in the absence of an increase in diastolic pressure (see Fig. 18.38). Chronically, elevated blood pressure is associated with an increased risk of damage to kidney, heart and brain as well as other diseases (atherosclerosis). Chronically elevated blood pressure is a sign rather than a disease itself, and in most cases of hypertension (so-called essential hypertension) the underlying cause is rarely diagnosed. Pulmonary hypertension is an entirely separate disease, and is discussed in Chapter 19.

The components of the normal blood pressure control system can be manipulated by drugs so as to treat hypertension. Blood pressure is controlled by an integrated neuronal and hormonal control system (Fig. 18.39). This regulates blood pressure via alterations in:

- Blood volume.

Classification of blood pressure based on the report of the 1993 Joint National Committee

Category	Systolic (mmHg)	Diastolic (mmHg)
Normal†	<130	<85
High normal	130–139	85–89
Hypertension		
Stage 1 (mild)	140–159	90–99
Stage 2 (moderate)	160–179	100–109
Stage 3 (severe)	180–209	110–119
Stage 4 (very severe)	≥210	≥120

† Optimal blood pressure with respect to cardiovascular risk is less than 120 mmHg systolic and less than 80 mmHg diastolic

Fig. 18.38 Classification of blood pressure based on the report of the 1993 Joint National Committee. Values are from the 5th report of the JNC on detection, evaluation, and treatment of high blood pressure. Isolated systolic hypertension is defined as a systolic blood pressure of 140 mmHg or more and a diastolic blood pressure of less than 90 mmHg and staged approximately.

- Cardiac output.
- Peripheral vascular resistance.

The primary therapeutic objective in the treatment of hypertension is a reduction of the sign itself (the high blood pressure) by drugs whose mechanisms of action at the system level are: altered blood volume, cardiac output, and peripheral vascular resistance. There is an expectation that a reduction of blood pressure will limit the development of subsequent organ pathology.

The tissue targets for antihypertensive drugs are:

- The sympathetic nerves, which release the vasoconstrictor norepinephrine.
- The kidney, which regulates blood volume.
- The heart, which generates cardiac output.
- The arterioles, which determine peripheral vascular resistance.
- Endothelial cells, which regulate circulating levels of the endogenous hypertensive and hypotensive agents such as angiotensin II and nitric oxide, respectively.
- The CNS, which senses the blood pressure and controls its set point by regulating some systems involved in blood pressure control.

Hypertension can be classified into essential (or primary) hypertension and secondary hypertension

Primary hypertension is an elevation of blood pressure with no apparent cause. It accounts for 90–95% of all cases and usually occurs in adulthood, typically at ages above 40 years. Several risk factors are associated with primary hypertension, including a genetic predisposition, obesity, high alcohol con-

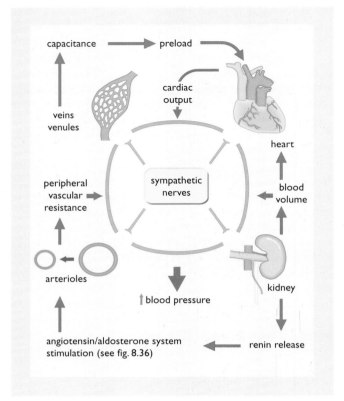

Fig. 18.39 Factors involved in blood pressure control. Determinants of blood pressure are cardiac output, determined by heart rate and stroke volume. Cardiac output depends on the amount of blood returning to the heart, which in turn depends on vein and venule capacitance (preload) and blood volume (under the control of the kidneys). Peripheral vascular resistance is determined by the arterioles.

sumption, and physical inactivity. Some of these may represent additional systems targets for antihypertensive drugs.

Secondary hypertension accounts for 5–10% of all cases and, by definition, is due to an identifiable cause, for example renovascular disease, which elevates blood pressure by activating the renin–angiotensin–aldosterone system (Fig. 18.40). A variety of endocrine diseases (e.g. pheochromocytoma, an adrenal medulla tumor that secretes excessive epinephrine) may also cause secondary hypertension.

Hypertension

- Hypertension is commonly diagnosed when the diastolic pressure is consistently found to be higher than 90 mmHg
- Blood pressure can be raised by increased cardiac output, increased peripheral resistance, or increased blood volume
- Primary hypertension has no apparent cause
- Secondary hypertension results from another disease such as pheochromocytoma

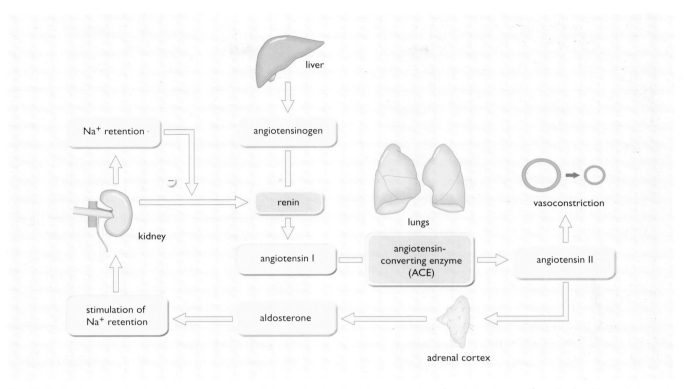

Fig. 18.40 Renin–angiotensin–aldosterone system. Release of renin stimulates conversion of angiotensinogen (from the liver) to angiotensin I, which in turn is converted to angiotensin II under the influence of angiotensin-converting enzyme. Angiotensin II leads to vasoconstriction, release of aldosterone (adrenal cortex), and Na+ retention. The latter increases blood pressure but reduces renin release, so the system is a homeostatic process.

Both primary and secondary hypertension can be classified by the degree of increased cardiovascular risk and the extent to which blood pressure is elevated

In most patients, treatment of hypertension is a lifetime project to reduce cardiovascular risk over many years. In some patients typically with markedly elevated blood pressure, it may also be necessary to decrease blood pressure over the course of hours or days. These relatively uncommon situations are often called hypertensive emergencies or urgencies respectively.

In most patients with hypertension the blood pressure increases progressively over months to years. As a result, an increased risk of cardiovascular disease develops slowly over a period of years (Fig. 18.41). The resultant loss of vascular elasticity and compliance then contributes to the establishment of chronic hypertension. Consequently, therapy involves long-term control of blood pressure.

In hypertensive emergencies the generally much larger increase in blood pressure, typically over a shorter period of time, may lead to immediately life-threatening target organ damage in heart, aorta, brain or kidneys (Fig. 18.42). In this situation the pharmacotherapeutic objective is to control blood pressure within minutes or hours. In treated patients, hypertensive emergencies are becoming increasingly rare as therapy improves, but emergencies may occur if the therapy is inadequate, if the patient stops taking their medication because they falsely think they are 'well,' or if the patient is undiagnosed

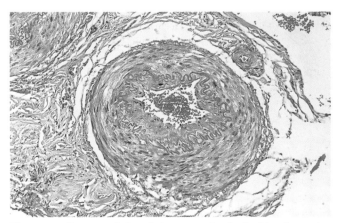

Fig. 18.41 Changes of chronic hypertension in the blood vessel wall. These occur slowly over time. Medial smooth muscle cells migrate into the intima so that the intima becomes thicker. (Courtesy of Dr Alan Stevens and Professor Jim Lowe.)

and has never been treated. The presentation involves high, and rising, blood pressure and signs of end-organ damage, e.g. encephalopathy. If an emergency occurs it is important to reduce the blood pressure quickly by intravenous drug administration, but carefully and in stages (usually chosen arbitrarily) to avoid low cerebrovascular pressure and cerebral ischemia (Fig. 18.43).

397

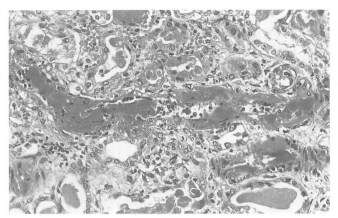

Fig. 18.42 Changes of accelerated hypertension in the blood vessel wall. Accelerated hypertension damages the blood vessel wall. Damage to the endothelial lining leads to adhesion and activation of platelets and release of various mediators (platelet-activating factor, thromboxane A₂, serotonin, ADP, thrombin). (Courtesy of Dr Alan Stevens and Professor Jim Lowe.)

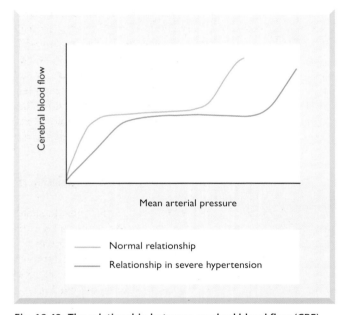

Fig. 18.43 The relationship between cerebral blood flow (CBF) and mean arterial pressure (MAP). In severe hypertension, particularly in emergency hypertension, a rapid reduction of MAP may cause an excessive reduction in CBF, cerebral ischemia, and possibly stroke.

Treatment of hypertension

Nondrug treatment is the ideal first-choice therapy. Patients with hypertension are advised to avoid activities that may predispose to cardiovascular disease. The major recommendations are:

- To exercise.
- To reduce body weight if overweight.
- In some cases, to restrict dietary salt intake.
- To stop smoking.
- To restrict ethanol intake in some patients.
- To treat lipoprotein disorders carefully.

Classes of drugs used for treating hypertension

- Diuretics
- Sympatholytics
- Direct-acting vasodilators
- Calcium antagonists
- Renin–angiotensin cascade inhibitors (including the angiotensin II receptor antagonist, losartan)

All antihypertensive drugs have adverse effects. Although this is true of all diseases to a greater or lesser extent, adverse effects are particularly important in the treatment of hypertension since most hypertensive patients are free of symptoms for most of the time (except during an emergency). It is only when secondary complications such as a stroke ensue that the disease becomes symptomatic. Therefore, any adverse drug effect, no matter how trivial, will make the patient feel worse. This explains why compliance is notoriously poor in long-term treatment of hypertension.

The pharmacotherapeutic response in the treatment of hypertension is a reduction in blood pressure to an acceptable level (typically to less than 140/90 mmHg, or even less than 130/80 mmHg in patients with diabetes or renal disease). This can be achieved by diverse system, tissue, cellular, and molecular mechanisms of drug action using a wide range of therapeutic options. Choice of drugs is influenced by demonstration of beneficial effects on clinically important end-points (for example thiazide diuretics and β adrenoceptor antagonists), cost, tolerability in individual patients, and by concomitant disorders (such as congestive heart failure or diabetes which mandate use of angiotensin-converting enzyme inhibitors as primary drugs).

Five classes of drug are currently used, but the classification is heterogeneous since some of the classes comprise drugs grouped in terms of their molecular mechanism of action, and others in terms of tissue or system mechanism of action. The choice of drug therapy may be influenced by the type of hypertension and any other clinical condition a patient may have.

The least toxic drug that can control the blood pressure should be used first

The first choice of drug is based on the general principle that the least toxic drug that can achieve effective control of the blood pressure should be used first (so as to maximize patient compliance). Several different types of drug may be chosen as an initial form of therapy according to the individual patient's presentation (Fig. 18.44). If that drug is inadequate, then it should be changed to one of another class, or a drug of another class should be used in addition to the first drug. The latter approach is often sufficient to achieve benefit because several class combinations may produce additive effects. In many guidelines for the treatment of hypertension, produced by learned societies around the world, a thiazide diuretic or a β adrenoceptor antagonist are frequently the recommended drugs

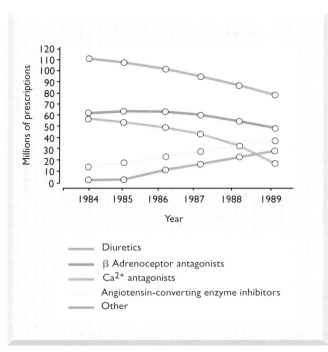

Fig. 18.44 Number of antihypertensive prescriptions in the US, 1984–1989.

for initial use in the long-term treatment of hypertension. This is typically based on the demonstrated clinical efficacy of these drugs in preventing adverse cardiovascular events (such as stroke) and also their established safety record and generally low cost to patients. ACE inhibitors such as lisinopril are increasingly used as an alternative to diuretics or β adrenoceptor antagonists, especially because they are generally well tolerated and have therapeutic advantages in patients with diabetes or congestive heart failure. Calcium antagonists have been shown to be effective in preventing adverse cardiovascular events in patients with isolated systolic hypertension. Other classes of antihypertensive drugs such as α_1 adrenoceptor antagonists, drugs that inhibit sympathetic nervous system activity, or arterial vasodilators such as hydralazine and minoxidil, are less frequently used. Multiple drug combinations are sometimes needed in patients with severe hypertension.

Generally, there is little difference between patient populations in terms of the ability of the different classes of drug to reduce blood pressure acutely. However, certain groups of people are more responsive in the long term to certain classes of drugs than others. For example, the Caucasian population responds better than people of African origin to adrenoceptor antagonists and ACE inhibitors, whereas the elderly population responds better than the young to calcium antagonists and diuretics. However, variation in drug responses is greater from individual to individual than between populations.

The ultimate aim of therapy is to reduce the increased mortality found in the hypertensive population. The few drugs that have been shown to achieve this include thiazide diuretics and ACE inhibitors. There are suggestions that some classes of drugs may increase, rather than decrease, mortality.

Diuretics are useful antihypertensives but their benefit may be unrelated to diuresis

The pharmacology of diuretics is discussed in detail in Chapter 17. Three types of diuretic are used in hypertension:

- Thiazides.
- Loop diuretics.
- Potassium-sparing agents.

Diuretics were once thought to lower blood pressure via a tissue mechanism involving increased water excretion in the kidney, which leads to a reduction of plasma volume, extracellular fluid volume, and cardiac output. However, there are several reasons for questioning this, the most important of which is that, for a range of diuretic drugs, antihypertensive activity is not directly proportional to diuretic activity:

- Thiazides are relatively effective antihypertensive agents, but are only moderately effective diuretics.
- Loop diuretics are relatively ineffective antihypertensive agents (in patients with normal renal function) but are powerful diuretics.

So, although diuresis has been the conventional explanation for the beneficial effect provided by diuretics in hypertension, there is increasing awareness that their molecular and tissue mechanisms of action in hypertension are not well understood.

Recently, it has been suggested that diuretics (especially the thiazides) may produce their effects in hypertension by modulating the activity of K^+ channels. ATP-regulated K^+ channels in resistance arterioles may be activated by thiazides. This molecular action leads to membrane hyperpolarization, which opposes smooth muscle Ca^{2+} entry and contraction and, at the system level, reduces peripheral vascular resistance.

Thiazides are the most commonly used antihypertensive diuretics

Thiazide diuretics (e.g. bendrofluazide, hydrochlorothiazide) and thiazide-like drugs which are sulfonamide derivatives, such as chlorthalidone, are actively transported by a probenecid-sensitive secretory mechanism into the proximal renal tubule. As diuretics, this group of agents acts on the luminal membrane of the cortical diluting segment of the distal convoluted tubule (see Chapter 17). If the diuretic effect of thiazides were responsible for their antihypertensive effect, the dose–response relationship for these two effects would be superimposble. This is not the case (Fig. 18.45), reinforcing the concept that another action is responsible for the antihypertensive effect. On the other hand, thiazides lose effectiveness in patients with moderate renal insufficiency.

Thiazides may cause male sexual dysfunction. Since hypertension (in the elderly male) is commonly associated with impotence, the prevalence and impact of this adverse effect are difficult to determine. Relatively high doses of thiazide diuretics may induce hyperuricemia, and have somewhat adverse effects on serum concentrations of lipids and glucose.

Hypokalemia may occur as an adverse effect of long-term thiazide treatment

One cellular action of thiazides is associated with a characteristic adverse effect: an increase in Na^+ concentration in the distal

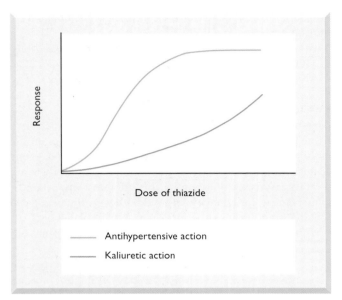

Fig. 18.45 Dose–response relationship for thiazide antihypertensive agents and blood pressure (antihypertensive action) and as a diuretic (shown here as effect on K⁺ excretion, the kaliuretic action). The lack of overlap of the curves suggests that the two effects may not be related.

convoluted tubule impairs K^+ reabsorption, since K^+ reabsorption is mediated here by Na^+/K^+ ATPase and therefore depends on an appropriate Na^+ gradient to allow Na^+/K^+ exchange. Thus, thiazide diuretics may cause an increase in K^+ excretion (kaliuresis) and possibly hypokalemia. However, if appropriately low doses of thiazides are used in the treatment of hypertension, these potential changes may not be clinically significant. Marked hyperkalemia induced by low doses of a thiazide diuretic in a patient with hypertension may prompt the suspicion that the patient has underlying primary hyperaldosteronism. Fortunately, the maximum antihypertensive effect of thiazides occurs with very low doses of 25–50 mg/day. Hypokalemia, should it occur, may give rise to, or exacerbate pre-existent, cardiac arrhythmias. Potassium supplements (oral potassium chloride) may be used to avoid hypokalemia. Alternatively, potassium-sparing drugs may be given in combination with thiazides.

Thiazides may induce an increase in plasma renin (owing to increased removal of blood Na^+ as a consequence of diuresis) and therefore formation of angiotensin II and release of aldosterone. As aldosterone contributes to K^+ loss from the kidney, this action therefore contributes to the hypokalemic effect of thiazides. Concomitant use of a β adrenoceptor antagonist or an ACE inhibitor reduces plasma renin activity or plasma angiotensin II activity, respectively. This can ameliorate the aldosterone-dependent component of the hypokalemic effect of thiazides. In addition, ACE inhibitors potentiate the hypotensive effects of thiazides.

Diuretic-induced hypokalemia may be avoided by using potassium-sparing diuretics

Avoidance of hypokalemia may be achieved by using so-called potassium-sparing diuretics. These act at the cortical collecting duct, where exchange of Na^+ for K^+ and H^+ ions occurs via an exchanger that is regulated by endogenous aldosterone (see Chapter 17):

- Drugs such as amiloride and triamterene act at the luminal membrane. Their molecular mechanism is blockade of Na^+ channels and noncompetitive antagonism of aldosterone.
- Spironolactone is a reversible competitive antagonist of aldosterone at its intracellular receptor in the luminal membrane of the cortical collecting duct. It is generally not used in the treatment of primary hypertension due to potentially severe adverse effects, especially in male patients where it interferes with testosterone synthesis and action.

The role of diuresis in mediating the antihypertensive effect of these drugs is highly questionable since triamterene is not an antihypertensive drug despite having a diuretic effect similar to antihypertensive agent, amiloride.

In general, when predictable adverse effects are anticipated and avoided, diuretics are well tolerated as antihypertensive agents, with only 10% of patients stopping therapy during long-term treatment.

Sympatholytics are a heterogeneous group of drugs that reduce blood pressure by a variety of actions in the cardiovascular system

The activity of the sympathetic nervous system plays a pivotal role in the acute regulation of blood pressure (Fig. 18.39). Sympatholytic drugs lower blood pressure by inhibiting one or more component of this activity. This system mechanism of action may be achieved in a variety of different ways:

- Some drugs act on the vasomotor center in the brain to reduce the tone of the sympathetic system tone centrally.
- Other drugs act peripherally on adrenergic neurotransmission at pre- or postsynaptic sites or on receptors activated by circulating epinephrine and neurally released norepinephrine.

Many sympatholytic agents possess both a direct and an indirect tissue mechanism of action, since they may directly affect nervous tissue function which then affects cardiac, vascular, or other tissue function. Others, such as β adrenoceptor antagonists, act directly on norepinephrine and epinephrine receptors in the cardiovascular system. Below, the sympatholytics are described in an order that reflects their selectivity of action as sympatholytics and not in relation to the frequency of their use as antihypertensive agents, which is described for each type of drug within each subsection.

Nonselective sympatholytics (i.e. ganglion blockers and adrenergic neuron blockers) are rarely used today because of their adverse effects.

β Adrenoceptor antagonists are the second most widely used group of antihypertensive drugs after diuretics

The mechanism of action of β adrenoceptor antagonists, as a class, in the treatment of hypertension is not known with certainty. These drugs have a range of molecular and tissue effects, and the benefit achieved with each drug may depend upon its own specific properties:

- The molecular mechanism of action is generally regarded to be competitive antagonism of β_1 adrenoceptors, although β_2 adrenoceptor antagonism may also contribute to the benefit achieved with some drugs. This uncertainty is not resolved.
- The cellular mechanism is not known, largely because controversy still exists with respect to the molecular mechanisms of action. The cellular effects of β_1 and β_2 antagonism are known, however, and are described below.
- The tissue mechanism of action is likewise unclear. β Adrenoceptor antagonists may act in the CNS to reduce sympathetic tone (see. Fig. 18.46), in the heart to reduce heart rate and cardiac output, and in the kidney to reduce renin production. A common feature of their action in hypertension is a reduction in peripheral resistance, but it is not clear how this effect occurs.

There are numerous different β adrenoceptor antagonists in clinical use (Fig. 18.47). They differ in their ability to block β_1 adrenoceptors in the heart and CNS versus β_2 receptors in the bronchi and peripheral blood vessels.

Atenolol and metoprolol are selective β_1 adrenoceptor antagonists used in hypertension

Historically, the term 'cardioselective' has been used to describe β_1 selective adrenoceptor antagonists, although these agents will affect any tissues that express β_1 adrenoceptors. Cardioselective β_1 adrenoceptor antagonists such as atenolol and metoprolol antagonize the effects of norepinephrine and epinephrine on heart rate, but have less effect on the airways than nonselective β adrenoceptor antagonists. Nonetheless, since β_1 versus β_2 selectivity is only relative (less than eightfold), these drugs are not safe enough to use in asthmatics, except under special circumstances (i.e., when no other antihypertensive is tolerated but some form of drug therapy is essential).

Pindolol is an antihypertensive β_1 adrenoceptor partial agonist

Some partial agonists at β_1 adrenoceptors are used in the treatment of hypertension (e.g. pindolol). These drugs inhibit excess β_1 adrenoceptor activity during sympathetic hyperactivity, but achieve an overall β_1 agonist effect when the sympathetic tone is low. Historically these drugs have been described as 'β_1 blockers with intrinsic sympathomimetic activity.' However, this description is imprecise as the agents are quite specifically partial agonists, as defined in Chapter 3. The β_1 adrenoceptor partial agonists reduce blood pressure to a similar degree to β_1 adrenoceptor antagonists, but evoke less reduction in resting heart rate. This may be advantageous if the patient is receiving, for an unrelated condition, concurrent treatment that widens the QT interval, since bradycardia exacerbates QT widening, and this can precipitate *torsades de pointes* (see page 367). Aside from this, the clinical significance of partial agonism is unknown. Also, in contrast with β_1 adrenergic antagonists, partial agonists have not been shown to be beneficial in the secondary prevention of myocardial infarction.

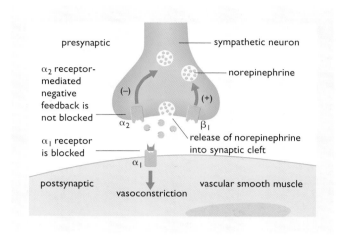

Fig. 18.46 Antagonism at postsynaptic α_1 adrenoceptors.
Prazosin (α_1 antagonist) prevents vasoconstriction by norepinephrine. Further effects of norepinephrine are reduced by a feedback mechanism since presynaptic α_2 adrenoceptors are not blocked by prazosin and so the α_2 adrenoceptors can be occupied by norepinephrine, thereby activating a negative feedback pathway.

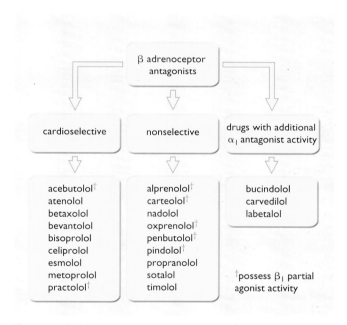

Fig. 18.47 β Adrenoceptor antagonists classified according to cardioselectivity and partial agonist activity.

Labetalol and carvedilol are nonselective α_1 and β_1 adrenoceptor antagonists used in hypertension

Drugs such as labetalol and carvedilol are nonselective α_1 and β_1 adrenoceptor antagonists. The ratio of extent of β_1 to α_1 antagonism elicited by submaximal dosage (that typically encountered therapeutically) is 10:1 for carvedilol and 4:1 for labetalol. These drugs, like pindolol, lower blood pressure via a reduction in peripheral vascular resistance with no change in heart rate or cardiac output. Carvedilol has other molecular actions that may be relevant to its additional role in treatment of heart failure (page 386).

β Adrenoceptor antagonists have a favorable risk–benefit ratio when used to treat hypertension

Although β adrenoceptor antagonists do not usually have serious adverse effects, these may be sufficient to impair compliance:

- β₁ Adrenoceptor antagonism can exacerbate CHF by reducing cardiac output. (Note that paradoxically some β₁ adrenoceptor antagonists at low dosage are now being used to treat CHF; see page 393).
- β₂ Adrenoceptor antagonism (the basis for 'non-cardioselective' actions) may lead to bronchospasm (meaning that these drugs are contraindicated in asthmatics) and lower the recovery from hypoglycemia in patients with diabetes mellitus.

Interestingly, the benefit of these drugs in secondary prevention of myocardial infarction in hypertensive patients may outweigh the risks for many patients with concomitant chronic obstructive pulmonary disease or type II diabetes.

Sudden discontinuation of β₁ adrenoceptor antagonists can cause angina pectoris and myocardial infarction

Discontinuation of some β₁ adrenoceptor antagonists can cause rebound sympathetic stimulation of the heart, leading to angina pectoris and myocardial infarction. It is recommended that if a β₁ adrenoceptor antagonist is ineffective or poorly tolerated, the patient should be gradually weaned off it, rather than abruptly transferred to other agents.

α₁ Adrenoceptor antagonists are beneficial in hypertensive patients with benign prostate hyperplasia (BPH)

Prazosin was the first selective agent with the molecular mechanism of postsynaptic α₁ adrenoceptor antagonism. Prazosin and newer analogs such as terazosin and doxazosin (Fig. 18.48) act directly on the effector component of the sympathetic neuroeffector junction, namely α₁ adrenoceptors, which are expressed in abundance in arteriolar resistance vessels where they mediate a vasoconstrictor tone. The tissue mechanism of action of α₁ adrenoceptor antagonists is therefore the inhibition of this tone. This reduces peripheral vascular resistance. Norepinephrine normally limits its own neuronal release by acting on presynaptic α₂ receptors (negative feedback). Drugs that block α₂ receptors, therefore, tend to increase norepinephrine release from sympathetic nerve terminals. In the heart, unrestricted norepinephrine release causes excess stimulation of postsynaptic β₁ adrenoceptors and tachycardia. Consequently nonselective α (α₁ and α₂) antagonists are not useful antihypertensives. Because prazosin has selectivity for α₁ receptors, the negative feedback mechanism remains intact, meaning that the drug's therapeutic effectiveness is not compromised by tachycardia (see Fig. 18.46).

α₁ Adrenoceptor antagonists can modify plasma lipid levels

α₁ Adrenoceptor antagonists can modify the plasma levels of low density lipoprotein (LDL) cholesterol, and apoprotein B, so that overall LDL cholesterol levels are reduced as well as very low density lipoprotein (VLDL) levels and total triglyceride levels. These agents also increase high-density lipoprotein (HDL) cholesterol levels and therefore reduce one of the risk factors associated with coronary artery disease (see Chapter 15), although the clinical relevance of this is unknown.

Prazosin is given twice a day, whereas doxazosin and terazosin require only once-daily administration because of their long plasma half-life, which affords better patient compliance. Other uses of prazosin are described in Chapter 22.

Urapidil is an α₁ adrenoceptor antagonist with additional 5-HT₁ₐ agonist activity. The latter action in the CNS (medulla) causes a reduction in sympathetic tone. Consequently urapidil can lower blood pressure without eliciting the reflex tachycardia typically seen with other α₁ adrenoceptor antagonists.

Prazosin-like drugs					
Drug	Main uses	Usual doses (mg/day)	Plasma half-life (h)	Metabolism and elimination	Adverse effects
Prazosin	Hypertension Congestive heart failure Raynaud's phenomenon	3–7.5 p.o.	4	Hepatic metabolism 50% first pass	Hypotension (rare); exacerbated by hyponatremia
Terazosin	Hypertension	1–20 p.o.	12	Hepatic metabolism 50% first pass Biliary/fecal elimination	Dizziness, headache, nasal congestion (all rare)
Doxazosin	Hypertension Congestive heart failure Benign prostatic hyperplasia	2–16 p.o.	19–22	Hepatic metabolism Low first pass Biliary/fecal elimination	Similar to terazosin

Fig. 18.48 Prazosin-like drugs. (p.o., orally)

Adverse effects of α_1 antagonists include postural hypotension, dizziness, weakness, fatigue, reflex tachycardia (except urapidil) and headaches, but little sedation, dry mouth, or ejaculation failure

α_2 Adrenoceptor agonists are not generally preferred drug choices for treating hypertension

Centrally acting α_2 adrenoceptor agonists such as clonidine, guanfacine, guanabenz and α methyldopa mimic the auto-inhibitory effects of norepinephrine on sympathetic activity without producing sympathomimetic effects (Fig. 18.49). The reason for this is their relative selectivity for α_2 receptors. The mechanisms of action are as follows:

- The molecular mechanism of action is α_2 adrenoceptor agonism (Fig. 18.50).
- The direct tissue mechanism of action is a reduction in the activity of the vasomotor center in the brain, leading to a fall in sympathetic nervous activity.
- This leads to a secondary tissue mechanism of action, a reduction in peripheral resistance as a result of arteriolar relaxation. However, with maintained therapy, a reduction in heart rate and cardiac output appear to be the predominant effects, especially with clonidine.

Clonidine is a widely used α_2 agonist (guanabenz and guanfacine have a similar molecular action), whereas α methyldopa is a pro-drug which is metabolized via a two-step enzymatic process in the CNS to α methylnorepinephrine (Fig. 18.51), which is an α_2 agonist. In the CNS, α methylnorepinephrine stimulates the vasopressor centers in the brainstem, which results in a reduction of sympathetic outflow. Because renal blood flow is well maintained with α methyldopa, it has been widely used in hypertensive patients with renal insufficiency or cerebrovascular disease. α Methyldopa is also recommended for use in hypertensive pregnant women because it has no adverse effects on the fetus despite crossing the blood–placenta barrier.

Adverse effects of this group of drugs are sedation (more so with clonidine and guanabenz than guanfacine), dry mouth, orthostatic hypotension (particularly in the elderly), male sexual dysfunction (impotence), and galactorrhea. α Methyldopa is now used very infrequently owing to more serious adverse

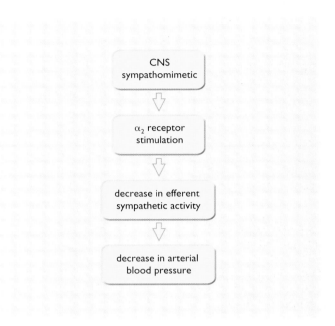

Fig. 18.50 α_2 **Agonism decreases sympathetic activity and consequently reduces blood pressure.**

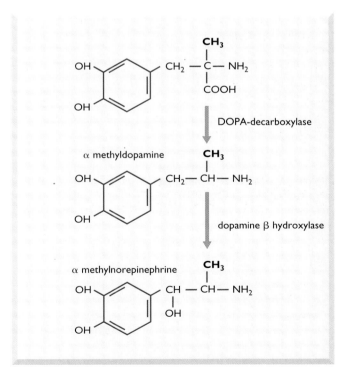

Fig. 18.51 Metabolism of α methyldopa to α methylnorepinephrine. Note that CH_3 is absent in DOPA, the endogenous precursor to dopamine, which is metabolized, by the same enzymes, to norepinephrine.

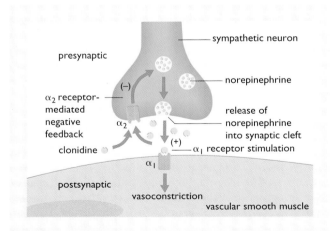

Fig. 18.49 Presynaptic α_2 agonism. This prevents the release of norepinephrine and subsequent postsynaptic α_1 agonism. Clonidine is an α_2 selective agonist. If the postsynaptic receptor is β_1, this, in the heart, mediates tachycardia.

effects (including diffuse parenchymal injury in the liver resembling the effects of viral hepatitis and, rarely, fever and hemolytic anemia).

The use of clonidine in hypertensive patients has been associated with a rapid rebound of blood pressure to pre-treatment levels when the treatment is stopped abruptly. This can cause withdrawal symptoms, including tachycardia, restlessness, and sweating. The rebound of blood pressure may be treated by reintroducing the drug or using a peripherally acting α_1 adrenoceptor antagonist to prevent sympathetic nervous system-mediated peripheral vasoconstriction. These adverse effects can be avoided by gradually decreasing the dose of clonidine over time.

Clonidine is available as a transdermal preparation that may provide control of blood pressure for up to 7 days with the potential for fewer adverse effects. However, adverse effects of the patch on the skin may be troublesome.

Adrenergic neuron blockers are rarely used in the treatment of hypertension, but have interesting pharmacology. The adrenergic neuron blockers, reserpine and guanidine derivatives such as guanethidine, act through different molecular and cellular mechanisms to achieve a similar tissue response.

▨ Reserpine has adrenergic neuron blocking actions resulting in arteriolar vasodilation and a reduced cardiac output

Reserpine is transported into peripheral sympathetic nerve terminals by uptake-1 (a mechanism for norepinephrine re-uptake into nerves) and its mechanisms of action are as follows:

- Its molecular mechanism of action is inhibition of the norepinephrine pump (an ATP and Mg^{2+}-dependent uptake molecule) located on the storage vesicles for norepinephrine in the neuronal cytoplasm.
- Its cellular mechanism of action is a reduction of the norepinephrine content of neuronal storage vesicles.
- Its direct tissue mechanism of action is a reduction of nerve action potential-mediated release of norepinephrine from sympathetic nerve terminals.
- Its indirect tissue mechanism of action is arteriolar vaso-dilation and reduced cardiac output.

Reserpine can reduce blood pressure effectively. However, a percentage of patients experience severe psychologic depression, and so use of this drug has declined. This adverse effect is dose-dependent so can be avoided by careful titration of dosage, starting from 0.1 mg/day or less.

▨ Guanethidine has two molecular and cellular mechanisms acting in parallel to achieve adrenergic neuron block

Guanethidine and related guanidine compounds including guanadrel, bethanidine, and debrisoquin are, like reserpine, transported into peripheral sympathetic nerve terminals by uptake-1. However, their molecular and cellular mechanisms of action differ from those of reserpine. In fact, two molecular and cellular mechanisms act in parallel to reduce the activity of the sympathetic nervous system:

- One molecular mechanism is competition with norepinephrine for the intracellular norepinephrine pump (an ATP- and Mg^{2+}-dependent uptake molecule). The drugs are actually taken up and stored in the adrenergic vesicles in preference to norepinephrine. The associated cellular mechanism of action is a reduced content of norepinephrine in the storage vesicles, and the direct tissue mechanism of action is a reduction of nerve action potential-mediated release of norepinephrine from sympathetic nerve terminals.
- The second molecular mechanism is binding to the inner surface of the neurolemma. The associated cellular mechanism is reduction of the fusion between storage vesicles and the neurolemma, known as the true 'adrenergic neuron blocking' action. The associated tissue mechanism of action is a reduction of nerve action potential-mediated release of norepinephrine from sympathetic nerve terminals. The tissue mechanism is a reduction in cardiac output as a result of a reduction in heart rate.

Reserpine and the guanidine analogs share two common adverse effects. These are:
- Postural hypotension.
- A generalized block of sympathetic neurotransmission.

Postural hypotension is a sudden fall in blood pressure on suddenly standing up. It results from a loss of the sympathetic-mediated reflex arterial and venous constriction in the lower body that normally occurs on standing. There is venous pooling of blood in the lower limbs (giving a reduction in preload) and a fall in cardiac output via the Starling mechanism (see section on Heart failure, page 386), which may cause fainting. Because of this, and the availability of newer safer drugs, guanethidine is now used only for patients with severe hypertension who are unresponsive to other drugs.

▨ Ca^{2+} Antagonists are increasingly used in the treatment of hypertension

These drugs fall into three main groups, based on their chemical structure (see page 380):
- The 1,4-dihydropyridines, nifedipine, nicardipine and amlodipine, are the most vascular-selective group and the most effective antihypertensive Ca^{2+} antagonists.
- The phenethylalkylamine, verapamil, and the benzothiazepine, diltiazem, are less vascular-selective and may also affect the AV node, causing AV block. Verapamil and diltiazem are therefore associated with cardiac conduction problems, especially when given to patients receiving β_1 adrenoceptor antagonists.

Elderly hypertensive patients respond well to calcium antagonists. However, people of African origin are less responsive. In general, Ca^{2+} antagonists have a rapid onset of action and reduce blood pressure within half an hour of administration. Occasional adverse effects include a throbbing headache, palpitations, sweating, tremor, and flushing (due to vasodilation), which occur with rapid-onset formulations, but are almost absent with the slow-onset, long-acting formulations which are strongly preferred. The main adverse effect with verapamil is constipation, but more importantly both verapamil and diltiazem can have negative inotropic effects in patients with pre-existing cardiac failure, and are therefore contra-indicated in such patients. Nifedipine and amlodipine do not do this (their adverse effects are discussed in the section on Treatment of stable angina, page 380).

Importantly, despite their ability to control hypertension, there is a growing awareness that Ca^{2+} antagonists may actually increase mortality in patients with hypertension, although the mechanism by which this occurs is unknown.

DIRECT-ACTING VASODILATORS Agents that dilate arterioles by a molecular mechanism that is not α_1 adrenergic receptor antagonism or L-type Ca^{2+} channel blockade have traditionally been called 'direct-acting vasodilators.' This was once a convenient shorthand for indicating that at the time the molecular (and often the cellular) mechanisms of action were unknown. Although these have now largely been resolved, the term 'direct-acting' has been retained. These agents are increasingly used for the treatment of hypertensive emergencies.

▨ Hydralazine is a third-line drug for mild to moderate hypertension

Hydralazine is the only direct-acting vasodilator drug used in treating mild to moderate hypertension, usually as a second- or third-line drug. It is also still used as a parenteral treatment in hypertensive emergencies and in hypertensive pregnant patients, because of a long safety record in this setting.

The molecular and cellular mechanisms of action of hydralazine are to increase cGMP following activation of guanylyl cyclase, resulting in relaxation of smooth muscle in precapillary resistance vessels and thereby reducing blood pressure by a reduction in peripheral resistance (see Fig. 18.2).

Hydralazine, in doses in excess of 200 mg/day, is associated with a lupus-like syndrome in some patients.

▨ Minoxidil is useful for severe hypertension with renal failure

Minoxidil is highly effective in reducing blood pressure, especially in severe hypertension and if there is renal failure. Diazoxide is similar to minoxidil, but is rarely used except in emergencies because of its adverse effects.

Minoxidil is a more effective vasodilator than hydralazine and produces dilation of resistance vessels. It works at the molecular level by activating ATP-sensitive K^+ channels leading to the hyperpolarization of the smooth muscle sarcolemma, and subsequently the Ca^{2+} influx via the L-type Ca^{2+} channels is reduced. Minoxidil is given once or twice a day, and is very effective in patients with severe hypertension and renal insufficiency. Like hydralazine, it should also be given in combination with diuretics and adrenergic receptor antagonists, to prevent reflex increases in cardiac output and fluid retention which may be profound in some patients.

A common adverse effect of minoxidil is facial hair growth, which limits the use of this drug in women but has resulted in its use to treat male-pattern baldness.

▨ Renin–angiotensin cascade modulators

The inactive decapeptide angiotensin I is converted to the active octapeptide angiotensin II by ACE (see Fig. 18.40). A reduction

---

Angiotensin-converting enzyme inhibitors

- Alacepril
- Benazepril
- Cilazapril
- Perindopril
- Quinapril
- Ramipril
- Zofenopril
- Delapril (clinical trials)
- Moexipril (phase III clinical trials)
- Spirapril (US new drug application)
- Trandolapril

---

in blood pressure may be achieved by blocking ACE activity or angiotensin II receptors. ACE inhibitors have the following mechanisms of action:

- The molecular mechanism of action is inhibition of ACE activity.
- The resultant cellular mechanism of action is reduced angiotensin II synthesis and reduced metabolism of some vasodilating kinins (such as bradykinin).

ACE inhibitors are useful for all types and severities of hypertension, and are widely used. They also reduce mortality. They are classified chemically on the basis of whether they contain sulfhydryl, carboxyl or phosphinyl moieties.

▨ Captopril, which interacts with ACE via its sulfhydryl moiety, was the prototype ACE inhibitor

Angiotensin II has a variety of effects that contribute to elevating blood pressure (Fig. 18.52). It constricts arterioles and stimulates aldosterone release from the adrenal cortex; in turn, aldosterone stimulates Na^+ reabsorption in the kidney (see use of spironolactone, page 400). As a result of reducing the synthesis of angiotensin II, captopril has two main tissue mechanisms of action: it causes vasodilation and reduces Na^+ retention.

Other commonly used ACE inhibitors are lisinopril (the most commonly used in the USA), enalapril, benazepril, cilazapril, ramipril, and quinapril (all of which interact with ACE via their carboxyl moieties), and fosinopril (which interacts with ACE via its phosphinyl moiety) (see Fig. 18.37). The carboxyl-containing ACE inhibitors (enalapril, lisinopril, etc.) have a slower onset and longer duration of action than captopril. Many ACE inhibitors are pro-drugs. The suffix '-at' is used to denote the active metabolite of ACE inhibitors. For example, enalapril and ramipril are metabolized to their active metabolites, enalaprilat and ramiprilat.

▨ ACE inhibitors may alter the balance between the actions of angiotensin II and bradykinin

Surprisingly, chronic use of ACE inhibitors is associated with a recovery in the blood concentration of angiotensin II, but blood

405

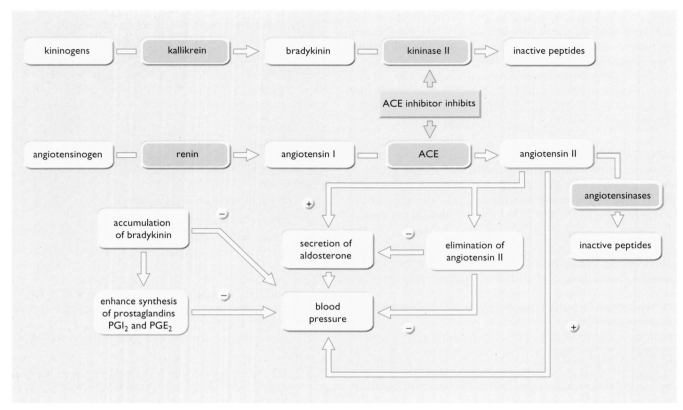

Fig. 18.52 Effects of angiotensin-converting enzyme (ACE) inhibitors. ACE inhibitors reduce angiotensin II (vasoconstrictor) concentrations and elevate bradykinin (vasodilator) concentrations. The accumulation of bradykinin shown in the lower part of the figure results from the action of the ACE inhibitors on kininase II. Note, kininase II and ACE are actually the same enzyme (peptidyl-dipeptidase).

pressure levels remain low. This suggests that additional mechanisms may be responsible for the antihypertensive effects. One possibility is an alteration of plasma bradykinin concentration. ACE catalyzes the inactivation of bradykinin, which is an endogenous vasodilator. The pharmacotherapeutic effects of ACE inhibitors may therefore be related to altering the balance between the actions of angiotensin II, bradykinin and possibly other kinins (see Fig. 18.52).

The tissue responses to ACE inhibitor are:
- A reduction in peripheral resistance with little change in heart rate or cardiac output.
- A reduction in Na$^+$ retention secondary to altered aldosterone levels.

ACE inhibitors are as effective as diuretics or β_1 adrenoceptor antagonists in treating hypertension. However, when ACE inhibitors are used concomitantly with a diuretic, overall therapeutic effectiveness may be better than that for either drug when used alone. This may result in part because the ability of diuretics to adversely activate the renin–angiotensin system is ameliorated by ACE inhibitors.

Inhibition of angiotensin II activity may cause a substantial reduction in renal perfusion pressure

Experimental and clinical evidence suggests that the reduction in efferent arteriolar resistance resulting from a reduction in angiotensin II actions following treatment with ACE inhibitors

may be useful in patients with renal dysfunction, particularly those with diabetic nephropathy or a reduced renal functional mass. This is because inhibition of angiotensin II activity may cause a substantial reduction in perfusion pressure. As a result, renal failure may develop in these patients.

ACE inhibitors are associated with few adverse effects (which increases patient compliance). One unusual adverse effect is a characteristic cough that is believed to be a consequence of the actions of bradykinin, the metabolism of which is inhibited by ACE inhibitors (see Chapter 19). This adverse effect appears to be least marked with fosinopril, which is structurally distinct from other ACE inhibitors.

ANGIOTENSIN II RECEPTOR ANTAGONISTS The prototype drug, saralasin, was discovered in the 1970s, but it is unsuitable for therapeutic use. Since it is a peptide it is not orally active and, when administered intravenously, it is immunogenic. More recently, compounds that are not peptides and are orally active have been developed. These novel nonpeptide angiotensin II receptor antagonists include losartan, candarsatan, and the investigational compound EXP3174.

Losartan has been approved for use in the treatment of hypertension in the USA. It differs from ACE inhibitors in that it does not directly affect bradykinin degradation. It is not yet known whether this confers advantages in terms of effectiveness and adverse effect profile compared with those of ACE inhibitors. However, the incidence of cough appears to be less compared with that for ACE inhibitors. The angiotensin II antagonists are currently being compared with ACE inhibitors for their relative effects on mortality in hypertension and CHF in man. At present, the ability of ACE inhibitors to elevate levels of bradykinin and other kinins is believed to contribute to overall drug actions, but the nature and importance of this compared with inhibition of angiotensin II production is uncertain. This is pharmacotherapeutically interesting since, if kinin elevation mediates part of ACE inhibitor benefit, the notion of replacing ACE inhibitors with selective angiotensin II antagonists would be flawed.

COMBINATION TREATMENT A useful pharmacotherapeutic approach for controlling elevated blood pressure is to use two or more drugs in combination. By combining drugs with different mechanisms of action the doses may be reduced, thereby reducing the adverse effects. The β adrenoceptor antagonist–diuretic combination is the most common combination strategy.

β Adrenoceptor antagonists and Ca^{2+} antagonists (dihydropyridine Ca^{2+} antagonists only) are usually well tolerated when used in combination, provided that care is taken with the dosage. Occasionally, the combination of nifedipine with β adrenoceptor antagonists is associated with bradycardia and heart failure owing to synergism of their effects (one mediated via cardiac β_1 adrenoceptor antagonism and the other via ventricular L-type Ca^{2+} antagonism).

Diuretics and ACE inhibitors (e.g. hydrochlorothiazide and perindopril) provide an effective combination for treating arterial hypertension that is well tolerated in many patients with mild to moderate hypertension. The advantage of combining diuretics and ACE inhibitors is an additive effect in reducing blood pressure. The mechanism has been mentioned earlier (page 400).

The combination of ACE inhibitors and Ca^{2+} antagonists is also effective at lowering blood pressure and is usually well tolerated.

Ca^{2+} antagonists and diuretics in combination do not usually have additive effects.

Using β_1 adrenoceptor antagonists with Ca^{2+} antagonists other than the dihydropyridines is dangerous

Using β_1 adrenoceptor antagonists in combination with nondihydropyridine Ca^{2+} antagonists (e.g. verapamil) is dangerous since these combinations have been reported to cause asystole, severe bradycardia, and hypotension, because of the combination of molecular mechanisms described above. Each lowers cardiac intracellular Ca^{2+}, an effect that reduces myocardial contractility. Dihydropyridines such as nifedipine do not do this because they are so highly vascular-selective that they do not affect cardiac tissue to any great extent.

EMERGING THERAPY FOR THE TREATMENT OF HYPERTENSION
Renin inhibitors are a new class of drugs that reduce angiotensin II levels. Several renin inhibitors have been developed with high potency and long duration of action. However, the oral bio-

---

> **Mechanisms of action of the major classes of antihypertensive drugs**
>
> - Thiazide diuretics increase Na^+ excretion and transiently reduce blood volume, but the mechanism by which they reduce blood pressure is uncertain
> - Sympatholytics reduce the ability of the sympathetic nervous system to raise blood pressure
> - Vasodilators relax vascular smooth muscle and reduce peripheral resistance
> - Angiotensin-converting enzyme (ACE) inhibitors reduce peripheral resistance and blood volume with no effect on heart rate

availability of currently available agents is too low to achieve effective plasma concentrations in humans.

Endopeptidase-24.11 is an enzyme that hydrolyzes the polypeptide atrial natriuretic peptide (ANP). ANP has diuretic, natriuretic, and vasodilator properties; it is released following changes in atrial volume or pressure, and therefore plays a role in regulating blood pressure. Theoretically, inhibition of endopeptidase-24.11 should reduce ANP degradation and thereby increase circulating levels of ANP. This form of drug treatment may prove beneficial in patients with hypertension. However, there are few clinical data to support the suggested proposal that drugs of this group are antihypertensive agents. This is probably due to their poor bioavailability or the low potency of agents tested so far. Recent data suggest that this group of drugs may have most benefit in patients with volume-dependent hypertension or low-renin hypertension.

TREATMENT FOR HYPERTENSIVE EMERGENCIES Hypertensive emergencies are situations in which the target organ damage is so extensive and acute that the patient's life is in immediate jeopardy. There is no particular level of blood pressure that provides the diagnosis but this depends on the clinical presentation. Some examples of hypertensive emergencies include hypertensive encephalopathy, dissecting aortic aneursym, pulmonary edema, myocardial ischemia, and accelerated renal failure due to hypertensive nephropathy. Treatment is summarized in Fig. 18.53.

Sodium nitroprusside is a direct acting vasodilator used in hypertensive emergencies

Sodium nitroprusside is given intravenously to produce a controlled rapid reduction in blood pressure during a hyper-

---

> **Hypertensive emergency**
>
> - Occurs when mean arterial pressure is an immediate threat to life
> - Intravenous nitroprusside is an efficacious drug in this setting

tensive emergency. It has a short half-life of 30–40 seconds. Sodium nitroprusside is a profound arterial and venous dilator (Fig. 18.53). The molecular mechanism of action for its effect is brought about by a second messenger, nitric oxide (NO; see Fig. 18.2). It is a pro-drug that spontaneously degrades to NO inside smooth muscle cells. NO increases cGMP in vascular smooth muscle cells by stimulating cytosolic guanylyl cyclase activity (see Fig. 18.21, page 379).

Sodium nitroprusside achieves a rapid onset of action and efficacy. An infusion can be used to reduce blood pressure rapidly, but it is important to monitor the blood pressure constantly. This is because nitroprusside can cause an abrupt fall in blood pressure, resulting in hypoperfusion of vital organs; dose must be titrated carefully, depending on the blood pressure response.

■ *Ganglion-blocking drugs are used only for emergency hypertension*

Trimethaphan is a nicotinic receptor antagonist with relative selectivity for the nicotinic receptors found in autonomic ganglia. It is used only for emergency hypertension associated with a dissecting aortic aneurysm. When given intravenously it produces generalized antagonism of both parasympathetic and sympathetic ganglia (i.e. gastric motility ceases, the bladder fails to empty, etc.) and is therefore unsuitable for maintenance therapy of hypertension.

OTHER TREATMENTS OF ACUTELY HIGH BLOOD PRESSURE A very high blood pressure on its own, in the absence of acute illness, does not usually require parenteral therapy, which can be dangerous. Patients with a less severe emergency can be given oral drug treatment. Any class of drug may be used, but the four classes most commonly used are:
- Diuretics.
- β Adrenoceptor antagonists.
- Ca^{2+} antagonists.
- ACE inhibitors.

Drugs used in hypertensive crises	
Vasodilators	**Onset of action (min)**
Nitroprusside	Immediate
Diazoxide	2–4
Hydralazine	10–20
Enalaprilat	15
Nicardipine	10
Sympatholytics	
Trimethaphan	1–5
Esmolol	1–2
Labetalol	5–10

Fig. 18.53 Drugs used in hypertensive crises. The drugs are shown in order of preference based on their rapidity of action.

Adverse effects of drugs on the heart		
Drug	**Adverse effects**	**Comments**
Doxorubicin	Cardiopathy	Total dose must be limited
Ibuprofen and related drugs	Elevation of blood pressure	Not a major concern
Cocaine/ amphetamines	Elevation of blood pressure	Dangerous effect of abuse

Fig. 18.54 Adverse effects of drugs on the heart.

Adverse effects of drugs on the heart
Some examples are listed in Fig. 18.54.

PATHOPHYSIOLOGY AND DISEASES OF BLOOD VESSELS

A variety of diseases involve a generalized or localized impairment of blood flow to specific tissues or organs and are grouped together here as peripheral vascular disease.

In most cases the specific molecular, cellular, and tissue mechanisms of action of the drugs used to treat peripheral vascular diseases are described elsewhere in this book. Specifically, the pharmacology of agents that dilate arterioles (e.g. Ca^{2+} antagonists) is described in the section on hypertension (see page 398), and antithrombotic drugs are described in the section on unstable angina (see page 381) and Chapter 13. Blood vessel diseases for which drug therapy is not used have not been discussed.

 Principles of treatment of peripheral vascular disease

- Drugs are targeted at the perfusion deficit and at the underlying cause (e.g. vasospasm) if known
- Thrombolytics are used if thrombosis has impaired perfusion
- Arteriodilators are used if vasospasm has impaired perfusion

Arterial disease
Peripheral vascular disease affecting the arteries can be caused by a number of pathologic processes:
- Arteriosclerosis is one of the pathologic processes that leads to peripheral vascular disease (Fig. 18.55).
- Dystrophic calcification of the media is observed in Mönckeberg's sclerosis, which is common in the major lower limb arteries of the elderly and is most common in people with diabetes mellitus.
- Cystic medial necrosis or degeneration describes mucoid degeneration of the collagen and elastic tissue of the media, often with cystic changes, and occurs predominantly in elderly patients with hypertension. Indeed, peripheral vascular disease is a feature commonly associated with long-standing hypertension.

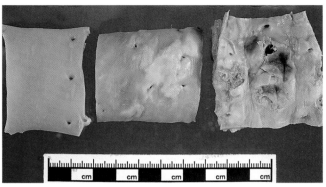

Fig. 18.55 Arteriosclerosis is characterized by thickening and hardening of walls of arteries and arterioles. The earliest changes are small fatty streaks (F), which are visible as pale areas beneath the endothelium in the aortic segment on the left. The central segment shows pearly white fibrolipid plaques (P), and the segment on the right shows advanced ulcerated plaques with adherent fibrin–platelet thrombus (T). (Courtesy of Dr Alan Stevens and Professor James Lowe.)

In patients with pre-existing peripheral vascular disease, aspirin and dipyridamole are effective in delaying the progression of the disease to thrombosis so may be used as prophylaxis. It is presumed that:

- Aspirin prevents thrombosis (see Chapter 13).
- Dipyridamole prevents thrombosis and dilates arterioles (see Chapter 13).

CHRONIC ISCHEMIA of the legs and intermittent claudication (limping) may arise as a consequence of atheromatous disease involving the aorta, iliac arteries, and/or any other peripheral vessels. Treatment is directed towards prophylaxis against thrombosis and comprises low-dose aspirin therapy (325 mg/day) and surgery. The molecular mechanism of action of aspirin is through cyclo-oxygenase inhibition as described in Chapter 16. The cellular mechanism of action is inhibition of the prothrombotic products of cyclo-oxygenase, especially thromboxane A_2, and the tissue response is inhibition of platelet aggregation.

ACUTE ISCHEMIA of the legs can be caused by arterial thrombi, but also occurs when stasis thrombi dislodge from the atria when atrial fibrillation is terminated. The only treatment is surgery, but prophylaxis with heparin or other anticoagulants is advisable before any elective termination of atrial fibrillation.

VASCULITIS is a broad term signifying inflammation within and surrounding blood vessels, caused by immune complex deposition. Arteries, venules, or capillaries affected by inflammation show necrosis and infiltration by lymphocytes and eosinophils, resulting eventually in ischemia of the related tissue. The different forms of vasculitis include systemic necrotizing vasculitis (e.g. polyarteritis nodosa, allergic angiitis), hypersensitivity vasculitis (e.g. serum sickness, Henoch–Schönlein purpura), and those associated with cardiac transplant rejection. These diseases are discussed in Chapter 20).

TAKAYASU'S SYNDROME is a rare condition, except in Japan. It is characterized by a vasculitis involving the aortic arch as well as other major arteries. Although glucocorticosteroids are used to treat this disease, heart failure and cerebrovascular accidents may eventually supervene. The molecular and cellular mechanisms of action of glucocorticosteroids are described in Chapter 16.

RAYNAUD'S DISEASE is an isolated condition in which bouts of intense arteriolar vasoconstriction occur in the arteries supplying the fingers or toes, and it is usually precipitated by cold or vibration.

Initially, treatment includes avoidance of exposure to cold and stopping smoking. More severe symptoms may require vasodilator treatment. In each case the tissue response of the drugs discussed below is to cause arteriolar vasodilation, although their efficacy may be modest for this disease.

α_1 Adrenoceptor antagonists such as prazosin may be used to reduce the vasospasm, but are not selective in their action on the vessels in spasm and can adversely lower blood pressure. The molecular mechanism of action of α_1 antagonists is antagonism of α_1 adrenoceptors, and the cellular mechanism is the same as for the treatment of hypertension (see page 402).

Direct-acting vasodilators (e.g. nitroglycerin and nitrates) are also used. These pro-drugs are converted to NO, which activates guanylyl cyclase leading to an elevation in cGMP (the cellular response; see Fig. 18.21).

Calcium antagonists such as diltiazem and nifedipine are also used. The molecular mechanism of action of diltiazem and nifedipine is blockade of L-type Ca^{2+} channels, and the cellular response is a reduction in Ca^{2+} entry and the cascade of events that leads to vasoconstriction (see section on treatment of hypertension, page 404).

In four separate clinical trials investigating the use of nifedipine in Raynaud's phenomenon, the majority of patients improved symptomatically. Nifedipine is more effective than prazosin and can be given by mouth before cold exposure to avoid attacks.

ACE inhibitors are also used. Their molecular mechanism of action is to inhibit the conversion of angiotensin I to angiotensin II, and the cellular mechanism of action is to prevent the formation of the vasoconstrictor substance, angiotensin II (see Fig. 18.40).

Prostacyclin may also be a beneficial treatment of Raynaud's disease because it causes vasodilation.

 Local treatment is needed for peripheral vascular disease

Drugs that prevent or disperse thrombosis or relieve vasospasm to treat peripheral vascular disease act locally. This is in contrast to the treatment of coronary artery disease, in which vessel dilation at distant sites is effective by reducing preload or afterload

409

Venous disease

The two main peripheral vascular diseases affecting the veins are varicose veins and venous thrombosis (including thrombophlebitis).

VARICOSE VEINS DEVELOP WHEN VEINS LOSE THEIR ELASTICITY AND BECOME ENGORGED WITH BLOOD. They are treated by injection or surgery. Sodium tetradecyl sulfate is injected into the vein as sclerotherapy. It causes inflammation of the intima and thrombus formation, which usually occludes the vein. The subsequent formation of fibrous tissue results in complete occlusion and subsequent loss of the vein.

VENOUS THROMBOSIS consists predominantly of coagulated blood with a small component of platelet aggregation. Superficial thrombophlebitis is a local superficial inflammation of the vein wall with secondary venous thrombosis. Superficial thrombophlebitis is treated with NSAIDs, including aspirin, because the inflammatory process rather than the tendency for thrombosis is the primary tissue target. Hyaluronidase is used to improve the circulation in superficial thrombophlebitis. It is a spreading or diffusing enzyme that modifies the permeability of connective tissue by hydrolyzing hyaluronic acid. This temporarily decreases the viscosity of the cellular cement and promotes the diffusion of injected fluids or of localized transudates or exudates.

In deep vein thrombosis a thrombus forms in a vein, commonly deep in the leg. Any inflammation is secondary. It is necessary to inhibit formation of the thrombus rather than direct therapy towards the secondary inflammation. The important secondary aim of treatment is to prevent pulmonary embolism resulting from entrapment of the dislodged venous thrombus in the pulmonary circulation (a goal similar to that in the ancillary treatment of atrial fibrillation).

Large doses of the anticoagulant heparin (or low molecular weight fragments such as enoxaparin) can be given as prophylaxis in the event of venous thrombosis for 1 week to 3 months. Heparin initiates anticoagulation but has a short duration of action. It inhibits the reactions that lead to the clotting of blood and formation of fibrin clots and, in combination with antithrombin III, inhibits thrombosis by inactivating activated factor X and inhibiting the conversion of prothrombin to thrombin (a mechanism described in more detail in Chapter 13). Heparin will not disperse an established thrombus.

Oral anticoagulants such as warfarin are given if a venous thrombus remains localized. Warfarin, another prophylactic agent, antagonizes the ability of vitamin K to facilitate the synthesis of clotting factor II, VII, IX, and X (see Chapter 13). However, it takes at least 49–72 hours for these anticoagulant effects to develop. Heparin and warfarin can cause inappropriate bleeding, so careful titration between effective and adverse doses is required.

Streptokinase is used in the treatment of established thrombi, and is followed by anticoagulant prophylaxis to prevent recurrence. It acts with plasminogen to produce an 'activator complex,' which converts plasminogen to plasmin.

 Venous thrombosis and its treatment

- Venous peripheral vascular disease is characterized by vascular inflammation and thrombosis
- Treatment of superficial thrombophlebitis is targeted towards inflammation, using nonsteroidal anti-inflammatory drugs
- Treatment and prophylaxis of deep vein disease is directed towards the thrombosis
- Heparin and warfarin are used as prophylaxis against thrombosis
- Streptokinase is used to disperse established thrombi

Plasmin degrades fibrin clots as well as fibrinogen and other plasma proteins. The section on blood clotting (see Chapter 13) may be read for further details.

Infections of the cardiovascular system

The general principles of treatment of infections are discussed in Chapters 8–10. Here, attention is drawn to the aspects of treatment of infection that are particular to the cardiovascular system.

INFECTIVE ENDOCARDITIS involves the endocardium or vascular endothelium. It is the most common infection of the cardiovascular system. It is common in drug addicts and in people with cardiac valve insufficiency. Occasionally it occurs as an acute infection, but more commonly it runs an insidious course and is known as subacute bacterial endocarditis (Fig. 18.56). Infective endocarditis is rare in the UK and USA (6–7 cases/100,000 population), but more common in developing countries. It occurs most commonly on rheumatic or congenitally abnormal valves as well as on a prolapsed mitral valve and in calcified aortic valve disease. However, normal valves may be involved, particularly after injection by addicts of nonsterile drugs. Virtually every form of microbiologic agent, including fungi, rickettsiae, and chlamydiae, have been shown to cause infective endocarditis. Most cases are, however, bacterial in origin with *Streptococcus viridans*, *Strep. faecalis*, and *Staphylococcus aureus* being the most common organisms.

If infective endocarditis is caused by *Strep. viridans* or *Strep. faecalis*, treatment is with penicillin G and gentamicin. If *Staph. aureus* is responsible, floxacillin and either fusidic acid or gentamicin are used. Infective endocarditis may occur following dental surgery as a result of bacteria from the oral cavity entering the blood stream, and so penicillin prophylaxis is used, and started 7 days before surgery.

MYOCARDITIS is inflammation of the heart, characterized by fever and heart failure, and is caused by infections with viruses, bacteria or parasites. A leukocytic infiltrate in the myocardium can be observed, followed by resultant nonischemic necrosis or degeneration of myocytes. Most cases of viral myocarditis are thought to be caused by enteroviruses (coxsackie, influenza, rubella, polio, adenovirus, echovirus) and are difficult to treat

megistus. There is an initial local lesion at the site of entry, followed by bouts of parasitemia and fever. Damage to the heart is caused by the toxins released by the parasite and by inflammatory cells.

There are two clinically distinct presentations of this disease:

- Acute Chagas' disease, which mainly affects children and is mild in most individuals. Damage to the heart results from a direct invasion of the myocardial cells by the parasite and the subsequent inflammatory events.
- Chronic Chagas' disease, which is characterized by damage to the heart muscle resulting from an autoimmune reaction induced by *T. cruzi* parasites and mediated by cytotoxic T cells.

Over 80% of patients with the acute form, and slightly more with the chronic form, are eventually cured of the infection.

Nifurtimox is the drug of choice for acute Chagas' disease, with benznidazole as an alternative drug that is effective against nifurtimox-resistant *T. cruzi*. Nifurtimox and benznidazole are not available in the UK. Nifurtimox exerts its trypanocidal action by forming free radicals. The free radicals react with molecular oxygen to form superoxide anions, hydrogen peroxide, and hydroxyl free radicals. Trypanosomes are susceptible to these reactive intermediates, which cause lipid and DNA peroxidation, because these organisms contain no catalase or glutathione peroxidase to inactivate the toxic products. Primaquine eliminates tissue infection and prevents the development of the blood (erythrocytic) forms of the parasite.

Adverse effects of benznidazole and nifurtimox include gastrointestinal upsets and rashes. Nifurtimox is highly toxic to human cells, but limited selectivity is achieved because the rates of radical formation are much lower in human cells than in trypanosomes. Nifurtimox may also cause anorexia, tremors, paresthesia, polyneuritis, and transient leukopenia. The adverse effects of primaquine are predominantly gastrointestinal.

PERICARDITIS is inflammation of the pericardium which surrounds the epicardial surface of the heart. Inflammation of the pericardium is usually secondary to a variety of cardiac diseases, systemic disorders, or metastases from neoplasms arising in remote sites. Pericarditis has numerous etiologies, but coxsackie viral infection is the commonest cause.

Anti-inflammatory medication such as oral aspirin, naproxen, or indomethacin is used to treat pericarditis. However, if it is severe or recurrent, systemic glucocorticosteroids may be necessary.

KAWASAKI'S DISEASE is a generalized vasculitis causing extensive damage to the vessels of the heart, which can be fatal. Although the etiology is unknown, current evidence suggests that it is probably not an autoimmune disease, but may be triggered by a virus. During the acute phase, Kawasaki's disease may be characterized by medium and large vessel arteritis, arterial aneurysms, valvulitis, and myocarditis. Of particular concern are coronary artery aneurysms, which may precipitate thrombosis or rupture. Lymphocyte and macrophage activation is evident in this disease. Experimental studies have shown the presence of antibodies that can kill endothelial cells previously

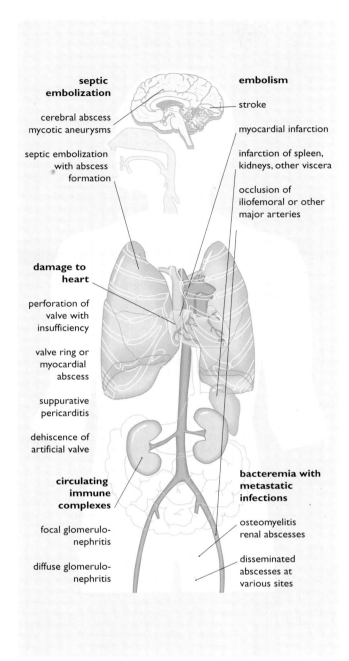

Fig. 18.56 The potential complications of infective endocarditis. (Modified from Bisno et al., *Hospital Practice* 1986; **21**: 139.)

with drugs. However, myocarditis may also be caused by bacterial infection (exotoxin produced by *Corynebacterium*, *Rickettsia*, *Chlamydia*, *Coxiella*) and protozoa (*Trypanosoma cruzi*, *Toxoplasma gondii*).

CHAGAS' DISEASE (American trypanosomiasis) is a protozoal infection that causes myocarditis. It is caused by the intracellular protozoan parasite, *T. cruzi*, and is the most frequent cause of heart failure in Brazil and neighboring Latin American countries. The parasite is transmitted by various insects including *Triatoma infestans*, *Rhodnius prolixus*, and *Panstrongylus*

treated with interleukin-1 or tumor necrosis factor. The function of these antibodies in the disease process is unknown: they may simply be a marker of the disease or they may have a pathogenic role.

Patients with Kawasaki's disease can be classified according to their relative risk of myocardial ischemia, on a scale of 1–5. No therapy is recommended until level 3, at which small- to medium-sized solitary coronary artery aneurysms are observed. Aspirin is then prescribed. Level 4 is characterized by the presence of one or more giant coronary artery aneurysms or multiple small- to medium-sized aneurysms without obstruction, and is treated with aspirin with or without the addition of warfarin. Patients considered to have the highest risk of myocardial infarction have evidence of coronary artery obstruction and are classified as level 5. They are treated with aspirin with or without the addition of warfarin, as well as Ca^{2+} antagonists to reduce myocardial oxygen demand.

Recent studies have found that the use of intravenous gammaglobulin therapy before the 10th day of the illness has reduced the morbidity from Kawasaki's disease and the apparent incidence of coronary artery abnormalities. Gamma-globulin contains antibodies against various viruses present in the population. The antibodies are directed against the virus envelope and can 'neutralize' some viruses and prevent their attachment to host cells.

RHEUMATIC FEVER is an inflammatory disease that occurs in children and young adults and is common in the Middle East, Far East, and Eastern Europe. It occurs in a small proportion of individuals (those who have a significant antibody response to streptococcal proteins) several weeks after a pharyngeal infection with group A streptococcus, at which stage autoantibodies against the heart can be detected (Fig. 18.57). There is evidence to suggest that carbohydrate antigens on the streptococci cross-react with an antigen on the heart valves and myocardium. Rheumatic fever is therefore though to develop as a result of an abnormal host immune response, both cellular and humoral, triggered by streptococcus A. It is likely that the disease is due

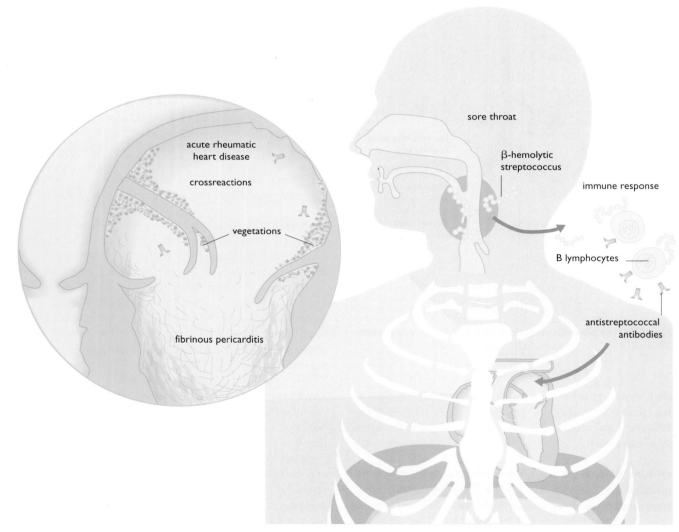

Fig. 18.57 Pathogenetic sequence and main morphologic features of acute rheumatic heart disease. Acute rheumatic fever often causes mitral valvulitis characterized by a linear arrangement of vegetations along the line of closure of the leaflets.

to a complex inter-relationship between the genetics of the host's immune system and the streptococcus bacillus.

The treatment of rheumatic fever initially involves eradication of residual streptococcal infections with a single intramuscular injection of benzathine penicillin or oral phenoxymethylpenicillin four times daily for 1 week. High-dose salicylate therapy inhibits cyclo-oxygenase activity and is given to the limit of tolerance determined by the development of tinnitus. If there is carditis, systemic glucocorticosteroids can be given.

Recurrences are common if there is persistent cardiac damage and are prevented by the continued use of oral phenoxymethylpenicillin daily or by monthly injections of benzathine penicillin, until the age of 20 years, or for 5 years after the last attack.

FURTHER READING

Cardiovascular therapeutics and experimental therapeutics are large and fast moving fields. The best way to stay in touch is to scan the journal *Circulation* (American Heart Association) for review articles and publications on multicenter clinical trials. There are many of these. Therefore we refer here primarily to more general and established reference texts and articles.

Cleophus TJ, Zwinderman AH. Beta-blockers and heart failure: meta-analysis of mortality trials. *Int J Clin Pharm Ther* 2001; **39**: 383. [An up to date appraisal of the topic.]

Connolly S et al. Effect of prophylactic amiodarone on mortality after acute myocardial infarction and in congestive heart failure: Meta-analysis of individual data from 6500 patients in randomised trials. *Lancet* 1997; **350**: 1417. [An appraisal of an unusual but very important cardiovascular drug.]

Domanski MJ et al. Effect of angiotensin converting enzyme inhibition on sudden cardiac death in patients following acute myocardial infarction. A meta-analysis of randomized clinical trials. *J Am Coll Cardiol* 1999; **33**: 598. [A recent appraisal.]

Fozzard HA, Haber E, Jennings RB, Katz AM, Morgan HE (eds). *The Heart and Cardiovascular System*. New York: Raven Press; 1995. [This two-volume book contains some excellent chapters written by researchers who have been at the forefront of their field.]

Heidenreich PA et al. Meta-analysis of trials comparing beta-blockers, calcium antagonists, and nitrates for stable angina. *JAMA* 1999; **281**: 1927. [A recent appraisal of the topic.]

Hosenpud JD, Greenberg BH (eds) *Congestive Heart Failure: Pathophysiology, Diagnosis and Comprehensive Approach to Management*. New York: Springer Verlag; 1994. [An excellent textbook that details the basic pathophysiology, pharmacologic therapy, and clinical approach to management of congestive heart failure.]

La Rosa JC et al. Effect of statins on risk of coronary disease: a meta-analysis of randomized controlled trials. *JAMA* 1999; **282**: 2340. [A recent appraisal.]

Pahor M et al. Health outcomes associated with calcium antagonists compared with other first-line antihypertensive therapies: a meta-analysis of randomised controlled trials. *Lancet* 2000; **356**: 1949.

Pater C. The current status of primary prevention in coronary heart disease. *Curr Controlled Trials Cardiovasc Med* 2000; **2**: 24–37. [An overview that highlights the limitations of current approaches—pharmacologic and other—to the leading cause of death in the developed world. This article undermines the notion that we have a broad range of truly effective drugs, which explains why much in the present chapter is circumspect and tentative: just because drugs are 'used,' it doesn't mean they are necessarily 'effective'.]

Saito I, Saruta T. Large, long-term, randomized trials and meta-analysis of therapy of patients with hypertension. *Jap J Clin Med* 1997; **55**: 2086. [A recent appraisal of the topic.]

Swales JD (ed.) *Textbook of Hypertension*. Oxford: Blackwell Scientific; 1994.

Task Force of the Working Group on Arrhythmias of the European Society of Cardiology. The Sicilian Gambit: A new approach to the classification of antiarrhythmic drugs based on their actions on arrhythmogenic mechanisms. *Circulation* 1991; **84**: 1831–1851. [This is a reappraisal of the state of antiarrhythmic therapy after a landmark clinical trial.]

Chapter 19

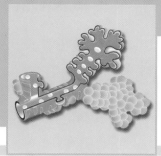

Drugs and the Pulm... System

PHYSIOLOGY OF THE PULMONARY SYSTEM

■ *Blood is oxygenated and carbon dioxide removed by the pulmonary system*

The body's metabolic processes use large quantities of oxygen and produce large amounts of carbon dioxide. The oxygen-absorbing surface of the lung (the gas-exchange surface) is therefore large (80 m²). It can fit into the body because it is folded and shaped into a branching tree-like system of air-conducting tubes (bronchi and bronchioles), which end in millions of tiny sacs called alveoli (Fig. 19.1).

Respiration is controlled by spontaneous rhythmic discharges from the respiratory center in the medulla of the brain, which is regulated by higher centers in the brain and vagal afferents from the lungs (Fig. 19.2) and influenced by:

- Changes in blood pCO_2, which activate chemoreceptors in the medulla.
- Changes in blood pO_2, which activate chemoreceptors in the aortic arch and carotid bodies.

■ *Airway smooth muscle tone is produced by parasympathetic, sympathetic, and nonadrenergic noncholinergic nerves and circulating epinephrine*

Airway smooth muscle is innervated by:

- The parasympathetic nervous system via the vagus nerve (cranial nerve X), and airway smooth muscle tone is

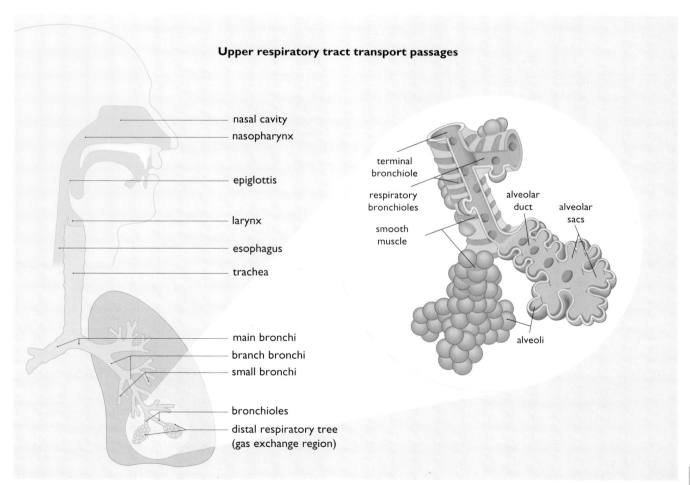

Upper respiratory tract transport passages

- nasal cavity
- nasopharynx
- epiglottis
- larynx
- esophagus
- trachea
- main bronchi
- branch bronchi
- small bronchi
- bronchioles
- distal respiratory tree (gas exchange region)

- terminal bronchiole
- respiratory bronchioles
- smooth muscle
- alveolar duct
- alveolar sacs
- alveoli

Fig. 19.1 Structure of the respiratory tract.

415

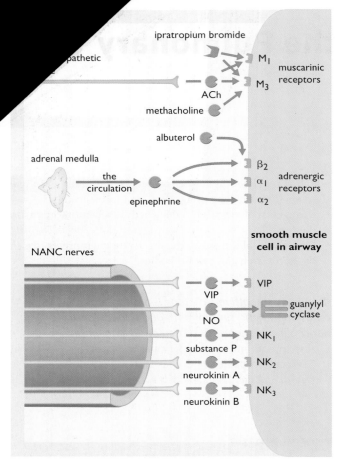

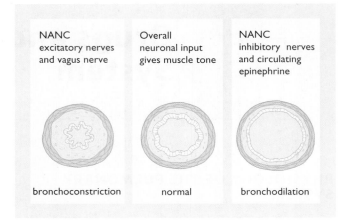

Fig. 19.3 Bronchial smooth muscle tone. Bronchial smooth muscle tone depends upon the balance between the parasympathetic input, circulating epinephrine, nonadrenergic, noncholinergic (NANC) inhibitory nerves, and sympathetic innervation of the parasympathetic ganglia.

Noninfectious diseases of the respiratory tract

- The most common diseases are asthma, allergic rhinitis, chronic bronchitis and cystic fibrosis
- Asthma is an inflammatory disease
- Cystic fibrosis is a genetic disease
- Cough is usually a symptom of an underlying disease

Fig. 19.2 Airway smooth muscle tone and innervation.
A constrictor tone is provided by the vagus nerve and release of acetylcholine (ACh). This is blocked by the mixed M_1/M_2 antagonist, ipratropium bromide. Methacholine challenge, to assess for asthma, activates these receptors. Epinephrine relaxes airway smooth muscle by activating β_2 receptors. This is mimicked by the therapeutic drug, albuterol. The other features of the figure, including vasoactive intestinal polypeptide (VIP) activation of VIP receptors, nitrergic release of nitric oxide (NO), and activation of various neurokinin (NK) receptors, all part of the nonadrenergic noncholinergic (NANC) system, may represent targets for future drug development.

[VIP]) used by the nonadrenergic noncholinergic (NANC) nerves of this system (see Fig. 19.2) producing smooth muscle relaxation and bronchodilation.

Bronchial smooth muscle relaxation (bronchodilation) is also produced by circulating epinephrine (adrenaline) binding to β_2 adrenoceptors on the muscle (see Fig. 19.2). Although the bronchial smooth muscle has little or no direct sympathetic innervation, there is a sympathetic supply to the parasympathetic ganglia.

Airway smooth muscle tone therefore depends on the balance between the:
- Parasympathetic input.
- Inhibitory influence of circulating epinephrine.
- NANC inhibitory nerves.
- Sympathetic innervation of the parasympathetic ganglia (Figs 19.2, 19.3).

PATHOPHYSIOLOGY AND DISEASES OF THE PULMONARY SYSTEM

Pulmonary disease can cause coughing, wheezing, shortness of breath, and abnormal gas exchange
Coughing, wheezing, shortness of breath, and abnormal gas exchange can result from:
- Changes in airway smooth muscle tone (e.g. bronchial asthma).

Drugs that alter respiration

- Narcotic analgesics, barbiturates, certain H_1 receptor antagonists, and ethanol cause respiratory depression
- Doxapram is a respiratory stimulant and is used for patients in ventilatory failure
- Respiratory stimulants are believed to stimulate both carotid chemoreceptors and the respiratory center
- They should be used with caution as they may have unwanted effects on the CNS such as convulsions, and their efficacy is uncertain

generated by acetylcholine acting on muscarinic receptors (Fig. 19.2).
- The so-called 'third nervous pathway,' with the neurotransmitters (nitric oxide and vasoactive intestinal polypeptide

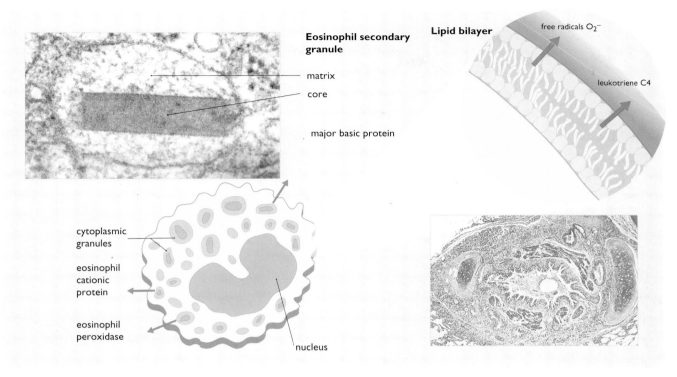

Fig. 19.4 Cytotoxic mediators released by eosinophils lead to epithelial damage. Infiltrating eosinophils release cytotoxic mediators, including major basic protein, eosinophil peroxidase, and eosinophil cationic protein from their granules. Certain inflammatory mediators can be released from the lipid bilayer upon eosinophil activation. Lower right, a section of asthmatic airway showing the pathophysiologic changes. (Courtesy of Dr Alan Stevens and Professor James Lowe.)

- Vascular congestion of the upper respiratory tract (e.g. rhinitis).
- Mucous plugging (e.g. chronic bronchitis).

Bronchial asthma

Bronchial asthma is a chronic inflammatory disease of the airways that causes acute bronchospasm and dyspnea
Bronchial asthma is a common disease, affecting up to 20% of the population in some countries. Its associated morbidity and mortality are rising in most countries despite increasing use of anti-asthma drugs.

The characteristic clinical features of bronchial asthma are associated with a chronic inflammatory response in the airways involving local lymphocyte and eosinophil accumulation, which is evident following bronchoalveolar lavage (BAL), on biopsy and at autopsy. It is thought that the granules of infiltrating eosinophils release cytotoxic mediators (Fig. 19.4), which damage the respiratory ciliated epithelium. The tissue damage is associated with increased airway irritability (bronchial hyperresponsiveness), which causes coughing and wheezing in response to stimuli that do not normally provoke such responses (Fig. 19.5).

Bronchial hyperresponsiveness may result from exposure of sensory nerves beneath the damaged epithelium (Fig. 19.6). Activation of these nerves on exertion or the exposure to environmental irritants results in local axon and vagal reflexes, which can produce bronchoconstriction, mucus secretion, and airway vasodilation (Fig. 19.6).

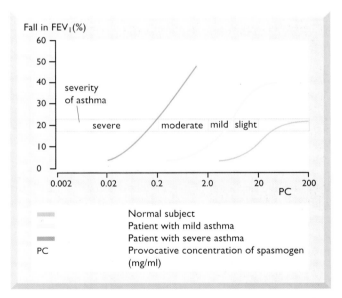

Fig. 19.5 Bronchial hyperresponsiveness. People with bronchial asthma have bronchial hyperresponsiveness, which causes them to cough and wheeze in response to stimuli that would not provoke such responses in normal subjects. Clinically, this hyperresponsiveness can be demonstrated by measuring the change in lung function, which is shown by a reduction in FEV_1 (forced expiratory volume in one second) in response to an inhaled spasmogen such as histamine or methacholine. Increased irritability is observed with increasing disease severity.

417

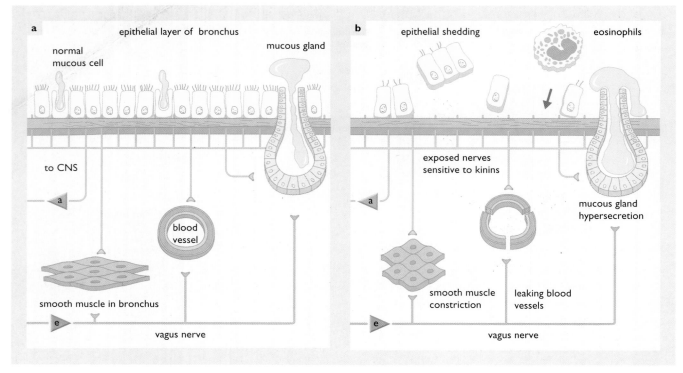

Fig. 19.6 Mechanism of bronchial hyperresponsiveness. This may result from exposure of sensory airway nerves following damage to the ciliated epithelial layer by cytotoxic mediators released by infiltrating eosinophils, which may then become hypersensitive as a result of exposure to inflammatory mediators such as prostaglandins and cytokines. (a) Normal lung; (b) asthmatic lung.

Bronchodilators and anti-inflammatory drugs are used in the treatment of asthma

Bronchodilators

Acute reversible bronchospasm contributes to the characteristic wheezing of asthma. It is readily treated by three different classes of bronchodilator drugs: β_2 adrenoceptor agonists, anti-cholinergics, and xanthines.

β_2 ADRENOCEPTOR AGONISTS are the most widely prescribed drugs for the treatment of the bronchoconstriction in asthma and are available by inhalation from a metered-dose inhaler or nebulizer, systemically as well as orally (Fig. 19.7). Short-acting β_2 adrenoceptor agonists for the acute relief of bronchospasm include albuterol, terbutaline, and fenoterol. Epinephrine, isoproterenol, isoetharine and metaproterenol are sometimes

used but are not selective for β_2 receptors, having various degrees of activity at α receptors and β_1 receptors, which are essentially unwanted effects. Most β_2 agonists are available as racemic mixtures, but recently the single R-albuterol has been introduced into clinical practice.

β_2 Adrenoceptor agonists relax airway smooth muscle through the activation of adenylyl cyclase. They are excellent functional (physiologic) antagonists of the bronchoconstriction caused by a wide range of stimuli. One of the drawbacks of albuterol, terbutaline and fenoterol, however, has been their short biologic half-life (2–3 hours), but a variety of long-acting β_2 adrenoceptor agonists have now been introduced that produce bronchodilation for up to 15 hours. Long-acting β_2 adrenoceptor agonists include salmeterol, aformoterol, and bambuterol. The prolonged action of salmeterol is believed to be due to the presence in the molecule of a long lipophilic tail, which binds to an 'exoreceptor' in the vicinity of the β_2 adreno-ceptor on airway smooth muscle. These long-acting drugs are intended for long-term prevention of asthma attacks, but are not recommended for acute relief, particularly salmeterol, which has a delayed onset of action. They are particularly useful for treating nocturnal asthma.

The adverse effects of β_2 adrenoceptor agonists include tremor and hypokalemia, and, when given in excessive amounts, tachycardia. The adverse effects of β_2 adrenoceptor agonists are reduced when they are inhaled and this is the preferred route of administration.

Clinical features of bronchial asthma

- Acute attacks of dyspnea associated with acute airway obstruction due to contraction of airway smooth muscle
- Mucus hypersecretion, which may lead to mucus plugging
- Airway inflammation
- Bronchial hyperresponsiveness

β₂ Agonists

β₂ Agonists	Route of administration	Dose range	Half-life (hours)
Albuterol	Oral: Extended release	2 mg/12 hours pediatric 4–8 mg/12 hours adult	5–6
Terbutaline	Oral: Tablets	5 mg 3 times daily for adults and children over 12 years 2.5 mg 3 times daily for children 6–12 years	3–4
	Injection: Subcutaneous	0.255 mg (0.25 ml) for adults and children over 12 years 0.006–0.01 mg/kg for children 6–12 years	3–4
	Inhalation: Micronized metered dose	2 inhalations of 0.2 mg separated by a 60-second interval every 4–6 hours for adults and children over 12 years	3–4
Fenoterol	Inhalation: Aerosol	1–2 inhalations (0.1 mg) up to 3 times daily in adults 1 inhalation (0.1 mg) up to 3 times daily for children over 6 years 1–2 inhalations (0.2 mg) up to 3 times daily in adults	6–7
Aformoterol	Inhalation: Breath-activated inhaler Breath-activated Dry Powder	1–2 capsules (12 μg) twice daily 6–12 μg twice daily in adults	
Salmeterol	Inhalation: Aerosol Powder	2 inhalations of 21 μg twice a day for adults and children over 12 years 1 inhalation of 50 μg twice daily for adults and children over 4 years	17 17
Isoproterenol	Inhalation: Aerosol Solution	1–2 inhalations of 0.131 mg up to 5 times a day in adults and children 5–15 deep inhalations of a 1:200 dilution of a 0.5% solution administered via a nebulizer in adults and children	
Bambuterol	Oral	10–20 mg daily at night in adults	

Fig. 19.7 β₂ Agonists.

ANTICHOLINERGICS Muscarinic receptor antagonists cause bronchodilation by binding to muscarinic receptors on airway smooth muscle and thereby preventing the action of acetylcholine released from parasympathetic nerves in the vagus nerve. Anticholinergics do not therefore prevent all types of bronchospasm, but are particularly effective against irritant-induced changes in respiratory function. Muscarinic receptor antagonists also decrease mucus secretion.

Currently available muscarinic receptor antagonists do not discriminate between M_2 and M_3 receptors (Fig. 19.8), and it is likely that M_2 autoreceptor antagonism on cholinergic presynaptic terminals may reduce the effectiveness of the antagonism at M_3 receptors on smooth muscle. Selective M_3 receptor antagonists could therefore be an important therapeutic advance.

Muscarinic antagonists include ipratropium bromide, oxitropium bromide, tiotropium bromide, and atropine (Fig. 19.9). The first two drugs are used clinically in many countries by the inhaled route to reduce the systemic adverse effects otherwise associated with this class of drugs. When inhaled they are poorly absorbed into the circulation from the lung, do not cross the blood–brain barrier, and have few adverse effects. Maximum bronchodilation is usually observed from 30 minutes after administration and they last for up to 5 hours. However, their efficacy in asthma is usually modest compared with their efficacy in chronic obstructive pulmonary disease (COPD) (see below).

XANTHINES have been widely used in the treatment of asthma since the start of the twentieth century following observations that 'strong coffee' relieved the symptoms of asthma. Coffee, tea, and chocolate-containing beverages contain naturally occurring xanthines such as caffeine and theobromine. The main xanthine used clinically is theophylline, which is sometimes used as theophylline ethylenediamine salt (aminophylline). Another xanthine preparation that is occasionally used is elixophylline. Xanthines are usually given orally, but are rapidly metabolized, and have a short biologic half-life. However, this

Plasma xanthine concentrations should therefore be measured routinely. Aminophylline can be given as a slow intravenous infusion with a loading dose for acute severe asthma.

For treatment of acute asthma in patients not receiving theophylline products, a loading dose of 5 mg/kg should be administered and maintained at 4 mg/kg every 6 h in young children (1–9 years), 3 mg/kg every 6 h in children (9–16 years) and smokers, 3 mg/kg every 8 h in nonsmoking adults, and 2 mg/kg in older patients.

Drug interactions are important as the serum theophylline concentration can be increased (barbiturates, benzodiazepines) or decreased (cimetidine, erythromycin, ciprofloxacin, allopurinol) by a variety of drugs. These interactions can cause variations in serum theophylline levels between patients, so the dose of theophylline must be titrated to suit the individual. Initially start at the lowest dose and if tolerated and adequate control of symptoms is not achieved then the dose can be increased in stages up to the maximum dosage recommended. An interval of 3 days must be left between increases in dosage to allow for serum levels to stabilize. In the case of acutely ill patients the serum levels should be monitored every 24 h. In all cases the dose should be adjusted to give a serum concentration of 5–15 μg/ml.

Sustained-release preparations are not suitable for the treatment of acute asthma, which should be treated with other medications or an immediate-release preparation.

For the treatment of nocturnal asthma the medication should be given at 8pm and serum theophylline levels should be monitored. It is preferable to titrate the dose with small increments allowing 3 days between increments increasing the dose only if it is tolerated and no adverse effects become apparent.

Xanthines are believed to produce bronchodilation by inhibiting a family of enzymes called phosphodiesterases (Fig. 19.10). These enzymes take part in the metabolism of the second messengers involved in relaxing airway smooth muscle (i.e. cAMP and cGMP). In particular, inhibition of phosphodiesterase 3 and 4 in airway smooth muscle leads to intracellular accumulation of cAMP and therefore smooth muscle relaxation (see Figs 19.10, 19.11).

Anti-inflammatory and prophylactic drugs

Anti-inflammatory drugs may resolve existing bronchial inflammation and/or prevent subsequent inflammation in asthma. Most anti-inflammatory drugs prevent subsequent inflammation and are therefore classed as prophylactic drugs for asthma. Since anti-inflammatory drugs do not cause bronchodilation, they are not recommended for acute asthma attacks.

GLUCOCORTICOSTEROIDS are the best established anti-inflammatory drugs for the treatment of the chronic inflammatory process underlying asthma. They inhibit inflammatory cell infiltration into the airways and reduce edema formation by acting on the vascular endothelium. Their mechanism of action is discussed in detail in Chapter 16.

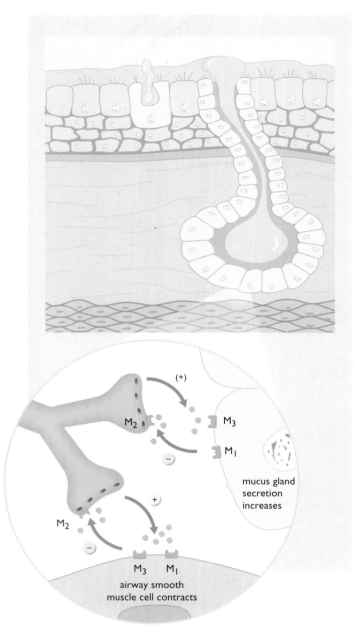

Fig. 19.8 Action of acetylcholine (ACh) on airway smooth muscle.
ACh released from parasympathetic neurons acts on M_1 and M_3 muscarinic receptors on airway smooth muscle and submucosal glands to bring about muscle constriction and mucus secretion. In addition, some of the released ACh acts on presynaptic M_2 muscarinic receptors on the nerve terminal to reduce further release of ACh. These M_2 receptors are known as 'autoreceptors.'

limitation is overcome by using 'slow-release' preparations, which will maintain effective plasma concentrations over 16–18 hours.

The major problem with using xanthines as bronchodilators is that they have a very narrow therapeutic window, consequentially plasma concentrations over 10 μg/ml are required for effective bronchodilation, but plasma concentrations over 20 μg/ml are associated with an increased likelihood of adverse effects, including nausea, cardiac arrhythmias, and convulsions.

420

Muscarinic receptor antagonists

Muscarinic receptor antagonists	Route of administration	Dose range	Half-life (hours)
Ipratropium bromide	Oral inhalation: Aerosol	20–80 µg 3 or 4 times daily in adults and children over 12 years 20–40 µg 3 times a day in children 6–12 years 20 µg 3 times daily	
	Dry powder Nasal inhalation: Nasal spray	20–80 µg 3 or 4 times daily in adults 42 µg in each nostril 2–3 times daily	
Oxitropium bromide	Oral inhalation: Aerosol	200 µg 2–3 times daily in adults	2–4
Tiotropium bromide	Oral inhalation: Aerosol		10

Fig. 19.9 Muscarinic receptor antagonists.

Classification of phosphodiesterase isozymes

Family	Isozyme	Tissue	Inhibitors
1	Ca²⁺/calmodulin dependent	Brain, airway smooth muscle	Vinpocetine Theophylline
2	cGMP stimulated	Heart, vascular smooth muscle, platelets, airway smooth muscle	Theophylline
3	cGMP inhibited	Lymphocyte, platelets, heart, vascular smooth muscle, airway smooth muscle	Milrinone Theophylline
4	cAMP selective	Inflammatory cells (neutrophil, macrophage, mast cell, eosinophil, lymphocyte) airway smooth muscle, heart, brain, striated muscle	Rolipram Theophylline Cilomilast Ruflumilast
5	cGMP selective	Trachea, platelets, vascular smooth muscle	Zaprinast Theophylline Sildenafil

Fig. 19.10 Classification of phosphodiesterase isozymes.

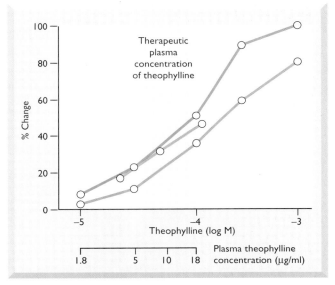

Fig. 19.11 Effects of theophylline at therapeutic concentrations. Percentage change in FEV$_1$ (red), percentage inhibition of airway smooth muscle relaxation (green), or percentage inhibition of phosphodiesterase activity in airway smooth muscle (purple) in relation to plasma concentrations of theophylline (µg/ml) or theophylline concentration (logM in an isolated tissue experiment). (Adapted with permission from Rabe et al. *Eur Resp J* 1995; **289**: 600–603.)

Glucocorticosteroids can be given prophylactically by inhalation to achieve a local anti-inflammatory effect without causing systemic adverse effects. Inhaled glucocorticosteroids used for bronchial asthma include triamcinolone, beclomethasone, budesonide, and fluticasone. Oral glucocorticosteroids may be required for severe asthma unresponsive to inhaled glucocorticosteroids, and usually prednisone, methylprednisolone, or prednisolone is prescribed (see Fig. 19.12).

Both oral and intravenous glucocorticosteroids are useful in the treatment of acute severe asthma. However, oral glucocorticosteroids have systemic adverse effects involving suppression of the hypothalamus–pituitary axis (see Chapter 15 and Fig. 19.12). Chronic use can lead to a variety of serious adverse effects, including stunting of growth in children (see Chapter 15 and Fig. 19.12).

Glucocorticosteroids for asthma

Glucocorticosteroids	Route of administration	Dose range	Drug interactions
Beclomethasone	Nasal inhalation aerosol	1 inhalation (42 µg/inhalation) in each nostril 2–4 times a day in adults and children over 12 years 1 inhalation (42 µg/inhalation) in each nostril 3 times a day in children 6–12 years	
	Suspension	1–2 inhalations (42 µg/inhalation) in each nostril twice a day in adults and children over 12 years 1 inhalation (42 µg/inhalation) in each nostril twice a day in children 6–12 years	
	Oral inhalation Aerosol	2 inhalations (42 µg/inhalation) given 3 or 4 times a day in adults and children over 12 years 1–2 inhalations (42 µg/inhalation) 3 or 4 times a day in children 6–12 years	
	Aerosol	2 inhalations (84 µg/inhalation) twice daily in adults and children over 12 years 2 inhalations (84 µg/inhalation) twice daily in children 6–12 years	
	Dry powder	200 µg twice daily or 100 µg 4 times daily in adults and children over 12 years 50–100 µg 2–4 times daily in children	
Budesonide	Nasal inhalation Nasal inhaler	256 µg daily either 2 sprays per nostril twice daily or 4 sprays per nostril once daily in adults and children over 6 years	Cytochrome P-450 3A inhibitors
	Nasal spray	64 µg per day (one spray of 32 µg per nostril once daily) in adults and children over 6 years	Cytochrome P-450 3A inhibitors
	Oral inhalation Dry powder	200–400 µg twice daily in adults and 200 µg twice daily in children previously maintained with bronchodilators alone 200–400 µg twice daily in adults and 200 µg twice daily in children previously maintained with inhaled corticosteroids 400–800 µg twice daily in adults and 400 µg twice daily in children previously maintained with oral corticosteroids	Cytochrome P-450 3A inhibitors Ketoconazole
	Aerosol	200 µg twice daily in adults and children	Cytochrome P-450 3A inhibitors
Fluticasone	Oral inhalation Dry powder	100 µg twice daily in adults and children over 12 years and 50 µg twice daily in children 4–7 years previously maintained with bronchodilators alone 100–250 µg twice daily in adults and children over 12 years and 50 µg twice daily in children 4–7 years previously maintained with inhaled corticosteroids 1000 µg twice daily in adults and children over 12 years previously maintained with oral corticosteroids	Cytochrome P-450 3A inhibitors
	Aerosol	88 µg twice daily in adults previously maintained with bronchodilators alone 88–220 µg twice daily in adults previoulsly maintained with inhaled corticosteroids 880 µg twice daily in adults previously maintained with oral corticosteroids	Cytochrome P-450 3A inhibitors
	Intranasal Nasal spray	220 µg/day given once or twice a day in adults 100–200 µg/day given once a day in children 4 years and older	Cytochrome P-450 3A inhibitors
Mometasone	Intranasal Nasal spray	200 µg/day given once a day in adults and children over 12 years 100 µg/day given once a day in children 6–12 years	

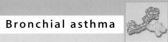

Glucocorticosteroids for asthma (Continued)

Glucocorticosteroids	Route of administration	Dose range	Drug interactions
Triamcinolone	Oral inhalation Aerosol	200 µg 3–4 times a day in adults and children over 12 years 100–200 µg 3–4 times a day in children 6–12 years	
	Nasal inhalation Nasal spray Systemic	220 µg once a day in adults and children over 6 years	
	Oral tablets	8–16 mg/day	Phenytoin Phenobarbitone Primidone Rifampin Carbamazepine Aminoglutethimide Ephedrine Diuretics Antihypertensives Estrogens Anticholinesterases Cardiac glycosides Hypoglycemics Oral anticoagulants NSAIDs Salicylates Live vaccines Amphotericin Acetazolamide Carbenoxolone Methotrexate Cyclosporine Erythromycin Azole antifungals
	Intramuscular injection	2.5–60 mg/day	As above
Dexamethasone	Systemic Oral	0.75–9 mg/day	See triamcinolone
Prednisone	Systemic Oral	5–60 mg/day	See triamcinolone

Methylprednisolone	Systemic
	  Oral
	  Intramuscular injection
	  Intravenous infusion
		4–48 mg/day
		4–48 mg/day
		
		30 mg/kg over 30 minutes every 4–6 hours for 48 hours
			See triamcinolone
			As above
			
			As above

Cortisone	Systemic
	  Oral
	  Intramuscular injection
		25–300 mg/day
		25–300 mg/day
			See triamcinolone
			As above

Fig. 19.12 Glucocorticosteroids for asthma.

🔑 **Drugs for asthma**

- All β adrenoceptor agonists promote bronchodilation
- The principal action of glucocorticosteroids is suppression of the inflammatory response
- Xanthines combine bronchodilator and anti-inflammatory properties
- Muscarinic receptor antagonist-induced bronchodilation is occasionally useful

---

⚠️ **Drugs that modify serum theophylline concentrations**

- Drugs that increase serum theophylline concentrations include:
  Oral contraceptives
  Erythromycin
  Ca^{2+} antagonists
  Cimetidine (but not ranitidine)
- Drugs that decrease serum theophylline concentrations include:
  Rifampin
  Phenobarbital
  Phenytoin
  Carbamazepine

XANTHINES not only produce bronchodilation, as described above, but also inhibit inflammatory cell activation and infiltration in the airways of asthmatics. Furthermore, xanthine withdrawal from some asthmatics after chronic treatment leads to a worsening of asthma, even in patients taking glucocorticosteroids. The anti-inflammatory effects are associated with plasma concentrations lower than those required to produce bronchodilation (5–10 mg/ml). Such findings have led to a reappraisal of the place of xanthines in the treatment of asthma (Fig. 19.11), particularly because:

- Xanthines are administered orally, which greatly enhances patient adherence compared with that for inhaled drugs.
- Low plasma concentrations of theophylline have fewer adverse effects.

The anti-inflammatory action of xanthines may be mediated through inhibition of phosphodiesterase 4, the isozyme found predominately in inflammatory cells (see Fig. 19.10). Recent evidence suggests that theophylline, which is an established agent for the treatment of acute bronchospasm in asthmatics, may be effective when used at low doses for long-term maintenance treatment in asthmatics as a result of this anti-inflammatory action.

CROMOLYN SODIUM, KETOTIFEN, AND NEDOCROMIL SODIUM are anti-allergic drugs used prophylactically in the treatment of bronchial asthma. Cromolyn and nedocromil sodium are active by inhalation. Ketotifen is orally active and is used worldwide except in the US. The mechanisms of action of these prophylactic drugs are not clearly understood, but cromolyn sodium was originally thought to be a 'mast cell stabilizer,' so preventing the release of histamine and other inflammatory mediators (see Chapter 16). It is now clear that this action is not the only effect of these prophylactic drugs. They are capable of affecting many inflammatory cell types including alveolar macrophages, thereby preventing inflammatory cell recruitment into the airway wall. In addition, cromolyn sodium and nedocromil sodium can depress the exaggerated neuronal reflexes triggered by irritant receptors in the airways, probably by suppressing the response of exposed irritant nerves (see Fig. 19.6). This action has led to their use in the treatment of 'asthmatic cough.'

Drugs affecting leukotriene synthesis and actions

ZAFIRLUKAST AND MONTELUKAST are orally active cysteinyl-leukotriene receptor antagonists that antagonize the actions of LTC_4 and LTD_4 on airway smooth muscle and vascular endothelium. They are particularly effective in patients with aspirin-induced asthma. They are also very effective in treating exercise-induced asthma and are available as once-a-day formulations which may improve adherence which is a major clinical problem in the treatment of asthma. Zileuton is an orally active inhibitor of the synthesis of cysteinyl-leukotrienes and other 5-lipoxygenase metabolites derived from arachidonic acid metabolism (see Fig. 16.10) which has also been shown to have a modest clinical effect in the treatment of asthma.

Cyclosporine analogs

Cyclosporine has been successfully used in the treatment of immune disorders involving lymphocytes (see Chapter 16) and has recently been shown to have some clinical benefit in asthmatics resistant to therapy with glucocorticosteroids. However, it has considerable adverse effects and so there is a growing interest in finding safer analogs of this drug to use in the treatment of asthma and other diseases.

■ *Anti-inflammatory treatment is used much earlier in asthma now than in the past*

As asthma is a chronic inflammatory disease of the airways, and not just a disease associated with bronchoconstriction, a number of organizations and societies around the world including the National Institutes of Health in the United States, the World Health Organization, the Canadian Thoracic Society, the British Thoracic Society, and the Australasian Thoracic Society have issued guidelines on the optimal treatment of bronchial asthma. These are based on a stepwise approach, but stress the need for anti-inflammatory treatment much earlier in the disease than has been used in the past.

Chronic obstructive pulmonary disease

Chronic bronchitis and emphysema often occur together in heavy smokers, a condition referred to as chronic obstructive pulmonary disease (COPD). Chronic obstructive pulmonary disease is an airways disease associated with chronic bronchitis, and in the later stages, emphysema. COPD mainly occurs in smokers. Chronic bronchitis is defined in functional terms as a disorder associated with the excessive production of sputum

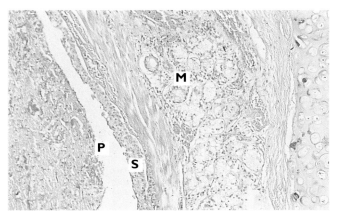

Fig. 19.13 Chronic bronchitis. The main abnormality is hypersecretion of mucus, which plugs the airway (P). Hypersecretion is associated with hypertrophy and hyperplasia of bronchial mucus-secreting glands (M). The Reid index, which is the ratio of gland:wall thickness in the bronchus, is increased in chronic bronchitis. Inflammation is typically absent, although excessive mucus production is frequently associated with the development of coincidental respiratory tract infections, leading to secondary inflammation. Squamous metaplasia (S) is common in patients who have persistent or recurrent superimposed infections. (Courtesy of Dr Alan Stevens and Professor James Lowe.)

Adverse effects of anti-asthma drugs

- β_2 Adrenoceptor agonists may cause tremor and their long-term use may worsen the underlying disease
- Xanthines cause tremor, tachycardia, and gastrointestinal irritation
- Oral glucocorticosteroids should be reserved for patients who do not adequately respond to other therapy, because they have a wide spectrum of adverse effects
- Aerosol glucocorticosteroids cause fewer adverse effects than oral glucocorticosteroids, and mainly overgrowth of Candida in the mouth and hoarseness

and cough, daily or on most days. Airway obstruction is the result of luminal narrowing and mucus plugs, and may lead to secondary respiratory infection (Fig. 19.13). Typically, chronic bronchitis causes alveolar hypoventilation, hypercapnia, and hypoxia, although some patients hyperventilate in order to avoid severe hypoxia. Secondary pulmonary hypertension may develop and lead to right heart failure (cor pulmonale). Patients typically have a productive cough, sputum production, breathlessness on exertion, and airway obstruction. Respiratory infection is common and can worsen the progress of the disease.

■ *Bronchodilators, mucokinetic drugs, and antibiotics are used to treat chronic bronchitis*

Bronchodilators

β_2 **ADRENOCEPTOR AGONISTS** (short- and long-acting) are used to treat breathlessness on exertion in chronic bronchitis,

but with this condition they are generally less effective than in the treatment of bronchial asthma because less of the airways obstruction is due to abnormal airway smooth muscle contraction.

XANTHINES are used in the treatment of chronic bronchitis, particularly for their effects on airway smooth muscle. They also have central nervous system (CNS) effects, leading to increased alertness, which may be important in chronic bronchitis, and can increase diaphragm contractility.

Mucokinetic drugs

N-**ACETYLCYSTEINE** breaks the disulfide bonds that hold mucus glycocoproteins together and thereby reduce the viscosity of mucus. N-Acetylcysteine and a related drug ambroxol have been shown to have some clinical benefit in the treatment of COPD. Other mucokinetic agents include guaifenesin, potassium iodide and even saline.

MUSCARINIC RECEPTOR ANTAGONISTS are the mainstay of therapy for chronic bronchitis because they can reduce much of the bronchospasm associated with smoking and the subsequent inhalation of irritants. Their ability to reduce mucus secretion in the airway by antagonizing acetylcholine acting on muscarinic receptors in mucus glands is also very beneficial (see Fig. 19.8).

Antibiotics

Patients with chronic bronchitis commonly get secondary bacterial infections colonizing the sputum. Antibiotics are therefore often prescribed for these patients and are discussed in more detail in Chapter 9 and below.

PDE4 inhibitors

Selective phosphodiesterase inhibitors inhibit the PDE4 isoenzyme present in most inflammatory cells. Recent clinical studies have suggested that the orally active PDE4 selective inhibitors, roflumilast and cilomilast, show clinical benefit in the treatment of COPD and to a lesser extent in asthma.

Adult respiratory distress syndrome

Adult respiratory distress syndrome (ARDS) is an acute life-threatening condition. It results from increased leakiness of the pulmonary capillary network leading to hypoxia, reduced lung compliance, alveolar infiltrates, and noncardiogenic pulmonary edema. It is common in patients with sepsis, who account for 50% of ARDS cases. The mortality rate of ARDS is approximately 60–70%.

■ *Current therapy for ARDS is inadequate*

No drug specifically prevents the onset of ARDS or lessens its lethality. However, there are promising studies in animals and case reports of emerging therapies for the future including monoclonal antibodies directed against cytokines, PAF, TNF, and IL-1 receptor antagonists.

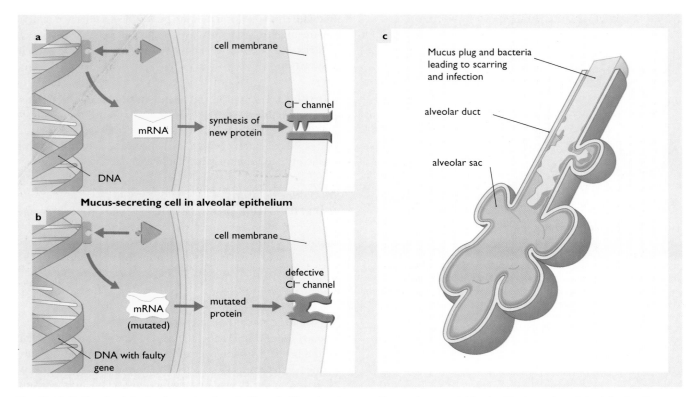

Fig. 19.14 Pathophysiologic elements of cystic fibrosis. Mutations in a specific protein essential for the Cl⁻ channel result in defective Cl⁻ clearance and water resorption. This results in thick and viscous secretions in ducted organs.

Cystic fibrosis

■ *Cystic fibrosis is caused by mutations in specific proteins essential for apical Cl⁻ clearance*

Cystic fibrosis is an inherited disease that starts early in childhood and affects the airways and ducts in various organs, principally the lungs, pancreas, and sweat glands. Patients with cystic fibrosis have mutations in specific proteins essential for apical Cl⁻ clearance (Fig. 19.14). This results in defective Cl⁻ clearance and excessive Na⁺ reabsorption and, as a consequence of osmotic changes, excessive water reabsorption. The defect results in thick and viscous secretion in ducted organs, typically in the airways of the lung, and ducts of the pancreas and sweat glands in homozygotes. In the lungs this gives rise to areas in which inspired air is poorly circulated, and the subsequent bacterial infection (involving *Staphylococcus aureus*, *Pseudomonas aeruginosa*, or other organisms) results in irreversible lung damage (bronchiectasis). Analogous processes involving retained secretions occur in the other organs.

■ *Mucokinetic drugs, antisecretory agents, antibiotics, and physiotherapy are used to treat cystic fibrosis*

The recent discovery of the nature of the genetic defect underlying cystic fibrosis has increased the chance of developing effective therapies, including gene therapy, to produce a true cure. At present, gene therapy is not available.

People with cystic fibrosis have a markedly reduced life expectancy, but it can be significantly extended by aggressive therapy with drugs and physiotherapy (Fig. 19.15). Current therapy of the pulmonary effects centers on:

Therapeutic approaches to cystic fibrosis	
Problem	**Approach**
Defective gene	Replace
Defective gene product	Add
Increased Na⁺ reabsorption	Increase Na⁺ excretion (amiloride)
Thick stagnant mucus	Expectorants, mucolytics, DNAases, physical therapy
Bacterial infection (*Staphylococcus aureus, Pseudomonas aeruginosa*)	Antibiotics
Irreversible lung damage	Lung transplant

Fig. 19.15 Therapeutic approaches to cystic fibrosis.

• Thinning secretions and thereby keeping airways and organ ducts patent.
• Combating opportunistic infections.

The purulent mucus secreted by people with cystic fibrosis is characteristically yellow and rich in DNA tangles (from killed cells), which has led to the use of DNAases to loosen secretions further (see below).

Mucokinetic drugs and antisecretory agents

Respiratory tract fluid secretion is reduced by muscarinic receptor antagonists. A variety of other drugs will increase the movement of fluid and reduce its viscosity.

- Expectorants increase the fluidity of the secretions and thereby improve the productivity of coughing. Typical expectorants include glyceryl guaiacolate, which can be given orally, and menthol and camphor, which are given as a vapor, but the effectiveness of these agents is limited. Potassium iodide may have better expectorant properties.
- Mucolytic agents decrease the viscosity of secretions. N-Acetylcysteine breaks the disulfide bonds that help pack the mucin molecule and thereby make it more viscous. However, it has many adverse effects including nausea, vomiting, stomatitis, and rhinorrhea.
- Agents that break down DNA tangles (e.g. recombinant DNAases given by aerosol) have recently been shown to be effective in the treatment of cystic fibrosis.

Antibiotics

The typical bacteria found in the lungs of patients with cystic fibrosis are *S. aureus* (early in the disease) and *P. aeruginosa*. Pneumonia is therefore particularly common. The first-line antibiotics used to treat this are gentamicin, tobramycin, or amikacin together with one of the following: ciprofloxacin, ticarcillin, imipenen, ceftazidime, and piperacillin. Tobramycin is often given as an aerosol. If there is excessive lung damage the patient may require a lung transplant.

Nonspecific cough

Coughing is a valuable reflex, but may require treatment if it becomes distressing and exhausting

Cough is a reflex triggered by mechanical or chemical stimulation of the upper respiratory tract, or by central stimuli (Fig. 19.16). It is a protective mechanism that serves to expel foreign bodies and unwanted material from the airways (Fig. 19.17). However, coughing is sometimes both useless and distressing

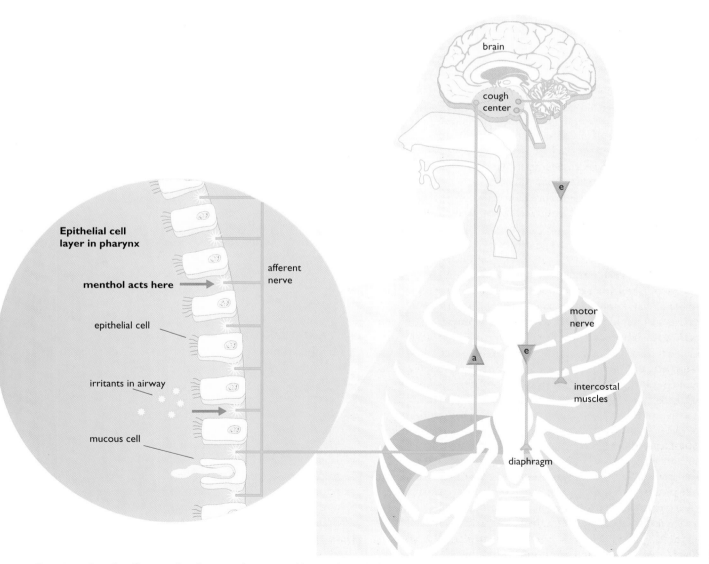

Fig. 19.16 Cough reflex arc. Coughing may be triggered by mechanical, chemical, or central stimuli. (a, afferent nerves; e, efferent nerves)

427

Causes of cough				
Mechanical	**Inflammatory**	**Extrathoracic**	**Abnormal cough reflex**	**Central**
Bronchitis	Asthma	Postnasal drip	Viral infection	Psychogenic
Pneumonia	Viral infection	Esophageal reflux	Asthma	
Cystic fibrosis and asthma	Pollutants	Middle ear disease	ACEI	
Tumor, granuloma, blood, edema	ACEI		Idiopathic	
Foreign body	Interstitial disease			

Fig. 19.17 Causes of cough. (ACEI, angiotensin-converting enzyme inhibitor) (Adapted with permission from Fuller. *Cough.* In: Crystal and West. *The Lung.* New York: Raven Press; 1991.)

and can psychologically and physically exhaust the patient. Cough suppression is then indicated.

As a reflex mechanism, a cough involves an arc (see Fig. 19.16) with sensor, central, and efferent components. The exact nature of the sensory receptors for cough are unknown. However, anatomically, cough-sensitive nerves extend from the larynx to the division of the segmental bronchi. The exact pathway of afferent fibers involved in cough and the exact location of the CNS relay (cough center) are also unknown. The efferent pathway for cough involves the intercostal and phrenic nerves. Abrupt contraction of the respiratory muscles leads to an explosive rise in intrathoracic pressure, which forces air out of the alveoli and through the airways.

■ *The sensor and central components of the reflex arc are targets for drugs used to suppress cough*

Drugs to suppress cough reduce either:

• Receptor activation and therefore the activity in afferent nerves.
• The sensitivity of the 'cough center.'

Drugs that reduce receptor activation

A variety of agents act at peripheral sites. These drugs act directly in some way to reduce the sensitivity of 'cough receptors' to substances such as irritant chemicals and autacoids, which activate the receptors.

MENTHOL VAPOR inhalation reduces the sensitivity of peripheral cough receptors in animals. This probably also occurs in humans. Sucking lozenges impregnated with menthol or eucalyptus oil will also reduce the tendency to cough.

TOPICAL LOCAL ANESTHETICS such as benzocaine, bupivacaine or lidocaine applied to the pharynx and larynx, can reduce the sensitivity of the 'cough receptors' in these areas to irritant chemical or physical stimuli. These are typically used to treat the cough associated with bronchoscopy and in patients who are refractory to other cough therapies.

BENZONATATE is taken orally and is thought to act on both peripheral and central receptors. It is probably less effective

than codeine (see below) and is chemically related to the local anesthetic tetracaine. It is available in the US, but not Canada.

Drugs that reduce the sensitivity of the 'cough center'

THE OPIOIDS Morphine and codeine possess central antitussive actions by virtue of their agonist actions on opiate receptors in the cough center. This action can be separated from other opioid effects. Codeine is usually used therapeutically in proprietary 'cough mixtures' in some countries but not the US.

Dextromethorphan is the d-isomer of methyl ether opiate, levorphanol, and is devoid of analgesic properties. It is as effective as codeine as a cough suppressant, but very high doses can cause CNS depression.

Chlophedianol is generally less effective than codeine. High doses can produce CNS effects such as excitation and nightmares.

Rhinitis and rhinorrhea

■ *Rhinitis and rhinorrhea are manifestations of mucosal inflammation in the nose*

Rhinitis is acute or chronic inflammation of the nasal mucosa, while rhinorrhea is characterized by the production of excessive watery nasal secretions by the nasal mucosa. Both occur mainly as the result of either:

• A viral infection of the nasal mucosa.
• An interaction between antigens and tissue-bound IgE antibodies within the nasal mucosa.

These interactions lead to increased nasal mucosal blood flow, or blood vessel permeability, or both. As a result, the volume of the nasal mucosa increases and inspiration of air through the nasal passages becomes more difficult.

The blood supply to the nasal mucosa includes extensive collaterals and venous sinuses to provide sufficient blood flow to keep the nasal mucosa warm and moist. The most important physiologic controlling mechanism for nasal blood flow is sympathetic neural tone, though autacoids also play a role (Fig. 19.18). Sympathetic activity reduces rhinitis and rhinorrhea, clears the nasal passages, and facilitates breathing. Sympatholytic drugs (adrenergic neuron blockers and α adrenoceptor antagonists) can cause nasal congestion.

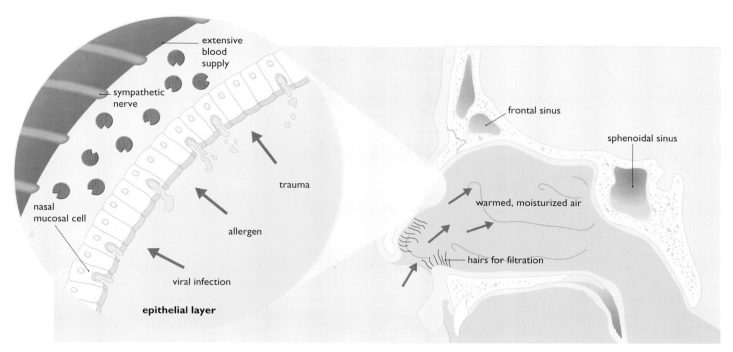

Fig. 19.18 Mechanisms of rhinitis and rhinorrhea. Sympathetic input is the most important physiologic controlling system regulating the extensive blood supply to the nasal mucosa. Fluid hypersecretion occurs in response to a variety of stimuli.

■ *H₁ receptor antagonists (antihistamines), anti-inflammatory drugs, and nasal vasoconstrictors are used to treat rhinitis and rhinorrhea*

There are a variety of targets at which drugs can be aimed to suppress rhinitis and control rhinorrhea (Fig. 19.19). Ideally, rhinitis should be controlled by targeting its cause. However, no treatment is effective against viral infections (e.g. the common cold) and they remain a therapeutic challenge. Immunologic reactions release autacoids such as histamine, which is one of the final mediators of rhinitis and the accompanying sneezing, and control can be achieved in the following ways:

• The immune reaction can be moderated by a local application of glucocorticosteroids sprayed directly onto the nasal mucosa.

• The next level of control is to prevent the antibody interaction resulting in release of autacoids.

Targets in the treatment of rhinitis and rhinorrhea

Target	Treatment
Nasal blood flow	Vasoconstrictors
Anti-inflammatory	Glucocorticosteroids
Suppression of mediator release	Cromolyn sodium
Mediator receptor blockade	H₁ receptor antagonists Leukotriene antagonists

Fig. 19.19 Targets in the treatment of rhinitis and rhinorrhea.

• Cromolyn sodium can be applied to the nasal mucosa to inhibit the release of histamine and other autacoids from mast cells and other inflammatory cells.

The hypersecretory phase of rhinitis can be prevented or reduced by using a drug to vasoconstrict the nasal mucosa, and α adrenoceptor agonists (sympathomimetics) are most commonly used for this purpose.

H₁ receptor antagonists

The major autacoid released during an allergic reaction in the nasal mucosa is histamine, which acts on the nasal mucosa, predominantly via H₁ receptors. H₁ receptor antagonists (see Chapter 16) are therefore useful in the treatment of allergic rhinitis. It cannot be assumed that there is no H₂ receptor involvement, but there have been no reports that H₂ receptor antagonists are effective against allergic rhinitis, even though the vasodilation associated with rhinitis may have an H₂ mediated component.

Anti-inflammatory drugs

GLUCOCORTICOSTEROIDS have marked anti-inflammatory actions. They also produce many adverse effects, including excessive suppression of the immune system, exacerbation of infections, and suppression of the adrenocortical axis, which are mainly seen following oral administration (see Chapter 15). Most of these adverse effects can be avoided if smaller doses are applied regionally or topically, although this can be associated with a local suppression of the immune reaction, giving rise to the possibility of subsequent local infection.

The most widely used glucocorticosteroids applied topically to the nasal mucosa are triamcinolone, beclomethasone, budesonide, and fluticasone, which are regularly sprayed as an aerosol into the nostril.

CROMOLYN SODIUM suppresses the release of autacoids from inflammatory cells involved in an allergic reaction (see Chapter 16). It is used to reduce the itching associated with rhinitis and sneezing and is available as a suspension to be applied topically to the nasal mucosa using an aerosol dispenser.

Sympathomimetic decongestants

The inflammatory and hypersecretory processes of the nasal mucosa involve active vasodilation. Therefore, one approach to control hypersecretion is to oppose vasodilation with vasoconstriction, which is effectively achieved by the administration of α adrenoceptor agonists (see Chapter 14). These drugs act upon α adrenoceptors in the nasal mucosa, decreasing its volume and resistance to movement of air. This may be due to activation of receptors on venous capacitance vessels. Activation of α adrenoceptors, possibly α_2, in nutrient arteries may lead to vasoconstriction of these vessels, possibly damaging the mucosal layer. The α adrenoceptor agonists were introduced as nasal decongestants many years before there was much knowledge of the subtypes of α adrenoceptors. Systematic attempts to evaluate selective agonists for their efficacy as decongestants might be useful.

α Adrenoceptor agonists will produce a degree of nasal vasoconstriction and decongestion when taken orally, but commonly cause generalized vasoconstriction and a tendency to elevate blood pressure. Nevertheless, drugs such as phenylephrine are included in proprietary (over-the-counter) oral mixtures for the treatment of rhinitis and rhinorrhea.

Emerging drugs

LEUKOTRIENE RECEPTOR ANTAGONISTS have been shown to be effective against allergic rhinitis in clinical trials.

Respiratory infections

The respiratory tract is a warm, moist environment lined with epithelial tissue that encounters inspired air laden with pathogens (see Fig. 19.1). Invading organisms include viruses, bacteria, fungi, and parasites.

Most common infections of the respiratory tract are due to viruses and bacteria. Some infections are relatively innocuous (e.g. the common cold), while others can be life-threatening (e.g. viral or bacterial pneumonia). The ease with which infection occurs in the respiratory tract varies according to the health of the individual. For example lung infection with *Pneumocystis carinii* is common in patients with the acquired immunodeficiency syndrome (AIDS). Furthermore, certain organisms invade only certain parts of the tract.

The respiratory cavity is liable to infection by bacteria, viruses, and fungi. Viral infection is usually self-limiting, although it leaves the tissue susceptible to secondary infection by bacteria and fungi. *Candida albicans* of the oral cavity is the most common fungal infection and follows a disturbance of immune status (e.g. systemic immunosuppression therapy or aerosol treatment of asthma with glucocorticosteroids).

Factors determining the use of antibiotics

- Clinical presentation of infection
- Identity of the infecting organism and its risk to the patient
- Sensitivity of the organism to individual antibiotics
- Likelihood of emergence of resistance
- Accessibility of drugs to the organism
- Availability of an effective antibiotic
- Adverse effects of effective antibiotics
- Pharmacodynamics and pharmacokinetics
- Pharmacoeconomics

Fig. 19.20 Factors determining the use of antibiotics.

Antibiotics can lead to the development of resistant organisms

Although many infections of the respiratory tract are self-limiting and leave little residual damage, others can cause permanent damage and chronically reduce the capacity of the lungs. Inappropriate use of antibiotics in the treatment of pulmonary bacterial infections (Fig. 19.20) carries a risk to both the patient and society because of the possible development of resistant organisms. In the absence of life-threatening infection, the choice of antibiotic is based on the identity of the invading organism and its sensitivity to available antibiotics. The organism must therefore be cultured and its antibiotic sensitivity determined. However, some organisms produce such a characteristic pattern of infection that clinical diagnosis and choice of therapy can be based on clinical presentation alone.

The existence of a range of antibiotics sharing similar properties has given rise to the concept of first-line, second-line, and third-line therapy based on specificity and selectivity for the different bacteria. First-line therapy refers to agents of first choice. Second-line therapy is used if the infection is not effectively treated by the first-line therapy, or if the patient cannot tolerate the first-line therapy.

Antibiotics used for specific respiratory tract infections

EPIGLOTTITIS The cephalosporin derivatives cefuroxime, cefotaxime, and ceftriaxone are used to treat life-threatening epiglottitis due to *Haemophilus influenzae* (type B), with chloramphenicol as a second-line drug. Chloramphenicol is effective, but can cause a lethal aplastic anemia (incidence approximately 1/30,000).

PHARYNGITIS There are no effective drugs to treat infectious inflammation of the pharynx due to viruses. Streptococcal group A bacteria produce the most troublesome infection and penicillins (V initially) are first-line antibiotics. Erythromycin is second-line therapy and cephalexin third-line (Fig. 19.21).

LARYNGITIS AND ACUTE RHINITIS with the common cold are viral infections. They are usually not treated, although the secondary bacterial infection that may occur can be treated with antibiotics. It is generally accepted that prescribing antibiotics

Treatment of bacterial pharyngitis

Type of infection	Group A streptococci		
In adults	**First-line**	**Second-line**	**Third-line**
	Penicillin V	Erythromycin	Cephalexin, clarithromycin
In children	Penicillin V, amoxicillin, pivampicillin	Erythromycin estolate	Cephalexin

Fig. 19.21 Drug treatment of bacterial pharyngitis.

specifically for viral infections of the upper respiratory tract is poor medical practice because of the risk of encouraging the development of resistant organisms.

SINUSITIS A variety of organisms are responsible for sinusitis in adults including *Streptococcus pneumoniae*, *H. influenzae*, *Micrococcus catarrhalis*, streptococci, Gram-negative bacilli, anaerobes, and respiratory viruses. Amoxicillin is generally the first-line antibiotic, while trimethoprim/sulfamethoxazole, rifampin, cefuroxime axetil, cefaclor, cefixime, amoxicillin/clavulanate are second-line. Trimethoprim, doxycycline, and clarithromycin are third-line.

Children with acute sinusitis, with or without perforation, due to infection with bacteria such as *S. pneumoniae*, *H. influenzae*, *M. catarrhalis*, group A streptococci, *Staphylococcus aureus*, Gram-negative bacilli, or anaerobes, are given amoxicillin and pivampicillin as first-line, while trimethoprim/sulfamethoxazole and cefuroxime axetil are second-line. Trimethoprim and clarithromycin are third-line.

BRONCHITIS There are no effective therapies for viral infections of the bronchi.
- If the bronchitis is mild to severe and bacterial in origin (i.e. due to *Mycoplasma pneumoniae*, *S. pneumoniae*, *Chlamydia pneumoniae*) first-line antibiotics are tetracycline and erythromycin. Second-line antibiotics are doxycycline and clarithromycin.
- If an adult presents with a mild to moderate acute exacerbation of chronic bronchitis following infection with organisms such as *S. pneumoniae*, *H. influenzae*, *M. catarrhalis* or *M. pneumoniae*, the first-line antibiotics are tetracycline, trimethoprim/sulfamethoxazole and amoxicillin, and second-line are doxycycline, cefuroxime axetil, cefaclor, amoxicillin/clavulanate, and clarithromycin.
- If bronchitis is accompanied by moderate to extensive underlying lung disease due to *S. pneumoniae*, *H. influenzae*, *M. catarrhalis* or *M. pneumoniae*, the first-line antibiotics are trimethoprim/sulfamethoxazole, cefaclor, cefuroxime axetil, amoxicillin/clavulanate, and any one of the above. The second-line antibiotics are floxacillin and ciprofloxacin.
- If there is an acute infective exacerbation of chronic bronchitis in the presence of bronchiectasis and infection due to *H. influenzae*, *S. pneumoniae*, *M. catarrhalis* or *Pseudomonas aeruginosa*, the first-line antibiotics are tetracycline and, trimethoprim/sulfamethoxazole. The second-line antibiotics are floxacillin, ciprofloxacin, cefaclor, cefuroxime axetil,

amoxicillin/clavulanate, and any one of the above with erythromycin or clarithromycin.

PNEUMONIA is an infection of the alveoli and small bronchioles that can involve the pleura (pleurisy). It can occur in a variety of situations and treatment varies according to the situation (Fig. 19.22).

In bronchopneumonia the primary infection is centered on the bronchi and spreads to involve adjacent alveoli, which become filled with an acute inflammatory exudate. Affected areas of lung become consolidated, at first in a patchy distribution involving only the lobules but, if untreated, the consolidation becomes confluent and involves one or both lobes. This pattern of disease is most common in infancy and old age, and predisposing factors include debility and immobility. Immobility leads to retention of secretions, which gravitate to the dependent parts of the lungs and become infected; bronchopneumonia, therefore, most commonly involves the lower lobes. The causative organisms depend upon the circumstances predisposing to infection.

Macroscopically, affected areas of the lung are firm and airless, and have a dark red or gray appearance in bronchopneumonia. There may be pus in peripheral bronchi. Histologically, there is acute inflammation of the bronchi and the alveoli contain an acute inflammatory exudate. The pleura is commonly involved, leading to pleurisy.

If the pneumonia is treated, recovery usually involves focal organization of the lung by fibrosis. Common complications include lung abscess, pleural infection, and septicemia.

WHOOPING COUGH is a potentially debilitating condition resulting from infection with *Bordetella pertussis*, and children can

Antibiotics

- Antibiotics should not be used to treat viral respiratory infections
- Different antibiotics act at different stages in bacterial growth and development
- Combinations of antibiotics may be synergistic and prevent the occurrence of resistant bacteria
- The full course of any antibiotic treatment must be completed or resistance is likely to develop

431

Treatment of bacterial pneumonia

Type of infection

Adults	First-line	Second-line
When community acquired and mild to moderate disease. No comorbidity S. pneumoniae, M. pneumoniae, C. pneumoniae, H. influenzae	Tetracyline, erythromycin	Doxycycline, clarithromycin
With comorbidity. Mixed infections with S. pneumoniae, H. influenzae, oral anaerobes, Gram-negative bacilli, S. aureus, Legionella sp.	Cefaclor, cefuroxime axetil, amoxicillin/clavulanate or any of these plus erythromycin or clarithromycin	
When community acquired severe disease in hospital, with or without comorbidity S. pneumoniae, H. influenzae, Legionella sp., M. pneumoniae, S. aureus, C. pneumoniae. Comorbidity pathogens: anaerobes, Gram-negative bacilli	Cefuroxime axetil, cefuroxime, cefotaxime, ceftriaxone, or any of these plus erythromycin or clarithromycin ± rifampin	Trimethoprim/sulfamethoxazole plus erythromycin
With severe disease in intensive care environment S. pneumoniae, H. influenzae, Legionella sp., Gram-negative bacilli, P. aeruginosa, S. aureus, M. pneumoniae, C. pneumoniae	Erythromycin ± rifampin plus one of ciprofloxacin, imipenem, or ceftazidime	
In institutionalized elderly patients with mild to moderate disease S. pneumoniae, H. influenzae, oral anaerobes, Gram-negative bacilli, S. aureus, Legionella sp.	Trimethoprim/sulfamethoxazole, cefaclor, cefuroxime axetil, amoxicillin/clavulanate, or any one of the above ± erythromycin or clarithromycin	
With severe disease S. pneumoniae, H. influenzae, oral anaerobes, Gram-negative bacilli, S. aureus, Legionella sp.	Cefaclor or cefuroxime axetil or amoxicillin/clavulanate or ceftriaxone or combinations, penicillin or amoxicillin plus ciprofloxacin	Ciprofloxacin plus clindamycin
Children With mild disease S. pneumoniae, S. aureus, streptococci Group A, M. pneumoniae, H. influenzae	Amoxicillin, pivampicillin, erythromycin estolate	Trimethoprim/sulfamethoxazole, clarithromycin, erythromycin/ sulfisoxazole, amoxicillin/clavulanate, cefixime, cefaclor, cefuroxime axetil chloramphenicol ± erythromycin or clarithromycin
With severe disease S. pneumoniae, S. aureus streptococci Group A, M. pneumoniae, H. influenzae	Cefuroxime ± erythromycin estolate or clarithromycin	Trimethoprim/sulfamethoxazole, clarithromycin, erythromycin/ sulfisoxazole, amoxicillin clavulanate, cefixime, cefaclor, cefuroxime axetil, chloramphenicol ± erythromycin or clarithromycin

Fig. 19.22 Treatment of bacterial pneumonia.

be vaccinated against it. Erythromycin (the estolate is preferred for children) is the first-line antibiotic, while trimethoprim/ sulfamethoxazole is second-line and tetracycline, amoxicillin, and ampicillin are third-line.

Tuberculosis

Tuberculosis is a bacterial infection with unique characteristics that make it difficult to treat. Infections with the mycobacteria (*Mycobacterium tuberculosis*) responsible for tuberculosis are more common where there is crowding and poverty. With the general improvement in world economies, housing, and hygiene, the incidence of tuberculosis, particularly in the wealthier countries, decreased remarkably in the latter half of the twentieth century, but the disease has recently increased in

Antitubercular drugs

- Mycobacteria readily develop drug resistance
- The main antitubercular drugs are isoniazid, rifampin, streptomycin, ethambutol, and pyrazinamide
- Drug combinations are always required in the treatment of tuberculosis

incidence and importance. Much of the increase is associated with AIDS, and strains of tubercle bacillus resistant to previously effective therapy continue to emerge.

M. tuberculosis can infect tissue other than respiratory tissue (e.g. brain and intestine), and the mycobacteria can be found in both closed and caseous cavity lesions and in macrophages. Often the disease is self-limiting and the mycobacteria are sealed in a calcified lesion, where they remain dormant. This prevents spread of the infection, but also prevents drugs from readily penetrating to the bacterium. Therefore, there is a risk of subsequent rupture of the lesion and renewed infection. An additional complication of the dormant phase is that anti-mycobacterial drugs act on actively growing organisms. Such features mean therapy must be continued for 9–18 months and combinations of drugs are used. Prophylactic therapy is required for the contacts of people with active disease. The main therapeutic aim is to achieve the lowest relapse rate possible, which is ideally less than 5%.

For a detailed description of drugs used to treat tuberculosis see Chapter 9. Briefly, combinations of drugs are used for extended periods. The major drugs for nonresistant tuberculosis are isoniazid, rifampin, ethambutol, pyrazinamide and streptomycin. Other useful drugs include capreomycin, cycloserine, ethionamide and para amino salicylic acid.

Treatment of tuberculosis

- The first-line treatment of tuberculosis is a combination of rifampin, isoniazid, and pyrazinamide
- Treatment is usually for 6 months and the pyrazinamide may be discontinued after 2 months

Hypersensitivity pneumonitis

Hypersensitivity pneumonitis (allergic alveolitis) is a lympho-cytic and granulomatous interstitial pneumonitis caused by type III and IV hypersensitivity reactions to repeated inhalation of a variety of antigens. Farmer's lung, caused by repeated inhalation of dusts in hay containing thermophilic actinomycetes, is the prototype of this disorder. The etiologic agents are most commonly thermophilic actinomycetes, fungi, or animal proteins inhaled in large quantities.

Hypersensitivity pneumonitis is characterized by the development of a cough, fever, chills, malaise, and dyspnea in a previously sensitized person (6–8 hours after exposure to the antigen), bilateral inspiratory crackles on auscultation, and poorly defined patchy or diffuse infiltrates on the chest radio-

graph. Pulmonary function tests show a restrictive pattern with decreased lung volumes, decreased diffusion capacity, and hypoxemia. Neutrophilia and an increase in C-reactive protein are common following exposure to the antigen.

Precipitating antibodies against the causative antigen are usually demonstrated in the serum of patients with hyper-sensitivity pneumonitis, and bronchoalveolar lavage consistently demonstrates an increase in T cells in lavage fluids (predominantly the $CD8^+T_C$ cell subset). In patients with very recent exposure to antigen, however, the $CD4^+T_H$ cells in lavage fluids may be increased.

MANAGEMENT The most effective treatment of hypersensitivity pneumonitis is avoidance of the offending antigen or environment. Dust control or use of protective masks to filter the offending dust particles in contaminated areas may also be effective. Glucocorticosteroids are the drug treatment of choice and markedly reduce the pulmonary inflammatory process.

Allergic bronchopulmonary aspergillosis

Allergic bronchopulmonary aspergillosis (ABPA) occurs in asthmatic patients and is an eosinophilic pneumonia resulting from an allergic reaction to Aspergillus fumigatus. The presence of A. fumigatus growing in the bronchial lumen provokes an allergic response in the airways and parenchyma. Type I and III (and possibly type IV) hypersensitivity reactions are involved in the pathogenesis. Histopathologic studies reveal eosinophilic infil-trations of the pulmonary parenchyma with a bronchiocentric infiltration of lymphocytes, plasma cells, and monocytes. ABPA is clinically characterized by bronchial asthma, which is usually long standing, pulmonary infiltrates, sputum production, blood eosinophilia, an immediate wheal and flare skin test, precipitating antibody in the serum to A. fumigatus, and high levels of total (and specific) IgE.

MANAGEMENT Treatment with glucocorticosteroids and other antiasthmatic drugs (theophylline, sympathomimetics) usually controls the asthma attacks, resolving the inflammatory process and allowing expectoration of the mucus plugs and A. fumigatus. Glucocorticosteroid therapy leads to decreased serum IgE levels and the pulmonary infiltrates disappear. A long-term main-tenance dose of prednisone (7.5–15 mg/day) may be needed to prevent the development of progressive irreversible disease. Inhaled beclomethasone dipropionate is also useful. Antifungal agents are not effective in resolving the inflammatory process. Immunotherapy with extracts of A. fumigatus is contraindicated because it produces bothersome local reactions and may cause exacerbation of symptoms.

Pulmonary embolism

In addition to its role in gas exchange, the vast surface area of the pulmonary vasculature also acts as a filter of blood since it is the first capillary network encountered by venous blood and is thus uniquely positioned anatomically for the entrapment of particulate matter that would otherwise enter the arterial circulation. Microentrapment probably goes on regularly but in some cases there can be marked embolism of the pulmonary

433

circulation that can lead to significant alteration in both pulmonary and cardiac function, and even death. Venous thromboembolism is relatively common with an estimated 140,000 deaths per year in the US. There are also individuals with chronic cor pulmonale resulting from chronic unresolved emboli.

The goal of treatment of venous thromboembolism is the prevention of recurrent, fatal pulmonary embolism. Heparin is initially used with doses adjusted to maintain the APTT within therapeutic levels (see Chapter 13). Heparin treatment is normally maintained for 5–10 days and is usually simultaneous with warfarin administered orally. Newer, low molecular weight heparin fractions are increasingly used in the treatment of venous thromboembolism in place of unfractionated heparin as they have the advantage of fixed-dose subcutaneous administrations without monitoring or dose adjustment and with a comparable or lower risk of hemorrhage. Meta-analysis of various trials also suggests that prophylactic treatment with antiplatelet drugs (see Chapter 13) reduces the incidence of deep vein thrombosis and pulmonary embolism.

Pulmonary hypertension

Primary pulmonary hypertension is rare, but secondary pulmonary hypertension is more common and results from a variety of causes such as connective tissue destruction, pulmonary embolism, COPD, fibrosing lung disease, and from the increased use of anorectic drugs such as aminorex fumarate and more recently dexfenfluramine hydrochloride.

Vasodilator drugs

Pulmonary hypertension is primarily treated with vasodilators, although there is still no consensus as to which vasodilator is best. In primary pulmonary hypertension, treatment is with calcium channel blockers, the most commonly used drugs being nifedipine and diltiazem (see Chapter 18). They are active acutely and are useful in identifying patients who will respond to long-term vasodilator treatment. Their relatively long half-lives mean that it takes up to 12 h to complete an acute vasodilator assessment, and as these drugs are able to affect all vascular beds, systemic vasodilation and hypotension are common side effects. If there is no acute response to calcium channel blockers, continuous i.v. infusion of prostacyclin (PGI_2) should be started. PGI_2 has a 3-minute half-life which makes it ideal for assessment of pulmonary hypertension. However, this also means PGI_2 must be infused continuously for chronic treatment making it expensive. PGI_2 also has many adverse effects including systemic hypotension, nausea, headache, flushing and abdominal pain, all of which resolve with a reduction in the infusion rate. Such side effects may be reduced by aerosolizing PGI_2. Infusion of PGI_2 should be 1 ng/kg/min and increased by 1–2 ng/kg/min until there is a positive response or appearance of adverse effects, with a maximum dose in adults of 12 ng/kg/min. Stable orally active PGI_2 analogs such as iloprost and beraprost have also shown positive clinical benefit.

Recently, inhaled nitric oxide has been shown to be effective in the treatment of pulmonary hypertension via pulmonary vasorelaxation. It has a great advantage over other vasodilator drugs in being selective regarding pulmonary hypertension as it has minimal effects on systemic blood vessels when inhaled. It is cheap, has a rapid onset of action (albeit very short-lived in the presence of O_2) and minimal adverse effects acutely. However, it requires the availability of a metered gas delivery system and careful environmental monitoring since some NO metabolites, such as NO_2, are toxic.

Adenosine is another potent vasodilator, which increases cAMP in vascular smooth muscle, and it can be useful for the assessment of vasodilator treatment of primary pulmonary hypertension. Adenosine has a very short half-life (10 sec) and is cheaper than PGI_2. It does, however, cause significant coronary vasodilation and reduced systemic vessel resistance.

O_2 is a selective pulmonary vasodilator and should be considered in all patients with pulmonary hypertension who are hypoxic at rest or who desaturate with exercise. This is particularly important in patients with raised pulmonary artery pressure resulting from COPD. 15–17 hours per day O_2 treatment in all patients has been shown to provide a marked improvement in disease progression and morbidity in patients with COPD. This selective effect of O_2 is by virtue of its effect on hypoxic pulmonary vasoconstriction.

Other drugs used for the treatment of pulmonary hypertension

The cardiac glycosides such as digoxin have been widely used to treat pulmonary hypertension although there is no consensus as to the benefit they bring. Symptomatic benefit has also been shown with sublingual isoproterenol, and both dopamine and dobutamine have been suggested to be useful in the event of acute deterioration of right ventricular function. Diuretics are also useful in right heart failure to reduce excessive right ventricular preload and to counteract the edema associated with pulmonary hypertension, although there is no evidence that these drugs alter survival.

Drugs with adverse effects in patients with respiratory disease
β Adrenoceptor antagonists

$β_2$ Adrenoceptor antagonists such as propranolol, with its potent capacity to block $β_2$ adrenoceptors, are strictly contraindicated in patients who have bronchial asthma because they precipitate severe bronchoconstriction, which may be lethal. This adverse effect results from the dependence of asthmatics on circulating epinephrine and/or the innervations of parasympathetic ganglia by sympathetic nerves as inhibitory mechanisms to offset vagal tone, which tends to reduce airway diameter. β Adrenoceptor antagonist eyedrops can also induce life-threatening asthma attacks in asthmatic subjects.

Angiotensin-converting enzyme inhibitors

Angiotensin-converting enzyme (ACE) inhibitors such as captopril and enalapril are used increasingly in the treatment of hypertension and congestive heart failure. However, ACE inhibitors such as captopril can induce coughing in some patients with concomitant allergic airway diseases. The mech-

Adverse effects of drugs used for respiratory diseases other than asthma and infection

- *Mucokinetic drugs have relatively few adverse effects*
- *The opioids are the only cough suppressants with a major adverse effect (i.e. the potential for drug abuse and social withdrawal)*

Adverse effects of antibiotics

- *The principal adverse effect of penicillin and cephalosporins is allergy*
- *The principal adverse effect of aminoglycosides is renal toxicity*
- *The principal adverse effects of sulfonamides are allergy and skin photosensitivity*
- *The principal adverse effects of antitubercular drugs vary with the drug*

anism is believed to be local generation of bradykinin because ACE inhibitors inhibit peptidyl peptidase enzymes involved in the metabolism of bradykinin in addition to inhibiting the conversion of angiotensin I to angiotensin II. The concentration of bradykinin in the lung can then become elevated and stimulate the afferent receptors, initiating cough. ACE-induced coughing is effectively treated with cromolyn sodium.

Nonsteroidal anti-inflammatory drugs

Approximately 20% of people with asthma can develop severe bronchoconstriction following ingestion of nonsteroidal anti-inflammatory drugs (NSAIDs). The mechanism is not fully understood, but may relate to the generation of lipoxygenase metabolites of arachidonic acid because it can be inhibited by 5-lipoxygenase inhibitors. NSAIDs, including aspirin, must therefore be used with caution in patients with asthma.

FURTHER READING

Antiplatelet Trialists Collaboration. Collaborative overview of randomized trials of antiplatelet therapy III. Reduction in venous thrombosis and pulmonary embolism by antiplatelet prophylaxis among surgical and medical patients. *Br Med J* 1994; **308**: 235–246.

Barnes PJ. Neural control of the lung. *Am Rev Resp Dis* 1993; **134**: 1289–1314. [A detailed review of the biology of the neural mechanisms involved in regulating the biology of the lung.]

Barnes PJ. Anti-inflammatory therapy for asthma. *Ann Rev Resp Med* 1993; **44**: 229–249. [This review provides an in-depth discussion of recent advances in the treatment of bronchial asthma.]

Barnes PJ, Chung KF and Page CP. Inflammatory mediators of asthma: an update. Pharmacological Reviews 1998; **50**(4): 515–596. [A comprehensive review of the inflammatory mediators involved in bronchial asthma and the implication for new therapies.]

Holgate S (ed.) *Immunopharmacology of the Respiratory System*. London: Academic Press; 1995. [An up-to-date review of the immunologic mechanisms contributing to lung disease.]

Karlsson JA, Fuller RW. Pharmacological regulation of cough reflex—from experimental models to antitussive effects in man. *Pulmonary Pharmacology & Therapeutics* 1999; **12**: 215–228. [An excellent overview of the pharmacology of cough.]

Nadel JA, Murray J (eds) *Textbook of Respiratory Medicine*, 2nd edn. London: WB Saunders; 1994. [An excellent textbook written by two distinguished American authors covering the clinical aspects of respiratory medicine.]

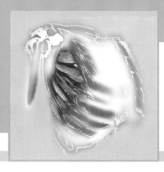

Chapter 20

Drugs and the Musculoskeletal System

PHYSIOLOGY OF THE MUSCULOSKELETAL SYSTEM

The musculoskeletal system protects vital structures and is responsible for a variety of mobility-related functions. The integrity of the musculoskeletal system depends on interactions between skeletal muscles, which usually cross joints and move the bones to which they are attached. Joints link two or more bones and provide a low-friction surface on which bones can move. Muscle function is controlled by voluntary and involuntary discharges from the motor cortex in the central nervous system (CNS). Muscle tone is modulated by spinal reflexes at the level of the spinal cord where the motor nerve exits.

The skeleton is made up of a series of bones and joints that maximize range while maintaining stability. The two types of bone are:

- Cortical compact bone (80%), which provides strength when torsion is the dominant force, is dense, and is the main component of long bones.
- Trabecular bone (20%), which resists compressive forces, is found at the end of long bones, and makes up the major component of the vertebral body.

There are also two types of joint:

- A synovial (true) joint (e.g. the knee joint) allows extensive movement. Its stability is maintained by ligaments as well as muscles that pass across it.
- A fibrocartilaginous joint (e.g. the sacroiliac joint) maximizes joint stability, but limits movement of the skeleton.

PATHOPHYSIOLOGY AND DISEASES OF THE MUSCULOSKELETAL SYSTEM

Osteoporosis

Osteoporosis is a thinning of normal bone with aging, but may be accelerated by a premature natural or surgical loss of ovarian

Bone diseases

- Can cause fractures and pain
- Osteoporosis is characterized by a reduced quantity of bone
- Osteomalacia is characterized by a lack of mineralization
- Paget's disease is characterized by the production of abnormal bone

function, medications (e.g. glucocorticosteroids), or lifestyle factors (e.g. alcohol, smoking). It is a common disorder in women and may result in forearm, hip, and spinal fractures. The increasing morbidity and mortality due to osteoporosis in Europe and North America reflect the increasingly aging population.

An assessment of bone density using imaging studies provides the best estimate of fracture risk

Bone quality is normal in osteoporosis, but its quantity is reduced (Fig. 20.1). The balance between formation (a function of osteoblasts) and bone resorption (a function of osteoclasts) determines whether the amount of bone increases or decreases over time. Bone mass is determined by the net effect of these two active ongoing processes. It increases from birth to about 30 years of age in both men and women (Fig. 20.2), and then slowly declines, with a more rapid decline in women in the early postmenopausal years.

Bone formation and resorption can be semiquantified by histomorphologic analysis on bone biopsy or indirectly assessed using markers of bone formation and resorption. Serum Ca^{2+} concentrations and Ca^{2+}-regulating hormones are normal.

Osteomalacia and rickets

Osteomalacia is a relatively uncommon condition of bone in which there is decreased mineralization of new bone matrix (Fig. 20.3). In children this lack of calcification may result in growth failure and deformity and is called rickets. Adults may present with bone pain, proximal myopathy, or fractures with minor trauma.

Osteomalacia is most commonly due to acquired vitamin D deficiency. Biochemical markers include hypocalcemia, a secondary elevation of PTH concentration, and a low plasma 25-hydroxyvitamin D concentration. Other less common hereditary types of osteomalacia also occur.

The major source of vitamin D is the skin, where it is produced by a photochemical reaction. It is also contained in food, particularly fortified milk. Individuals who lack exposure to sunlight because of climate, type of clothing, or institutionalization (such as long-term geriatric care) are at risk of vitamin D deficiency (see Chapter 27).

Paget's disease of bone

Paget's disease is a bone condition that presents with bone pain, skeletal deformity, neurologic complications, or fractures. The incidence is highly variable: it is common in Central Europe,

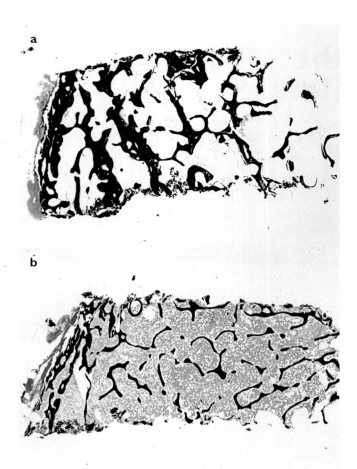

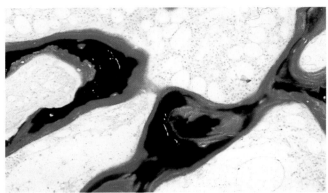

Fig. 20.3 Osteomalacia. Micrograph of iliac crest bone embedded in acrylic resin without previous decalcification from a patient with osteomalacia. There is a broad zone of unmineralized osteoid (red) and a central zone of mineralized bone (black) in this section stained by the von Kossa's silver technique. (Courtesy of Dr Alan Stevens and Professor Jim Lowe.)

Fig. 20.1 Osteoporosis. (a) Micrograph of a resin section of a bone biopsy from the iliac crest showing normal cortical and trabecular bone stained with a silver method, which makes calcified bone show up as black. (b) Micrograph of bone from a patient with osteoporosis. When compared with (a), which shows the bone mass of a healthy patient of the same age, it is clear that the cortical zone is narrower and that the trabeculae are thinner and less numerous. (Courtesy of Dr Alan Stevens and Professor Jim Lowe.)

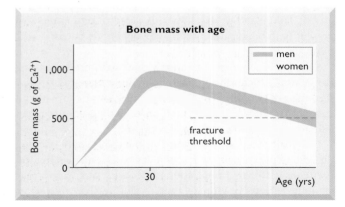

Fig. 20.2 Bone mass with age.

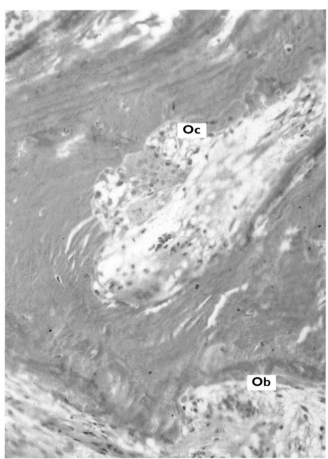

the UK, Australia, New Zealand, and the US, and rare in Africa, the Middle and Far East, and Scandinavia.

The pathology reveals excessive bone resorption and formation (Fig. 20.4) and there are three phases: osteolytic,

Fig. 20.4 Paget's disease. Micrograph of a resin-embedded, Gouldner-stained section from a patient with active Paget's disease. There is uncontrolled osteoclast (Oc) resorption of a bone, and osteoblasts (Ob) are attempting to fill in sites of recent osteoclast erosion in an adjacent site. (Courtesy of Dr Alan Stevens and Professor Jim Lowe.)

osteoblastic, and quiescent. All three patterns may be present in one patient at the same time. The presence of inclusion bodies on histopathology has led to the suggestion that the disease may have a viral origin.

Osteoarthritis

Osteoarthritis is the most common joint disease. It is characterized pathologically by a loss of articular cartilage, bone remodeling and hypertrophy, subchondral bone sclerosis, and bone cysts. It may be the result of either:

- Excessive loads on the joint.
- The presence of abnormal cartilage or bone.

The most characteristic feature of osteoarthritis is gradual progressive cartilage loss. The early biochemical changes with osteoarthritis include 1) a reduction of glycosaminoglycan content in cartilage (with lower chondroitin sulfate, keraton sulfate and hyalouronic acid), 2) increased enzymes that break down cartilage (matrix metalloproteinase), and 3) increased water content. The increased enzyme activity of matrix metalloproteinase is partly responsible for the breakdown of proteoglycan and collagen. The chondrocyte initially is stimulated to increase the number of chondrolytes and also produce cytokines such as interleukin-1 (IL-1) and tumor necrosis factor alpha (TNF-α). Naturally occurring small proteins are present to inhibit these catabolic enzymes. The pathophysiologic changes cause the localized pain that initially occurs with use and is relieved with rest, but which later occurs with minimal activity or movement. Joint stiffness, which is characteristic of inflammatory arthritis, is minimal or short lived.

Rheumatoid arthritis

Rheumatoid arthritis is a chronic inflammatory disease of joints that results in joint pain, swelling, and destruction. It affects an estimated 1% of the adult population throughout the world. Progression of the disease results in joint destruction, deformity, and significant disability.

Rheumatoid arthritis is characterized by chronic inflammation in the synovium, which lines the joint. The synovium is inflamed, with an accumulation of polymorphonuclear leukocytes in the superficial layers and mononuclear cells (CD4-positive T lymphocytes and plasma cells) beneath the lining cell layer and deep in the synovial tissues. With disease progression there is massive synovial hypertrophy, with invasion by both inflammatory cells and fibroblast-like cells. Fibrovascular tissue known as 'pannus' invades and destroys both bone and cartilage. Mediators of inflammation control the inflammatory synovitis, cartilage breakdown and bone erosions. Pro-inflammatory cytokines including TNF-α, IL-1, granulocyte–macrophage colony stimulating factor (GM-CSF), IL-6, and chemokines are produced in the rheumatoid joint. In addition cytokines that are anti-inflammatory, IL-4 and IL-10, are present and may suppress the inflammatory state. Drugs such as soluble IL-1 receptor antagonist (IL-1ra) can be further considered as anti-inflammatory molecules (Fig. 20.5). TNF-α has direct effects on synovitis, osteoclasts and chondrocytes. Intense research in recent years has led to specific biologic therapies that are now in clinical use. Further promising

therapies will likely continue to emerge. Current blocking agents that have been studied in rheumatoid arthritis include infliximab and etanercept (discussed later). Many other biologic therapies are being studied in early clinical trials.

Rheumatoid arthritis is associated with a variety of non-articular clinical syndromes including vasculitis, subcutaneous nodules, interstitial pulmonary fibrosis, pericarditis, mononeuritis multiplex (vasculitis of peripheral nerves), Sjögren's syndrome (inflammation of the salivary and tear glands), Felty's syndrome (splenomegaly and leukopenia), and ocular inflammation.

Early diagnosis and intervention with disease-modifying agents may reduce the significant associated morbidity of rheumatoid arthritis. The treatment of rheumatoid arthritis involves the use of anti-inflammatory drugs and other disease-modifying agents.

Gout and other types of crystal arthritis

Gout is a common disease characterized by the precipitation of monosodium urate crystals in tissues

Gout predominantly affects men in their thirties and forties, but also occurs in postmenopausal women. The clinical manifestations include acute inflammatory arthritis (acute gout), chronic articular and periarticular inflammation, uric acid kidney stones (urolithiasis), and gouty nephropathy, which is rare. Hyperuricemia is common, but unless associated with symptoms and signs should not generally be treated.

Uric acid production and secretion is usually balanced to keep the tissue uric acid concentration below values at which urates precipitate and crystals form (Figs 20.6, 20.7). Genetic and environmental factors may affect both the production and renal secretion of uric acid. Hyperuricemia is associated with obesity, diabetes mellitus, hypertension, and renal insufficiency, and treatment with thiazide diuretics and low-dose salicylates.

Uric acid overproduction, which is seen in 10% of individuals with gout, can be associated with inherited enzyme deficiencies or myeloproliferative disorders. A reduced renal clearance of uric acid is responsible for the remaining 90% of cases. Decreased renal excretion of urate is associated with chronic renal failure, lead nephrology, ketoacidosis, hypothyroidism and diabetes insipidus.

Calcium pyrophosphate dihydrate (CPPD) deposition disease and hydroxyapatite deposition

Calcium pyrophosphate dihydrate (CPPD) deposition disease has been reported in association with a variety of conditions and may result in acute inflammation (pseudogout) or joint degeneration. Pseudogout is a relatively common disease with clinical features indistinguishable from those of acute gout. The characteristic acute inflammatory response involves neutrophils reacting to calcium pyrophosphate crystals. The tissue inflammation responds to the same medical treatment as gout. Hydroxyapatite deposition may result in acute joint inflammation, periarticular inflammation, and subcutaneous tissue deposition. It is frequently associated with osteoarthritis, but the importance of apatite crystals in the pathogenesis of osteoarthritis is not clear.

439

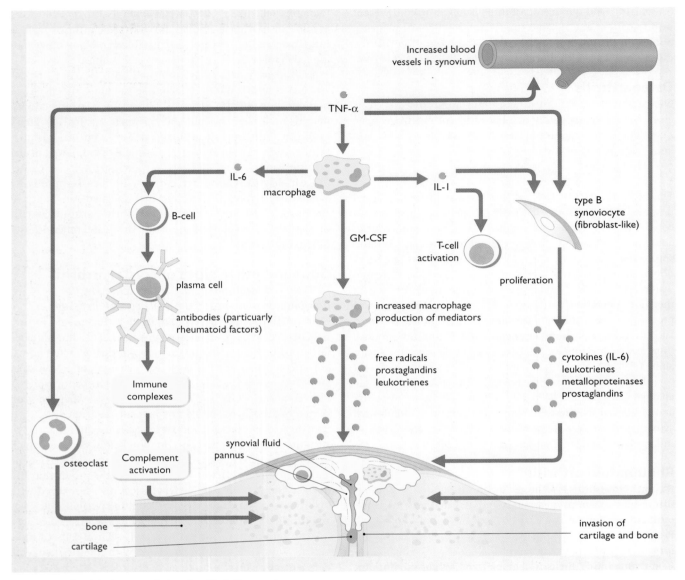

Fig. 20.5 Role of TNF-α on cells involved in inflammation.

Systemic lupus erythematosus

Systemic lupus erythematosus (SLE) is an autoimmune disease that affects approximately 1 in 1000 individuals. It is more prevalent in young females. Its associated morbidity and mortality are decreasing in most parts of the world as a result of early recognition and treatment. Associated complications are higher in poorer socio-economic groups, and the incidence of SLE is higher in certain individuals of African, Hispanic, or Asian descent. SLE is characterized by a variety of clinical features, which include skin and musculoskeletal manifestations. Renal, pulmonary, serosal, neuropsychiatric and reticuloendothelial involvement are less common, but potentially more serious. Pathologic findings include inflammation, blood vessel abnormalities, and immune complex deposition.

The immunologic disturbance includes antibodies to a variety of 'self' tissues. Antinuclear antibodies (ANA) against components of the cell nucleus are most common. The contri-

bution of ANA to the clinical events is unclear because of the presence of antibodies in nondisease states and because the target antigen in the nucleus would normally be protected from antibody binding. The immune disturbance promotes B cell hyperactivity to both self and foreign antigens. Activation of an antibody response to a foreign antigen such as a virus may be a triggering mechanism.

Seronegative spondyloarthropathies

Seronegative spondyloarthropathies are a group of inflammatory types of arthritis characterized by common clinical features and associated to a varying degree with the HLA-B27 gene. Sacroiliitis is the characteristic feature of this disorder that includes ankylosing spondylitis, psoriatic arthritis, reactive arthritis, and the arthritis associated with inflammatory bowel disease.

Pathologically, granulation tissue erodes the fibrocartilaginous joint, resulting eventually in ossification and possible

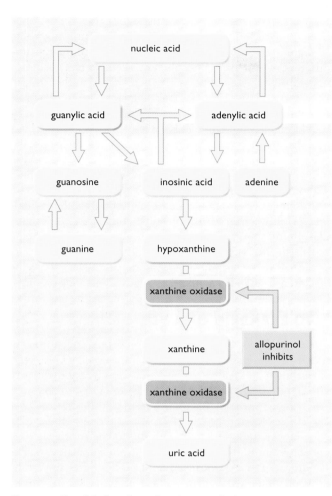

Fig. 20.6 Simplified outline of purine metabolism.

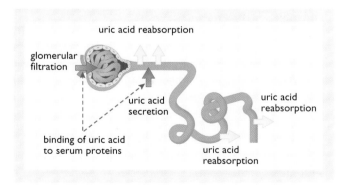

Fig. 20.7 Uric acid secretion and reabsorption in kidney.
Uricosuric agents block uric acid reabsorption in the proximal tubules.

bony fusion. Inflammation similar to the inflammatory process of rheumatoid arthritis may involve the peripheral synovial joints. Enthesitis (inflammation of tendinous insertions to bone) is another characteristic feature. Extra-articular features include ocular inflammation, cutaneous inflammation, and occasionally cardiac involvement.

DRUGS USED TO TREAT MUSCULOSKELETAL DISEASES

Drugs for osteoporosis

Drugs used to treat osteoporosis in postmenopausal women include hormone replacement therapy, calcitonin, bisphosphonates, selective estrogen receptor modulators (SERMs), calcium, and vitamin D.

Hormone replacement therapy

Estrogen replacement therapy (ERT) at the time of the menopause inhibits the effect of osteoclasts on bone resorption (see Chapter 15). It therefore slows bone loss and may actually increase bone quantity in the first few years following cessation of normal ovarian function. It can be provided orally, by injection, or transdermally, as estrogens and their esters are easily absorbed through the skin, mucous membranes, and gastrointestinal tract. The different routes of administration have different pharmacokinetics and other properties. Oral estrogen (e.g. conjugated equine estrogen, estrone sulfate, and micronized estradiol-20β) is the most widely prescribed drug to treat postmenopausal osteoporosis.

Estrogens circulate in the blood in association with sex hormone binding globulin and albumin and, like other steroid hormones, act in the cell nucleus. They diffuse passively through cell membranes and bind to the nuclear estrogen receptor found in estrogen-responsive tissues. Following activation, the estrogen receptor binds to specific DNA sequences that result in transcription of adjacent genes. Recent research has determined that there are at least two types of estrogen receptors: alpha and beta. Estrogen has been shown to bind to the alpha receptor and forms an estrogen-receptor complex which thus binds to the Estrogen Response Element. The alpha receptor is located in reproductive tissues including breast and endometrium. The beta receptor is predominant in non-reproductive tissues including bone, liver and the cardiovascular system. This partly explains why estrogen and estrogen-like substances have different effects in different tissues.

■ *The decision to start ERT and patient adherence to therapy depend not only on its effect on bone but also on its other clinical effects*

ERT will relieve vasomotor symptoms if given in the first few years of the menopause. Usually treatment can be tapered, but occasionally long-term treatment is required. ERT inhibits bone loss and may initially increase bone density. In addition, it influences lipoprotein metabolism (see Chapter 15), resulting in decreased low density lipoprotein (LDL) cholesterol and increased high-density lipoprotein (HDL) concentrations, thereby potentially protecting against cardiovascular disease. Some clinical studies have shown a reduced rate of myocardial infarction, decreased mortality from cardiovascular disease, and an overall reduction in total mortality in postmenopausal women who receive ERT. However, a 4-year prospective study in postmenopausal women with a history of heart disease has shown increased cardiovascular events with estrogen replacement at 1 year of study. There is a trend towards reduced events in the last 3 years of this study. Results of definitive prospective

441

studies are still pending. Transdermal estrogen usually controls postmenopausal symptoms and osteoporosis, but has less effect on lipoproteins.

Progesterone should be considered for all patients started on ERT who have not had a hysterectomy, because it will reduce the significantly increased risk of endometrial cancer associated with ERT to below the native risk. Unopposed estrogens should only be given to women who have had a hysterectomy and therefore have no risk of developing endometrial hyperplasia. The addition of cyclic progesterone therapy usually results in the continuation of monthly menstruation, but menstrual bleeding can be reduced by using lower doses or continuous progesterone. Continuous use of progesterone inhibits endometrial proliferation and reduces the risk of endometrial cancer, but can cause 'breakthrough bleeding.' There is some evidence that progesterone diminishes the favorable effect of estrogens on the lipoprotein profile. Progesterone can be given orally, transdermally, or by injection. Common oral progesterones used include medroxyprogesterone, norethindrone, and micronized progesterone.

Calcitonin

Calcitonin, a 32-amino acid peptide that directly inhibits osteoclasts, can slow bone loss. It acts on a calcitonin receptor that is expressed in a variety of cells, but most importantly osteoclasts. There is homology between this receptor on osteoclasts and the parathyroid hormone (PTH) receptor on osteoblasts. The cell surface calcitonin receptor is coupled to adenylyl cyclase so that its activation increases the intracellular concentration of cAMP, resulting in an inhibitory effect on the osteoclasts. Calcitonin may exert an effect on the osteoblasts, but this is less clear.

Oral calcitonins are ineffective because they are broken down by aminopeptidases and proteases in the gastrointestinal tract. Parenteral calcitonin is well absorbed, but this inconvenient route of administration limits its widespread use. Intranasal calcitonin is therefore used instead: although it is not well absorbed, with low peak plasma concentrations, it is more practical and has wider patient acceptance. Recent randomized controlled trials of nasal calcitonin have demonstrated an improved bone density of 1–2% over 2 years. One study has demonstrated reduction of vertebral fractures with nasal spray calcitonin 200 IU daily, but not at 400 IU daily. Injected calcitonin at higher doses (50–100 IU/day) has analgesic properties and is frequently used in patients with severe pain due to recent vertebral compression fractures.

Intranasal or subcutaneous calcitonin can be given to produce beneficial effects on the bone without causing serious systemic adverse effects. Marine (salmon or eel) calcitonins are usually used because they are many times more potent than human calcitonin. Minor adverse effects include flushing and gastrointestinal symptoms (nausea, vomiting, or diarrhea). Neutralizing antibodies may develop which inhibit calcitonin's actions.

Bisphosphonates

Bisphosphonates are analogs of pyrophosphate, but have a carbon rather than an oxygen atom. The P–C–P structure allows for many variations by changing the side chains on the carbon atom. Small changes in the side-chain structure can result in significant physicochemical, biologic, and therapeutic differences, and every phosphonate needs to be considered individually.

Bisphosphonates have a strong affinity for calcium phosphate and act exclusively in calcified tissues. The mechanism of bisphosphonate inhibition of bone resorption is unclear. It was postulated that it was physicochemical, but a direct cellular effect may be more important. Unlike calcitonin, which has an immediate effect on resorption, bisphosphonates take about 48 hours to block resorption.

Different bisphosphonates have significantly different antiresorptive potency, the potencies of etidronate, clodronate, tiludronate, pamidronate, alendronate, and risedronate being 1, 10, 10, 100, 1000, and 5000, respectively.

Oral absorption of most bisphosphonates is at best 1–10% of a given dose. They should never be given with milk products, food, or at the same time as Ca^{2+} supplements, as this further inhibits absorption by up to 90%.

Recent large prospective studies in osteoporosis have shown that at least three bisphosphonates (etidronate, alendronate, risedronate) increase bone density by 4–9% over the first 3 years of treatment and reduce vertebral fractures by approximately 50%. If given continuously, etidronate can cause osteomalacia. This can be avoided by intermittent administration over 2 weeks with periods of several weeks to 3 months off the drug. Bone biopsy studies up to 7 years after cyclic etidronate have not shown mineralization defects. Bisphosphonates such as alendronate and residronate do not have this effect and can be given continuously.

Alendronate 10 mg daily or risedronate 5 mg daily have shown significant improvement in bone density in 3-year prospective placebo controlled trials. Fracture reduction is 50% for a single further vertebra fracture and up to 90% reduction in multiple vertebral fractures.

Recently studies have supported taking bisphosphonates such as alendronate in larger doses (35–70 mg) orally once weekly. The advantage is that patients are less inconvenienced than in taking bisphosphonates daily and then waiting 30–120 minutes for a meal.

The most common clinical adverse effects of bisphosphonates are gastrointestinal (heartburn, nausea, abdominal pain). However short-term upper endoscopy studies show incidence of gastric ulcers to be 4–14%. Much less frequent but often mentioned is the concern of erosive esophagitis. It is recommended to take these medications with water and then to avoid lying supine for 30 minutes.

Bisphosphonates are slowly released from the skeleton and may have actions on bone tissue for years. There is some concern that this prolonged action may have an undetermined accumulative effect 10–20 years later. Most experts are reluctant to use bisphosphonates in very young people for this reason.

Selective estrogen receptor modulators

Selective estrogen receptor modulators (SERMs) are drugs that have tissue-specific effects in different areas: similar to estrogen

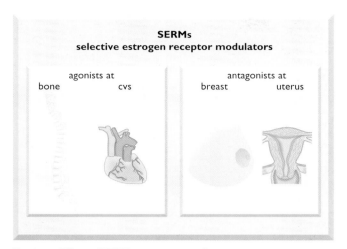

SERMs
selective estrogen receptor modulators

agonists at		antagonists at	
bone	cvs	breast	uterus

Fig. 20.8 Effect of SERMs on estrogen tissues.

in bone and cardiovascular system but not in other tissues such as breast and endometrium (Fig. 20.8). SERMs are believed to act competitively on the alpha estrogen receptor and may function as competitive inhibitors in tissues with alpha receptors. They bind to beta estrogen receptor complex and have agonist effects in tissues where these beta estrogen receptors predominate. The drug tamoxifen has been studied and shown to prevent the recurrence of breast cancer, likely due to antiestrogen effects. It also showed benefit in protecting against osteoporosis and cardiovascular disease, but has been found to increase the incidence of endometrial cancer. Raloxifene is a benzothiophene derivative that is also a SERM. The raloxifene-estrogen receptor complex binds to a unique area of DNA, different from the estrogen-response element, to produce estrogen-antagonist effects in some tissues and agonistic action in others. Long-term clinical trials of 3 years with raloxifene 60 mg/d have shown improvement of bone density of the hip (2–3%) and lumbar spine (3–4%). Fracture studies have shown reduction of new vertebral fractures by approximately 50%. In these same studies there was no evidence of increased risk of endometrial cancer and an improvement in the lipoprotein profile. These studies also show a highly significant reduced risk of breast cancer taking raloxifene compared to patients taking placebo.

Adverse effects include an increased risk of venous thromboembolic events similar to estrogen. Also, women noted a slight increase in hot flushes and leg cramps.

Other therapies

Calcium supplements have a small beneficial effect on preventing bone loss. Calcium, in the form of either dietary Ca^{2+} or oral Ca^{2+} supplements, is inexpensive and safe and should be recommended to all patients to slow bone loss. It is recommended that postmenopausal women have a Ca^{2+} intake of more than 1500 mg daily.

Vitamin D analogs facilitate Ca^{2+} absorption from the gastrointestinal tract and may have an effect on both bone resorption and formation. However, their efficacy in reducing the risk of fractures remains to be determined.

Tibolone is a synthetic C-19 steroid compound with weak hormonal properties. In animal studies tibolone has 1/50th the potency of ethinyl estradiol, 1/8th that of norethisterone, and much less androgenic potency. Tibolone does not stimulate the endometrium and at a daily dose of 2.5 mg reduces vasomotor menopausal symptoms. In clinical trials tibolone at 1.25 mg and 2.5 mg/day has had favorable effects in biochemical markers of bone resorption (urinary C telepeptides) and bone formation (serum osteocalcin). Short-term studies have shown increases in bone mass in the spine and prevention of bone loss in the forearm in postmenopausal women. Long-term studies are needed to demonstrate fracture reduction.

PTH hormone analogs used in cyclic doses are being evaluated in clinical trials. They stimulate osteoblasts and thereby result in increased bone formation. Although they can only be given by injection, they may be a highly effective treatment for increasing bone in the first few years after menopause.

Drugs for osteomalacia

Vitamin D is used to treat and prevent osteomalacia. Vitamin D-deficient osteomalacia responds well to vitamin D, 25-hydroxyvitamin D, 1α-hydroxyvitamin D, or 1,25-dihydroxyvitamin D. Patients with osteomalacia may also respond to sun exposure. In the US, dairy products are fortified with vitamin D and osteomalacia is relatively rare.

Drugs for Paget's disease

Drugs used to treat Paget's disease of bone include analgesics, calcitonin, and bisphosphonates.

SIMPLE ANALGESICS (aspirin, acetaminophen) are often used for pain due to Paget's disease. Nonsteroidal anti-inflammatory drugs (NSAIDs) also reduce the pain, but do not reduce the long-term complications.

CALCITONIN inhibits resorption and can reduce pain by a variety of potential mechanisms. Marine (salmon and eel) calcitonins are more potent than human calcitonin, but can be associated with the development of antibodies, resulting in resistance to treatment. The treatment needs to be given subcutaneously to achieve adequate blood concentrations to be effective in reducing bone pain. These high doses (50–100 IU/day) are commonly associated with adverse effects including cutaneous flushing and gastrointestinal effects.

BISPHOSPHONATES are an effective treatment of Paget's disease and currently are the mainstay of treatment. They reduce the turnover of both 'pagetic' and normal bone (see page 442). Large studies with alendronate and risedronate in Paget's disease have shown that they effectively reduce the activity of pagetic bone. The doses used are generally higher than the daily dose used for osteoporosis. Gastrointestinal intolerance is the main adverse effect and tends to be a larger clinical concern at the higher doses used in Paget's disease.

In patients that are not able to tolerate alendronate or risedronate because of GI adverse effects, then intravenous pamidronate infusions over a few hours can be effective.

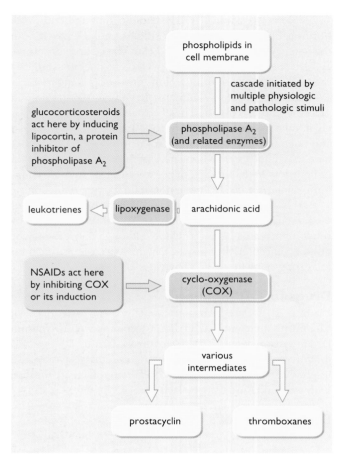

Fig. 20.9 **Arachidonic acid and its metabolites.** (NSAIDs, nonsteroidal anti-inflammatory drugs)

Drugs for osteoarthritis

Drug treatment of osteoarthritis includes analgesics and non-steroidal anti-inflammatory drugs.

ANALGESICS, particularly acetaminophen, often relieve the pain of osteoarthritis and are the preferred drug therapy. Data from large clinical studies show the effectiveness of analgesics in comparison to NSAIDs in osteoarthritis, showing they are as effective. Narcotic analgesics generally should only be used for short periods, intermittently, or for acute flares.

NSAIDs are frequently used to treat patients with osteoarthritis. They are effective analgesics and can also treat any associated inflammation, but have no major effect on the underlying process. NSAIDs inhibit cyclo-oxygenase, the enzyme that converts arachidonic acid to prostaglandins (Fig. 20.9). However, currently available NSAIDs have minimal effect on lipoxygenase, the enzyme that plays an important role in transforming arachidonic acid to leukotrienes. NSAIDs also have other immunoregulatory effects, but these are not thought to be clinically significant.

NSAIDs are associated with a high incidence of gastro-intestinal adverse effects. The most common GI adverse effects are nausea, vomiting, dyspepsia, abdominal pain and diarrhea.

Nonsteroidal anti-inflammatory drugs

	Maximum recommended doses	Approximate half-life (hours)
NSAIDs		
Diclofenac	150 mg/day	1–2
Etodolac	1200 mg/day	5–10
Fenoprofen	2400 mg/day	2
Ibuprofen	3200 mg/day	2
Indomethacin	150 mg/day	2
Ketoprofen	300 mg/day	5(?)
Ketorolac	40 mg/day	5
Meloxicam	15 mg/day	1–3
Nabumetone	2000 mg/day	22
Naproxen	1500 mg/day	15
Oxaprozin	1800 mg/day	24–48
Piroxicam	20 mg/day	30–60
Sulindac	400 mg/day	7–15
Tolmetin	1800 mg/day	7
Coxibs		
Celecoxib	400 mg/day	10
Rofecoxib	50 mg/day	15–20

Fig. 20.10 **Nonsteroidal anti-inflammatory drugs.**

Less common but more clinically significant are gastric ulcers and GI tract bleeding. Studies comparing different NSAIDs need to evaluate both efficacy and adverse effects at the dose used. Unfortunately many studies fail to compare equivalent doses of NSAIDs. Traditional NSAIDs include ibuprofen, naproxen, ketoprofen, flurbiprofen, indomethacin, ketorolac, nabumetone, oxaprozin, piroxicam, sulindac, and tolmetin (Fig. 20.10).

Recently it has been recognized that there are two different cyclo-oxygenase enzymes that convert arachidonic acid to prostaglandins. The cyclo-oxygenase (COX) enzyme exists in two isoforms. COX-1 produces a class of prostaglandins that are important in normal physiologic functions including gastrointestinal mucosal protection, and regulation of platelet function and renal cells. COX-2 enzymes are inducible in disease states and are responsible for pain and inflammation. The COX-2 isoform also has an important function in renal tissue.

> *Adverse effects of nonsteroidal anti-inflammatory drugs*
>
> - *Gastrointestinal tract: gastric irritation, peptic ulcers, bleeding, perforation*
> - *Kidney: decreased renal blood flow, decreased creatinine clearance, increased blood pressure, rarely interstitial nephritis or nephrotic syndrome*
> - *CNS: headaches, confusion, tinnitus, aseptic meningitis (rare)*
> - *Hematopoietic system: bleeding, inhibited platelet adhesion (irreversible effect with aspirin persisting 10–12 days)*

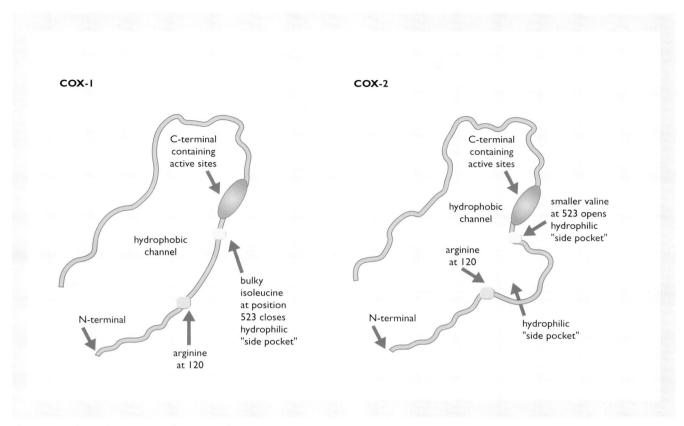

Fig. 20.11 Schematic structure of COX-1 and COX-2 enzyme.

The structures of COX-1 and COX-2 have considerable homology, but because of a number of amino acid differences, drugs have been developed recently with selectivity for the COX-2 isoform (Figs 20.11–20.13).

In recent years celecoxib and rofecoxib are two new drugs that have been designated as class 'coxibs', drugs that are highly selective for inhibiting the COX-2 enzyme (Fig. 20.14). Large clinical trials with these two drugs have demonstrated similar efficacy in reduction of pain as compared to traditional NSAIDs such as ibuprofen, naproxen, and diclofenac. Early clinical trials have shown an apparent reduction in gastrointestinal adverse effects such as gastric ulcers. Increasingly celecoxib and rofecoxib are used to treat osteoarthritis after a good trial of nonpharmacologic measures and adequate doses of acetaminophen (2–4 g/day) have been insufficient.

Adverse effects of coxibs include minor GI side effects, but more importantly it is recognized that coxibs lead to a similar risk of aggravating hypertension, renal insufficiency and congestive heart failure to that of traditional NSAIDs.

In one large trial comparing rofecoxib to naproxen it was observed that there was a higher number of myocardial infarctions in the rofecoxib treated patients. This observation can possibly be explained by the fact that coxibs do not have an antiplatelet effect. It is recommended that if patients are at high risk of cardiovascular events then aspirin or other antiplatelet agents need to be added.

Treatments for osteoarthritis

- Mechanical devices to relieve stress in the joint
- Analgesics
- Anti-inflammatory drugs
- Surgical intervention

Drugs for rheumatoid arthritis

Drugs used in the treatment of rheumatoid arthritis can be categorized on the basis of their therapeutic effects, primarily based on their symptomatic or anti-inflammatory actions compared with their capacity to induce a remission or delay progress of the disease and associated joint destruction. The treatment of patients with rheumatoid arthritis is based on an understanding of the biology and natural history of the disease coupled with the results of clinical trials. Joint damage often occurs soon after the development of the disease. This has led to interest in using powerful drugs with the potential to modify disease progress early in the course of rheumatoid arthritis (Fig. 20.15). Acetaminophen, aspirin, NSAIDs and new coxibs have been the initial treatment; however, these drugs provide symptomatic relief rather than prevent joint destruction. In addition, glucocorticoids have been used to suppress exacerbation of

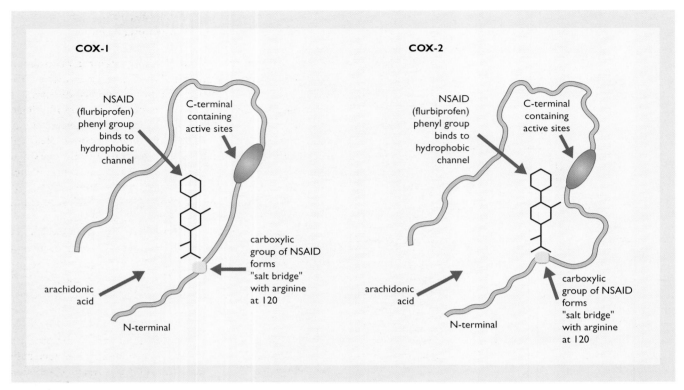

Fig. 20.12 Classical NSAIDs block both COX-1 and COX-2 enzyme.

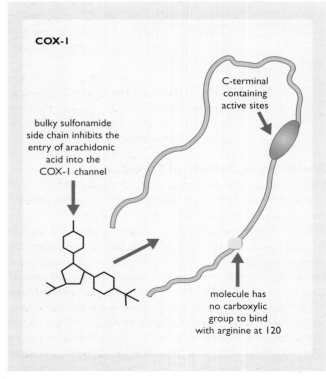

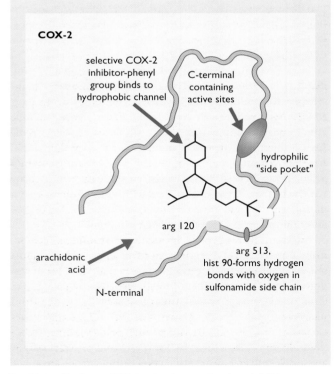

Fig. 20.13 Schematic demonstration of coxib or COX-2 selective inhibitor having less effect on COX-1 enzyme.

Fig. 20.14 Coxibs or COX-2 selective medications inhibit prostaglandin production from arachidonic acid.

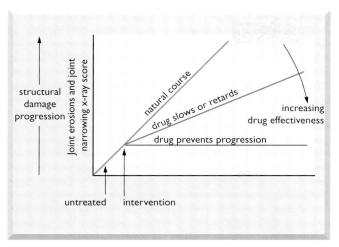

Fig. 20.15 Early intervention will reduce joint damage.

joint inflammation. On the other hand, there is now a large group of drugs with very different structures and actions that are termed disease modifying antirheumatic drugs (DMARDs) since they inhibit progression of the disease. Important examples of DMARDs include antimalarials, methotrexate, gold, D-penicillamine, sulfasalazine, azathioprine, cyclosporine, leflunomide, etanercept and infliximab. In recent years there is a growing trend to treat rheumatoid arthritis aggressively with early potent DMARDs.

■ *Anti-inflammatories inhibit the cyclo-oxygenase enzyme (COX-1 and COX-2) resulting in decreased prostaglandin synthesis.*
The three main classes are:
* Salicylates (acetylated and nonacetylated).
* NSAIDs.
* Coxibs.

ASPIRIN is an acetylated salicylate that is an effective and inexpensive anti-inflammatory drug. It is distinct from other NSAIDs because it is an irreversible cyclo-oxygenase inhibitor as it acetylates the active site in the cyclo-oxygenase enzyme. The salicylates have been commonly used to treat rheumatoid arthritis in the past and frequently continue to be used by patients and physicians because of their low cost. Enteric coated aspirin and nonacetylated salicylates are better tolerated than aspirin on the gastrointestinal tract. Typically doses are given 3–4 times a day, usually with meals to minimize adverse effects on the stomach. Absorption is usually rapid and complete but may be delayed with enteric coated preparations or sustained released preparations. Aspirin is converted to an active metabolite with a long half-life. At relatively low doses, aspirin is eliminated by typical first order kinetics. At higher doses salicylates exhibit zero order kinetics with a constant amount of active drug metabolized per unit time (see Chapter 4). Clinically this is important in that high doses of aspirin can be given twice daily if desired. However, at high doses when toxicity appears it may be of prolonged duration. The maximum concentration should be 200–300 mg/ml; it is not often

necessary to measure serum concentrations as adverse effects (GI, decreased hearing or tinnitus) usually limit doses.

NSAIDs have, in the last two decades, been the mainstay of treatment to reduce symptoms of rheumatoid arthritis but, like salicylates, they do not alter the progression of disease. The selection of a particular NSAID is often based on physician experience and knowledge of the correct dose and schedule. If symptoms are not controlled then the physician will suggest the dose be increased with caution to the maximal recommended dose (see Fig. 20.10). Failure of response after an adequate trial of a minimum of two weeks warrants consideration of a second NSAID. Various NSAIDs can be tried until the patient has adequate or optimal control of symptoms.

The addition of a second NSAID or a combination of an NSAID and salicylates is not recommended as this results in additive risk of GI adverse effects. Physicians need to educate patients about this risk as often over the counter (OTC) medications containing salicylates or NSAIDs are used without consultation.

COXIBS which are selective COX-2 enzyme inhibitors are increasingly used as the medication of choice to reduce pain and swelling in inflammatory arthritis. The doses used are often maximal recommended doses. As the dose of coxibs is increased, there is an increased risk of adverse effects including edema, increased blood pressure, and reversible renal insufficiency.

LOW-DOSE GLUCOCORTICOIDS The common adverse effects of glucocorticosteroids depend on the dose and duration of treatment. In addition to bruising and skin thinning, a major long-term concern is bone loss. The need to use the minimum dose of glucocorticosteroids should be emphasized to the patient.

Intra-articular glucocorticosteroids are highly effective, have fewer systemic adverse effects than oral treatment, and are used if only one or two joints are affected. The major risk is the potential to introduce joint infection and the possible risk of accelerating joint cartilage destruction.

■ *If active rheumatoid arthritis is not controlled with nonsteroidal anti-inflammatory drugs or low-dose glucocorticosteroids, other antirheumatic drugs should be considered*
Clinically useful agents include antimalarials, sulfasalazine, injectable gold salts or oral gold, penicillamine, methotrexate, azathioprine, cyclosporine, leflunomide, etanercept, and infliximab. Severe active rheumatoid arthritis is usually treated with one or more of these disease-modifying drugs in addition to an NSAID and/or low-dose prednisone. Second-line treatments may be considered for mild, moderate and severe disease. Antimalarials may be considered for mild disease or used in conjunction with a second agent for moderate or severe disease. Methotrexate is usually the initial treatment for moderate or severe disease. Sulfasalazine may be considered instead of methotrexate based on adverse effect concerns. The recent

447

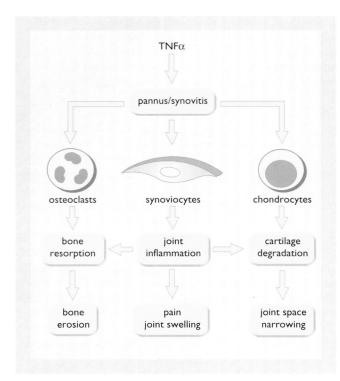

Fig. 20.16 Role of TNF-α in rheumatoid arthritis.

introduction of leflunomide has decreased the use of gold, azathioprine, penicillamine, and cyclosporine. The newer biological agents against TNF-α that include etanercept and infliximab are increasing considered if there is not good response to therapy with less expensive treatments, if adverse effects limit use of other treatments, or if rapid disease remission is considered a priority (Fig. 20.16).

ANTIMALARIALS Hydroxychloroquine and chloroquine are examples of antimalarials used to induce remission or help reduce inflammation in rheumatoid arthritis. However, although antimalarials are thought to be the least effective disease-modifying agents, they have the lowest toxicity. The dose should be maintained for a trial of 6 months to determine their effectiveness. Color vision and peripheral vision should be monitored from 6–12 months, depending on the dose.

The anti-inflammatory mechanism of action of chloroquine and hydroxychloroquine is unclear. There is some evidence that they interfere with a wide variety of leukocyte functions. They may inhibit IL-1 production by macrophages, lymphoproliferative responses, and cytotoxic responses of T lymphocytes. At high doses (which are now rarely used) they also have an inhibitory effect on DNA synthesis.

SULFASALAZINE Sulfasalazine is frequently used in the UK as the first-choice disease-modifying agent, but is used less commonly in the US. It is thought to be as effective as gold, but probably has fewer adverse effects. Sulfasalazine is a combination of 5-aminosalicylic acid linked covalently to sulfapyridine. It is poorly absorbed orally, but is cleaved to its active components by colonic bacteria. It is believed that sulfapyridine is absorbed systemically and is possibly responsible for its therapeutic effect. Sulfapyridine is eventually excreted in the urine. The mechanism of action is unclear, but there is some evidence that it reduces natural killer cell activity and alters other lymphocyte functions.

The adverse effects are primarily caused by sulfapyridine. Severe reactions include acute hemolysis in individuals with glucose-6-phosphate dehydrogenase deficiency, and rarely agranulocytosis. Rashes occur in 20–40% of patients. Other adverse effects include nausea, fever, and arthralgias.

GOLD Intramuscular gold salts have historically been the formulation for rheumatoid arthritis in the US. Adverse effects include dermatitis, proteinuria, and bone marrow suppression. Monitoring should include a complete blood count and urinalysis before each injection. Oral gold preparations have been available for a number of years; they appear to be less effective than injectable gold. There are two parenteral gold salts available, gold sodium thiomalate and aurothioglucose, and one oral form, namely auranofin.

Gold salts are taken up by reticuloendothelial cells (i.e. in the bone marrow, lymph nodes, liver, and spleen), and in these tissues they impair macrophage function and cytokine activity. Other possible mechanisms of action include inhibition of prostaglandin synthesis, interference with complement activation, cross-linking of collagen, and inhibition of lysosomal activity.

PENICILLAMINE Oral penicillamine, which is a chelator of heavy metals, has been a useful agent in the treatment of rheumatoid arthritis and its effectiveness is comparable to that of injectable gold. It is well absorbed orally (40–70%), although food will decrease its absorption. It is metabolized in the liver and is excreted in the urine and feces.

The mechanism of action of penicillamine in rheumatoid arthritis is unclear. It suppresses autoantibodies to IgM and has other effects on immune complexes. (The main disadvantage of penicillamine is its many and varied adverse effects.)

METHOTREXATE Methotrexate is a folic acid antagonist that is effective in the treatment of rheumatoid arthritis if given orally or parenterally in weekly doses of 5–25 mg/week (see Chapter 16). The mechanism of action is not clearly understood.

Adverse effects of penicillamine

- *Cutaneous: macular or papular rashes, urticaria, pemphigoid, lupus erythematosus, dermatomyositis*
- *Hematologic: fatal hematologic reactions are rare but include thrombocytopenia, leukopenia, agranulocytosis, aplastic anemia*
- *Renal: reversible proteinuria in the nephrotic range*
- *Unusual adverse effects: acute pneumonitis, myasthenia gravis (with long-term treatment)*
- *Less serious effects: nausea, other gastrointestinal effects, transient anosmia*

However, it decreases inflammatory cells in the synovium, and this may prevent erosion and joint damage. There is concern that methotrexate is associated with liver damage with cumulative doses over 1.5 g. In patients with certain coexisting diseases, including alcoholic liver disease, obesity, and diabetes mellitus, the increased risk of liver toxicity may warrant avoidance of the drug. Monthly complete blood counts and measurement of liver enzymes and serum albumin concentrations are recommended. If there are persistent elevations of liver enzyme concentrations, or hypoalbuminemia, methotrexate should be discontinued and appropriate investigations done to determine the cause of the liver disease. Investigations might include a liver biopsy to look for evidence of early fibrosis or cirrhosis, which warrants permanent discontinuation of methotrexate. Other common adverse effects of methotrexate include nausea, oral ulcers, hair loss, acute pneumonitis, (1−2%) and bone marrow suppression.

AZATHIOPRINE Azathioprine is an orally active purine analog that is cytotoxic to inflammatory cells (see Chapter 16). Treatment may be necessary for 3−6 months to be clinically effective. As azathioprine can cause serious adverse effects, including bone marrow suppression and liver toxicity, close monitoring is necessary.

LEFLUNOMIDE Leflunomide is an isoxazole immuno-modulatory agent which inhibits dihydro-orotate dehydro-genase, an enzyme important in the synthesis of pyrimidine. As a result of its action it has antiproliferative activity and an anti-inflammatory effect. Leflunomide has been shown to inhibit the *de novo* synthesis of uridine. After oral administration, leflunomide is metabolized to its active metabolite which is responsible for all of its activity. Leflunomide may be given orally in a loading dose of 100 mg/day for 3 days to attain rapid steady-state concentrations. Maintenance dosing would take an estimated 2 months to achieve this concentration. The active drug is extensively bound to albumin (>99%) in healthy subjects. The active metabolite is eliminated by further metabolism and excreted in the biliary system and urine.

Large clinical trials indicate that leflunomide is effective in decreasing joint swelling and tenderness over 12 months. Studies have compared leflunomide to placebo, methotrexate and sulfasalazine. Responses were evident by 1 month with stabilization of clinical response by 6 months. Leflunomide showed similar clinical improvement to both methotrexate and sulfasalazine.

The main concern about toxicity is elevation of liver enzymes. Increases of transaminase (ALT + AST) are usually less than twofold, and revert rapidly to normal with discontinuation of the drug. If elevation is twofold, but less than threefold, dose reduction can be considered. In the presence of persistent elevations greater than threefold, liver biopsy should be considered if treatment is continued. Methotrexate demonstrated pharmacologic interaction with leflunomide, and used together there is potential concern of increased hepatotoxicity. There is no apparent increased risk of malignancy but further long-term studies are needed. Women of childbearing potential

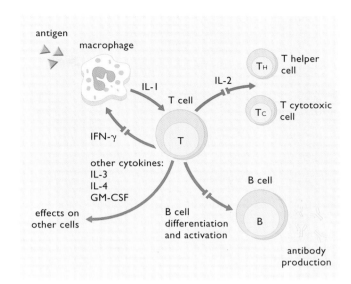

Fig. 20.17 Effects of cyclosporine on the immune system.
Cyclosporine acts at a number of levels, denoted by breaks in arrows. (GM-CSF, granulocyte/macrophage colony stimulating factor; IFN-γ, interferon-γ; IL-1, interleukin-1) (Adapted with permission of Novartis, from *Sandorama Special* 2, Sandoz Medical Publications, 1993.)

should use reliable contraception methods. Although there are no controlled studies in pregnant women, animal studies suggest there could be a risk of fetal death or teratogenic effects. In situations where rapid drug elimination is warranted, a drug elimination schedule using cholestyramine three times a day for several days can be employed, presumably efficacious on account of an enterohepatic circulation of the drug.

CYCLOSPORINE The importance of lymphocytes in the inflammatory response in rheumatoid arthritis provides a theoretic basis for trials of cyclosporine and its analogs in the treatment of rheumatoid arthritis, as cyclosporine is known to influence lymphocyte function (Fig. 20.17, see Chapter 16). There is recent evidence that, despite potential toxicity, cyclosporine may control resistant synovitis in selected patients.

ETANERCEPT Etanercept is a genetically engineered fusion protein of two identical chains of a recombinant human TNF receptor with the P 75 monomer fused to the Fc domain of human IgG1. This protein binds and inactivates TNF which has direct effects on synoviocytes, osteoclasts and chondrocytes (Fig. 20.16). It is many times more effective in binding TNF than natural, soluble TNF receptors. Sequestration of TNF by etanercept inhibits cell lysis.

Etanercept is given by a subcutaneous injection twice a week. The medial half-life is 115 hours (range 98−300).

There is little information on the effect of renal or hepatic impairment in the drug's literature. Etanercept can be used safely with salicylates, NSAIDs, analgesics, glucocorticoids and methotrexate.

Etanercept has shown reduced joint pain and swelling in a number of clinical trials as measured in terms of the American College of Rheumatology (ACR) criteria of response over a

12-month period. Studies compared to methotrexate show a similar reduction in joint space narrowing but etanercept has demonstrated less progression of erosion over a 2-year period.

Serious allergic adverse reactions are uncommon with etanercept. In clinical trials allergic reactions were reported in less than 2% of patients. However, local injection site reactions were common (37%) and included: erythema, itching, pain or swelling. These reactions were described as mild to moderate and generally did not lead to discontinuation of etanercept. In clinical trials that were placebo controlled, 4% of patients treated with etanercept had a serious adverse event compared to 5% of placebo treated patients. Patients developing an infection should be monitored carefully; and with a serious infection or sepsis, etanercept should be at least temporarily discontinued.

INFLIXIMAB Infliximab is a chimeric IgG1 anti-TNF-α monoclonal antibody. This molecule binds the soluble cytokine TNF-α and also binds membrane bound TNF-α, leading to loss in functioning TNF-α. It is a synthetic product made from both a human and mouse component. Clinical studies have shown the half-life to be 8–12 days, and it can be detected in the circulation for approximately 50 days. Treatment consists of an intravenous induction dose and maintenance doses every few weeks (4–8 weeks). Efficacy studies have shown that infliximab, if used with low-dose methotrexate in rheumatoid arthritis, will significantly prevent disease progression in the first 2 years of treatment. Radiographic studies have shown little progression in joint erosion and joint space loss, and in higher doses have demonstrated reversal of joint erosion.

The safety profile of infliximab has been demonstrated in a number of clinical trials and in over 50,000 treated patients. In 5% of patients early hypersensitivity reactions may be observed during or shortly after infusions. Reactions include hypotension, urticaria, and shortness of breath. Mild reactions usually can be treated with slowing of infusion rates and pre-medication with antihistamines. Serious infections have occasionally been observed in patients taking infliximab. Patients that have a new infection while taking infliximab should be monitored closely. Treatment should be held or discontinued with a serious infection or sepsis. Recently it has been recognized that patients may reactivate dormant TB infections. Some patients treated with infliximab develop antibodies against the drug, referred to as human anti-chimeric antibodies (HACA). The presence of HACA is associated with a higher rate of infusion reactions. Concomitant administration of methotrexate or azathioprine results in a lower incidence of these antibodies. Therefore, in rheumatoid arthritis, it is recommended patients be treated with concomitant oral weekly methotrexate.

ANAKINRA is a recombinant IL-1 receptor antagonist (IL-1ra). This protein results in a notable reduction of macrophages and lymphocytes in synovial tissue on biopsy. Anakinra is given by daily subcutaneous injections up to 150 mg/day. In large multinational clinical trials in rheumatoid arthritis, anakinra has been shown to be effective as monotherapy and in combination with methotrexate in reducing joint pain and swelling. Similarly to etanercept and infliximab, it also significantly reduces radiographic joint narrowing and erosions. Serious adverse effects are rare. Injection site reactions are common (over 40%) at higher daily doses (150 mg/day) but result in discontinuation in fewer than 5% of patients.

Drugs for crystal arthritis

Drugs used to treat acute crystal arthritis include nonsteroidal anti-inflammatory drugs, colchicine, and glucocorticosteroids.

NSAIDs are usually started at the first sign of an acute attack of crystal arthritis and continued until the signs of inflammation resolve. Most commonly indomethacin is started in a dose of 50 mg three times a day and then slowly tapered over 10–14 days. Other NSAIDs that may be effective include diclofenac, ketoprofen, tolmetin, naproxen, celecoxib and rofecoxib. Good clinical efficacy studies are lacking comparing different NSAIDs in acute crystal arthritis. The pharmacology and adverse effects of NSAIDs are discussed above.

COLCHICINE is effective in acute gout and other types of crystal arthritis. It penetrates inflammatory cells and migrates into the microtubular system where it has a direct inhibitory action on the microtubules so that the inflammatory cells lose their ability to respond. Colchicine disrupts the structure of tubulin which impairs the capacity of inflammatory cells to move to the site of inflammation (chemotaxis) and decreases phagocytosis. The maximal dose of 6 mg (10 tablets) over 24 hours should not be exceeded and then no further colchicine should be given for the next 7 days. Intravenous colchicine should be used rarely, if at all. Colchicine toxicity is increased with renal impairment.

Adverse effects include gastrointestinal toxicity, with nausea, vomiting, and diarrhea in up to 80% of individuals at higher doses. Colchicine has also been associated with bone marrow suppression, renal failure, disseminated intravascular coagulation, hypocalcemia, seizures, and death. Rarely, chronic use is associated with a neuromuscular disorder resembling polymyositis. An overdose of colchicine may be fatal, in part due to disruption of intestinal epithelial cells which ordinarily turn over rapidly.

GLUCOCORTICOSTEROIDS may be an effective treatment in acute crystal arthritis including gout when alternatives, including NSAIDs or colchicine, are not tolerated or are contraindicated. Options include oral prednisone or intravenous or intra-articular glucocorticosteroids (often useful when only one or two joints are involved). Intramuscular adrenocorticotropin hormone (ACTH, corticotropin) which also stimulates secretion of adrenal androgens in addition to glucocorticoids, offers no known advantage over glucocorticosteroids.

Regulating serum uric acid concentrations provides an effective method of preventing recurrent episodes of gout
Initial preventive management of gout should include weight and blood pressure control, a low purine diet (red meats or seafood) and avoidance of medications that can contribute to

hyperuricemia. Drugs such as low-dose aspirin, ethanol, thiazide diuretics, cyclosporine, and ethambutol can decrease urate clearance.

Increasing uric acid excretion

Blood uric acid concentration can be decreased by increasing clearance of uric acid (uricosuric agents) or by decreasing uric acid synthesis (xanthine oxidase inhibitors). Measurement of the amount of uric acid excreted in the urine should be done prior to using a uricosuric drug. Increasing uric acid clearance in patients overproducing uric acid could result in production of uric acid stones in the urine.

URICOSURIC AGENTS are the treatment of choice for individuals who:

- Have diminished renal clearance of uric acid (i.e. do not overproduce uric acid).
- Do not have renal stones or renal dysfunction, as increasing renal excretion of uric acid could transiently increase risk of worsening stone disease.
- Have had a previous reaction to a xanthine oxidase inhibitor.

Uricosuric agents such as probenecid and sulfinpyrazone block the reabsorption of filtered and secreted uric acid in the renal tubules leading to increased clearance of uric acid and a subsequent decrease in its plasma concentration (see Fig. 20.7). Probenecid blocks tubular reabsorption of organic anions such as uric acid and decreases serum urate levels. The most common adverse effects are rash and gastrointestinal upset. Sulfinpyrazone is a congener of phenylbutazone, and similarly blocks urate reabsorption in the renal tubule. The most frequently reported adverse effects of sulfinpyrazone are gastrointestinal, including nausea and aggravation of peptic ulcer disease. Blood dyscrasias including aplastic anemia have been reported but are rare.

Inhibition of uric acid synthesis

Allopurinol is a xanthine oxidase inhibitor; it competitively binds to the enzyme which controls the last two steps in purine metabolism, of both adenine and guanine, to uric acid.

ALLOPURINOL is useful for lowering uric acid in patients with:

- Uric acid overproduction.
- Nephrolithiasis.

Allopurinol is commonly preferred to a uricosuric agent by patients because of the ease of administration. The typical dose is 300 mg/day orally, but may need to be increased to 600–800 mg/day. The dose must be decreased if glomerular filtration is decreased, and should be less than 200 mg/day when the creatinine clearance is 10–20 ml/min (0.20–0.33 ml/s).

The adverse effects of allopurinol are not dose-related; the relatively minor problems include headaches, dyspepsia, and diarrhea. A pruritic rash develops in 5% of patients. Rarely, a syndrome of hypersensitivity to allopurinol may occur with fever, renal failure, and toxic epidermal necrolysis which can be life threatening and precludes the further use of this drug.

Allopurinol is readily absorbed, with 80% being bioavailable within 2–6 hours. It is oxidized by xanthine oxidase to oxypurinol. Both allopurinol and oxypurinol inhibit xanthine oxidase, thereby decreasing the conversion of hypoxanthine and xanthine to uric acid. The advantage is that these precursors of uric acid are readily soluble and excreted in the urine (see Fig. 20.6).

Drug interactions with allopurinol are common. For example, allopurinol interferes with:

- The metabolism of other purine analogs such as azathioprine and 6-mercaptopurine and the doses of these drugs need to be reduced by 25–50% when allopurinol is given.
- Hepatic inactivation of other drugs, including that of oral anticoagulants. Prothrombin activity must be closely monitored if allopurinol is given, and the dose of oral anticoagulant may need adjusting.

Drugs for systemic lupus erythematosus

Treatment of systemic lupus erythematosus involves anti-inflammatory and immunosuppressive drugs.

Classification of drugs used for systemic lupus erythematosus	
Mild disease	Nonsteroidal anti-inflammatory drugs Glucocorticosteroids (low-dose prednisone) Antimalarials Methotrexate
Severe disease	Glucocorticosteroids (high-dose prednisone, methylprednisolone) Azathioprine Alkylating agents (cyclophosphamide)
Investigational	Cyclosporine Immune globulin

Fig. 20.18 Classification of drugs used for systemic lupus erythematosus.

GLUCOCORTICOSTEROIDS The symptoms and signs of acute inflammation in the skin and joints in SLE are readily treated with glucocorticosteroids (Fig. 20.18). Options include:

- Topical preparations for inflammatory rashes.
- Low-dose oral therapy for mild disease.
- Higher-dose oral or pulse intravenous infusions for severe and life-threatening disease.

The mechanism of action of glucocorticosteroids is unclear. They have a direct effect on the bone marrow cells, resulting in demargination of circulating neutrophils (neutrophilia) and, at the same time, leukopenia, with fewer circulating eosinophils and monocytes. At high doses, glucocorticosteroids inhibit cytokine release and action. They have minimal effect on lymphokine production and cytotoxic, helper, and suppressor activity of T cells. High-dose glucocorticosteroids may act by inducing the synthesis of a peptide that inhibits phospholipase A_2, which controls both prostaglandin and leukotriene production (see Chapter 16).

The dose is chosen to minimize the risk of adverse effects yet provide adequate drug to suppress the inflammatory

451

response. Oral prednisone or prednisolone is used in preference to other longer-acting oral drugs such as dexamethasone and is usually given in a single morning dose. Prednisone is available in convenient doses (5 mg tablets) to facilitate dose increases or reductions. Adverse effects of glucocorticosteroids include skin thinning and bruising, central obesity, muscle wasting, hypertension, glucose intolerance, and osteoporosis.

ANTIMALARIALS are particularly effective treatment for cutaneous lesions and inflammatory arthritis in patients with SLE. Once they have been started and have produced clinical benefit, their discontinuation may result in a recurrence of disease manifestations. Antimalarial drugs include hydroxychloroquine, quinacrine, and chloroquine; their pharmacology is discussed in Chapter 11. The first two drugs are used extensively in many countries, while chloroquine is a less expensive but less well tested alternative. The relative safety of antimalarials makes them attractive drugs for early intervention. Common adverse effects include nonspecific symptoms, cutaneous rashes, and gastrointestinal complaints. Less frequently there are CNS reactions. Retinal toxicity is the major clinical concern, but is rarely seen at low doses of antimalarials. Visual field and color vision should be tested at baseline and then every 6 months or as recommended by an ophthalmologist.

AZATHIOPRINE (see Chapter 16) is widely used for many of the manifestations of SLE including renal disease to reduce requirements for glucocorticosteroids. Azathioprine reduces inflammation in lupus nephritis and improves renal function. However, it has potentially major adverse effects, including bone marrow suppression. Significant hepatic toxicity has been observed, but is usually reversible if the medication is discontinued. It is not clear whether azathioprine increases the risk of malignancy, particularly hematopoietic and lymphoreticular malignancy.

ALKYLATING AGENTS are the most effective agents after glucocorticosteroids for treating life-threatening SLE (Fig. 20.19). They inhibit the activation and division of inflammatory cells (see Chapter 16). Cyclophosphamide is usually added to high-dose glucocorticosteroids to treat severe SLE that is either life threatening or does not respond to glucocorticosteroids and azathioprine. The dose of glucocorticosteroid should be reduced slowly following clinical improvement. Cyclophosphamide is a more effective treatment of diffuse lupus nephritis than other treatments.

Cyclophosphamide has significant adverse effects (see Chapter 16).

Drugs for seronegative arthritis

NONSTEROIDAL ANTI-INFLAMMATORY DRUGS are the most widely used drugs for treating the inflammation of seronegative spondyloarthropathies.

The most effective NSAIDs including indomethacin, diclofenac, naproxen, tolmetin, celecoxib, and rofecoxib are often recommended first. Other NSAIDs may be effective and can be tried if the above are not effective or are associated with

Drugs affecting inflammation and the immune system		
	Disease indication	**Adverse effects**
Antimalarials	RA, SLE	Retinopathy
Gold salts	RA	Dermatitis GI symptoms Proteinuria
Penicillamine	RA, scleroderma	Dermatitis GI symptoms Proteinuria
Methotrexate	RA, psoriasis Polymyositis Dermatomyositis SLE	Myelosuppression Pneumonitis Ulcerations Hepatotoxicity
Sulfasalazine	RA Inflammatory bowel disease	Dermatitis GI symptoms Hepatitis
Azathioprine	RA, SLE Polymyositis Transplantation	Myelosuppression GI symptoms Hepatotoxicity
Cyclophosphamide	Vasculitis SLE	Myelosuppression Alopecia GI symptoms Infertility Hemorrhagic cystitis Malignancy
Cyclosporine	RA Transplantation SLE Psoriasis Uveitis	Hypertension Renal toxicity Neurotoxicity Hepatotoxicity
Glucocorticosteroids	RA SLE Transplantation Vasculitis Connective tissue disease	Cushing's syndrome Osteoporosis Cataracts Ulcers
Leflunomide	RA	Myelosuppression GI symptoms Liver
Etanercept	RA	Rash Infection
Infliximab	RA	Rash Infection Hypersensitivity reaction
Anakinra	RA	Injection site reaction

Fig. 20.19 Drugs affecting inflammation and the immune system. (GI, gastrointestinal; RA, rheumatoid arthritis; SLE, systemic lupus erythematosus)

adverse effects. Although various clinical trials suggest that certain NSAIDs are more effective than others, clinical experience and familiarity with doses is probably more important than selecting any one NSAID.

GLUCOCORTICOSTEROIDS do not affect the long-term outcome of seronegative spondyloarthropathies, but might be beneficial in low doses to control symptoms. Sulfasalazine, which is frequently used to treat rheumatoid arthritis, may control the peripheral arthritis in this disease. All drugs used to treat rheumatoid arthritis can be used to treat psoriatic arthritis.

■ *Some common drugs have adverse effects on the musculoskeletal system*

Low-dose aspirin (less than 2 g/day) can raise serum uric acid levels by interfering with the excretion of uric acid in the renal tubule. These doses of aspirin are commonly used to prevent cardiovascular events including myocardial infarct and stroke. Considerations for treatment would include switching to sulfinpyrazone or adding allopurinol if acute attacks are severe or frequent.

Hydralazine has been commonly used to treat hypertension in the past and may be used to treat select patients with congestive heart failure. In up to 50% of patients antinuclear antibodies (ANA) may be found in the blood of patients taking hydralazine long term. Individuals who are slow acetylators (see Chapter 4) or take relatively large doses are more likely to develop an SLE-like syndrome that includes rash, arthralgia, and fever. With the development of this syndrome there should be rapid withdrawal of the drug. Usually symptoms resolve but they may require treatment with steroids and sometimes the symptoms will be prolonged.

Glucocorticoids are commonly used to treat both musculoskeletal and non-musculoskeletal immune disorders. Unfortunately, they cause osteoporosis and steroid myopathy. The mechanism of glucocorticoid osteoporosis is multifactorial including: direct inhibition of osteoblasts, increased calcium urinary excretion, and decreased GI calcium absorption. Preventative measures include minimizing the dose and duration of glucocorticoid use, encouraging appropriate calcium and vitamin D supplementation, weight bearing exercises and consideration of drugs used in the treatment of osteoporosis. The best studied medications to prevent glucocorticoid-induced osteoporosis are alendronate and risedronate (see Osteoporosis, page 437).

Glucocorticoids may induce muscle atrophy and weakness. If this complication develops, an exercise program may improve general function but dose reduction is the only treatment that will provide long-term benefit.

The statins are synthetic lipid-lowering agents that may be associated with both myalgias and myositis. In clinical studies elevations of CPK have been reported in up to 5% of patients. Rarely patients develop an acute myopathy with severe proximal muscle weakness and marked elevations of CPK. The risk of myopathy is increased with concomitant use of fibrate and other lipid-lowering treatments including niacin. Patients starting therapy should be advised of this risk and should

Organisms causing septic arthritis	
Non-gonococcal	Gram-positive (65–85%) Gram-negative bacilli (10–15%) Mixed aerobic and anaerobic (5%) Mycobacteria and fungi (<5%)
Neisseria gonorrhoeae	

Fig. 20.20 Organisms causing septic arthritis.

promptly report unexplained muscle pain, tenderness or weakness. Usually symptoms remit with prompt withdrawal of the drug.

Musculoskeletal infections
Septic arthritis

Septic arthritis is characterized by fever, pain, swelling, and a reduced joint range. In sexually active individuals there should be a high index of suspicion for *Neisseria gonorrhoeae*. Otherwise, most cases are caused by Gram-positive organisms (*Staphylococcus aureus* and streptococci, Fig. 20.20). Important host factors include:

- Underlying joint disease (rheumatoid arthritis, osteoarthritis).
- Chronic illnesses (diabetes mellitus, chronic renal failure).
- Alcohol abuse.
- Drugs (glucocorticosteroids, cytotoxics, intravenous drug abuse).
- Extra-articular infections (urinary tract, skin).

Most joint infections are single, but 20% are polyarticular.

Early effective management is important to prevent muscle contractures and, more importantly, joint destruction. If infection is suspected, the joint should be promptly aspirated and the fluid analyzed for manifestations of infection. Treatment involves the use of appropriate antibiotics and an effective method of drainage (e.g. arthroscopy, arthrotomy, repeated needle aspiration). Initial selection should be based on the patient's age and any associated diseases, and the Gram stain. The regimen can be adjusted at 24–48 hours when the culture results are available, and later modified when the sensitivities are known. Suggested initial antibiotic regimens (see Chapter 23) include:

- Intravenous methicillin or cloxacillin with or without an intravenous aminoglycoside.
- Intravenous imipenen.
- Intravenous ceftriaxone.

Parenteral antibiotics produce excellent synovial and intra-articular antibiotic concentrations. Intra-articular antibiotics are not needed.

The duration of therapy is determined by the clinical response, the effectiveness of drainage, and the organism. Streptococcal infection can usually be effectively treated with 2 weeks of intravenous therapy followed by 2–4 weeks of oral high-dose treatment. Staphylococcal infections may require longer treatment. Convincing clinical studies comparing short versus long (i.e. 2–6 weeks) periods of intravenous antibiotic therapy are not available.

453

Osteomyelitis

Bacteria can invade bone in a variety of ways: as a result of direct trauma, surgery, or extension from a soft tissue infection, and in the blood. The resulting osteomyelitis may present acutely, subacutely, or chronically with bone pain, fever, and leukocytosis. Patients with sickle cell disease are 100 times more likely to present with osteomyelitis than the general population. Bone destruction with periosteal elevation may be seen radiographically. Abscess and sinus formation may occur. A bone scan is the most commonly used primary diagnostic tool for evaluating osteomyelitis in both adults and children. The diagnosis is often made late clinically so it is important to recognize early imaging findings.

Treatment includes:

- Splinting to prevent fractures.
- Consideration of surgical drainage.
- Intravenous antibiotics.

Prosthetic joint infections

Prosthetic joint infections are increasingly common, but are difficult to diagnose and treat. Over 100,000 total hip replacements are carried out each year in the US and one of the main clinical concerns is the risk of bacterial infection of the prosthetic implant. Such an infection may occur early postoperatively (i.e. within a year) or be a late complication and result from a bacteremia. Skin contaminants are isolated from early postoperative infection (i.e. *Staphylococcus epidermidis, S. aureus,* anaerobes). Late infections are usually due to staphylococci, streptococci and Gram-negative bacilli. There is increasing concern about the emergence of methicillin-resistant *S. aureus* (MRSA).

■ *All bacteriologically confirmed infections should be treated with high-dose intravenous antibiotics, appropriate surgical debridement, and reimplantation*

Six weeks of high-dose intravenous antibiotics alone results in low rates of cure (i.e. less than 20%). Adding antibiotic to the cement at the time of revision surgery may be beneficial. Results are further improved by carrying out a two-stage revision procedure, with a temporary prosthesis for 6 weeks to several months and then permanent reimplantation.

Prophylactic perioperative antistaphylococcal antibiotics are believed to prevent infection if used in a short course starting immediately before surgery and continuing 24–72 hours after surgery. In addition, antibiotics are often used empirically in the first 3–6 months following joint replacement to prevent prosthetic joint infection with procedures such as dental surgery and genitourinary manipulation, but this topic needs further study.

FURTHER READING

Choy EH, Panayi GS. Cytokine pathways and joint inflammation in rheumatoid arthritis. *N Engl J Med* 2001; **344(12)**: 907–916.

Fung HB, Kirschenbaum HL. Selective cyclooxygenase-2 inhibitors for the treatment of arthritis. *Clin Ther* 1999; **21(7)**: 1131–1157.

Kleerekoper M, Schein JR. Comparative safety of bone remodeling agents with a focus on osteoporosis therapies. *J Clin Pharmacol* 2001; **41(3)**: 239–250.

O'Dell JR. How is it best to treat early rheumatoid arthritis patients? *Baillieres Best Pract Res Clin Rheumatol* 2001; **15(1)**: 125–137.

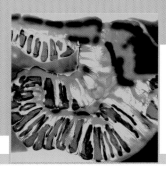

Chapter 21

Drugs and the Gastrointestinal System

PHYSIOLOGY OF THE GASTROINTESTINAL SYSTEM

The alimentary tract is a smooth muscle tube lined internally by an epithelium that varies in structure depending on its functions. Functions of the alimentary tract include:

- Food ingestion.
- Breaking food up into small portions.
- Converting large food molecules into smaller molecules (amino acids, small peptides, carbohydrates, sugars, and lipids) by enzymes and other secretions so that they can be absorbed into the blood and lymph circulation. Most of the small molecules are then transported to the liver where they are used as building blocks for essential proteins, carbohydrates, and lipids.
- Excretion of undigested and previously digested matter as waste products.
- Water and electrolyte balance.
- Regulation of hormone secretion in various segments of the alimentary tract to enable controlled digestion and excretion.

■ The esophagus transports undigested fragmented food from the pharynx to the stomach where digestion begins

The esophagus is about 25 cm long and opens into the stomach at the esophagogastric junction. The stomach is a dilated portion of the digestive tract where the fragmented food is retained while it is macerated and partially digested.

The gastric epithelium secretes hydrochloric acid, digestive enzymes, and mucus. It also contains hormone-secreting cells. The acid and digestive enzymes convert food into a thick semi-liquid paste (chyme), while mucus lubricates ingested food and protects the stomach from the corrosive effects of the acid and enzymes.

■ The liver is a metabolic, secretory, and immunologic organ

The liver's metabolic role includes:

- Anabolism and catabolism of many endogenous substances, including glycogen and hemoglobin.
- Metabolism of many drugs and foods.

The metabolic and secretory systems metabolize, transport, or secrete endogenous and exogenous chemicals, and can be modified by chemicals, including drugs. The Kupffer cells of the liver play an important role in immune responses.

The liver is also part of the biliary tract. It manufactures and secretes bile, which is collected by the bile ducts and stored in

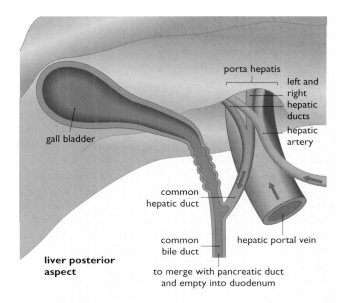

Fig. 21.1 The liver has two blood supplies. The liver is supplied by the systemic circulation via the hepatic artery to serve the nutritional needs of the hepatic cells. It is also supplied by the portal vein, which delivers blood that has already perfused the upper intestine.

the gallbladder, from where it is discharged into the duodenum to aid fat digestion.

The liver has two blood supplies (Fig. 21.1). Blood from these supplies then flows into the hepatic venous system and hepatic vein.

■ The liver is exposed to drugs that enter the circulation from any site of administration

All substances, including drugs, absorbed from the upper intestine are carried immediately to the liver by the portal vein, while substances in the systemic circulation can reach the liver through the hepatic artery. Drugs given orally can therefore have a double exposure to the liver via the portal vein and the systemic circulation. Drugs can also be secreted into the bile, which is excreted via the bile duct into the lumen of the duodenum. The drug can then be reabsorbed and reach the liver again via the portal vein. This phenomenon is called enterohepatic circulation of drugs. (See Chapter 4 for further details.)

■ *The large intestine comprises the cecum, the ascending, transverse, and descending and sigmoid colon, and the rectum*

The main function of the large intestine is to convert the liquid small intestinal contents to solid indigestible waste material (feces) by extensive reabsorption of water and soluble salts from the bowel contents. Mucin is required to lubricate the bowel contents as they pass along the bowel.

PATHOPHYSIOLOGY AND DISEASES OF THE GASTROINTESTINAL SYSTEM

Peptic ulcer disease

Peptic ulcer disease results when the normal balance of factors that damage or protect the gastrointestinal mucosal barrier is disturbed. Pathologic factors that are associated with peptic ulcer disease are shown in Fig. 21.2. Other acknowledged risk factors for peptic ulcer disease are genetic predisposition, smoking and stress. *Helicobacter pylori* plays a significant role in the pathogenesis of gastritis, peptic ulcer disease, and gastric cancer.

Peptic ulcer disease is chronic, recurs, and affects at least 10% of the population in developed countries. A considerably higher percentage of the population suffers from dyspeptic symptoms without having ulcers (nonulcer dyspepsia). Of the adult population worldwide, 50–80% is infected with *H. pylori*, which, if untreated, can persist for decades. However no more than 10–20% of infected people develop peptic ulcer disease

Causes of damage to the gastrointestinal mucosal barrier and treatment

Cause of damage	Treatment
Helicobacter pylori infection	Antibiotics plus PPI or H$_2$ antagonists
Increased acid	Reduced by PPI, H$_2$ antagonists, or prostaglandins
Reduced thickness of mucus layer	Heal ulcer, prostaglandins and sucralfate stimulate mucus secretion
Reduced bicarbonate	Prostaglandins and sucralfate stimulate
Increase in type I pepsin	Increase stomach pH, bind to Al^{3+} salts or sucralfate
Decreased mucosal blood flow	Increase prostaglandins, sucralfate increases blood flow
NSAID-induced ulcer erosion potential	NSAID withdrawal or COX-2 selective NSAID or substitute with an NSAID with a low erosion potential combined with a prostaglandin analog

Fig. 21.2 Causes of damage to the gastrointestinal mucosal barrier and treatment. (NSAID, nonsteroidal anti-inflammatory drug; PPI, proton pump inhibitor)

or neoplasia, although many more may have low-grade gastritis. An essential point is that almost all patients with gastritis and duodenal ulceration, and 80–90% of patients with gastric ulcers, have an *H. pylori* infection in their gastric antrum.

Risk factors for acquiring *H. pylori* infection are under investigation. There appears to be a positive relationship with better economic conditions in childhood, but others report a positive relationship with crowded living conditions and growing up in rural areas. The methods of transmission are uncertain: contact with animals and contaminated sewage are possibilities.

The additional factors that cause infected individuals to develop clinical disease may involve the relative virulence of different strains of *H. pylori*, genetic differences in the host, age at which the host acquired the infection, and compounding environmental factors. The importance of each of these factors is poorly understood. The virulent strains of *H. pylori* causing cytotoxicity and peptic ulcer are associated with the gene termed vacA, but this relationship is far from absolute.

■ *Treatment of peptic ulcer disease should include eradication of* H. pylori

To reduce the incidence of recurrence of peptic ulcer associated with *H. pylori* infection, treatment regimens must include eradication of *H. pylori*, and many practitioners argue that such a regimen should be included for all cases of peptic ulcer disease. Recurrence of duodenal ulceration, after healing, can be as high as 80% within 1 year when *H. pylori* eradication is not part of the treatment, but less than 5% when *H. pylori* is eradicated. If *H. pylori* eradication is not part of the treatment, recurrence can be reduced by maintenance doses of acid secretion inhibitors. The best practice, now and in the future, for eradication of *H. pylori* is still an evolving issue, partly because of the development of resistance to the main antibiotics used. Currently a variety of regimes that constitute 'triple therapy' are utilized as 'best' therapy, ensuring a relatively simple regime and adequate adherence. Other 'dual therapy' regimes with a proton pump inhibitor (PPI) plus one antibiotic give erratic success rates and are no longer recommended. The United States Food and Drug Administration recommends metronidazole or amoxicillin plus clarithromycin plus a PPI given twice daily for 14 days. The choice of metronidazole or amoxicillin may depend on the local patterns of *H. pylori* resistance. Eradication rates of greater than 90% should be expected with the best triple regimes. Some European studies have shown eradication rates of more than 90% with 7-day dosing using 'triple regimes' but other studies have required 14 days of therapy to achieve these levels of eradication. There appears to be little to choose between particular PPIs on the grounds of efficacy or side effects.

In resistant cases, however, a PPI has also been used as part of 'quadruple therapy' with both amoxicillin and clarithromicin plus metronidazole. There is little doubt that a PPI improves the ability of antibiotics to eradicate *H. pylori*, perhaps by increasing gastric pH, and improving antibiotic stability and absorption.

Combinations of the H$_2$ receptor antagonist ranitidine with bismuth (see below) are also available and there have been

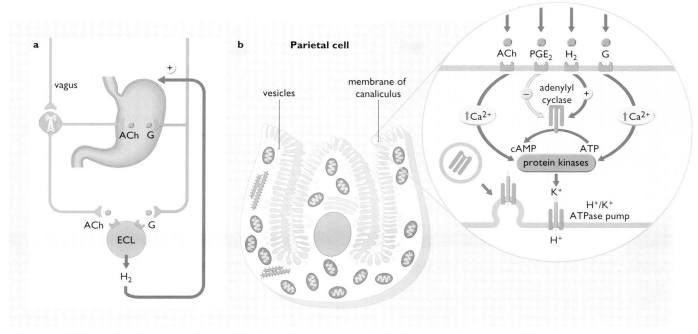

Fig. 21.3 Acid secretion from the parietal cell. (a) Gastrin (G) and acetylcholine (Ach) stimulate the parietal cell directly to increase acid secretion, and also stimulate the enterochromaffin-like (ECL) cells to secrete histamine, which then acts upon the H_2 receptors of the parietal cell (b). The H^+/K^+ ATPase pump is in tuberovesicles, which fuse with the canalicular membrane upon stimulation and release H^+ into the lumen; Cl^- is transported into the lumen by a separate carrier system. The parietal cell also has receptors for prostaglandin (PG) E_2 and their stimulation inhibits acid secretion.

reports of good success rates when this formulation is given with clarithromycin.

General drawbacks with these regimes are:

- Problems with compliance.
- The rapid development of resistance, particularly to metronidazole.
- An adverse response to alcohol with metronidazole.
- Adherence problems particularly if a quadruple regime is used.

Gastric acid secretion inhibitors

Gastric acid secretion depends on the activation of gastrin, H_2, and muscarinic type 3 (M_3) receptors. Parietal cells (Fig. 21.3) are located in the oxyntic glands of the gastric mucosa. Their unique acid pump is contained within vesicles in the cytosol. Cell stimulation leads to insertion of these vesicle membranes into the canalicular membranes, thereby enabling acid secretion. During stimulation, vesicles are depleted, but their number is restored when there is no acid secretion. Acid secretion depends on the activation of three main receptors on the basolateral membrane of the parietal cell:

- Gastrin receptors, which respond to gastrin secreted from the G cells in the antrum.
- H_2 receptors, which respond to histamine secreted from the enterochromaffin-like (ECL) cells that lie close to the parietal cell.
- M_3 receptors on the parietal cell, which respond to acetylcholine released from neurons innervating the parietal cell. These enteric neurons also synapse at interneurons in which the muscarinic receptor appears to be an M_1 subtype.

Muscarinic and gastrin receptors are found on ECL cells as well as on parietal cells and ECL receptor stimulation leads to increased histamine release. Stimulation of the different parietal cell receptors acts through various signal transduction mechanisms (see Fig. 21.3) to stimulate acid secretion. Histamine stimulates the adenylyl cyclase system, while gastrin and acetylcholine both increase intracellular Ca^{2+}, but by different mechanisms.

▣ *Proton pump inhibitors and H_2 receptor antagonists inhibit acid secretion by the parietal cell*

PROTON PUMP INHIBITORS Peptic ulcers treated with gastric acid inhibitors heal rapidly, but recurrence is common unless *H. pylori* is eliminated. The first proton pump inhibitor marketed was omeprazole and a range of structurally modified benzimidazoles are now marketed (Fig. 21.4). They inhibit the H^+/K^+-dependent ATPase proton pump that controls H^+ secretion from the parietal cell into the secretory canaliculi (see Fig. 21.3). They inhibit acid secretion by more than 90% and frequently produce achlorhydria. PPIs have limited *H. pylori*-suppressing activity, but when given alone do not effectively eradicate *H. pylori*. PPIs have been shown conclusively to be more effective at healing ulcers than the H_2 receptor antagonist famotidine, which inhibits acid secretion by about 60%. PPIs inhibit the final common point (the Na^+/K^+ ATPase pump) in acid secretion induced by the histamine, gastrin and acetylcholine dependent pathways (90% inhibition). With H_2 antagonists the acetylcholine and gastrin pathways are not inhibited.

PPIs are inactive pro-drugs and are converted at acid pH in the canaliculi to sulfenamide, which combines covalently with

457

Proton pump inhibitors (PPIs)

Drug	Bioavailability (%)	Elimination	Half-life (hours)	Comments
Omeprazole	45	Hepatic metabolism	0.5–1	Differences between the PPIs in clinical effectiveness are small but limited data show a higher healing rate with esomeprazole
				Esomeprazole is available in Sweden and is a single isomer of omeprazole
Lansoprazole	85	Hepatic metabolism	<2	Pantoprazole does not inhibit P-450 enzymes while other PPIs do but to a variable extent
				PPIs are metabolized in part by cytochrome (CYP)2C19, a P-450 isoform that is subject to genetic polymorphism. However, the importance of genetically related control of PPI metabolism to clinical management is not yet clear
Pantoprazole	77	Hepatic metabolism	1	Duration of action of PPIs far outlasts their half-lifes but rabeprazole has a shorter duration of action as its action on the proton pump is partially reversible
Rabeprazole	~52	Hepatic metabolism	1–2	The AUC of all drugs increases in liver disease but dosage adjustment is not necessary
				Esomeprazole is the first to be licensed for 'on-demand' treatment of esophageal reflux disease where patients will take it as necessary to control symptoms.
Esomeprazole	64–90		1.5	All PPIs have some ability to inhibit *Helicobacter pylori in vitro*

Fig. 21.4 Proton pump inhibitors. (AUC, area under curve)

SH groups on the H^+/K^+ ATPase. They are given as enteric-coated and slow-release formulations to prevent sulfenamide formation in the stomach lumen. Sulfenamide, unlike omeprazole, does not readily cross biologic membranes, and therefore it accumulates in the canaliculi of parietal cells; because of this, and the unique nature of the pump, PPIs have little action on ion pumps elsewhere in the body. PPIs have a considerably longer duration of action than H_2 antagonists and are given once daily. Their long duration of action is due to their irreversible inhibition of the H^+/K^+ ATPase pump. Rabeprazole however does have a shorter duration of action than other PPIs (Fig. 21.4).

The danger of long-term acid suppression with a PPI has been debated. Atrophic changes have been reported in the gastric corpus after 36 months of treatment in some patients with gastroesophageal reflux disease (GERD), especially if gastritis was present before PPI administration. In such a situation there was also a marked increase in ECL cell hyperplasia. However, with more than 10 year's experience of the use of PPIs, their long-term safety appears more secure.

H_2 **RECEPTOR ANTAGONISTS** including cimetidine, ranitidine, famotidine, and nizatidine, competitively block histamine-induced acid release by the parietal cell (Fig. 21.5). Suppression

H_2 receptor antagonists used in peptic ulcer disease

Drug	Bioavailability (%)	Elimination	Half-life (hours)	Comment
Cimetidine	60–70	Renal	1–3	Inhibits P-450 enzymes
Ranitidine	50	Renal/liver	2–3	No effect on P-450 enzymes
Famotidine	40–50	Renal/biliary	3–4	No effect on P-450 enzymes
Nizatidine	95	Renal	1.5	No effect on P-450 enzymes
Ranitidine bismuth citrate	(ranitidine 50; bismuth—)	Renal/liver	2–3	Dissociates in gastric fluid to ranitidine and bismuth; bismuth has negligible absorption, slow renal excretion

Fig. 21.5 H_2 receptor antagonists used in peptic ulcer disease.

Antiulcer drugs and drugs used for GERD

- *Overall, proton pump inhibitors (PPIs) and H₂ antagonists have a low incidence of adverse effects*
- *Cimetidine and omeprazole, but not ranitidine, nizatidine, or famotidine, inhibit cytochrome P-450 liver enzymes. Cimetidine and omeprazole reduce the metabolism of drugs such as warfarin, theophylline, phenytoin, and 'ecstasy'*
- *H₂ antagonists rarely cause gynecomastia*
- *PPIs cause hypergastrinemia*
- *PPIs increase the risk for Campylobacter infection tenfold in patients over 45 years of age*
- *Sucralfate interacts with tetracyclines, cimetidine, digoxin, and phenytoin*
- *Bismuth produces a black tongue and stools*

Drugs for peptic ulcer and gastroesophageal reflux disease (GERD)

- Acid suppression enhances *Helicobacter pylori* eradication by antibiotics
- *H. pylori* eradication reduces ulcer recurrence rates
- Proton pump inhibitors (PPIs) suppress acid secretion more than H₂ antagonists
- Sucralfate and bismuth can increase prostaglandin, mucus and bicarbonate secretion and reduce the number of *H. pylori*
- Omeprazole is the drug of choice for GERD

of acid secretion is less than with a PPI because only the histamine component is inhibited. Although this is sufficient to result in ulcer healing in a high percentage of patients, they are uniformly less effective than PPI. Night-time administration is particularly important for ulcer healing because acid buffering is less at night. The dosage is either twice daily, or a single dose at night for 4–8 weeks. Cimetidine and famotidine are now available without prescription in some countries in packs containing only 2 weeks' supply for the treatment of dyspepsia. The unrestricted use of cimetidine and omeprazole needs careful consideration because their inhibition of cytochrome P-450 hepatic enzymes can lead to reduced metabolism of drugs that are detoxified by this enzyme system.

When gastrointestinal erosions result from nonsteroidal anti-inflammatory drug (NSAID) consumption, PPIs are effective in preventing erosion formation and appear to be more effective than H₂ receptor antagonists

Other drugs used in peptic ulcer disease

MISOPROSTOL is an analog of prostaglandin (PG) E₁. Endogenous PGE₂ and PGI₂ are important for maintaining the integrity of the gastroduodenal mucosal barrier (Fig. 21.2) and synthesis of the endogenous concentrations of PG required for

mucosal barrier integrity is thought to be via pathways involving the cyclo-oxygenase type I (COX-1) enzyme. Nonsteroidal anti-inflammatory and antipyretic drugs such as aspirin inhibit COX-1 (see Chapter 16) and thereby reduce mucosal, and possibly parietal cell PG synthesis, resulting in erosions and reduced healing of peptic ulcers and increased acid secretion. However recent studies suggest that COX-2-derived prostaglandins may also be involved in maintaining the mucosal barrier and ulcer healing. NSAIDs that have a greater selectivity for inhibition of COX-2 than COX-1 such as celocoxib and rofecoxib produce lower levels of gastrointestinal damage than the less selective NSAIDs (see Chapter 16). However, gastrointestinal damage is not completely eliminated by substituting these drugs for older NSAIDs. Misoprostol can be used to heal and prevent NSAID-induced damage when co-prescribed with an NSAID. Misoprostol has a half-life of 0.3 hours and is rapidly metabolized during the first pass to misoprostol acid. Its effects are shown in Fig. 21.2. Its unwanted effects are diarrhea and abdominal cramps; it may cause uterine contractions and should be avoided in pregnancy. Menorrhagia and postmenopausal bleeding may also occur. Although misoprostol replaces the prostaglandins that have been depleted by NSAIDs, some reports suggest that its effectiveness is no better than H₂ antagonists for treating or preventing NSAID-induced erosions.

SUCRALFATE is an aluminium polymer with sucrose octasulfate. In an acid environment, aluminium is released and its anionic form binds to tissues in the ulcer base creating a protective barrier. It undergoes minimal systemic absorption in healthy individuals, but it can accumulate in renal impairment. Sucralfate has antacid activity. It increases mucosal blood flow, mucus, PG, and bicarbonate secretion, and decreases pepsin activity (see Fig. 21.2). Sucralfate also reduces the number of H. pylori and the adherence of H. pylori to the gastric mucosa and this may explain the lower recurrence rate with its use. Sucralfate has to be taken orally four times daily and its aluminium content causes constipation.

BISMUTH CHELATE binds to the ulcer base and has favorable actions, similar to those of sucralfate, on bicarbonate, pepsin, mucus and PG secretion. It is rarely given alone, but forms part of the classic triple therapy regimen for treating peptic ulcers associated with H. pylori infection. However, it has been largely superseded and is now reserved for resistant cases. It is only moderately lethal to H. pylori when given alone and in such a situation it will eradicate the bacteria in only 20% of cases. It is given orally four times daily. Bismuth is minimally absorbed and the small amounts that are absorbed are eliminated slowly in the urine. In renal disease the failure to eliminate the small absorbed amounts could produce encephalopathy and, for this reason, administration is limited to 6 weeks.

PIRENZEPINE is a muscarinic M₁ receptor antagonist acting on receptors in the enteric nervous system and to a lesser extent on M₃ receptors on parietal cells. The type of muscarinic receptor present on the ECL cell is uncertain. Pirenzepine

Antacids used in peptic ulcer disease

Antacid	Salt	Unwanted effects	Comments
Aluminum	Hydroxide	Constipation	For all antacids medication up to four times daily is required
Magnesium	Carbonate/trisilicate	Diarrhea	Reduces the pH-dependent actions of pepsin; Al^{3+}, Mg^{2+} bind and inactivate pepsin
Calcium	Carbonate	High dose hypercalcemia	Facilitates ulcer healing but controlled studies are limited; slower healing rate than H_2 antagonists or PPI
Aluminum/magnesium and calcium/magnesium complexes	Hydroxide/carbonate		
Sodium	Bicarbonate	Alkalosis on prolonged use	Raising gastric pH with antacids or H_2 antagonists and PPIs may damage pH-sensitive enteric coatings on formulations of other drugs
Alginic acid preparations	Aluminum/magnesium complex plus alginic acid	(See GERD, below)	

Fig. 21.6 Antacids used in peptic ulcer disease. (PPI, proton pump inhibitor; GERD, gastroesophageal reflux disease)

inhibits acid and pepsin secretion, but this class of drug is relatively unpopular as a first choice because there is a high incidence of anticholinergic side effects (dry mouth and blurred vision).

ANTACIDS consist of Al^{3+} and Mg^{2+} salts, and less commonly Na^+ and Ca^{2+} salts, and are used for nonulcer dyspepsia and gastroesophageal reflux disease (GERD) (Fig. 21.6) (see below). They neutralize acid and increase gastric pH. A maintenance regimen of antacid can reduce the recurrence rate of duodenal ulcers over 1 year when compared with a placebo, and in one study was as effective as a maintenance regimen of H_2 receptor antagonists. For other actions, see Fig. 21.6.

Gastroesophageal reflux disease (GERD)

One in 10 people have GERD in which stomach and duodenal contents reflux into the esophagus. This can lead to an inflamed esophageal mucosa (esophagitis). Chronically this esophagitis can progress to erosive esophagitis and transformation of the esophageal mucosa into a columnar gastric-type mucosa (Barrett's metaplasia). The latter is a premalignant condition leading to esophageal adenocarcinoma. GERD reflux is often associated with gastric distension, a transiently reduced lower esophageal sphincter pressure, and diminished esophageal peristalsis, although in severe erosive esophagitis reflux may occur in the absence of reduced lower esophageal sphincter pressure. As a result of these associations, the injurious low pH gastroduodenal contents reside in the esophagus for damaging lengths of time because of the tendency for the reflux to move upwards. This upward movement in people with GERD is in contrast to what happens in people without GERD, where reflux results in increased esophageal peristalsis and rapid emptying of the esophagus. Neutralization of the esophageal contents by

esophageal and salivary secretions is an important protective mechanism. In addition, nonadrenergic noncholinergic (NANC) control may also be important, partly through the involvement of nitric oxide and cholecystokinin, which induce relaxation of the lower esophageal sphincter.

There is an uncertain and complex relationship between *H. pylori* and GERD. Some studies have shown that the symptoms of GERD may actually worsen in some patients when *H. pylori* is eliminated. Further studies are required to clarify this dichotomy.

ACHALASIA In this condition, there is a significant reduction in nitrergic neurons in the sphincter, and lower esophageal sphincter pressure is increased. This raised pressure can be reduced by local administration of botulinum toxin which acts to deplete parasympathetic neurons of their acetylcholine (see Chapter 14).

◾ *Drugs used to treat gastroesophageal reflux disease increase gastrointestinal motility, sphincter pressure and reduce acid and bile secretion*

Treatment regimens for GERD depend on the severity of the disease (Fig. 21.7). Occasional uncomplicated GERD (heartburn) is most often treated by self-medication, frequently with H_2 receptor antagonists or antacids.

PROTON PUMP INHIBITORS (PPIs) are the drugs of choice in moderate/severe GERD symptoms and esophagitis. Many independent clinical trials have now shown the superiority of PPIs over H_2 antagonists or sucralfate. As a generalization, PPIs relieve symptoms in days and heal esophagitis in 4–8 weeks. It does not appear, however, that raising esophageal pH results in a real risk of occurrence of malignancy.

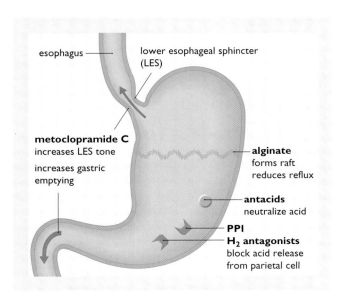

Fig. 21.7 The sites of action of drugs used to treat gastroesophageal reflux disease (GERD). (PPI, proton pump inhibitors)

H_2 **ANTAGONISTS** Although these are now thought to be less effective than PPI in GERD, a 12-week course of H_2 antagonists produced healing in up to 75% of patients with erosive esophagitis. This rate was not improved with 24 weeks of treatment. However, other studies contend that the effects of H_2 antagonists are purely symptomatic and do not produce healing.

ANTACIDS AND ALGINIC ACID For uncomplicated esophagitis (heartburn) Mg^{2+} and Al^{3+} antacids can be given in combination with alginic acid, an inert substance that foams in acid and forms a raft on the stomach contents, thereby reducing reflux. The foaming raft has a high pH, but much of the benefit of these preparations may be derived from the antacid constituents. Alginates are also available in combination with cimetidine.

PROKINETIC (MOTILITY-PROMOTING) DRUGS In GERD, a prokinetic drug that increases gastric motility and thus empties the stomach more quickly may ameliorate the symptoms, particularly when they are mild. Prokinetic drugs are not used alone in GERD, but as adjuncts to PPI and H_2 antagonist drug therapy. Metoclopramide and domperidone are dopamine type 2 (D_2) receptor antagonists and 5-hydroxytryptamine (5-HT) receptor stimulants. Although, as a result of animal studies, metoclopramide is thought to act on $5\text{-}HT_4$ interneurons in the stomach enteric nervous system, resulting in acetylcholine release, increased gastric motility, and an increased rate of gastric emptying, there is no firm evidence that this is the site of action in humans. However, the prokinetic effect on the human stomach plus an action in increasing lower esophageal sphincter tone is probably the mechanism of its beneficial effect in GERD (see Fig. 21.7). There is little evidence that it can heal the eroded esophagus. Metoclopramide also has anticholinergic

and central nervous system (CNS) effects as a result of blocking dopamine receptors. Domperidone, a D_2 antagonist that does not cross the blood–brain barrier, is a suitable alternative to metoclopramide. Metoclopramide and domperidone are also used for treating nausea and vomiting, and further details are discussed below.

Constipation

Regulation of normal gastrointestinal motility involves the CNS, the enteric nervous system, and gastrointestinal hormones. There are many causes of constipation, but ultimately it results from an absence of propagating contractions in the colon, which may be associated with either decreased or increased segmenting contractions. In some patients there may be abnormalities of propulsion in just the proximal or distal parts of the colon. Normal defecation of formed stools can vary from three times a day to only once every 3 days.

The incidence of severe chronic constipation, excluding that due to organic disease or an iatrogenic cause, is not known, but it is significantly greater in women than in men. The definition of constipation is also clouded, it is sometimes described as an altered frequency of defecation, and sometimes as difficult defecation.

■ *Constipation is managed by dietary improvement, eliminating any drugs that can cause constipation, excluding the presence of underlying pathology, and laxatives*

Laxatives

The mechanisms of action of laxatives are illustrated in Fig. 21.8, and more details about commonly used laxatives are given

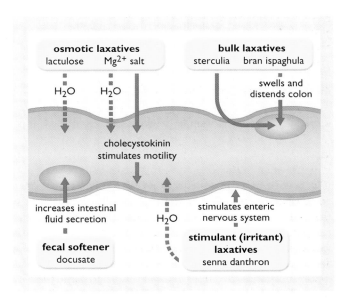

Fig. 21.8 Mechanism of action of laxatives. Bulk laxatives absorb water and on swelling slowly distend the colon and increase peristaltic motility; osmotic laxatives enhance peristalsis by osmotically increasing the bowel fluid volume; stimulant (irritant) laxatives stimulate the enteric nervous system; fecal softeners increase intestinal fluid secretion.

Drugs used for the treatment of constipation*

A variety of bulk-forming laxatives including bran, ispaghula, sterculia, methylcellulose	*
Senna	Minimal absorption: action takes up to 12 hours given orally and less than 2 hours rectally
Bisacodyl	Administered orally or rectally Minimal absorption but relatively quick action after 6–8 hours orally but less than 60 minutes rectally
Lactulose	Poorly absorbed orally and broken down to active acids in the colon Takes 1–2 days to act
Docusate	Surfactant action. Minimally absorbed. Acts in up to 3 days
Magnesium sulfate	Acts within 6 hours. Up to 30% absorbed. Renal elimination
Danthron	An animal carcinogen restricted for use in the terminally ill Liver damage
Sodium picosulfate	Used only as a preoperative bowel preparation

* Because most drugs are minimally absorbed in most situations, plasma levels are insignificant. Side effects of all these preparations are flatulence, cramps and abdominal discomfort; individual unwanted effects are described in the text.

Fig. 21.9 Drugs used for the treatment of constipation*.

in Fig. 21.9. Laxatives are widely misused in some societies for many reasons, including eating disorders where they are used to reduce caloric intake. Sometimes the use of laxatives may disguise the presence of underlying disease (e.g. obstruction).

BULK LAXATIVES Constipation and diarrhea can be treated with bulk provided in the form of dietary fiber. Unprocessed fiber (e.g. bran from unprocessed wheat or citrus sources) forms a readily available nondigestible source of bulk-forming laxative that can be used if sufficient fiber cannot be obtained from a normal balanced diet. It may take several days for full effectiveness to be seen and may cause flatulence. Dietary fiber acts by absorbing water and promoting bacterial growth, since as it swells it distends the colon and increases peristaltic motility. Other bulk laxatives include preparations of ispaghula husk, sterculia gum, and methylcellulose, which are available in more palatable forms than unprocessed fiber and are gluten-free; some preparations are also sugar-free. They have essentially the same action as bran, but sterculia contains polysaccharides, which are broken down by bacteria, and the resulting fatty

acids can have an additional osmotic effect. Fiber is thought to normalize stool texture, and is also used to treat patients with loose stools (see page 464).

OSMOTIC LAXATIVES are widely prescribed. They are poorly absorbed and increase the small and large bowel fluid volume by osmosis and as a result increase peristaltic motility.

Lactulose is widely used and is a semisynthetic disaccharide of galactose and fructose. It passes unchanged to the colon and is then broken down by bacteria to lactic and acetic acids, which act osmotically to increase fluid volume and lower pH. It is effective within 2–3 days. Mg^{2+} salts and Na^+ acid phosphate are used less often than lactulose; they are poorly absorbed and are osmotically active. Mg^{2+} also increases the synthesis of cholecystokinin, which increases colon motility and fluid secretion into the lumen.

STIMULANT CONTACT OR IRRITANT LAXATIVES should not be given over the long term. They have limited or restricted uses and can cause long-term pathologic problems. They act within hours and include:

- Senna, which is a plant alkaloid obtained from plantains. The constituent anthroquinones are hydrolyzed by gut bacteria to yield glycosides and subsequently anthracenes. These stimulate the enteric nervous system and alter fluid balance across the gut wall to promote propulsive motility.
- Bisacodyl, which is a diphenolic compound similar to phenolphthalein that can be given rectally for a rapid response.
- Danthron, which has similar properties to senna, but is carcinogenic in animal studies and is reserved for use only in the terminally ill.
- Sodium picosulfate, which is frequently used for bowel preparation before endoscopy or surgery.

The mechanisms of action of this group of drugs are poorly understood, but it has been suggested that they damage intestinal cells and weaken intercellular junctions. They also stimulate PG, cAMP, and possibly cholecystokinin, and vasoactive intestinal polypeptide (VIP) synthesis. These changes can all affect fluid balance and motility.

Chronic use of the anthroquinone laxatives can lead to melanosis coli, a black discoloration of the colonic mucosa, which can persist for years. Chronic administration of stimulant laxatives can also lead to the development of a 'cathartic colon,' which is a progressive deterioration of colon function that can exacerbate an existing bowel dysfunction.

FECAL SOFTENERS Docusate is dioctyl sodium sulfosuccinate. It has detergent properties, increases intestinal fluid secretion, and has weak stimulatory activity on intestinal motility. It relieves constipation within 1–2 days.

PROKINETIC DRUGS Bethanechol, metoclopramide, and naloxone can stimulate colon motility, but descriptions of their use in the treatment of severe chronic constipation are insubstantial and require further clarification.

Chronic laxative use

- Chronic use of stimulant (irritant) laxatives can lead to the development of a 'cathartic colon' with reduced propagative motility, dilation, and exacerbation of any underlying disease
- Can damage the enteric nervous system
- Can lead to electrolyte imbalance

Diarrhea

There are many causes of diarrhea including:

- An existing chronic disease (e.g. loss of functioning mucosa in inflammatory bowel diseases and gut resections, motor abnormalities of irritable bowel syndrome, malabsorption diseases, endocrine abnormalities such as thyrotoxicosis).
- Infectious agents.
- Drugs.
- Psychologic factors.

Acute secretory diarrhea usually results from an infection.

Acute infectious diarrhea is extremely common and usually lasts just a few days. A common cause is acute viral gastroenteritis, and in children a rotavirus is usually the identified cause. In many cases, particularly adults, viral causes are often not identified, but bacterial pathogens such as *Campylobacter* are commonly cultured.

Worldwide, acute diarrhea (mainly of infectious origin) causes up to five million deaths every year as a result of dehydration. Approximately 85% of these deaths are in children less than 2 years of age and many could be prevented by simple measures. In Britain about 12 children younger than 1 year of age die each year from infectious diarrhea, while 20% of all health service consultations in the UK are for children less than 2 years of age with acute diarrhea.

The vigor of treatment for acute diarrhea depends upon the differential diagnosis and the patient's age. Young children are particularly prone to dehydration as 15% of the body weight turns over each day as water. Classifying enteropathogenic bacteria according to whether or not they invade the intestine is also important when deciding upon treatment (Fig. 21.10).

- Generally invasive bacteria cause bloody, relatively small volume diarrhea.
- Adhesive but noninvasive enterotoxigenic bacteria produce toxins, which can increase cAMP or cGMP and result in a massive secretion of Cl$^-$ followed by water and Na$^+$ secretion. The molecular mechanism of cholera toxin action involves the ADP-ribosylation of the α subunit of Gs. After this covalent modification, the GTPase activity of this subunit is lost, leading to prolonged action of adenylyl cyclase by GTP-αs. More than 1 liter of fluid can be lost every hour, but with effective rehydration the infection tends to be short lived.

It needs to be borne in mind that diarrhea along with vomiting (see below) is a part of the body's defense mechanism for ridding itself of invading organisms.

Approximately 20% of travelers abroad suffer an acute episode of diarrhea. It is estimated that the predominant infectious causes are noninvasive *E. coli* (40%), *Shigella* (10%), *Campylobacter jejuni* (3%), protozoa (5%), and viruses (10%), while no pathogen is isolated in about 22%. This pattern is quite different from that of home-acquired pathogens.

Rotavirus is the most important pathogen causing dehydrating diarrhea in infants in both developed and developing countries. In the USA there are an estimated 3.5 million cases of rotavirus diarrhea every year among infants, and up to 125 related deaths. Worldwide there are an estimated 800,000 deaths from rotavirus-related gastroenteritis. Successful vaccines against some strains are being evaluated.

Pathologic features of some enteroinfective organisms that cause diarrhea

Infective organism	Mechanism	Volume of diarrhea
Rotavirus	Damages small bowel villi	+ (watery stools)
Adhesive enterotoxigenic bacteria *Escherichia coli* *Salmonella enteritidis*[1] Cholera	Noninvasive. Adhere to brush borders of intestinal absorptive cells. Secrete enterotoxins that alter fluid electrolyte transport and increase prostaglandin activity. Stimulate enteric nervous system	++ (watery stools) ++ (watery stools) +++ (watery stools)
Invasive bacteria *Shigella*[1] *E. coli*[1,2] *Salmonella typhimurium* *Campylobacter jejuni*[1]	Invade epithelium. Secrete enterotoxins. Cause inflammation and tissue destruction. Some move between epithelial cells	Bloody stools

[1] Sometimes causes vomiting
[2] Some strains

Fig. 21.10 Pathologic features of some enteroinfective organisms that cause diarrhea. (The mechanisms stated are generalizations. Each bacterium uses distinct mechanisms to penetrate the epithelium and produce damage and diarrhea.)

■ *The mainstay of treatment of acute diarrhea is the correction of dehydration and not the reduction of stool fluid output*

Rehydration therapy

Oral rehydration therapy (ORT) is the first priority in the treatment of acute diarrhea of all causes, and promptly administered oral formulations save many lives. In many cases, particularly those of viral origin, oral rehydration is the only therapy needed, but intravenous therapy is needed if there is a severe electrolyte imbalance. ORT will not immediately reduce the volume of diarrhea, but absorption of the administered electrolytes leads to correction of the electrolyte imbalance, fluid balance and acidosis, while the body systems eliminate the pathogens. The success of this will depend upon the nutritional and physical status of the patient. There are several oral formulations (in powder form).

THE WORLD HEALTH ORGANIZATION (WHO) ORAL REHYDRATION THERAPY recommended formulation contains:
- NaCl   3.5 g/liter (Na$^+$ 90 mmol/liter).
- KCl   1.5 g/liter (K$^+$ 20 mmol/liter).
- NaCitrate   2.9 g/liter (citrate 30 mmol/liter).
- Chloride   (80 mmol/liter).
- Glucose   20 g/liter (111 mmol/liter).

OTHER FORMULATIONS contain considerably less Na$^+$ than this WHO formula, which can sometimes produce hypernatremia, and formulations containing less Na$^+$ (approximately 50 mmol/liter) should probably be used in developed countries. Clearly, a source of uninfected drinkable water is required for reconstituting the solutions. The correct amount of water must be added to avoid worsening the dehydration if the solutes are too concentrated. In fact, the WHO formulation is slightly hypertonic. Some formulations contain HCO$_3^-$ rather than citrate, but these tend to deteriorate in hot conditions. More recently, formulations that produce a hypotonic solution, containing a glucose polymer have been tested; this reduces volume loss by about 30% when compared with no treatment. Glucose is necessary because it facilitates Na$^+$ absorption via the Na$^+$/glucose cotransporter, and this also increases water absorption. Other formulations that replace glucose with amino acids or even cooked cereal have also been used, with similar results to those of the WHO formulation.

Drugs used to treat diarrhea

Many drugs have an antidiarrheal action because they alter intestinal propulsive motility and increase the time for fluid absorption; however, only a small number are commonly used for acute infective diarrhea. Not only do these drugs enhance absorption by slowing transit time, but some also accelerate absorption as a separate action.

OPIATE-LIKE ANTIDIARRHEAL AGENTS include:
- Diphenoxylate and loperamide, which are congeners of meperidine.
- Codeine, which is a congener of morphine.

They act on μ opiate receptors in the myenteric plexus and possibly on 5-HT receptors; and by modulating acetylcholine release they reduce peristaltic activity, but enhance segmental activity and tone, and increase transit time. They may also enhance absorption by acting on opiate receptors. Although these drugs have been available for many years, it is difficult to gain a consensus about their use, which has been largely based on individual preference and divergent advice.

Patients with viral gastroenteritis or traveller's diarrhea generally require no antidiarrheal treatment, but opiates can reduce the duration of diarrhea by about 12 hours. Some reports suggest that these drugs should not be given for infections caused by enteroinvasive bacteria such as *Shigella* (Fig. 21.10) because they delay clearance of the organism, prolonging the diarrhea and accompanying fever, but other reports state that this is of little clinical consequence.

Co-phenotrope is a combination of diphenoxylate and atropine. It can produce the typical antimuscarinic adverse effects of blurred vision and dry mouth and there is little evidence to suggest that the combination has advantages. Diphenoxylate has a half-life of 2–3 hours, is metabolized by liver enzymes, and does not readily penetrate the blood–brain barrier.

Loperamide has relatively selective actions on the gut, having a half-life of 10–12 hours because of enterohepatic recycling, thereby extending the drug concentration in the gut. Diphenoxylate and loperamide may cause constipation, cramps and drowsiness, paralytic ileus and abdominal bloating. See Chapter 14 for details of unwanted effects of codeine.

STOOL MODIFIERS such as the absorbent clay, kaolin, are given in combination with morphine. Kaolin has a bulking action, improving stool consistency. Other bulking agents, such as wheat bran, increase stool viscosity. It is critical that fluid and electrolyte balance is maintained when bulking agents are used. Kaolin may also absorb toxins, although this effect is largely anecdotal.

ANTIBIOTIC treatment of diarrhea should be undertaken sparingly. It is rarely required for the treatment of communally acquired infectious diarrhea in developed communities because this is likely to be self-limiting and viral in origin. Tetracycline can be given for severe cholera and for *Salmonella typhimurium*, although substantial outbreaks of infections can be resistant, as happened with a cholera outbreak in the Ruandan refugee

> ### Opiate antidiarrheals
>
> - *Codeine and diphenoxylate, but not loperamide, cross the blood–brain barrier and produce euphoria and respiratory depression, particularly in children*
> - *Can delay clearance of enteroinvasive bacteria such as Shigella, but some investigators suggest that this is of little clinical consequence*
> - *Chronic use of opiates can cause paralytic ileus and toxic megacolon*

camps in Tanzania in 1994. *Shigella* can be treated with ampicillin, although again there are marked individual variations, with a high level of resistance in some strains, and alternative antibiotics may be necessary. *Campylobacter jejuni* is sensitive to erythromycin or ciprofloxacin. (Antibiotics are discussed in detail in Chapter 9.)

The indiscriminate use of broad-spectrum antibiotics has led to a high level of resistance in many enteropathogenic bacteria. The use of antibiotics that destroy the normal flora as well as the pathogen may allow overgrowth of organisms such as *Clostridium difficile*, which can cause serious pseudomembranous colitis requiring treatment with either metronidazole or vancomycin. Commonly used drugs that can cause diarrhea or constipation are shown in Fig. 21.11.

Irritable bowel syndrome

Irritable bowel syndrome (IBS) is a disorder resulting in recurrent abdominal pain and either diarrhea or constipation, resulting in relatively poorly defined subclassifications of diarrhea-dependent or constipation-dependent IBS. Other nongastrointestinal symptoms such as lethargy, urinary frequency, anxiety, depression may also accompany intestinal symptoms. IBS is said to occur in up to 15% of the population.

Drugs for diarrhea and constipation
• Rehydration is of prime importance in diarrhea
• Opiates decrease peristalsis and increase overall gut tone
• Antibiotics should be necessary only for specific infectious diarrheas such as cholera
• Mechanisms of actions of laxatives include an osmotic effect, bulking, irritation, stimulation of the enteric nervous system, and fecal softening
• Bulk laxatives act within days, but irritant laxatives act within hours

Patients usually have hypersensitivity particularly in the colon but a clear pathophysiologic etiology is so far obscure; a psychological component may be relevant. The drug treatment of IBS is at present relatively nonspecific as befits its unknown etiology. The evidence base for the effectiveness of drugs is weak and the placebo component of treatment is high. Drugs used in IBS are listed in Fig. 21.12.

Drugs used to treat IBS

Antispasmodic agents such as mebeverine and dicyclomine act by direct effects and by inhibiting muscarinic receptors. Mebeverine and dicyclomine are well absorbed, have short half-lifes, and are metabolized in the liver. Diarrhea and constipation can be managed with antidiarrheal agents or laxatives (see above).

GASTROINTESTINAL SEROTONIN RECEPTOR AGONISTS AND ANTAGONISTS The role of serotonin (5-HT) in gastrointestinal function is complex. The gut contains a multitude of 5-HT receptor subtypes that differ in their distribution. Receptors may be situated on enteric interneurons or on different neuronal cell membranes. The stimulation of the same receptor subtype sited at different locations in gastrointestinal tract can result in opposite actions on motility. 5-HT can affect both gastrointestinal motility and epithelial cell electrolyte and water secretions.

Drugs that can cause diarrhea or constipation	
Constipation	**Diarrhea**
Al^{3+} salts	Mg^{2+} salts
Anticholinergics	Erythromycin
Antidepressants	Ampicillin
Fe^{3+} preparations	Prokinetics
Antispasmodics	Theophylline
Opiates	Indomethacin
Ca^{2+} antagonists	Fe^{3+} preparations
Sympathomimetics	Levodopa
	Propranolol
	Parasympathomimetics

Fig. 21.11 Drugs that can cause diarrhea or constipation.

Drugs used in the treatment of irritable bowel syndrome (IBS)			
Drug*	**Action**	**Half-life (hours)**	**Comment**
Mebeverine	Direct effect on smooth muscle	2.5	
Dicyclomine	Antimuscarinic and direct effect	9–10	Antimuscarinic side-effects
Tegaserod	5-HT$_4$ receptor agonist		Trials have shown variable effectiveness in women with constipation-predominant IBS.
Antidepressants			See Chapter 14

* The precise use of all of these agents in IBS is still being evaluated. Another 5-HT$_4$ agonist, prucalopride, is under development

Fig. 21.12 Drugs used in the treatment of irritable bowel syndrome.

Tegaserod is a partial 5-HT$_4$ agonist and is effective in the treatment of the constipation-predominant form of irritable bowel syndrome. It is too early to be certain about the long-term benefit of these drugs.

ANTIDEPRESSANTS The use of tricyclic and selective serotonin reuptake inhibitors in IBS are being examined but further studies are required to clearly define their roles.

Inflammatory bowel disease

The incidence of inflammatory bowel disease (IBD), which includes ulcerative colitis (UC) and Crohn's disease (CD), is about 1/10,000/year. The etiologies of UC and CD are unknown, but there is considerable overlap between the two conditions. Multifocal infarction and infection with *Mycobacterium* and other pathogens have been implicated, but their relevance is far from clear. Products of nonpathogenic intestinal flora may also play a role. Genetic factors, environmental conditions, and alterations in the mucosal immune system are also thought to be involved.

IBD follows a course of flare-ups (with chronic intestinal inflammation, which may be accompanied by fever and anemia) and periods of remission. Frequent, bloody, loose stools and abdominal pain are common, and patients are prone to infection.

■ *Aminosalicylates, glucocorticosteroids, and immunosuppressants are used to treat inflammatory bowel disease*

AMINOSALICYLATES such as sulfasalazine are widely used in the treatment of CD and UC to maintain remission. They have only limited use for treating acute relapses. Sulfasalazine is broken down by gut flora, mainly in the cecum and colon, to the active component 5-aminosalicylate (5-ASA) and sulfapyridine, which appears to cause the adverse effects of nausea, toxic effects on red cells, and oligospermia. The mechanism of action of 5-ASA is unknown. The use of sulfasalazine to treat CD is largely limited to where 5-ASA is released (i.e. colonic involvement) (see Fig. 21.13).

Mesalamine is 5-ASA and olsalazine is two molecules of 5-ASA linked by a diazo bond, which is cleaved in the colon. They have a lower incidence of adverse effects than sulfasalazine, but olsalazine tends to cause diarrhea in some patients.

Aspirin worsens IBD and should be avoided.

GLUCOCORTICOSTEROIDS are widely used to treat relapses of IBD. Their mechanism of action as anti-inflammatory drugs is covered in Chapters 15, 16, and 19. They are of limited use in maintaining remission. Their adverse effects (see Chapter 15) on the endocrine system have led to the development of locally acting, poorly absorbed glucocorticosteroids such as budesonide.

TNF-α antibody

Infliximab is the first monoclonal antibody approved for Crohn's disease. TNF-α is involved in the synthesis of pro-inflammatory cytokines such as IL1 and resultant eosinophil and neutrophil infiltration and activation. Infliximab is given intravenously, and a course of intermittent injections with gaps of several weeks between can induce remission for several months. Its long-term safety is still being investigated. Infliximab is also being used in the treatment of arthritis (Chapter 13). Etanercept is another TNF-α antibody that is

	Drug	Half-life (hours)	Comment
Drugs used for the treatment of inflammatory bowel disease			
Aminosalicylates	Sulfasalazine (5-ASA≡sulfapyridine)	5-ASA 4–10	Cleaved in colon to active 5-ASA
	Mesalamine (5-ASA)	0.5–1	Given as enteric formulation
	Olsalazine (5-ASA≡5-ASA)	1	Cleaved in colon to release active 5-ASA
	Balsalazide (5-ASA≡4-amino-benzoyl-β-alanine (inert carrier)	Not known	Cleaved in colon to release active 5-ASA Systemic absorption is slow and variable
TNF-α antibody	Infliximab	9.5 days	Given intravenously
Corticosteroids	Budesonide Prednisolone	2 18–36	Budesonide has limited gastrointestinal absorption See Chapters 15 and 19 for details
Immunosuppressives	Azathioprine Cyclosporin A	3–5 27	See Chapter 16 for details See Chapter 16 for details
Antibiotics	Metronidazole	6–9	See Chapter 9 for details

Fig. 21.13 Drugs used for the treatment of inflammatory bowel disease.

Drugs and inflammatory bowel disease

- Aminosalicylates such as mesalamine and olsalazine maintain remission
- Glucocorticosteroids are effective for acute relapses of the disease
- Poorly absorbed glucocorticosteroids (e.g. budesonide) have little effect on the hypothalamic–pituitary–adrenal axis
- Nonsteroidal anti-inflammatory drugs exacerbate inflammatory bowel disease

approved for arthritis and is currently being studied for inflammatory bowel disease.

IMMUNOSUPPRESSANTS can be useful in the treatment of IBD:

- Azathioprine and 6-mercaptopurine reduce the need for glucocorticosteroids and are particularly useful for glucocorticosteroid-refractory and glucocorticosteroid-dependent patients, but it is several months before their effect becomes evident.
- Cyclosporine produces improvement in symptoms within 2 weeks, but has to be given as a high-dosage intravenous administration because oral therapy is ineffective.
- Methotrexate appears to be beneficial in some patients, but its usage and benefits require further evaluation.

Other new therapies under consideration include interferon-γ and anti-CD4 antibody. Treatment with 5-lipoxygenase inhibitors, nicotine, and short-chain fatty acids has also been reported.

🔲 *The antibiotic metronidazole is useful for treating some resistant patients and in treating anal fistulae*

PATHOPHYSIOLOGY AND DISEASES OF THE LIVER

Jaundice

Jaundice is a yellowing of the skin and conjunctiva. It is produced by increased serum concentrations of bilirubin, which result in the deposition of bilirubin and its metabolic products in the skin and other organs. Causes of increased serum bilirubin concentrations include:

- Increased formation of bilirubin due to increased breakdown (hemolysis) of red blood cells so that bilirubin production exceeds the capacity of the liver to metabolize it.
- Inadequate bilirubin metabolism in the liver due to congenital abnormalities, or disease of the liver parenchyma.
- Obstruction to bile outflow from the liver so that bilirubin 'spills' into the blood.

Many drugs can cause jaundice by one or more of these mechanisms (Fig. 21.14).

There is no specific drug treatment for jaundice.

Congenital liver disease

The three congenital diseases of the liver of particular note in pharmacology are Wilson's disease and hemochromatosis (see

Mechanism of action of some drugs that cause jaundice

Mechanism	Drug	Comment
Hemolysis (increased bilirubin production)	Antimalarials Sulfonamides Aspirin Phenacetin	Occurs in people with glucose-6-phosphate dehydrogenase (G6PD) deficiency
	Cephalosporins Methyldopa	Immunologic basis
Altered hepatic bilirubin uptake	Rifampin	
Hepatotoxicity	Carbon tetrachloride	
	Acetaminophen overdose	Treat with *N*-acetylcysteine
	Tetracycline	Avoid in pregnancy
Diffuse hepatocellular damage	Tricyclic antidepressants	Uncommon
	Isoniazid	Related to dose and patient's age
Intrahepatic cholestasis	Anabolic steroids Phenothiazines	
	Erythromycin	Incidence probably not related to type of salt used (e.g. estolate)

Fig. 21.14 Mechanisms of action of some drugs that cause jaundice.

below), because drug treatment is useful, and Dubin–Johnson syndrome, which can alter liver metabolism of drugs.

WILSON'S DISEASE (HEPATOLENTICULAR DEGENERATION) is a rare (1/million population) autosomal recessive trait in which there is defective copper excretion into the bile. This leads to an accumulation of copper in the tissues, including the brain, resulting in neurologic and hepatic dysfunction.

Treatment involves the use of drugs that chelate copper (usually penicillamine, see Chapter 29) and promote its removal from the body.

DUBIN–JOHNSON SYNDROME is characterized by hyper-bilirubinemia and jaundice because the liver is unable to secrete conjugated bilirubin efficiently. This results from a congenital impairment of an ATP-dependent transport system that is specific for a variety of multivalent organic anions, including conjugated bilirubin. Drugs such as oral contraceptives are also metabolized by this method and should be avoided by individuals with Dubin–Johnson syndrome.

Acquired liver disease

CHEMICAL-INDUCED LIVER DISEASE Many chemicals are toxic to the liver (e.g. halogenated hydrocarbons such as carbon tetrachloride). Ethanol is the most commonly ingested hepato-toxic substance and chronic excess intake produces a fatty liver and cirrhosis (see Chapter 29).

LIVER INFECTIONS Hepatitis A, B, and C, are among the most common infectious diseases, and their consequences can include cirrhosis and possibly carcinoma of the liver. They are best controlled by the prophylactic use of specific vaccines.

Parasitic infections such as *Schistosoma mansoni*, *Echinococcus*, *Ameba histolytica*, and *Chlonorchis sinesis* occur in the liver, and can be treated with the appropriate antiparasitic agents (see Chapter 11).

Drugs and the liver
Drugs in biliary colic

Biliary colic is pain resulting from spasm of the gallbladder or common hepatic duct due to stones interfering with the passage of bile or otherwise initiating spasm. Biliary colic is characterized by spasmodic, cramping pain, typically in the right upper quadrant of the abdomen. Stones in the hepatic common duct (choldedocholithiasis) occur in 15–20% of patients with chronic cholelithiasis, i.e. stones collecting in the gallbladder itself. Common duct obstruction due to choledo-cholithiasis is one of the causes of jaundice. The pain of biliary colic often requires a narcotic analgesic for its relief. Meperidine frequently is chosen because of morphine's ability to produce spasm of the smooth muscle of gallbladder, the duct or its sphincters that is liable to make the pain worse. It is not clear that meperidine is less likely than morphine to produce such spasm. A nonsteroidal anti-inflammatory drug, e.g. diclofenac given rectally or intravenously can lessen pain presumably by reduction of prostaglandin synthesis in the duct and hence reducing spasm. Once the pain is controlled, more definitive measures such as radiologically controlled manipulation of an obstructing stone or surgical intervention can be implemented. There is risk of cholangitis (inflammation in the bile ducts) and antibiotics should be administered as necessary. Their use, however, must be accompanied by procedures directed toward the removal of any obstruction in the bile duct.

Hemochromatosis

This is an autosomal recessively inherited disease in which excess iron is deposited in peripheral tissues including the liver. In 85% of people with hereditary hemochromatosis in the United States, there is missense mutation in the HFE gene that regulates synthesis of HFE protein. (The latter is related to the HLA proteins involved in immune responses.) A defect in HFE protein (which ordinarily binds to transferrin, see Chapter 13) results in loss of the control of iron absorption across the intestinal mucosa. Absorption of iron normally is regulated in the intestinal mucosa so that when ferritin stores are high, absorption is markedly reduced. The body has no mechanism for excretion of iron. In hemochromatosis the control of absorption is defective, excess iron is absorbed, iron overload occurs and iron is deposited in systemic tissues including the liver. Such deposition can result in hepatic cellular damage and cirrhosis. Treatment is repeated phlebotomies (drawing off blood) to reduce iron load in the body, but sometimes an iron chelator such as deferoxamine (see Chapter 29) is necessary to remove excess iron from the body.

Cirrhosis

Cirrhosis is a result of injury to hepatocytes characterized by development of fibrotic tissue in the liver and raised pressure in the hepatic portal venous system. This in turn leads to production of varices (varicose veins) at the sites of major anastomoses between the portal and systemic venous systems, namely in the mucosa of the distal esophagus and anal canal. Severe, life-threatening bleeding readily occurs from these varices and constitutes a major problem in cirrhosis. The increased portal venous pressure plus altered metabolism of aldosterone by damaged hepatocytes also results in accumu-lation of fluid in the peritoneal cavity, a condition known as ascites. Esophageal varices and ascites are hallmarks of cirrhosis of the liver. The commonest cause of cirrhosis of the liver is excessive intake of ethanol but infection with hepatitis virus B or more often hepatitis virus C also are frequent causes.

The management of liver cirrhosis includes controlling acute bleeding from intestinal varices, reducing the frequency of recurrence of bleeding and reducing accumulation of ascitic fluid.

Drugs used in cirrhosis of the liver

BLEEDING VARICES Varices at the lower end of the esophagus or anal canal can bleed massively periodically. The amount of bleeding during such an episode often can be reduced by administration of somatostatin or its analogs. Somatostatin (see Chapter 15) has largely been replaced by longer-acting analogs such as octreotide or vapreotide in the treatment of bleeding varices. Following intravenous administration, octreotide has a plasma half-life of 1.5 hours and vapreotide of 30 minutes, compared with 1–3 minutes for somatostatin. These drugs are given as an intravenous bolus followed by an infusion for 2 to 3 days. The mechanisms involved in their therapeutic effect are not certain. They seem to lessen bleeding by reducing visceral blood flow, possibly by producing vasocontriction of the intestinal vasculature due to their interaction with somatostatin receptor subtypes 2 and 5 in these blood vessels. Somotostatin receptors are G protein-coupled receptors that inhibit cyclic AMP production.

Patients with bleeding because of coagulopathies due to impaired synthesis of clotting factors by the liver generally require infusions of fresh frozen plasma (see Chapter 13).

REDUCTION OF RECURRENT BLEEDING The frequency of recurrent bleeding from esophageal varices can be reduced by daily oral administration of certain β adrenoceptor antagonists, including propranolol and nadolol. The mechanism for this prophylactic effect of these drugs is uncertain. Indeed, since it is not clear that this effect is solely due to β adrenoceptor antagonism, it may well not be a class effect, i.e. an action shared by all β adrenoceptor antagonists. Consequently, it is prudent for the therapist to employ the specific β adrenoceptor antagonists that have been demonstrated in clinical trials to have efficacy in this situation. The aim is to reduce portal venous pressure and so lessen the chance of bleeding from the varicose veins in the mucosa of the esophagus and anal canal. Some patients require procedures to either ablate the esophageal varices or to divert blood flow in order to decrease portal pressures.

TREATMENT OF ASCITES Ascites is the presence of increased amounts of fluid in the abdominal cavity. Ascitic fluid accumulates in part because of increased portal venous pressure, but in many patients with cirrhosis there is also decreased plasma oncotic pressure (osmotic pressure due to proteins) because of reduced albumin production by the cirrhotic liver. Both the increased portal pressure and decreased plasma oncotic pressure unbalance fluid movements into and out of the blood vessels of the gut and peritoneum. The net effect is increased passage of fluid out of the vasculature (transudation) into the extracellular space and increased extracellular fluid, in particular, in the abdominal cavity. In turn, this reduces intravascular plasma volume which induces secondary hyperaldosteronism. Increased aldosterone tends to restore intravascular volume towards normal by promoting marked salt retention by the kidneys, associated with loss of potassium into the urine. Unfortunately, this adaptation is at the cost of increasing total body sodium and water, increasing ascites, and often peripheral edema. Ascitic fluid is prone to infection, decreases patient mobility and may compress the lower lobes of the lung when massive. While treating ascitic patients with drugs has not been shown to prolong life, it may delay complications and improve their quality of life.

DIURETIC THERAPY OF ASCITES Patients with ascites should ideally sharply decrease sodium in their diet; however, this can be difficult and is generally insufficient to prevent excessive salt retention by the kidneys. Consequently, diuretics are often required to decrease formation of ascitic fluid and peripheral edemea in patients with liver disease. Diuresis induced by spironolactone, an aldosterone antagonist in the kidney (see Chapter 17), is an important part of treatment. Spironolactone inhibits sodium retention in the distal tubule as well as decreasing potassium wasting by the kidneys. Furosemide, a 'loop' diuretic can be added if the diuresis produced by spironolactone is inadequate. In addition, ascitic fluid can be drawn off (a paracentesis). The aim of therapy is to reduce the amount of transudation of fluid into the peritoneal cavity, i.e. to reduce the accumulation of ascitic fluid.

Drugs or fluid removal must be utilized with caution: intravascular volume constriction can lead to hypotension and kidney failure. Also, electrolyte imbalance can precipitate hepatic encephalopathy.

Drug therapy of hepatic encephalopathy

Hepatic encephalopathy is a complex syndrome that occurs in many patients with severe liver failure; it is characterized by changes in mental functioning that may be profound, ultimately leading to coma. The pathogenesis of hepatic encephalopathy is uncertain but it has been associated with changes in ammonia concentrations and alterations in GABA receptor activation, as well as changes in neurotransmitters in the brain. Patients with portal hypertension may be at increased risk for hepatic encephalopathy, likely due to diversion of gastrointestinal venous drainage directly into the peripheral circulation without going through the liver.

Management of patients with hepatic encephalopathy includes general measures such as correcting plasma electrolyte disturbances, avoiding plasma volume contraction, avoiding high protein intake, and minimizing the use of psychoactive drugs, all factors that can precipitate clinical deterioration. While the pathogenesis of the disorder is not clearly understood, specific drug therapy of hepatic encephalopathy is aimed at decreasing ammonia production.

Neomycin is an antibiotic with very low systemic bioavailability. It is probably efficacious in the treatment of hepatic encephalopathy by diminishing the number of microorganisms in the gut that have urease activity. This diminishes the liberation of ammonia. Neomycin rarely causes toxicity to the kidney or ears (as may occur with other aminoglycosides) on account of its poor oral absorption.

Lactulose is a sugar not readily absorbed by the small intestine. In the colon, it is metabolized to a variety of organic acid molecules; the increased production of hydrogen ions lowers the pH of the colonic contents, converting ammonia (NH_3) to ammonium (NH_4^+). NH_4^+ is then trapped in the lumen of the colon and consequently does not reach the peripheral circulation. The oral dose of lactulose is titrated to produce several loose stools per day. Excessive dosage of lactulose may cause severe diarrhea, which can worsen hepatic encephalopathy by promoting intravascular volume contraction and electrolyte disturbances such as hyponatremia.

Viral liver infections

Hepatitis B is a disease transmitted by the body fluids of a person secreting the virus, and by blood, blood products or equipment contaminated by the virus. It can be treated with famciclovir (see Chapter 8) but is best treated prophylactically by immunization, particularly in children and in people at high risk of infection such as healthcare workers.

Hepatitis C infection is common: antibodies to hepatitis C are present in about 8% of the population of the United States, and chronic liver disease, cirrhosis and liver failure frequently occur in this population. Its mode of transmission is not clear but includes transmission by body fluids, including by needle-sharing. Treatment of active and chronic hepatitis C is still evolving but includes the use of interferons, often accompanied by use of the antiviral agent, ribavirin (see Chapter 8).

PATHOPHYSIOLOGY AND DISEASES OF THE BILIARY TRACT

Bile consists of approximately:
- 65–90% bile salts (e.g. cholic acid, deoxycholic acid, chenodeoxycholic acid, and lithocholic acid, coupled to glycine or taurine).
- 5–25% cholesterol.
- 2–25% phospholipids.
- Bilirubin, fatty acids, electrolytes, and water.

There is a tendency for stones to form in the bile (cholelithiasis) and this is frequently accompanied by inflammation of the gallbladder (cholecystitis).

Cholelithiasis

The chemical nature of gallbladder stones varies widely, and only stones formed from cholesterol can be dissolved by drugs. Such stones are particularly common when there has been rapid weight loss (e.g. during treatment of morbid obesity).

The naturally occurring bile acid ursodiol (ursodeoxycholic acid) is the oral agent of choice for dissolving cholesterol stones. It has largely superseded chenodiol (chenodeoxycholic acid), which is associated with liver toxicity and diarrhea. Ursodiol:
- Decreases cholesterol secretion into the bile.
- May decrease cholesterol absorption from the intestine.
- May increase bile flow.

The net effect is a reduced cholesterol concentration in the bile and a tendency for dissolution of existing cholesterol stones. Cholesterol synthesis is not decreased. Ursodiol can cause diarrhea, nausea and vomiting, anxiety and depression.

CHOLECYSTITIS Since the inflammation of cholecystitis is caused by stones and bacterial infection, the definitive treatment is an appropriate antibiotic followed by surgery. Pain associated with cholecystitis can be severe, and morphine is usually required to control it. Patients with cholecystitis also need adequate intravenous fluids, as nausea and vomiting are common and can be severe.

PATHOPHYSIOLOGY AND DISEASES OF THE PANCREAS

The pancreas is an endocrine and exocrine organ that secretes insulin and glucagon into the blood and digestive enzymes into the duodenum.

PANCREATIC INFLAMMATION can be acute or chronic.
- Acute pancreatitis is a medical emergency and treatment is supportive, i.e. parenteral fluids and relief of pain, (see Chapter 14) and relief of nausea (see below).
- Chronic pancreatitis is associated with ethanol ingestion and ethanol should therefore be avoided. There can be a lack of pancreatic digestive enzymes (see Cystic fibrosis, below, for treatment).

DIABETES MELLITUS is characterized by a relative lack of the endocrine secretion of insulin and/or resistance to insulin (see Chapter 15).

CYSTIC FIBROSIS is a multisystem disorder in which secretory mechanisms are impaired, and in which the respiratory system is most affected (see Chapter 19). It is associated with a lack of pancreatic digestive enzymes, as in chronic pancreatitis. Pancreatic enzymes (lipase, amylase, and proteinase) are therefore given orally to aid fat, starch, and protein digestion. The formulations are acid-resistant so that the enzymes reach the duodenum intact.

NAUSEA AND VOMITING

Nausea frequently precedes the act of vomiting, but either may occur alone

Nausea is a highly subjective and peculiarly unpleasant sensation, normally felt in the throat or stomach as a sinking sensation in the epigastrium. Acute nausea is a temporarily unpleasant sensation that precludes other mental and physical activity and is usually relieved by an emetic episode. Chronic nausea severely reduces the quality of life.

Nausea is usually accompanied by a vasomotor (autonomic nervous system) disturbance causing pallor, sweating, and relaxation of the lower part of the esophagus and abdominal muscles. The latter tends to increase tension on the gastric and esophageal muscles, stimulating afferent nerve endings that may induce the sensation of nausea. The upper small intestine then contracts and this is closely followed by contraction of the pyloric sphincter and the pyloric portion of the stomach. These changes result in emptying of the contents of the upper jejunum, duodenum, and pyloric portion of the stomach into the fundus and body of the stomach, which are relaxed. The cardiac sphincter, the esophagus, and the esophageal sphincter are also relaxed. The gastrointestinal system is therefore prepared for retching and vomiting, which is reflex in origin and serves to remove the contents of the upper gastrointestinal tract from the body. This is useful for removing toxic material from the gut, but such an action does not provide an adequate explanation for most causes of emesis.

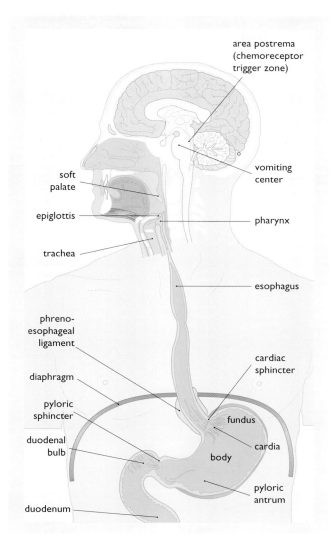

Fig. 21.15 The major visceral and central structures involved in the emetic reflex.

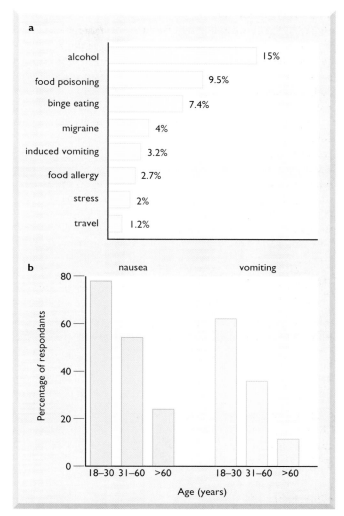

Fig. 21.16 Causes and incidence of nausea and vomiting. (a) The percentage of participants from an otherwise healthy population in the UK reporting vomiting from different causes. (b) The percentage of individuals in each group who reported nausea or vomiting at least once during the previous 12-month period.

■ *The emetic reflex involves a series of highly coordinated changes in gastrointestinal motility and respiratory movements*

Emesis is initiated by a deep and sharp inspiration and is immediately followed by reflex closure of the glottis and a raising of the soft palate, thereby preventing the passage of vomitus into the lungs and nasal cavity (Fig. 21.15). The abdominal muscles then contract in the rhythmic manner of 'retching' movements, which compress the stomach between the contracted diaphragm and abdominal organs. The inevitable increase in intragastric pressure causes evacuation of the stomach contents through the relaxed esophagus; definite antiperistalsis in the stomach itself is rarely observed. This profile of activities varies in the infant, in whom the abdominal muscles and diaphragm do not apparently play a role in, for example, regurgitation of an oversize meal; instead, the reverse peristalsis is produced by contraction of the stomach muscles alone. Reverse peristalsis originating in the upper bowel may itself be a direct cause of nausea and vomiting.

■ *Nausea and/or vomiting may result from single or, more usually, multifactorial stimuli*

The most frequent causes of nausea and emesis in an otherwise healthy population are shown in Fig. 21.16.

Pivotal events in nausea and emesis

- Relaxation of the esophagus, esophageal sphincter, cardiac sphincter, and fundus and body of the stomach
- Contraction of the upper small intestine and pyloric stomach, emptying their contents into the relaxed stomach
- Deep inspiration and closure of the glottis and raising of the soft palate
- Rhythmic contraction of the diaphragm and abdominal muscles to compress the stomach and evacuate its contents via the mouth

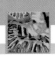

GASTROINTESTINAL IRRITATION is a frequent inducer of nausea and emesis and is produced by:

- Stimulation of mechanoreceptors by distension or obstruction in the gut.
- Stimulation of chemoreceptors responsive to bacterial endotoxins.
- The accidental or deliberate ingestion of toxic materials such as alcohol or a wide range of therapeutic agents (e.g. NSAIDs and antibiotics).

Projectile vomiting, an unusual type of vomiting of considerable force, may be observed in infants and results from pyloric stenosis.

MOTION SICKNESS Explanations of motion or movement sickness are centered around the sensory conflict that can occur between discordant visual, vestibular (the semicircular canals and otolith organs), and proprioceptive input. An essential function of the vestibular system is the development of compensatory eye movements to stabilize the retinal image of an earth-fixed visual target in the presence of head movement. This reflex is inappropriate when the visual world shares the same movement as that of the head and generates sensory conflict.

PREGNANCY SICKNESS Approximately 85% and 52% of pregnant women experience nausea and vomiting, respectively, during the first trimester. The incidence of such 'morning sickness,' which can actually occur at any time of the day, then sharply declines with the duration of pregnancy (Fig. 21.17). A very small number of women, perhaps 1/1000, show the continued vomiting of hyperemesis gravidarum. The cause of nausea and vomiting in pregnancy is unknown, but probably involves a number of factors including:

- Altered gastric function (e.g. delayed gastric emptying).
- Changes in intra-abdominal pressure.
- Metabolic changes.
- Changes in hormone function.
- Psychogenic influences.

INTRACRANIAL PATHOLOGY A sudden bout of vomiting associated with severe headache may be a consequence of a raised intracranial pressure resulting from an intracranial hemorrhage or a severe inflammatory response. It may be produced by a direct influence on the central structures coordinating the vomiting reflex, with additional inputs from nociceptors in vascular smooth muscle. Migraine (see Chapter 14) is more common and is characterized by severe unilateral headaches associated with gastrointestinal disturbances, nausea, and vomiting.

METABOLIC DISORDERS A wide variety of metabolic disorders (see Chapter 15) can induce nausea and vomiting (e.g. hypoglycemia or uremia).

PSYCHOGENIC TYPES OF NAUSEA AND RETCHING OR VOMITING include:

- Chronic psychogenic vomiting (or more commonly retching), which usually occurs on getting up or just after breakfast; it may persist for years.

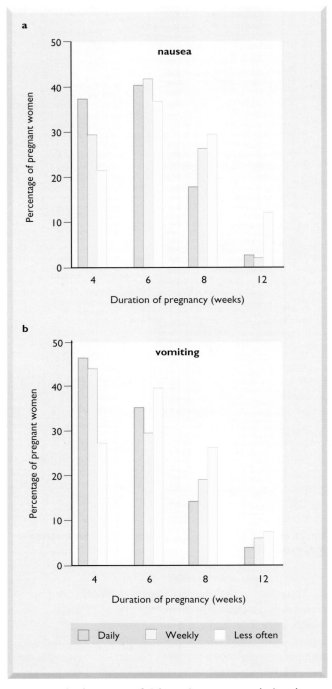

Fig. 21.17 The frequency of sickness in pregnancy during the first trimester. The majority of women who experienced daily symptoms of nausea and vomiting reported that the onset of their symptoms occurred within 4–6 weeks of their last menstruation.

- Nervous dyspepsia, which describes a feeling of satiety, abdominal discomfort, nausea, and vomiting associated with psychoneurotic features such as anxiety, irritability, and weight loss.
- Anorexia nervosa and bulimia, which have a well-established psychopathology and in which retching and/or vomiting is a symptom of serious psychiatric illness.

- Certain sights, smells, or feelings, which can trigger revulsion or fear that can cause immediate nausea and vomiting.
- Anticipatory nausea and vomiting, which occurs in up to 30% of patients with cancer and results from inadequate control of chemotherapy-induced emesis. It is a learned response and the patients associate their emetic treatment with the hospital and its personnel. Associated 'stimuli' (e.g. the hospital or nurses) can trigger emesis on sight.
- Anxiety, which predisposes to nausea and emesis.

PAIN The severe discomfort of somatic or cardiac pain or the intense pain caused by distension of the bile or urethral ducts can induce nausea and vomiting.

DRUG- AND RADIATION-INDUCED EMESIS Many compounds can induce emesis and the major classes of drugs that predictably induce nausea and vomiting include:
- Cancer chemotherapy and radiation.
- Apomorphine, levodopa, and ergot derivatives (e.g. bromocriptine, lergotrile) with dopamine agonist properties, used in the treatment of Parkinson's disease.
- Morphine and related opioid analgesics.
- Cardiac glycosides such as digoxin.
- Drugs enhancing 5-HT function.
- Miscellaneous agents (e.g. heavy metals, ipecacuanha alkaloids, veratrum alkaloids).

Many cytotoxic treatments cause dose- and regimen-related severe nausea and vomiting (Fig. 21.18). Nausea and vomiting induced by radiation is also related to the dose used and to the area and extent of the body irradiated. In addition, cytotoxic or radiation treatment frequently causes severe disruption to the gastrointestinal tract where products of tissue destruction may be released and a local inflammatory response may influence vagal afferent nerve endings within the gut to trigger the emetic reflex. The release of 5-HT from the enterochromaffin cells provides an important example. Such substances may be transported in the blood and, with the cytotoxic agents themselves, directly stimulate the central components mediating the emetic reflex.

Apomorphine, levodopa, and ergot derivatives with dopamine agonist properties, used in the treatment of Parkinson's disease, act mainly by directly stimulating the

central chemoreceptor mechanisms. They also induce gastric stasis.

Morphine and related opioid analgesics have probably the most complex mechanisms of action of any drugs that cause nausea and vomiting. Acute administration of such agents to opioid-naive patients frequently induces nausea and sometimes vomiting. However, tolerance develops rapidly to such effects and the first treatment antagonizes the emetic effects to a second opioid injection or other emetogens. The emetic potential may be mediated in the chemoreceptor trigger zone (CTZ), whereas the 'broad-spectrum' antiemetic effect may be mediated downstream from the CTZ and close to the 'vomiting center.' The antiemetic effect may relate to an endogenous tone exerted by opioids from the enkephalin, dynorphin, or the pro-opiomelanocortin series. The ability of narcotic antagonists such as naloxone to precipitate nausea or vomiting supports this hypothesis.

Cardiac glycosides such as digoxin can induce abdominal pains, nausea, and vomiting. This probably relates to a central action on the CTZ and an irritant action within the gastrointestinal tract, which may be worsened by a cardiac arrhythmia.

Drugs enhancing 5-HT function (e.g. 5-hydroxytryptophan, the precursor of 5-HT, or selective serotonin reuptake inhibitors (SSRIs) such as fluoxetine and paroxetine; see Chapter 14) have been reported to induce nausea and occasionally vomiting. This may relate to increased 5-HT activity in both the brain and intestine.

When administered orally, heavy metals such as copper sulfate, zinc sulfate, antimony, and mercuric chloride have an irritant action in the gut, triggering the emetic reflex via vagal and splanchnic nerves. Some of these agents may also directly stimulate the central mechanisms. The ipecacuanha alkaloids also stimulate peripheral and central mechanisms, while veratrum alkaloids stimulate the nodose ganglia of the vagus to trigger the emetic reflex.

POSTOPERATIVE NAUSEA AND VOMITING (PONV) provides one of the best examples of the multifactorial nature of nausea and vomiting. It may be triggered by:
- Inhalational agents, particularly nitrous oxide, which are variably associated with PONV.
- Intravenous anesthetics and spinal anesthesia.

Emetic potential of chemotherapeutic drugs

Severely emetogenic in almost all patients	Moderately emetogenic	Least emetogenic
Cisplatin	Mitomycin C	5-Fluorouracil
Mustine	Procarbazine	Cytarabine
Cyclophosphamide	Nitrosoureas	6-Mercaptopurine
Dacarbazine		Bleomycin
Doxorubicin		Vinblastine
		Vincristine

Fig. 21.18 Emetic potential of chemotherapeutic drugs.

Major stimuli of nausea and vomiting

- Gastrointestinal irritation
- Motion sickness
- Hormone disturbance
- Intracranial pathology
- Metabolic disorders
- Psychogenic factors
- Pain
- Drugs and radiation
- Endogenous toxins

- Certain types of surgery, particularly gynecologic, pediatric strabismus, and abdominal surgery. The latter can cause stretching, distension, or tissue damage (i.e. gastrointestinal irritation).
- Pain resulting from surgery or disease.
- Hypoxia, hypotension, and carbon dioxide retention.
- Clumsy movement of the patient in the recovery room or ward or following day-case surgery, causing a labyrinthine disturbance.
- Certain pre- or postoperative drug treatments (e.g. opioid analgesics).
- Psychogenic factors such as anxiety.
- A high body weight.
- Sex and age. The risk of PONV is three times higher in adult females than in adult males, and children are twice as susceptible as adults.

Individual responses to many emetic stimuli vary widely

Even the simple introduction of a spatula into the mouth to facilitate oral examination will immediately provoke a 'gagging' reflex in some people. Approximately 70% of women suffer PONV following gynecologic surgery, but it is not possible to identify those at risk. Patients who have had nausea and vomiting following previous surgery are likely to experience it again. Furthermore, women who experience pregnancy sickness are much more likely to develop nausea and vomiting in response to any hormonal disturbance (e.g. the contraceptive pill) or to traveling, and with migraine (Fig. 21.19). Also, people who have an emetic response to a first drug challenge are likely to show a similar response to a subsequent challenge (i.e. individuals tend to have consistent responses). A simple enquiry may therefore identify people at greater risk (those who have a lower emetic threshold). These people are particularly likely to develop nausea and vomiting under emotional strain.

The frequency and intensity of episodes of nausea and vomiting vary enormously

A single short-lived bout of emesis induced by a single psychogenic stimulus is quite different from the intense, intractable,

The number of women who reported sickness with oral contraceptives, travel, or migraine and the relationship to vomiting in pregnancy

Pregnancy sickness	Oral contraceptive sickness	Travel sickness	Migraine sickness
Vomiting	30 (70%)	77 (63%)	45 (65%)
No vomiting	13 (30%)	46 (37%)	24 (35%)

Fig. 21.19 The number of women who reported sickness with oral contraceptives, travel, or migraine, and the relationship to vomiting in pregnancy. There was a higher than expected incidence of vomiting during pregnancy in these groups of women than in women who had no sickness.

and devastating nausea and vomiting caused by highly emetogenic chemotherapy. The first is unpredictable and therefore untreatable by drugs, but the latter can now be efficiently managed in most patients.

The consequences of vomiting pose different problems to patient and clinician

To the patient, either a brief or persistent period of vomiting is always of concern. However, a brief period of vomiting in an otherwise healthy individual generally poses little medical risk, whereas, in the postoperative patient, even a brief but powerful period of retching or vomiting can cause tissue rupture. Not only will persistent nausea and vomiting incapacitate the patient, but the persistent vomiting may result in the loss of hydrochloric acid, leading to alkalosis and dehydration.

Persistent nausea or vomiting may be symptoms of an underlying disease

Persistent nausea or vomiting may be indicative of gastrointestinal, neurologic, or metabolic disorders that require direct treatment, and it may be desirable to withhold antiemetic therapy until a diagnosis has been made.

Both central and peripheral systems mediate nausea and emesis

The causes of emesis provide vital clues to the stimuli influencing the emetic reflex, although the precise circuitry and transmitter mechanisms mediating the reflex remain largely unknown. However, key structures and pathways are now being identified, based on the results, obtained almost exclusively from animals, of central and peripheral nerve lesions, intracerebral injection of drugs into discrete brain regions, and electrophysiologic stimulation of discrete brain regions (Figs 21.20, 21.21.).

THE CHEMORECEPTOR TRIGGER ZONE (CTZ) is a key structure in mediating nausea and vomiting and is located within the area postrema, a circumventricular organ located at the caudal end of the fourth ventricle. It lacks an effective blood–brain barrier and is therefore ideally suited for detecting emetic agents in both the systemic circulation and the cerebrospinal fluid (CSF). A lesion of the CTZ abolishes the emetic response to many emetogens. The area postrema has numerous afferent and efferent connections with the underlying structures, the subnucleus gelatinosus and nucleus tractus solitarius. These brain regions are also important structures in the emetic reflex and, with the area postrema, receive vagal afferent fibers from the gastrointestinal tract, which is a major source of emetic stimuli.

THE 'VOMITING CENTER' is a second major 'structure' mediating nausea and vomiting and is more accurately described as a collection of effector nuclei rather than a discrete brain area. It receives major inputs from:
- The CTZ.
- The gut, of a vagal and sympathetic form.
- The cardiovascular system.

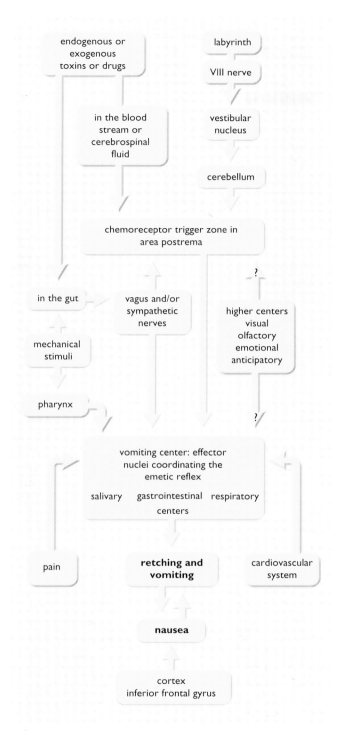

Fig. 21.20 The major emetic stimuli, pathways, and structures mediating the emetic reflex and nausea.

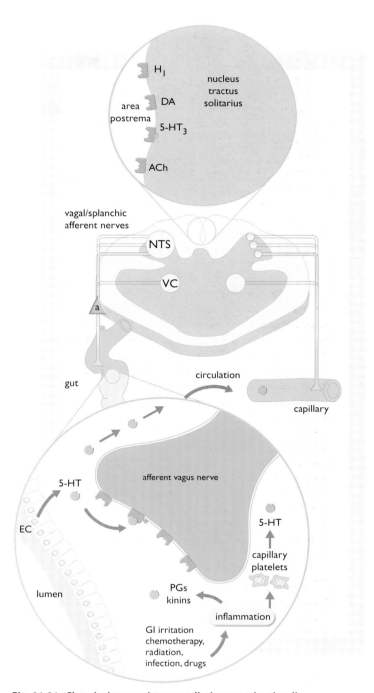

Fig. 21.21 Chemical transmitters mediating emetic stimuli.
Stimuli in the gastrointestinal tract cause nausea and vomiting via neuronal (vagus nerve) and blood-borne influences on the central chemoreceptor trigger zone in the area postrema and nucleus tractus solitarius (NTS) and the 'vomiting center' (VC). 5-hydroxytryptamine (5-HT) released from the enterochromaffin cells (ECs), and possibly platelets acting on 5-HT$_3$ receptors, may play a major role, along with inflammatory mediators released in the vicinity of afferent nerve endings. (GI, gastrointestinal; PGs, prostaglandins)

- A variety of limbic brain nuclei (e.g. the olfactory tubercle, amygdala, hypothalamus, and ventral thalamic nucleus). Electrical stimulation of all these structures can induce emesis. The latter nuclei may be involved in olfactory, emotional/ anticipatory, hormonal/stress, and pain-induced vomiting, respectively. The location of the visual inputs to the emetic circuitry remains unknown.

THE BRAIN REGIONS THAT PRODUCE THE SENSATION OF NAU-SEA have been difficult to determine, since nausea is a subjective experience and animal models are not available. However, noninvasive magnetic source imaging has recently revealed that there is neuronal activation in the cortex in the inferior frontal gyrus, in volunteers nauseated by ipecacuanha or vestibular stimulation. The activation caused by ipecacuanha, but not by vestibular stimulation, was antagonized by the 5-HT receptor antagonist, ondansetron (see below). This brain area may therefore be important in the perception or sensation of nausea.

◼ Retching, vomiting, or regurgitation occasionally constitute a medical or surgical emergency

Retching, vomiting, or regurgitation occasionally needs emergency treatment for example:

- When induced by major intracranial pathology or intestinal obstruction.
- In infants, where fluid loss may cause dehydration.
- When the force of retching or vomiting tears esophageal tissue.
- In emergency surgery, when the patient has recently had a meal and therefore has a high risk of developing aspiration pneumonia. This is an important cause of death in pregnant women.
- In patients with a defective gag reflex, who have a high risk of developing aspiration pneumonia.
- When it is due to hyperemesis gravidarum.

◼ The preferred treatment of nausea and vomiting is removal of the cause

Treatment of the cardiovascular pathology in migraine with the 5-HT$_1$ receptor agonist sumatriptan will relieve the neurologic manifestations, headache, gastrointestinal effects, and nausea and vomiting, despite sumatriptan's having no direct effect on the emetic reflex (Fig. 21.21).

◼ Antiemetic therapy can be life-saving for patients with cancer

Patients with cancer will more readily accept or continue with what may be a curative course of chemotherapy if they are given effective antiemetic therapy. More aggressive chemotherapy regimens with a greater chance of eradicating the tumor can now be given without producing an unacceptable incidence of nausea and vomiting.

Drugs used for the symptomatic relief of nausea and vomiting (Fig. 21.22)

Symptomatic control of nausea and vomiting involves using drugs and procedures that affect the emetic reflex.

Although acute nausea itself poses no medical problem, it is a very distressing symptom and can cause as much suffering as pain. Indeed, a bout of retching or vomiting may be welcomed by the patient because it terminates the feeling of nausea. Persistent nausea usually leads to a loss of appetite, a reduced food intake, malnutrition, and serious debilitation, requiring prompt medical treatment.

There are now at least four major groups of compounds to control nausea and emesis. Procedures and treatments that alleviate retching and vomiting generally prevent nausea.

Inadequate control of the first bout of nausea and vomiting may compromise the treatment of later episodes.

Drugs used for the symptomatic relief of nausea and vomiting include:

- 5-HT$_3$ receptor antagonists.
- Dopamine receptor antagonists.
- Muscarinic receptor antagonists.
- Histamine H$_1$ receptor antagonists.
- Sedatives and hypnotics.
- Phenothiazines.

Dopamine receptor antagonists

Dopamine and dopamine receptors are found in high concentrations in the area postrema, the dorsal motor nucleus of the vagus nerve, and the nucleus tractus solitarius. The traditional view has been that apomorphine, levodopa (via dopamine), lergotrile, bromocriptine, and other dopamine agonists used in the treatment of Parkinson's disease induce nausea and vomiting by stimulating dopamine receptors in the CTZ. Dopamine receptor antagonists block such receptors and thereby prevent nausea and emesis.

SPECIFIC DOPAMINE RECEPTOR ANTAGONISTS (e.g. **HALOPERIDOL AND FLUPHENAZINE**) The use of these drugs is limited in two ways:

- First, they do not inhibit nausea and emesis induced by stimuli other than dopamine agonists (although droperidol is used in PONV, see below).
- Second, they have major adverse effects of motor impairment, severe akinesia and muscle rigidity, and dystonias (muscle spasm) caused by striatal dopamine receptor blockade, particularly in young people.

The adverse effects are less with domperidone and sulpiride because they are less able to penetrate the blood–brain barrier in the striatal areas, but can easily access structures such as the area postrema, which lack a blood–brain barrier.

METOCLOPRAMIDE is a dopamine receptor antagonist that has been widely used as an antinauseant/antiemetic for gastrointestinal disorders and migraine and, in much higher doses, for cancer chemotherapy- and radiation-induced sickness. Its unusual and established ability to facilitate gastric emptying

Drugs used for the treatment of nausea and vomiting

	Drug	Half-life (hours)	Bioavailability (%)	Elimination	Comments
Dopamine receptor antagonists	Chlorpromazine	8–35	Highly variable via oral route, 10–37	Hepatic metabolism	Given orally, rectally or by intramuscular injection; strong anticholinergic and α-adrenergic blocking activity, sedation, hypotension. Antipsychotic. Extrapyramidal side-effects. Low systemic bioavailability due to extensive presystemic metabolism. There are possibly more than 100 metabolites which vary widely from one person to another
	Domperidone	12–16	93	Gut wall and liver	Given orally or rectally; low bioavailability (about 15%). Penetrates CNS poorly. Low CNS effect. Stimulates lower esophageal sphincter and gastric emptying. Used in gastroesophageal reflux disease. Can cause hyperprolactinemia. Used for gastroesophageal reflux disease
	Metoclopramide	3–5	>90	Hepatic metabolism + renal	Given orally or by intramuscular injection or intravenous injection; bioavailability 40–100%. Crosses blood–brain barrier. Indications as for domperidone. Causes drowsiness, hyperprolactinemia. Renal failure may alter pharmacokinetics
	Perphenazine	9		Metabolism	Given orally; low oral bioavailability (30–40%). Indications and side-effects as chlorpromazine but less anticholinergic and α-adrenoceptor blocking activity
	Prochlorperazine	6–7	>80	Hepatic metabolism	Given orally, rectally or by deep intramuscular injection; variable absorption of oral doses. Indications and side-effects as for perphenazine. Extensive first-pass metabolism
	Trifluoperazine	7–18		Metabolism	Given orally; oral bioavailability has not been defined; numerous metabolites formed. Indications and side-effects as for perphenazine but weaker anticholinergic and α-adrenergic blocking activity
	Droperidol	12–16	75	Hepatic metabolism	Undergoes enterohepatic recirculation. May enhance the absorption of drugs administered concomitantly
Antimuscarinics	Dimenhydrinate	2.4–8	72	Hepatic	May inhibit CYP ZD6. Peak plasma concentrations amongst caucasian subjects are greater than in orientals who have higher mean volumes of distribution and 70% greater mean clearance values
	Hyoscine (scopolamine)	8		Metabolism	Given orally for motion sickness and vertigo; not as effective for treatment of nausea from other causes; drowsiness; less active than atropine on heart, bronchial, and gastrointestinal smooth muscle
Antihistamines	Cinnarizine	3		Metabolism	Given orally for motion sickness. Mechanism of action is speculative; sedative
	Cyclizine	20		Metabolism	Given orally for motion sickness and vertigo; acts by H₁ receptor blockade but also muscarinic blocking activity. CNS depressant, sedative
	Dimenhydrinate	3.5		Metabolism	Given orally for motion sickness and vertigo. Anticholinergic; CNS depressant, sedative

Drugs used for the treatment of nausea and vomiting (Continued)

	Drug	Half-life (hours)	Bioavailability (%)	Elimination	Comments
Antihistamines	Promethazine	7–14	>80	Hepatic metabolism	Given orally; a phenothiazine having antihistamine (H₁ receptors) anticholinergic and weak antidopaminergic actions; sedative. Extensive first-pass metabolism, probably with biliary excretion being the major route of excretion
5-HT₃ receptor antagonists	Granisetron	3–9	41–66	Hepatic metabolism (+ some renal)	Given orally or by intravenous injection or infusion; oral bioavailability is 40–70%. Given alone or with dexamethasone. Central and peripheral mechanisms of action, constipation, headache. Variable metabolism by P-450 enzymes. Particular use in reducing nausea and vomiting induced by chemotherapy or radiotherapy. CYP 3A appears to be involved in metabolism
	Ondansetron	3	59	Hepatic metabolism	Given orally, rectally, by intramuscular injection or by slow intravenous infusion. Other details as for granisetron
	Tropisetron	6–7		Metabolism	Given by slow intravenous injection or infusion followed by oral dosage. Other details as for granisetron
	Dolasetron	0.13–0.25 (mean 7; see Comment)	>85	Hepatic metabolism	There is extensive presystemic metabolism to produce an active metabolite (MDL 74156), and following oral administration the plasma concentrations of dolasetron are low
Drug sedatives, hypnotics, and nabilone	Barbiturates, e.g. pentobarbital	20–30	100	Hepatic	Half-life is shorter following chronic dosing, due to autoinduction of metabolism
	Benzodiazepines, e.g. diazepam	30	100	Hepatic	Peak plasma concentrations achieved at 15 to 90 minutes in adults and 15 to 30 minutes in children; a secondary peak occurs at 6 to 12 hours due to enterohepatic recirculation. There are active metabolites with plasma half-lifes of 30 to 200 hours or longer in patients over 65 years of age
	Chloral hydrate	8–12 (See Comment)	100	Hepatic	Chloral hydrate is reduced to an active metabolite trichloroethanol
	Cannabis (delta 9-tetrahydrocannabinol)	20–36	Low	Hepatic	Converted to an active metabolite 11-hydroxy-delta 9-tetrahydrocannabinol

Fig. 21.22 Drugs used for the treatment of nausea and vomiting.

and intestinal activity may contribute directly to its anti-nauseant/antiemetic actions in gastrointestinal disorders and migraine. However, such actions do not reflect a dopamine receptor blockade, but more probably an agonist action at the 5-HT$_4$ receptor. Furthermore, its ability to prevent chemotherapy- or radiation-induced emesis when used in exceptionally high doses is more readily attributed to its low potency 5-HT$_3$ receptor antagonism (see below).

Muscarinic receptor antagonists (see Chapter 14)

Scopalamine is the most effective remedy for motion sickness of all types, although nausea and vomiting induced by extreme changes in motion and space travel remains an intractable problem, and it fails to control all types of movement sickness (e.g. due to severe vestibular disturbance). Scopalamine has a greater central depressant effect than atropine and its antiemetic action is attributed to a blockade of muscarinic cholinergic receptors in the area postrema or associated nuclei of the dorsal vagal complex. Scopalamine is also a potent inhibitor of gastrointestinal movements and relaxes the gastrointestinal tract, and these effects may make a modest contribution to the antiemetic action.

Adverse effects of scopalamine include sedation and predictable autonomic adverse effects with increase of dose (e.g. blurred vision, urinary retention, decreased salivation). The sedation and blurred vision preclude its use by airline pilots, train, bus, and car drivers, and those operating machinery.

Histamine H$_1$ receptor antagonists

Antihistamines used for motion sickness include buclizine, cyclizine, dimenhydrinate, meclizine, and promethazine. Their antiemetic actions are attributed to a central blockade of H$_1$ receptors in the area postrema and possibly underlying structures. However, most antihistamines are also potent muscarinic receptor antagonists, and this behavior may make an important contribution to their antiemetic actions. Indeed, chlorpheniramine, which is an H$_1$ receptor antagonist that fails to block centrally mediated cholinergic effects, does not inhibit motion sickness. Whatever the contribution of H$_1$ and ACh receptor blockade to the antiemetic potential, a sedative capability may also contribute to the effect, although this is less or absent for cinnarizine. However, some antihistamines that cause sedation are not antiemetic and in addition sedation can be a dangerous adverse effect in those operating machinery or driving vehicles. The H$_1$ receptor antagonists may play some role in the treatment of PONV and pregnancy sickness.

5-HT$_3$ receptor antagonists

Ondansetron, granisetron, and tropisetron are all 5-HT antagonists and the most recently introduced antiemetic agents. Their ability to antagonize chemotherapy- and radiation-induced emesis was first established in animal models in 1986. Their efficacy relates to blockade of 5-HT$_3$ receptors, which are located in high density:

- In the area postrema and nucleus tractus solitarius.
- On vagal afferent nerve endings in the gut.

It is hypothesized that severely emetogenic regimens such as cisplatin cause gastrointestinal tissue disruption, which initiates the release of 5-HT from the enterochromaffin cells within the mucosa. 5-Hydroxyindoleacetic acid, the metabolite of 5-HT, can then be detected in increased amounts in the urine. It is hypothesized that the release of 5-HT stimulates 5-HT$_3$ receptors located on vagal afferent nerve endings and trigger vagus nerve firing to initiate the emetic reflex. The 5-HT$_3$ receptors within the area postrema/nucleus tractus solitarius lie on the vagus nerve terminals, since they disappear if the vagus is cut (Fig. 21.21).

Ondansetron and the other 5-HT$_3$ receptor antagonists control nausea, retching, and vomiting in patients with cancer receiving emetogenic treatments, especially during the acute phase (i.e. day 1 of treatment); the symptoms are completely controlled in 70% of patients and there is reduced vomiting in the others. However, on the second and subsequent days (i.e. a 'delayed phase') the antiemetic effects are less pronounced and the addition of a glucocorticosteroid is needed to produce a maximally efficacious antiemetic regimen. Dexamethasone or methylprednisolone are now frequently used in combination with ondansetron or other 5-HT$_3$ receptor antagonists to secure optimal control, even on the first day of treatment. This is vitally important for the patient with cancer, since the development of almost any nausea and vomiting during treatment can lead to a learned 'anticipatory nausea,' which is characterized by nausea and vomiting at all future treatments and even at the sight of the nursing staff or hospital where the treatment was initially given. Such anticipatory nausea is resistant to all drug treatments, including the 5-HT$_3$ receptor antagonists.

The 5-HT$_3$ receptor antagonists have no effect on motion sickness or apomorphine-induced vomiting. They will, however, block the vomiting induced by ipecacuanha. Ondansetron has also been shown to antagonize:

- The nausea induced by morphine.
- The nausea and gastrointestinal adverse effects of SSRIs.

Its use in the treatment of other causes of gastrointestinal irritation is being investigated.

ADVERSE EFFECTS OF 5-HT$_3$ RECEPTOR ANTAGONISTS 5-HT$_3$ receptor antagonists have a remarkable safety profile, their use being accompanied by a small incidence of headache, constipation, and a sensation of warmth or flushing.

MAJOR ADVANTAGES OF 5-HT$_3$ RECEPTOR ANTAGONISTS are that they are not sedative, they do not interact with other drugs, and they do not cause generalized autonomic adverse effects, endocrine changes, or motor impairments. This contrasts with the endocrine and motor impairments induced by metoclopramide, which blocks dopamine and 5-HT$_3$ receptors, at the same concentration. Before the availability of ondansetron, the most effective control of chemotherapy- and radiation-induced vomiting had been achieved by the empirical use of exceptionally high doses of metoclopramide.

■ Ondansetron is the drug of choice in the treatment of PONV

The lack of interaction between 5-HT$_3$ receptor antagonists and other drugs prompted the use of ondansetron in the treatment of PONV, for which it is as efficacious as any of the existing remedies (e.g. cyclizine, droperidol), but does not produce their adverse effects. Also, ondansetron does not adversely affect the course of anesthesia or postoperative recovery. It is effective in approximately 60% of patients. Its mechanism of action is thought to relate to a central and peripheral 5-HT$_3$ receptor blockade to attenuate the overall influence of the many factors triggering PONV.

Phenothiazines

Agents such as chlorpromazine, promethazine, prochlorperazine, and trimeprazine have a mixed pharmacology as antagonists at muscarinic, histaminergic, dopaminergic, adrenergic, and serotonergic receptors. Nausea and vomiting that fails to respond to specific pharmacologic treatments may sometimes respond to this multireceptor blockade (e.g. pregnancy sickness, PONV). As the mechanisms mediating most types of nausea and vomiting are not clear, but there may be many different contributary stimuli, the use of a 'mixed' pharmacologic approach is logical.

Sedatives and hypnotics

Vomiting is blocked by anesthesia and lesser degrees of CNS depression, which may attenuate a low emetic threshold that would normally trigger intractable nausea and vomiting. Barbiturates and chloral hydrate have been used, but benzodiazepines are a more contemporary treatment and have the advantage of causing amnesia to prevent recall of a highly distressing event. However, caution is needed as the potential for vomiting or aspiration, in the presence of reduced consciousness with a reduction or loss of reflex closure of the trachea, can be catastrophic.

Ancillary treatments of nausea and vomiting

Movement disturbance and visual, olfactory, and emotional psychogenic factors are potent but variable emetic stimuli and can be expected to contribute to the development of nausea and vomiting in many, and perhaps most, patients. For example:

- The residual vomiting of patients with cancer placed on an open ward after 5-HT$_3$ receptor antagonism could well be partly psychogenic rather than an exclusively chemotherapy-induced vomiting.
- The sight, sound, or smell of just one other patient who is vomiting is sufficient to trigger the same response in others.

Arrangements should therefore be made to avoid, obviate, or reduce the likelihood of such occurrences.

The apparent effectiveness of histamine H$_1$ receptor antagonists in pregnancy sickness in some patients may reflect a vestibular stimulus from disturbed movement. If so, alternative approaches might be considered to reduce movements. This is particularly important in the pregnant patient, in whom drug treatments should not be used unless unavoidable, because of the risk of teratogenicity.

■ *Nausea and vomiting is often best managed using a combination of ancillary and drug treatments*

Since individuals have such marked variations in their response to emetic stimuli, and the various stimuli contributing to

---

> 🔑 **Treating nausea and vomiting**
>
> - Medical, surgical, or psychiatric procedures are used to alleviate the cause
> - Provide an environment for the patient to adopt a supine position with no visual, olfactory, vestibular, or emotional precipitants of nausea or vomiting
> - Pharmacologic blockade at specific neurotransmitter receptor sites within the vomiting reflex
> - Psychologic procedures to offer relaxation and reassurance and relieve anxiety
> - Advice about modifying eating habits
> - Acupuncture at the Neiguan point (the sixth point on the pericardial meridian)

nausea and vomiting may differ between patients, there is probably no absolute antiemetic regimen for any one clinical presentation (e.g. pregnancy sickness, PONV). Many clinical presentations of nausea and vomiting are potentially multifactorial and therefore the use of ancillary and combined drug treatments should be considered to achieve optimal control. Psychogenic stimuli and vestibular disturbance should be reduced to a minimum with nondrug treatments, and then residual symptoms of motion sickness should be treated with antihistamines or scopolamine, and gastrointestinal irritation with 5-HT$_3$ receptor antagonists. Potential antinausea/antiemetic regimens are shown in Fig. 21.23.

Therapeutic induction of vomiting

This has three aims:

- To administer an emetic agent such as apomorphine with a drug of abuse or an aldehyde dehydrogenase inhibitor with alcohol, so that the unpleasant act of nausea and vomiting is associated with drug abuse. Aversion therapy of this nature is of doubtful value and there is a risk of inappropriate drug interactions.
- To include subemetic doses of apomorphine or other emetic agents in proprietary products such as methadone and acetaminophen, to ensure that accidental or deliberate overdose will produce a dose of emetogen sufficient to empty the stomach contents.
- To use mechanical stimuli (e.g. a finger in the pharynx) or irritant solutions (e.g. saline, ipecacuanha), administered orally as an emergency procedure, to trigger the gagging and emetic reflex and empty the stomach following the ingestion of toxic material. This is carried out only if there is no erosion of the gastrointestinal tract and gastric lavage is not feasible.

Future developments in antiemetic therapy

A disadvantage of present antiemetic therapy is that different antiemetic agents are needed to treat vomiting arising from different stimuli, which appear to influence many different peripheral and central mechanisms. Present research is aimed at inhibiting the 'vomiting center' more directly, to stop the emetic reflex at its final output. The goal is to develop a

The treatment of nausea and vomiting

Cause of nausea and vomiting	Symptomatic and other treatments	Adverse effects
In all cases reduce psychogenic and vestibular stimuli to a minimum and give appropriate reassurance		
Gastrointestinal irritation	Ondansetron Metoclopramide Phenothiazines	Headache, constipation, and warmth or flushing Extrapyramidal adverse effects Anticholinergic adverse effects and sedation
Motion sickness	Hyoscine or antihistamine	Anticholinergic adverse effects and sedation
Pregnancy sickness	Advice on diet and dangers to the fetus of using drugs	Teratogenicity
If nausea or vomiting remains unacceptable use phenothiazine, antihistamine, or ondansetron		
Chronic psychogenic retching/vomiting	Psychiatric referral: no useful drug treatment	
Severe pain	Opioid analgesics	Respiratory depression, constipation
Dopamine agonist therapy in the parkinsonian patient	Domperidone, sulpiride; adjust dose of dopamine agonist	
Parkinsonian patients are exceptionally sensitive to neuroleptic-induced extrapyramidal adverse effects		
Morphine and opioid compounds	Phenothiazine Ondansetron	Anticholinergic adverse effects and sedation Headache, constipation, and warmth or flushing
Cardiac glycosides	Reduce dose of cardiac glycoside	
Drugs enhancing 5-HT function (e.g. SSRIs)	Ondansetron; adjust dose of 5-HT agonist	Headache, constipation, and warmth or flushing
Cancer chemotherapy/radiation treatment	Ondansetron/granisetron/tropisetron plus glucocorticosteroid	Headache, constipation, and warmth or flushing
Pyloric stenosis	Scopolamine butylbromide before surgery	Anticholinergic adverse effects
Postoperative nausea and vomiting	Ondansetron	Headache, constipation, and warmth or flushing

Fig. 21.23 The treatment of nausea and vomiting. (5-HT, 5-hydroxytryptamine; SSRIs, selective serotonin reuptake inhibitors)

treatment that can block all forms of vomiting (i.e. a 'broad-spectrum' antiemetic). For example, in animals, substance P antagonists block vomiting caused by all agents so far examined. However, it will be essential, if any such therapies are to be of significant clinical value, that they also antagonize nausea.

FURTHER READING

Bell SJ, Kamm MA. The clinical role of anti- TNFalpha antibody treatment in Crohn's disease. *Aliment Pharmacol Ther* 2000; **14**: 501–514.

Camilleri M. Clinical evidence to support current therapies of irritable bowel syndrome. *Aliment Pharmacol Ther* 1999; **13**: 48–53.

Farthing MJ. Irritable bowel syndrome: new pharmaceutical approaches to treatment. *Baillière's Best Pract Res Clin Gastroenterol* 1999; **13**: 461–471.

Farthing KJ. Diarrhoea: a significant worldwide problem. *Int J Antimicrob Agents* 2000; **14**: 65–69.

Graham DY. Therapy of *Helicobacter pylori*: current status and issues. *Gastroenterology* 2000; **118**: S2–S8.

Hoffman JC, Zeitz M. Treatment of Crohn's disease. *Hepatogastroenterology* 2000; **47**: 90–100.

Kenny GNC. Risk factors for postoperative nausea and vomiting. *Anaesthesia* 1994; **49** (Suppl): 6–10. [Illustrates the different stimuli that may trigger emesis.]

Ladabaum U, Hasler WL. Novel approaches to the treatment of nausea and vomiting. *Dig Dis* 1999; **17**: 125–132.

Maton PN, Burton ME. Antacids revisited: a review of their clinical pharmacology and recommended therapeutic use. *Drugs* 1999; **57**: 855–870.

Metz DC, Kroser JA. Helicobacter pylori and gastroesophageal reflux disease. *Gastroenterol Clin N Am* 1999; **28**: 971–985.

Miller AD. Physiology of the brain stem emetic circuitry. In: Bianchi AL, Grélot L, Miller AD, King GL (eds) *Mechanisms and Control of Emesis, vol 223*. Colloque INSERM: John Libbey Eurotext; 1992, pp. 41–50. [Indicates the brain systems mediating emesis.]

Millward-Sadler GH, Wright R, Arthur MJP (eds) *Liver and Biliary Disease (I and II)*. London: WB Saunders; 1992. [These are a classic pair of books for understanding the basic sciences and correlates in liver disease.]

Naylor RJ, Rudd JA. Emesis and antiemesis. In: Hanks GW, Sidebottom E (eds) *Cancer Surveys: Palliative Medicine—Problem Areas in Pain and Symptom Management, vol 21*. Cold Spring Harbor Laboratory: Cold Spring Harbor Laboratory Press; 1994, pp. 117–135. [A review of drug-induced emesis and its treatment.]

Rizk AN, Hesketh PJ. Antiemetics for cancer chemotherapy-induced nausea and vomiting. A review of agents in development. *Drugs RD* 1999; **2**: 229–235.

Stot JRR. Prevention and treatment of motion sickness in man. In: Bianchi AL, Grélot L, Miller AD, King GL (eds) *Mechanisms and Control of Emesis, vol 223*. Colloque INSERM: John Libbey Eurotext; 1992, pp. 203–211. [A review of the prevention and treatment of motion sickness in man.]

Walsh JH, Peterson WL. The treatment of *Helicobacter pylori* infection in the management of peptic ulcer disease. *N Engl J Med* 1995; **333**: 984. [This article outlines the current thinking in the treatments of ulcer disease.]

Welage LS, Berardi RR. Evaluation of omeprazole, lansoprazole, pantoprazole, and rabeprazole in the treatment of acid-related diseases. *J Am Pharm Assoc* 2000; **40**: 52–62.

Whitehead SA, Holden WA, Andrews PLR. Pregnancy sickness. In: Bianchi AL, Grélot L, Miller AD, King GL (eds) *Mechanisms and Control of Emesis, vol 223*. Colloque INSERM: John Libbey Eurotext; 1992, pp. 297–306. [An account of the factors contributing to pregnancy sickness.]

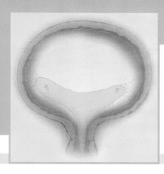
Drugs and the Genitourinary System

The genitourinary system can be conveniently subdivided into organs involved in the storage and controlled voiding of urine (e.g. bladder and urethra) and those involved in male and female reproductive physiology (e.g. ovaries, uterus, testes and vas deferens). Although the prostate is functionally part of the latter system, as the abnormal pathophysiology of this gland manifests clinically as a voiding disorder, it is discussed in this chapter in the context of its role in the micturition reflex.

PHYSIOLOGY OF THE LOWER URINARY TRACT

■ *The micturition reflex is an integrated response that results in the controlled voiding of urine*

The lower urinary tract includes the detrusor muscle, the trigone and urethra (Fig. 22.1). Under normal circumstances both autonomic and central pathways control the micturition reflex.

The lower urinary tract is innervated by the parasympathetic, somatic and sympathetic nervous systems (Figs 22.2, 22.3). The innervation of the detrusor smooth muscle is predominantly cholinergic with the neurotransmitter, namely acetylcholine, activating postsynaptic muscarinic receptors to produce bladder contraction and emptying. Of the known muscarinic subtypes so far identified, it is the M_3 receptor that is primarily involved in the activation of bladder contraction. In contrast, the adrenergic innervation of the detrusor is relatively sparse and the neurotransmitter, norepinephrine, produces relaxation, largely via β_2 adrenoceptors. It is assumed that sympathetic activity during bladder filling facilitates urine storage by relaxing the detrusor and thereby increasing functional bladder capacity although its physiologic significance in humans appears very limited. Ultimately, however, distension of the detrusor will initiate the micturition reflex (Fig. 22.2).

a

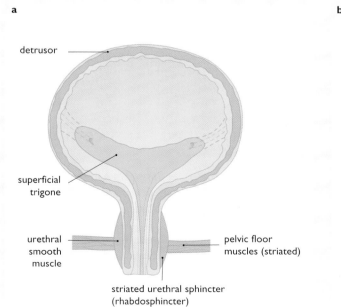

b

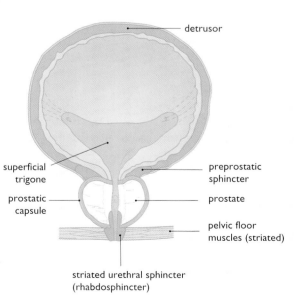

Fig. 22.1 Structure of the lower urinary tract in women (a) and in men (b).

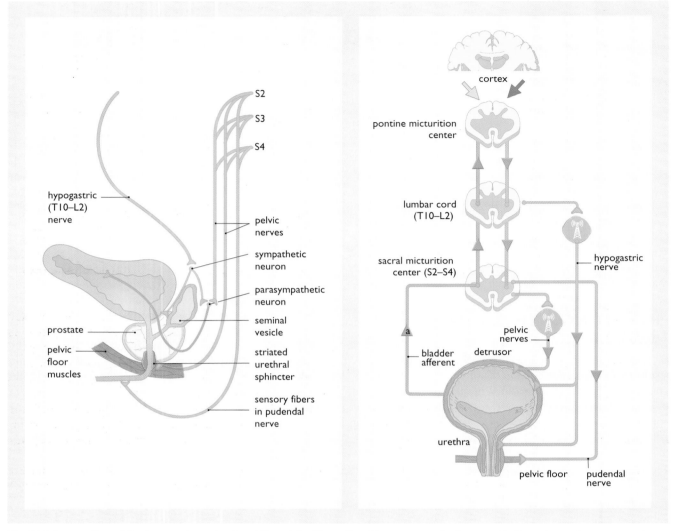

Fig. 22.2 Innervation of the lower urinary tract and the micturition reflex. The parasympathetic, sympathetic, and somatic nervous systems supply the lower urinary tract through the pelvic, hypogastric, and pudendal nerves. The afferent branch of the micturition reflex runs in the spinal cord via the dorsal root ganglia to the pontine micturition center which is under voluntary control. The efferent branch runs from the pontine micturition center to the sacral micturition center, from which the preganglionic nerves run to the pelvic plexus and then to the bladder to cause contraction. At the same time, the efferent branch inhibits the hypogastric and pudendal nerves, leading to relaxation of the outflow region and the pelvic floor.

Normally, continence is maintained by counterbalancing actions within the urogenital sinus. The major outflow conduits of trigone and urethra have a rich adrenergic innervation. During filling, the norepinephrine released by tonic sympathetic nervous activity acts on α_1 adrenoceptors to maintain urethral closure. The urethra also contains a striated muscle component, located in the external urethral sphincter (rhabdosphincter) that together with the pelvic floor muscles plays an important role in maintaining continence.

In males the urethra has to pass through the prostate. Urethral resistance can be profoundly altered by the size of the prostate and/or the tone of the surrounding peri-urethral smooth muscle. The contractile state of the prostatic smooth muscle is determined by the action of norepinephrine on α_1 adrenoceptors.

PATHOPHYSIOLOGY AND VOIDING DISORDERS

Urinary incontinence results from a failure to store urine properly. In males this is usually associated with an enlargement of the prostate (benign prostatic hyperplasia; BPH)

Overall, micturition disorders can be subdivided into two major categories, i.e. those associated with abnormal storage or abnormal voiding.

Urinary incontinence

Urinary incontinence is common, occurring in over 10% of the adult female population. It is defined as an objectively demonstrable involuntary loss of urine (Fig. 22.4) and the

Receptor functions in the lower urinary tract

Detrusor

- Contraction-mediating muscarinic (M_3) receptors dominate functionally
- Relaxation-mediating β adrenoceptors ($β_2$ adrenoceptors) dominate over contraction-mediating α adrenoceptors ($α_1$ adrenoceptors)

Urethra

- Contraction-mediating α adrenoceptors ($α_1$ adrenoceptors) dominate functionally over relaxation-mediating β adrenoceptors ($β_2$ adrenoceptors)
- Muscarinic receptors, but function is unknown

Prostate

- Contraction-mediating α adrenoceptors ($α_1$ adrenoceptors) dominate in the prostatic stroma, and may contribute to the increased outflow resistance found in benign prostatic hyperplasia (i.e. the 'dynamic' component of obstruction)
- Muscarinic receptors localized to the epithelium may have a secretory function

Fig. 22.3 Receptor functions in the lower urinary tract.

Types of urinary incontinence

Urge incontinence
- Motor urge incontinence (involuntary detrusor contractions)
- Sensory urge incontinence

Hyper-reflexia: involuntary detrusor contractions associated with neurologic disorders (e.g. multiple sclerosis, trauma)

Stress incontinence: defective urethral closure mechanism
- Defective transmission of intra-abdominal pressure to the proximal urethra
- Lack of estrogen

Benign prostatic hyperplasia: lower urinary tract symptoms, usually associated with bladder outlet obstruction, secondary to prostatic enlargement and often accompanied by detrusor instability.

Fig. 22.4 Common types of urinary incontinence in males and females.

condition has a major impact on patient quality of life. It has been calculated that more pads and diapers are sold for adult incontinence in the USA than for pediatric use. Urinary incontinence in the elderly plays an important role in prompting nursing home admission.

Stress incontinence is the involuntary loss of urine in the absence of detrusor contraction and occurs when the intra-vesical (intra-bladder) pressure exceeds the urethral pressure. For example, in some women who have had babies, this can be provoked by stimuli such as coughing, sneezing, laughing or exercise. The primary cause is a change in position of the urethra from a mainly intra-abdominal structure to being partially extra-abdominal (Fig. 22.5).

Urinary urge incontinence is the involuntary loss of urine in association with a strong desire to void or urgency. It can be subdivided into motor urge incontinence and sensory urge incontinence. Motor urge incontinence is associated with detrusor overactivity and/or decreased detrusor compliance, determined by urodynamic measurements. Overactivity is

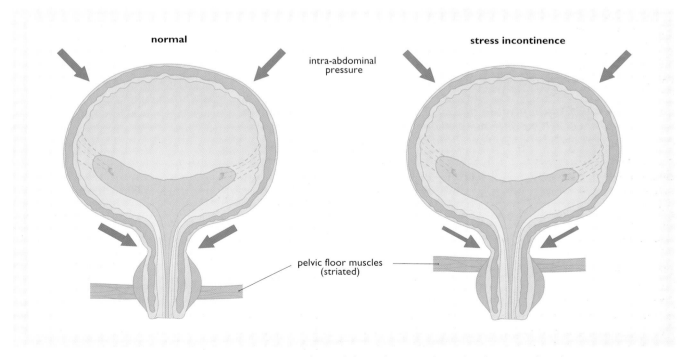

Fig. 22.5 Stress incontinence. There is defective transmission of intra-abdominal pressure (arrows) to the proximal urethra.

Drugs used to treat incontinence

Urge incontinence and hyper-reflexia
Antimuscarinic drugs
Drugs with mixed actions
Antidepressants
α_1 Adrenoceptor antagonists
β_2 Adrenoceptor agonists
Desmopressin

Stress incontinence
α Adrenoceptor agonists
Estrogens (in postmenopausal women)

Benign prostatic hyperplasia
α_1 Adrenoceptor antagonists
5α-reductase inhibitors
Combinations

Fig. 22.6 Drugs used to treat the symptomatology of incontinence in males and females.

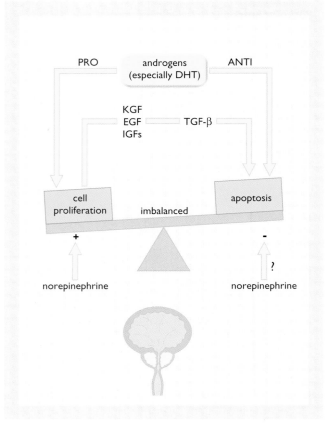

Fig. 22.7 Representation of some of the major factors controlling tissue proliferation and apoptosis. (DHT, dihydrotestosterone; EGF, endothelial growth factor; IGFs, insulin growth factors; KGF, keratinocyte growth factor; TGF-β, transforming growth factor β.)

characterized by involuntary detrusor contractions during the filling phase that may be spontaneous or provoked and which the patient cannot suppress completely. Detrusor overactivity can develop as a consequence of outflow obstruction (usually BPH), inflammation and irritative disorders of the prostate and bladder (e.g. prostatitis and interstitial cystitis), or the cause may be unknown.

Many patients may be suffering from both stress and urinary urge incontinence and are therefore best diagnosed as experiencing mixed incontinence. Hyper-reflexia describes the condition of uncontrolled detrusor contractions associated with neurologic disorders.

The medical management of these disorders, summarized in Fig. 22.6, is described in more detail below.

■ *Treatment of both urinary urge incontinence and hyper-reflexia is directed towards decreasing detrusor muscle activity and increasing bladder capacity*

Benign prostatic hyperplasia (BPH)

■ *The symptoms of BPH are often associated with an enlarged prostate and bladder outflow obstruction*
Benign prostatic hyperplasia (BPH) is the most frequently diagnosed neoplastic disease in the ageing male, affecting

---

🔑 Treatment of urinary incontinence and urinary retention

- Treatment of a failure to store urine (urinary incontinence) is aimed at decreasing detrusor activity, increasing bladder capacity, or increasing outlet resistance
- Treatment of a failure to empty urine (urinary retention) is aimed at increasing detrusor activity or decreasing outlet resistance

---

approximately 85% of men over 50 years of age and requiring them to consult their physician. By the ninth decade of life, 50% of all American men require treatment for symptomatic relief of the lower urinary tract symptoms (LUTS) associated with BPH. Clinically, BPH is characterized by prostatic enlargement and the accompanying symptoms of bladder outlet obstruction, such as urinary incontinence on one hand, and, on the other hand, urinary retention. Rarely, however, with the advent of effective management, will this be sufficiently severe for urinary retention to occur.

Although the molecular processes involved in the pathogenesis of BPH are not completely defined. It is clear that there is a heavy dependence on androgenic factors and in particular the 5α-reduced metabolite of testosterone, dihydrotestosterone (DHT) (Fig. 22.7).

The development of LUTS secondary to prostatic enlargement is thought to be caused by static (mechanical) and dynamic components of urethral restriction. The mechanical component arises from the physical obstruction of urinary outflow caused by urethral constriction, induced by the mass of the enlarged gland. The dynamic component is related to the variations in smooth muscle tone in the fibromuscular stroma, prostate capsule and bladder neck. This peri-urethral smooth

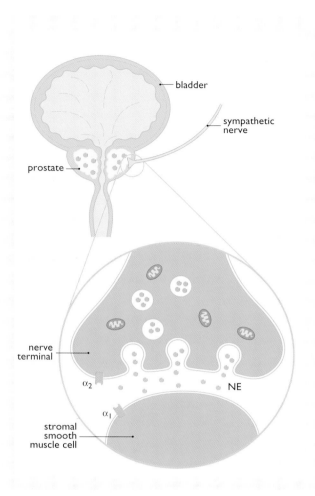

Fig. 22.8 Sympathetic innervation of the human prostate showing the location of α_1 and α_2 adrenoceptors. Norepinephrine (NE) is released from sympathetic nerve terminals to act on post-junctional α_1 receptors.

muscle tone varies according to the degree of sympathetic nervous system activity. Norepinephrine released from the nerve terminals acts on post-junctional α_1 receptors (Fig. 22.8). The resultant increase in muscle tone increases urethral resistance and reduces the flow of urine. Nonetheless, the mechanisms involved in sustaining symptoms such as urgency, frequency and nocturia in men with BPH is complex and may involve neural mechanisms that persist even when the functional obstruction to urine flow is relieved.

The drugs used to treat BPH are summarized in Fig. 22.6 and described below.

Drugs used in the treatment of BPH symptoms act by either reducing the tone in prostatic smooth muscle or by 'shrinking' the prostate

Drug treatment of incontinence and BPH

In most cases medical management is directed towards provision of acute symptomatic relief rather than affecting the underlying etiology or disease progression

Drug therapy of urinary urge incontinence and hyper-reflexia

The mainstay in the management of urinary urge incontinence is the use of antimuscarinic agents. These drugs act to decrease detrusor activity and increase bladder capacity

The parasympathetic nervous system is fundamentally involved in producing contractions in normal and overactive bladder. The link with abnormal bladder pathophysiology forms the rationale for the use of muscarinic antagonists (antimuscarinics) in the treatment of urinary urge incontinence; these drugs have been shown to have clinical efficacy. Unfortunately the role of the parasympathetic nervous system in normal bladder physiology accounts for one of the major limitations in their use. At doses only slightly higher than providing benefit, antimuscarinics can produce almost complete bladder paralysis and/or urinary retention.

The other major limitation of the first generation of antimuscarinics is that their antagonism of muscarinic receptors in other organs may lead to troubling adverse effects, such as a high incidence of dry mouth. This can be sufficiently severe that the patients can neither speak, masticate, or swallow, and is the major reason for noncompliance. Other classical antimuscarinic side effects, e.g. blurred vision, constipation, and drowsiness, may occur at clinically effective doses.

OXYBUTYNIN Although both of the prototypic antimuscarinics, atropine and hyoscine, have been used, oxybutynin, as one of several formulations, is the most commonly prescribed antimuscarinic for the treatment of urinary urge incontinence (Fig. 22.9). The efficacy of oxybutynin is well documented in several well-designed placebo-controlled studies. Despite its adverse event profile it has become the drug of choice. Although the drug has direct smooth muscle relaxant properties, these only occur at much higher concentrations (500 times) than the antimuscarinic actions. It is therefore likely that at therapeutic plasma concentrations oxybutynin acts only on antimuscarinic receptors.

Molecular biologists have identified five antimuscarinic receptor subtypes (M_1–M_5). However the last two subtypes have not yet been shown to have any functional correlate. When considered in relation to the three pharmacologic subtypes identified (M_1, M_2, M_3), oxybutynin has some selectivity (10-fold) for M_1 and M_3 over M_2. The receptor type involved in the bladder is the M_3 subtype. However, the salivary glands also contain M_3 receptors. This probably accounts for the dry mouth observed at effective doses of the standard formulation of oxybutynin. An improved benefit–adverse effect profile has been shown in carefully controlled clinical trials for a novel, extended-release formulation of oxybutynin (XL). This exemplifies the potential impact of altered pharmacokinetics on the overall profile of a drug in man.

Oxybutynin is a tertiary amine that is well absorbed, but undergoes an extensive first-pass metabolism. It has very low bioavailability (6%) in volunteers that probably accounts for large inter- and intra-patient variability in response. The half-life is 2 hours which is less than optimal and a three times daily

487

Clinical profiles of commonly used forms of antimuscarinics

Parameter	Drug	
	Tolterodine	Oxybutynin (long-acting formulation)
Mechanism of action	Muscarinic receptor antagonist with high affinity for urinary bladder ($M_3 = M_2 = M_1$)	Muscarinic receptor antagonist ($M_3 > M_1 \gg M_2$)
Claim	Overactive bladder with symptoms of urinary frequency, urgency or urge incontinence	Overactive bladder with symptoms of urinary frequency, urgency or urge incontinence
Efficacy • Voided volume reduction per micturition • Reduction in number of incontinence episodes per day • Percentage achieving continence	20% vs 10% placebo 50% vs 35% placebo 35%	25% vs 10% placebo 55% vs 30% placebo 40–45%
Pharmacokinetics	$t_{1/2}$ 3–9 h	$t_{1/2}$ 12–17 h
Adverse events	Dry mouth 39% Headache 13% Dizziness 9% Constipation 7% Hypertension 2%	Dry mouth 61% Constipation 13% Somnolence 12% Headache 10% Diarrhea 9% Nausea 9%
Contraindications	Urinary retention GI disturbances Glaucoma	Urinary retention GI disturbances Glaucoma
Dosing schedule	Oral b.i.d.	Oral q.d.

Fig. 22.9 Clinical profiles of commonly used forms of antimuscarinics.

or more frequent regimen must be used to give good 24-hour cover with the standard release formulation.

An active metabolite of oxybutynin, N-desethyl oxybutynin, occurs at much higher plasma concentrations and could make a major contribution to the overall clinical profile. The pharmacology of the parent drug and metabolite are, however, similar.

The bulk of patients experience classical antimuscarinic side effects (dry mouth, constipation, blurred vision, and drowsiness) when taking oxybutynin, although it is capable of bringing patients back to dryness and reducing frequency and severity of incontinent episodes. There have been attempts in small clinical studies to reduce adverse effects by delivering the drug locally (intra-vesically).

A novel extended-release formulation of oxybutynin is available and undoubtedly circumvents one of the problems of the conventional formulation, i.e. the requirement for repeat daily dosing. Early clinical data would tend to indicate that the adverse effect profile is improved compared to the standard formulation. This could be anticipated from the more consistent 24-hour plasma drug concentrations or could be due to a different metabolic profile. A comparison of the pharmaco-kinetic profiles of the immediate-release (IR oxybutynin) and extended-release (XL oxybutynin chloride) forms of oxybutynin is shown in Fig. 22.10. The improved clinical profile of the XL formulation can be completely rationalized on the basis of these pharmacokinetic differences, the XL formulation resulting in a much smoother 24-hour profile with less peak to trough variability.

OTHER ANTIMUSCARINICS The clinical profile of antimus-carinics, at least with respect to efficacy, is an attractive one. Apart from the novel formulation of oxybutynin discussed above, another 'new generation' drug, tolterodine, has reached the market. The overall pharmacologic and clinical profile are summarized in Fig. 22.9. Tolterodine is effective but also produces the classical antimuscarinic adverse effects. Although it has been predicted that the drug will have a superior clinical profile over oxybutynin, the pharmacological basis for this improvement is difficult to understand at this point. Tolterodine appears to have similar activities for all three muscarinic subtypes. Only carefully controlled comparative studies will determine whether the profiles of the two drugs are different and indeed a recent comparison between tolterodine and the

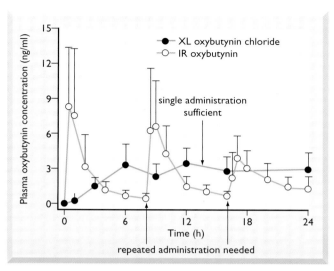

Fig. 22.10 Oxybutynin plasma concentrations following a single oral dose of XL oxybutynin (15 mg) or IR oxybutynin (5 mg) administered every 8 hours.

immediate release form of oxybutynin, suggests there is little difference between the two.

The first antimuscarinic selectively targeting the M_3 subtype, darifenacin, is undergoing late stage clinical development. However, as salivary secretion is also M_3-mediated, it is perhaps unwise to speculate that darifenacin will offer a major clinical advantage.

Several other agents with antimuscarinic (emepronium and propantheline) or mixed antimuscarinic and smooth muscle relaxant properties (e.g. dicyclomine) are available. In general they possess the expected antimuscarinic adverse effect profile and are not suitable for once-a-day dosing.

OTHER AGENTS Several tricyclic antidepressants have beneficial effects in patients with detrusor overactivity, but imipramine is the only one that has been relatively widely used. It is now mainly used in the treatment of nocturnal enuresis in children with a more restrictive use in bladder overactivity in the elderly.

Imipramine has complex pharmacologic actions including antagonism of muscarinic receptors (see Chapter 14). Whether this or its action as an inhibitor of monoamine uptake accounts for its action in detrusor instability is not known. The therapeutic use of tricyclic antidepressants, including imipramine, can cause serious cardiovascular side effects (e.g. orthostatic hypotension and arrhythmias). Children appear particularly sensitive. Obviously the benefit/risk ratio should be considered in each case (see Chapter 14 for more information about imipramine and related drugs).

Desmopressin is a synthetic vasopressin analog, acting on V_2 receptors to produce a pronounced antidiuretic effect. It has virtually no vasopressor actions which are mediated via V_1 receptors (see Chapter 17). It produces a substantial reduction in nocturnal urine production and is an established short-term treatment for enuresis in children. Desmopressin also reduces

the frequency of nocturia in men with BPH and in patients with multiple sclerosis, and may be of value in some adults with detrusor overactivity.

Stress incontinence

⬜ *The medical management of stress incontinence is aimed at increasing outlet resistance*

Moderate or severe stress incontinence is usually treated by a relatively trivial and successful corrective surgical procedure. Traditionally pharmacologic management is restricted to patients with mild to moderate symptomatology, and patients who have not responded adequately to behavioral modifications e.g. pelvic floor exercises. The objective is to increase outflow resistance. Theoretically, this can be achieved by increasing the low intra-urethral pressure or by improving the functionality of the urethral mucosa.

α ADRENOCEPTOR AGONISTS α adrenoceptor agonists elevate intra-urethral pressure. The most widely used is ephedrine. However, in addition to acting as an α_1 adrenoceptor agonist, ephedrine also acts on β receptors and acts as an indirect sympathomimetic by releasing norepinephrine from nerve terminals. As a result it can elevate blood pressure and cause sleep disturbances, tremor and palpitations. There is some evidence that tachyphylaxis (tolerance) can occur on long-term administration. In the USA phenylpropanolamine has been used as an alternative. Phenylpropanolamine is no longer available over the counter (OTC) in the USA; i.e., it requires a drug prescription.

ESTROGENS The beneficial effects of estrogen include induction of proliferation of the urethral mucosa with subsequent improvement in the mucosal augmentation of outflow resistance. In addition estrogens increase the effect of α agonist stimulation of urethral smooth muscle contractility. Ultimately, the ideal therapy could involve co-administration of an estrogen and an α agonist. Conventionally, estrogens are administered in the form of a sustained-release ring.

Benign prostatic hyperplasia

⬜ *The medical management of BPH is directed towards either reducing the size of the prostate using 'prostate shrinkers' or towards reducing the contractile tone in the area of the prostate surrounding the urethra using α_1 receptor-selective antagonists*

Medical management is used routinely in cases of mild to moderate prostatism. In patients with severe symptomatology or urinary retention, surgery is the preferred option. A potential treatment algorithm is shown in Fig. 22.11.

The development of the symptoms of BPH is generally considered to arise from prostatic enlargement causing urethral restriction and bladder outflow obstruction. There are two components to the obstruction. There is the mechanical component arising from the physical obstruction induced by the enlarged prostatic mass, and a dynamic or fluctuating component related to the variations in smooth muscle tone in the prostate (see Fig. 22.8). Treatment modalities therefore aim

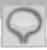

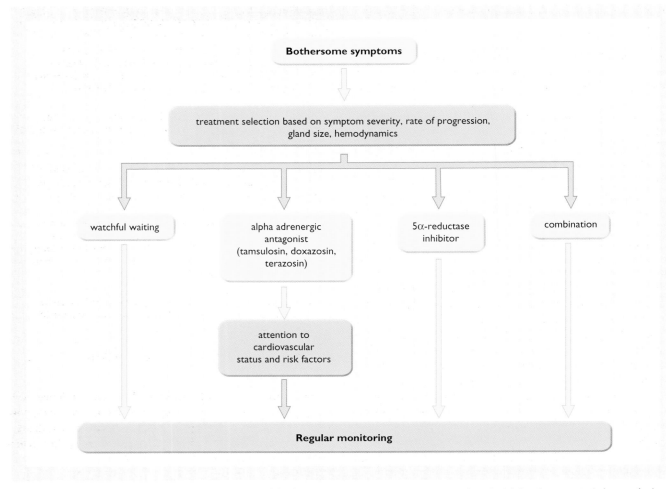

Fig. 22.11 Treatment options for the management of the lower urinary tract symptoms associated with benign prostatic hyperplasia.

either to reduce the mechanical obstruction or to induce relaxation of the peri-urethral prostate smooth muscle.

PROSTATE SHRINKERS Although many factors are involved in prostatic proliferation, the androgens, particularly dihydrotestosterone (DHT), have a prime role (Fig. 22.7). A critical concentration of androgen is required to maintain the benign growth pattern and androgen deprivation results in significant involution of the glandular epithelial component of the prostate.

Finasteride is a drug specifically developed to inhibit the enzyme 5α-reductase that controls the production of DHT from testosterone. As anticipated, the drug has been shown to reduce circulating DHT concentrations to values almost as low as those found in castrated males. In several studies, consistent with the androgen dependency theory, a reduction in prostate size was observed in BPH patients treated with finasteride (5 mg) for periods of a year or more. In these long-term studies the need for surgery and incidence of urinary retention was reduced by up to 50%. Once again this is consistent with an effect of finasteride on gland size and/or growth. Disappointingly, however, in most studies finasteride has little demonstrable effect on BPH symptoms experienced by patients,

and certainly no effect over the first six months. The major adverse effect associated with the use of finasteride is a reduction in libido in up to 15% of patients. This is perhaps not surprising when considered in relation to the well documented relationship between androgens and male sexual activity.

An alternative lower dose (1 mg) formulation of finasteride has been marketed for the treatment of male pattern baldness. The growth of certain types of hair is dependent on circulating and intra-follicular DHT levels. Although the prime form of the isozyme in the hair follicle is 5α-reductase 1, it is assumed that the generalized effect of finasteride on systemic androgens accounts for the benefit.

There are two isoforms of 5α-reductase, 5α-reductase 1 and 2. Finasteride inhibits only the latter, the major isoform in prostatic tissue. It has been argued that one of the limitations of finasteride is that circulating DHT produced by extraprostatic 5α-reductase 1 (in e.g. skin, liver, and fibroblasts) can maintain prostatic growth. On this basis several dual isozyme inhibitors are undergoing evaluation. The most advanced of these is dutasteride which is in phase III clinical development. However, in the absence of any long-term clinical data it is not known whether dual isozyme inhibitors offer any clinical advantage over finasteride and indeed, with respect to androgen depletion-related side effects, whether they may be more problematic.

α1 ADRENOCEPTOR SELECTIVE ANTAGONISTS (BLOCKERS) In contrast to finasteride, patients taking α_1 receptor antagonists experience improvement in symptomatology that is almost immediate.

Since the initial use of phenoxybenzamine established the efficacy of α receptor antagonism in BPH, preferable drugs, initially prazosin, and then subsequently several other α_1 receptor selective antagonists (e.g. alfuzosin, doxazosin, indoramin, tamsulosin and terazosin) have become available and now represent the mainstay of BPH therapy. The pharmacologic and clinical characteristics of this class of drugs are summarized in Fig. 22.12.

All data has been reviewed on several occasions by the α receptor antagonist committee of the WHO International Consultation on BPH; this group has come to the conclusion that differences between α receptor antagonists are largely restricted to pharmacokinetic properties, i.e. at full α-blocking doses all have equivalent efficacy and similar adverse effect profiles. On this basis the following summary of the key features of terazosin can be considered representative of the class, unless otherwise indicated. However, as indicated below, tamsulosin may differ to some extent from this profile.

Since the discovery of α_1 and α_2 receptors, our understanding of adrenoceptor pharmacology has increased substantially (Fig. 22.13). Three native α_1 adrenoceptor subtypes have now been identified with molecular cloning and are known to be located in the prostate; the α_{1A}, α_{1B} and α_{1D} subtypes have

Summary of key features of α blockers

Alfuzosin. Has equal affinity for α_{1A}, α_{1B} and α_{1D} subtypes. Is available in immediate-release and sustained-release formulations with half lifes of between 3 and 11 h dependent on formulation. Tends to be used either q.d. or b.i.d.

Doxazosin. Longest half life of all α blockers (16–22 h) has equal affinity for all 3 subtypes. Is used for co-morbid treatment of hypertension

Prazosin. Although widely used still because of low generic cost, creates problems with patient compliance due to t.i.d. dosing and marked first dose orthostasis

Tamsulosin. Has been claimed to be 'uroselective' and has slightly higher affinity for prostatic α_{1A} receptor subtype than the α_{1B} and α_{1D} subtypes. Only available as one dose 0.4 mg which can create problems for physicians. Marketed as once daily dosing with $t_{1/2}$ of 16 h

Terazosin. Pharmacological and clinical profile identical to doxazosin and also used as part of a treatment schedule for hypertension in several countries

Fig. 22.12 Summary of key features of α blockers.

high affinity for prazosin. There is also some evidence indicating that there is an α_{1L} receptor which has relatively low affinity for this drug. Many investigators consider that the α_{1A} subtype present in the peri-urethral stroma is the prime determinant of prostatic tone.

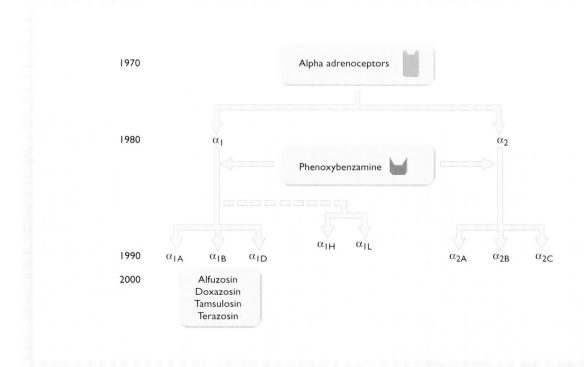

Fig. 22.13 Summary of adrenoceptor pharmacology.

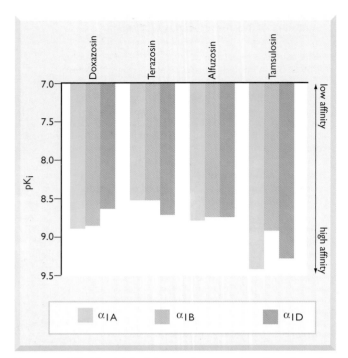

Fig. 22.14 **Affinities (pKi) of doxazosin, terazosin, alfuzosin and tamsulosin for the cloned** α_{1A} **(green),** α_{1B} **(orange) and** α_{1D} **(purple) adrenoceptor subtypes.**

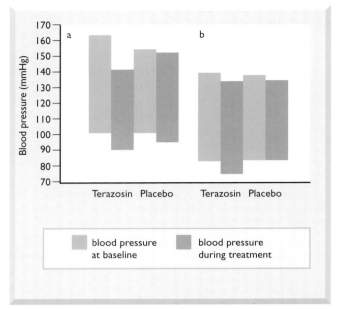

Fig. 22.15 **Effect of terazosin on blood pressure in (a) hypertensive and (b) normotensive patients.** Data show blood pressure at baseline (orange) and after treatment (purple).

As a class, α_1 receptor antagonists have been shown to be safe and effective in the treatment of the symptoms associated with BPH. Both obstructive and irritative symptoms are improved and patients notice the benefit within the first few weeks. The observed changes in urinary flow and residual volume are consistent with an effect in urethral resistance. While it is clear that urine flow rates generally increase, some of the symptoms, such as urgency, frequency and nocturia, may improve by mechanisms that are not completely clear, i.e. not necessarily due to improved urine flow rates. Prazosin has been used in this context for several years but its dosing regimen, and the first-dose orthostatic hypotension arising from rapid absorption, limit its clinical utility. Terazosin was the first selective α_1 antagonist specifically developed to overcome these shortcomings. Terazosin has similar affinity for the α_{1A}, α_{1B} and α_{1D} subtypes (Fig. 22.14) and is therefore considered to have a balanced profile. In addition terazosin can be distinguished from prazosin on the basis of physicochemical differences that result in a more gradual onset of action (less first-dose orthostasis) and a much longer plasma half-life, consistent with once-a-day use.

Although terazosin was developed, as were most α antagonists, as an antihypertensive agent, the drug has relatively little effect on normotensive blood pressure (Fig. 22.15). In other words, there are antihypertensive drugs (lower elevated blood pressures) that have relatively little effect on normal blood pressure. On occasion, however, terazosin and related drugs can cause postural hypotension. The major class-related adverse effects include dizziness, fatigue, somnolence and headache. Most patients with dizziness do not have postural hypotension.

Most of the adverse effects are relatively mild and may be transient, not requiring discontinuation of the drug. The clinical database of terazosin extends to over 3 billion patient-days and show that the drug is well tolerated. Several long-term studies show that the efficacy of terazosin is maintained for up to 7 years with no evidence of tachyphylaxis.

Medical management of BPH—the future

Until recently the α_{1A} subtype was considered to be the most important subtype in the alleviation of the symptoms of BPH. For several years the pharmaceutical industry have been developing agents that selectively target this subtype; the assumption has been that efficacy would be maintained or improved and that the cardiovascular adverse effects (presumed to be α_{1A} and α_{1D} receptor mediated) would be decreased. However, clinical trials to date have been disappointing both with respect to efficacy and adverse effect improvement. While at relatively low doses, tamulosin's likelihood of causing postural hypotension may be less than that of other α_1 receptor antagonists, it may not be as efficacious as other drugs at these doses. It is now considered likely that, to maximize efficacy, blockade of not only α_{1A} but also other α_1 receptor subtypes is required. It may be that α_1 receptors outside the prostate, for example in the bladder or in the spinal cord/CNS, may be involved in producing some of the symptoms of BPH.

A potentially logical combination would be the use of finasteride and an α receptor antagonist. Such a combination would produce the rapid symptom improvement from the α_1 receptor antagonist and also affect the underlying etiology; it has been conjectured that such a combination might have additive benefits. However, clinical trials to date do not appear to support the expense associated with the use of such com-

Treatment of benign prostatic hyperplasia

- α_1 adrenoceptor antagonists are widely used and provide rapid (2 weeks) improvement in symptoms. All tend to be associated with some degree of cardiovascular side effects (dizziness, headache and fatigue)
- 5α-reductase inhibitors are used particularly in patients with larger glands. As would be anticipated, the 'prostate shrinking' action takes some time to develop. Benefit may not be apparent for up to 1 year

Plant extracts used in the management of benign prostatic hyperplasia

- *Hypoxis rooperi* (South African star-grass)
- *Urtica* spp. (Stinging nettle)
- *Sabal serrulatum* (Dwarf palm)
- *Serenoa repens B* (American dwarf palm)
- *Cucurbita pepo* (Pumpkin seed)
- *Pygeum Africanum* (African plum)
- *Populus tremula* (Aspen)
- *Echinacea purpurea* (Purple coneflower)
- *Secale cereale* (Rye)

Fig. 22.16 Plant extracts used in the management of benign prostatic hyperplasia. Efficacy and safety are uncertain.

Yearly incidence and death rates for various cancers in the US

Origin	Incidence	Deaths
Urinary tract		
Prostate	200,000	38,000
Testes	6800	325
Bladder	51,200	10,500
Kidney	27,600	11,300
Others		
Gastrointestinal	220,000	120,000
Lung	172,000	153,000

Fig. 22.17 Yearly incidence and death rates for various cancers in the US.

binations, the added clinical benefit appearing to be minimal. An α_1 receptor antagonist is sufficient in most cases.

It is intriguing to note that there is an increasing use of plant extracts (phytotherapy) by BPH patients (Fig. 22.16). It is estimated that extracts of saw palmetto (*serenoa repens*) sell in excess of $3 billion per annum. It is obvious from the use of this type of nutraceutic that safety and efficacy are a major issue for patients (see Chapter 30).

PROSTATE CANCER

Early stage and metastatic prostate cancer can be treated with hormone modulating therapy. Usually surgery, in combination with drug and radiotherapy, is required to effect a cure

Although prostate cancer is the third most common cause of cancer death in men in most developed countries (Fig. 22.17), there is a surprising lack of consensus concerning its management, particularly the treatment of localized lesions. The principal reason is the difficulty in predicting which lesions will progress to the detriment of the patient as opposed to those that will remain localized and asymptomatic within the individual's lifespan. In other words, many men die with prostate cancer rather than as a result of it. However, as the death rate from competing mortalities is now falling and the incidence of clinical prostatic disease is increasing, the challenge is to identify and treat effectively the life-threatening lesions in the most efficient manner. Unfortunately, in most countries only

about 30% of prostate cancers are diagnosed when still confined within the gland. It is easier to treat localized than metastatic disease.

In the early neoplastic stage, prostate cancer is androgen dependent. On this basis, hormone therapy is used in conjunction with surgery and radiation therapy.

Androgen action on prostatic cells can be modulated in a variety of ways. Clinically, medical castration with a GnRH analog is as effective as orchiectomy

Testosterone secretion is dependent on the actions of LH and FSH (Fig. 22.18). Traditionally inhibition of secretion has been achieved, initially surprisingly, using GnRH (LHRH) analogs that act as partial agonists in stimulating secretion of LH and FSH. Although GnRH analogs cause a temporary increase in circulating LH and FSH concentrations, subsequently there is a substantial decrease in testosterone concentrations. This is due to desensitization of GnRH receptors in the pituitary (see Chapter 3 for discussion of desensitization of responses mediated by cell surface receptors). The long-term effect is that plasma testosterone levels are decreased to values close to those of castrated men. The transient increase in testosterone levels has been called the 'flare phenomenon,' because of the theoretical risk of stimulation of metastatic growth of the tumor. For this reason, it is often recommended that for the first 4 weeks of GnRH analog therapy, adjunctive treatment with an anti-androgen (see below) should be employed. A new generation of 'super agonists' such as abarelix, which may be relatively free of the initial hormone elevation, are under development. In most countries GnRH therapy is the front line in the medical management of prostate cancer (Fig. 22.19). The available analogs are leuprolide, buserelin and goserelin. All three are available as a 3-monthly injectable depot formulation suitable for administration in the primary care setting. All GnRH analogs produce a major detrimental effect on sexual function. The pharmacodynamic and pharmacokinetic properties of the various drugs and their formulations are shown in Fig. 22.20.

493

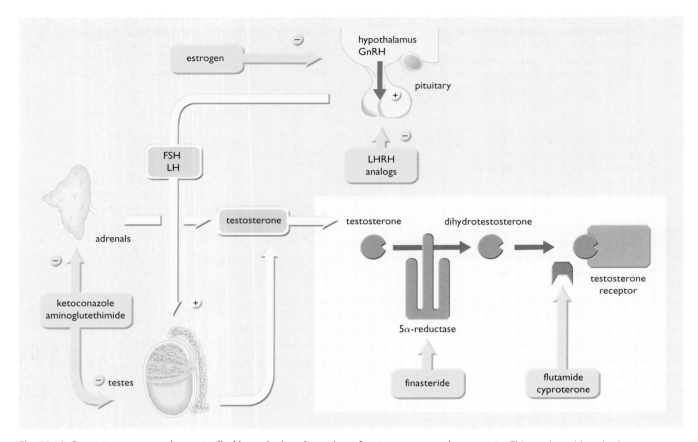

Fig. 22.18 Prostate cancer can be controlled by reducing the action of testosterone on the prostate. This can be achieved using a variety of methods. Release of the gonadotropin releasing hormone (GnRH) from the hypothalamus can be inhibited by estrogens, while the effects of luteinizing hormone releasing hormone (LHRH) to release FSH and LH can be blocked by LHRH analogs. Alternatively, testosterone synthesis can be inhibited by ketoconazole and aminoglutethimide, while the conversion of testosterone to its prostate-activating derivative, dihydrotestosterone, can be prevented by 5α-reductase inhibitors such as finasteride. Another approach is to block the testosterone receptor with flutamide or cyproterone.

Commonly used treatments for localized and metastatic prostate cancer	
Treatment	**Status**
Watchful waiting	Localized
Radical radiotherapy	Localized
Radical prostatectomy	Localized

Androgen blockade
  Bilateral orchiectomy
  LHRH analogs
  Bilateral adrenalectomy
	Metastatic

Fig. 22.19 Commonly used treatments for localized and metastatic prostate cancer.

■ Anti-androgens act locally within the prostate to block the growth stimulating actions of dihydrotestosterone (DHT)

Although shown to be effective, unfortunately—owing to the primary mechanism of action on inhibiting androgen action—the effects can be self-limiting. As a class, anti-androgens block not only the androgen receptor at the level of the prostate, but also within the hypothalamopituitary complex. At this level, androgens normally exert a self-regulating negative feedback influence. As a result of the central androgen receptor blockade, LH secretion is enhanced and testosterone biosynthesis is increased.

■ Other methods of achieving androgen blockade have been evaluated.

Estrogens, particularly diethylstilbestrol (DES), inhibit the release of GnRH from the hypothalamus, thereby reducing LH and FSH release and decreasing testosterone production. Although inexpensive, DES is associated with significant cardiovascular toxicity, erectile dysfunction and gynecomastia. In most circumstances, DES is no longer first-line therapy for prostate cancer.

Finasteride is a competitive inhibitor of 5α-reductase, the enzyme that converts testosterone to DHT in the prostate (see BPH section above). Several studies have confirmed that finasteride produces substantial reductions (65–75%) in circulating DHT levels. Although the drug is used in the treatment of BPH, its utility in prostate cancer remains unproven.

Commonly used drugs and treatment regimens for prostate cancer

	Agent	Dose	Side-effects
LHRH analogs	Leuprolide Goserelin Buserelin	Monthly (soon 3-monthly)	Hot flushes Impotence ↓Libido
Non-steroidal anti-androgens	Flutamide Nilutamide Bicalutamide	250 mg t.d.s. 300 mg/day 150 g/day	Gynecomastia Diarrhea
Progestogenic anti-androgens	Cyproterone acetate	100 mg t.d.s.	Fluid retention Impotence
Estrogens	Diethylstilbestrol	2–5 mg/day	Impotence Gynecomastia Cardiovascular toxicity

Fig. 22.20 **Commonly used drugs and treatment regimens for prostate cancer.**

Finasteride only inhibits one isoform, 5α-reductase 2. To maximize the clinical benefit in prostate cancer (and indeed in BPH), it may be necessary to inhibit both 5α-reductase isoforms. An inhibitor of 5α-reductase 1 and 2, dutasteride, currently in clinical development, may offer some advantages.

ERECTILE DYSFUNCTION

Over the last decade, the management of erectile dysfunction has been revolutionized with the advent of effective pharmacologic therapies

Erectile dysfunction (ED) (regrettably previously known as impotence, a word which has an inappropriate connotation), is defined as the consistent inability to achieve and/or maintain an erection sufficient for satisfactory sexual activity. The causes of ED are multifactorial, with psychological, neurologic, endocrinological, vascular, traumatic and iatrogenic components potentially playing a role. ED is usually defined as psychogenic, organic or mixed.

Potential risk factors include ageing, smoking, hypertension, hyperlipidemia, diabetes mellitus, vascular disease, depression and a variety of drugs (Fig. 22.21). ED may have a major impact on the quality of life for many men and their partners. The probability of ultimately having some form of ED for men aged 40 years or over is almost 55%.

The erectile process is an integrated vascular response. Mainly, erection involves relaxation of cavernosal smooth muscle whereas detumescence involves contraction

The erectile process in the penis is a complex series of integrated vascular events culminating in the accumulation of blood under pressure and end organ rigidity. An erection can only occur when the smooth muscles of the arteries and sinusoids in the penis (Fig. 22.22) have relaxed. The erectile tissue then fills with blood at arterial pressure. The resultant increase in intra-corporal pressure expands the relaxed tra-

Drugs that can cause erectile dysfunction

Class of drug	Specific drugs
Antihypertensives	Clonidine, methyldopa, hydrochlorothiazide, β adrenoceptor antagonists
Psychotropics	Monoamine oxidase inhibitors, tricyclic antidepressants, phenothiazines, benzodiazepines
CNS depressants	Sedatives, narcotics, ethanol, anxiolytics
Miscellaneous	Atropinics, estrogens, cimetidine, anticancer drugs

Fig. 22.21 **Drugs that can cause erectile dysfunction.** These drugs cause erectile dysfunction either indirectly by actions within the central nervous system or directly by actions on the smooth muscle of the penis or on penile innervation.

becular walls against the tunica albuginea. Compression of the plexus of subtunical arteries follows, reducing venous outflow (the veno-occlusive mechanism); this increases pressure within the corpora and gives a rigid penis. Detumescence occurs through the reversal of this process and follows contraction of penile smooth muscle.

Although erection depends on a local vascular event, the process relies on the integration of neuronal and hormonal mechanisms at various levels of the neuroaxis

The overall tone of the cavernosal smooth muscle represents the integrated response to many different pathways and systems (Fig. 22.23). In essence these can be considered to be either: extrinsic, involving spinal or supraspinal pathways, and classical neurotransmission across neuroeffector junctions; or, paracrine

495

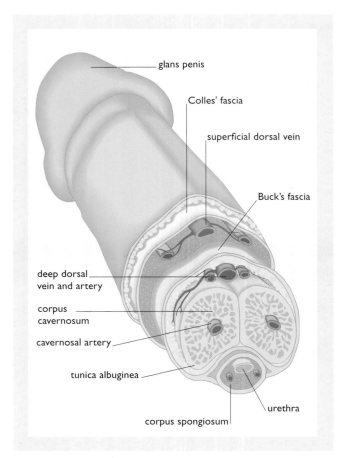

Fig. 22.22 Structure of the penis. The procreative function of the penis depends upon erection, which results from dilation of the cavernosal artery and filling of the corpora cavernosa and corpus spongiosum with arterial blood. The various fascias, particularly the tunica albuginea, prevent excessive dilation of the penis and limit venous drainage. Both arterial dilation, increasing flow, and reduction of venous outflow are important for maintaining erection.

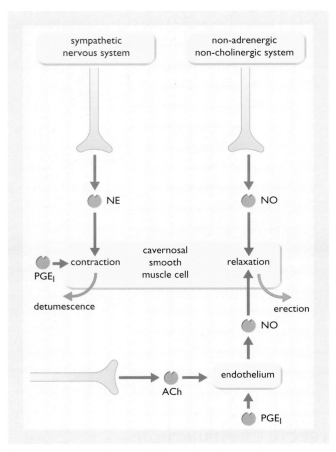

Fig. 22.23 Autonomic control of erection. The use of pharmacologic agents to produce cavernosal smooth muscle relaxation. Smooth muscle tone is the prime determinant of the degree of erection. NO, nitric oxide; NE, norepinephrine; ACh, acetylcholine; PGE_1, prostaglandin E_1.

Neurotransmitters involved in penile smooth muscle contractility	
Relaxation	**Contraction**
• Acetylcholine • Nitric oxide • Vasoactive intestinal polypeptide • Prostaglandin E_1 • Calcitonin gene-related peptide	• Norepinephrine • Endothelin-1 • Neuropeptide Y • ATP

Fig. 22.24 Neurotransmitters involved in penile cavernosal smooth muscle contractility.

or autocrine local control systems involving various neuromodulator substances.

Almost certainly, ED occurs when an imbalance is created in the integrated response. Not surprisingly, the autonomic nervous system, i.e. the sympathetic noradrenergic and the nonadrenergic noncholinergic (NANC) nitric oxide (NO)-containing nerve fibers, provides the local control for normal erections. The neurotransmitters/neuromodulators controlling smooth muscle tone are shown in Fig. 22.24. However, the erectile process is unique among visceral functions in that there is an absolute requirement for central neural input to ensure normal function.

Of particular interest in understanding drug action is the NANC system. On sexual stimulation, the neuromodulator nitric oxide (NO) is released and acts postjunctionally to activate an intracellular enzyme cascade (Fig. 22.25). NO is produced by the precursor L-arginine, which is converted by the enzyme nitric oxide synthase. Within the cavernosal smooth muscle cells, NO increases production of cyclic guanosine monophosphate (cGMP). cGMP decreases intracellular calcium concentrations which leads to relaxation of the smooth muscle. Tissue engorgement and erection follow. Subsequently cGMP is broken down, predominantly by an enzyme, phosphodiesterase type 5 (PDE5), which accounts in part for detumescence. However, detumescence is more directly controlled by activity in the sympathetic nervous system. Released norepinephrine acts on postjunctional α_1 adrenoceptors, producing contraction of the corporal smooth muscle leading to increased venous outflow and detumescence.

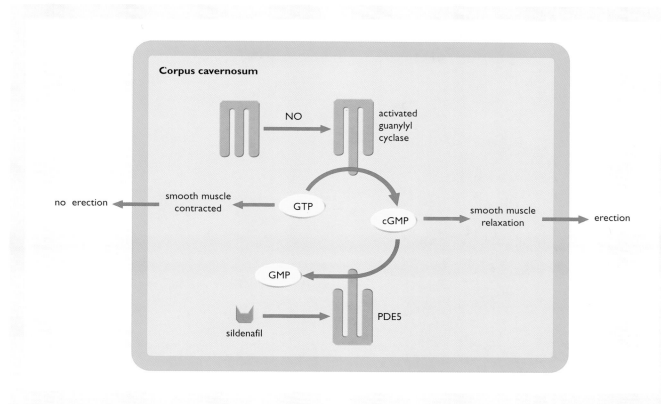

Fig. 22.25 The control of smooth muscle contraction and relaxation, and erection, in human corpus cavernosum. The effects of sildenafil are shown. cGMP, cyclic guanosine monophosphate; GMP, guanosine monophosphate; GTP, guanosine triphosphate; NO, nitric oxide; PDE5, phosphodiesterase type 5.

Pharmacotherapy

▓ *Prior to initiation of therapy a full diagnostic investigation must be completed*

An algorithm for the management of patients with ED is shown in Fig. 22.26. Subsequent to clinical evaluation and diagnosis of ED, a variety of management options are now available, dependent on patient preference. An obvious starting point is the modification of potentially reversible causes of the condition. In its simplest form, this can involve lifestyle modification, e.g. stress reduction, dietary changes, smoking cessation or establishing more effective control of blood glucose in diabetics. In other cases involving an iatrogenic basis for the ED (Fig. 22.21), discontinuation or modification of ongoing therapy can achieve considerable success. More commonly, interventional therapy is needed. This can range from pharmacologic agents, psychotherapy, minimally invasive procedures such as vacuum devices, to more invasive procedures such as surgery.

▓ *Drugs can act peripherally, or centrally, to initiate or augment erections*

Since the pioneering self-injection studies of Brindley in the 1970s, the use of pharmacologic agents to produce cavernosal smooth muscle relaxation and thereby erection has increased dramatically. Traditionally vasorelaxant substances such as papaverine and phenoxybenzamine have been administered by direct intracavernosal injection. As monotherapy their use has

been largely discontinued, owing largely to the relatively high incidence of penile fibrosis and penile fibrotic nodules. In several countries a Trimix strategy is widely used. This involves the injection of a combination of a mixture of phentolamine, papaverine and prostaglandin E_1 (PGE_1). The pharmacologic synergy (Fig. 22.27) of these agents reduces the doses required for each drug separately and appears to result in a corresponding reduction in the incidence of penile fibrosis. However, the use of PGE_1 as monotherapy exceeds the use of all other injectables.

PGE_1 (alprostadil) is poorly absorbed orally and is broken down rapidly on entering the blood stream so that systemic concentrations are quite low. This necessitates the use of local delivery systems, usually intracavernosal. The response rate and magnitude of the response are excellent. Alprostadil (5–20 μg) is effective across a wide range of etiologies, with up to 70% of men reporting full erections. The most common adverse effect and the reason for discontinuation of therapy is pain at the site of injection in up to a third of patients. In long-term studies the incidence of fibrotic episodes is relatively low (<1%). Until the arrival of sildenafil, intracavernosal alprostadil was the preferred treatment option for most patients.

In an attempt to reduce the incidence of pain at the injection site an intra-urethral delivery system has been developed for alprostadil. However, compared to the intracavernosal form the efficacy is reduced (responder rate and magnitude of response). There is also a relatively high incidence of urethral burning and

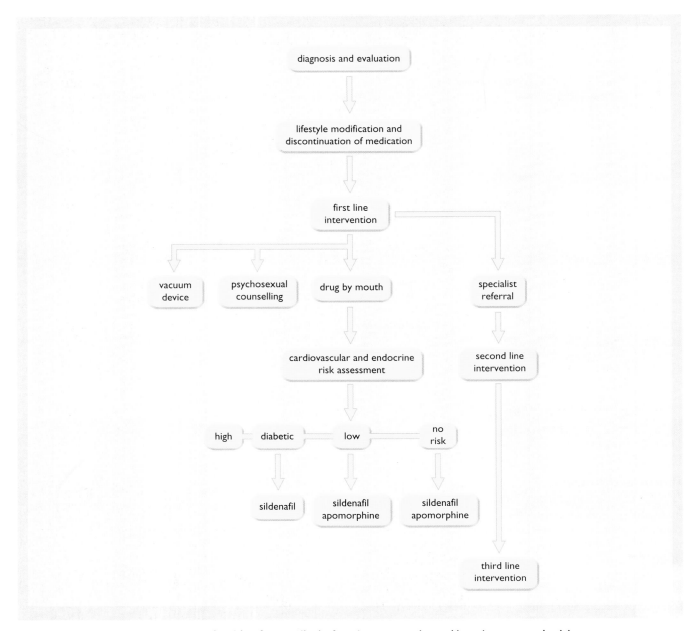

Fig. 22.26 Decision-making treatment algorithm for erectile dysfunction commonly used by primary care physicians.

Actions on cavernosal smooth muscle

Papaverine: Direct relaxation of cavernosal smooth muscle due to an action on intracellular calcium levels. May also be a contribution from inhibition of PDE

Phentolamine: Secondary affect on cavernosal smooth muscle tone. In this situation, blocks the postjunctional (α_1) actions of norepinephrine in corpus cavernosum (see Fig. 22.23)

Prostaglandin E$_1$: Prime action is intracellular on calcium mobilization, but there may also be a prejunctional action affecting neurotransmitter release

Fig. 22.27 Actions on cavernosal smooth muscle.

itching due to the active system and the insertion of the delivery system.

Sildenafil is the first orally active agent for the treatment of ED

The arrival of sildenafil in the marketplace has revolutionized the management of ED. The impact of effective and relatively safe therapy can be seen in terms of patient consultations. Prior to sildenafil it was calculated that less than 2% of ED sufferers were prepared to talk about their disorder. Since sildenafil became available, 18% of sufferers have presented to a physician.

Sildenafil is a potent inhibitor of PDE5 (Fig. 22.28). As a consequence, under certain conditions, this will augment the effects of intracorporal cGMP by inhibiting the breakdown of this nucleotide (Fig. 22.29). The drug only works under

PDE isozymes in human tissues

PDE isoform	Substrate	Effect of cGMP on hydrolysis of cAMP	Tissue localization	Tissue	Geometric mean IC_{50} (nM)*
PDE1	cGMP > cAMP	No effect	Brain, heart, kidney, liver, skeletal muscle, vascular and visceral smooth muscle	Cardiac ventricle	280
PDE2	cAMP, cGMP	Stimulation	Adrenal cortex, brain, corpus cavernosum, heart, kidney, liver, visceral smooth muscle, skeletal muscle	Corpus cavernosum	68,000
PDE3	cAMP	Inhibition	Corpus cavernosum, heart, platelets, vascular and visceral smooth muscle, liver, kidney	Corpus cavernosum	16,200
PDE4	cAMP	No effect	Kidney, lung, mast cells, heart, skeletal muscle, vascular and visceral smooth muscle	Skeletal muscle	7200
PDE5	cGMP	Not relevant	Corpus cavernosum, platelets, skeletal muscle, vascular and visceral smooth muscle	Corpus cavernosum	4
PDE6	cGMP	Not relevant	Retina	Retina (cone) Retina (rod)	34 38

cAMP, cyclic adenosine monophosphate; cGMP, cyclic guanosine monophosphate; PDE, phosphodiesterase.
*The IC_{50} is the concentration of sildenafil required to inhibit enzyme activity by 50%.

Fig. 22.28 PDE isozymes in human tissues.

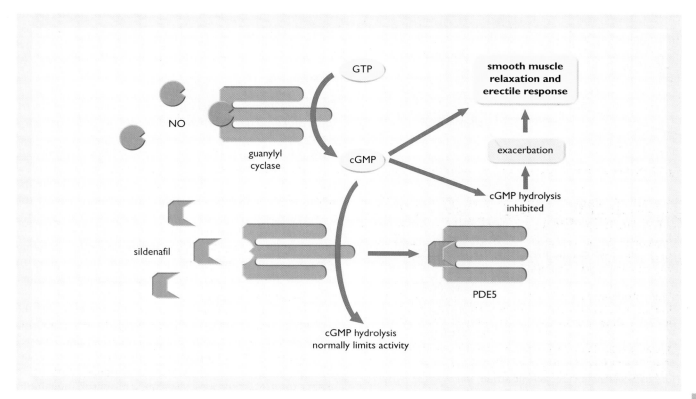

Fig. 22.29 Sildenafil—mechanism of action. The role of PDE5 and PDE5 inhibitors (sildenafil) in the erectile process. (NO, nitric oxide; GTP, guanosine triphosphate; cGMP, cyclic guanosine monophosphate; PDE5, phosphodiesterase type 5.)

conditions of sexual stimulation. Overall, therefore, sildenafil acts to restore the natural response to sexual stimulation.

Sildenafil is rapidly absorbed with onset of action within an hour. The pharmacokinetic half-life is 4–6 hours. However, owing to the relatively high plasma concentration achieved over the therapeutic dose range (25, 50 and 100 mg) the functional or pharmacodynamic half-life is much longer, with some patients experiencing erections up to 36 hours after a single dose.

Sildenafil is effective across a wide range of ED etiologies (Fig. 22.30). Roughly 65–70% of patients will get an erection although the response in diabetics is somewhat lower. It is pertinent to note that some patients switch from sildenafil to intracavernosal injection as the quality of the erection (largely rigidity) is better with the injectable. In the majority of cases the convenience and spontaneity of the oral form offer considerable advantages.

The major adverse effects of sildenafil appear to be cardiovascular, i.e. headache, flushing and nasal stuffiness. These are all likely to be as a consequence of inhibition of PDE5 and as such a 'class effect.' The dysphagia/dyspepsia observed particularly at high doses is also likely to be due to inhibition of PDE5, in this case in the lower esophageal sphincter. In some cases the patients appear to self co-administer nonsteroidals and H$_2$ antagonists, to attenuate headache and dyspepsia, respectively.

Sildenafil also produces transient visual disturbances in the form of subtle changes in colour perception (blue aura) in up to 5% of patients. This is almost certainly due to the relatively poor selectivity that sildenafil has for PDE5 over PDE6; the latter being involved in retinal vision transmission.

As well as enhancing the response of endogenous (naturally occurring) NO, sildenafil will also augment the response to drugs that activate NO synthesis; these are primarily nitroglycerin, isosorbide methylnitrate or other nitrate-based medications. This drug interaction can result in life-threatening hypotension due to profound NO mediated vasodilation. For this reason, the use of sildenafil is absolutely contraindicated in patients taking these medications. In addition, amyl nitrate, which is sometimes used illicitly, should never be combined with sildenafil. Since the nitrate interactions are as a consequence of PDE5 inhibition, the use will be contraindicated with other members of this class of drugs for ED.

Sildenafil is eliminated predominantly by cytochrome P-450 isozymes (CYP3A4) in the liver. Clearance of the drug may be decreased in the elderly and in patients with renal or hepatic insufficiency, although dose adjustment is not generally required. Inhibitors of CYP3A4, such as cimetidine, ketoconazole and erythromycin, decreased the clearance of sildenafil. There is some evidence that sildenafil will alter the response to vasoactive agents such as amlodipine and ACE inhibitors, and this may not be a class effect. Certainly the issue of cardiovascular risk is foremost in patients' minds when taking sildenafil, and this may have had negative impact on the use of this drug.

Novel PDE5 inhibitors, less likely to have the visual disturbance-inducing PDE6 effects, are currently in development.

■ *Drugs can induce erections by central actions. The key to successful drug development is establishing cardiovascular safety*

Many patients with ED have concomitant cardiovascular disease that may or may not have been diagnosed. Over the last few years the management of ED has been revolutionized with the advent of an oral agent, sildenafil. However, as we enter the twenty-first century, it has become apparent that many patients still do not seek treatment. At least in part this is due to concerns about the safety of current therapies. Existing therapies employ mainly peripheral and direct routes to vasodilate the penile vasculature. However, there are other options (Fig. 22.31).

Sildenafil or intracavernosal drugs act to augment either the NO system or to attenuate the counterbalancing sympathetic noradrenergic system. However, it is the CNS that initiates signaling to the penis and integrates the overall response; i.e. the CNS has a prime role in the normal sexual response. To exploit this CNS control mechanism, a novel sublingual (SL) formulation of the dopamine agonist, apomorphine, has been developed specifically for the treatment of patients with ED.

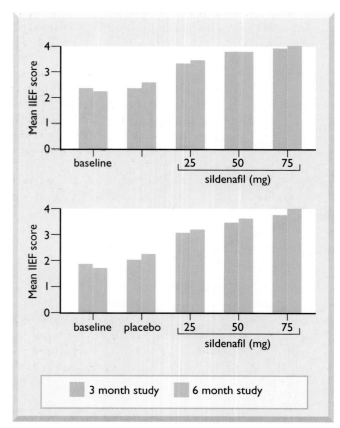

Fig. 22.30 Sildenafil's erectogenic action. Improvement in the ability to (a) achieve and (b) maintain an erection, at the end of a 3-month (orange) or 6-month (green) study, as assessed by patients using the International Index of Erectile Function (IIEF) Questionnaire.

Classification of agents used to treat erectile dysfunction

Locus	Description	
	Initiator	Conditioner
Central	Apomorphine	Testosterone
Peripheral	PGE₁ Triple mix	Sildenafil

Fig. 22.31 Classification of agents used to treat erectile dysfunction.

Treatment of the patient with erectile dysfunction

- Patient management has been revolutionized with the development of orally active sildenafil. The drug acts by inhibiting PDE5
- Sildenafil, like the earlier vasoactive drugs that were injected intracavernosally, acts locally. An alternative approach is to alter the control of the erectile process by an action in the CNS. Apomorphine SL, a centrally acting dopamine agonist, has also been shown to be highly effective

Apomorphine SL was marketed in Europe in June 2001 and is awaiting approval in the USA.

Overall, the clinic data show that apomorphine (2 and 3 mg) is effective across the broad etiological causes of ED in patients that present to specialist and primary care physicians. The profile of rapid (<20 min) restoration of normal sexual function and good tolerability should ensure that apomorphine becomes a welcome addition to the therapeutic management of the ED patient.

URINARY TRACT INFECTIONS (UTI)

Urinary tract infections (UTIs) are among the most common infections encountered in medical practice
Many antimicrobial drugs are excreted unchanged in the urine at high concentrations. For this reason low and relatively non-toxic doses of many antibiotic classes are effective in urinary tract infections.

Urinary tract pathogens

- *Escherichia coli*
- *Staphylococcus saprophyticus*
- *Klebsiella/Enterobacter*
- *Proteus*
- *Pseudomonas*
- Enterococci
- *Staphylococcus epidermidis*

The great majority of urinary bladder infections (cystitis) are caused by single bacterial species. Amongst these, *E. coli* is by far the most common, accounting for up to 85% of general or community-based infections. Such infections typically are sensitive to a wide range of antibiotics. Nosocomial infections, however, are often due to more resistant pathogens and may require parenteral antibiotics. Historically, a colony count of >10⁵/ml was considered the criterion for UTI. However, it is now recognized that half of all women with symptomatic infections have much lower counts. In addition the presence of pyuria (white blood cells in the urinary sediment) correlates poorly with the diagnosis of UTI. Consequently, identification of these cells in the urine is, alone, not sufficient for diagnosis.

Ascending infection from the urethra is the most common route of infection. Women are particularly at risk because the female urethra is short and the vagina becomes colonized with bacteria. Sexual intercourse is a major precipitating factor in young women and the use of diaphragms and spermicidal creams (which also alter normal vaginal flora) further increase the risk of cystitis. Pyelonephritis (infection of a kidney) most commonly occurs from the ascent of infection up the ureter. Hematogenous (blood-borne) spread to the urinary tract is rare with the exception of tuberculosis and cortical renal abscesses. Equally rare is spread from the lymphatics. Occasionally, direct extension from other organs may occur, e.g. in inflammatory bowel disease.

Soft tissue infections (pyelonephritis and prostatitis) require intensive therapy, typically from 2–4 weeks or even longer, while mucosal infections (e.g. cystitis) may require a few days of therapy depending on the antibiotic selected.

Prophylactic antibiotic therapy may be given to prevent recurrence. Women who have more than three episodes of cystitis are considered candidates for prophylaxis. Only selected antimicrobial agents are suitable for prophylaxis. Optimally they must eliminate pathogens from fecal or introital reservoirs and not cause bacterial resistance. The most commonly used is a mixture of trimethoprim and sulfamethoxazole.

Urinary tract infections can be broken down into individual disorders, particularly:
- Acute cystitis.
- Acute pyelonephritis.
- Acute bacterial prostatitis.
- Chronic bacterial prostatitis.
- Nonbacterial prostatitis.
- Acute epididymitis.
- Prostatodynia.

A summary of the antibiotic treatment regimens is shown in Fig. 22.32. In addition, all forms of prostatitis and prostatodynia are generally treated with α receptor antagonists such as doxazosin or terazosin at doses similar to those used in the treatment of BPH.

DRUGS AND THE UTERUS

The control of human parturition is unclear. However, drugs that modify the progress of labor and delivery are frequently used in obstetrics

Therapy for urinary tract infections

Diagnosis	Antibiotic	Route	Duration
Acute pyelonephritis	Ampicillin, 1 g every 6 hours, and gentamicin, 1 mg/kg every 8 hours	i.v.	21 days
	Trimethoprim–sulfamethoxazole, 160/800 mg every 12 hours	Orally	21 days
	Ciprofloxacin, 750 mg every 12 hours	Orally	21 days
	Ofloxacin, 200–300 mg every 12 hours	Orally	21 days
Chronic pyelonephritis	Same as for acute pyelonephritis, but duration of therapy is 3–6 months		
Acute cystitis	Trimethoprim–sulfamethoxazole, 160/800 mg, two tablets	Orally	Single dose
	Cephalexin, 250–500 mg every 6 hours	Orally	1–3 days
	Ciprofloxacin, 250–500 mg every 12 hours	Orally	1–3 days
	Nitrofurantoin (Macrocrystals), 100 mg every 12 hours	Orally	7 days
	Norfloxacin, 400 mg every 12 hours	Orally	1–3 days
	Ofloxacin, 200 mg every 12 hours	Orally	1–3 days
Acute bacterial prostatitis	Same as for acute pyelonephritis		21 days
Chronic bacterial prostatitis	Trimethoprim–sulfamethoxazole, 180/800 mg every 12 hours	Orally	1–3 months
	Ciprofloxacin, 250–500 mg every 12 hours	Orally	1–3 months
	Ofloxacin, 200–400 mg every 12 hours	Orally	1–3 months
Acute epididymitis			
Sexually transmitted	Ceftriaxone 250 mg as single dose plus:	i.m.	10 days
	Doxycycline, 100 mg every 12 hours	Orally	
Non-sexually transmitted	Same as for chronic bacterial prostatitis	Orally	3 weeks

Fig. 22.32 Therapy for urinary tract infections.

Physiology

Uterine smooth muscle is characterized by a high level of spontaneous electrical and contractile activity. The contractile activity is initiated by rises in intracellular calcium concentrations. The uterus has parasympathetic and sympathetic innervation, either of which can induce increased uterine activity, via muscarinic and α_1 receptors respectively. However, activation of β adrenoceptors in the uterus exerts a major inhibitory action on uterine motility, a feature that can be exploited clinically. This is analogous to β adrenoceptor-mediated smooth muscle relaxation in blood vessels. Several other inhibitory and stimulatory factors and processes have been described for the uterus (Fig. 22.33). The major excitatory factors include oxytocin, prostaglandins E_2 and $F_{2\alpha}$ and 5-HT. The tone of uterine smooth muscle is influenced by circulating estrogens.

Human parturition is the result of a complex, and incompletely understood, interaction between fetal and maternal endocrine systems. Undoubtedly both oxytocin and prostaglandins are involved but the precise roles remain undefined.

Drugs that increase uterine motility

■ *The main uses of these drugs are: to induce or augment labor in selected individuals, to control postpartum hemorrhage, and for therapeutic abortion*

Uterine-stimulating agents are frequently used to induce labor in situations where continuation of pregnancy is considered to be of greater risk to the mother or fetus than the risk of delivery or pharmacologic induction. These situations include diabetes, isoimmunization, hypertensive states, intrauterine growth reduction and placental inadequacy. In some cases not discussed here, Cesarean section may be the optimal approach to delivering a well baby. With medical therapy, the drug of choice is oxytocin given as an intravenous infusion. When employed at term, oxytocin usually initiates labor. Occasionally the uterus can be stimulated to an extent where sustained tetanic contractions can occur. In this potentially adverse situation where the placental circulation can be compromised,

Drugs and endogenous factors that can profoundly influence uterine smooth muscle

Excitation	Inhibition
• Muscarinic agonist	• B_2 Adrenoceptor agonist
• α_1 Adrenoceptor agonist	• Calcium channel blocker
• Oxytocin	
• PGE_2 or $F_{2\alpha}$	
• 5-HT	

Fig. 22.33 Drugs and endogenous factors that can profoundly influence uterine smooth muscle.

withdrawal of the drug or even administration of a β_2 adreno-ceptor agonist to inhibit uterine motility may be necessary. Terbutaline or ritodrine are the drugs of choice. Oxytocin is also used to augment labor if the progress is considered to be too slow.

After delivery of the fetus, it is desirable to have the uterus firm and active to reduce the incidence and magnitude of post partum hemorrhage. If uterine stimulation is required, a low dose of oxytocin may be used. If the desired uterine tone can be achieved, an intramuscular ergot alkaloid (ergonovine or methylergonovine) may be used to sustain uterine stimulation. However, these agents should not be used in hypertensive patients as their pronounced serotoninergic (5-HT) activity could induce further blood pressure elevation. An additional problem is that long-term use of both alkaloids can reduce lactation. Alternatively, intramuscular injection of 15-methyl $PGF_{2\alpha}$ (carboprost) may be tried. The ergot alkaloids are seldom used alone owing to the pronounced vasoactive effects associated with their serotoninergic actions. When used, usually relatively low doses are given and in combination with low doses of prostaglandins, thereby optimizing uterine actions and minimizing the degree of cardiovascular risk.

Uterine stimulants have also been used to induce therapeutic abortions. Abortion during the first trimester has traditionally been accomplished by means of suction curettage. However, for this stage of pregnancy there is increasing use of RU 486 or mifepristone. Mifepristone is a 19-norsteroid-progesterone antagonist that inhibits the action of endogenous progesterone on the uterus. The creation of an endocrine imbalance results in a potent abortifacient action. RU 486 is usually co-administered with a prostaglandin and causes abortion of the fetus in 99% of cases.

Mifepristone is a substituted 19-norsteroid (Fig. 22.34). The antiprogestational activity of mifepristone results from a competitive interaction with progesterone on the progesterone receptor. The endometrial and myometrial effects of progester-one are thereby blocked and termination of pregnancy results.

Following oral absorption the drug is rapidly absorbed with C_{max} occurring within 90 minutes. The drug is 69% bioavailable

and the elimination half-life is 18 hours. Mifepristone is metabolized by CYP-450 3A4 and as such activity may be increased by co-administration of other similar metabolizers. This is particularly relevant considering the target population may be taking azole antifungals, which are known to undergo metabolism by this route.

In general termination results from a 3-day daily dosing regimen of 200 mg mifepristone supplemented often by oral misoprostol on day 3. Normally in the period following ingestion, as a consequence of the primary pharmacology, the patient may need medication for uterine cramps and gastro-intestinal symptoms.

Beyond the second trimester several alternative approaches are available. These are primarily prostaglandin based, involving vaginal suppositories of PGE_2 or intramuscular $PGF_{2\alpha}$.

Drugs that decrease uterine motility

Therapeutically drugs that inhibit uterine contractions are used to delay or prevent premature labor, or to slow or arrest labor in order to undertake other procedures

Preterm (premature) labor is that which begins before the 37th week of pregnancy. It is responsible for a large fraction of neonatal illnesses and death due to inadequate fetal develop-ment. Despite major advances in neonatal care, retention of the fetus to full term is preferred in most instances. It is not always possible to determine whether premature labor is imminent. At least half of women presenting with premature but regular contractions will stabilize on bed rest. When this is insufficient, a tocolytic agent may be tried, generally when the gestation period is between 20 weeks and 34/36 weeks.

The preferred agents are the β_2 receptor agonists, particularly terbutaline and ritodrine. Both are available for oral and parenteral administration. As might be anticipated these β_2 agonists can produce quite marked cardiovascular changes, particularly tachycardia and increased cardiac output. In addition, long-term administration can result in hyperglycemia and as such their use in insulin-dependent diabetics may be difficult. A similar reduction in uterine motility can be achieved with calcium channel blockers. The relatively short-acting nifedipine has achieved some use in this context. There is little evidence from controlled clinical trials that these therapies actually improved fetal outcome.

β_2 Agonists have also been used to suppress uterine con-tractions under other circumstances. These include the allevi-ation of fetal distress during transport of the mother to hospital and during preparation for an operative delivery. Such a delivery may be necessitated by breech presentation, prolapsed cord or partial placental displacement.

FURTHER READING

Andersson K-E. The pharmacology of lower urinary tract smooth muscle and penile erectile tissues. *Pharmacological Reviews* 1993; **45**: 253–308. [Overview of overall autonomic control.]

Andersson K-E, Lepor H and Wyllie MG. Prostatic α_1-adrenoceptors and uroselectivity. *Prostate* 1997; **30**: 202–215. [Describes basic research into adrenoceptor subtypes.]

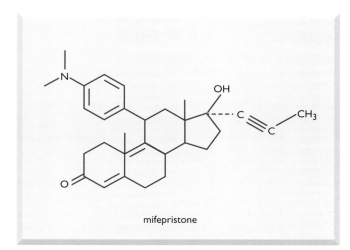

Fig. 22.34 Chemical structure of mifepristone.

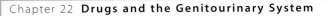

Eri LM and Tveter KJ. Alpha blockade in the treatment of symptomatic benign prostatic hyperplasia. *J Urology* 1995; **154**: 923–934. [Good clinical summary of α adrenoceptor antagonists.]

Naylor A. Endogenous neurotransmitters mediating penile erection. *Br J Urol* 1998; **81**: 424–431. [Covers cavernosal second messenger systems.]

Oesterling JE. Benign prostatic hyperplasia: a review of its histogenesis and natural history. *Prostate Supplement* 1996; **6**: 67–73. [Covers endocrine control of prostate growth.]

Wein AJ. Pharmacologic options for the overactive bladder. *Urology* 1998; **51** (Suppl 2A): 43–47. [Good summary of treatment options.]

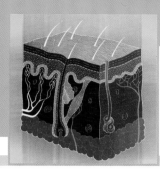

Chapter 23

Drugs and the Skin

PHYSIOLOGY OF THE SKIN

Skin protects the body against the environment and prevents excessive loss of protein, electrolytes, water, and heat. It is one of the largest organs, with a surface area of approximately 1.8 m^2, and accounts for 16% of body weight. It is composed of epidermis, dermis, and subcutis (Fig. 23.1).

PATHOPHYSIOLOGY AND DISEASES OF THE SKIN

The treatment of skin damage produced by trauma or disease is aimed at:
- Healing or eliminating the disease.
- Replacing or amplifying normal skin function.

Skin treatment preparations therefore include:
- Preparations aimed at the specific disease state.
- Preparations that increase protection from the environment and prevent loss of protein, electrolytes, water, and heat.

Although skin disease can be disfiguring and affect the quality of life, it is rarely life threatening. The risk–benefit ratio of any treatment must be considered when deciding on therapy. There are a number of skin disorders for which there is no safe and effective treatment, but under such circumstances the importance of camouflage creams and wigs must not be overlooked.

▓ *Drugs used to treat skin disease are ideally not absorbed beyond the skin*

Treatment applied to the skin may be designed for use in skin disease or the skin may act as a transdermal delivery system (see Chapter 5). Cutaneously applied drugs are delivered by a variety of vehicles, including ointments, creams, pastes, powders, aerosols, gels, lotions, and tinctures (Fig. 23.2). The choice of vehicle depends on:
- The solubility of the active drug.
- The ability of the vehicle to hydrate the stratum corneum and therefore enhance penetration.
- The stability of the drug in the vehicle.
- The ability of the vehicle to retard evaporation from the surface of the skin. This is greatest for ointments, and least for tinctures.

However, absorption of the drug depends on:
- Body site (e.g. drug absorption is low from the palms and soles, higher from the scalp and face, and very high from the scrotum and vulva).

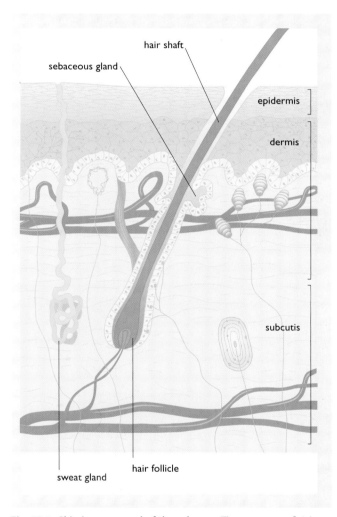

Fig. 23.1 Skin is composed of three layers. The most superficial layer of the skin is the epidermis, which varies in thickness from site to site. Beneath this lies the dermis, composed of collagen and some elastic fibers. The subcutis is the deepest layer of the skin and consists mainly of adipose tissue intersected by fibrocollagenous septa.

- Skin hydration (e.g. oil-in-water emulsions and occlusive dressings).
- Skin condition (e.g. damage due to inflammation or burns increases absorption).

Increasing the concentration gradient across the skin increases the mass of drug transferred per unit time. The ability of the skin to act as a reservoir for drugs must be considered when

Vehicles used for topically applied skin preparations

Vehicle	Physical and chemical properties	Use	Commercial examples
Ointments	Thicker than creams		
Water-soluble	Mixtures of polyethylene glycols to form macrogels; consistency can be varied; easily washed off	Lubricants; burn dressings; to improve the penetration of active drugs (e.g. hydrocortisone) into the skin	Macrogels and polyethylene glycol mixtures
Emulsifying	Allow evaporation; mix with water and skin exudate		Emulsifying ointment
Nonemulsifying	Do not mix with water; act as occlusive dressings, therefore enhancing hydration and drug penetration, and softening crusts, but preventing evaporation and heat loss	Chronic dry skin conditions, but are difficult to remove except with oil or detergents, and are rather messy and inconvenient	Paraffin ointment Simple ointment
Creams	Emulsion of oil in water or water in oil		
Oil in water	Vanish easily; washable; mix with serous discharge. Some contain a surface tension reducing agent	Cosmetically acceptable; a vehicle for water-soluble substances	Aqueous cream, cetomacroglycol
Water in oil	Act like oils (i.e. do not mix with serous discharge and aid skin hydration)	More cosmetically acceptable than ointments because they vanish easily, and are easy to apply; can be used on hairy areas; a vehicle for fat-soluble substances	Oily cream, zinc cream
Pastes	Thick, semi-occlusive ointment containing insoluble powders; very adhesive and can absorb some discharge		Zinc compound paste
Powders	Absorbent, but can cause crusting if applied to exudates; reduce friction between skin surfaces and have a cooling effect by increasing the effective surface area of the skin	A vehicle for antifungal powders	Zinc starch, talc
Gels	Semi-solid colloidal solutions or suspensions		
Lotions	Main component is water; evaporation of the water cools the skin and the subsequent vasoconstriction reduces inflammation	Can be used in hairy areas and in the presence of exudation	
Shake lotions	A means of applying powder to the skin, with additional cooling due to evaporation	Should not be used if there is much exudate	Calamine lotion

Fig. 23.2 **Vehicles used for topically applied skin preparations.**

determining dosing schedules, as drugs with a short systemic half-life may have a longer local half-life in the skin.

Although topical treatment is attractive for treating skin disease in terms of the risk–benefit ratio, many conditions require systemic therapy. The retinoids were specifically designed to treat skin diseases, but many other systemic agents used in the treatment of skin disease were originally developed for other conditions.

SKIN DISEASES

Skin disease accounts for 10–20% of all consultations in general practice. The most common skin complaints are dermatitis and eczema (5% of population), acne (1%), urticaria (1%), psoriasis (0.5%), viral warts (>1%), and skin cancer approximately 0.1% per year.

ECZEMA AND DERMATITIS

Eczema and dermatitis are interchangeable terms and describe a pattern of inflammation in the skin characterized by the presence of intercellular edema (spongiosis) in the epidermis rather than a single disease (Fig. 23.3). Although the unqualified term is often used to denote atopic eczema, eczema can also arise as the result of contact with irritants, e.g. strong acids, or contact allergens, e.g. nickel; hypersensitivity to *Pityrosporum* yeast (seborrheic dermatitis); local factors such as venous stasis (varicose eczema); or hypersensitivity reactions to drugs.

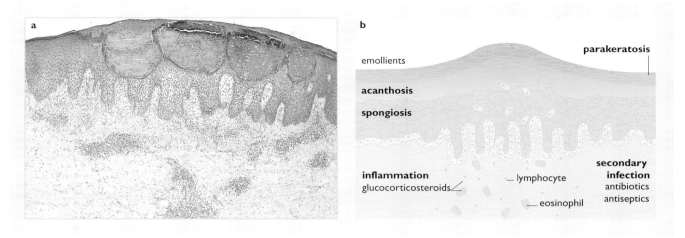

Fig. 23.3 Eczema. (a) Eczema is characterized histologically by epidermal spongiosis, permeated by an inflammatory infiltrate, predominantly of monocytes. (Courtesy of Dr P. McKee.) (b) Sites of drug action in eczema: emollients help to reduce transepidermal water loss, which is increased as a result of spongiosis; glucocorticosteroids are anti-inflammatory and vasoconstricting, and reduce keratinocyte cell division.

Rational treatment of eczema includes attempts to remove or minimize the above triggers as well as drugs aimed at reducing inflammation (corticosteroids, cyclosporine, azathioprine). The damage of the skin caused by the inflammation results in increased transepidermal water loss which can be partially corrected by the use of topical and bath emollients. Soap substitutes are used to minimize irritation of the damaged skin and antihistamines are used to reduce itching and hence further destruction of the skin surface by scratching.

Glucocorticosteroids (see also page 515)

Topical glucocorticosteroids are the mainstay of treatment of atopic eczema. They are anti-inflammatory and vasoconstricting, and reduce keratinocyte cell division. They are classified into four groups (Fig. 23.4), according to their vasoconstricting potency, which correlates remarkably well with their clinical efficacy.

Note that the different salts of hydrocortisone have very different potencies. Dermatologists therefore avoid nonspecific prescribing of glucocorticosteroids. The fluorinated glucocorticosteroids are particularly potent and are absorbed systemically. It is claimed that the newer glucocorticosteroids fluticasone propionate and mometasone fumarate are potent topical glucocorticosteroids with less systemic absorption.

Systemic steroids are rarely necessary in the treatment of atopic eczema, even in adults. They show relative lack of efficiency, tachyphylaxis and rebound and can interfere with growth particularly during the adolescent growth spurt. Glucocorticoids are discussed in detail in Chapter 16.

Cyclosporine

The efficacy of cyclosporine in atopic eczema was discovered by chance in patients undergoing organ transplantation who had coexistent eczema. Clinical trials in both adults and children have shown efficacy which is often rapid in onset but the condition relapses within weeks of stopping therapy. It is

Glucocorticosteroids and their vasoconstricting potencies	
Mild potency	Hydrocortisone 0.1, 0.5, 1, 2.5% Hydrocortisone acetate 1% Fluocinolone acetonide 0.0025% Methylprednisolone acetate 0.25%
Moderate potency	Hydrocortisone with urea Alclometasone dipropionate 0.05% Betamethasone valerate 0.025% Clobetasone butyrate* 0.05% Deoxymethasone 0.05% Fluocinolone acetonide 0.00625% Fluocortolone hexanoate 0.1% , 0.25% Fluocortolone pivalate 0.1%, 0.25% Flurandrenolide 0.0125%
Potent	Hydocortisone butyrate 0.1% Beclomethasone dipropionate 0.025%, 0.05% Betamethasone valerate 0.1% Budesonide 0.025% Deoxymethasole 0.25% Diflucortolone valerate 0.1% Flucloronide 0.025% Fluocinolone acetonide 0.025% Fluocinonide 0.05% Fluticasone propionate 0.05% Mometasone furoate 0.1% Triamcinolone acetonide 0.1%
Very potent	Clobetasol propionate 0.05% Diflucortolone valerate 0.3% Halcinonide 0.1%

Fig. 23.4 Glucocorticosteroids and their vasoconstricting potencies.

currently recommended in adults for short-term treatment of severe atopic eczema which has failed to respond to conventional therapy.

507

Cyclosporine acts mainly on T lymphocytes, but may also have a direct effect on DNA synthesis and proliferation in keratinocytes. Cyclosporine is discussed in detail in Chapter 15.

Patients need careful evaluation prior to starting cyclosporine, particularly with regard to renal function. Cyclosporine blood levels are not routinely measured in patients with skin diseases as the doses used (maximum 5 mg/kg) are well below those typically used in organ transplantation. Patients taking cyclosporine are advised to avoid excess sun exposure, UVB or PUVA therapy (because of the well established excess of skin cancers in patients who have had transplants which may in part be attributable to immunosuppressive therapy).

Cyclosporine is used for psoriasis more widely than for atopic eczema. It is indicated for severe psoriasis where conventional therapy is ineffective or inappropriate. Cyclosporine is beneficial in psoriatic arthropathy (see Chapters 16 and 20) and can be used in conjunction with methotrexate to minimize the toxicity and cumulative dose of each agent.

The value of cyclosporine in a variety of rare and severe dermatoses, such as pyoderma gangrenosum, is being evaluated.

Azathioprine

Azathioprine is a cytotoxic immunosuppressant which is used in unresponsive atopic eczema both as a steroid sparing agent and alone. (See Chapters 12 and 16 for more information about azathioprine.)

Emollients

Creams and ointments that improve skin hydration are called emollients. Ointments are generally greasy preparations which are insoluble in water and anhydrous, and are more occlusive than creams. Some newer ointments have both a hydrophilic and lipophilic component while others are water soluble ointments. Emollients reduce the excess transepidermal water loss, a feature of eczema, as evidenced by surface electrical capacitance, measurement of transepidermal water loss, and moulding of skin surface replicas. Thus they help restore barrier function but do not have an anti-inflammatory effect. They can soothe itching by their cooling effect but this is a transient benefit. There is some evidence that they reduce the susceptibility of eczematous skin to irritants.

Emollients form the mainstay of treatment of ichthyosis. Preparations containing urea and propylene glycol, which improve penetration, have been shown to be superior to other emollients in lamellar ichthyosis. Emollients are also useful in the treatment of other dry scaly skin conditions such as psoriasis.

There is a wide selection of commercially available emollients, containing a variety of ointments and creams (see Fig. 23.2), some of which are very greasy and can be too occlusive, while others are more water soluble and creamy, but less hydrating and need more frequent application. A mixture of soft white paraffin and liquid paraffin in equal parts is a thick emollient, whereas many of the cream formulations are thin emollients. Patient preference is an important consideration since these agents need to be used regularly and persistently. In practice this is influenced by stinging on application, ease

of application, appearance on the skin (is it obviously greasy?), smell, duration of action, effect on clothing, and ease of removal.

Bath emollients are similar to emollients in action and are designed for addition to the bath water to prevent skin drying while bathing.

Soap substitutes

Creamy cleansers are preferred to soaps in patients with atopic eczema, as the detergent in soaps can be both irritant and drying.

Antihistamines

H_1 antagonists are widely used in the treatment of atopic dermatitis in an effort to alleviate the itch (see Chapter 16). Although many clinical trials have suggested that the beneficial effect of antihistamines is due to their sedative effect (inhibiting scratching) some of the newer antihistamines, e.g. cetirizine, may have anti-inflammatory properties which may be relevant to their action in atopic dermatitis.

Antihistamines are the mainstay of treatment of urticaria and are also useful in the management of acute anaphylaxis and angioedema. In the treatment of urticaria, the choice of agent depends on the need for sedation, which is often desirable in acute urticaria but not in the chronic form.

For prolonged treatment, patients prefer longer-acting drugs. Astemizole is the longest-acting H_1 antagonist, but like terfenadine interacts with drugs commonly used in primary care (e.g. erythromycin) to produce prolongation of the QT interval, and this must be considered when using these agents. Loratadine is a long-acting antihistamine that appears not to produce these interactions.

Histamine H_2 antagonists have sometimes been advocated in urticaria but the evidence regarding their efficacy is conflicting. They have more recently been used at high dosage to treat viral warts but the results of clinical trials to date have been variable.

Approaches to the treatment of eczema are summarized in Fig. 23.3.

Acne

▨ Acne is a disease of the pilosebaceous unit

Acne is characterized by comedones (keratin plugs in the sebaceous duct opening), inflammatory papules, pustules, nodules, cysts, and scars. The rash occurs where there is a high density of pilosebaceous glands (e.g. on the face, back, and chest). Androgenic stimulation of the sebaceous glands at puberty accounts for the high prevalence of acne at puberty, and the active pilosebaceous follicles are heavily colonized by *Propionibacterium acnes*. The mechanism for keratin plug formation is poorly understood, but is thought to be pivotal. Continued gland secretion then results in swelling of the glands and ducts, with nodule and cyst formation and the induction of an inflammatory response, which produces inflammatory papules and pustules. Approaches to the treatment of acne are shown in Fig. 23.5.

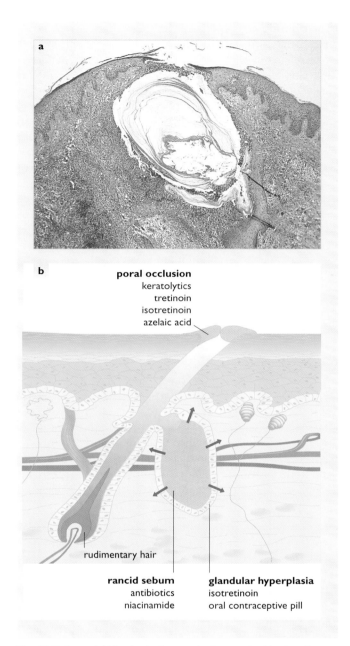

Fig. 23.5 Acne. (a) Histologically, acne is characterized by keratin plugs (comedones) which block the sebaceous follicle, so that sebum cannot escape. The sebaceous glands are often hyperplastic, and there can be an intense neutrophil influx. (Courtesy of Dr P. McKee.) (b) Sites of drug action in acne.

Keratolytics

Topical keratolytics (e.g. salicylic acid, sulfur) are used in acne to reduce pore occlusion which is characteristic of acne.

SULFUR although of proven efficacy is rarely used because of its smell.

SALICYLIC ACID is soluble in alcohol but only slightly soluble in water. It is thought to act by solubilizing the cell surface proteins that keep the stratum corneum intact, resulting in desquamation. It is keratolytic at a concentration of 3–6%. Higher concentrations can destroy tissues.

Salicylic acid is absorbed percutaneously, and 1 g of 6% salicylic acid results in plasma concentrations of approximately 0.5 mg/dl (0.04 mmol/liter). Salicylism and death have been recorded after topical application but the threshold for toxicity is 30–50 mg/dl (2.17–3.62 mmol/liter). Such concentrations are unlikely to be achieved with keratolytic concentrations (3–6%) but should be borne in mind with higher, destructive concentrations, especially in children.

Adverse effects include urticarial and anaphylactic reactions in patients who are sensitive to salicylates.

Clinical uses other than acne include destruction of viral warts in concentrations of 16–40%, use in conjunction with topical steroids to increase skin penetration (concentrations of approx 10%), and in conjunction with benzoic acid in Whitfield's ointment which is fungicidal.

AZELAIC ACID is a saturated nine-carbon-atom dicarboxylic acid. It was originally obtained by the oxidation of oleic acid by nitric acid but it can also be obtained by fermentation by a variety of micro-organisms.

The observations that the *Pityrosporum* fungus can oxidize oleic acid to azelaic acid in culture, and that azelaic acid is a competitive inhibitor of tyrosinase, led to studies to test the hypothesis that this acid was responsible for the hypo-pigmentation which characterizes pityriasis versicolor and therefore might have a role in hyperpigmentation disorders.

In subsequent studies azelaic acid was shown to have a beneficial effect in melanosis due to hyperfunction of pro-liferative melanocytes but to lack a de-pigmenting effect on normal skin. In patients being treated for melasma those with co-incident acne noticed improvement. Subsequent research has demonstrated that azelaic acid has:

- Anti-enzymatic and antimitochondrial activity: it is a reversible inhibitor of cytochrome P-450 reductase and 5 α-reductase and can reversibly inhibit some enzymes of the respiratory chain as well as being a competitive inhibitor of tyrosinase. It also has an inhibitory effect on anaerobic glycolysis.
- Antimicrobial and antiviral effect: in culture azelaic acid inhibits both aerobic and anaerobic micro-organisms including *P. acnes*, and an inhibitory effect on vaccinia virus replication has been shown.
- Effect on tumoral cells in culture: a dose-dependent effect on proliferation and viability of melanoma cells, lymphoma and leukemia derived cell lines while not affecting normal cells in culture.

In acne, inhibition of aerobic respiration and anaerobic glycolysis are thought to be important in its effects on micro-organisms, and the reduction of cellular energy formation in keratinocytes may be relevant. Azelaic acid is keratolytic and comedolytic and in part normalizes the disturbed terminal differentiation of keratinocytes in the follicle infundibulum. It is available as a topical cream for the treatment of acne.

Furthermore, anaerobic glycolysis is thought to be important in sebaceous glands, so that there may be an additional direct effect on sebaceous gland activity.

Azelaic acid is well tolerated. Benefit is often not seen for up to 4 weeks and treatment should be continued for several months.

In pigmentary disorders the primary effect of azelaic acid is thought to be the reduction of cellular energy formation. It has been shown to be as effective as hydroquinone 4% in this regard.

BENZOYL PEROXIDE penetrates the stratum corneum and follicular openings unchanged, but is converted to benzoic acid in the epidermis and dermis. It has several actions:

- Germicidal—having an effect on the reduction in facial microbial flora equal to that of systemic tetracycline.
- Keratolytic.
- Comedolytic.
- Anti-inflammatory.
- Sebostatic? (subject of some controversy).

Adverse effects of benzoyl peroxide include irritation with increasing concentrations, and sensitizing properties: up to 1% of patients develop a contact allergic dermatitis. Bleaching of hair, skin and clothing can be unacceptable.

In addition to its use in acne, benzoyl peroxide has been used in combination with miconazole, where it is said to increase efficacy, and a 20% lotion has been used to promote rapid re-epithelialization of wounds.

Mild keratolytics are also used to enhance the emollient effect of a cream or vehicle (e.g. urea). Stronger keratolytic therapy is used for conditions such as viral warts.

Niacinamide

Niacinamide is the amide of vitamin B_3. Physiologically, it is converted to nicotinamide adenine dinucleotide (NAD) or the dinucleotide phosphate (NADP), both of which function as coenzymes (see Chapter 27). Niacinamide is thought to act by electron scavenging, inhibition of phosphodiesterase, and/or increased tryptophan conversion to serotonin. It also has direct effects on inflammatory cells, inhibiting neutrophils, suppressing lymphocyte transformation, and inhibiting mast cell histamine release. Niacinamide may be a useful treatment for acne. Clinical trials to date suggest that topical niacinamide gel is as effective as topical clindamycin for mild to moderate acne, and represents a nonantibiotic treatment that appears to be well tolerated. In acne its main effect seems to be inhibition of cyclic AMP phosphodiesterase and lymphocyte transformation, which may inhibit epithelial proliferation in the pilosebaceous unit.

Antibiotics (see Chapter 9)

TOPICAL ANTIBIOTICS Topical administration of antibiotics for acne (Fig. 23.6) has been shown to be equi-effective to benzoyl peroxide or tretinoin, but their long-term use risks the emergence of resistant organisms.

SYSTEMIC ANTIBIOTICS Oral antibiotics (Fig. 23.7) are more effective than topical antibiotics in the treatment of acne. Treatment should be continued for a minimum of 6 months but some improvement should be evident at 3 months. If there is no improvement consider changing antibiotic as resistant strains of P. *acnes* are increasingly common, particularly to

Topical antibiotics—acne

Antibiotic	Efficacy	Other issues affecting choice
Clindamycin	1% clindamycin phosphate = oral minocycline and tetracyline = 5% benzoyl peroxide gel • topical tetracycline • < topical niacinamide	
Erythromycin	Only lipid soluble formulations—propionate or stearate—are effective 2% erythromycin gel = 1% clindamycin phosphate 1.5% erythromycin solution = 1% clindamycin phosphate solution	Erythromycin resistance common
Erythromycin with zinc castor oil in oily cream 1:9		May delay emergence of resistance
Erythromycin with benzoyl peroxide		May delay emergence of resistance
Tetracyclines	Effective and considered cosmetically acceptable by 90% patients	Tetracycline resistance common Stain clothing and skin

Fig. 23.6 Topical antibiotics—acne.

Systemic antibiotics—acne

Antibiotic	Advantages	Disadvantages
Tetracyclines	Antibiotic of choice. Bacteriostatic at high doses; at low doses affect bacterial function	Not recommended under the age of 12 because of discoloration of teeth. Avoid in pregnancy and breastfeeding
• Oxytetracycline		Chelates with calcium-containing food, so needs to be taken with water half an hour before food otherwise there is reduced absorption
• Minocycline	Compliance improved by once-daily dosage, as better absorbed	Can cause hyperpigmentation due to deposition of drug in skin
• Doxycycline	Compliance improved by once-daily dosage, as better absorbed	Photosensitivity dose-related
Erythromycin	Bacteriostatic Can be used in patients who may become pregnant or breastfeeding	
Trimethoprim	Equi-effective to tetracycline Reserved for third-line treatment	
Clindamycin	Useful because of lipid solubility	Not to be used routinely because of risk of pseudomembranous colitis

Fig. 23.7 Systemic antibiotics—acne.

erythromycin, tetracycline, and doxycycline. Some of the therapeutic effect of these antibiotics is due to nonbacterial effects which include:

- Enzyme inhibition, e.g. *Corynebacterium acnes* lipase.
- Modulation of chemotaxis.
- Modulation of lymphocyte function.
- Modulation of cytokines, especially IL-1α expression.

Retinoids (Fig. 23.8)

Retinoids include vitamin A and its derivatives, and have potent effects on:

- Cell differentiation, which they induce.
- Cell growth, inducing hyperplasia, hypergranulosis, and decreased numbers of tonofilaments and desmosomes in the epidermis. The latter effect is thought to account for the keratolytic effect.
- The immune response, stimulating cell-mediated cytotoxicity and acting as an adjuvant to stimulate antibody production to antigens that were not previously immunogenic. They also reduce neutrophil migration, although the mechanism for this is not known.

Intracellularly, retinoids stabilize lysosomes, increase ribonucleic acid polymerase activity, increase incorporation of thymidine into DNA, and increase prostaglandin (PG) E$_2$, cAMP and cGMP concentrations. The action of retinoids is mediated by retinoic acid receptors (RARs) which are members of the thyroid/steroid superfamily of receptors. The RARs bind retinoids and DNA, and function as transcription factors initiating transcription (see Chapter 27).

Retinoids

	Drug	Disease
1st Generation	Retinol Tretinoin Isotretinoin	Acne
2nd Generation	Etretinate Acitretin	Psoriasis (and other papulosquamous diseases)

Fig. 23.8 Retinoids.

TOPICAL RETINOIDS (Fig. 23.9) Tretinoin is the acid form of vitamin A (i.e. retinoic acid). It is formed by oxidation of the alcohol group in vitamin A alcohol, with all four double bonds in the side chain in the transconfiguration. It is insoluble in water, but soluble in many organic solvents. It is available topically for use in acne, where its efficacy is attributed to decreased cohesion between epidermal cells and increased epidermal cell turnover. It is thought that this helps remove comedones, and convert closed comedones to open comedones.

The main adverse effect is skin irritation, but patients also should be warned to avoid exposure to ultraviolet light while using tretinoin as it appears to increase the tumorigenic potential of ultraviolet light in animal studies.

A regular application of 0.05% tretinoin cream for a minimum of 4 months improves the appearance of photo-

Topical retinoids

Drug name	Advantages	Mode of action
Tretinoin Retinoic acid 0.01–0.05 in cream or gel		Binds to cytosolic retinoid acid-binding protein (RAR) with high affinity. Binds all nuclear receptors
Isotretinoin 0.05%	= Benzoyl peroxide and topical tretinoin	
Adapalene	More effective with less irritation than tretinoin. Only topical retinoid with significant anti-inflammatory effect	Does not bind cytosolic retinoid RAR and binds RAR β and α selectively in nucleus

Fig. 23.9 Topical retinoids.

damaged skin, and is licensed for the treatment of mottled hyperpigmentation and fine wrinkling caused by chronic sun exposure.

ORAL RETINOIDS Isotretinoin is a synthetic retinoid that is now available for systemic and topical use. Its main effect seems to be to reduce the size and function of the sebaceous glands, and a 4–6-month course is highly effective in the treatment of acne in the majority of patients.

Isotretinoin is well absorbed, extensively bound to plasma proteins, and eliminated. It is given at a dose of 0.5–1 mg/kg.

The adverse effects of isotretinoin resemble the effects of hypervitaminosis A, producing dry skin and mucous membranes, and epidermal fragility. Rarely, visual disturbances, hair thinning, myalgia and arthralgia, and raised liver enzymes have been reported. Cutaneous complications include photosensitivity, allergic vasculitis, granulomatous lesions, and acne

Treatment of acne

- Keratolytics should be used as first-line therapy
- If a systemic antibiotic is needed, tetracyclines are indicated in children over 12 years of age, but should not be given to children under 12 because of their effects on maturing teeth
- Oxytetracycline should be given before minocycline because of the rare reaction to minocycline involving liver, joints, and fever
- In children under 12 years of age erythromycin is the systemic drug of choice
- In adults, tetracyclines should be given in preference to erythromycin as erythromycin is used for life-threatening infections such as *Mycoplasma pneumoniae*
- Antibiotic resistance to *Propionibacterium acnes* is as high as 40% in patients with acne referred to hospital

fulminans. Isotretinoin can cause benign intracranial hypertension (BIH), so frequent or unusual headaches are an indication to stop treatment and investigate as appropriate. As tetracyclines can also cause BIH, the two drugs should not be given together. Triglyceride concentrations increase during treatment, but with normal initial concentrations this increase is rarely sufficient to stop therapy and is reversible on stopping treatment.

■ *Isotretinoin is teratogenic and should be given to women of child-bearing age only after appropriate counseling and with adequate contraception*

Psoriasis

Psoriasis is a genetically determined hyperproliferative disorder that can be triggered by infection, trauma, drugs, ultraviolet light, and stress, and rarely by hypocalcemia. Psoriatic skin turns over in seven days rather than the normal 56 days. It is characterized by:

- Thickened skin plaques with superficial scales.
- Capillary dilation in the papillary dermis.
- An inflammatory infiltrate, predominantly of lymphocytes, in the dermis.
- A neutrophil infiltrate in the epidermis.

The capillary dilation may be an initiating event or an attempt to nourish the hyperproliferating skin. The precise contribution of the inflammatory cells to the clinical disease is not clear.

Approaches to the treatment of psoriasis are shown in Fig. 23.10.

Treatment for patients with psoriasis must be individualized. For localized disease, topical therapy is often sufficient. Vitamin D analogs are rapidly becoming first-line treatment not least because they are clean, nonstaining, nonsmelling preparations which afford a cosmetic advantage over tar and anthralin preparations. However, these preparations need to be applied accurately to affected sites and if the percentage of body area affected is large, the potential to disturb systemic calcium homeostasis needs to be considered. Anthralin (see below) is still the least toxic agent and offers the potential benefit of inducing remission. However, it is very messy to use and irritation can be a problem particularly in the fair skinned. Most

Adverse effects of isotretinoin

- *Teratogenicity*
- *Dry skin and mucous membranes*
- *Epidermal fragility*
- *Rarely, visual disturbances, hair thinning, myalgia and arthralgia, and raised liver enzymes*
- *Allergic vasculitis*
- *Granulomatous lesions*
- *Acne fulminans*
- *Benign intracranial hypertension*
- *Increased triglyceride concentrations*

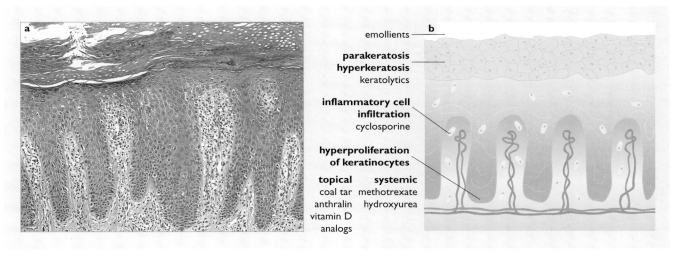

Fig. 23.10 Psoriasis. (a) Psoriasis is characterized by epidermal acanthosis, with clubbed papillae, suprapapillary thinning with dilation of the capillaries, and hyper- and parakeratosis. Lymphocytes predominate in the dermis, whereas neutrophils may form microabscesses in the epidermis. (Courtesy of Dr P. McKee.) (b) Sites of drug action in psoriasis.

patients requiring anthralin are treated in daycare centers or as inpatients, so that a time commitment is required from the patients to be worthwhile. Tar preparations often offer the best compromise between efficacy, ease of application, and tolerable mess and smell.

In patients with more widespread disease, combination therapy—in particular with light therapy—is often instigated. Again to be effective phototherapy demands committed patients, as treatment regimes involve visits to the hospital twice a week for 6–8 weeks.

In patients with associated psoriatic arthropathy, and in patients where the extent of the disease is causing great disability, systemic therapy may be contemplated. All systemic agents used for psoriasis—methotrexate, hydroxyurea, cyclosporine, and acitretin—have potentially serious adverse effects and the decision to embark on such treatment needs to be reached after careful discussion with patients, and with well defined clinical justification.

Vitamin D

The naturally occurring active metabolite of vitamin D_3, 1α 25 dihydroxyvitamin D_3 (calcitriol), and two synthetic analogs—calcipotriol and tacalcitol—are effective when applied topically in psoriasis

Vitamin D analogs inhibit epidermal proliferation, induce terminal keratinocyte differentiation, and have anti-inflammatory properties *in vitro* and *in vivo*.

Vitamin D receptors (VDRs) are found in keratinocytes, melanocytes, Langerhans' cells, dermal fibroblasts, monocytes, and T lymphocytes in normal skin. They belong to the large family of structurally related ligand-inducible transcription factors, which includes the retinoid receptors and thyroid hormone receptors (see Chapters 15 and 27).

In psoriasis, there is increased expression of VDRs in the basal and suprabasal layers of the epidermis, as well as a marked increase in the density of VDR positivity in intra-epidermal and perivascular T cells and macrophages.

The effects of vitamin D analogs include:

- Inhibition of T cell proliferation by blocking the transition of T cells from the early to the late G1 phase of the cell cycle.
- Inhibition of the release of various cytokines, including interleukin (IL)-2, IL-6, IL-8, interferon (IFN)-γ, tumor necrosis factor (TNF)-β, and granulocyte–macrophage colony stimulating factor (GM-CSF).
- A reduction in the capacity of monocytes to stimulate T cell proliferation and lymphokine release from T cells.
- Reduced neutrophil accumulation in psoriatic skin.

The mechanism of action of these analogs is not yet elucidated. The goal is to develop analogs that induce the expression of the vitamin D-responding genes governing Ca^{2+} homeostasis and analogs that induce expression of the vitamin D-responding genes influencing the keratinocyte cell cycle.

Clearly, for the treatment of skin disease, such analogs should optimally affect the cell cycle and have a minimal effect on systemic Ca^{2+} homeostasis.

CALCIPOTRIENE is a vitamin D_3 analog (a side-chain modification of 1α 25-dihydroxyvitamin D_3). It is available for the topical treatment of psoriasis as a cream, ointment, and scalp solution. It is effective alone, and has been shown to have a sparing effect when used with ultraviolet light treatment, cyclosporine, methotrexate, and retinoids. Calcium metabolism is not affected at doses of less than 100 g/week.

Calcipotriene has become the drug of choice for mild to moderate psoriasis. Its non-staining formulation greatly improves patient compliance compared with that for coal tar and anthralin preparations. It causes facial irritation in some patients. Calcipotriene has also been reported to be of benefit in the treatment of other dyskeratotic states and pityriasis rubra pilaris.

TACALCITOL (1α 24-dihydroxyvitamin D$_3$) has recently become available in the UK for the topical treatment of psoriasis. It is applied once daily, and in clinical trials was tolerated on the face and in the flexures.

Anthralin

The anti-psoriatic component of goa powder was identified as chrysarobin, an easily oxidizable reduction product of chrysophanic acid, in 1878. The synthetic chrysarobin substitute, anthralin, was introduced in 1915.

One of the challenges of anthralin formulation has been achieving a compound which is stable in the reduced active form over long periods while permitting it to oxidize rapidly within the tissue. This has traditionally been achieved using zinc and salicylic acid paste, although newer cream formulations and liposomal formulations have been developed.

One of the limitations of anthralin compounds is that they cause irritation and staining. Anthralin is unique because it can lead to remission of psoriasis.

Anthralin is available as a cream (0.1–2%) and ointment (0.1–2%) for home use. The treatment is usually applied for 30–60 minutes (short-contact anthralin therapy) and then removed. Anthralin paste is largely confined to hospital use and can be applied for 24 hours or for shorter time periods. Anthralin must be applied to a test area first before treating the whole body, as patient tolerance varies. The strength of anthralin is gradually increased (e.g. doubling concentrations every 3–5 days). Therapy is discontinued when the plaques have flattened. Anthralin inevitably stains the skin and this stain can be removed with a keratolytic agent. It also stains clothing. Anthralin can be used in combination with light therapy, and coal tar baths (Ingram regimen).

No systemic toxicity has been reported with anthralin. However, it is irritant to normal skin and therefore must be applied accurately to the plaques of psoriasis.

Tar preparations

Therapeutic tars are products of the destructive distillation of wood, coal, or bitumen. They are highly complex mixtures with some 10,000 constituents. Petroleum tars have no therapeutic importance.

WOOD TARS (OIL OF CADE, BEE, BIRCH, AND PINE) are available as ointments, pastes, and alcohol paints. They may sensitize, but do not photosensitize.

BITUMINOUS TARS were originally obtained from the distillation of shale deposits containing fossilized fish. Some have a high sulfur content. They are less effective than coal tars and do not photosensitize.

COAL TAR is a black fluid with a characteristic smell. Different methods of distilling heated coal have been used to try to remove its color and odor. Coal tar modifies keratinization but its mechanism of action is poorly understood. The high boiling-point tar acids (phenolics) may be responsible for its therapeutic effect, possibly by releasing lysosomes in the granular layer. Coal tars are also antipruritic (and are therefore used for eczema as well as psoriasis), mildly antiseptic, and photosensitizing. Refined tars are less phototoxic, but phototoxicity is directly related to therapeutic efficacy in psoriasis.

The carcinogenicity of pitch and heavy tar fractions is well established, but malignant tumors are extremely rare in relation to tar therapy. A few cases of genital cancer have been reported, but a recent study with a 25-year follow up has shown that the incidence of skin tumors in patients using coal tar is not increased.

The photosensitizing potential of coal tars is exploited in the Goeckerman regimen (i.e. combination therapy with ultraviolet light B) for psoriasis, which reduces epidermal DNA synthesis, possibly by forming cross-links between opposite strands on the DNA double helix.

The most common adverse effect is an irritant folliculitis. Phototoxicity and contact allergic dermatitis can also occur.

Acitretin

Acitretin is the main active metabolite of etretinate; etretinate is an aromatic retinoid with a slow terminal elimination phase of several months.

Acitretin was developed in the hope that its decreased lipophilicity and reduced elimination half-life (50 hours rather than 80 days for etretinate) would be an advantage particularly in women of child-bearing potential as the retinoids are highly teratogenic. However, in some patients reversed metabolism of acitretin to etretinate has been demonstrated, so that pregnancy must be avoided for at least 2 years after the ingestion of acitretin, like its predecessor, etretinate.

Acitretin is used in the treatment of psoriasis, particularly erythrodermic and generalized pustular psoriasis, at doses of 0.5–1 mg/kg. Higher doses are needed for chronic plaque psoriasis, but its use in combination therapy with psoralen plus ultraviolet light A (PUVA) or ultraviolet light B is increasing because it has an ultraviolet light-sparing effect.

Acitretin has a narrow therapeutic window and at doses of 1 mg/kg adverse effects are common. Dryness of the lips, eyes, and mucous membranes are frequent as is desquamation of palms and soles and skin burning sensations. Hair loss, nose bleeds and paronychia are often a nuisance and may limit the dose. More serious adverse effects include musculoskeletal effects resembling diffuse idiopathic skeletal hyperostosis. Prior and periodic radiographic screening is therefore advised for long-term use. As with isotretinoin, liver function and lipids need regular monitoring.

In patients who cannot tolerate doses of acitretin which are sufficient to control their disease, combination therapy can be considered. Acitretin has been used in combination with tar, dithranol, UVB and PUVA. Combination with methotrexate has been reported in difficult cases but these drugs pose potential interactions with increased blood levels of methotrexate and combined effects on liver toxicity. However, it is sometimes necessary to continue acitretin in a patient until the therapeutic effects of methotrexate are established as this takes 6 to 8 weeks.

It has been claimed that tumors, including solar keratoses, kerato-acanthoma, epidermodysplasia verruciformis, basal cell epithelioma (BCE) and leukoplakia, sometimes clear following treatment with isotretinoin or etretinate. The use of retinoids in preventing skin tumors in high-risk patients, such as those with xeroderma pigmentosum and transplant patients, is currently being investigated in ongoing trials.

Methotrexate

Methotrexate exerts a strong antimitotic effect on keratinocytes by inhibiting DNA synthesis by competitive inhibition of dihydrofolate reductase (see Chapter 16). At doses used in the treatment of psoriasis, methotrexate also inhibits neutrophil chemotaxis. It is administered once a week for the treatment of psoriasis. Patients taking methotrexate must refrain totally from alcohol. Renal, hepatic, and bone marrow function must be assessed prior to, and during, methotrexate treatment, and note should be taken of potential drug interactions (see Chapters 17 and 28).

CYCLOSPORINE (see Eczema above)

Photo(chemo)therapy

UVB therapy is effective in many patients with psoriasis. Other patients require stronger, PUVA photochemotherapy (psoralens + UVA). Psoralens are photoctivated chemicals that intercalate with DNA, forming cyclobutane adducts with pyrimidine in bases on subsequent exposure to ultraviolet light A. This forms the basis of PUVA photochemotherapy. This is an established treatment for psoriasis and mycosis fungoides, and clinical trials are being conducted to investigate its use in vitiligo.

Drugs acting on hair

FINASTERIDE at 1 mg/ml has recently been launched for the treatment of male androgenic alopecia (see Chapter 22 for description of finasteride).

TOPICAL MINOXIDIL reverses androgenic alopecia in some patients. Its mechanism of action is unknown and its effect on androgenic alopecia is not permanent, with hair loss occurring within 4–6 months when it is stopped.

CYPROTERONE ACETATE in conjunction with ethinyl estradiol is used to prevent the progression of androgenic alopecia in females.

Cyproterone acetate is the treatment of choice for female hirsutism. It is an anti-androgen and:
* Decreases adrenal androgen secretion.
* Competes with both testosterone and dihydrotestosterone for the androgen receptor.
* Inhibits the 5α-reductase enzyme.
* Inhibits luteinizing hormone secretion by its progestational effects.

A dose of 2 mg daily is sufficient, and it is usually given in combination with an estrogen to ensure regular menstrual bleeding. An improvement may not be evident for 6–12 months. A male fetus will probably be feminized if a pregnancy occurs when cyproterone acetate is used alone.

LUTEINIZING HORMONE RELEASING HORMONE ANALOGS may improve hirsutism in patients with high androgen levels of ovarian origin.

DRUGS THAT MODIFY INFLAMMATORY RESPONSES IN THE SKIN

Glucocorticosteroids

The efficacy of glucocorticosteroid required depends on:
* The skin disease (e.g. very potent for lichen planus).
* The site to be treated (e.g. mild to moderate only for facial application).
* The age of the patient (e.g. the indications for a potent glucocorticosteroid in a child are limited).

In general, very potent glucocorticosteroids should be given to adults only under specialist supervision and should not be prescribed for children without consultation with a specialist. Glucocorticosteroid penetration varies with:
* Body site. It is higher when applied to the genitals, face, and scalp than when applied to the trunk and limbs.
* State of the skin. It is enhanced by erythema or erosion.
* Occlusion, which increases penetration at least tenfold.
* The vehicle used. Ointments produce higher penetration than creams.
* Concentration of drug. A high concentration produces higher penetration than a low concentration, but penetration is not proportional to the concentration difference (e.g. increasing the concentration of hydrocortisone tenfold results in a fourfold increase in penetration).

◾ *Intralesional glucocorticosteroids are used for keloid and hypertrophic scars, chondrodermatitis nodularis helicis, and acne cysts*

Local injection is also sometimes helpful in alopecia areata and hypertrophic lichen planus that has not responded to topical glucocorticosteroids.

Intralesional administration of glucocorticosteroids overcomes the limited penetration of topical glucocorticosteroids and is used to provide a high local concentration of glucocorticosteroid. Relatively insoluble glucocorticosteroids (e.g. triamcinolone acetonide, triamcinolone diacetate, triamcinolone hexacetonide, betamethasone acetate–phosphate) are used to achieve high local doses, which are gradually released for 3–4 weeks. The injections must be limited to 1 mg per site to avoid local skin atrophy.

◾ *Topical glucocorticosteroids are indicated in the treatment of inflammatory skin disorders and are a vital part of the acute treatment of most forms of dermatitis (eczema)*

The potency of topical glucocorticosteroid used must be titrated to the disease severity and the minimum effective strength determined for each patient. In seborrheic dermatitis, a combination of glucocorticosteroids and antipityrosporal agents is useful to calm the eczema, but antipityrosporal agents used early in relapse should be sufficient.

Topical glucocorticosteroids are useful in the treatment of flexural psoriasis, but should not be used as a first-line treatment elsewhere as a rebound exacerbation of the disease occurs on withdrawal. It is not uncommon for patients to require increasing doses of glucocorticosteroids to control the disease. If very potent glucocorticosteroids are then withdrawn, generalized pustular psoriasis can ensue, which is a medical emergency and often requires systemic treatment with agents such as methotrexate (see page 177).

Potent topical glucocorticosteroids are used short-term in the treatment of vitiligo and alopecia areata, but should not be continued for more than 4 weeks.

A trial of topical glucocorticosteroids is worthwhile for sarcoidosis, discoid lupus erythematosus, and pemphigus, although systemic treatments are often necessary.

■ *Systemic glucocorticosteroids are used for severe acute dermatoses, pemphigus, pemphigoid, and lichen planus*

Systemic glucocorticosteroids are used only for severe dermatologic diseases because the treatment benefits must outweigh the risks of long-term use (see Chapter 12). They are indicated for:

- Severe acute dermatoses such as anaphylaxis, acute contact allergic dermatitis, acute autoimmune connective tissue diseases and generalized vasculitis, and generalized drug eruptions.
- Chronic disabling disorders such as pemphigus and pemphigoid.
- Severe lichen planus.
- Pyoderma gangrenosum.
- Sarcoidosis.
- Various other unusual dermatoses.

■ *All the adverse effects of systemic glucocorticosteroids can be observed if there is significant systemic absorption of topical glucocorticosteroids*

Local adverse reactions include worsening and spread of any infection (viral, bacterial, and fungal). Skin atrophy, striae, hirsutism, acne, and depigmentation may occur with long-term use, and the application of potent glucocorticosteroids on the face induces a 'perioral dermatitis.'

Antimalarial drugs

Hydroxychloroquine, chloroquine, and mepacrine have a beneficial effect on discoid and systemic lupus erythematosus, polymorphic light eruption, and solar urticaria, and there is some evidence of a therapeutic response in cutaneous sarcoidosis and porphyria cutanea tarda. Their mechanism of action in these disorders is unknown, but they have been shown to:

- Inhibit prostaglandin synthesis, chemotaxis, and hydrolytic enzymes.
- Stabilize membranes.
- Bind to DNA.

Sulfa drugs

Dapsone is the drug of choice for leprosy, and is also used in the treatment of dermatitis herpetiformis, immunobullous disorders, and numerous other rare dermatoses (see Chapter 9). Its mechanism of action is unclear, although neutrophils and immune complexes seem to play a part in the diseases influenced by the drug. Patients taking dapsone must be monitored for signs of hemolysis and methemoglobinemia because hemolytic anemia is a common adverse reaction and, although rare, methemoglobinemia can be a rapidly fatal complication.

Other sulfa drugs having some of the useful effects of dapsone are sulfapyridine and sulfamethoxypyridazine.

Other drugs modifying the immune response

COLCHICINE is an alkaloid derived from the autumn crocus that:

- Inhibits neutrophil and monocyte chemotaxis, collagen synthesis, and mast cell histamine release.
- Increases collagenolysis.
- Arrests mitosis in metaphase and is therefore antimitotic.

Colchicine has been used in the treatment of a variety of dermatologic diseases characterized by leukocyte infiltration of the skin, including Behçet's syndrome, psoriasis, palmoplantar pustulosis, dermatitis herpetiformis, Sweet's syndrome, necrotizing vasculitis, childhood dermatomyositis, and systemic sclerosis.

Adverse effects include gastrointestinal disturbances, which are very frequent in patients taking relatively large doses of colchicine.

THALIDOMIDE is an immunomodulatory drug whose activities are not well characterized but may involve decreasing concentrations of TNF-α. It is used for the treatment of recalcitrant aphthous ulceration, especially in patients with HIV, and has been beneficial in the treatment of pyoderma gangrenosum and Behçet's syndrome. It is efficacious in erythema nodosum leprosum.

Adverse effects include teratogenicity which may be profound: the drug is contraindicated in any woman who might become pregnant. Patients need to be closely monitored in order to detect neuropathy at an early stage, ideally while the problem is subclinical.

The kinetics of thalidomide are not well characterized; it has a half-life of 3–5 hours.

ORAL CONTRACEPTIVES Combination contraceptive pills containing cyproterone acetate, ethinyl estradiol, and desogestrol are 'acne-friendly,' unlike most other contraceptive pills which tend to aggravate acne.

ALKYLATING AGENTS AND ANTIMETABOLITES Drugs such as alkylating agents and antimetabolites (see Chapter 28) are used in dermatology only if the disease is sufficiently disabling to justify the risks of their use (Fig. 23.11).

Alkylating agents and antimetabolites and their dermatologic disease indications

Drug	Uses
Cyclophosphamide	Pemphigus, pemphigoid Wegener's granulomatosis Lupus erythematosus Polymyositis Mycosis fungoides Histiocytosis X
Chlorambucil	Mycosis fungoides Behçet's disease Lupus erythematosus Wegener's granulomatosis Glucocorticosteroid-resistant sarcoidosis Sézary syndrome
Mustine injection	Mycosis fungoides
Dacarbazine injection	Metastatic malignant melanoma
Methotrexate (given weekly; caution in the elderly and in renal impairment)	Psoriasis Reiter's syndrome Pityriasis rubra pilaris Ichthyosiform erythroderma Sarcoidosis Pemphigus/pemphigoid Glucocorticosteroid-resistant dermatomyositis
Hydroxyurea (less effective than methotrexate)	Psoriasis
Azathioprine (glucocorticosteroid-sparing agent)	Pemphigus/pemphigoid Lupus erythematosus Dermatomyositis Wegener's granulomatosis Actinic reticuloid Pityriasis rubra pilaris Intractable eczema in adults
Bleomycin	Squamous cell carcinoma Mycosis fungoides and other lymphomas Viral warts (intralesional)
Melphalan	Scleromyxedema
Cyclosporine	Psoriasis Atopic dermatitis Pemphigus/pemphigoid Mycosis fungoides/ Sézary syndrome
5-Fluorouracil	Solar keratoses (topical) Keratoacanthoma (intralesional)

Fig. 23.11 Alkylating agents and antimetabolites and their dermatologic disease indications. Their use is justified only if the disease is sufficiently disabling.

DRUGS THAT PROTECT THE SKIN FROM ENVIRONMENTAL DAMAGE

Sunscreens

The growing incidence of melanoma and non-melanoma skin cancers and skin ageing has been associated with exposure to ultraviolet light. Sunburn before 10 years of age is a major risk factor for malignant melanoma. Photosensitivity can be a manifestation of some diseases and the use of certain drugs. These conditions are best prevented by sun avoidance or using physical barriers to solar penetration, such as clothing. If exposure is unavoidable chemical sunscreens can be used to minimize exposure. The topical use of sunscreens reduces the risk of sunburn and probably prevents squamous cell carcinoma of the skin when used mainly during unintentional sun exposure. However, the use of sunscreens to extend the duration of intentional sun exposure may negate any beneficial effect on preventing melanoma skin cancer.

Sunscreens are classified as either absorbent or reflectant:
- Absorbent sunscreens are photo-absorbing chemicals and can be categorized according to their predominant active wavelength (Fig. 23.12).
- Reflectant sunscreens are inert minerals such as titanium dioxide, zinc oxide, red petroleum, and calamine, which are cosmetically less attractive because they are greasy and sticky and do not vanish on the skin.

Commercial preparations contain these ingredients in various proportions.

In practice, the sun protection of a sunscreen is about half that suggested by the skin protection factor (SPF)

The efficacy of a sunscreen is expressed as the skin protection factor (SPF), which is the ratio of the time required to produce minimal erythema with a sunscreen to the time required to produce minimal erythema without a sunscreen. However, the

Absorbent sunscreens and the predominant wavelength screened

Cinnamates	UVB
para-Aminobenzoic acid	UVB
Salicylates	UVB
Benzophenones	UVA
Camphor	UVA
Dibenzoylmethane	UVA
Aminobenzoates (padimate O)	UVB
Anthralin	UVA

Fig. 23.12 Absorbent sunscreens and the predominant wavelength screened. (Ultraviolet [UV] A, 320–360 nm; UVB, 290–320 nm)

amount of drug applied in the laboratory to determine such protection is much greater per unit area than the same amount applied in practice and it is difficult to make allowances for loss of the sunscreen with sweating and swimming so that the sun protection of a sunscreen is about half that suggested by the SPF in practice. Therefore:

- If the SPF is less than 10, the sunscreen is only mildly protective.
- If the SPF is 10–15, the sunscreen is moderately protective.
- If the SPF is higher than 15, the sunscreen will provide appreciable protection.
- If the SPF is higher than 25, the sunscreen will provide almost full protection, as required by patients with photosensitivity.

Sunscreen preparations have been refined to increase cosmetic acceptability, water resistance, durability, and effectiveness. However, the active ingredients, the base, the fragrances, and the stabilizers can all cause irritant, allergic, phototoxic, or photoallergic adverse reactions.

Antiviral agents (see also Chapter 8)

Acyclovir cream can be used for primary or recurrent labial herpes simplex (cold sores) and for genital herpes simplex infections.

Penciclovir cream is a newer topical antiviral preparation which is licenced for labial herpes simplex infection. Both agents need to be used as early as possible in the outbreak and one study showed shortening of an attack by a mean of only 0.7 days using acyclovir cream.

Systemic therapy is recommended for vaginal or buccal infections and for herpes zoster. In addition to reducing viral shedding and aiding healing, there is good evidence that early antiviral treatment lessens the incidence of postherpetic neuralgia which can be very disabling. Acyclovir is variably absorbed when orally administered. Consequently, in severe disease and in eczema herpeticum, parenteral administration is recommended. Prior to the development of antiviral agents, eczema herpeticum carried a significant mortality, and long-term eye damage caused considerable morbidity.

■ *In adults, valacyclovir, a pro-drug which ensures much better bioavailability of acyclovir, has largely superseded acyclovir*

Antiviral therapy can be life-saving for both chickenpox/shingles and herpes simplex infections in immunocompromised patients, and is sometimes used in this population for prophylaxis. It is generally inappropriate to treat immunocompetent patients with chickenpox in whom the disease is milder.

Systemic acyclovir, valacyclovir, and famciclovir decrease healing time and sometimes abort attacks of genital herpes. They are also useful for the treatment of varicella zoster infections (i.e. chickenpox, shingles). In shingles, administration of antiviral therapy within 72 hours of onset of the rash, shortens the duration of pain as well as of the rash, and reduces the incidence, severity, and duration of chronic pain (postherpetic neuralgia). The risk of visual complications

of zoster affecting the ophthalmic branch of the Vth cranial nerve is also reduced by prompt treatment. Prophylactic acyclovir is indicated for immunocompromised patients, and patients who develop recurrent erythema multiforme after herpes infections.

Antibacterial agents
Topical antibiotics (Fig. 23.13 and see Chapter 9)
Topical antibiotics are used in the treatment of acne (see above).

Fusidic acid is active against *Staphylococcus aureus* on the skin and can be used to treat early superficial skin infections such as impetigo and folliculitis although systemic antibiotics are often necessary in these conditions. Fusidic acid resistance develops relatively rapidly, but a pause from the use of the drug leads to re-colonization with fusidic acid-sensitive species. Mupirocin is also active against *S. aureus* including MRSA but for this reason should probably be reserved for the treatment of MRSA.

Nasal carriage of *S. aureus*, which can be the source of recurrent skin staphylococcal infection, can be treated with neomycin and chlorhexidine. Nasal mupirocin can be used for resistant organisms. Silver sulfadiazine is often used in the prevention and treatment of infection in burn wounds. This is a sulfonamide and some absorption occurs if extensive areas are treated (monitor for pancytopenia). Argyria has also been reported after prolonged use.

Topical metronidazole is used in the treatment of rosacea.

Systemic antibiotics
The large majority of patients with cellulitis give the typical history of severe flu-like symptoms preceding by 12–36 hours any symptoms in the affected part, which then becomes red, warm and swollen, characteristic of streptococcal infection. The drug of choice is *systemic* penicillin. Rarely, staphylococcal infection causes cellulitis in debilitated, immunodeficient or diabetic patients; in these cases anti-staphylococcal antibiotics should *accompany* the penicillin. Erythromycin should be used for patients who are penicillin allergic. Despite adequate antibiotic therapy, the signs may take several weeks to resolve. The temptation to change antibiotic therapy if the cellulitis is not spreading should be resisted. The time to resolution is least in patients who are treated adequately as soon as symptoms develop. Patients who have had one episode of cellulitis should be warned that they are at increased risk of a second attack and that antibiotic therapy should be sought immediately. Consideration should be given to continuing penicillin V longer term, e.g. 250 mg b.d. for 3–6 months, as second, and indeed, sequential attacks of streptococcal cellulitis are so common.

Antifungal agents
There are many topical and systemic antifungal agents for the treatment of skin, hair, and nail infections with fungi and yeasts (see Chapter 10).

Antiseptic agents (Fig. 23.14)
These may obviate the need for antibiotics.

Activities and uses of topical antibacterial drugs used in dermatology and their complications

Drug	Activity spectrum	Uses	Complications
Bacitracin	Gram-positive organisms, anaerobic cocci, *Neisseria*, tetanus bacilli, diphtheria bacilli	Nasal staphylococcal carriers	Resistance with long-term use Contact allergic dermatitis Rarely contact urticaria
Gramicidin (available only in combination with neomycin, polymyxin, bacitracin, and nystatin)	As for bacitracin		Rarely contact allergic dermatitis
Mupirocin	Most Gram-positive aerobic bacteria including methicillin-resistant *Staphylococcus aureus* (MRSA)	Impetigo, nasal staphylococcal carriage	May cause irritation of nasal mucosa (contains propylene glycol)
Polymyxin B sulfate	Gram-negative organisms including *Pseudomonas*, *Escherichia coli*, *Enterobacter*, and *Klebsiella*	Used in compound antibiotic preparations	Neurotoxic and nephrotoxic if systemically absorbed, therefore to be avoided in open wounds or denuded skin Contact dermatitis uncommon
Neomycin	Gram-negative organisms including *E. coli*, *Proteus*, *Klebsiella*, and *Enterobacter*		Serum concentrations rarely detectable Contact dermatitis common with cross-sensitivity to streptomycin, kanamycin, paromomycin, gentamicin
Gentamicin	As for neomycin, but more effective against *Pseudomonas*, and active against staphylococci and group A hemolytic streptococci		Use of topical gentamicin should be limited because of concerns about the emergence of resistance Neurotoxic, nephrotoxic, and ototoxic if absorbed Detected in plasma if applied to a large skin area, especially if denuded skin
Clindamycin	*Propionibacterium acnes*	Acne	10% absorption Rarely pseudomembranous colitis Skin irritation with alcohol vehicle, less with gel
Erythromycin Erythromycin in combination with benzoyl peroxide Erythromycin in combination with zinc acetate	*P. acnes*	Acne	Resistance increasing Combinations are claimed to reduce emergence of resistant strains
Metronidazole		Rosacea	Drying, burning, stinging
Tetracyclines (tetracycline, meclocycline)	*P. acnes*	Acne	Temporary yellow staining of skin Photosensitivity has not been a problem, but phototoxic Contraindicated in pregnancy, and in renal and hepatic disease

Fig. 23.13 Activities and uses of topical antibacterial drugs used in dermatology and their complications.

Antiparasite preparations (Fig. 23.15)

Aqueous preparations of these drugs are preferred in the treatment of scabies as the alcoholic lotions are irritant. A single application is usually sufficient, but an application on two or three consecutive days is needed for hyperkeratotic scabies. All members of the household must be treated at the same time. Applications are usually applied from the neck down, but treatment of the scalp, face, and neck is recommended for children under 2 years of age, elderly patients, immuno-compromised patients, and those for whom a previous treatment has failed. Benzyl benzoate may require up to three applications on consecutive days.

Antiseptic agents

Drug name	Uses	Comments
Chlorhexidine	Antiseptic skin cleanser	Alcoholic solutions not suitable before diathermy
Benzalkonium chloride	Antiseptic skin cleanser	
Triclosan	Antiseptic skin cleanser	
Potassium permanganate 1:10,000 solution	Antiseptic skin cleanser, astringent	
Cetrimide	Disinfectant and detergent properties	Occasional sensitizer
Hydrogen peroxide	Disinfectant used for deep wounds and ulcers	
Streptokinase–streptodornase and dextranomer preparations	Aid ulcer desloughing, which helps eradicate local infection	
Povidone iodine	Disinfectant, less irritant	Caution in pregnancy, breast feeding and renal impairment. Application to large wounds or severe burns may produce systemic effects such as metabolic acidosis, hypernatremia and renal impairment. Avoid regular use in patients with thyroid disease or those receiving lithium therapy. Rarely sensitivity
Hexachlorophene	Irritant	Avoid in neonates and large raw surfaces Avoid in pregnancy Can cause sensitivity and, rarely, photosensitivity
Chlorinated solutions, e.g. dilute hypochlorite solution		No longer recommended because of irritancy, bleaches clothing

Fig. 23.14 Antiseptic agents.

Antiparasite preparations

Drug	Disease	Mechanism	Adverse effects
Lindane	Scabies (head lice resistance high so no longer recommended) Crab lice		Avoid in pregnancy, breast feeding mothers, patients with low body weight, young children, and those with a history of epilepsy
Malathion	Scabies: kills both adult lice and ova *in vitro* Head lice Crab lice	Organophosphate cholinesterase inhibitor	
Permethrin	Scabies Lice (but resistance increasing)	Neurotoxic	
Benzyl benzoate			Irritant, avoid in children
5% precipitate of sulfur in petrolatum			Rarely used because of odor and staining It is a possible alternative for treating pregnant women and infants
Carbaril	Head lice		

520

Fig. 23.15 Antiparasite preparations.

Patients should be told that the itch of scabies can persist for several weeks and that itching does not necessarily indicate treatment failure.

For head lice, both malathion and carbaril should be used as lotions rather than shampoos, and left in contact with the scalp for 12 hours. Aqueous formulations are preferred for asthmatic patients and small children to avoid alcoholic fumes. The treatment should be repeated after 7 days to kill lice emerging from any eggs that might have survived the first application.

For crab lice, treatment should be applied to the whole body for 12 hours, and repeated 7 days later.

Insect repellents

These agents repel insects primarily by vaporization of the active ingredients diethyltoluamide and dimethyl phthalate. The duration of action is limited by the rate of vaporization and washing and rubbing off. Few preparations currently available are effective for more than a few hours. Allergic reactions can develop, especially with prolonged use.

Barrier preparations

Barrier creams have been developed to protect the skin from irritants (e.g. in industry, for patients with dermatitis). They rely on:
- Water-repellent substances (e.g. silicones).
- Soaps.
- Impermeable deposits such as titanium, zinc, and calamine. Their efficacy is limited because they must be removable by washing and cannot be so occlusive that they block pores and follicles. They have a role in protecting skin from discharges and secretions and are used for diaper rash and colostomies.

Bandages and dressings

A variety of bandages and dressings are prescribable and play an important role in the management of skin problems. Medicated bandages impregnated with zinc paste, with or without coal tar/ichthammol are useful in the management of eczema, acting as an emollient, antipruritic, and barrier to scratching. Bandages containing calamine and clioquinol and fabric dressings impregnated with povidone-iodine, chlorhexidine, framycetin, sodium fusidate, and paraffin are also available.

Silicone gel sheets are clear, soft, and semi-occlusive, and conform well to awkward contours of the body. They have a role in the treatment of hypertrophic scars. Their mechanism of action is not fully understood: pressure, temperature of the scar, and oxygen tension within the scar are not involved, and it is currently believed that the gel may work by promoting scar hydration.

DRUGS ACTING ON SKIN CONSTITUENTS
Drugs acting on keratinocytes

UREA makes creams and lotions feel less greasy, increases the hydration of the stratum corneum (concentration, 2–20%), and is a keratolytic (20%). A concentration of 30–50% urea with occlusion can be used to soften the nail plate before nail avulsion.

Urea appears to act by modifying prekeratin and keratin, leading to increased solubilization. It may also cleave the hydrogen bonds that keep the stratum corneum intact. It is absorbed percutaneously, but is a natural product of metabolism, and is excreted in the urine without systemic toxicity.

Adverse effects include irritation and stinging, especially with occlusion and in the perineal area.

SALICYLIC ACID Low concentrations (up to 2%) of salicylic acid are used in the treatment of acne (see above). Higher concentrations (up to 50%) can be used to eradicate warts and calluses, but are contraindicated in patients with diabetes mellitus or peripheral vascular disease because they can induce ulceration. Salicylic acid is absorbed percutaneously, and 1 g of 6% salicylic acid results in plasma concentrations of approximately 0.5 mg/dl (0.04 mmol/liter).

PROPYLENE GLYCOL is keratolytic at a concentration of 40–70% and is useful in the treatment of hyperkeratotic conditions such as palmoplantar keratoderma, psoriasis, pityriasis rubra pilaris, and hypertrophic lichen planus. Propylene glycol also increases the water content of the stratum corneum. This hygroscopic characteristic encourages the development of an osmotic gradient through the stratum corneum, increasing the hydration of the outermost layers and drawing water out of the inner layers of the skin. Propylene glycol can be used alone or in a gel with 6% salicylic acid. It has the advantage of minimal absorption, and what is absorbed is oxidized in the liver to lactic acid and pyruvic acid, which are then used in general metabolism. Its major adverse effect is irritancy, and it can cause contact allergic dermatitis.

PODOPHYLLUM RESIN is an alcoholic extract of *Podophyllum peltatum*, and is used in the treatment of condyloma acuminatum and plantar warts. Podophyllotoxin and its derivatives are cytotoxic agents that act on the microtubule proteins of the mitotic spindle, preventing normal assembly of the spindle and arresting epidermal mitoses in metaphase. The tincture needs to be applied accurately to the wart tissue to prevent severe erosion of the surrounding normal skin, and allowed a contact time of 2–3 hours (possibly increasing to 6–8 hours if tolerated) for 3–5 applications only. If this is not successful, alternative treatment modalities should be considered as the resin is absorbed and distributed in lipids, including those in the central nervous system. If extensive areas need treatment they should be treated in sections to minimize absorption, particularly from intertriginous areas and large moist warts.

Adverse effects include nausea, vomiting, muscle weakness, neuropathy, and even coma and death. Local irritation is common. Podophyllum resin is contraindicated during pregnancy because of its possible cytotoxic effects on the fetus.

Drugs acting on glands

See Isotretinoin and Niacinamide.

521

Drugs acting on nerves

■ *Topical nonsteroidal anti-inflammatory drugs and capsaicin can relieve pain*

Local pain can be transiently relieved by topical nonsteroidal anti-inflammatory drugs (NSAIDs) (see Chapter 7), while capsaicin (0.075%) cream is licensed for the treatment of post-herpetic neuralgia. Capsaicin is a naturally occurring alkaloid found in fruits and capsicum. Crude extracts of capsicum or capsicum oleo-resin contain small amounts of capsaicin and a number of co-capsaicinoids, which are thought to cause the counter-irritant erythematous reaction that accompanies the application of these extracts. Capsaicin itself acts by depleting sensory C fibers of neuropeptides, particularly substance P. It is not a traditional counter-irritant and does not induce vasodilation.

Recently, capsaicin has also been reported to activate vanilloid receptors on sensory nerves and it is possible that this activation renders the vanilloid densensitized to endogenous activators which include low pH, heat and certain lipid mediators generated during the inflammatory process.

■ *Topical applications relieve itch, partly by a cooling effect*

Phenol, menthol, and camphor are often added to topical applications to relieve itch and probably act as weak local anesthetics. Calamine, astringents such as aluminum acetate and tannic acid, and coal tar also have some topical antipruritic effect.

■ *Itch may be relieved systemically by histamine H_1 antagonists (see eczema)*

Hypnotics, chlorpromazine, trimeprazine, and sedative anti-depressants are sometimes helpful in the treatment of pruritus, possibly because they alter the perception of itch.

CAMOUFLAGE CREAMS

Camouflage creams contain titanium dioxide in an ointment base with a variety of color shades that can be matched to the site and skin color of the patient. The best results are achieved by camouflage consultants.

FURTHER READING

Dutz JP, Ho VC. Immunosuppressive agents in dermatology. An update. *Dermatol Clin* 1998; **16**: 235–251. [Review.]

Leppard L, Ashton R. *Treatment in Dermatology*. Oxford: Radcliffe Medical Press; 1993. [Aimed at undergraduates and nonspecialists, explaining the rationale for treatment of skin diseases.]

Shelley W, Shelley ED. *Advanced Dermatologic Therapy*, 2nd edn. Philadelphia: WB Saunders; 2001. [Detailed review of treatment of skin diseases.]

Williams LC, Nesbitt LT Jr. Update on systemic glucocorticosteroids in dermatology. *Dermatol Clin* 2001; **19**: 63–77. [Review.]

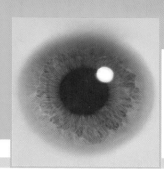

Chapter 24

Drugs and the Eye

BIOLOGY OF THE EYE AND PRINCIPLES OF DRUG USE FOR THE EYE

Structure and physiology of the eye

The eye focuses images from the external world onto the retina and converts them into electrical signals, which are then perceived by the brain. As vision is a major sense, a large area of the brain is used for processing this information, which is produced by two outposts of the central nervous system, the retinae. The retinae are contained within the eyeballs and are connected to the rest of the central nervous system by the optic nerves.

The eyeball is a spherical organ of about 25 mm in diameter. It contains a lens and two fluid-filled chambers, and is enclosed by the following four layers of specialized tissue (Fig. 24.1):

- The cornea and sclera.
- The uveal tract (iris, ciliary body, and choroid).
- The pigment epithelium.
- The retina.

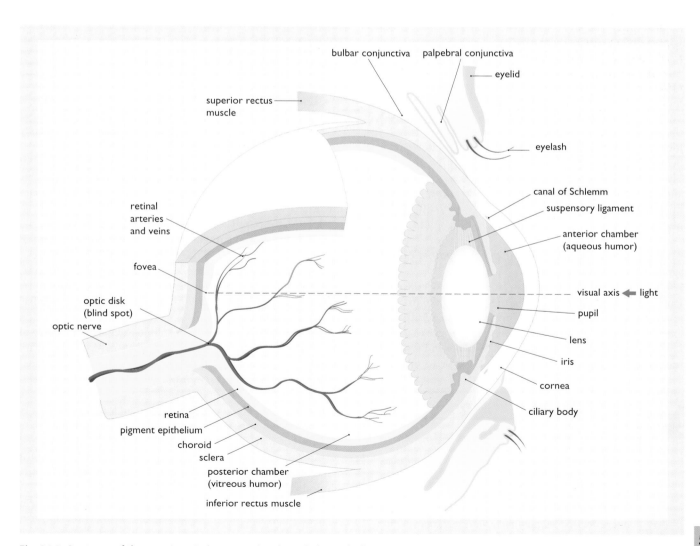

Fig. 24.1 Anatomy of the eye. A vertical cross-section through the eyeball.

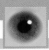

The most anterior part of the eye around the eyeball is the bulbar conjunctiva, which also lines the inside of the eyelid where it becomes the palpebral conjunctiva.

The cornea is a transparent tissue at the front of the eye that allows light to enter the eyeball and contains fine sensory fibers. The majority of the eye's refractive power is at the air/corneal interface. The sclera is a continuation of the cornea and is the tough protective coat of the eye (the white of the eye), while the uveal tract is a layer of tissue beneath the sclera. From the front of the eye to the back, the uveal tract forms the iris (a pigmented smooth muscle), the ciliary body, and the choroid (a vascular bed beneath the retina). The retina is the neural tissue containing the eye's photoreceptor cells (rods and cones) and forms the innermost layer of the eyeball. To reach these photoreceptor cells, light must travel through the cornea, a fluid-filled anterior chamber, the lens, a fluid-filled posterior chamber, and the cellular layers of the retina. Obviously, all these tissues must be transparent to allow the light to pass through, and any condition that reduces the transparency of any of them will reduce visual capability.

■ The eye is moved within the orbit by six extraocular muscles

The six extraocular muscles are:

- The medial and lateral rectus muscles on either side of the eye.
- The superior rectus and oblique muscles above the eye.
- The inferior rectus and oblique muscles below the eye.

These striated muscles are controlled by the motor neurons of the oculomotor, trochlear, and abducens nerves (the third, fourth, and sixth cranial nerves, respectively), and are unusual because they contain fibers that are multiply innervated. The majority of mammalian striated fibers have between one and three neuromuscular end-plates. Multiply innervated fibers, such as the rectus muscle, can have up to 80 end-plates per fiber.

■ Pupil size is controlled by light, parasympathetic and sympathetic stimulation

High light levels reaching the retina lead to constriction (miosis) of the pupil (the hole in the center of the iris), while low light levels lead to dilation (mydriasis). In addition, light entering one eye causes the pupil of the other eye to constrict. This is known as the consensual pupil response and is produced by the brain. It only occurs if the brain is able to process the

---

 Causes of mydriasis (pupil dilation)

- Low light levels**
- Drugs that block muscarinic acetylcholine receptors in the iris**
- Sympathetic stimulation*
- Drugs that activate α_1 adrenoceptors in the iris (α_1 adrenoceptor agonists)*

*Weak dilation
**Strong dilation

Causes of miosis (pupil constriction)

- High light levels**
- Parasympathetic stimulation**
- Drugs that activate muscarinic acetylcholine receptors in the iris**
- Drugs that activate opioid receptors in the central nervous system**
- Drugs that block α_1 adrenoceptors in the iris (α_1 adrenoceptor antagonists)*

*Weak constriction
**Strong constriction

---

visual information it receives from the retina. This response is therefore a useful diagnostic tool for assessing brain damage in comatose or unconscious patients, and many doctors carry a small torch to test for it.

The parasympathetic nervous system maintains the tone of the iris and, when stimulated, causes miosis, while sympathetic stimulation (the 'fright, flight, and fight' response) causes mydriasis.

The dilator pupillae (the radial smooth muscle of the iris) is innervated by sympathetic fibers from the superior cervical ganglion. As elsewhere in the body, the sympathetic nervous system's neurotransmitter is norepinephrine, which acts on α_1 adrenoceptors resulting in pupil dilation. Drugs that are α_1 adrenoceptor agonists therefore contract the dilator pupillae and cause mydriasis (Fig. 24.2).

The constrictor pupillae (the sphincteric smooth muscle of the iris) is innervated by parasympathetic fibers from the ciliary ganglion. The parasympathetic nervous system's neurotransmitter acetylcholine acts on muscarinic receptors in the constrictor pupillae. Like adrenoceptor agonists, drugs that block muscarinic acetylcholine receptors are therefore also mydriatics (i.e. produce mydriasis).

Drugs that are clinically useful and cause miosis are confined to muscarinic agonists and are called miotics. Adrenoceptor antagonists such as phentolamine are miotics, but have little clinical value in the eye.

Some drugs act at the level of the central nervous system to alter pupil size, for example an opioid receptor agonist, such as morphine, which produces the characteristic 'pinhole' pupil.

⚠ Neuromuscular blockers and the eye

- *Multiply innervated muscle tonically contracts in response to depolarizing neuromuscular blockers such as succinylcholine (see Chapter 26), and intraocular pressure may therefore increase*
- *In the normal eye this may not be a problem because succinylcholine is short acting*
- *If the eye has a penetrating injury the ocular contents may prolapse*

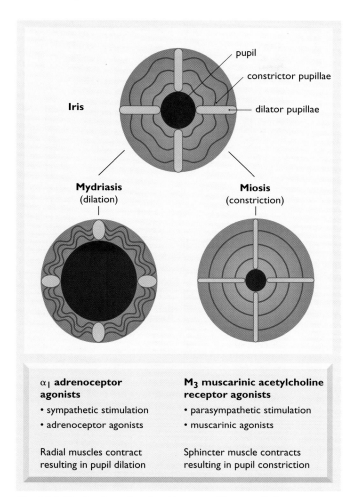

Fig. 24.2 Mechanisms involved in controlling pupil size.

α_1 adrenoceptor agonists	M$_3$ muscarinic acetylcholine receptor agonists
• sympathetic stimulation	• parasympathetic stimulation
• adrenoceptor agonists	• muscarinic agonists
Radial muscles contract resulting in pupil dilation	Sphincter muscle contracts resulting in pupil constriction

In the figure the labels read: pupil, constrictor pupillae, Iris, dilator pupillae, Mydriasis (dilation), Miosis (constriction).

Accommodation is the mechanism that focuses the image on the retina

Accommodation is the ability of the eye to change its refractive power, which is a measure of how strongly it can bend a path of light. Refractive power is usually measured in units called diopters. The majority of the refractive power of the eye is located at the air/corneal interface and this is fixed. However, a small proportion of the refractive power is variable, owing to the ability of the lens to change its radius of curvature.

The lens is suspended in the eyeball from the ciliary muscle by suspensory ligaments. When the ciliary muscle relaxes, the suspensory ligaments are taut, stretching the lens into an ellipsoid shape. The low radius of curvature of the lens focuses distant objects onto the retina (far or distant vision). When the ciliary muscle contracts as a result of parasympathetic stimulation (i.e. acetylcholine acting on muscarinic receptors), the suspensory ligaments relax, and the lens takes up a more spherical shape. The curvature of the lens therefore increases and focuses near objects onto the retina (near vision). The contraction of the ciliary muscle for near vision explains why eyes get 'tired' after reading for long periods of time.

During accommodation for near vision, the pupil constricts, confining the light rays to the center of the lens to reduce spherical aberration and improve the quality of the image. This is the accommodation pupil reflex. Drugs that antagonize the accommodative event are often termed 'cycloplegics' and are exclusively muscarinic antagonists. There are no adrenergic receptors in the ciliary muscle and accommodation is not therefore altered by sympatholytics or sympathomimetics.

The ability to accommodate (i.e. of the order of 12 diopters) in youth and young adulthood gradually decreases with age, because the lens becomes less flexible. By the age of 50 years, the accommodative power of the lens reduces to 1 or 2 diopters. This is why older people are generally 'long sighted' and need reading glasses. This natural condition of aging is termed 'presbyopia.'

Aqueous humor production is a continuous process

The anterior chamber of the eyeball is filled with a watery fluid called aqueous humor, which is continually produced by the blood vessels in the ciliary body at a rate of 3 ml/day. It flows first into the posterior chamber and then through the pupil into the anterior chamber (Fig. 24.3). The majority of the aqueous humor drains into the episcleral veins via the trabecular meshwork and the canal of Schlemm, but some 10% drains through the uveoscleral outflow into the circulation by a trans-scleral route. The rate of production and drainage of aqueous humor is responsible for maintaining the intraocular pressure, which is normally 12–20 mmHg.

The production of aqueous humor is indirectly related to the blood pressure and the rate of blood flow in the ciliary body. As elsewhere, activation of α_1 adrenoceptors constricts the blood vessels in the ciliary body. Circulating epinephrine acting on β adrenoceptors on the ciliary body increases the production of aqueous humor. However, there may also be α_2 adrenoceptors located on the ciliary body that reduce aqueous formation as well as on presynaptic adrenergic nerve terminals which reduce release of norepinephrine onto the ciliary body.

The enzyme carbonic anhydrase is important for aqueous humor formation. Its role in the eye is similar to that in the kidneys or other organs where fluid movement is involved. The composition of aqueous humor is similar to that of blood plasma; however, the protein content (10 mg/100 ml) is much lower than in plasma (6000 mg/100 ml) so that the aqueous humor fluid is transparent rather than translucent. Also, aqueous humor is not purely an ultrafiltrate of plasma because it has a higher bicarbonate and ascorbic acid content. This difference in composition suggests that it is produced by an active secretion process. This point is important in understanding how one class of drugs (carbonic anhydrase inhibitors) acts to reduce its production (see page 533).

Smooth muscle contraction is the key to many physiologic events in the eye

Pupil dilation and constriction, constriction of the blood vessels, and contraction of the ciliary muscle depend on the contraction of smooth muscle. Although these events are controlled by different branches of the autonomic nervous system using different neurotransmitters and receptors, their

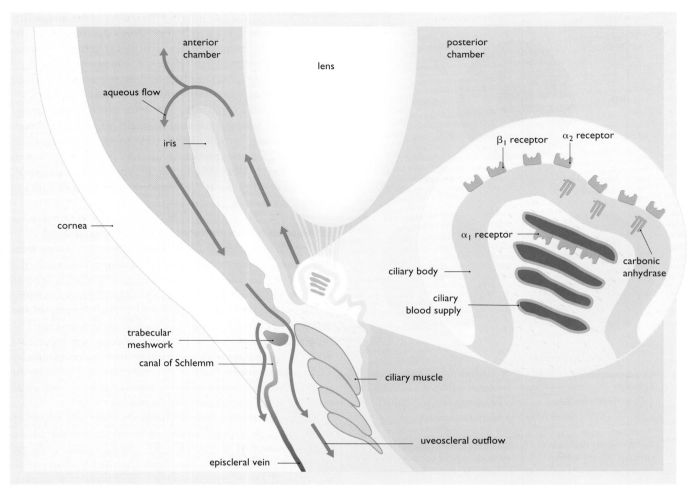

Fig. 24.3 Production and drainage of aqueous humor. The inset shows the location of α and β adrenoceptors and the enzyme carbonic anhydrase, which are all molecular targets for drugs that reduce the production of aqueous humor.

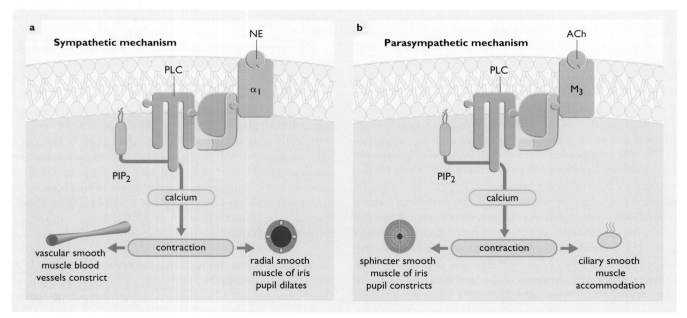

Fig. 24.4 Cellular transduction pathway in smooth muscle. Activation of α_1 adrenoceptors (α_1) by norepinephrine (NE) or M_3 muscarinic receptors (M_3) by acetylcholine (ACh) leads to activation of G proteins, which stimulate inositol-1,4,5-trisphosphate (IP_3) production from phosphatidyl bisphosphate (PIP_2) by the enzyme phospholipase C (PLC). IP_3 releases Ca^{2+} from intracellular Ca^{2+} stores, and the Ca^{2+} then activates calmodulin–myosin light chain kinase and triggers contraction.

cellular transduction systems are similar. Both α_1 adrenergic receptors and M_3 muscarinic acetylcholine receptors activate G proteins which in turn activate the enzyme phospholipase C (PLC) leading to muscle contraction (see Chapter 3) (Fig. 24.4).

The retina converts light into electrical signals

The retina is part of the central nervous system embryologically and can be considered as an extension of the brain. It receives oxygen and metabolic requirements from the choroid plexus behind and the retinal blood vessels in front, and is the only place where the circulatory system of the brain can be viewed directly. The macula lutea with the fovea at its center are areas characterized by their high density of photoreceptor cells and absence of retinal blood vessels. The sharpest images are therefore produced on this part of the retina, and the resulting visual images sent to the brain are the most detailed and of the highest quality.

The retina is a well-ordered layered structure of nerve cells. The two types of photoreceptor (rods and cones) are located next to the pigment epithelium and perform different functions:

- Rods are only active at low light levels.
- Cones are only active at high light levels and are also responsible for color vision.

These photoreceptors convert light into electrical signals using the opsin family of proteins as light detectors. The signals are then sent back towards the vitreous humor through bipolar cells and to retinal ganglion cells, the axons of which make up the optic nerve, which connects with the brain. Other cells in the retina include amacrine, horizontal, and interplexiform cells, which are involved in the considerable image processing that goes on in the retina. The perception of light by the brain requires the conversion of light into an electrical signal in photoreceptor cells, promoting them to modulate release of their neurotransmitter which then causes activation of neural pathways that ultimately impinge on the visual cortex in the occipital lobes.

The regulation of release of glutamate, the neurotransmitter for photoreceptor cells involves a sequence of steps (Fig. 24.5). In the eye, the enzyme guanylyl cyclase (GC) continuously converts guanosine triphosphate (GTP) to cyclic guanosine monophosphate (cGMP). On the other hand, cGMP is eliminated by conversion to GMP by phosphodiesterase (PDE) enzymes. PDEs constitute a gene family; various examples are shown in Fig. 22.28. The PDE of importance in rod photoreceptors is the type 5 isoform. In the dark, the type 5 PDE has relatively low activity, leading to accumulation of cGMP.

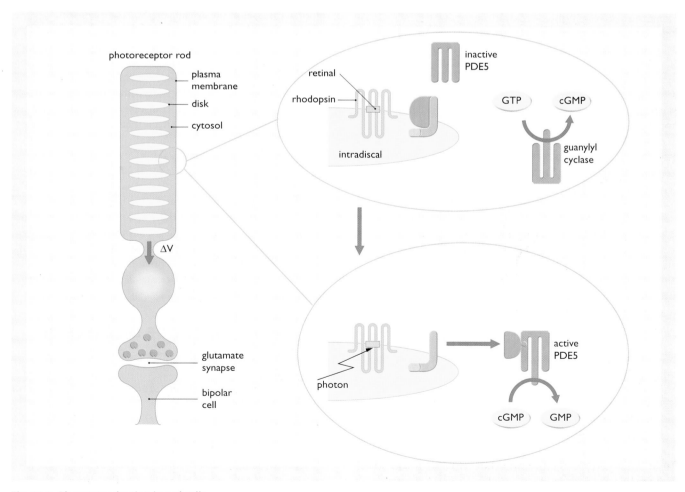

Fig. 24.5 Phototransduction in rod cells.

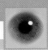

Regulation of cGMP concentrations is critical to the signaling mechanisms of rod photoreceptor cells. The light receptor is a protein termed rhodopsin: interestingly, its structure is similar to that of a typical G protein-coupled receptor (Chapter 3). Rhodopsin has a critical 11-cis retinal functional group: when a photon of light interacts with the retinal moiety, there is a conformational change in rhodopsin. See Chapter 27 for information about 11-cis retinal, the active form of vitamin A in the eye. The conformation change in rhodopsin in turn activates a specific G protein termed transducin (Gt). Transducin has similar overall structure to G proteins coupled to typical hormone and drug receptors (Chapter 3). The α subunit of transducin separates from the anchoring β/γ subunits leading to activation of the type 5 PDE and a consequent fall in cGMP concentrations in these cells.

In the plasma membranes of photoreceptor cells reside a special class of ion channels which require cGMP to bind to them in order to open (cGMP-gated channels). In the presence of cGMP, these channels allow the entry of cations such as Na^+ and Ca^{2+} into the photoreceptor cells (so-called dark current) leading to depolarization of these cells. As for most neuronal cells, depolarization causes the opening of voltage-gated calcium channels at the presynatic terminal prompting the release of the cell's neurotransmitter, in this case glutamate. Consequently, in the absence of light (i.e., dark), since photoreceptor cells contain relatively high concentrations of cGMP, the cells are depolarized and are releasing neurotransmitter.

Conversely, in the presence of light, the type 5 PDE is activated, increasing the conversion of cGMP to the inactive GMP molecule; i.e., there is a fall in the cGMP concentration. Consequently, the cGMP-gated ion channels carrying the dark current close and the photoreceptor cell hyperpolarizes, leading to closure of voltage-gated calcium channels at the presynatic terminal and a reduction in glutamate release. Therefore in the presence of light, photoreceptor cells have low cGMP concentrations, are hyperpolarized and are not releasing their neurotransmitter glutamate. Therefore, at the first synapse of the visual system, light is signaled by a decrease in glutamate release. However, the next cells in the signaling chain, namely bipolar cells, fall broadly into two classes. ON-bipolar cells are cells which respond to the cessation of neurotransmitter by depolarizing; on the other hand, OFF-bipolar cells respond to the cessation of glutamate stimulation by hyperpolarizing. Therefore the retina at a very early stage in visual processing actively codes both light and dark in parallel 'ON' and 'OFF' channels.

■ *Different areas of the visual field have different functions*
Although the image produced by the central vision of the macula lutea and fovea is the most detailed, the visual field extends to some 200° binocularly. Most of the peripheral retina is concerned with detecting movement and triggers the eye to center on a new visual stimulus. For example, if someone walks into the peripheral visual field of someone who is reading, the reader may detect the movement, but will only identify who has entered their visual field if they look up and center their fovea on the person's face.

Diseases of the eye and methods of treatment			
Disease	**Drugs**	**Surgery**	**None**
Open-angle glaucoma	✓	–	–
Closed-angle glaucoma	✓	✓	–
Inflammation and allergic conditions	✓	–	–
Squints and oculomotor disorders	✓	✓	–
Tear deficiency	✓	–	–
Infections	✓	–	–
Detached retina	–	✓	–
Cataracts	–	✓	–
Retinitis pigmentosa	–	–	✓
Amblyopia	–	–	✓
Retinopathy	–	–	✓

Fig. 24.6 Diseases of the eye and methods of treatment.

Peripheral vision is also responsible for low light vision as most of the rod photoreceptors, which are responsible for night vision, are located outside the fovea. Loss of peripheral vision is termed 'tunnel vision' and is often associated with genetic retinal disease such as retinitis pigmentosa. Other diseases such as glaucoma and diabetes mellitus can also have effects that alter the visual fields.

DISEASES OF THE EYE

There are many eye diseases, some of which are listed in Fig. 24.6, but only those that can be treated by drugs are discussed in this chapter. Despite claims, there is no clear clinical evidence that any drug treatment or vitamin supplementation prevents or cures cataracts, age-related maculopathy or genetic retinal dystrophy. Drug therapy of glaucoma, inflammation of the eye, oculomotor disorders, tear deficiency and infections of the eye are presented in this chapter.

PATHOPHYSIOLOGY OF DISEASES OF THE EYE

Glaucoma
■ *Glaucoma is caused by poor drainage of aqueous humor and can cause blindness*
Glaucoma is characterized by:
- An increase in intraocular pressure to over 21 mmHg.
- Fundus changes, in particular optic disk 'cupping.'
- Visual field changes.
If untreated, it permanently damages the optic nerve and this can cause blindness. The two main types of glaucoma are

Drugs used to treat glaucoma

Type	Mechanism	Drug example	Comments
Decrease aqueous humor formation			
β Adrenoceptor antagonists	Block β_1 receptor on ciliary body	Timolol maleate	First-line treatment
α Adrenoceptor agonist	Agonist of prejunctional α_2 receptors and/or α_1 (vasoconstrictor) receptors on ciliary vessels	Apraclonidine	
Carbonic anhydrase inhibitors	Block carbonic anhydrase and reduce bicarbonate formation	Acetazolamide	
Increase drainage of aqueous humor			
Miotics	Activate muscarinic receptors on the iris and ciliary muscle causing pupil constriction and ciliary muscle contraction, which may improve uveoscleral outflow	Carbachol	
Prostaglandin analogs	A $PGF_{2\alpha}$ analog increases uveoscleral outflow	Latanoprost	Recently introduced

Fig. 24.7 Drugs used to treat glaucoma.

open-angle (simple) and closed-angle glaucoma. The angle referred to is the filtration angle formed between the iris and the cornea.

Open-angle and closed-angle glaucoma
Open-angle glaucoma is a chronic disease that is primarily treated with drugs. The primary defect is reduced drainage of the aqueous humor into the canal of Schlemm. There is evidence that this can be a congenital defect. The two rationales behind the drug treatments used for this disease are to reduce the production of aqueous humor or to increase its drainage (Fig. 24.7). Closed-angle glaucoma results from forward ballooning of the peripheral iris (iris bombé) so that it touches the back of the cornea, thereby reducing the flow of aqueous humor between the cornea and the iris.

Tear deficiency
The tear film on the cornea contains three layers, a thin superficial lipid layer suspended above an aqueous layer which in turn is above a mucous layer. Deficiencies in any of these layers can lead to a condition known as 'dry eye.' Ocular disease and drugs can cause tear deficiencies which can also occur in a number of systemic diseases. For example tear deficiency in association with rheumatoid arthritis is termed Sjögren's syndrome. A number of clinical tests can be used to assess symptoms relating to dry eyes. Fluorescein or rose bengal staining of the cornea may indicate aqueous and mucous deficiency, respectively. Other tests measure the stability of the tear film and the functioning of the lacrimal glands.

Inflammation and allergy
As shown in Fig. 24.1 the eye is constructed of different layers of tissue and all can become inflamed owing to infection (bacterial or viral), allergy, chemical burn or unknown factors (idiopathic). Inflammation of the conjunctiva is termed conjunctivitis. Similarly keratitis, uveitis, scleritis, and neuritis

describe inflammation of the cornea, uveal tract, sclera, and nerves respectively. It is of course possible that more than one tissue becomes inflamed at any one time. Systemic disease can become manifest or complicated by inflammatory symptoms in the eye. Reiter's syndrome is characterized by arthritis, urethritis and conjunctivitis. The effect inflammation has on the eye depends on the extent, the duration, and which tissues are involved. For example if the cornea becomes inflamed it may lose its transparency and therefore affect vision. While inflammation is generally associated with pain, this is not always the case.

Squint and oculomotor disorders
Disorders involving the control of muscles around the eye and those controlling the eyelids are usually termed neuro-ophthalmic disorders. For example blepharospasm is characterized by repetitive blinking which can lead to an involuntary spasm of eyelid closure. The cause of blepharospasm is often unknown but may involve a neurochemical abnormality in the central nervous system. Squint (strabismus) on the other hand involves the lack of control of the extraocular muscles and if seen in young children needs to be treated early on to prevent degradation of vision known as amblyopia. The autoimmune systemic disease myasthenia gravis causes a weakening of skeletal muscles: the ocular muscles are most often involved (90% of cases) (see Chapter 14). Ocular symptoms include ptosis (involuntary eye closure) and diplopia (double vision due to dysfunctional ocular muscles).

PROPERTIES OF DRUGS USED IN THE EYE

■ *Drugs applied to the eye must be uncharged to cross the cornea*
In order to act within the eye, all drugs applied topically to the eye must cross the cornea. They must therefore be lipophilic or uncharged. The ocular penetration of a weakly basic

Ophthalmic preparations

- Most drugs mentioned in this chapter are available as specific ophthalmic preparations (e.g. eye drops or creams)
- As the majority of eye drugs are applied locally, the risk of systemic adverse effects is minimized but not completely avoided
- Some locally applied drugs can cause systemic adverse effects
- Slow-release formulations may reduce the risk of adverse effects

or acidic drug can be improved if the pH is appropriately adjusted to produce a larger proportion of uncharged drug (see Chapter 4). However, drug solutions do not need to be isotonic compared to lacrimal secretions (tears).

Most drugs for the eye are available as sterile eye drop preparations and care must be taken not to contaminate them or cause cross-contamination from one eye to the other. Single-use eye drops should be used, if possible.

 Melanin in the iris binds some drugs and affects their action

The action of some drugs is related to eye color, which is produced by the content of the pigment melanin in the iris. Black or dark brown irises contain significantly more melanin than green, gray, or blue irises. Melanin binds a variety of drugs such as atropine and such drugs can therefore take longer to act and have longer-lasting effects if the patient has a dark iris. Care is

Eye color and drugs

- Iris pigmentation can affect the onset and duration of action of many drugs applied to the eye
- Black and brown irises contain more pigment (melanin) than green, gray, or blue irises
- The more pigment in the iris, the more drug can bind to it, resulting in a slower onset and longer duration of action

needed to avoid overdosing patients with highly pigmented irises.

Some drugs used to treat eye disease can alter eye color
Chronic application of epinepherine can cause the deposition of a type of black melanin pigment (adrenochrome deposits) formed by the oxidation and polymerization of the drug. Latanoprost can increase the pigmentation of the iris, particularly in people with mixed colored irises. This effect may be particularly striking when only one eye is being treated with the drug.

Preservatives in eye drops may cause allergic reactions
Many substances are used as preservatives in eye drops and may cause allergic responses in susceptible individuals. The preservative benzalkonium chloride should be avoided in patients using soft contact lenses as it can accumulate in the lens and may induce toxic reactions.

Drugs used in ophthalmic diagnosis

Muscarinic antagonists are used for mydriasis
Many systemic and retinal diseases can be diagnosed by looking at the fundus, and drugs that dilate the pupil (mydriatics) improve the view of the fundus. The most effective class of such drugs is that of muscarinic antagonists (Fig. 24.8), and the particular drug used is chosen according to its duration of action and whether cycloplegia is required. They all act by blocking the muscarinic receptors in the iris and ciliary muscle, thereby antagonizing the parasympathetic control of these muscles. Cyclopentolate and atropine are the preferred drugs for producing cycloplegia in children.

Adrenergic receptor agonists such as epinephrine and phenylephrine hydrochloride also dilate the pupil, but only to a small extent and they do not cause cycloplegia.

Local anesthetics are used to produce corneal anesthesia
The cornea is a particularly sensitive tissue and it is therefore commonly anesthetized in ophthalmic diagnosis because intraocular pressure measurement (tonometry) involves placing a device on the cornea for a short period of time. Such anesthesia is provided by a group of chemically related drugs, the

Mydriatic and cycloplegic drugs

Drug	Maximum effect time (minutes)	Recovery time (hours)	Mydriatic effect	Cycloplegic effect
Muscarinic antagonists				
Atropine sulfate	40	240	+++	+++
Scopolamine	30	200	+++	+++
Homatropine	30	40	+++	++
Cyclopentolate	60	20	+++	+++
Tropicamide	30	5	+++	++
α_1 Adrenergic agonist				
Phenylephrine	30	3	+	none

Fig. 24.8 Mydriatic and cycloplegic drugs.

Corneal local anesthetics

Drug	Duration of action	Use	Comments
Tetracaine	10 minutes	Minor surgery	Widely used
Benoxinate	10 minutes	Tonometry	Widely used Formulated with fluorescein
Proparacaine	11 minutes	Tonometry Minor surgery	Less stinging, useful in children
Lidocaine	50 minutes	Tonometry Minor surgery	Formulated with fluorescein

Fig. 24.9 Corneal local anesthetics.

local anesthetics (Fig. 24.9), which may also be used for minor eye operations. The mechanisms of action of these compounds are explained in Chapter 14.

▪ Fluorescent dyes are used to detect foreign bodies

Fluorescent dyes (Fig. 24.10) such as fluorescein sodium and dichlorotetraiodofluorescein (rose bengal) are instilled into the eye to detect corneal lesions or foreign bodies. Rose bengal is only taken up by injured or infected cells, and is therefore useful for detecting corneal damage and viral infections.

Treatment of glaucoma

Glaucoma is in fact a term to describe the loss of retinal ganglion cell function, which results in reduced visual abilities and ultimately blindness. Historically this has been linked with an elevated intraocular pressure (IOP). Nonetheless, loss of these cells can occur without rise in IOP (normal tension glaucoma) or a rise in IOP can occur without damage (ocular hypertension). However the lowering of IOP is the mainstay of glaucoma treatment although the ultimate goal is to prevent and reverse reduced visual function. In other words, IOP is a surrogate end-point in treating patients to avoid loss of visual function.

β Adrenergic antagonists used for glaucoma

Drug	Relative potency	Half-life (hours)	β$_1$-selective	Ocular discomfort
Timolol	5	4	No	++
Betaxolol	1	16	Yes	+++
Carteolol	10	5	No	0
Levobunolol	15	6	No	++
Metipranolol	2	2	No	+

Fig. 24.11 β Adrenergic antagonists used for glaucoma.

Drugs that reduce production of aqueous humor

The first line of treatment is usually a β adrenoceptor antagonist. Beta receptor antagonists selected for use topically on the eye are typically devoid of the local anesthetic properties of some of these drugs. For example, propranolol is not used to treat glaucoma since it has local anesthetic effects at the locally high concentrations that are achieved with topical drug administration, which would disadvantageously anesthetize the cornea. Examples of non-selective β adrenoceptor antagonists used topically in the treatment of glaucoma include carteolol, levobunolol and timolol; these drugs have similar affinities for both β$_1$ and β$_2$ adrenoceptors (Fig. 24.11) (see Chapter 18 for more information about β adrenoceptor antagonists). These drugs decrease the rate of aqueous humor formation by blocking β adrenoceptors in the ciliary body, presumably by decreasing the action of circulating epinephrine as well as norepinephrine released by the sympathetic nerve supply to the ciliary body. Selective β adrenoceptor antagonists such as betaxolol hydrochloride (β$_1$ selective) have also been shown to reduce intraocular pressure effectively. Betaxolol may be tolerated in patients with a history of reactive airways disease (e.g. asthma) presumably due to its selectivity on β$_1$ receptors although caution and close monitoring is required if therapy with betaxolol is used in these patients.

Aqueous humor formation may also be decreased by α adrenoceptor agonists (Fig. 24.12). Epinephrine is not very effective because it is poorly absorbed from the surface of the eye: also, it is rapidly metabolized by enzymes such as

Fluorescent dyes

Dye	Excitation	Emission	Use
Fluorescein sodium	480 nm (blue)	520 nm (yellow-green)	Tonometry Epithelial/corneal defects Aqueous leaks
Dichlorotetraiodofluorescein (Rose bengal)	White light	Pink/magenta	Corneal damage Viral infections

Fig. 24.10 Fluorescent dyes.

α Adrenergic agonists used for glaucoma

Drug	Receptor subtype	Adverse effects not expected from mechanism of action	Comments
Epinephrine	α and β	Black cornea	Endogenous neurohormone
Dipivefrin	α and β		Pro-drug of epinephrine (see Fig. 24.13)
Clonidine	α₂		Little used due to systemic adverse effects
Apraclonidine	α₂	Conjunctivitis Dermatitis	Less systemically active analog of clonidine
Brinonidine	α₂	Fatigue Drowsiness	Recently introduced

Fig. 24.12 α Adrenergic agonists used for glaucoma.

β Adrenoceptor antagonists

Topical application of β adrenoceptor antagonists may lead to systemic drug absorption; consequently their use is generally contraindicated in patients with:

- *Asthma*
- *Obstructive airways disease*
- *Bradycardia*
- *Heart block*
- *Heart failure*

---

monoamine oxidase. This problem can be overcome by using the pro-drug dipivefrin hydrochloride. (A pro-drug is a substance that is not itself biologically active, but is metabolized by the body into an active substance.) Dipivefrin hydrochloride is more lipophilic, and once in the eye it is converted to epinephrine, the active metabolite, by the action of corneal esterase enzymes (Fig. 24.13). The mechanism by which epinephrine (dipivefrin) lowers intraocular pressure is controversial. One possibility is that it acts on ciliary body β₂ receptors decreasing the production of aqueous humor. However, administration of epinephrine initially actually increases intraocular pressure (as might be predicted by the fact that β adrenergic antagonists

Fig. 24.13 The pro-drug dipivefrin.

decrease IOP); it is only with chronic use that a lowering in IOP occurs. This time-course raises the possibility that epinephrine acts by desensitizing β adrenergic responses in the eye (see Chapter 5 for discussion of desensitization). A second hypothesis is that long-term use of epinephrine causes a reduction of the blood supply to the ciliary body by activating α_1 adrenoceptors expressed in arteries, leading to vaso-constriction with consequent decrement in the rate of for-mation of aqueous humor.

The use of apraclonidine is generally confined to extreme or acute cases of raised intraocular pressure as with chronic use it can cause an allergic-type conjunctivitis or dermatitis in about 40% of patients. It is a derivative of the α_2 adrenoceptor agonist clonidine (see Chapter 18). The mechanism of action of apraclonidine, like epinephrine, in lowering IOP is unclear. A number of possibilities have been proposed:

- Activation of α_2 adrenoceptors in the ciliary body to reduce aqueous humor formation directly.
- Activation of α_1 adrenoceptors to reduce ciliary blood flow in a manner similar to epinephrine. Although apraclonidine is an α_2 selective agonist, at high concentrations it may also activate α_1 receptors.
- Activation of presynaptic α_2 'autoreceptors' leading to decreased norepinephrine release and therefore reduced aqueous humor production due to diminished postsynaptic β receptor stimulation.

Its adverse effects include those expected from its mechanism of action as an α receptor agonist: hyperemia, eyelid retraction, vasoconstriction of the conjunctiva (blanching), and mydriasis.

Carbonic anhydrase inhibitors are drugs that are efficacious when administered orally in patients with glaucoma (Fig. 24.14). The conversion of carbon dioxide and water to carbonic acid (and therefore bicarbonate) is catalyzed by the enzyme carbonic anhydrase. This conversion in the absence of carbonic anhydrase is slow and is speeded up some 10,000-fold depend-ing on the isoform of the enzyme. As the production of aqueous humor depends on the active transport of bicarbonate and Na^+ ions, reducing the activity of carbonic anhydrase

decreases aqueous humor production. Acetazolamide is a syn-thetic sulfonamide developed in the 1950s and is an effective agent in reducing IOP. However, because of its adverse effects, it is not well tolerated. Adverse effects, particularly in the elderly, include paresthesia, hypokalemia, a lack of appetite, drowsiness, and depression. Adverse effects from acetazolamide have been diminished by the development of a slow-release formulation of the drug. This may be due to the fact that peak concentrations of the drug obtained with the slow-release formulation in plasma are about 1/3 of those obtained with the ordinary tablet, although the duration of peak concen-trations is prolonged with the slow-release form of the drug (see Chapter 4 for discussion of pharmacokinetics). A further decrement in the adverse effects of carbonic anhydrase in-hibitors has been the topical administration of drugs in this class directly on the eyes. Topical carbonic anhydrase inhibitors, such as dorzolamide, act by inhibiting a particular isoform of carbonic anhydrase (CA-II) found in the ciliary body (and also in red blood cells). Furthermore, dorzolamide works well in combination with β adrenoceptor antagonists or miotics.

Drugs that increase the drainage of aqueous humor

Miotics (Fig. 24.15) may, to some degree, assist in the drainage of aqueous humor, possibly by increasing the uveoscleral outflow. Miotics have the obvious adverse effect of constricting pupils, which may impair vision in the dark. Of more concern is the chronic accommodative spasm induced by these drugs

Miotics used for glaucoma

Drug	Action	Comments
Carbachol	Mixed muscarinic and nicotinic agonist	
Pilocarpine	Muscarinic agonist	Slow-release formulation

Fig. 24.15 Miotics used for glaucoma.

Carbonic anhydrase inhibitors used for glaucoma

Drug	Route of administration	Isozyme-selective	Pharmacokinetics Onset	Peak	Duration	Comments
Acetazolamide	Oral Parenteral Slow-release capsules	No	1 hour	2–6 hours	>7 hours	Bone marrow suppression Aplastic anemia Anaphylactic shock
Dichlorphenamide	Oral	No	2 hours	2 hours	6 hours	Anorexia Confusion
Methazolamide	Oral	No	1 hour	2–3 hours	12 hours	Malaise Fatigue
Dorzolamide HCl	Topical	Yes CA-II		2 hours		Lower systemic adverse effects Better patient adherence

Fig. 24.14 Carbonic anhydrase inhibitors used for glaucoma.

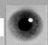

Osmotic agents used for acute, severe increases in intraocular pressure					
Drug	**Route of administration**	**Pharmacokinetics** Onset	Peak	Duration	**Comments**
Glycerin	Oral	15 minutes	45 minutes	5 hours	Metabolized
Isosorbide	Oral	30 minutes		5 hours	Not metabolized
Mannitol	Intravenous	30 minutes	60 minutes	6 hours	Agent of choice
Urea	Intravenous	30 minutes		5 hours	Little used

Fig. 24.16 Osmotic agents used for acute severe increases in intraocular pressure.

which may lead over time to blurred vision and headaches. These adverse effects occur in most patients, but usually decrease with time in older patients. Slow-release formulations of miotics (e.g. modified-release of pilocarpine, a muscarinic cholinergic agonist) are available to minimize these adverse effects in younger patients, as unlike eye drops, slow-release formulations do not produce a high initial concentration in the eye.

Recently a novel class of drug has been introduced to increase drainage of aqueous humor. Latanoprost is a prostaglandin analog which increases uveoscleral outflow by mimicking the action of prostaglandin $F_{2\alpha}$ (Fig. 24.7). It is thought to act by relaxing the ciliary muscle followed by a longer-term action of remodeling of the extracellular matrix.

Effectiveness of drugs used to treat glaucoma

In comparative studies the systemic carbonic anhydrase inhibitors are as effective as the α adrenergic agonists and better that the β receptor antagonists at reducing IOP. However, clinical effectiveness is not the only driving force dictating the choice of drugs, as a consideration of the adverse effects and the nature of the patients are also required.

Clinical management of open-angle glaucoma

There is no evidence-based consensus for the treatment of glaucoma. Usually drug therapy is initially by the use of a β adrenoceptor antagonist. However, if the target reduction in intraocular pressure is not achieved then a miotic or α adrenergic agonist might be added. It may seem strange to use both β receptor antagonists and α receptor agonists in the same patient, but as described above, these drugs likely act via different mechanisms to reduce intraocular pressure and so may have additive effects. Typically, systemically administered carbonic anhydrase inhibitors are used as third line agents as they may have important adverse effects. Better tolerated topical carbonic anhydrase inhibitors such as dorzolamide may become more widely used. Latanoprost gives further scope for treatment of resistant cases of raised IOP. In the end the choice of drug may depend on individual patient characteristics; for example β receptor antagonists may be contraindicated in patients with asthma or congestive heart failure. In the young, and in patients with increased risk of retinal detachment, miotics should be used with caution.

Closed-angle glaucoma

In emergency situations, drug treatment is used to reduce the peripheral ballooning and so lower the acute rise in intraocular pressure. Mannitol, an osmotic diuretic administered intravenously, or glycerin given orally, increase the osmolarity of the blood and can rapidly decrease markedly elevated intraocular pressure which is an immediate threat to vision (Fig. 24.16). Topical miotics such as pilocarpine or carbachol can sometimes tauten the iris and temporarily promote some decrement in IOP (Fig. 24.15). Hyperosmotic agents lower IOP by reducing vitreous volume. The increase in plasma osmolarity following administration of a hyperosmotic agent causes a net movement of water from the vitreous into intraocular blood vessels. A reduction of around 10% of the volume of the anterior chamber is produced which reduces IOP and may also deepen the anterior chamber allowing posterior movement of the iris. This is particularly useful in cases of closed-angle glaucoma.

A permanent cure is produced by laser surgery. An yttrium–aluminum–garnet (YAG) laser is used to form a hole in the iris (iridectomy) to increase the flow of aqueous humor.

Treatment of inflammation and allergy

Inflammation of the eye is treated with a short course of glucocorticosteroids

Local intraocular inflammation and uveitis (inflammation of the uveal tract) can be treated with a short course of glucocorticosteroids, which are the first line of treatment for local inflammation. Their mechanism of action is explained in Chapter 15. However, these drugs are for short-term use only. With prolonged use they may cause 'steroid glaucoma' or cataracts. They should therefore only be given under close ophthalmologic supervision. Examples of glucocorticosteroids in clinical use today are listed in Fig. 24.17. Systemic

---

Mydriatics and glaucoma

- Mydriatics may be hazardous in patients suspected of closed-angle glaucoma as they may exacerbate the condition
- Pupil dilation and paralysis of the ciliary muscle reduce the drainage of aqueous humor

Glucocorticosteroids for the eye

Drug	Relative anti-inflammatory activity	Use
Betamethasone	25	Short-term treatment of inflammation
Clobetasone butyrate		Short-term treatment of inflammation
Dexamethasone	25	Short-term treatment of inflammation
Fluorometholone	25	Short-term treatment of inflammation
Hydrocortisone acetate	1	Short-term treatment of inflammation
Prednisolone	4	Effective for anterior segment inflammation
Rimexolone	4	Postoperative inflammation Uveitis

Fig. 24.17 Glucocorticosteroids for the eye.

glucocorticosteroids may be appropriate for severe eye disease such as scleritis, episcleritis, and blinding uveitis.

A correct diagnosis is essential: glucocorticosteroids will worsen an inflamed eye produced by a dendritic ulcer resulting from a herpes simplex virus infection and may lead to blindness or even loss of the eye.

Allergic conditions such as allergic conjunctivitis can be treated with H₁ antihistamines such as antazoline or other mast cell stabilizing drugs such as cromolyn sodium or nedocromil

Glucocorticosteroids

- *Topical glucocorticosteroids used long term can cause cataracts and glaucoma*
- *Glucocorticosteroids can cause blindness if used when there is local herpes infection*

sodium (Fig. 24.18). Topical glucocorticosteroids may also be needed for severe allergy.

Treatment of tear deficiency

A variety of drugs can be used as artificial tears to prevent dry eyes becoming painful and prevent damage to the cornea. Examples are listed in Fig. 24.19. Acetylcysteine is a mucolytic that can be used to break up mucoid secretions in the eye, which are often associated with a poor tear film over the eye.

Treatment of squint and oculomotor disorders

Some extraocular and eyelid muscle disorders can be treated with botulinum toxin

Some neuromuscular disorders of the extraocular muscles (squints) and eyelids (blepharospasms) can be treated with botulinum toxin A. This is one of the toxins produced by the bacterium *Clostridium botulinum*, which causes some forms of food poisoning leading to potentially generalized muscle paralysis. However, therapeutic injection of skeletal muscles with botulinum toxin causes only local effects. Over a period of about 3 days after such an injection, the muscle relaxes and stays relaxed for up to 6 weeks. Botulinum toxin A blocks acetylcholine release from the motor nerve terminals (Fig. 24.20). Botulinum toxin A has enzymatic activity and cleaves proteins that are necessary for docking and fusion of acetylcholine vesicles to the presynaptic nerve terminal membranes. In particular SNAP-25 is cleaved and the only way the release of acetylcholine can return is with the synthesis of new

Other anti-inflammatory drugs for the eye

Drug	Mechanism of action	Use
Antazoline sulfate	H₁ histamine receptor antagonist	Allergic conjunctivitis
Azelastine hydrochloride	H₁ histamine receptor antagonist	Seasonal allergic conjunctivitis
Emedastine (recently introduced)	H₁ histamine receptor antagonist	Seasonal allergic conjunctivitis
Levocabastine	H₁ histamine receptor antagonist	Seasonal allergic conjunctivitis
Lodoxamide	Mast cell stabilizer (calcium channel blocker?)	Allergic conjunctivitis
Nedocromil sodium	Mast cell stabilizer (calcium channel blocker?)	Allergic conjunctivitis Vernal keratoconjunctivitis
Sodium cromoglicate	Mast cell stabilizer (calcium channel blocker?)	Allergic conjunctivitis Vernal keratoconjunctivitis

Fig. 24.18 Other anti-inflammatory drugs for the eye.

Substances used for tear deficiency

Compound	Use	Comments
Acetylcysteine	Tear deficiency Impaired mucus production	Mucolytic agent
Carbomers (polyacrylic acid)	Dry eye conditions Unstable tear film	
Hydroxyethylcellulose	Tear deficiency	
Hypromellose	Tear deficiency	
Liquid paraffin	Dry eye conditions	
Polyvinyl alcohol	Tear deficiency	
Povidone	Dry eye conditions	
Sodium chloride	Irrigation	
Zinc sulfate	Astringent	Little used

Fig. 24.19 Substances used for tear deficiency.

proteins, which explains the long duration of the effect. To ensure correct needle placement for the injection it is recommended that the procedure is performed with a special needle that allows recording of the electromyogram (EMG) at the same time. For example, by weakening the muscles surrounding the eye, involuntary spasms of these muscles can be prevented in patients with recurrent spasms.

The skeletal muscle autoimmune disease myasthenia gravis may weaken the muscles of the eyelids as well as the extraocular muscles. Systemic administration of anticholinesterase drugs such as neostigmine bromide and pyridostigmine bromide relieves the ocular and other symptoms (see Chapter 14).

DRUGS THAT HAVE ADVERSE EFFECTS ON THE EYE

Lacrimators

Lacrimators are drugs that are not used therapeutically. They cause intense irritation of the cornea and conjunctiva, for example tear gases such as orthochlorobenzylidenemalononitrite (CS gas) and sprays containing extracts of chilli peppers, capsaicin (Mace). CS gas is used as an harassing agent for controlling civil disorders, and in some countries these substances are legally available for use in personal protection.

These compounds activate vanilloid (capsaicin) receptors, which are found on sensory nerves and are nonselective cation

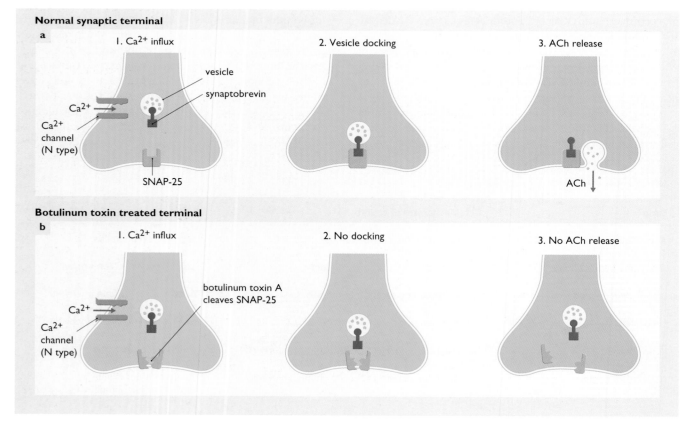

Fig. 24.20 The cellular mechanism of action of botulinum toxin. Botulinum toxin prevents vesicle docking and acetylcholine (ACh) release from motor nerves. It does this by cleaving synaptosomal-associated protein (SNAP-25), which is an important docking protein and has a molecular weight of 25 kDa.

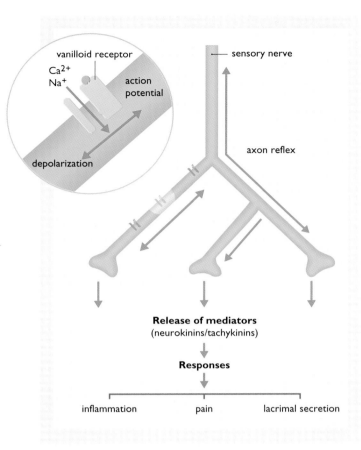

Fig. 24.21 Mediator release by lacrimators and related substances. The axon reflex caused by capsaicin agonists results in mediator release from sensory fibers leading to pain, inflammation, and glandular secretions.

channels. Activation of the receptor opens the ion channel, allowing the flow of Na^+ and Ca^{2+} ions into the nerve; this depolarizes the nerve and can generate action potentials. The action potentials can then travel both orthodromically and antidromically along the fibers, depolarizing many nerve

terminals (Fig. 24.21). A variety of mediators (neurokinins and tachykinins, which cause pain, inflammation, and lacrimal gland secretion) are then released from sensory nerve terminals in response to the stimulation. This sensation can be duplicated by touching the eyes after cutting up chilli peppers, and the sensory nerve receptors were therefore named after this 'lacrimator' in chilli peppers (i.e. capsaicin).

Cataractogenic drugs

When the lens becomes opaque it is called a cataract. Drugs that can cause cataracts include:

- Locally applied drugs such as glucocorticosteroids when given long term.
- Systemic drugs such as the phenothiazines (used to treat schizophrenia, see Chapter 14) (Fig. 24.22).

Retinopathic drugs

A number of systemically administered drugs can cause retinopathy. Ingestion of as little as 10 g of methanol, which is often found in illicit spirits such as moonshine and poteen, may damage retinal ganglion cells. The axons of these cells form the optic nerves and the resulting damage can cause blindness. The damage occurs because an enzyme in the retina that normally converts retinal to retinal as part of the normal pigment (rhodopsin) cycle, converts methanol to formaldehyde. Formaldehyde rapidly reacts with proteins (which is why it is used as a tissue fixative) and damages many cells, but particularly the retinal ganglion cells. Methanol poisoning is discussed in Chapter 29.

Chloroquine, which was first used as an antimalarial drug and is now used for rheumatoid conditions, can cause reversible cataracts and also irreversible and very characteristic 'bull's eye' retinopathy. However, if the dose is kept below 250 mg/day this adverse effect is less common.

Indomethacin, ethambutol, tamoxifen, and phenothiazines are some of the other drugs that have adverse effects on the retina or the optic nerve. In some cases these retinal adverse effects are dose dependent. For example, retinal toxicity is rare

Systemic drugs that have adverse effects on the eye					
Drug	Use	Chapter	Cataracts	Retinopathy	Optic neuropathy
Chloroquine	Antimalarial	25	✓	✓	–
Phenothiazines	Antipsychotic	7	✓	✓	–
Tamoxifen	Anticancer	28	–	✓	–
Methanol	Recreational	29	–	–	✓
Ethambutol	Antitubercular	11	–	–	✓
Indomethacin	Anti-inflammatory	17	–	✓	–
Oxygen	Neonatal care	–	–	✓	–

Fig. 24.22 Systemic drugs that have adverse effects on the eye.

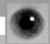

 Drugs that have adverse effects on the eye

- Cataracts can be caused by some locally applied drugs (e.g. echothiophate)
- Cataracts can be caused by some systemically applied drugs (e.g. chloroquine)
- Retinopathies can be caused by some systemically applied drugs (e.g. tamoxifen)

if the dose of ethambutol is kept below 15 mg/kg/day. (It is prudent to arrange for ophthalmologic monitoring of patients taking these drugs.)

A specific problem of premature infants, who are often placed in a high-oxygen environment to aid their survival, is retrolental fibroplasia. This is produced by the inappropriate growth of blood vessels into the vitreous humor and is triggered by abrupt removal from a high-oxygen environment. The growth of these vessels can distort the retina, leading to visual defects and blindness.

EYE INFECTIONS

Infections of the eye are commonly bacterial

Infections of the eye are commonly of bacterial or viral origin.

- Bacterial blepharitis and acute infective conjunctivitis are treated with topical antibacterial drops or creams.
- Gonococcal conjunctivitis requires both topical and systemic antibacterial therapy.
- Corneal ulcers and keratitis require specialist treatment involving the subconjunctival administration of antibiotics.
- Endophthalmitis is caused by infection and inflammation at the back of the eye and is a medical emergency. It may require intraocular injections of antibiotics.

Fungal eye infections are rare, but may occur in agricultural workers and require specialist treatment.

A wide range of antibacterial drugs are available (Fig. 24.23) for treating eye infections. Most can be used as broad-spectrum antibiotics, but some are reserved for specific infections.

Adverse effects associated with antibacterial drugs are minimal, and usually comprise transient stinging and itching. Chloramphenicol, the most widely used antibiotic, has been rarely associated with aplastic anemia, and ciprofloxacin is best avoided in children because it is particularly liable to cause local burning and itching sensations. The mechanisms of action of these drugs are discussed in Chapter 9.

There are fewer antiviral drugs available for ophthalmic use. Acyclovir is used to treat corneal ulcers caused by herpes simplex infection, and ganciclovir is used to treat cytomegalovirus infection of the eye, which occurs in patients with AIDS. The mechanisms of action of these drugs are discussed in Chapter 8.

Antibacterial drugs used for eye infections

Drug	Use	Comments
Chloramphenicol	Broad spectrum	Drug of choice
Chlortetracycline	Chlamydial infections Trachoma	
Ciprofloxacin	Broad spectrum Corneal ulcers	
Framycetin sulfate	Broad spectrum	
Fusidic acid	Staphylococcal infections	
Gentamicin	Broad spectrum *Pseudomonas aeruginosa* infections	
Lomefloxacin	Broad spectrum	Recently introduced
Neomycin sulfate	Broad spectrum	
Ofloxacin	Broad spectrum *Pseudomonas aeruginosa* infections	
Polymyxin B sulfate	Broad spectrum	
Propamidine isethionate	Acanthamoeba keratitis	Little value in bacterial infections

Fig. 24.23 Antibacterial drugs used for eye infections.

FURTHER READING

Bartlett JD, Jaanus SD. *Clinical Ocular Pharmacology*, 4th edn. London: Butterworth Heinemann; 2001. [A major work for reference].

Denniston A, Reuser T. The use of botulinum toxin in ophthalmology. *Hosp Med* 2001; **62**: 477–479. [A review of botox therapy used in ophthalmology.]

Dowling JE. *The Retina: an Approachable Part of the Brain*. Cambridge, Mass: Harvard University Press; 1987. [An excellent book on the retina, written by a leading retinal scientist.]

Fraunfelder FT, Fraunfelder FW. *Drug Induced Ocular Side Effects*, 5th edn. London: Butterworth Heinemann; 2000. [A major work for reference.]

Zimmerman TJ, Kooner KS, Sharir M, Fechter RD. *Textbook of Ocular Pharmacology*. Philadelphia: Lippincott-Raven; 1997. [A major work for reference.]

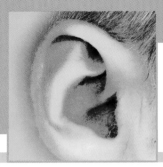

Chapter 25

Drugs and the Ear

PHYSIOLOGY OF THE EAR

■ *The ear is a sensory organ that detects sound and head position and movement*

The outer ear collects sound waves and directs them to the tympanic membrane, which, with the middle ear ossicular chain, amplifies sound vibration and transforms it into fluid shifts within the inner ear (Fig. 25.1). The organ of Corti in the cochlea (Fig. 25.2) contains sensory receptor hair cells (Fig. 25.3), which are set into motion by vibration of the cochlear duct basement membrane. Hair cell motion displaces the hair cell stereocilia projecting from the cell apex. This results in cellular depolarization produced by an inward cation current (Ca^{2+}, Na^+) entering the apical end of the hair cell. The hair cell then releases a chemical transmitter from its basal end, leading to stimulation of the afferent bipolar neurons of the auditory nerve and their central connections. Stereocilial deflection in the opposite direction results in hair cell hyperpolarization, which inhibits basal neurotransmitter release and suppresses auditory neurons activity. Stereocilial oscillation therefore produces a train of excitatory and inhibitory impulses within the auditory nerve with the same frequency characteristics as the original sound.

Balance depends on inputs from the vestibular, visual, and proprioceptive sensory systems to the balance centers of the brain. The peripheral vestibular system (Fig. 25.4) consists of:

• The otolithic organs, the utricle and saccule, which sense linear acceleration.

• The semicircular canals, which sense angular acceleration or rotation.

The sensory input from these organs is critical for maintaining equilibrium and stabilizing gaze with head movement. Depending on head position or movement, vestibular hair cells

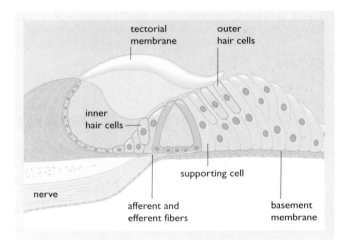

Fig. 25.2 The organ of Corti. Movement of the basement membrane results in shearing between the hair cells (fixed in their supporting cells) and the tectorial membrane.

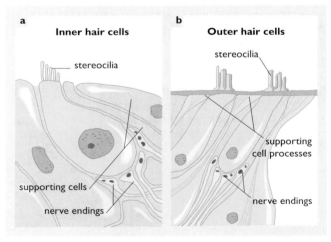

Fig. 25.3 Cochlear hair cells. There are two types of cochlear hair cells: (a) inner hair cells, which synapse with afferent nerve endings, and (b) outer hair cells, which synapse with efferent nerve endings.

Fig. 25.1 Structure of the ear (transverse section). The ear senses sound as well as head position and motion.

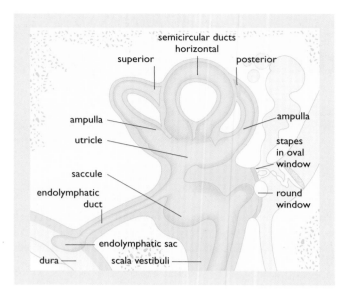

Fig. 25.4 The peripheral vestibular system. The peripheral vestibular system includes the semicircular canals (which sense rotary acceleration) and the otolithic organs, the utricle and saccule (which sense linear acceleration).

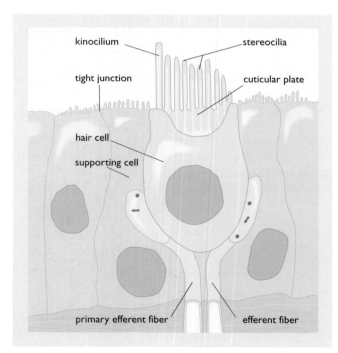

Fig. 25.5 The vestibular hair cells. In addition to having stereocilia, vestibular hair cells have a motile kinocilium. Stereocilial deflection towards the kinocilium results in hair cell depolarization, while deflection away from the kinocilium results in hair cell hyperpolarization.

(Fig. 25.5) are either depolarized or hyperpolarized. Depolarization increases the basal release of neurotransmitter and the resting firing rate of the associated vestibular afferent neuron. Hyperpolarization has the opposite effect. Head movement and position are therefore resolved into stimulatory increases or

Etiology of hearing loss		
Conductive hearing loss		**Sensorineural hearing loss**
Congenital	Acquired	Noise-induced
Atresia of pinna and canal	Otitis externa	Otosclerosis
Abnormalities of the middle ear	Otitis media, acute and chronic (perforated tympanic membrane)	Infections (e.g. measles, mumps)
	Otosclerosis	Acoustic neuroma
		Autoimmune
		Drug-induced (NSAIDs, antibiotics, antineoplastics, loop diuretics)

Fig. 25.6 Hearing loss due to problems with the conductive and/or neuronal portion of the ear.

inhibitory decreases of the resting firing rate of the vestibular nerve and its central connections.

PATHOPHYSIOLOGY AND DISEASES OF THE EAR

The main symptoms of ear disorders are hearing loss, tinnitus, vertigo, pain, pressure, and itchiness.

Hearing loss

Hearing loss may be conductive (resulting from disorders of external or middle ear sound conduction) or sensorineural (resulting from abnormalities of the inner ear sensory cells and their central connections) (Fig. 25.6). Drugs which induce hearing loss affect the sensorineural pathway.

Infections

Ear infections are extremely common and involve the outer ear (otitis externa), middle ear (otitis media), or inner ear (labyrinthitis).

Otitis externa

Otitis externa is a bacterial or fungal infection of the soft tissue of the external ear canal. Common bacterial causes include *Pseudomonas aeruginosa*, *Proteus mirabilis*, staphylococci, streptococci, and various Gram-negative bacteria. *Candida* and *Aspergillus* species are the most common fungal causes. Most pathogens are inhibited by an acidic medium, and a solution of equal parts of vinegar and isopropyl alcohol prevents otitis externa. All infected debris and pus must be removed from the ear (otic toilet) before starting any medication. Moisture should be avoided.

Treatment of otitis externa

Infection	*Pseudomonas aeruginosa, Proteus mirabilis, Staphylococcus aureus*	
First-line: mild	Second-line: moderate	Third-line: severe
Polymyxin/neomycin hydrocortisone otic solution	Dicloxacillin (p.o.), cephalexin, ciprofloxacin	Cefazolin (i.v.), dicloxacillin, ciprofloxacin, other quinolones

Fig. 25.7 Treatment of otitis externa. (i.v., intravenous; p.o., oral)

First-line medical therapy includes topical preparations combining an antibiotic and glucocorticosteroid, such as neomycin with polymyxin and hydrocortisone. Polysorbate, gentian violet or nystatin may be used as topical antifungal agents. Dicloxacillin, cephalexin, trimethoprim–sulfamethoxazole, or ciprofloxacin are given orally for progressive cellulitis of the external ear canal, while intravenous cefazolin, dicloxacillin, or ciprofloxacin may be needed for severe cases. A prolonged course of combination antipseudomonal therapy is required for invasive skull base osteitis, preferably aztreonam with clindamycin or a combination of ciprofloxacin with one of the following: ticarcillin, piperacillin, ceftazidime, imipenem, gentamicin, tobramycin, or amikacin (Fig. 25.7).

Otitis media

Acute purulent otitis media is a bacterial infection of the middle ear. The usual pathogens are *Streptococcus pneumoniae*, *Haemophilus influenzae*, and *Moraxella catarrhalis*. There is an increasing incidence of antibiotic-resistant bacteria.

First-line therapy should include amoxicillin or erythromycin plus a sulfonamide or trimethoprim–sulfamethoxazole. Second-line therapy is directed at a possible β lactamase-producing organism and may include amoxicillin–clavulanate, cefaclor, cefuroxime, cefixime, or clarithromycin (Fig. 25.8).

OTITIS MEDIA with an effusion is the presence of (usually sterile) fluid in the middle ear and may follow acute otitis media or occur independently. It usually clears spontaneously but, if not, a two-week course of amoxicillin or trimethoprim–sulfamethoxazole can promote fluid clearance. Use of nasal sprays containing steroids to promote drainage by opening the Eustachian tubes can also be useful.

CHRONIC OTITIS MEDIA is defined by the presence of a perforated tympanic membrane in the presence of middle ear infection. Bacteria that cause active infection in the presence of a perforation include *P. aeruginosa*, *Proteus* spp., staphylococci, Gram-negative organisms, and anaerobes (*Klebsiella* spp., *E. coli*, *B. fragilis*). Treatment includes ear drops with neomycin and polymyxin and an oral agent such as trimethoprim–sulfamethoxazole or cephalexin, though amoxicillin–clavulanate or ciprofloxacin with metronidazole may be required. If pseudomonas is the cause of persistent otorrhea, combining two different ear drops, one containing ciprofloxacin and the other an aminoglycoside (gentamicin, tobramycin), may be effective. Aminoglycosides can cause ototoxicity when applied to the middle ear, but this is rare in the presence of active infection.

Treatment of otitis externa

- The external ear must be thoroughly cleaned before starting antibiotic therapy
- A combination ear drop is first-line therapy
- Severe infections may require parenteral antibiotics and narcotic analgesics

Drugs used to treat otitis media

- *Frequent use of antibiotics in young children can cause gastrointestinal upset and thrush*
- *Aminoglycoside-containing ear drops can be ototoxic in the presence of middle ear inflammation*
- *Repeated use of antibacterial ear drops predisposes to secondary fungal infection*

Treatment of acute purulent otitis media

Infection	*Streptococcus pneumoniae, Haemophilus influenzae, Moraxella catarrhalis*	
First-line: p.o.	Second-line: p.o.	Third-line: i.v.
Amoxicillin, erythromycin with sulfonamide, trimethoprim–sulfamethoxazole	Amoxicillin–clavulanate, cefaclor, cefuroxime, cefixime, clarithromycin	Third generation cephalosporins or quinolones (surgical intervention)

Fig. 25.8 Treatment of acute purulent otitis media. (i.v., intravenous, p.o., oral)

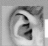

Suppurative labyrinthitis

Bacterial infection of the spaces of the inner ear causes profound cochlear and vestibular destruction and loss of both hearing and vestibular function in the affected ear. Intralabyrinthine infection results from:

- Spread of otitis media via the round or oval windows.
- A labyrinthine fistula.
- Lateral extension of meningitis through the cochlear aqueduct and cribriform plate at the lateral end of the internal auditory canal.

If infection is due to otitis media, treatment includes surgical drainage and intravenous antibiotics (ceftriaxone for acute otitis media, nafcillin with ceftazidime plus metronidazole for chronic otitis media). If infection is due to meningitis, the appropriate intravenous antibiotic (see Chapter 9) should be given. Whether concurrent intravenous glucocorticosteroids reduce the incidence of post-meningitis hearing loss is controversial.

Hearing loss

■ *Ototoxic drugs are common causes of hearing loss and must always be considered* (see below)

Otosclerosis

Otosclerosis is characterized by idiopathic circumscribed endochondral otic capsule bone destruction and replacement with vascular bone and then dense lamellar bone. Characteristic sites include the anterior oval window niche, which results in stapes footplate fixation and a conductive hearing loss. Sensorineural hearing loss can result from a focus of otosclerosis adjacent to the endolymphatic space.

Epidemiologic studies indicate a lower incidence of otosclerosis in regions with high fluoride concentrations in drinking water. However, the only widely recognized indication for using fluoride is progressive sensorineural hearing loss with a high risk of otosclerosis on taking the patient's history or upon examination. Calcium, 2–3 g daily, should be administered along with the fluoride.

Sudden sensorineural hearing loss

Sudden sensorineural hearing loss (SSHL) is usually unilateral, progresses within hours to days, and is associated with tinnitus and, less frequently, vertigo. There are a variety of causes (Fig. 25.9). If a specific cause cannot be identified it is thought to result from a viral infection, vascular disorder, or inner ear membrane rupture.

SSHL is a medical emergency and, if specific etiologies have been excluded, many clinicians recommend a moderate course of glucocorticosteroids tapered over 10 days to 2 weeks, although the efficacy of this treatment is not established. The best treatment responses appear to occur in patients with moderate hearing losses who start glucocorticosteroids within 10 days. Treatment is not required for mild hearing loss, which routinely recovers spontaneously, and there is no established benefit for severe hearing loss. Other agents used to treat SSHL include vasodilating drugs, plasma expanders, and carbogen (5% CO_2, 95% O_2), but there is no convincing evidence that these are effective.

Conditions causing sudden sensorineural hearing loss	
Classification	**Example**
Congenital	Mondini's deformity
Acquired Physical factors	Barotrauma, electrical, concussion, temporal bone fracture, perilymph fistula
Chemical factors Metabolic	Diabetes mellitus, hyperlipidemia, hypothyroidism (Pendred's syndrome)
Ototoxic medications	Anti-inflammatory drugs, antibiotics, antineoplastics, loop diuretics
Infections and inflammation	Viral infection (measles, mumps, herpes zoster), bacterial infection (syphilis, mycoplasma, meningitis), chronic granulomatous disease (sarcoidosis)
Vascular	Vasculopathies, coagulopathies, emboli, migraine
Immunologic	Cogan's syndrome
Neoplastic	Acoustic neuroma, carcinoma
Idiopathic	Multiple sclerosis

Fig. 25.9 Conditions causing sudden sensorineural hearing loss.

Autoimmune hearing loss

Autoimmune sensorineural hearing loss typically affects young adults, is slowly progressive over months, and is not accompanied by other systemic disease or hereditary defects. It appears to be due to an autoimmune reaction to a specific inner ear antigen. There is no vertigo, but more severe disease causes ataxia in dim light.

Treatment depends on the severity of the hearing loss, likelihood of autoimmune dysfunction, and the patient's general medical condition. For more severe and bilateral cases, prednisone for 2–4 weeks is the treatment of choice. A second immunosuppressive agent may be needed if:

- There is a good response and hearing recovers but the patient becomes chronically dependent on glucocorticosteroids to maintain hearing.
- There is a strong suspicion that autoimmunity is the cause. Cyclophosphamide, methotrexate, or penicillamine can be effective, but the patient must be closely monitored for adverse effects.

Tinnitus

Tinnitus is the perception of sound in the absence of an external source. It may be:

- Objective and result from sounds generated within the body, which are audible to an observer.
- Subjective and characterized by an auditory sensation in the absence of a physical sound.

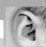

Causes include musculoskeletal and vascular sounds producing objective tinnitus, and disorders of the peripheral and central auditory systems, which usually produce subjective tinnitus. The cause may be known (e.g. noise-induced, presbycusis). The first symptom of drug-induced ototoxicity often is tinnitus. NSAIDs, antibiotics and antineoplastic agents are the most commonly involved drugs. Most patients also have an irreversible high-frequency sensorineural hearing loss.

Once an underlying disease has been excluded, the goal is to relieve the annoyance that tinnitus causes. If it is mild, patients may simply need information about its cause and benign nature. Masking (the use of a noise generator to 'cover over' the subjective sound) is the prime treatment. Medication, and behavioral modification, may be needed for intractable tinnitus. Medications include:

- Local anesthetics (procaine, lidocaine).
- Benzodiazepines (diazepam, alprazolam, clonazepam).
- Baclofen.
- Tricyclic antidepressants (amitriptyline).

The mechanism of local anesthetic control of tinnitus probably involves neuron plasma membrane Na^+ channel blockade, and the principal site is probably central at the level of the cochlear nerve and its brainstem connections. Lidocaine has dramatically suppressed tinnitus in some patients, but must be given intravenously.

Benzodiazepines improve the patient's emotional response to tinnitus, but are also thought to suppress tinnitus directly. In some patients this may be due to insufficient inhibitory activity in the ascending auditory system. Benzodiazepines may act by enhancing the activity of the inhibitory neurotransmitter γ-aminobutyric acid (GABA).

Other medications used with varying success for tinnitus include tricyclic antidepressants such as amitriptyline.

Vertigo

Vertigo is the hallucinatory perception of movement and can result from disorders of the peripheral or central vestibular systems.

Peripherally induced vertigo is usually the more severe and associated with other aural symptoms such as hearing loss or tinnitus. It is produced by:

- Benign positional vertigo, which is either spontaneous or secondary to head trauma, occurs with motion of the head, and usually lasts less than 30 seconds. There is a sensation of rotary motion, either of the world moving or one moving in the world. Malpositioning of otoliths is presumed to

trigger an attack. It is treated by systematic head maneuvers and positioning to try to re-position the otoliths of the inner ear.
- Constant, often permanent, hypofunction of the affected labyrinth, for example acute vestibular neuronitis, suppurative labyrinthitis, and vestibular trauma.
- Transient fluctuations in vestibular neuron activity such as Ménière's disease and recurrent vestibulopathy.

Centrally induced vertigo may be associated with signs of brainstem or cerebellar pathology. Medical treatment of vertigo is aimed at stabilizing pathologic fluctuations in peripheral vestibular function and promoting central compensation if there is a permanent decrease in vestibular function.

Vestibular neuronitis and vestibular trauma

Vestibular neuronitis results in an acute decrease in vestibular function, which may be mild and reversible or profound and permanent. Symptoms include severe vertigo which can be accompanied by nausea. It is probably caused by a virus of unknown type. Vestibular trauma can have a similar range of severity, depending upon whether there has been a brain concussion, total destruction of the vestibular structures, or division of the vestibular nerve.

Central adaptation must begin during the first month after onset. Patients must remain active, as forced inactivity may predispose to incomplete adaptation and permanent ataxia. Antinauseants such as dimenhydrinate may be needed for severe nausea, and the vestibular suppressants used for acute Ménière's disease (see next section) can be used sparingly. No medication specifically promotes central adaptation.

Ménière's disease and recurrent vestibulopathy

Ménière's disease is a peripheral vestibular disorder associated with intermittent overaccumulation of endolymphatic fluid (endolymphatic hydrops). It causes episodes of severe rotary vertigo that continue for hours, hearing loss, tinnitus, and a pressure sensation in the ear. Initially these symptoms occur in 'attacks,' but eventually the condition 'burns out,' leaving the patient with a stable severe sensorineural hearing loss and a permanent, usually well-compensated, decrease in peripheral vestibular function.

Ménière's disease is managed with medication, diets to restrict Na^+ intake and prevent hydrops, and physical therapy to adapt to the loss of vestibular function. Medications include:

- Diuretics (hydrochlorothiazide, furosemide) to limit endolymphatic fluid accumulation.
- Vestibular suppressants (sedatives, antihistamines, anticholinergics, narcotics).
- Vasodilating drugs.
- Aminoglycosides to ablate peripheral vestibular function.

Hydrochlorothiazide prevents recurrent vertigo in many patients. The doses range from 10 to 50 mg daily; if the dose is greater than 25 mg, attention must be paid to the possibility of potassium depletion by repeated measurements of serum K^+ and high potassium diet. Meclizine moderates acute attacks, and it is likely that this occurs via its capacity to antagonize

> ### Anti-tinnitus drugs
>
> - *Tocainide is the only local anesthetic that can be given orally, but it can have serious adverse effects on the heart*
> - *Benzodiazepines should be used sparingly because they can be habituating*
> - *Tricyclic antidepressants have antimuscarinic and cardiac adverse effects (see Chapter 14)*

543

Drugs for Ménière's disease

- Hydrochlorothiazide reduces endolymph production
- Meclizine has anticholinergic effects
- Benzodiazepines are both vestibular suppressants and cerebral sedatives
- Aminoglycosides induce a stable decrease in vestibular function

Drugs used to treat Ménière's disease

- *Diuretic therapy can cause K^+ depletion, hyperglycemia, and hyperlipidemia, and exacerbate gout*
- *Severe permanent ataxia and oscillopsia can follow streptomycin treatment of bilateral Ménière's disease if it produces a total loss of vestibular function*
- *Intratympanic gentamicin treatment is associated with a 10–20% incidence of hearing loss*

muscarinic cholinergic receptors rather than H_1 histamine receptors. This is an example of a drug known to be in one class (antihistamine) which actually has its therapeutic benefit through another mechanism common to a different class of compounds (drugs identified as specific anticholinergic compounds). If an attack becomes severe, a benzodiazepine such as diazepam or lorazepam not only provides sedation but also acts directly on the medial and lateral vestibular nuclei to suppress otolithic and semicircular canal activity. More specific anticholinergic medications such as scopolamine have limited use because their adverse effects are more profound than those of meclizine. Some parenteral narcotics (e.g. fentanyl, droperidol) are potent vestibular suppressants and are occasionally needed for an acute, incapacitating attack.

Chemical ablation of vestibular function may be indicated for recurrent incapacitating vertigo that cannot be controlled by medications; the patient, with physician guidance, must decide if it would be easier to cope with a permanent, medically induced loss of vestibular function. Streptomycin can be given parenterally for active disease in both ears, and is carefully titrated to a point of symptom control, but all peripheral vestibular function must not be ablated as this can cause incapacitating oscillopsia and ataxia. For unilateral Ménière's disease, gentamicin can be injected directly into the middle ear, from where it is actively transported across the round window into the labyrinthine fluids. Here, it probably acts on dark cells (thought to be important in the production of endolymph) and has a toxic effect on the vestibular hair cells. Most patients adapt well after unilateral destruction of vestibular function and have no further disabling spells of vertigo.

Recurrent vestibulopathy, also known as vestibular Ménière's disease, presents with similar recurrent vertigo, but with no auditory symptoms. The vertigo is typically more benign than that of Ménière's disease and is usually controlled with similar medication.

Facial nerve palsy

Bell's palsy is acute unilateral facial weakness or paralysis without an identifiable cause, though herpes simplex virus type I has been implicated. Herpes zoster oticus (HZO) is acute facial paralysis with pain and varicelliform lesions, which often involve the conchal bowl, the concave central portion of the external ear. It is probably due to varicella-zoster virus infection of the geniculate ganglion and often there is eighth cranial nerve involvement, producing a profound sensorineural hearing loss and vestibular loss. Edema traps the facial nerve as it passes through the narrow fallopian canal, resulting in ischemia and neural dysfunction.

The use of glucocorticosteroids to treat acute facial paralysis is controversial. They are not indicated for incomplete facial paralysis, as this usually recovers fully without medication. If used for complete facial paralysis in Bell's palsy or HZO, they should be given within the first 10 days at a moderate dose, which is then tapered.

Acyclovir (acycloguanosine), a nucleoside analog that inhibits viral DNA replication (see Chapter 8), reduces functional deficits in immunocompromised patients with HZO but has no proven benefit for Bell's palsy. Ideally, treatment should be started as soon as possible after symptoms develop, up to about 72 hours after onset.

OTOTOXIC DRUGS

Four clinically important classes of drugs cause inner ear toxicity (Fig. 25.10). Both hearing and balance usually are affected. Tinnitus is an additional feature that often accompanies drug-induced ototoxicity.

Analgesics and antipyretics

The tinnitus characteristic of salicylate-induced ototoxicity often is accompanied by hearing loss. The mechanism of salicylate ototoxicity is not fully understood. However, salicylates accumulate within extracellular fluid compartments and reduce prostaglandin synthesis within the stria vascularis by inhibiting cyclooxygenase, which catalyzes the first step in prostaglandin synthesis from arachidonic acid. This causes vasoconstriction within the stria vascularis, ischemia, and

Classification of ototoxic medications

Class	Examples
Analgesics and antipyretics	Salicylates, quinine
Antimicrobials	
Aminoglycoside antibiotics	Gentamicin, neomycin
Glycopeptide antibiotics	Vancomycin
Macrolide antibiotics	Erythromycin
Antineoplastics	Cisplatin
Loop diuretics	Furosemide, ethacrynic acid

Fig. 25.10 Classification of ototoxic medications.

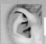

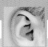

inhibition of the cochlear nerve action potential. Salicylate ototoxicity occurs at serum concentrations over 0.35 mg/ml and is reversible within 48–72 hours of salicylate withdrawal.

Antimicrobials

Aminoglycoside antibiotics have adverse effects on the kidney and inner ear: streptomycin and gentamicin are more vestibulotoxic; kanamycin, tobramycin, and amikacin have more effect on cochlear hair cells. Gentamicin-induced ototoxicity can be demonstrated in approximately 5% of patients treated with this drug. Netilmicin has a reported prevalence of hearing loss in 1 per 250 patients and vestibular toxicity in 1 per 150 patients. Aminoglycosides first bind to the outer surface of the hair cell membrane and disturb Ca^{2+} membrane channels. They then bind to phosphatidylinositol bisphosphate on the inner surface of the cell membrane. Interference with intracellular Ca^{2+} and polyamine-regulated processes causes additional membrane damage, which eventually leads to cell death by apoptosis. Reversible ototoxicity can occur; however, severe, irreversible and untreatable hearing deficits are common. As patients requiring aminoglycosides often have debilitating medical conditions, early complaints of 'dizziness' and tinnitus may be overlooked, especially in a bed-bound patient. Permanent disabling vestibulotoxicity often is only recognized when the mobile patient complains of:

- Movement intolerance.
- Oscillopsia (difficulty in stabilizing gaze during head movement).
- Ataxia.

The best management is to identify patients with an increased risk (Fig. 25.11) and to minimize their exposure by monitoring serum drug concentrations (see Chapters 4 and 9) and switching to non-ototoxic antibacterials as soon as possible. Measurement of auditory function, such as by sequential audiometry, is a good way to detect ototoxicity of any drug. Hearing can be reduced even with blood concentrations that are within the range usually considered normal. The concentration of an aminoglycoside in the cochlear perilymph is both time- and plasma concentration-dependent. Therefore use of these antibiotics should be at the lowest effective dose for the briefest possible time.

Glycopeptide antibiotics such as vancomycin are increasingly used clinically on account of increasing incidence of resistance of certain bacteria. Their mechanism of ototoxicity is not clear, but the pattern with outer hair cell loss preceding inner hair cell loss is similar to that seen with aminoglycosides, likely due to apoptosis.

High-frequency sensorineural hearing loss, 'blowing' tinnitus, and vertigo can follow large intravenous doses of erythromycin, a macrolide antibiotic which inhibits bacterial protein synthesis by binding to the 50S ribosomal subunit. Patients with an increased risk include those with hepatic or renal failure or legionnaires' disease, and the elderly. The mechanism of this ototoxicity is unknown, but it is reversible on drug withdrawal.

Antineoplastics

Cisplatin's ototoxic effect is probably due to local production of oxidants such as NO and induction of apoptosis with resulting labyrinthine hair cell degeneration. Cisplatin is primarily cochleotoxic, causing degeneration of the outer hair cells, spiral ganglion cells, and cochlear neurons, with relative sparing of the vestibular system. The morphologic changes within the inner ear are similar to those of aminoglycoside ototoxicity. The outer hair cells of the basal turn of the cochlea are the most susceptible. Carboplatin also produces dose-dependent hearing loss, thought to result from generation of oxidative free radicals and subsequent apoptosis of cochlear cells.

Diuretics

Loop diuretics (furosemide and ethacrynic acid) inhibit Cl^- reabsorption at the distal loop of Henle and promote extracellular fluid excretion. Within the inner ear they inhibit cell membrane K^+ transport within the stria vascularis and are principally cochleotoxic. Like aminoglycosides, loop diuretics have adverse effects on both the kidney and inner ear, and the toxic effects of these two medications can be synergistic. There is an increased risk of toxicity if the drug is given too rapidly by bolus injection, or if the patient is elderly or has renal failure. Tinnitus, hearing loss, and vertigo may occur within minutes and can be reversible if the medication is withdrawn immediately.

Factors that increase risk of aminoglycoside ototoxicity
Impaired renal function
Prolonged course of treatment (over 10 days)
Concomitant use of other nephrotoxic or ototoxic drugs (loop diuretics, high-dose erythromycin, vancomycin)
Advanced age
Previous aminoglycoside therapy
Pre-existing sensorineural hearing loss

Fig. 25.11 Factors that increase risk of aminoglycoside ototoxicity.

FURTHER READING

Alberti P, Ruben R (eds) *Otologic Medicine and Surgery*. New York: Churchill Livingstone; 1988. [A comprehensive text with thoughtful reviews of many otologic topics.]

Fairbanks D. *Pocket Guide to Antimicrobial Therapy in Otolaryngology—Head and Neck Surgery*, 7th edn. Alexandria, VA: The Americal Academy of Otolaryngology—Head and Neck Surgery Foundation, Inc.; 1993. [A handy quick reference.]

Jackler R, Brackman D (eds) *Neurotology*. St. Louis: Mosby; 1994. [A recent text with excellent basic science and thorough clinical reviews.]

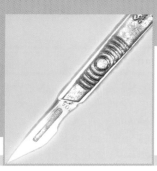

Chapter 26

Drug Use in Anesthesia and Critical Care

PATHOPHYSIOLOGY OF SURGICAL INJURY AND CRITICAL ILLNESS

General and local anesthesia make surgery possible. The purpose of surgery is:
- To repair, remove or replace damaged or diseased tissues.
- To remove healthy tissue, as in organ donation for transplantation, or deliver babies as in obstetrics.

To perform modern surgery requires anesthesia (general or local).

▨ The history of anesthesia contains many lessons

Prior to the discovery and introduction of drugs that produced the state now known as anesthesia, there was little that could be done to alleviate the pain and fear of surgery. Surgery has been practiced for millennia, but all that could be done to reduce the pain and fear was to dose the patient with ethanol and/or opium. While these two drugs reduce pain and consciousness they do not produce anesthesia, a word coined by Oliver Wendell Holmes in 1847 to describe the ability of ether and nitrous oxide to produce unconsciousness, and allow surgery to be performed without the reactions associated with pain and awareness (general anesthesia). Only 40 years later, with the introduction of local anesthetic drugs, was it realized that surgery could also be performed without pain if the surgical area was anesthetized with an appropriate local anesthetic.

Some actions of one of the first anesthetic drugs, nitrous oxide (synthesized by Priestly in 1776), were described by Davy who in the 1790s, with others, recognized that nitrous oxide, and later ether, altered consciousness, and suggested that they could be used to produce unconsciousness as an aid in surgery. Unfortunately such prescience was not acted upon ('an idea before its time'). The use of either of the two chemicals to induce anesthesia did not occur until 1845 despite the fact that both were regularly used at parties, 'ether frolics,' to produce states of intoxication.

In the mid-1800s, as the intellectual climate in medicine began to change, a desire to make surgery painless developed. Thus began a systematic effort to introduce nitrous oxide and ether into medicine as general anesthetics. Major steps forward were made in the USA in 1845/6 by Wells and Morton. Wells introduced nitrous oxide into dentistry while Morton introduced ether into surgery. The story of how these two innovators introduced anesthetics into the clinic is a lesson in the trials and tribulations of medical innovators. In the UK Simpson

(1847), heartened by such studies, began a systematic search for new anesthetics. This search involved sniffing organic solvent vapors to test their effects on himself and his colleagues. Within a short period this search led to chloroform which became the anesthetic of choice in the UK for almost the next 100 years.

Well into the middle of the next century ether, nitrous oxide (available in steel cylinders in 1868) and chloroform were the mainstay of general anesthesia around the world. With their use a great deal of knowledge about anesthetics and the 'stages' of anesthesia was accumulated, and theories of anesthesia promulgated. However, newer and better agents were only slowly discovered. Each of the above drugs is far from ideal as a general anesthetic. Nitrous oxide lacks potency and can never be given at a concentration that produces anesthesia; ether has a slow onset of action and is irritating to the respiratory system as well as being potentially explosive; chloroform is more potent, and is not flammable, but can cause fatal cardiac arrhythmias and liver toxicity. The gas cyclopropane was discovered to be an anesthetic in 1929, but despite being explosive, was used for many years.

A number of events and discoveries changed the above situation. The discovery of the hypnotic effects of barbiturates led to thiopental, a barbiturate that rapidly produces a brief anesthesia when injected intravenously, a way of rapidly inducing general anesthesia. A revolution occurred with the introduction, by Raventos, of halothane, the first of the new halogenated hydrocarbon anesthetics, easy and safe to use by inhalation and not explosive. Such was the value of halothane that many of the newer drugs (see later) have been modeled upon it. Another significant step in anesthesia was the introduction of curare as a neuromuscular blocking drug. This allowed anesthesiologists to provide adequate muscle relaxation, reducing the need for high concentrations of general anesthetics.

> ### ABC approach for the unconscious patient
>
> - **Airway:** maintain patency
> - **Breathing:** ventilate and oxygenate
> - **Circulation:** compress chest to provide a pulse if not present, obtain intravenous access, administer fluids and drugs as required
> - **Defibrillate heart:** if necessary; diagnose and treat reversible causes

> ### Postoperative complications of surgery
>
> - **Circulation:** *bleeding, fluid loss, electrolyte imbalance, deep vein thrombosis, pulmonary embolism, pressure sores*
> - **Surgical wound:** *infection, separation*
> - **Gut:** *paralytic ileus, gastric ulceration, nutritional deficiency*
> - **Major organ failures:** *brain, lungs, heart, kidneys, liver*

The ability to control anesthesia had been helped by recognizing that patients inhaling ether progressed through four stages of anesthesia. The first stage was analgesia; the second, excitement, with loss of consciousness but heightened reflexes; the third, surgical anesthesia, in which reflexes disappear as the stage deepens. The final stage, medullary paralysis, was failure of respiration and vasomotor control, and death. Other anesthetics do not show exactly the same stages, but the stages give an idea of how anesthesia progressively acts on the CNS. Newer drugs are designed to pass rapidly through the early stages, especially stage two. Nowadays general anesthesia is used to produce loss of consciousness, analgesia, neuromuscular blockade and a degree of amnesia. These requirements generally require a mixture of drugs, rather than a single anesthetic.

Regional (local) anesthetics have a different history. Koller early in the last century recognized that cocaine blocked the sensation of touch in the eye and introduced its use in ocular surgery. Cocaine blocks sodium channels in nerves and thereby blocks the flow of both sensory and motor information through the nerves. With the synthesis of other local anesthetics (such as lidocaine in 1943) it became apparent that local anesthetics could be useful for certain types of surgery. A local area (e.g. skin) can be anesthetized if the local anesthetic is infiltrated into the area. Greater areas can be deprived of feeling if a major nerve is blocked, and even larger areas if a local anesthetic is placed in or near the spinal cord. The use of local versus general anesthesia varies from country to country.

Paradoxically, surgeons achieve healing by first inflicting injury. Of course surgery is different from accidental trauma, because the nature and extent of injury are carefully controlled and the body's responses are partially attenuated by anesthesia, i.e. the unconsciousness of general anesthesia is accompanied by a depression of the respiratory and cardiovascular responses to surgery. However, excessive pharmacologic depression of these responses can in turn lead to injury of critical organs, especially in patients with limited respiratory and cardiovascular reserves. As a result, cardiorespiratory monitoring and treatment strategies during anesthesia parallel the 'ABC' approach used to resuscitate critically ill patients in the intensive care unit.

The injury response to surgery

The suppression by anesthetics of the physiologic responses to surgery is probably beneficial, during the perioperative period.

The responses to tissue injury involve local changes and stimulation of the neurologic pathways with respiratory, cardiovascular, endocrine, metabolic and inflammatory components which have evolved to increase the chance of survival following life-threatening injury. For example (see Fig. 26.1):

- Local tissue factors lead to vasospasm and coagulation and so reduce bleeding.
- Increases in sympathetic activity compensate for reductions in the circulating blood volume.

However, the accelerated clotting cascade results in a systemic hyper-coagulating state whereas a large increase in catecholamine activity produces tachycardia and hypertension and an increased risk of angina, myocardial infarction and congestive heart failure. Anesthesia and postoperative acute pain control decreases the stress response and in turn reduces the cardiovascular risks in predisposed patients.

Other than bleeding, surgical injury is associated with significant fluid shifts when the abdomen is opened. Evaporative losses occur from the large serosal surface area of the intestines and fluid accumulation develops in the intestinal interstitial compartment as the so-called 'third space loss.' These fluid losses must be replaced perioperatively with crystalloid (salts in water) to avoid hypovolemia and hemodynamic instability. In the initial days following surgery, however, third space losses will shift back, expand the vascular compartment and predispose patients with heart disease to angina and heart failure. The neurologic response to surgery is proportional to the magnitude of nociceptive stimuli and tissue injury. For example, the response to intra-abdominal surgery is greater than the response to surgery of the extremities. Similarly, greater concentrations of anesthetics are required to suppress larger nociceptive stimuli.

Anesthetics and other perioperative drugs are therefore used to suppress pain, anxiety and awareness, to maintain oxygenation, hemodynamic stability and fluid balance, and to prevent sepsis. Anesthesia is an insensitivity to pain that involves suppression of either:

- Central neural processing (general anesthesia).
- The afferent sensory reflex (regional anesthesia).

PREMEDICATION PRIOR TO ANESTHESIA

Drugs are given before anesthesia for the following reasons: sedation, analgesia, antisialog effect (before 'awake' intubation with a fiberoptic bronchoscope), 'gastric prophylaxis' and

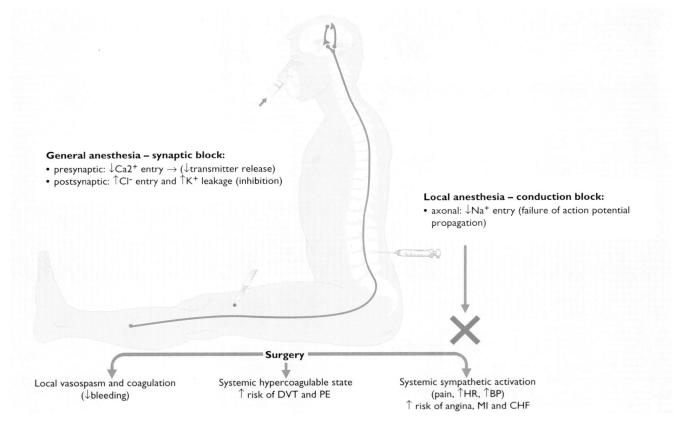

General anesthesia – synaptic block:
- presynaptic: ↓Ca2+ entry → (↓transmitter release)
- postsynaptic: ↑Cl⁻ entry and ↑K⁺ leakage (inhibition)

Local anesthesia – conduction block:
- axonal: ↓Na⁺ entry (failure of action potential propagation)

Surgery

Local vasospasm and coagulation (↓bleeding)

Systemic hypercoagulable state ↑ risk of DVT and PE

Systemic sympathetic activation (pain, ↑HR, ↑BP) ↑ risk of angina, MI and CHF

Fig. 26.1 Anesthetic suppression of the physiologic response to surgery.

coexisting disease treatment (Fig. 26.2). Prophylactic antibiotics, to prevent either wound infection or bacterial endocarditis, and prophylactic anticoagulation, to prevent deep vein thrombosis, may be ordered preoperatively by the surgeon. However, prophylactic anticoagulation should be postponed if epidural or spinal anesthesia is planned by the anesthesiologist because of the risk of epidural hematoma and spinal cord compression.

Premedication and airway techniques to prevent pulmonary aspiration

Anesthetics can induce regurgitation and vomiting with the risk of aspiration since the normal protective airway reflexes are obtunded. Recent food consumption therefore places patients at risk of pulmonary aspiration and death during anesthesia. Although the risk of pulmonary aspiration is reduced in elective surgery by preoperative fasting, postponing emergency surgery will not guarantee an empty stomach while pain and opioids reduce gastric motility.

To guard against this antacids are given to neutralize acid, histamine H_2 receptor antagonists and proton pump inhibitors to reduce acid production, while drugs which increase upper gastrointestinal tract motility aid physiologic emptying of the stomach. These drugs have been given before anesthesia to fasting patients with a history of gastroesophageal reflux but such premedication has limited success and is therefore not routinely used.

The best prevention of pulmonary aspiration during emerg-

ency surgery, other than using regional (local) anesthesia, involves one of the following two airway techniques: tracheal intubation with sedation and local anesthesia (awake intubation); or intubation as soon as intravenous anesthesia is sufficient and neuromuscular paralysis is induced (the rapid anesthesia–intubation sequence). The patient is still at risk for pulmonary aspiration when the gag reflex is obtunded, i.e. in the period between drug administration and successful intubation, and immediately after extubation, during recovery from anesthesia. Intubation in the conscious patient is not feasible in uncooperative patients, whereas rapid anesthesia–intubation can be a cardiovascular risk in the elderly and the critically ill.

Premedication to treat coexisting cardiorespiratory and endocrine disease

Chronic obstructive pulmonary disease and limited respiratory reserve predispose a patient to postoperative atelectasis, pneumonia, hypoxemia and ventilatory failure, especially after upper abdominal and thoracic surgery. Reversal of bronchospasm, treatment of chronic bacterial infection with bronchodilators, antibiotics and physiotherapy should be used for several days preoperatively if elective surgery is possible.

General anesthetics are myocardial depressants while epidural and spinal anesthesia cause vasodilation as a result of blockade of sympathetic nerves. Heart failure and hypovolemia must therefore be treated preoperatively to avoid the hypotensive effects of anesthesia. Similarly, angina, hypertension and arrhythmias should be pharmacologically controlled, and chronic medications, with the possible exception of diuretics, should be continued. Diuretic or adrenocorticosteroid-induced potassium depletion should be corrected over several days to minimize the perioperative risk of arrhythmias (see Fig. 26.3).

Drugs to be stopped, continued, or started preoperatively

	Drugs	Perioperative aims
STOP	Oral hypoglycemics	Avoid hypoglycemia and cerebral damage
	Monoamine oxidase inhibitors (MAOIs)	Avoid hypertensive crisis and hyperpyrexia
	Warfarin (e.g. for atrial fibrillation or prosthetic valve, convert to heparin and discontinue shortly before surgery)	Avoid excessive bleeding intraoperatively (with minimal increase in risk of cerebral embolism and stroke)
	Diuretics	Avoid hypovolemia and hypokalemia
CONTINUE	Opioids	Avoid preoperative pain
	Anticonvulsants	Avoid seizure
	Bronchodilators	Avoid bronchoconstriction
	Antihypertensives and cardiac drugs with exception of diuretics	Avoid hypertension, angina, congestive heart failure, arrhythmia
	Adrenocorticosteroids (increase dose)	Avoid adrenal insufficiency
	Insulin (decrease dose)	Avoid ketoacidosis
START	Histamine H_1 and H_2 receptor antagonists	Allergy prophylaxis in atopic patients
	Benzodiazepines	Provide anxiolysis and anterograde amnesia in frightened patients
	Bronchodilators (inhaled)	Avoid bronchoconstriction in stable asthmatics
	Anticholinergics	Avoid bradycardia in young children (cardiac output depends on the heart rate)
	Adrenocorticosteroids (increase dose)	Avoid adrenal insufficiency if drug history positive in past year
	Antacids, histamine H_1 receptor antagonists, gastric motility agents	Increase gastric pH and decrease gastric residual volume
	Antiemetics	Reduce risk of nausea and vomiting
	Heparin	Prevent deep vein thrombosis and pulmonary embolism
	Antibiotics	Prevent wound infection and subacute bacterial endocarditis

Fig. 26.2 **Drugs to be stopped, continued, or started preoperatively.**

Anesthetic interactions with pre-existing drug therapy

Body location	Drug	Anesthetic interaction
Brain	Acute alcohol intoxication	Potentiates general anesthetics
	Chronic alcohol abuse	Increases general anesthetic requirements
	Clonidine	Potentiates general anesthetics (but continue preoperatively to avoid intraoperative 'rebound' hypertension because of its short half-life)
Lung	Smoking	Pulmonary injury decreases oxygen transfer and carbon monoxide decreases blood oxygen capacity
	Past use of bleomycin	High F_iO_2 can precipitate adult respiratory distress syndrome
Circulation	Diuretics	Hypovolemia increases risk of hypotension and acute hypokalemia increases risk of arrhythmias during general anesthesia
	β Adrenoceptor agonists, bronchodilators	Potentiate arrhythmias from volatile inhaled anesthetics
	β Adrenoceptor antagonists	Potentiate myocardial depression from general anesthetics
	Ca^{2+} antagonists	Potentiate myocardial depression from general anesthetics
	Monoamine oxidase inhibitors (MAOIs)	Sympathetic stimulants or meperidine may precipitate hypertension and hyperpyrexia
	Past use of doxorubicin	Cardiomyopathy increases risk of heart failure from anesthesia
Neuromuscular junction	Aminoglycosides	Potentiate nondepolarizing neuromuscular blockers

Fig. 26.3 **Anesthetic interactions with pre-existing therapy.**

Fasting diabetic patients have a decreased need for oral hypoglycemic drugs and insulin. To avoid the possibility of excessively low blood glucose concentrations, oral diabetic drugs should be withheld on the morning of surgery and sometimes, depending upon the drug's duration of action, stopped 1 to 2 days preoperatively (e.g. chlorpropamide). Insulin-dependent diabetics require intravenous infusion of glucose and a reduction in their usual dose of insulin before surgery. If insulin is not provided, free fatty acids are mobilized from adipose tissues and metabolized to ketones by the insulin-deficient liver, resulting in life-threatening ketoacidosis. Adrenal insufficiency can occur at the time of surgical stress in patients who are taking adrenocorticoids. Parenteral replacement therapy should therefore be started on the morning of surgery and tapered as the postoperative stress resolves. Figure 26.2 gives examples of the drugs that should be stopped, continued, or started preoperatively.

GENERAL ANESTHETICS

General anesthetic drugs are classified on the basis of their route of administration (i.e. inhaled or intravenous). Inhaled general anesthetics include the inorganic gas nitrous oxide and several halogenated hydrocarbons that are volatile liquids at room temperature, such as ether, chloroform, halothane, methoxyflurane, enflurane, isoflurane, sevoflurane and desflurane. Intravenous anesthetics include thiopental and methohexital (barbiturates), propofol (phenolic compound), etomidate (carboxylated imidazole) and ketamine (phency-clidine derivative).

Molecular mechanism of action of general anesthesia

Many of the molecular actions of the intravenous anesthetics are mediated through interactions with specific receptors, whereas inhaled/gaseous anesthetics have nonspecific and indirect actions on ion channels. For example, the actions of the intravenous agents involve increased GABAergic inhibition (thiopental, propofol and etomidate) and/or decreased glutamatergic excitation (ketamine), whereas the actions of the inhaled agents include increased inhibition via K$^+$ channel leakage. At a cellular level, these ionic actions lead to depression of synaptic transmission, especially in the thalamus and cerebral cortex. It is important to note that all sensory stimuli, with the exception of olfaction, pass through the thalamus, and oscillating activity in thalamocortical neurons determines sleep and wakefulness.

The regional mechanisms by which general anesthetics induce unconsciousness and suppression of the motor and autonomic reflex responses to surgical stimuli, however, remain uncertain. There are at least two reasons for this uncertainty. The underlying basis of consciousness is not understood, and anesthesia consists of additional consequences that are difficult to quantify: analgesia, hypnosis and amnesia. In fact, the co-administration of two or more intravenous agents (including benzodiazepines and opioids) along with an inhaled anesthetic

provides the best hemodynamic control for major surgery. All of these various consequences are therefore referred to as components of 'balanced' anesthesia.

Clinical induction and maintenance of general anesthesia

■ *General anesthesia typically involves intravenous induction and inhalation maintenance, with or without opioids and neuromuscular blockers*

Changing a patient's consciousness from an alert to an anesthetized state involves a transition phase, induction (see Fig. 26.4). During induction airway, respiratory and circulatory reflexes are progressively depressed in a dose-related manner by anesthetics. Respiratory effects include a decreased ventilatory response to hypercarbia, and especially to hypoxemia. Circulatory effects involve depression of myocardial contractility, vascular smooth muscle tone and the autonomic nervous system. The ventilatory and cardiovascular depressive effects of anesthetics, however, are offset by the nociceptive stimulation of surgery.

There is no clinically useful monitor for grades of anesthesia. As a result cardiorespiratory stability is used to infer an absence of consciousness. Safe induction then requires careful airway and ventilatory control with frequent monitoring of pulse oximetry, capnometry and vital signs. Hemodynamic depression is managed firstly by ensuring adequate oxygenation and ventilation, and secondly, by treating unrecognized hypovolemia, cardiac ischemia or excess anesthetic. The use of slow induction (using either an intravenous infusion or a volatile inhaled anesthetic) instead of fast induction (using an intravenous bolus) does not necessarily improve safety. For example, neuro-excitation with vomiting, laryngospasm, cough and apnea can occur during slow transition between wakefulness and anesthesia. Although intravenous induction is preferred by adults, inhalation inductions are still used in children where access to a vein is restricted as a result of poor patient cooperation.

■ *Airway methods determine anesthetic selection which in turn affects airway and ventilatory control*

Manual methods for maintaining a patent airway produce painful stimuli and reflex muscle activity, which must be suppressed to reduce patient injury. When comparing the intensity of stimulation produced by airway manipulation, an oropharyngeal and a laryngeal mask produce the least, whereas an endotracheal tube produces the most stimulation. As a result, higher doses of intravenous anesthetics and opioids are used during an induction involving tracheal intubation. In addition, tracheal intubation generally requires the use of neuromuscular blockers (NMBs; see below) as summarized in Fig. 26.5.

■ *During the period when the patient is emerging from anesthesia (emergence), neither intravenous nor inhaled anesthetics provide residual analgesia*

Opioids (e.g., morphine, meperidine, fentanyl, alfentanil, sufentanil, remifentanil) are administered perioperatively in part to permit transition from anesthesia to a pain-free, but

551

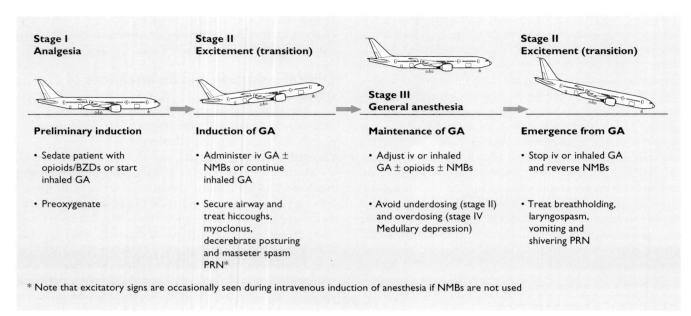

Fig. 26.4 Stages of anesthesia.

Airway and breathing decisions in general anesthesia		
Question	**Alternatives**	**Rationale**
Airway method?	**Face mask or laryngeal mask**	Less invasive but less reliable, short-duration procedure not requiring intubation
	Tracheal intubation	Requires neuromuscular blocker (NMB) and may cause trauma Maintains secure airway (e.g. head and neck surgery, surgery in the prone position) Protects lungs from aspiration (e.g. bleeding airway, recently ingested food or swallowed blood, hiatus hernia, bowel obstruction) Facilitates mechanical ventilation (e.g. anesthetic-, NMB- or opioid-induced respiratory failure)
Breathing method?	**Spontaneous**	Less invasive since inspiratory pressures are negative (positive in mechanical ventilation), but breathing may be inefficient. For short-duration procedure
	Mechanical	Treats respiratory failure and decreases oxygen consumption

Fig. 26.5 Airway and breathing decisions in general anesthesia.

awake, state. An additional benefit of opioid administration during anesthesia is a decreased need for intravenous and inhaled anesthetics and therefore less circulatory depression. Emergence can be complicated by excessive opioid administration, however, as opioids produce a dose-related respiratory depression (see Acute Pain Management).

Inhaled anesthetics
Recent history

Following the original discoveries discussed previously, and the introduction of halothane, the major advances have been the introduction of newer halogenated hydrocarbon vapor anesthetics. Enflurane and isoflurane were released in the 1970s and 1980s respectively. Further chemical refinements led to the release in the 1990s of two fluorinated hydrocarbon anesthetics, sevoflurane and desflurane. These newer inhaled anesthetics are associated with significantly faster induction and emergence times as well as lower risks of liver toxicity.

Pharmacokinetics and pharmacodynamics

How do inhaled anesthetics differ pharmacologically from intravenous anesthetics when viewed from their unique lung route for administration and elimination? Pharmacokinetically, inhaled agents do not need to be metabolized before being eliminated by the lung and are therefore preferred for maintaining anesthesia. Loss of drug via expired air allows for a rapid decrease in the quantity of anesthetic in the brain and the heart and reversal of the anesthetic effects.

Pharmacodynamically, inhaled anesthetics are administered at a specific gas or vapor concentration, rather than as a dose, since inspiration and expiration are inextricably linked. Because the partial pressure of an inhaled anesthetic in the lung and the brain are equal when a steady-state is reached, the gas concentration in the lung correlates with the brain concentration. By monitoring end-expiratory gas concentrations, plus hemodynamic responses, an anesthesiologist can assess graded 'dose'–response relationships during the fluctuating intensity of surgery. In contrast, brain concentrations of intravenous anesthetics cannot be estimated in this way in humans.

The end-expiratory anesthetic concentration (Minimum Alveolar Concentration or 'MAC' value) is used to predict anesthetic potency between different inhaled anesthetics and different patients. Analogous to the ED_{50} for a quantal 'dose'–response curve, MAC is the end-expiratory gas concentration that prevents movement in response to a surgical skin incision in 50% of subjects. MAC allows an assessment for different agents of relative potency in the brain and cardiovascular systems (see Fig. 26.6). For example, all inhaled anesthetics when given at 1.3 MAC prevent movement in 95% of patients, but their hemodynamic actions vary markedly. In addition, factors individual to different patients can increase or decrease MAC.

Nitrous oxide is typically administered in combination with a volatile anesthetic because of its low potency (MAC 105%) and poor blood solubility. This low potency limits the amount of N_2O that can be administered but the low blood solubility means that minimal amounts of nitrous oxide must be dissolved in the blood before equilibration occurs between the alveolar and arterial partial pressures. This translates into a faster induction and emergence.

Clinical use and toxicity

Following their introduction in the 1990s, sevoflurane and desflurane have replaced the use of halothane in children and isoflurane in adults, respectively. This probably occurred in part because of an increased need for reduced case turnover times. The newer drugs, sevoflurane and desflurane, have marginally reduced emergence times compared with halothane and isoflurane. Typically, halogenated hydrocarbon vapor anesthetics are administered in combination with nitrous oxide unless the patient has a pneumothorax, bowel obstruction or air embolism. With the administration of up to 70% inspired nitrous oxide, closed airspaces rapidly expand.

 The potency measure for inhaled anesthetics is MAC

- Minimum Alveolar Concentration (MAC) is the end-expiratory anesthetic concentration which abolishes response to a skin incision in 50% of patients
- 1.3 times MAC will prevent response in 95% of patients because of the very steep dose–response curve

---

 Inhalation anesthetic toxicities

- *Volatile induced hepatoxicity ('halothane hepatitis')*
- *Enflurane and sevoflurane nephrotoxicity due to fluoride as a metabolic product*
- *Nitrous oxide transient bone marrow depression, peripheral neuropathy (due to decreased B_{12} availability), abortions in operating room staff*

As a result, scavenging systems are used in the operating room

---

Comparative pharmacology of inhaled vapor anesthetics

	Halothane	Isoflurane	Sevoflurane	Desflurane
MAC	105%	1.2%	2%	6%
Respiratory irritation during inhaled induction	–	+	–	++
Heart rate	↓	↑↑	↑	↑↑
Blood pressure	↓	↓	↓	↓
Systemic vascular resistance	–	↓	↓	↓
Myocardial contractility	↓	–	–	–
Cardiac output	↓	–	–	–
Blood:gas partition coefficient*	2.5	1.5	0.69	0.42
Speed of onset (and recovery)	Slow	Medium	Rapid	Rapid
Metabolism	20%	0.2%	>2% (to fluoride)	<0.02%
Risk of 'hepatitis'	1:10,000?	Rare	Rare	Rare

*Blood:gas partition coefficient reflects solubility; higher numbers indicate higher solubility in blood relative to gas.

Fig. 26.6 Comparative pharmacology of inhaled vapor anesthetics.

In contrast to sevoflurane, desflurane is ill-suited for inhalation inductions since it causes coughing and breath-holding if administered too rapidly. Yet all vapor anesthetics produce dose-dependent decreases in airway resistance in animal models of bronchoconstriction. Sevoflurane is metabolized to fluoride and 'compound A' with a potential for renal toxicity whereas desflurane is essentially inert. All volatile inhaled anesthetics are contraindicated in patients genetically susceptible to malignant hyperthermia.

Intravenous anesthetics
History
After 50 years as the induction agent of choice, thiopental moved to second place in the 1990s as propofol was introduced. Large doses of fentanyl and sufentanil, alone, have been used for the past 25 years to induce and maintain anesthesia for cardiac surgery or for surgical patients with low cardiac output. However, postoperative ventilation is generally required. Ketamine's sympathetic stimulation is still desirable when inducing anesthesia in patients with circulatory shock, or acute bronchospasm, but hallucinations may occur during recovery.

Pharmacokinetics and pharmacodynamics of two anesthetics used routinely—thiopental and propofol
Due to high lipid solubility, thiopental is combined with sodium carbonate to make it water soluble, whereas propofol is formulated as an emulsion with Intralipid (a parenteral nutrition emulsion). However, high lipid solubility results in easy access to the CNS. Following an intravenous injection both drugs are rapidly distributed to the brain and unconsciousness occurs within 30 seconds, the so-called one 'arm to brain' circulation time. After injection, the concentration in the brain decreases as either drug redistributes to other highly perfused tissues with lower lipid content. In fact, redistribution, not metabolism, accounts for an 'ultrashort' duration of action and early awakening within 10 minutes from a single dose of thiopental or propofol.

The hepatic metabolism of thiopental is slow and therefore drug accumulation and slow awakening occurs with repeated administration. In contrast, propofol is rapidly metabolized and can therefore be used as an intravenous agent to both induce and partially maintain anesthesia for surgery. However, the slow metabolism of benzodiazepines and opioids makes their use as sole agents for i.v. anesthesia almost impractical because of greater postoperative drowsiness.

Clinical use and toxicity—thiopental and propofol
In addition to its use in anesthesia, thiopental is used in critical illness to stop seizures and to treat elevations in intracranial pressure. Thiopental is not used for conscious sedation since small doses lower pain thresholds and produce paradoxical excitement. In fact, insertion of a laryngeal mask airway following induction with thiopental requires the use of a neuromuscular blocker (NMB) to facilitate its insertion, and to prevent laryngospasm. With propofol, neuromuscular blockade is not required. Additional advantages with propofol are less postoperative drowsiness, and less nausea and vomiting,

Thiopental versus propofol for induction of anesthesia

- Thiopental is dissolved in bicarbonate solution
- Propofol is suspended in Intralipid
- Both have a very short duration of action
- Thiopental is rapidly redistributed but not rapidly metabolized
- Propofol is rapidly metabolized

making it especially suitable for daycare surgery. However, it costs more.

As is the case with inhaled anesthetics, thiopental and propofol cause some degree of respiratory depression as well as dose-dependent depression of cardiac output and arterial pressure. Intralipid (a parenteral food) is used as a solvent for propofol and this means that its use is contraindicated in those with egg or soya bean allergies. Thiopental is contraindicated in patients genetically susceptible to attacks of porphyria.

Neuromuscular blocking drugs and antagonists
Tracheal intubation generally requires the use of NMBs since laryngeal stimulation is associated with reflex closure of the vocal cords and resulting hypoxemia if intubation is not successful. Intubation secures an airway and facilitates mechanical ventilation (see Fig. 26.5). Neuromuscular blockade is also needed during abdominal or thoracic surgeries to prevent reflex-induced muscle contraction. Alternatively, reflex muscle responses can be suppressed by high concentrations of volatile inhaled anesthetics, but this is accompanied by circulatory depression. If NMBs are used, however, intubation and mechanical ventilation are of course needed.

Classification and history
NMBs block normal synaptic transmission at the neuromuscular junction as a result of actions on the nicotinic cholinergic receptor. Two types of receptor blockade determine the onset time, duration of action and adverse effects of NMBs. The two types of NMBs are known as depolarizing and nondepolarizing NMBs. The onset and duration of action of the latter class is significantly longer, making them more suitable for surgical relaxation than intubation. Although both types of NMBs were first used during general anesthesia in the 1940s (succinylcholine and d-tubocurarine, respectively), only new nondepolarizing NMBs have since been developed. These newer drugs include the aminosteroid compounds: pancuronium, vecuronium, and rocuronium; and the benzylisoquinolinium compounds: atracurium, cisatracurium, mivacurium. Figure 26.7 tabulates the actions and characteristics of the above NMBs.

Curare was a mixture of alkaloids isolated from South American arrow poisons. Claude Bernard, in a series of classic experiments (1856), showed that they blocked neuromuscular

Comparative pharmacology of neuromuscular blockers (NMBs)

	Succinylcholine	Pancuronium	Rocuronium
Class	Depolarizing	Nondepolarizing	Nondepolarizing
Time to intubation (mins)	<1	3–8	1.5
Duration (mins)	5	60–75	30–45
Histamine release	Slight	No effect	No effect
Kidney excretion (%)	0	80	30
Actions on nAChR (ganglion)	Stimulates	No effect	No effect
Actions on mAChR	Stimulates	Limited block	No effect

Fig. 26.7 Comparative pharmacology of NMBs.

transmission at the level of the nerve ending and not at the nerve or muscle. The most important of the curare alkaloids is tubocurarine, a quaternary ammonium compound that does not penetrate the CNS. Interestingly, the neuromuscular blocking properties of succinylcholine were not realized in 1906 in experiments testing its parasympathetic effects, as the test animals had been paralyzed with curare. Succinylcholine was developed specifically about 1950 as an NMB with a different mechanism of action and short duration.

Molecular mechanism of action

Understanding the actions of NMBs requires some understanding of neuromuscular transmission. Acetylcholine (ACh) in the nerve ending of the motor nerve is packed in vesicles (about 10,000 molecules). An action potential invading the end-plate opens N-type calcium channels and the resulting entry of calcium mobilizes the vesicles so as to release their contents into the junctional cleft. Most of these ACh molecules bind with nicotinic acetylcholine receptors (nAChR—an ionotropic receptor) to open the Na/K liquid-gated ion channel on which the nAChRs are located. Once ACh unbinds it is exposed to acetylcholinesterase and broken down. Therefore, most of the released ACh is not able to bind for a second time.

Molecular target for neuromuscular blocking drugs (NMBs) is the nicotinic acetylcholine receptor (nAChR)

- Nondepolarizing NMBs bind to ACh binding sites on nAChR without activating
- Depolarizing NMBs bind to ACh binding sites on nAChR and activate
- ACh competes with nondepolarizing NMBs for ACh binding site
- ACh adds to effects of depolarizing NMBs

The neuromuscular junction has a large safety margin in that end-plate potentials must be significantly reduced with nondepolarizing NMBs before weakness occurs. In clinical anesthesia, the twitch response to four electrical stimuli administered at a rate of two Hz (the so-called 'train of four') is monitored. Nondepolarizing blockade leads to an increasing reduction in the four twitches. In fact, in the presence of effective neuromuscular blockade for intra-abdominal surgery, only the first response can be elicited. This occurs because the train of four elicits a progressive decrease in the amount of ACh released (the number of quantal components) and therefore a progressive decrease in safety margin. Providing that two or more twitches have returned, blocking acetylcholinesterase enables ACh to act repeatedly on receptors to open channels with consequent increase in end-plate amplitude and transmission can be re-established; with excessive NMB, the increase in end-plate potential will be insufficient to re-establish transmission. It is important to note that inhaled vapor anesthetics and many other drugs have a small neuromuscular blocking action that is normally not manifested at clinical doses, but will enhance neuromuscular blockade by nondepolarizing NMBs.

The molecular mechanism of action of nondepolarizing NMBs involves binding to the acetylcholine recognition sites on the nicotinic acetylcholine receptors (nAChR) that have a pentameric structure forming a cluster around a central transmembrane pore. There are two acetylcholine-binding sites on the pentamer. When these are both occupied by acetylcholine the channel opens allowing Na and K to flow down their concentration gradients, resulting in depolarization of the end-plate of the skeletal muscle fiber and activation of voltage-dependent sodium channels to carry the excitation signal throughout the muscle fiber. These actions of ACh are very brief since it is exposed to acetylcholinesterase and broken down to inactive acetate and choline, the latter being recycled into the nerve ending. Tubocurarine blocks neuromuscular transmission by occupying the ACh binding site, without activating the receptor, and thereby denies ACh access.

Succinylcholine, which is chemically two ACh molecules linked through their acetyl groups, activates the nAChR when it binds to the ACh recognition site. In binding to the receptor succinylcholine acts as an ACh analog and thereby produces the same effects as ACh. ACh, which is rapidly broken down by the acetylcholinesterase in the synaptic cleft, has only a very short life in the cleft. On the other hand, succinylcholine is only broken down by the cholinesterase in the plasma and therefore remains at effective concentrations for much longer. As a result of the continued presence of the drug and activation of the nAChR there is maintained depolarization of the end-plate and desensitization of the voltage dependent sodium channel. In addition there is depolarization of the nAChR and hence neuromuscular transmission fails. A very similar neuromuscular block occurs if acetylcholinesterase is blocked and large doses of ACh are given to the end-plate.

The differences in the molecular mechanisms by which nondepolarizing and depolarizing NMBs produce their block is responsible for many of their characteristic actions. One of the major differences between the two is the fact that succinylcholine produces muscle fasciculations when it is given i.v. Fasciculations are unsynchronized contractions of whole motor units. These are associated with myalgia that persists up to days postoperatively. The predominant mechanism responsible for fasciculations is stimulation of the intrafusal muscles of the stretch receptors with consequent *reflex* activity of motor neurons. Interestingly intrafusal muscles are packed with nAChR as are the extraocular muscles of the eye. Contracture of the latter by succinylcholine can exacerbate glaucoma.

The use of succinylcholine is also associated with a rise in the serum potassium. This is normally not important but in those with recent burns, spinal cord injuries or myopathies it is much more marked. This is believed to be a result of denervation in the damaged area and a subsequent spread of receptors which when activated cause net loss of potassium from muscles.

In some people (1 in 2,000) there is a genetic determined lack of the plasma esterases responsible for the breakdown of succinylcholine and in such people neuromuscular block with succinlycholine lasts much longer. Where the level of the plasma esterase is reduced neuromuscular block lasts for up to 2 hours whereas in those with no enzyme paralysis lasts for many hours.

Pharmacokinetics and pharmacodynamics of two NMBs used routinely—succinylcholine and rocuronium

Succinylcholine is metabolized by plasma cholinesterase and therefore succinylcholine has a short plasma half-life of about 5 minutes. The pharmacodynamic half-life is the same as the plasma half-life since the nAChR and the end-plate recover within milliseconds. Thus, succinylcholine is useful when given intravenously for producing a short-lived neuromuscular block, ideal for intubation. However, either large or repeated administrations of succinylcholine will produce a so-called 'phase II' block. Although a phase II block resembles the block produced by nondepolarizing NMBs, the mechanism is unknown.

As a nondepolarizing NMB, rocuronium competes with ACh for postsynaptic nicotinic receptors and so produces paralysis without depolarizing the end-plate, or causing fasciculations or myalgia. After about 30 minutes, partial recovery from block occurs because of hepatic metabolism of rocuronium. Pharmacologic reversal of paralysis is then possible by administering an anticholinesterase (e.g., edrophonium, neostigmine or pyridostigmine) to decrease breakdown of acetylcholine and overcome the competitive block. Because the anticholinesterase also acts to elevate ACh at muscarinic cholinergic receptors (mAChR), a muscarinic receptor antagonist (e.g. atropine or glycopyrrolate) is given to prevent the effects of excessive mAChR stimulation (i.e. cardiac arrest, bronchospasm, excessive GI activity).

Clinical use and toxicity—succinylcholine and rocuronium

Since it has a rapid onset and short duration of action, succinylcholine is used for intubation by anesthesiologists and skilled critical care physicians. Succinylcholine is also used prior to electroconvulsive therapy and for the emergency treatment of post-extubation laryngospasm. The onset time of rocuronium (90 seconds) approaches that of succinylcholine, making this nondepolarizing NMB suitable for a rapid anesthesia–intubation sequence (see Premedication) when succinylcholine is contra-indicated. In contrast to succinylcholine, rocuronium's duration of action is intermediate.

Plasma esterase deficiency is a relative contraindication to the use of succinylcholine, whereas malignant hyperthermia or conditions at risk for a hyperkalemic response (see above) are an absolute contraindication. Comparatively, rocuronium has fewer disadvantages than succinylcholine and even other nondepolarizing NMBs. For example, rocuronium is not associated with decreases in blood pressure due to histamine release (as with the benzylisoquinolinium compounds, especially with d-tubocurarine) or increases in heart rate (as with pancuronium). Patients with myasthenia gravis (an autoimmune disease characterized by antibodies to the nAChR, nicotinic acetylcholine receptor), however, are extremely sensitive to all nondepolarizing NMBs.

REGIONAL ANESTHESIA

Regional anesthesia is an alternative to general anesthesia for major surgery on the extremities or the lower abdomen. The choice between regional and general anesthesia is based on the surgical procedure, the surgeon's skill and anesthetist's experiences, and the patient's medical status and preference. Regional techniques can be combined with general anesthesia to reduce the concentration of general anesthetic used (therefore their undesirable effects) and to improve postoperative analgesia. However, except for some specific surgeries (e.g. Cesarean section, transurethral prostatectomy, hip and knee surgery in the elderly, emergency surgery), regional anesthesia is not necessarily safer than general anesthesia. General anesthesia becomes necessary if regional anesthesia fails.

Local anesthetics
History, mechanisms of action and chemistry

Following the discovery of the topical anesthetic properties of naturally occurring cocaine in the late 19th century, procaine and lidocaine were synthesized in 1905 and 1943 respectively. These and other synthetic local anesthetics have a basic chemical pharmacophore of a lipophilic aromatic ring and a hydrophilic tertiary amine separated by a hydrocarbon chain. The hydrocarbon chain is linked to the lipophilic component by either an amide or an ester bond, thereby providing a chemical basis for local anesthetic classification. This classification is important because esters (e.g. cocaine, procaine, tetracaine, benzocaine) are metabolized by plasma and liver cholinesterase with the formation of a potential allergen, para-aminobenzoic acid (PABA). In contrast, amides (e.g. lidocaine, mepivacaine, bupivacaine, etidocaine, prilocaine and ropivacaine) are more slowly metabolized in the liver and rarely evoke allergic reactions. The main characteristics of the two major drugs are given in Fig. 26.8.

Local anesthetics block axonal conduction by virtue of blocking the neuronal voltage-gated sodium channels whose activation is responsible for action potential transmission along a nerve. Their site of action is believed to be at intracellular parts of the channel. They initially pass in their uncharged form through the nerve membrane but once inside the axon, the charged form binds to the channel to prevent its function. The small size, and lack of myelination, means that smaller nerve fibers, that is, those involved in pain and temperature conduction, are more sensitive to blockade than are the larger fibers responsible for touch or motor control.

The pKa, protein binding, and lipid solubility characteristics of local anesthetics influence their onset time, duration of action, and potency. As weak bases with pKa (8–9) values above physiologic pH (7.4), most local anesthetics are primarily in their charged form in normal tissue. As a result local anesthetics whose pKa is closet to pH 7.4 will have the fastest onset time, because only the uncharged lipid soluble form diffuses through tissues and crosses nerve membranes. Once inside the cell the charged form is thought to be the active form that blocks the channel.

The effect of pKa also explains why local anesthetics are ineffective if injected into an infected tissue, which is at an acidic pH. Local anesthetics with high protein binding attach strongly to the protein component of the nerve membrane lipid bilayer, and thereby have longer durations of action. Finally, lipid solubility influences potency, as well as paralleling protein binding in influencing duration of action.

Pharmacokinetics and pharmacodynamics

In addition to the above chemical influences, the duration of action of local anesthesia can be increased by adding a vasoconstrictor drug, such as epinephrine. However, epinephrine-containing solutions should neither be injected intracutaneously nor into a digit, an ear, the nose or the penis because of the risk of gangrene. In turn, systemic absorption of injected local anesthetic depends on the vascularity of the injection site and the presence of epinephrine, as well as the dose administered and the pharmacologic properties of the drug.

Clinical use and toxicity

To compensate for its lower potency, lidocaine is commercially supplied in higher concentrations than bupivacaine. Compared to bupivacaine, however, lidocaine has a faster onset time and a shorter duration of action. If a differential blockade occurs (i.e. pain transmission is blocked, but touch is preserved), pressure will be sensed during surgery. Unfortunately, an anxious patient will perceive any sensation as a failure of the local anesthetic. Conscious sedation (see below) can therefore facilitate the likelihood of success of regional anesthesia.

General anesthetic and resuscitative drugs, equipment and expertise should be immediately available when regional anesthesia is performed. Systemic toxicity of a local anesthetic

---

Comparative pharmacology of local anesthetics

	Lidocaine	Bupivacaine
Chemical classification	Amide	Amide
pKa	7.9	8.1
Onset	Rapid	Slow
Protein binding (%)	70	95
Duration after infiltration (hours)	1–2	4–8
Lipid solubility	2.9	28
Potency	1	4

Fig. 26.8 Comparative pharmacology of local anesthetics.

Postoperative complications of anesthesia

- **General anesthesia and/or opioids:** CNS (particularly respiratory) depression, nausea and vomiting, aspiration

- **Epidural and spinal anesthesia:** urinary retention, hypotension

- **Spinal anesthesia:** postural headache

- **Position during surgery:** peripheral nerve palsies

- **Succinylcholine:** muscle pain (myalgia) and raised serum potassium

- **Opioids:** cough suppression leading to pneumonia from retained secretions

can cause seizures and cardiovascular instability, whereas a high spinal anesthetic can produce acute respiratory failure and cardiac arrest. Besides accidental intravascular injection, the plasma concentration is determined by the relationship of absorption, redistribution and metabolism.

CONSCIOUS SEDATION

Conscious sedation with intravenous benzodiazepines, and/or propofol with or without opioids, allows many patients to tolerate unpleasant diagnostic and therapeutic procedures by relieving anxiety and pain and increasing the patient's acceptance of the procedure being performed. Ideally, the relief of anxiety and fear reduces the need for analgesics, allowing a sedated patient to cooperate and respond appropriately to oral command. Unfortunately, a patient may suddenly become unconscious owing to excessive intravenous sedation and/or the use of multiple drugs. In this situation, reflex pain withdrawal may be misinterpreted as wakefulness and inappropriately lead to further sedative administration. The unconscious state can be associated with airway obstruction or respiratory depression that must be rapidly managed to avoid hypoxemic brain damage and cardiac arrest. To minimize this risk, the preparation before the procedure involves fasting. Supplemental oxygen should be used routinely with a designated person monitoring a pulse oximeter, blood pressure and the patient's wakefulness using frequent oral commands, both during and following the procedure.

Intravenous benzodiazepines and antagonists

Intravenous benzodiazepines (e.g. diazepam or midazolam) are administered by intermittent bolus injection to provide conscious sedation during regional anesthesia and for critically ill patients in the intensive care unit. Benzodiazepines potentiate the action of the neuroinhibitory transmitter GABA, and these drugs often impair memory formation. Amnesia can be advantageous in the short term, but disadvantageous if persistent for several hours.

Benzodiazepine-induced respiratory or cardiovascular depression is generally minimal unless these drugs are combined with opioids or other CNS depressants. In the elderly, however, doses are reduced. Flumazenil, a competitive $GABA_A$-antagonist, is used to reverse excess sedation due to benzodiazepines. Repeated administration may be required since flumazenil has a shorter half-life than most benzodiazepines.

🔑 **Safety during intravenous sedation and analgesia**

- **Consciousness:** monitored by designated third person
- **Airway:** fasting to avoid aspiration if loss of consciousness occurs
- **Breathing:** supplemental oxygen and pulse oximetry
- **Circulation:** intravenous access for emergency drugs

POSTOPERATIVE PAIN MANAGEMENT

Following major surgery, uncontrolled acute pain has been associated with morbidity and even mortality. For example, hypoxemia and pneumonia can occur following thoracic and abdominal surgery if inadequate pain control restricts deep breathing and effective coughing. In addition, major tissue injury initiates the 'stress-response.' Depending on the magnitude of the tissue injury, and the status of the patient, acute pain management involves one or more of the following drugs and techniques: parenteral, epidural and/or intrathecal opioids; regional analgesia with local anesthetics; nonsteroidal anti-inflammatory drugs. Pain and opioids are discussed in detail in Chapter 14.

The adverse effects of opioids include nausea and vomiting, localized urticaria, pruritus, sedation and respiratory depression. Opioids impair the ventilatory response to carbon dioxide and eliminate the response to hypoxemia. Although the incidence of severe respiratory depression is low, close patient observation is mandatory since this complication can be life-threatening. Airway management equipment, oxygen, naloxone (an opioid antagonist), pulse oximetry and expertise should be available.

Intramuscular versus intravenous opioid administration

In comparison to the intravenous route, intramuscular administration of opioids is associated with a slower onset of action and a larger fluctuation in drug levels. Repeated intramuscular administration every 3 to 4 hours produces an alternating overdose–underdose cycle. The 'peak' phase is of analgesia with a high incidence of opioid adverse effects, while the 'trough' phase is inadequate analgesia (see Fig. 26.9).

When an initial intravenous bolus loading dose followed by continuous intravenous infusion of an opioid is used there

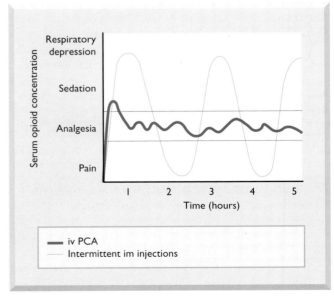

Fig. 26.9 Intramuscular versus intravenous morphine. (Adapted with permission of Dr Pat Sullivan from *Anaesthesia for Medical Students*, Ottawa Civic Hospital, 1999.)

are fewer adverse effects than with intermittent intravenous administration, and variations in plasma level of the opioid are decreased. However, assessment is still required, either to decrease the infusion rate during bed rest and sleep, or to administer 'top-up' injections in the prevention of 'break-through' pain during ambulation and physiotherapy.

Intravenous patient-controlled analgesia

Both patients and staff prefer intravenous patient-controlled analgesia (PCA). With nurse-controlled analgesia, for example, the patient must notify the nurse when pain is present and then wait for the preparation of each injection. PCA offers psychological control to the patient and a reduced workload to the nurse. The PCA device, so as to minimize the risk of an overdose, restricts the amount of opioid that can be self-administered. For example, the PCA machine will deliver a bolus dose on demand, but only if a pre-defined 'lockout' interval has elapsed since the last administration. In addition, a 4-hour dose limit can be programmed.

CRITICAL CARE

Prompt basic and advanced life support is critical to the unconscious patient. An unobstructed airway is of paramount importance since airway obstruction and hypoxemia can lead to brain damage, cardiac arrest or death, while in patients with intracranial space-occupying lesions, hypercarbia can produce cerebral vasodilation, increased intracranial pressure and further cerebral ischemia. Breathing must be maintained to ensure oxygen delivery and carbon dioxide elimination. If the patient remains unconscious, tracheal intubation is required to protect the airway from aspiration of gastric contents.

Patients with multiple traumas, or with critical illness, typically have impaired oxygen delivery (see Fig. 26.10). For example:
- Chest crush injuries or pneumonia cause atelectasis and 'hypoxic hypoxia.'
- Bleeding decreases oxygen-carrying capacity and leads to 'anemic hypoxia.'
- Inadequate blood flow due to circulatory failure produces 'ischemic hypoxia.'

Removal of carbon dioxide can also be impaired, for example, as a result of depressed ventilatory control due to head trauma, or ineffective respiration due to chest trauma. Initial management of critical illness includes routine oxygen therapy and close observation of vital signs.

Oxygen therapy and mechanical ventilation

Simple oxygen devices provide a variable fraction of inspired oxygen (F_iO_2) since oxygen is inspired along with room air.

Supplemental oxygen can be administered via nasal prongs (F_iO_2 0.24 to 0.4 with oxygen flows 1 to 6 liters/min) or vented mask (F_iO_2 0.4 to 0.6 with oxygen flows 5 to 8 liters/min). Since the development of pulse oximetry, air entrainment devices that deliver a restricted F_iO_2 are seldom used for patients with chronic carbon dioxide retention. Oxygen toxicity of the lung (and eye in premature neonates) may follow the use of a

> ### Monitoring for resuscitation and anesthesia
>
> - **CNS:** level of consciousness
> - **Airway and Breathing:** respiratory rate, pulse oximetry, expired capnometry, arterial blood gases
> - **Circulation:** heart rate, blood pressure, EKG, urine output

prolonged and high F_iO_2 (F_iO_2 1.0 for 12 hours for lung; higher sensitivity for eye).

Although the need for mechanical ventilation is often obvious in patients with severe head or chest trauma, a diagnosis of acute and progressive respiratory failure in patients with pre-existing cardiorespiratory disease can be difficult. An increasing respiratory rate and increasing pCO_2 and decreasing pO_2 in arterial blood may allow an early diagnosis before the development of a life-threatening emergency. Intubation and mechanical ventilation are not without risk in critically ill patients, as anesthesia is often needed, with resultant cardiovascular depression and decreased organ perfusion. Although anesthesia, neuromuscular blockade and the appropriate expertise are often required for intubation, opioids and benzodiazepines rather than NMBs are generally sufficient to allow mechanical ventilation following intubation.

Management of hemodynamic instability

Oxygen delivery depends on an intact circulation; therefore, inadequate tissue perfusion must be treated promptly. Acute circulatory failure is due to either (Fig. 26.11):
- Hypovolemia (decreased preload).
- Compromised cardiac function (decreased heart rate, very high heart rate, decreased contractility).

Septic shock resulting from the release of vasoactive substances is associated with hypovolemia because vasodilation and leaking capillaries decrease preload.

Management of hemodynamic instability requires measurement of heart rate, blood pressure and preload. While much hypovolemia is hemorrhagic in origin, nonhemorrhagic hypovolemia and cardiogenic circulatory failure can be a cause or also present. For example, an elderly patient with a bowel obstruction can become hypovolemic as a result of gastrointestinal fluid accumulation and sepsis; associated circulatory failure can then lead to tachycardia and coronary hypoperfusion, which in turn can produce acute heart failure.

Healthy adults can compensate for the rapid loss of up to 15% of their blood volume (i.e. 15% × 70 ml/kg) with an increased cardiac output. However, the necessary sympathetic reflexes can be depressed by anesthesia, resulting in a precipitous fall in blood pressure and tissue perfusion. Thus it is crucial to restore intravascular fluid volume prior to anesthesia. Most preoperative patients will develop signs of inadequate tissue perfusion once 30% of the blood volume has been lost. Clinical markers of progressive organ dysfunction are oliguria, tachycardia, hypotension, dyspnea, metabolic acidosis and mental changes such as agitation.

559

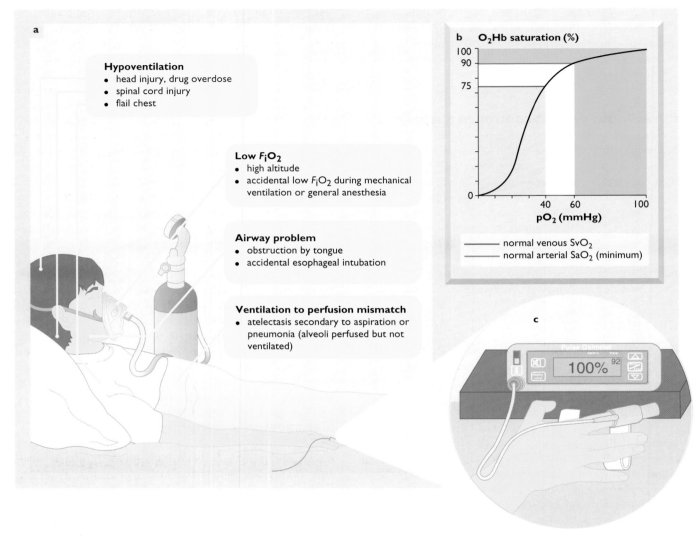

Fig. 26.10 Hypoxemia, oxygen saturation of hemoglobin, and clinical monitoring. (a) Possible causes of hypoxemia. Normal oxygenation requires sufficient inspired oxygen, a patent airway, an intact respiratory center, an innervated and stable chest wall, and ventilated and perfused alveoli. (b) Oxyhemoglobin (O₂Hb) dissociation curve and pulse oximetry. The O₂Hb dissociation curve describes the relation between the saturation of Hb with oxygen. The flat portion at the top of the sigmoid-shaped curve indicates near-maximal oxygen capacity. Saturation of Hb with oxygen is about 90% when pO₂ is 60 mmHg and about 100% when pO₂ is 100 mmHg or greater. (c) Pulse oximetry can provide a noninvasive monitor of oxygen content of arterial blood as well as pulsatile perfusion. However, pulse oximetry does not necessarily indicate circulatory adequacy. (SaO₂, percentage saturation of arterial Hb; pO₂, partial pressure of oxygen; SvO₂, percentage saturation of venous Hb)

Fluid therapy and blood transfusions

The initial treatment of acute circulatory failure is aimed at ensuring adequate intravascular volume. Severe circulatory failure with low brain and heart perfusion pressures requires the temporary use of inotropic drugs and vasopressor drugs at the same time as fluids (see below). Immediate surgical control is the best form of therapy for internal bleeding (e.g. that due to a ruptured ectopic pregnancy or ruptured aortic aneurysm).

CRYSTALLOID THERAPY When hypovolemia is diagnosed, fluid must be administered rapidly.

The solutions initially used should be 'crystalloids' that contain water and electrolytes at an isotonic concentration. Four times the estimated blood loss must be given as crystalloid to maintain an adequate blood volume, since there is a rapid distribution of ions and water from the intravascular compartment to the interstitial fluid compartment (see Fig. 26.12).

COLLOID AND BLOOD THERAPY If a patient with acute circulatory failure due to hypovolemia remains hypotensive, despite the administration of electrolytes, synthetic (e.g. pentastarch) or natural colloids may be required. Colloid solutions are of the same oncotic pressure and provide the same intravascular expansion as whole blood. Ideally, blood products should not be used for simple volume expansion because of the potential immunologic and infectious hazards of transfusions. Plasma and platelets should be used for coagulopathies and red blood cells to maintain arterial oxygen content.

Monitoring fluid replacement

Heart rate, blood pressure and urine output are useful parameters of the hemodynamic efficacy of fluid replacement. Sometimes invasive methods for assessing volume status (e.g.

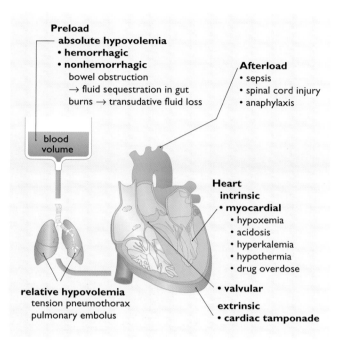

Fig. 26.11 Classification of acute circulatory failure. Clues to the correct diagnosis will be provided by the history, physical examination (CNS and pupil status; breath sounds and tracheal deviation; heart rate and flat or distended neck veins; temperature), pulse oximetry and electrocardiography.

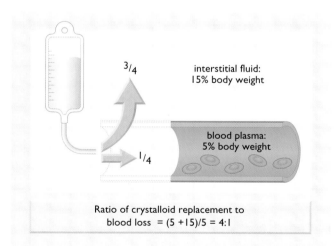

Fig. 26.12 Extracellular fluid compartments, blood loss, and crystalloid replacement. Water and electrolytes are freely diffusible between plasma and interstitial fluid through capillary pores. During bleeding, water and electrolytes are mobilized from the interstitial fluid into the circulation. Similarly, when replacing blood loss with normal saline or lactated Ringer's solution, three-quarters of the infused crystalloid will move from the circulation into the interstitial fluid. Therefore, the required crystalloid resuscitation volume is four times the blood loss.

central venous pressure and pulmonary arterial occluded pressure measurements) and cardiac output measurements are useful. The hemoglobin (Hb) concentration is an unreliable estimate of blood loss until there has been adequate fluid replacement and hemodilution. Once a steady state has been reached, however, a reduction of 10 g/liter Hb is equivalent to one unit of blood lost (500 ml whole blood, 300 ml packed red blood cells) in a 70 kg adult. Since donor blood is separated into individual components, replacement of 50% of the blood volume with crystalloid, non-plasma colloid, and packed red blood cells, can dilute clotting factors and platelets.

Drug therapy in advanced life support

If hypotension or a low urine output persists after adequate volume expansion, drugs are given for the associated medical problems. Such drug treatment may include:

- Vasopressor drugs for inadequate brain and myocardial perfusion pressures.
- Inotropic drugs, with or without afterload reduction for a low cardiac output.
- Antibiotics for sepsis.
- Sodium bicarbonate for acidosis.
- Dopaminergic doses of dopamine when urine output is low despite adequate perfusion pressures.

Once the patient's circulatory status has improved, the underlying cause must be identified and treated without delay. The useful drugs in this area are indicated in Fig. 26.13.

Targets in the treatment of acute circulatory failure	
Target	**Supportive treatment**
Basic life support	Oxygenation, ventilation, chest compressions and defibrillation if cardiac arrest
Preload	
Hypovolemia	Volume infusion with crystalloid and colloid
Low blood oxygen capacity	Packed red blood cells
Coagulopathy	Frozen plasma, platelets
Heart	
Bradycardia	Atropine, transcutaneous pacing, dopamine, epinephrine
Severe tachycardia	Pharmacologic slowing ± pharmacologic or electric cardioversion
Low cardiac output	Inotropes: ephedrine, dopamine, dobutamine
	Afterload reduction: sodium nitroprusside, nitroglycerin
Afterload	
Low brain and heart perfusion pressures	Vasopressors: phenylephrine, dopamine, epinephrine, norepinephrine

Fig. 26.13 Targets in the treatment of acute circulatory failure.

FURTHER READING

Guidelines 2000 for Cardiopulmonary Resuscitation and Emergency Cardiovascular Care: International Consensus on Science. *Circulation* 2000; **102** (8 Suppl). [A multi-authored consensus manual of both cardiac and noncardiac resuscitation.]

Stoelting RK. *Pharmacology and Physiology in Anesthetic Practice*, 3rd edn. Lippincott-Raven; 1999. [A reference textbook of the basic sciences most relevant to anesthesia patient care.]

Sullivan P (ed.) *Anaesthesia for Medical Students*, 2nd edn. Ottawa: DocuLink International; 1999. [A paperback handbook for medical students taking a clinical rotation in anesthesia.]

Chapter 27

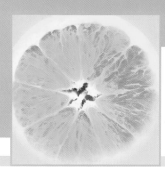

Drug Use in Disorders of Nutrition

Components of nutrition

- Water
- Carbohydrates
- Proteins
- Fats
- Vitamins
- Trace elements
- Indigestible fibers

Essential amino acids

- Histidine
- Isoleucine
- Leucine
- Lysine
- Methionine
- Phenylalanine
- Threonine
- Tryptophan
- Valine

Nutrition is required for growth, maintenance of body weight, support of physiologic functions and as a source of energy. Food provides the following components:

WATER Water should be provided ad libitum, to avoid dehydration. Under normal conditions water is lost from the body by four routes: feces (100 ml), perspiration and exhalation (600–1000 ml), and urine (1000–1500 ml). Losses of water may increase in severe diarrhea (2000–5000 ml) and fever (200 ml/day/1°C increase). The posterior pituitary gland secretes antidiuretic hormone to adjust urine osmolality in order to balance urine output so that total body loss of water essentially equals the intake of water over time.

CARBOHYDRATES Carbohydrates are polyhydroxyaldehydes or ketones or compounds that yield these derivatives on hydrolysis. Carbohydrates are contained in several forms according to their degree of polymerization:
- Monosaccharides, also called simple sugars, consist of a single unit (such as glucose, fructose, or galactose).
- Disaccharides are made of two units joined together (for example sucrose and lactose).
- Oligosaccharides consist of three to nine monosaccharide units.
- Polysaccharides (e.g. starch, cellulose) consist of many monosaccharide units. Polysaccharides are stored as glycogen.

Carbohydrates are important as an energy source and as precursors for the biosynthesis of many cellular components.

PROTEINS The building blocks of proteins are amino acids. The proteins in diet are digested to liberate essential and non-essential amino acids. Essential amino acids, known also as indispensable amino acids, must be provided in food since they cannot be synthesized in sufficient quantities in the body. There are nine essential amino acids: histidine, isoleucine, leucine, lysine, methionine, phenylalanine, threonine, tryptophan, and valine. In addition to these essential amino acids, growing infants require arginine. Amino acids are required for the synthesis of proteins and other molecules (for example peptide hormones and porphyrins), and as energy source. Amino acids can be a source for gluconeogenesis in the liver. Tissue proteins constantly undergo turnover, due to breakdown and resynthesis with various half-lifes. The requirements for nutritional proteins increase in many circumstances, such as during growth, and with burns or trauma.

FATS 98% of the fat supplied by nutrition is in the form of triacylglycerols (triglycerides), and the other 2% consists of phospholipids and cholesterol. Complete hydrolysis of triacylglycerols yields glycerol and free fatty acids. Fatty acids can be divided into two groups according to the number of double bonds: saturated (no double bonds) and unsaturated. Butyric acid and palmitic acid are examples of saturated fatty acids. Unsaturated fatty acids can be further subdivided according to the degree of unsaturation: monounsaturated acids (e.g. oleic acid) and polyunsaturated acids (e.g. linoleic acid, arachidonic acid). Linoleic acid is the only essential fatty acid as it must be provided in the food. Fats of plant origin usually are composed largely of unsaturated fatty acids and are liquid at room temperature. By catalytic hydrogenation during commercial food processing, known as 'hardening,' some of the double bonds are saturated and these oils are converted into solid fats.

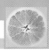

Fats serve as a major source of energy, owing to the high energy density as compared to that from carbohydrates or proteins. Fats are stored as lipid droplets in specialized cells called adipocytes, or fat cells. In addition to their energy value, fat content in the diet increases the palatability of food.

VITAMINS See below.

TRACE ELEMENTS See below.

INDIGESTIBLE FIBERS Indigestible fibers, consisting mainly of cellulose (non-starch polysaccharides), help to maintain proper motility of the gastrointestinal tract.

How energy is expressed

Energy provided by carbohydrates, proteins and fats is expressed in terms of kilocalories (kcal). One calorie is defined as the amount of heat required to raise the temperature of 1 g of water by 1°C (from 14.5°C to 15.5°C). Fats provide the highest energy yield (Fig. 27.1). Carbohydrates and fats spare proteins from being utilized as an energy source. Nutritional proteins serve primarily for the synthesis of tissue proteins, unless the intake of carbohydrates and fats is insufficient to provide adequate energy.

The average requirement of calorie intake of a healthy adult with light activity is about 2000 kcal. Several conditions influence requirement for intake and these include pregnancy, lactation, exercise, disease states, age and rate of growth. The elderly usually require reduced energy intake.

Total parenteral nutrition (TPN)

Clinical conditions may prevent patients from taking adequate food by mouth, e.g. unconsciousness, inability to swallow, inflammatory bowel disease, surgery, trauma, or malignant disease. These patients may need nutritional support which can be supplemented either by the enteral route (infusion of nutrient solutions into the upper gastrointestinal tract) or parenterally (infusion of nutrient solutions into the blood stream, using a peripheral vein). The term total parenteral nutrition (TPN) is used when parenteral nutrition serves as the sole source of nutrition. TPN solutions are concentrated hypertonic solutions, and owing to their high osmolarity, it is impossible to use peripheral venous lines because of the risk of thrombophlebitis. For this reason, TPN solutions are generally administered through a central venous line (superior vena cava, subclavian vein) because the greater flow in these veins dilutes the concentrated TPN solutions more rapidly. These solutions should provide the major components of nutrition: nitrogen source (essential and non-essential amino acids), energy source (dextrose), and fats (including the essential fatty acid, linoleic acid). For long-term administration of TPN solutions, vitamins and trace elements must be supplemented in sufficient amounts to prevent deficiencies. Fat is given in the form of lipid emulsions and these are administered either from the same container used for the other ingredients or from a separate container. The most common complication of TPN solutions is infection of the intravenous line.

EXAMPLES OF EXCESSIVE AND INADEQUATE CALORIC INTAKE

Obesity

Imbalanced food intake may lead to obesity (excessive calcoric intake compared to energy expenditure) or weight loss (complete or partial deprivation of caloric intake compared to energy expenditure). Obesity is a nutritional problem, with environmental, behavioral, socio-economic and genetic background, which affects about a third of the adult population in the Western world with increasing prevalence worldwide.

Energy provided by carbohydrates, proteins and fats	
Component	**Average energy yield (kcal/g)**
Carbohydrates	4
Proteins	4
Fats	9

Fig. 27.1 Energy provided by carbohydrates, proteins and fats. Average values are given due to the large variation in the chemical composition of these nutrients.

🔑 **Obesity increases the risk for**

- Cardiovascular system
  - Workload in the heart
  - Sudden death due to cardiac arrhythmias
  - Atherosclerosis
- Diabetes mellitus
  - Type II diabetes mellitus
- Cancer
  - Endometrial and postmenopausal breast cancer in women
  - Prostate cancer in man
  - Colonorectal cancer in men and women
- Pulmonary function
  - Sleep apnea
- Joint problems
  - Osteoporosis
  - Gout
- Skin problems
  - Acanthosis nigricans
  - Skin turgor and friability
- Endocrine system
  - Irregular and anovulatory cycles
  - Earlier menopause
  - Changes in thyroid hormone and its metabolism

Body mass index (BMI; kg/m²) as a measure of optimal body weight		
Undernutrition	**Normal weight**	**Overnutrition**
Severe <15.9 kg/m²		Overweight 25.0–29.9 kg/m²
Moderate 16–16.9 kg/m²	**18.5–24.9 kg/m²**	Obesity 30.0–39.9 kg/m²
Mild 17.0–18.4 kg/m²		Morbid obesitiy >40.0 kg/m²

Fig. 27.2 Body mass index (BMI) as a measure of optimal body weight.

Obesity develops over years and many obese children have the tendency to remain obese as adults. Obesity, resulting from positive energy balance, may be defined in terms of increased body weight or alternatively as increased total body fat. The cosmetic standard of thinness as well as the body weight itself (except for exceedingly high weight) are not of major concern. The most important problem is that obesity is associated with a three- to fourfold increase in morbidity for several medical complications such as cardiovascular diseases, hypertension, gallbladder disease, respiratory disease, osteoarthritis, and some types of cancer.

A clinically useful quantitative measure for overweight is based on the body mass index (BMI) which relates weight (in kilograms) and height (in meters) as weight/(height)². Overweight is defined as a BMI of greater than 25 and less than 30 kg/m². Obesity is defined as BMI equal to or greater than 30 kg/m² (Fig. 27.2). However, body fat distribution between central and peripheral compartments is also correlated with increased risk. Morbidity and mortality are highly associated with central distribution of body fat—ratio of waist circumference divided by hip circumference, >0.9 in women and >1.0 in men. Acceptable normal values for central distribution of body fat are <0.75 in women and <0.85 in men.

There are genetic determinants in the pathogenesis of obesity. The gene ab-gene and the protein leptin regulate food intake. Leptin, produced in adipose tissue, interacts with hypothalamic receptors to signal the filling of adipose tissue, and thereby regulate food intake and expenditure. Although increased levels of leptin have been detected in obese persons, the structure of the coding sequences of the leptin and its receptor genes are normal in most obese patients. The potential roles of these proteins in the pathogenesis of obesity in humans is presently unclear.

Control of body weight

Vital organs such as the brain, have a continuous demand for energy irrespective of the availability of food or frequency of meals. Since energy supply can not be guaranteed on a meal to meal basis, there exist metabolic and hormonal pathways which store energy (for example, as glycogen in liver) and utilize it when food is unavailable.

A small imbalance in caloric intake over a long period, e.g. a daily excess of 50 kcal, will produce a 2 kg weight gain over a year. The hypothalamus is an important site where energy intake and expenditure are regulated. Neural and endocrine signals originating from adipose tissue, neural, endocrine, and gastrointestinal systems are integrated in the hypothalamus. This is followed by afferent signals to higher centers (to produce feelings of hunger and satiety) and to the autonomic nervous system and pituitary gland to control energy expenditure (Fig. 27.3). Consequently, regulation of appetite and sensations of satiety are very complex processes that are controlled by both peripheral and central mechanisms.

Treatment of obesity

Since the development of obesity is a multifactorial problem, various strategies should be undertaken in treating overweight persons. The importance of treatment is highly dependent on several factors: the actual BMI, presence of central distribution of body fat, and the presence of other coronary risk factors. Individuals with associated risk factors should be considered for treatment when BMI values are equal to or higher than 27 kg/m². For most people, an initial loss in body weight is relatively easy to achieve, but ongoing weight loss and long-term maintenance is much more challenging. The average weight reduction with most of the available strategies does not exceed 10%. In fact, more than 90% of people who lose weight initially, regain the weight subsequently. Therefore, combined approaches for treatment are recommended and these should be undertaken on an ongoing basis.

BEHAVIORAL MODIFICATION Behavioral modification is an important strategy and is aimed at changing eating behavior and increasing awareness of overeating. Among other things, this may include:
- Daily recording of food intake.
- Advice on meal frequency.
- Advice on pace of eating.
- Removal of cues for overeating.
- Separation of eating from other activities.

EXERCISE It is crucial to adjust an exercise protocol to the specific patient based on motivation, and degree of overweight. The primary purpose of exercise in treating obesity is to increase energy expenditure while also improving cardiovascular fitness. Exercise should include activities such as walking and cycling, and should initially produce relatively low levels of energy expenditure. Daily, long-term low intensity exercise is

 Strategies for treatment of overweight and obesity

- Behavioral modification
- Exercise
- Diet
- Surgery
- Drug therapy

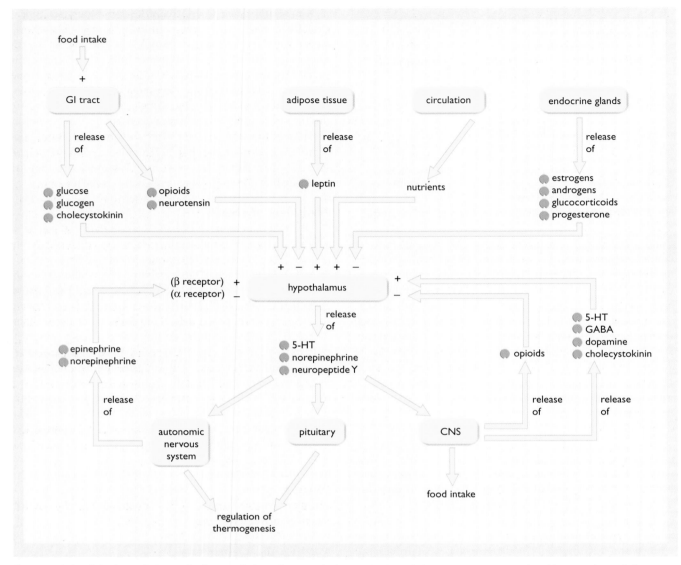

Fig. 27.3 Role of the hypothalamus in the regulation of energy balance. The hypothalamus integrates neural and hormonal signals from various organs and sends information to the central nervous system and the autonomic nervous system. The resulting output modifies food intake and thermogenesis. +, Chemicals that decrease appetite or increase energy expenditure; –, chemicals that increase appetite or decrease energy expenditure. (GI tract, gastrointestinal tract; PNS, peripheral nervous system; CNS, central nervous system)

as efficient as high intensity short-term exercise and decreases the risk of drop-out of patients due to lack of tolerance, and thereby improves the chances for long-term success.

DIET Weight reduction diet protocols designed for obese patients, are based on modifying the content of food with respect to fats, carbohydrates, proteins and fibers, aiming at reducing calorie intake. The average calorie intake requirement of a healthy adult is about 2000 kcal. Induction of a deficit of 500–600 kcal is tolerable and safe for most people and produces weight loss of about 0.5 kg/week. Reduction of calorie intake below 1000 kcal requires medical supervision. Any weight reducing protocol should provide sufficient essential nutrients, including vitamins and minerals. Within the framework of diet, the use of food substitutes may be helpful. Food substitutes are low-calorie chemicals which substitute for sugars and fats:

- **Artificial sweeteners** are widely used as low-calorie additives in food products and are also incorporated into 'diet' drinks. Some of these chemicals exceed the sweetness of sucrose by about 30–1000-fold. The most widely used sweeteners include saccharin sodium (×400), cyclamate sodium (×30), aspartame (×180), sucralose (×300–1000), acesulfame potassium (×200) and xylitol.
- **Fat substitutes** mimic fats for their palatable properties and maintenance of taste preference while decreasing fat content in the diet. Chemically, fat substitutes are protein-based, carbohydrate-based or fat-based molecules. Regular consumption of fat substitutes may produce gastrointestinal adverse effects, such as loose stools and abdominal cramps.

The most recent preparation of fat substitute approved by the FDA is olestra, a sucrose polyester, which contains 0 kcal/g because it is not absorbed. Since olestra may decrease absorption of fat soluble vitamins, olestra-containing foods are supplemented with vitamins A, D, E and K.

SURGERY Surgical treatments are aimed at reducing gastric volume by stapling the stomach. This measure is effective in producing long-term weight loss; nevertheless it is indicated primarily for highly selected, morbidly obese patients.

Pharmacotherapy

Obesity is a chronic disorder

Amphetamine has been used in the past to suppress appetite, but owing to toxicity and the potential for abuse, its use is not recommended. Likewise, dexfenfluramine and fenfluramine, inhibitors of serotonin reuptake, initially found to be effective treatment for long-term therapy, were withdrawn as their use was associated with valvular heart defects. Investigative drugs proposed for treatment include: a caffeine-ephedrine mixture which may increase calorie expenditure, opioid receptor antagonists naloxone and naltrexone, and bulk-forming substances such as methylcellulose. The therapeutic value of these compounds is likely limited and their general use is not recommended.

Two drugs approved for clinical use as anti-obesity agents are sibutramine and orlistat. A reduction of up to 10% in body weight is expected if these drugs are used continuously in conjunction with diet therapy and behavioral modification.

- Sibutramine
  - Serotonin and norepinephrine reuptake inhibitor.
  - Decreases appetite (food intake) and increases energy expenditure.
- Orlistat
  - A pancreatic lipase inhibitor.
  - Decreases fat absorption in the small intestine by inhibition of triglyceride digestion.

Sibutramine

MODE OF ACTION Sibutramine blocks reuptake of serotonin and norepinephrine in the CNS. Through poorly understood mechanisms, these effects may contribute to appetite (promote sense of satiety) and increase resting energy expenditure (increased metabolic rate).

DOSE The recommended starting dose is 10 mg/day. If an adequate rate of weight loss is not achieved within four weeks, the dose is generally increased to 15 mg/day.

PHARMACOKINETICS Absorption following oral administration is rapid. The drug undergoes extensive first-pass metabolism in the liver. Sibutramine is metabolized by cytochrome P-450 3A4 (CYP3A4) isoenzyme to yield two active metabolites: M1 (mono-desmethylsibutramine) and M2 (di-desmethylsibutramine). Both sibutramine and its metabolites are highly (>94–97%) bound to plasma proteins. Elimination is primarily renal. Pharmacokinetic data for sibutramine and the two active metabolites are presented in Fig. 27.4.

EFFECTIVENESS 7–10% reduction in body weight with preferential reduction in visceral fat. Maximal weight loss is achieved by 6 months, and maintained as long as the drug is continued.

ADVERSE EFFECTS Tachycardia, dry mouth, constipation, insomnia, increase in blood pressure. The drug is contraindicated in patients with heart disease, cerebrovascular disease, and poorly controlled hypertension.

DRUG INTERACTIONS Pharmacokinetic interactions with drugs that inhibit cytochrome P-450 3A4 (erythromycin, cimetidine, ketoconazole) are to be expected.

Orlistat

MODE OF ACTION Inhibits pancreatic lipase, and thereby decreases gastrointestinal absorption of fats.

DOSE 120 mg three times a day.

PHARMACOKINETICS There is a minimal absorption of orlistat following an oral dose. Plasma concentrations are generally low (<10 μg/L). Orlistat does not accumulate in plasma with long-term therapy. As would be expected, orlistat is mainly

Pharmacokinetic parameters following oral administration of sibutramine and orlistat

	Drug class	Pharmacokinetics			
		Bioavailability (%)	C_{max} (ng/ml)	t_{max} (hour)	$t_{1/2\beta}$ (hour)
Sibutramine M1 (active metabolite) M2 (active metabolite)	Serotonin reuptake inhibitor	>97%	 4 6	Sibutramine 1.2 3–4 3–4	Sibutramine 1.1 14 16
Orlistat	Lipase inhibitor	<1%	<10	2–4	1–2

Fig. 27.4 Pharmacokinetic parameters following oral administration of sibutramine and orlistat. C_{max} = maximum plasma concentration; t_{max} = time to C_{max}; $t_{1/2\beta}$ = elimination half-life.

eliminated in the feces (>95%) and only negligible amounts are excreted in the urine. Pharmacokinetic data for orlistat are presented in Fig. 27.4.

EFFECTIVENESS Up to 10% reduction in body weight has been observed in patients taking orlistat for up to 2 years in combination with a hypocaloric diet.

ADVERSE EFFECTS Owing to minimal oral absorption, systemic adverse effects are negligible. The major complaints are gastrointestinal adverse effects resulting from inhibition of fat absorption, and these include oily stool and fecal urgency. Potential long-term effects of unabsorbed lipids on intestinal function are not known.

CONTRAINDICATIONS None.

DRUG INTERACTIONS No observable drug interaction of orlistat with other medications. However, impaired absorption of fat-soluble vitamins is a concern.

Anorexia nervosa

Anorexia nervosa is an eating disorder which occurs most frequently during adolescence in healthy white females; more rarely, boys may develop this serious eating disorder. These youngsters typically develop distorted perception of their body image and are driven to achieve thinness at all costs. In order to accomplish this goal, they drastically restrict their food intake to a point of emaciation. A variant form of this disorder is bulimia nervosa, in which the youngsters indulge in excessive eating followed by induction of vomiting and intensive use of laxatives. Apart from severe loss of body weight (BMI <18 kg/m²) diagnosis is based on occurrence of amenorrhea (in girls) and false perception of body image.

The common clinical features in advanced cases include: cold intolerance, hypothermia, hypotension, bradycardia, ammenorrhea, loss of body fat, dry and yellow skin, hirsutism, edema, anemia, hypokalemia, and abnormal glucose tolerance. Treatment has limited efficacy with a mortality rate of about 5%. Only 50% of patients regain normal weight, while the others either remain underweight or continue to be anorexic.

Malnutrition to a point of cachexia is also common in a variety of chronic illnesses, including cancer, HIV infection, and chronic heart failure. Cachexia is expressed as a drastic reduction of body weight with loss of fat and lean tissue mass. Loss of appetite in these patients underlies the reduction in body weight. It has been suggested that cytokines, in general,

and tumor necrosis factor (TNF-α), in particular, contribute to development of cachexia. The mechanism by which TNF-α may exert its effect to reduce appetite may derive from inhibitory signals to the hypothalamus. Recent studies have suggested that patients with cachexia may benefit from oxandrolone, an anabolic agent, which moderates the loss of body weight.

VITAMINS

Vitamins are defined as structurally unrelated organic compounds that must be provided in small quantities in the diet. Although diet is the principal source, there are other sources: for example, vitamin D is synthesized in skin exposed to ultraviolet light, and vitamin K and biotin are synthesized by intestinal flora.

Vitamins differ from:
- Minerals, which are also nutrients required in small quantities, because minerals are inorganic substances.
- Essential amino acids, which are also organic nutrients, because essential amino acids are needed in large quantities.

The discovery of vitamins has important historical roots. The recognition of deficiency states, seen only rarely today, often led to the isolation of the individual vitamins.

Rickets, beriberi, and scurvy are examples of deficiency diseases which ultimately led to the discovery of vitamins D, B, and C, respectively.

Classification

Vitamins are a heterogeneous group of compounds with very different structures, sources, daily requirements, and modes of action. There are two major types based on solubility: water-soluble vitamins (e.g. vitamin B complex, vitamin C) and fat-soluble vitamins (e.g. vitamins A, D, E, and K) (Fig. 27.5). Subclassification of vitamins takes into account features other than solubility, for example storage capacity in the body, mode of action, and potential toxicity.

■ *The body's storage capacity for different vitamins varies*
The body's storage capacity is high for fat-soluble vitamins and

Diagnosis of anorexia nervosa

- BMI <18 kg/m²
- Amenorrhea
- Fear of becoming fat even when underweight
- Distorted perception of body image

Classification of vitamins	
Water-soluble vitamins	**Fat-soluble vitamins**
Vitamin C	Vitamin A

B complex vitamins
  Vitamin B₁ (thiamine)
  Vitamin B₂ (riboflavin)
  Vitamin B₃ (nicotinic acid)
  Vitamin B₆ (pyridoxine)
  Vitamin B₁₂ (cobalamin)
Pantothenic acid
Biotin
Folic acid
	Vitamin D
	
	Vitamin E
	
	Vitamin K

Fig. 27.5 Classification of vitamins. The two major groups based on solubility are water-soluble and fat-soluble vitamins.

Approximate body stores of vitamins	
Vitamin	**Body's storage capacity**
Vitamin B_{12}	3–6 years
Vitamin A	6–10 months
Vitamin D	2–4 months
Folic acid	1–3 months
Vitamin C	2–4 weeks
Vitamin B_3	2–4 weeks
Vitamin K	1–2 weeks
Vitamin B_1	1–2 weeks
Vitamin B_2	1–2 weeks
Vitamin B_6	1–2 weeks

Fig. 27.6 Approximate body stores of vitamins.

Mode of action of vitamins		
Co-enzymes	**Antioxidants**	**Hormones**
Vitamin B_1	Vitamin C	Vitamin A
Vitamin B_2	Vitamin E	Vitamin D
Vitamin B_3		
Vitamin B_6		
Vitamin B_{12}		
Vitamin K		
Biotin		
Folic acid		
Pantothenic acid		

Fig. 27.7 Mode of action of vitamins. Vitamins exert their effects in three main ways: as coenzymes, as antioxidants, and as hormones.

lower for water-soluble vitamins. An exception to this rule is the body's storage capacity for the water-soluble vitamin B_{12}, which is normally sufficient for about 3–6 years (Fig. 27.6).

■ *Some vitamins are more toxic than others*
Toxicity due to either long-term accumulation in the body or a short-term administration of a high dose is more likely with fat-soluble vitamins (e.g. vitamins A and D). Vitamin poisoning may occur when excessive amounts of various dietary supplements are consumed without adequate guidance.

Vitamin as therapy
■ *Vitamins maintain growth and normal body functions*
There are large variations in the daily requirements of the different vitamins. An inadequate supply is associated with specific deficiency diseases. Some people, such as pregnant women, alcoholics, and strict vegans have an increased risk of developing vitamin deficiency.

How vitamins work
Vitamins exert their effects in three main ways: as coenzymes, as antioxidants, and as hormones (Fig. 27.7).

■ *Most water-soluble vitamins act as coenzymes for specific enzymes*
Many enzymes are inactive without the presence of small amounts of substances called co-factors. These cofactors can be trace metals or organic molecules, and organic molecules that function as co-factors are called coenzymes. Coenzymes take part in the reaction being catalyzed. During the process they

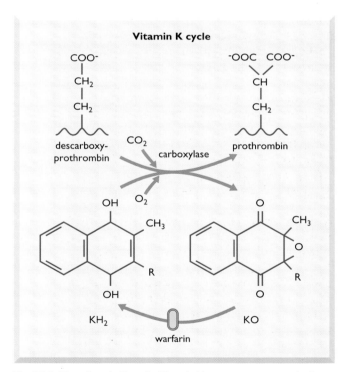

Fig. 27.8 The vitamin K cycle. Vitamin K acts as a coenzyme in the conversion of descarboxyprothrombin to prothrombin catalyzed by carboxylase. During the carboxylation process, vitamin K is converted to its inactive oxide and then metabolized back to its active form. The reductive metabolism of the inactive vitamin K epoxide back to its active hydroquinone form is warfarin sensitive. Warfarin and related drugs block the γ-carboxylation and this results in molecules that are biologically inactive for coagulation.

are transformed into an intermediate form and are subsequently generated back to their active form (Fig. 27.8). Most water-soluble vitamins act as coenzymes for specific enzymes.

569

Some vitamins act as antioxidants, others as hormones

Vitamin C and vitamin E function as antioxidants, while two fat-soluble vitamins, vitamin A and vitamin D, act as hormones. Specific binding sites (receptors) have been identified for vitamin A and vitamin D for exerting their hormonal activity.

Recommended dietary allowances and daily intake

Recommended dietary allowances (RDAs) of vitamins (as well as minerals and trace elements) have been established in most countries. RDAs are aimed at maintaining maximal stores of the vitamins without causing toxicity and are intended to meet the requirements of normal persons with respect to age and sex. The recommended daily intake has been based on a daily intake of 2000 kcal (Fig. 27.9). In the US, RDAs are published periodically by the Food and Nutrition Board, National Academy of Sciences, and National Research Council.

Interaction of vitamins with drugs and foods

There are several examples of common food interactions. For example, ingestion of large doses of vitamin C-containing fruits interferes with the absorption of vitamin B_{12}. Likewise, certain fish and blueberries may contain thiaminase, which inactivates vitamin B_1. In addition, egg white contains avidin, a glycoprotein, which prevents the absorption of biotin.

Drug–vitamin interactions are discussed in the appropriate sections for the individual vitamins. In general, long-term ingestion of unabsorbed lipids such as mineral oil (used as a laxative) may dramatically decrease the absorption of the fat-soluble vitamins and may lead to the related vitamin-deficiency diseases. Other drug–vitamin interactions include:

- Estrogen-containing oral contraceptives with vitamins B_1, B_2, and folic acid.
- Antibiotics (tetracyclines, neomycin) and sulfonamides with vitamins B_3, B_{12}, vitamin C, vitamin K, and folic acid.
- Anticonvulsants with vitamin D, vitamin K, and folic acid.
- Phenothiazines and tricyclic antidepressants with vitamin B_2.
- Diuretics with vitamin B_1.
- Isoniazid and penicillamine with vitamin B_6.
- Methotrexate with folic acid.

Vitamins as dietary supplements

Dietary supplements may contain over-the-counter drugs, plant extracts, and vitamins. These substances may have adverse effects and interact with drugs and foods if not used properly.

Vitamin pills are mostly consumed by children, the elderly, and exercising adults, and about 40% of the adult population in the US and Canada supplement their diet with vitamins daily.

The usefulness of vitamin pills for purposes other than correcting deficiency symptoms has not been established. An intake of fat-soluble vitamins at doses exceeding the RDA has a potential risk of producing hypervitaminosis. Ingestion of megadoses of vitamin C carries a risk of causing kidney stones, while immediate adverse effects, such as increased clotting tendency, may arise from vitamin K ingestion by patients taking a stable dose of warfarin.

WATER-SOLUBLE VITAMINS

Vitamin B_1 (thiamine)

Source

Vitamin B_1 is found in dried yeast, whole grains, whole brown rice, and wheat germ.

Functions

Thiamine, in the form of thiamine diphosphate (pyrophosphate), acts as a coenzyme in carbohydrate metabolism in reactions involving decarboxylation of α-ketoacids, such as pyruvate and α-ketoglutarate. Thiamine also acts as a coenzyme for the transketolase reactions of the hexose monophosphate shunt for using pentose. Selected reactions which require thiamine as a coenzyme are listed in Fig. 27.10.

Deficiency

The deficiency state of vitamin B_1 is beriberi (Fig. 27.11). This deficiency disease became more common with increasing consumption of polished rice prepared from brown rice by husking off the outer germ layer, which contains most of the vitamin B_1 activity. In the 1880s, dietary supplements of meat and grains were used to cure beriberi in sailors in the Japanese Navy. There are two forms of beriberi: dry and wet beriberi.

- Dry beriberi relates to nervous system deficiency resulting in a degenerative neuropathy characterized by general neuritis, paralysis, and atrophy of the muscles (see Fig. 27.11).

Daily vitamin requirements	
Vitamin A	5000 IU
Vitamin B_1	1.5 mg
Vitamin B_2	1.7 mg
Vitamin B_3	20 mg
Vitamin B_6	2 mg
Vitamin B_{12}	0.003 mg
Vitamin C	60 mg
Vitamin D	400 IU
Vitamin E	30 IU
Vitamin K	0.08 mg
Pantothenic acid	10 mg
Biotin	0.3 mg
Folic acid	0.4 mg
(Daily values based on 2000 kcal daily intake)	

Fig. 27.9 Daily vitamin requirements.

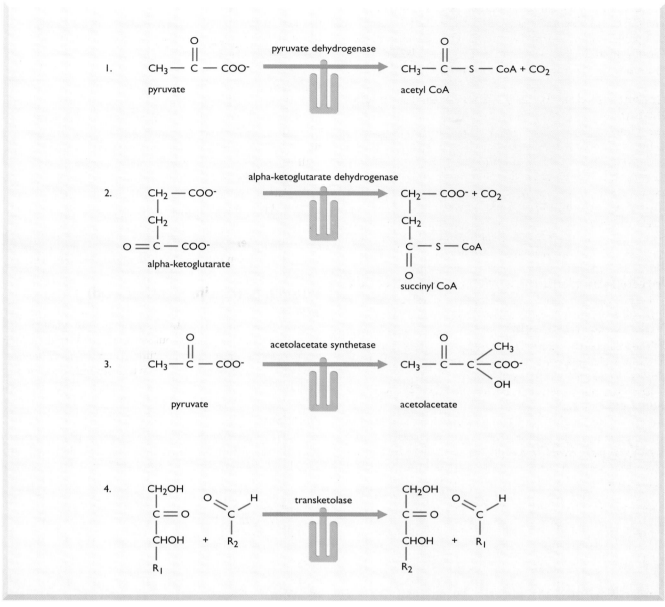

Fig. 27.10 Selected reactions which require thiamine as coenzyme.

- Wet beriberi describes involvement of the cardiovascular system resulting in edema partly due to myocardial insufficiency, palpitations, tachycardia, and an abnormal electrocardiogram.

Apart from insufficient intake, vitamin B_1 deficiency may result from heavy alcohol consumption, when it may cause Wernicke's encephalopathy and Korsakoff's psychosis. Infantile beriberi may result from a low content of thiamine in the breast milk of thiamine-deficient women.

Pharmacotherapeutic use

The main use of thiamine is to treat or prevent thiamine deficiency, especially in alcoholics. It may be infused intravenously in an emergency situation (e.g. in acute Wernicke's encephalopathy) at doses between 50–100 mg of thiamine. It has been observed that administration of glucose to asymptomatic thiamine-deficient individuals may precipitate acute symptoms. In the glycolytic pathway, glucose is catabolyzed through 10 successive enzyme-catalyzed reactions to yield pyruvate. Pyruvate is an essential intermediate involved in both catabolic reactions (conversion to carbon dioxide and water through the citric acid cycle) and anabolic reactions (e.g. for synthesis of the amino acid, alanine). The oxidative decarboxylation of pyruvate to acetyl-CoA is an irreversible reaction which consumes thiamine and may exhaust the body pool in vitamin-deficient patients, potentially precipitating encephalopathy. For this reason, whenever glucose is given to a patient suspected to be thiamine-deficient, this vitamin should be administered concomitantly.

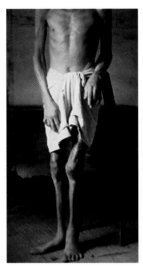

Fig. 27.11 Beriberi showing peripheral neuropathy. Some patients develop wrist drop and marked wasting of the lower extremities. (Courtesy of Dr A. Bryceson.)

Vitamin B$_2$ (riboflavin)
Source
Vitamin B$_2$ is found in yeast, organ meat such as liver, dairy products, and green leafy vegetables.

Functions
Riboflavin, in the form of flavin mononucleotide (FMN) or flavin adenine dinucleotide (FAD), acts as a coenzyme for various respiratory flavoproteins which catalyze oxidation–reduction reactions. The role of this vitamin is inherent to the ability of the isoalloxazine ring to accept up to two electrons donated by hydrogen atoms to form the appropriate reduced forms (Fig. 27.12). Energy is conserved in the reduced form of the coenzyme.

Deficiency
The symptoms of deficiency include sore throat, stomatitis, glossitis, cheilosis, seborrheic dermatitis, and in some cases corneal vascularization and amblyopia. Isolated deficiency of riboflavin is rare, and in most cases it occurs in combination with deficiencies of other water-soluble vitamins.

Phenothiazines, tricyclic antidepressants, and quinine (an antimalarial) inhibit flavokinase, which converts riboflavin to FMN, and may therefore increase requirements for riboflavin.

Pharmacotherapeutic use
Vitamin B$_2$ is given in a dose of 5–20 mg/day to treat deficiency.

Vitamin B$_3$ (niacin, nicotinic acid)
Source
Vitamin B$_3$ is found in meat, fish, legumes, and whole grains. Tryptophan may serve as a source for nicotinic acid (niacin) since it can be converted to nicotinic acid with an efficiency of 60:1 (i.e. 60 tryptophan molecules to form one nicotinic acid molecule).

Functions
Niacin is converted in the body into two physiologically active forms: nicotinamide adenine dinucleotide (NAD) and nicotinamide dinucleotide phosphate (NADP). The main

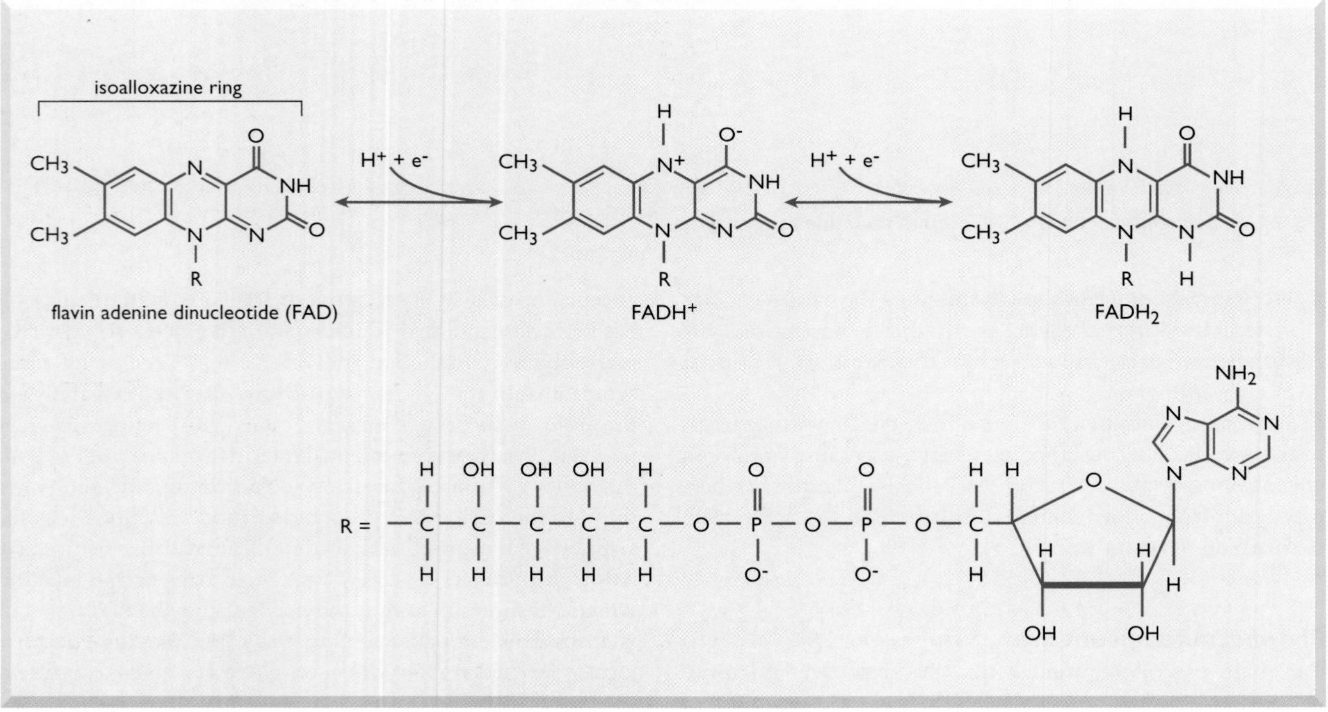

Fig. 27.12 Flavin adenine dinucleotide (FAD) and its reduced forms.

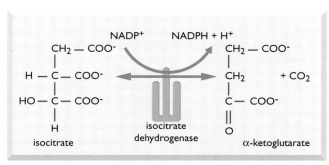

Fig. 27.13 Oxidative decarboxylation of isocitrate to form α-ketoglutarate requiring NADP as a coenzyme.

function of vitamin B_3 is in oxidation–reduction reactions using NAD or NADP. It is an essential coenzyme for many dehydrogenases in the Krebs cycle, for anaerobic carbohydrate metabolism, and for lipid and protein metabolism. For example, one of the reactions in the citric acid cycle requires NADP as a coenzyme for the oxidative decarboxylation of isocitrate to form α-ketoglutarate (Fig. 27.13).

Deficiency
Pellagra, the deficiency disease of vitamin B_3, was first described in 1735 by Casal as the *mal de la rosa* disease (i.e. sickness of the rose) because of the roughness and color of the skin. The term pellagra is translated from Italian as rough (*agra*) skin (*pelle*).

The primary symptoms of pellagra are dermatitis, diarrhea, and dementia (the three Ds). Pellagra is occasionally observed in populations who use corn as their major source of protein, as corn has a low tryptophan content.

Pharmacotherapeutic use
Niacin is effective for treating pellagra. It is also useful, in pharmacologic doses much greater than required as a vitamin, in the treatment of several types of lipoprotein disorders (see Chapter 12).

Toxicity
Niacin may produce unpleasant flushing and vasodilation when treating hyperlipidemia with pharmacologic doses. These effects may diminish over time or with the use of aspirin. Severe hepatotoxicity has been associated with the use of long-acting formulations of niacin used in the treatment of hyperlipidemias.

Vitamin B_6 (pyridoxine)
Source
Vitamin B_6 is found in meat, fish, legumes, dried yeast, and whole grains.

Fig. 27.14 Involvement of vitamin B_6 in two biochemical pathways. 1: Formation of GABA requiring glutamate. 2: Biosynthesis of 5-hydroxytryptamine (serotonin) requiring L-aromatic amino acid decarboxylase.

Functions

Vitamin B_6 in the form of pyridoxal phosphate is the coenzyme for a variety of essential reactions in the metabolism of certain amino acids (including decarboxylation, transamination and racemization), sulfur-containing and hydroxy-amino acids, and fatty acids. Impaired formation of γ-aminobutyric acid due to impaired glutamate decarboxylase is believed to cause the tendency to convulsions seen in vitamin B_6 deficiency. Two classical examples are given in Fig. 27.14 to illustrate the role of this vitamin in the biosynthesis of GABA and 5-hydroxytryptamine (serotonin).

Deficiency

Deficiency of vitamin B_6 may result from dietary insufficiency. It may also occur in patients being treated with penicillamine, oral contraceptives, and isoniazid. Isoniazid combines with pyridoxal to form pyridoxal hydrazone, which has no co-enzyme activity. Signs of deficiency include seborrhea-like skin lesions, anemia, neuropathy, and convulsions in infancy.

Pharmacotherapeutic use

Although vitamin B_6 is essential, clinical syndromes of isolated deficiency are rare and may be attributed to drugs–vitamin interaction. It may be given as an addition to the therapy of patients with other vitamin B complex deficiencies.

Toxicity

Long-term ingestion of excessive dosages of vitamin B_6 can cause peripheral neuritis.

Vitamin B_{12}
Source

Muscle meats, liver, and dairy products are the exclusive source of vitamin B_{12}. The dietary source of vitamin B_{12}, in these animal products, is derived microbially from normal gut flora.

Structure

The basic structure of vitamin B_{12} is complex. Dorothy Hodgkin was awarded the Nobel prize for elucidating this structure (Fig. 27.15). It consists of a corrin nucleus (a porphyrin-like ring structure with four reduced pyrrole rings linked to a central cobalt atom), 5,6-dimethylbenzimidazolyl nucleotide, and variable R groups. Different substitutions, covalently bound to the cobalt atom, result in different cobalamins (see Fig. 27.15). The active forms of vitamin B_{12} are 5-deoxyadenosylcobalamin and methylcobalamin.

Absorption

Dietary vitamin B_{12} is absorbed in the distal ileum by a receptor-mediated process. A prerequisite to vitamin B_{12} absorption is its combination with an intrinsic factor secreted into the lumen of the stomach by the parietal cells of the gastric mucosa. Once absorbed, vitamin B_{12} is transported to the various cells of the body, bound to a plasma glycoprotein, transcobalamin II. Excess vitamin B_{12} is stored in the liver, and only trace amounts are normally lost in the urine and stools.

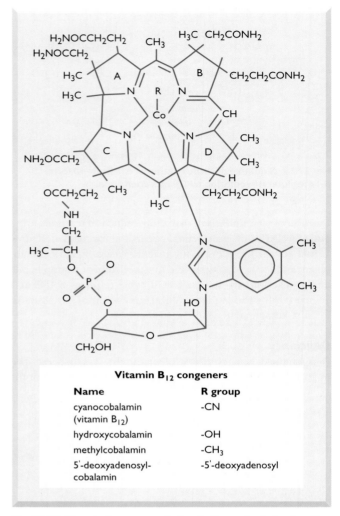

Vitamin B_{12} congeners	
Name	**R group**
cyanocobalamin (vitamin B_{12})	-CN
hydroxycobalamin	-OH
methylcobalamin	-CH_3
5'-deoxyadenosyl-cobalamin	-5'-deoxyadenosyl

Fig. 27.15 Chemical structure of vitamin B_{12} and cobalamins. The basic structure of vitamin B_{12} consists of a corrin nucleus (a porphyrin-like ring structure with four reduced pyrrole rings linked to a central cobalt atom), 5,6-dimethylbenzimidazolyl nucleotide and variable R groups. Different substitutions covalently bound to the cobalt atom result in different cobalamins.

There are sufficient stores in the liver to provide about 3–6 years' supply of the daily requirement of about 2–3 μg.

Functions

Vitamin B_{12} is vital for cell growth and mitosis. It is essential for the conversion of methylmalonyl coenzyme A (CoA) to succinyl CoA (Fig. 27.16) and for folate regeneration (Fig. 27.17). Accumulation of methylmalonyl CoA in vitamin B_{12} deficiency with the resulting synthesis of abnormal fatty acids and their incorporation into cell membranes may account for the neurologic manifestations of vitamin B_{12} deficiency.

The role of vitamin B_{12} in folate regeneration is the biochemical link between vitamin B_{12} and folic acid metabolism. This explains the functional deficiency of folic acid metabolites in vitamin B_{12} deficiency. In vitamin B_{12} deficiency there is an accumulation of 5-methyltetrahydrofolate due to impaired regeneration of folic acid, and this results in impaired DNA synthesis and megaloblastic anemia.

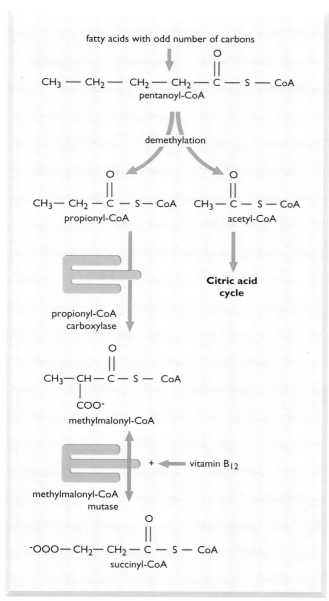

Fig. 27.16 Conversion of methylmalonyl CoA to succinyl CoA. The oxidative pathway of fatty acids with an odd number of carbons ends with an intermediate product, pentanoyl-CoA, which in turn is oxidized and cleaved to acetyl-CoA and propionyl CoA. Acetyl-CoA is oxidized via the citric acid cycle whereas propionyl-CoA is converted to succinyl-CoA. Methylmalonyl CoA mutase requires vitamin B_{12} as a coenzyme. Deficiency of vitamin B_{12} will result in accumulation of methylmalonyl-CoA and as a consequence, synthesis of nonphysiologic fatty acids containing an odd number of carbons.

Deficiency

Ever since the 1820s the disease pernicious anemia (deficiency of vitamin B_{12}) was associated with digestive or absorptive problems in the gastrointestinal tract. Vitamin B_{12} deficiency results mainly from impaired absorption due to one of the following:

* A deficiency of intrinsic factor.
* Defects in absorption of the vitamin B_{12}–intrinsic factor complex.

The most common causes of vitamin B_{12} deficiency are pernicious anemia (due to defective secretion of intrinsic factor following destruction of secretory cells in the stomach as a result of autoimmune disease), partial or total gastrectomy, malabsorption syndrome, inflammatory bowel disease, gastrointestinal resection, fish tapeworm infection, and a strict vegan diet.

Deficiency impairs DNA synthesis, cell division, and function, and so the effect is most apparent in tissues where cells are rapidly dividing (e.g. bone marrow, gastrointestinal epithelium). Megaloblastic anemia is the main hematologic finding. Other clinical features are sterility, organic brain syndromes (hallucinations, emotional lability, and dementia), spinal cord degeneration, and peripheral neuropathies.

Pharmacotherapeutic use

Treatment of vitamin B_{12} deficiency involves replacing vitamin B_{12} by injection and treating the cause, if possible.

Folic acid
Source

Folic acid is found in organ meat such as liver, dried yeast, and fresh green leafy vegetables.

Functions

Folic acid (pteroylglutamic acid) is composed of a pteridine ring, p-aminobenzoic acid (PABA), and glutamic acid. Once absorbed, it is reduced to tetrahydrofolic acid (THF), which acts as an acceptor of one-carbon units. Methotrexate blocks the conversion of folic acid to THF by binding to the enzyme tetrahydrofolate reductase. The role of vitamin B_{12} in folate regeneration is shown in Fig. 27.17. Folate cofactors are essential for the one-carbon transfer reactions necessary for DNA synthesis. Folic acid is a coenzyme for the:

* Conversion of homocysteine to methionine. As shown in Fig. 27.17, the conversion of homocysteine to methionine is highly dependent on folic acid and vitamin B_{12}, the deficiency of which lead to accumulation of homocysteine. Folic acid (and vitamin B_{12}) have been found to lower blood concentrations of homocysteine. Elevated concentrations of homocysteine in blood are associated with increased risk for atherosclerosis and ischemic heart disease. Folic acid supplementation may lower homocysteine blood concentrations; whether this lowers the risk of developing atherosclerosis and coronary heart disease remains to be determined.
* Conversion of serine to glycine.
* Synthesis of thymidylate (a rate-limiting step in DNA synthesis).
* Metabolism of histidine.
* Synthesis of purines.

Deficiency

In 1919, Sir William Osler showed that anemia associated with pregnancy differed from that caused by vitamin B_{12} deficiency. During the 1940s, folic acid was purified and synthesized and

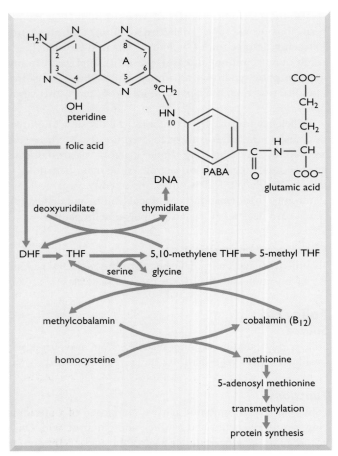

Fig. 27.17 Structure and regeneration of folic acid by vitamin B$_{12}$.
Folic acid is reduced first to dihydrofolic acid (DHF) and subsequently
to tetrahydrofolic acid (THF) by folate reductase. In the process serine
is converted to glycine, and THF accepts one carbon unit to form 5,10-
methylene THF. The latter can either be converted to 5-methyl THF, or
donate the methylene group to deoxyuridilate and revert to DHF.
Kinetically, the formation of 5-methyl THF is more favorable. The
transfer of the methylene group from 5,10-methylene THF to
deoxyuridilate is an essential step for DNA synthesis. 5-Methyl THF
must be transformed to THF to maintain the required supply of 5,10-
methylene THF. This is carried out by donating the methyl group to
vitamin B$_{12}$ to form methylcobalamin. This in turn donates the methyl
group to homocysteine, forming methionine. Methionine is then
transformed to 5-adenosylmethionine which is important for protein
synthesis. 5-Methyl THF accumulates in vitamin B$_{12}$ deficiency. The
methionine synthase pathway, the transformation of homocysteine to
methionine, has a key role in folate regeneration.

found to be responsible for this form and other origins of
megaloblastic anemia.

Folate deficiency is mainly expressed as megaloblastic
anemia, and is often seen in alcoholics and in people with
extensive small bowel disease. The daily requirement in normal
adults is approximately 100–200 μg. Pregnant or nursing
women require 200–500 μg or more daily.

Pharmacotherapeutic use

The usual oral dose is 1 mg/day for deficiency states. In
addition, prenatal supplements of folic acid are important in
preventing neural tube defects when given 3 months before
conception and during the first trimester. This is a challenging
issue from the public health perspective as this defect may have
occurred before a woman may realize that she is pregnant.

Toxicity

Large doses of oral folic acid may decrease the effect of anti-
epileptic medications. Correcting hematologic symptoms with
folic acid should always be preceded by a correct diagnosis
because, although large doses of folate will correct the anemia
of people with vitamin B$_{12}$ deficiency, it will not correct the
central nervous system damage, which will continue.

Pantothenic acid
Source

Pantothenic acid is widely distributed in both animal and
vegetable foods.

Structure

Pantothenic acid was the last nutrient to be listed as a vitamin.
Lipmann and Kaplan received the Nobel prize for elucidating
the function of CoA (Fig. 27.18). Pantothenic acid is an integral
moiety in CoA, which serves as a coenzyme for reactions
involving the transfer of acetyl groups.

Functions

This vitamin is an essential constituent of CoA and acyl carrier
protein (see Fig. 27.18). Coenzyme A serves as a cofactor for a
variety of reactions involving the transfer of two-carbon groups,
which are important in:

- Oxidative metabolism of carbohydrates.
- Gluconeogenesis.
- Degradation of fatty acids.
- Synthesis of sterols, steroid hormones, and porphyrins.

Deficiency

Symptoms resulting from a deficiency of pantothenic acid are
uncommon because it is so plentiful in foods, but may develop
in people with liver disease or who drink excessive alcohol.
They include paresthesia of the limbs, muscle weakness, and
'burning feet' syndrome.

Biotin
Source

Biotin is found in yeast, egg yolk, meat, and dairy products.
Intestinal microflora are an additional source. Egg white contains a glycoprotein called avidin, which binds tightly to biotin
and prevents its intestinal absorption. Avidin is denatured in
cooked eggs.

Functions

Biotin acts as a coenzyme in reactions involving carbon dioxide
fixation (carboxylation). Four carboxylases require biotin:
acetyl-CoA carboxylase, pyruvate carboxylase, methylcrotonyl
CoA carboxylase and propionyl CoA carboxylase. The biologically active form of biotin is biocytin, a complex in which

Fig. 27.18 Structural correlation between pantothenic acid and coenzyme A.

biotin is covalently linked to an ε-amino group of a lysine residue of the appropriate enzyme. For example, Fig. 27.19 illustrates the conversion of pyruvate to oxaloacetate.

Deficiency
Biotin defiency is rare, but may occur during long-term total parenteral nutrition (TPN), prolonged consumption of egg white and in individuals with multiple carboxylase deficiency. Symptoms include anorexia, nausea, vomiting, general lassitude, and a dry dermatitis.

Pharmacotherapeutic use
Large doses (5–10 mg/day) are usually given for deficiency.

Vitamin C
Source
Vitamin C is found in citrus fruits, tomatoes, potatoes, cabbage, and green peppers.

Structure
There are two active forms of vitamin C: L-ascorbic acid and dehydroascorbic acid. Ascorbic acid is easily oxidized to dehydroascorbic acid.

Absorption
Vitamin C is readily absorbed in the ileum by a Na^+-dependent carrier-mediated mechanism. It is stored in all tissues, with the highest concentrations in the adrenal and pituitary glands. In all tissues, ascorbic acid is reversibly converted to de-

hydroascorbic acid. The main metabolite is excreted by the kidneys as an oxalate salt. Massive doses of vitamin C may cause kidney stones and diarrhea.

Functions
Vitamin C acts as a reducing agent. It is required for:
* Collagen formation; without it, protocollagen does not cross-link properly, resulting in impaired wound healing.
* Synthesis of biogenic amines, norepinephrine, and epinephrine.
* Synthesis of carnitine, the carrier protein that facilitates the transport of fatty acids into mitochondria for β-oxidation.

Deficiency
Vitamin C deficiency is called scurvy and results from either increased requirements or a low intake. Scurvy (Fig. 27.20) became prevalent in the 1500s when long sea voyages became common. As a result, oranges and lemons were prescribed for long sailing voyages, and subsequently, in the 1740s, citrus fruits, which contain citric acid, were used to prevent scurvy. Scurvy is characterized by hemorrhages, loose teeth, gingivitis (see Fig. 27.20), and swollen joints. Albert Szent-Gyorgyi received the Nobel prize in part for his work leading to the discovery of Vitamin C.

Pharmacotherapeutic use
Doses of 100–1000 mg/day orally have been used to treat ascorbic acid deficiency disease. Large doses have been proposed as being useful for general well-being and in the treat-

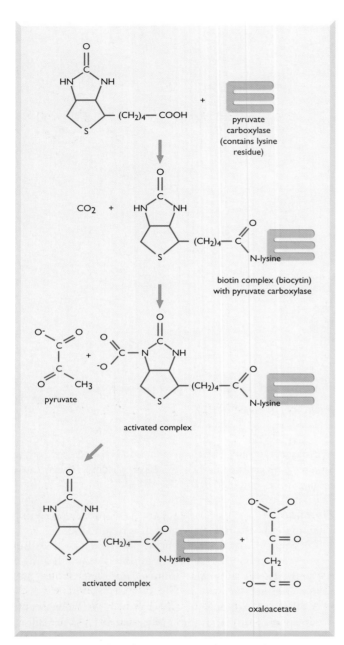

Fig. 27.19 Conversion of pyruvate to oxaloacetate by pyruvate carboxylase. This is a two-step reaction. At first, a carboxyl group derived from HCO_3^- is attached to biocytin, the biotin/carboxylase complex, where upon it is transferred to pyruvate.

ment of cancer; this issue has been very topical in the general news from time to time. However, there is no evidence to support this use of the vitamin; indeed, efficacy in cancer has not been demonstrated in controlled clinical trials.

Toxicity

There are two arguments against the use of megadoses of ascorbic acid. The first is the risk of oxalate formation in the kidneys, and the second is rebound scurvy, which may occur if megadoses have been taken for a long time and are then suddenly stopped.

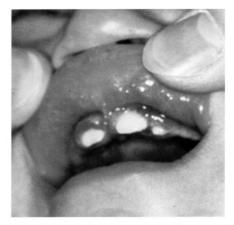

Fig. 27.20 Scurvy. Vitamin C deficiency is rare. Features of scurvy include severe gingivitis and loosening of the teeth. (Courtesy of Professor R. Waterlow.)

Clinically available retinoids		
Chemical name	**Alternative name**	**Clinical use**
Retinol		Vitamin A deficiency
Retinoic acid (all-*trans*)	Tretinoin	Acne (topical treatment)
Retinoic acid (13-*cis*)	Isotretinoin	Acne (systemic treatment)
Etretinate		Psoriasis

Fig. 27.21 Clinically available retinoids.

FAT-SOLUBLE VITAMINS

Vitamin A

Source

Vitamin A is found in fish liver oils, egg yolk, and green leafy or yellow vegetables.

Structure

Vitamin A refers to a group of retinoids and carotenoids. Retinoids include both naturally occurring and synthetic analogs of vitamin A (Figs 27.21 and 27.22).

Absorption

Retinoid esters are hydrolyzed in the intestinal lumen and absorbed by a carrier-mediated mechanism. The absorbed retinyl esters are taken up by the liver, hydrolyzed, and transported in the circulation bound to retinol-binding protein (RBD). This complex is taken up by various organs, especially the intestine, liver, and eye, where it binds to specific sites on the cell membrane. At certain sites, such as the retina, retinol is converted to 11-cis retinal and incorporated into rhodopsin (see below).

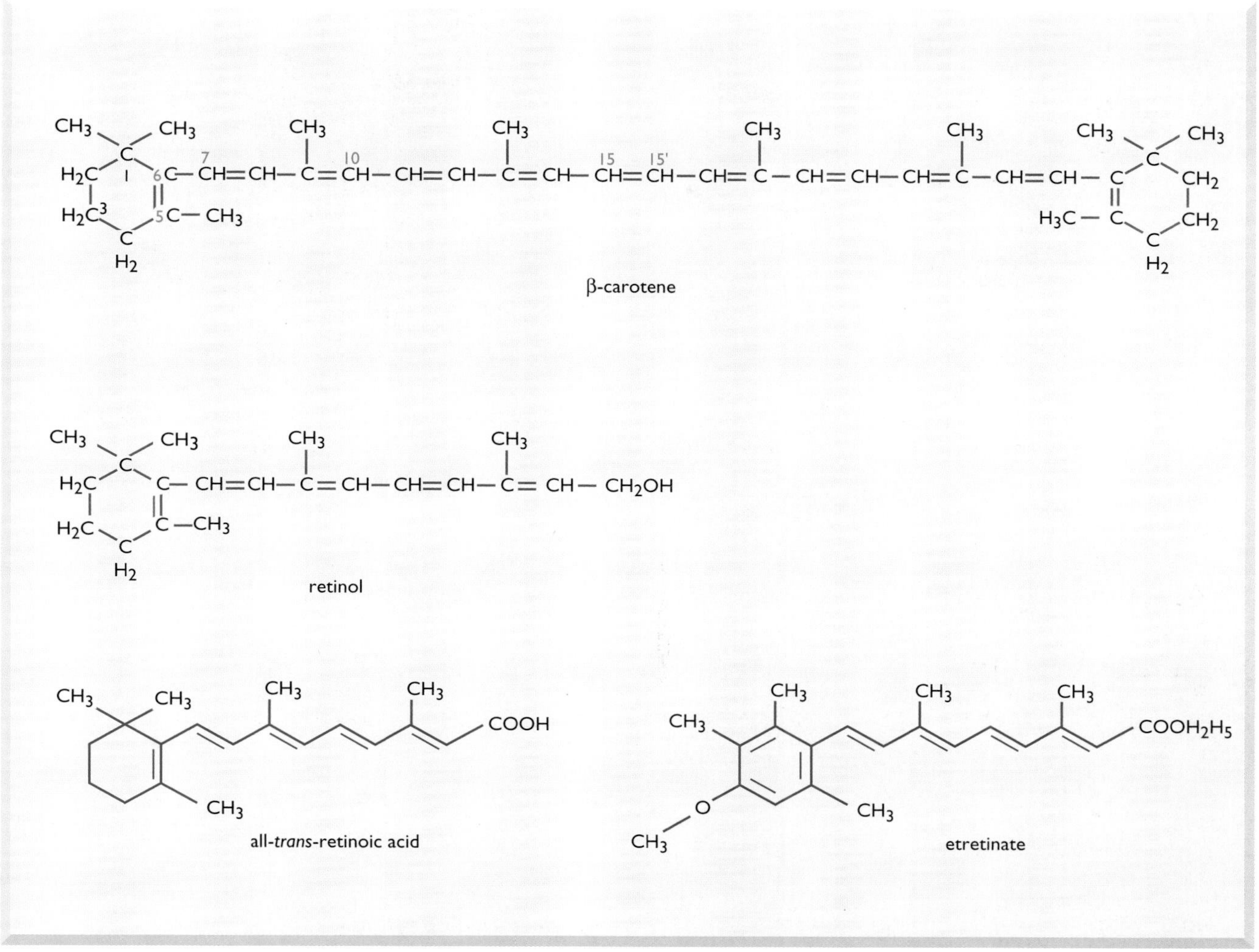

Fig. 27.22 Chemical structure of β-carotene and selected retinoids.

Functions

Vitamin A plays a role in:

- The photoreceptor mechanism of the retina.
- The integrity of epithelia.
- Lysosome stability.

THE PHOTORECEPTOR MECHANISM OF THE RETINA The role of vitamin A in vision is shown in Fig. 27.23. The retina contains two specialized receptors (rods and cones), which mediate photoreception. Cones are receptors for high-intensity light and are also responsible for color vision, whereas rods are sensitive to low-intensity light.

The active form of vitamin A in the visual system is 11-*cis* retinal. The photoreceptor protein contained in rods is opsin. The attachment of 11-*cis* retinal to opsin and the subsequent formation of rhodopsin, a typical G protein-coupled receptor, is required to absorb light. Absorption of a photon of light causes photodecomposition of rhodopsin and the formation of unstable conformational states, which lead to isomerization of 11-*cis* retinal to all-*trans* retinal and the dissociation of opsin. All-*trans* retinal can isomerize to 11-*cis* retinal and combine with opsin or be reduced to all-*trans* retinol. The activated rhodopsin interacts with transducin, a G protein, to stimulate a cyclic guanosine monophosphate (cGMP) phosphodiesterase, leading to decreased conductance of cGMP-gated Na^+ channels in the plasma membrane. This change produces membrane hyperpolarization and generation of an action potential in the ganglion cells, which is conducted to the brain via the optic nerve.

INTEGRITY OF EPITHELIA Vitamin A is important for initiating and controlling epithelial differentiation in mucosal and keratinized tissues.

ROLE IN CARCINOGENESIS Retinoids have inhibitory effects on cellular differentiation mechanisms and they might be useful in the treatment and prevention of certain human cancers. These effects are mediated through an interaction with nuclear retinoic acid receptors resulting in modulation of gene expression. Three retinoic acid receptor genes, named α, β, and γ, have been localized to human chromosomes 17, 3, and 12, respectively. These receptors belong to a receptor superfamily

579

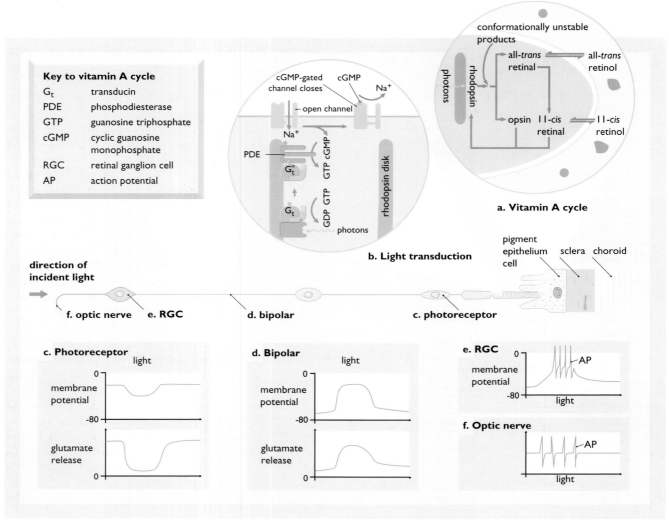

Fig. 27.23 Role of vitamin A in vision. The attachment of 11-*cis* retinal to opsin to form rhodopsin is required for the absorption of light(a). Absorption of a photon of light results in a photodecomposition of rhodopsin and formation of unstable conformational states, leading to isomerization of 11-*cis* retinal to all-*trans* retinal and the dissociation of opsin. All-*trans* retinal can isomerize to 11-*cis* retinal and combine with rhodopsin or be reduced to all-*trans* retinol. The activated rhodopsin interacts with transducin, a G protein, to stimulate a cGMP phosphodiesterase, leading to a decreased conductance of cGMP-gated Na$^+$ channels in the plasma membrane (b). This change produces membrane hyperpolarization and generation of an action potential in the retinal ganglion cells, which is conducted to the brain via the optic nerve (c–f).

that includes receptors for steroid hormones, thyroid hormones and calcitriol. All-*trans* retinoic acid was found to induce complete remission in 90% of patients with acute promyelocytic leukemia (APL). Likewise, isoretinoin was found to produce regression of oral leukoplakia provided the drug is administered chronically.

Deficiency

The link between night blindness and vitamin A deficiency became clear only relatively recently. During the 1900s and 1920s it was shown that a fat-soluble material in egg yolk and cod liver oil was essential to promote growth and cure night blindness. However, it was not until the 1930s that the structures of β-carotene and related compounds were elucidated.

On the other hand, vitamin A toxicity was observed in arctic explorers who consumed large amounts of polar bear livers.

Symptoms of vitamin A deficiency include xerophthalmia (dry and lusterless cornea and areas covering the eye, Fig. 27.24), keratomalacia (dryness and ulceration of the cornea, Fig. 27.25), Bitot's spot, and night blindness. The health and integrity of the skin is also decreased in vitamin A deficiency.

Deficiency can result from a low intake or from fat malabsorption due to a variety of diseases. Alcohol consumption may decrease the vitamin A stores in the liver.

Pharmacotherapeutic use

Retinoic acid (tretinoin, all-*trans* retinoic acid) is the acid form of vitamin A. It is an effective topical treatment for acne vulgaris

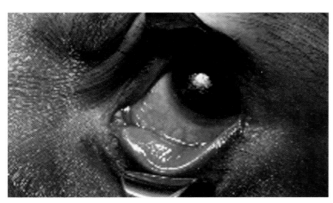

Fig. 27.24 Xerophthalmia. Vitamin A deficiency is a common cause of blindness in pre-school children in the tropics. The dryness of the cornea and conjunctiva gives the eye a dull hazy appearance. (Courtesy of Professor W. Peters.)

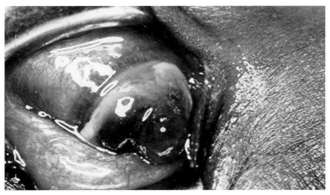

Fig. 27.25 Keratomalacia. This is a softening or coagulative necrosis of the cornea that occurs in chronic severe vitamin A deficiency. (Courtesy of Professor J. Waterlow.)

(see Fig. 27.21). A topical application of retinoic acid usually irritates the skin, producing dryness and erythema. These adverse effects are common during the first few weeks of therapy, and usually diminish with continued use.

A synthetic analog of vitamin A, 13-cis retinoic acid (isotretinoin), is effective orally and used for severe cystic acne (see Chapter 23). Common adverse effects resemble those of hypervitaminosis A. Teratogenicity is a major risk in pregnant women taking isotretinoin, and women of childbearing age must use effective contraception before starting retinoids. This risk may persist for months after therapy is stopped owing to prolonged residency of various retinoids in the body.

Another synthetic derivative of vitamin A, etretinate, is used topically for the treatment of psoriasis. Synthetic retinoids used in skin diseases have enhanced activity on epithelial differentiation combined with decreased systemic toxicity.

Toxicity

Hypervitaminosis A develops when the intake of retinoids greatly exceeds requirements. Symptoms include pruritus, dermatitis, skin desquamation, disturbed hair growth, fissures of the lips, headache, anorexia, fatigue, irritability, hemorrhage,

and congenital abnormalities. The adverse effects of systemic acne treatment described above essentially represent a state of hypervitaminosis A. As indicated above, retinoids such as isotretinoin should not be consumed by women who could become pregnant.

Vitamin D
Source

Vitamin D is found in fish liver oils, and egg yolk, and is synthesized in skin exposed to ultraviolet (UV) light. Essentially there are two sources of vitamin D:

- The diet provides vitamin D_3 (cholecalciferol) from animal sources and vitamin D_2 (ergocalciferol) from plant sources.
- Vitamin D_3 is synthesized in the skin from 7-dehydrocholesterol (produced in the wall of the intestine from cholesterol) by the action of UV light. Exposure of the face and hands to sunlight for 15 minutes is enough to supply the daily requirement of vitamin D. Dietary requirements of vitamin D are negligible for people who live in sunny areas or who spend much of their times outdoors. Vitamins D_2 and D_3 are equally effective as vitamins.

Structure and metabolic activation

Vitamin D is a family of sterol derivatives. It is a prehormone, which is converted in the body into a number of biologically active metabolites (Fig. 27.26). Vitamin D_3 is first converted to 25-hydroxyvitamin D_3 (25[OH]D_3, calcifediol) in the liver, and this is further converted in the kidneys to 1,25-dihydroxyvitamin D_3 (1,25[OH]$_2D_3$, calcitriol). A further metabolite with activity is 24,25-dihydroxyvitamin D_3 (24,25[OH]$_2D_3$); however, its physiologic role is less well understood.

Absorption

As with other fat-soluble vitamins, vitamin D is only optimally absorbed by the intestine when there is fat in the diet. After absorption, vitamin D_3 is transported in chylomicrons to the liver and stored with a carrier protein, vitamin D-binding protein. Vitamin D and its metabolites circulate in plasma bound to this protein. Excess vitamin D is stored in adipose tissue.

There are two major steps in the metabolism of vitamin D:
- The first process is 25-hydroxylation, which occurs in the liver.
- The second process is 1-hydroxylation in the kidney, which is stimulated by parathyroid hormone (PTH). A decreased ionized Ca^{2+} concentration in the plasma stimulates PTH secretion from the parathyroids (Fig. 27.27).

Biliary excretion is the major pathway of elimination, and 24-hydroxylation in the kidney is a preliminary step.

Functions

1,25[OH]$_2D_3$ acts as a hormone and plays an important role in Ca^{2+} homeostasis (see also Chapter 15). Together with PTH, it maintains plasma levels of Ca^{2+} by:
- Promoting intestinal absorption of Ca^{2+}.
- Increasing Ca^{2+} mobilization from bone.

581

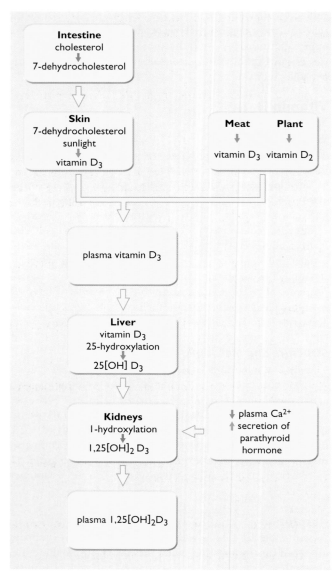

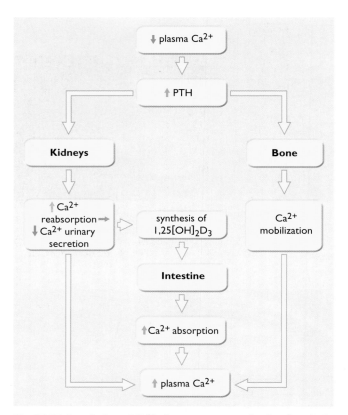

Fig. 27.27 Regulation of Ca²⁺ plasma concentration by vitamin D and parathyroid hormone (PTH). Vitamin D and PTH regulate plasma Ca²⁺ concentrations by acting on three main target tissues: intestine, kidney, and bone. A decrease in plasma Ca²⁺ concentration triggers increased secretion of PTH, which acts on the kidneys and bones. PTH in the kidneys promotes the synthesis of 1,25-dihydroxyvitamin D₃ (1,25[OH]₂D₃), which in turn increases gastrointestinal absorption of Ca²⁺. In other words, decreased plasma Ca²⁺ concentration leads to enhanced Ca²⁺ mobilization from bone, increased reabsorption in the kidneys, and facilitated absorption in the gut.

Fig. 27.26 Activation of vitamin D. Vitamin D (dietary and that synthesized in the skin) is converted in the body into a number of biologically active metabolites. Vitamin D₃ is first converted to 25-hydroxyvitamin D₃ (25[OH]D₃) in the liver, and this is further converted in the kidneys to 1,25-dihydroxyvitamin D₃ (1,25[OH]₂D₃).

- Decreasing Ca²⁺ excretion from the kidney (by enhancing renal reabsorption).

Physiologic concentrations of calcitonin have a negligible role in Ca²⁺ homeostasis in humans.

The concentrations of PTH and 1,25[OH]₂D₃ change in response to changes in calcium concentrations in plasma. These processes maintain plasma Ca²⁺ concentration at approximately 10.0 mg/100 ml.

Other functions of 1,25[OH]₂D₃ include:

- Enhanced bone formation by promoting osteoclast maturation and indirectly stimulating osteoclast activity.
- Cell differentiation.
- Inhibition of the growth of some carcinomas, especially breast cancer and malignant melanoma.

Deficiency

In the 1810s it was discovered that cod liver oil would cure rickets, the classical deficiency disease of vitamin D (Fig. 27.28a). The adult form of rickets is osteomalacia (Fig. 27.28b). Demineralization of bones results from the release of calcium into the plasma, which is triggered by PTH. People with a high risk of vitamin D deficiency include infants in whom dietary deficiency may be worsened by a lack of sunlight exposure, the elderly, and patients with renal failure in whom a deficiency of 1,25[OH]₂D₃ results from a lack of synthesis in the kidneys. Hypoparathyroidism and estrogen administration can decrease PTH levels and have similar effects. Fat malabsorption and alcohol consumption may also result in deficiency. The general signs of hypocalcemia are increased excitability including paresthesia, tetany, and increased neuromuscular excitability, laryngospasm, and convulsions.

Pharmacotherapeutic use

Plasma levels of Ca²⁺ provide the definition for hyper- and

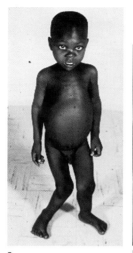
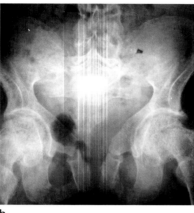

a   b

Fig. 27.28 Vitamin D deficiency. (a) Rickets causing gross deformity of the legs and pigeon chest in this boy. (Courtesy of Professor R. Hendrickse.) (b) Osteomalacia. The increased demands of pregnancy may result in gross deformity of the pelvis. (Courtesy of Dr G. D. Scarrow.)

hypocalcemic states. The pharmacotherapeutic uses of vitamin D (Fig. 27.29) are:
- To treat rickets (nutritional and metabolic), osteomalacia, and hypoparathyroidism. Metabolic rickets is usually treated with agents that do not require renal l-hydroxylation to become activated (e.g. calcitriol).
- To treat psoriasis when derivatives with no vitamin D activity (e.g. calcipotriol) may be used.
- Prevention and treatment of osteoporesis.

Toxicity

Hypercalcemia may be caused by excess vitamin D. Prolonged hypercalcemia produces initially reversible, but subsequently irreversible, renal damage and calcification of soft tissue, including that of the cardiovascular system. Hypervitaminosis

may be accompanied by growth retardation in children, fetal defects, reduced parathyroid function, and aortic stenosis.

Vitamin E
Source
Vitamin E is found in vegetable oils, wheat germ, leafy vegetables, egg yolk, margarines, and legumes.

Structure
α-Tocopherol is the most active of eight naturally occurring tocopherols with vitamin E activity. β-Tocopherol (wheat) and γ-tocopherol (corn and soya bean oils, margarines) are at least half as potent as the α form, whereas δ-tocopherol (sunflower oil) has almost no biologic activity.

Function
Vitamin E acts as an antioxidant, but this effect is of uncertain clinical significance.

Deficiency
Premature infants are at risk of vitamin E deficiency because there is poor transplacental transport.

Pharmacotherapeutic use
The only indication for vitamin E therapy is hemolytic anemia of the newborn.

Vitamin K
Source
Vitamin K is found in leafy vegetables, vegetable oils, and liver, and is synthesized by intestinal flora.

Structure
Vitamin K is a quinone derivative and there are two natural forms:
- Vitamin K_1 (phytonadione) is found in food.
- Vitamin K_2 (menaquinone) is synthesized by intestinal bacteria.

Forms of vitamin D and their clinical use

Name	Chemical name	Clinical use
Cholecalciferol	Vitamin D_3 (D_3)	Deficiency
Ergocalciferol	Vitamin D_2 (D_2)	Deficiency
Calcifediol	25-hydroxyvitamin D_3 (25[OH]D_3)	Deficiency
Calcitriol	1,25-dihydroxyvitamin D_3 (1,25[OH]$_2D_3$)	Deficiency
Secalcifediol	24,25-dihydroxyvitamin D_3 (24,25[OH]$_2D_3$)	None
Dihydrotachysterol		Deficiency
Calcipotriol		Psoriasis (experimental)

Fig. 27.29 Forms of vitamin D and their clinical use.

Vitamin K$_2$ is not a single compound, but a series of substances with varying lengths of side chain (n = 1–13); menaquinone-4 is the most biologically active form. Vitamin K$_3$ is a synthetic water-soluble derivative.

Functions

Vitamin K is essential for the formation of prothrombin and factors VII, IX, and X, which are glycoproteins with a number of γ-carboxyglutamic acid residues clustered at the N-terminal end of the peptide chain. Vitamin K is needed as a co-factor for this post-translational modification. During the carboxylation process, vitamin K is converted to its inactive oxide and then metabolized back to its active form (see Fig. 27.8). The reductive metabolism of the inactive vitamin K epoxide is warfarin sensitive. Warfarin and related drugs block the γ-carboxylation and this results in molecules that are biologically inactive for coagulation. Broad-spectrum antibiotics that alter gut bacterial flora decrease vitamin K production and can increase the effects of warfarin anticoagulation.

Deficiency

In 1935, Henrik Dam found that a factor was required to cure coagulation defects and this was named vitamin K ('koagulation factor').

Vitamin K deficiency causes hemorrhage due to prothrombin deficiency leading to a prolonged prothrombin time. Drug therapy with anticonvulsants (hydantoins) and antibiotics (neomycin) may result in a vitamin K deficiency. Newborns, especially those that are premature, are at risk of deficiency because of the low amount of vitamin K in breast milk and low intestinal synthesis. Fat malabsorption or dietary consumption of unabsorbed lipids such as mineral oil can also cause vitamin K deficiency.

Hepatic insufficiency precipitates the consequences of vitamin K deficiency as a result of the already compromised liver synthesis of coagulation factors.

Pharmacotherapeutic use

The major clinical use of vitamin K is to treat and/or prevent vitamin K deficiency, especially in newborns. It can be given parenterally to antagonize the effects of warfarin rapidly, but reversal of the anticoagulant effects is delayed owing to the time required to replenish the decreased plasma concentrations of vitamin K-dependent clotting factors.

Toxicity

Kernicterus, which is an abnormal accumulation of bilirubin in the central nervous system, may be caused by excess vitamin K.

TRACE ELEMENTS

Some elements, including certain metals, are essential for life. The most obvious example of such a metal is iron, without which, oxygen-carrying molecules and certain enzymes are unable to function. Iron is discussed in detail in Chapter 13. Other important elements such as potassium, sodium, magnesium, and iodine are discussed throughout the book.

Daily requirements of trace elements and minerals			
Daily requirements (mg)			
Trace elements		**Minerals**	
Chromium	0.12	Calcium	1000
Copper	2	Iron	15
Fluoride	2	Magnesium	400
Iodine	0.15	Phosphorus	1000
Manganese	2	Zinc	15
Molybdenum	0.075		
Selenium	0.075		

Fig. 27.30 Daily requirements of trace elements and minerals.

Some elements serve analogous functions to those of iron in terms of acting as essential co-factors for enzymes. These elements include the metals copper, zinc, selenium, manganese, molybdenum, and cobalt, as well as the ion fluoride.

Daily requirements of trace elements and minerals are listed in Fig. 27.30.

Deficiencies of trace elements

■ Copper deficiency has hematologic effects

Copper deficiency is very rare since the trace amounts required by the body occur in most foods. However, it can occur in Menkes' syndrome or following intestinal bypass surgery, or can be induced by an excessive intake of zinc. In copper deficiency, enzymes such as cytochrome oxidase are less active than normal, resulting in hematologic consequences such as leukopenia and mild anemia. Minute quantities (1–2 mg) of cupric sulfate added to the diet will resolve the deficiency.

■ Zinc deficiency affects nucleic acid metabolism

Zinc is important for nucleic acid metabolism and a lack of zinc is unusual because it is a common component of many foods. Genetic factors or inadequate parenteral nutrition can, however, cause deficiency. This results in a distinctive rash and a variety of unrelated conditions including hypogonadism, impaired wound healing, altered immune function, and depressed mental function. Oral zinc rapidly alleviates these symptoms. Zinc salts (acetate, gluconate) as lozenges were used for treating common cold with inconclusive results.

■ Selenium is a component of glutathione peroxidase

Selenium is an important component of glutathione peroxidase. Only microgram quantities (10–75 μg depending upon age) are required. This quantity is usually ingested in a normal diet, and so selenium deficiency is rare.

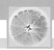

Whether reduced activity of glutathione peroxidase is associated with the myopathies (particularly cardiac) caused by selenium deficiency is unknown.

▓ Manganese deficiency can retard growth

Manganese plays an important role in mucopolysaccharide metabolism and deficiency can retard growth.

▓ Molybdenum deficiency produces symptoms of gout

Molybdenum deficiency produces symptoms of gout owing to its role in purine metabolism. In gout, urate crystals settle into the joints, and produce swelling of the joints accompanied with fevers.

▓ Fluoride deficiency leads to faulty tooth enamel and abnormal bone structure

Addition of fluoride to drinking water deficient in fluoride and to dental products, such as toothpaste, appears to reduce the incidence of caries in a population dramatically. This is a direct effect of fluoride's role in the development of tooth enamel.

Fluoride deficiency not only results in the production of faulty tooth enamel, but also causes abnormal bone structure. Where fluoride is not added to drinking water, the ingestion of fluoride tablets can be of value.

FURTHER READING

Guyton A (ed.) *Textbook of Medical Physiology*. Philadelphia: WB Saunders Company; 2000. [An excellent textbook on medical physiology.]

Lehninger AL (ed.) *Lehninger Principles of Biochemistry*. New York: Worth Publishers; 2000. [An excellent textbook on biochemistry.]

Quinn PJ (ed.) *Subcellular Biochemistry*, volume 30: Fat soluble vitamins. New York: Plenum Press; 1998. [Biochemical aspects of fat soluble vitamins.]

Rolfes SR, DeBruyne LK, Whitney EN (eds) *Life span Nutrition, Conception through Life*. New York: Wadsworth Publishing Company; 1998. [Detailed and comprehensive information on the role of vitamins in nutrition.]

Sherwood L (ed.) *Human Physiology: from Cells to Systems*. Thomson Publishing; 1997. [A well-written and highly illustrated textbook on human physiology.]

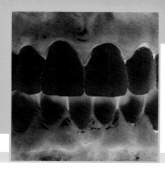

Chapter 28

Drug Use in Dentistry

PHYSIOLOGY OF THE ORAL CAVITY

The teeth and supporting tissues provide the initial digestive processes essential to all bodily activities. Chewing and swallowing are carried out by specialized oral tissues, such as the teeth, tongue, salivary glands, and muscles of mastication. The maxillary and mandibular dentition articulate via the temporomandibular joint in a specific pattern to generate the forces needed for mastication. Chewing pressures and oral sensations are mediated by the trigeminal nerve in response to information provided by proprioceptive nerves in the oral tissues.

The salivary glands produce more than a liter of saliva daily to lubricate the oral tissues, facilitate taste, and initiate the digestive process.

The teeth and other oral tissues

■ *Tooth structure, the oral mucosa, and the salivary glands are important in health and in dental disease*

The tooth crown is composed of a crystalline and highly mineralized (96%) calcified tissue, the enamel. Dentin, a less-mineralized tissue, forms the bulk of the tooth structure and protects the vital tooth pulp throughout the root length. The dental pulp contains loose connective tissue, blood vessels, and nerves. Odontoblasts, which produce the dentin, are found at the interface between the pulp tissue and dentin, with projections extending into the dentinal tubules. Finally, the root is covered with a calcified connective tissue structure, the cementum (Fig. 28.1). Carious lesions expanding into the dentin, or surgical removal of enamel during treatment, exposes the dentinal tubules to external stimuli and painful sensations.

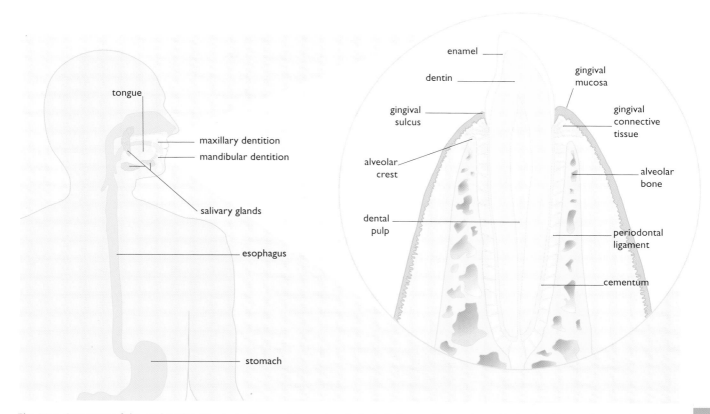

Fig. 28.1 Structure of the oral cavity. The major tissues of the oral cavity include the maxillary and mandibular dentition and supporting tissues, the tongue, and the salivary glands, all of which function together to initiate the digestion of food and nutrients.

Teeth are attached to the maxillary and mandibular alveolar bone by the supporting structures of the teeth, which are termed the periodontium. Alveolar bone is unique because its primary function is to support the teeth and it will gradually disappear as teeth are lost. The periodontal ligament is located between the alveolar bone and cementum, and contains fibers specifically arranged to connect the teeth with alveolar bone. This arrangement allows for subtle tooth movement in response to the forces of mastication.

Oral mucosa

The buccal mucosa is similar to other mucosal tissues, but the gingival mucosa in proximity to the teeth and covering the periodontium is a specialized mucosa. The mucosal attachment to the tooth, near the cemento-enamel junction, creates a ring of unattached gingival tissue, which forms a small space between the mucosa and tooth (i.e. the gingival sulcus or crevice). The depth of the gingival sulcus in relation to the height of the gingival attachment are important in the diagnosis and treatment of periodontal disease.

Salivary glands

Adequate salivary flow and composition are essential for maintaining healthy oral tissues. Saliva consists of water and mucin combined with minerals, enzymes, and immune components. It initiates digestion of some food stuffs, functions as a lubricant to protect mucosal tissues, and facilitates mastication. It is also involved in taste perception and caries prevention and as a factor influencing the microbial environment of the mouth.

DISEASES OF THE ORAL CAVITY

Dental plaque, caries, and gingivitis

◾ *Most dental diseases are associated with micro-organisms, infection, and the resulting inflammatory response*

Dental plaque

Caries and gingivitis are common dental diseases and are related to the formation of dental plaque. Plaque is a soft nonmineralized deposit consisting of micro-organisms in a glycoprotein matrix. It begins as a pellicle of salivary proteins adhering to the enamel surface. Oral micro-organisms colonize the pellicle forming the plaque, and can account for up to 70% of the plaque content. The varieties of plaque micro-organisms play a key role in the development of dental disease. If plaque is removed or reduced through regular dental hygiene practice, the incidence of dental caries, gingivitis, and periodontitis is significantly reduced. Plaque that has become mineralized is called dental calculus (tartar).

Dental caries

Dental caries or decay is probably the most universal and common of all reported dental diseases. Caries development is a time-dependent event involving a critical relationship between the host, plaque micro-organisms, metabolic acid production and diet. *Streptococcus mutans* is generally regarded as the most cariogenic micro-organism, but *Lactobacillus* species are also implicated in some types of carious lesions. Acid production associated with a combination of cariogenic micro-organisms and a cariogenic diet including sucrose or other rapidly digestible carbohydrates furthers the progression of demineralization and the development of carious lesions. Factors that reduce saliva production can also contribute to the development of dental caries (Fig. 28.2). Once caries reaches the dentinal tissues, it progresses in a more diffuse pattern.

Gingivitis (inflammation of the gingiva)

Gingivitis describes the inflammatory reaction of the gingival mucosa in close proximity to the teeth to a variety of etiologic agents including plaque micro-organisms.

- Plaque-associated gingivitis is common, particularly in people with poor oral hygiene. It is usually asymptomatic except for localized bleeding during brushing. If plaque and calculus deposits expand into the gingival crevice, the nature of the micro-organisms changes to an anaerobe-dominated bacterial population and leads to more serious infections of the periodontium.

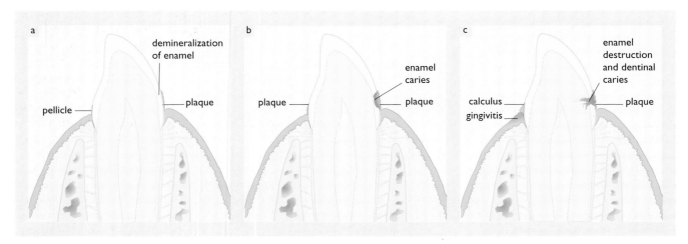

Fig. 28.2 Development of pellicle, plaque, calculus, and gingivitis and progression of dental caries. Colonization of dental plaque with cariogenic micro-organisms can progress to demineralization (a), enamel caries (b), and dentinal caries (c). Plaque bacteria can induce an inflammatory gingivitis.

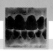

Diseases of the oral cavity

- Plaque is an important factor in dental disease
- Caries is the most common dental disease
- Gingivitis is the inflammatory reaction to plaque micro-organisms
- Preventive dental medicine can reduce the incidence of these diseases
- Early dental intervention is the key to controlling dental disease

- Acute necrotizing ulcerative gingivitis (ANUG) is an acute painful form of gingival infection associated with fusiform and spirochete organisms, with a clinical presentation very different from that of the inflammatory gingivitis of plaque. Ulcerated and highly inflamed gingival tissues are typically observed. Fever and lymphadenopathy may also be part of the acute presentation.

Systemic factors may also play a role in gingivitis.

Management

Dental plaque, caries, and gingivitis are three distinct presentations of dental disease, but are uniquely linked as a focus for preventive dental medicine.

▪ Removal of plaque and calculus (oral prophylaxis and scaling) from tooth surfaces is a major part of the overall preventive program

Over-the-counter (OTC) mouth rinses have limited benefits in controlling plaque and calculus. Chlorhexidine gluconate oral rinse reduces plaque bacteria and gingivitis with twice-daily use, but must be used in conjunction with appropriate dental treatment. Its use in other oral mucosal diseases is discussed later. Dentifrices containing other antibacterial agents, including triclosan and fluoride, are also promoted for plaque control. Calculus-control toothpastes containing pyrophosphate or zinc salts are designed to prevent supragingival calculus formation and do not affect existing calculus.

CHLORHEXIDINE GLUCONATE is a bisquanide, cationic agent with antibacterial action. The cationic portion of the molecule binds to negatively charged bacterial cell components altering cell osmotic dynamics with leakage of cellular ions. In higher concentrations, chlorhexidine is bactericidal as it causes precipitation of cellular contents. The spectrum of activity of chlorhexidine includes many Gram-positive and Gram-negative micro-organisms which have been implicated in dental disease. Examples are *S. mutans*, *Porphyromonas gingivalis*, *Prevotella intermedia*, *Bacteroides forsythus* and *Campylobacter rectus*.

Chlorhexidine is indicated for use as adjunctive treatment to prophylaxis and scaling to reduce plaque formation and for control of gingivitis. It is administered as an oral rinse (0.12% to 0.2%). Twice daily rinses (15 ml for 30 seconds and expectorated) are initiated after prophylaxis and scaling for use between dental appointments. Up to 30% of chlorhexidine is retained in the oral cavity after rinsing and is slowly released over 12 hours. The sustained action is believed to be related to binding to oral tissues, namely the hydroxyapatite of tooth enamel, the pellicle, the oral mucosa and salivary proteins. Rinsing with water, eating or drinking must be avoided for at least 30 minutes after use.

Because chlorhexidine is used topically, systemic side effects are rarely noted as limited amounts will be swallowed. Repeated use of chlorhexidine rinses is associated with discoloration of teeth and alteration of taste in some patients. The discoloration is superficial and easily removed by professional tooth polishing. Chlorhexidine is contraindicated in patients with a positive history of hypersensitivity to the drug.

▪ Treatment and prevention of dental caries includes plaque control and the use of systemic and/or topical fluorides

Fluoride in the water supply and in a multitude of dental products has significantly reduced the incidence of dental caries in children in developed countries, but dental caries in areas where fluoride is not available remains a major dental concern.

Treatment and prevention of dental caries includes:
- Removal of all carious lesions.
- Oral hygiene to reduce dental plaque.
- Dental sealants to cover pits and fissures in tooth structure.
- Cariogenic diet control.
- Systemic or topical fluorides.

SYSTEMIC AND TOPICAL FLUORIDES IN DENTISTRY The beneficial effect of fluoride in caries prevention was initially recognized in the 1930s. In many countries, multiple fluoride preparations are available for systemic or topical application to prevent dental caries. Maximum benefits accrue when fluoride use is coupled with a program of regular preventive dental care. Other uses of fluoride, depending on the product selected, include a reduction in tooth sensitivity due to exposed dentinal or cemental surfaces, remineralization of incipient carious lesions, and some reduction in gingivitis.

The anticariogenic action of fluoride is not completely defined, but may reside in the diverse effects of fluoride. Data show that fluoride interacts with the hydroxyapatite of enamel to produce fluorhydroxyapatite. This later compound is less soluble in acids originating from sugar metabolism by plaque bacteria. Fluoride has also been shown to decrease the population of *S. mutans*, and to interfere with metabolism in plaque bacteria. Other data show that fluoride promotes the remineralization of demineralized enamel in incipient carious lesions. Other sources of fluoride include a variety of fluoride rinses, dentifrices and gels and stannous fluoride solutions, all of which are intended for topical application.

Sodium fluoride tablets are available to supplement systemic fluoride ingestion in the presence of inadequate fluoridated water supplies. Fluoride is absorbed rapidly (80 to 90%) from the upper GI tract with peak blood levels occurring in approximately 30 minutes. It is widely distributed to calcified tissues, bone and teeth, with up to 50% of the daily intake deposited in calcified tissues. Renal clearance accounts for most of the excreted dose. Systemic fluorides are generally administered

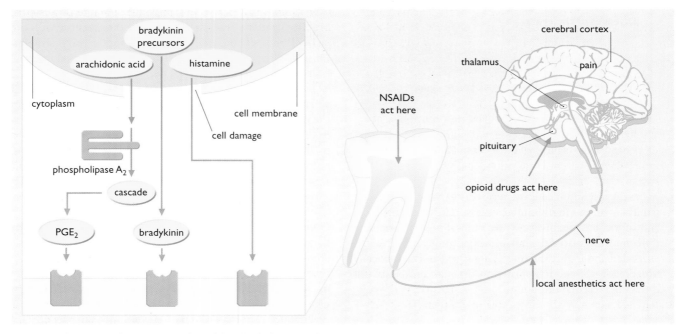

Fig. 28.3 Diagrammatic representation of the sites of action of opioids, nonsteroidal anti-inflammatory drugs (NSAIDs), and local anesthetic drugs when used for acute dental pain. Opioids act within the central nervous system to alter pain perception; aspirin and NSAIDs inhibit prostaglandin (PG) synthesis at the site of injury, and local anesthetics block transmission of the noxious stimulus.

with water or juice as dairy products substantially reduce fluoride absorption. Systemic fluoride should not be prescribed when the water content of fluoride exceeds 0.6 ppm. Daily sodium fluoride doses, which vary among countries, are established and published by various dental organizations. Fluoride supplementation must take into account the total daily amount of naturally ingested fluoride from all sources, the climate (in hot climates more water is consumed) and the patient's age, weight and physical status.

Adverse effects of supplemental systemic or topical fluorides are usually limited to gastrointestinal complaints associated with excessive fluoride ingestion, and occur infrequently. However, the use of prescribed fluorides and topical home fluoride products in very young children should be supervised to avoid excessive ingestion. Side effects include nausea with or without vomiting, excessive salivation and abdominal pain. Severe toxicity, requiring medical attention, may occur with accidental ingestion of larger amounts (10 to 20 mg in children). Chronic ingestion of excessive fluoride can lead to the development of dental fluorosis, an unsightly staining of the teeth.

Acute dental pain

Pain as a general topic, and the principles of its treatment are covered in detail in Chapter 14.

Acute pain associated with dental disease is probably the most common complaint of dental patients. Any injury to the oral tissues leads to the release of inflammatory mediators and signs of inflammation including pain. Prostaglandins have been implicated in the genesis of dental pain as their action is associated with sensitization of trigeminal afferent nerve endings to other inflammatory mediators, such as bradykinin

or histamine (Fig. 28.3). Acute oral pain is a symptom of many orofacial diseases including acute infection, mucosal lesions, obstructed salivary gland ducts, and tissue trauma.

Early carious lesions are often associated with acute transient pain that is readily alleviated by dental treatment. However, untreated carious lesions continue to destroy tooth structure, allowing oral micro-organisms to invade pulpal tissues. Pulpal infection leads to the development of painful inflammation or to an acute periapical abscess and persistent pain. If left untreated this infection can rapidly extend from the alveolar bone into adjacent soft tissues resulting in a cellulitis.

Determining the etiology of dental pain is sometimes complicated because pain can be referred from other tissues such as the sinuses, the ears, and temporomandibular joint.

◼ *Oral surgery, periodontal therapy, or other dental treatment can cause pain*

The pain caused by oral surgical intervention, periodontal therapy, or other dental treatment is invariably accompanied by inflammation and pain. Indeed, the fear of pain from dental treatment prompts many to avoid or defer treatment. Dental pain intensity can range from mild to severe depending on the individual patient, the disease presentation, and the type of dental treatment, and it can be as unbearable as any other type of pain. Acute pain following dental treatment is usually most intense during the first 12–24 hours after treatment and declines over the next 2–3 days.

Management

Management of acute orofacial pain begins with diagnosis and appropriate dental treatment. Systemically administered drugs, or local anesthetic drugs, either alone or in combination, are

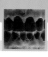
most frequently used for controlling acute orofacial pain, especially before and immediately after definitive dental treatment. Opioids with a favorable oral-to-parenteral effectiveness ratio are preferred, as is the oral route of administration. Acute orofacial pain of moderate intensity or greater can be effectively managed with opioid drugs. Opioids act centrally to modify pain perception by interacting with multiple opiate receptors and mimicking endogenous opioid peptides (see Chapter 14). Sedation and euphoria often accompany opioid analgesia as an added benefit in controlling the emotional component of pain. Opioids are rarely used alone for acute dental pain and are frequently combined with aspirin, NSAIDs or acetaminophen. Detailed discussion of these and related drugs and their use in acute pain syndromes is found in Chapter 20. Local anesthetic drugs with or without vasoconstrictors are essential for the control of pain during dental surgery and treatment. Vasoconstrictive drugs are used in combination with local anesthetics to prolong the duration of action by delaying absorption of the local anesthetic drug. A secondary benefit of the vasoconstrictive drug is local control of bleeding during soft tissue surgery. The pharmacology of local anesthetics is described in detail in Chapter 26.

Examples of local anesthetics/vasoconstrictors commonly used in dentistry:

Amide local anesthetics:
- Lidocaine with and without epinephrine.
- Mepivacaine with and without levonordefrin.
- Prilocaine with and without epinephrine.
- Etidocaine with epinephrine.
- Bupivacaine with epinephrine.
- Articaine with epinephrine.

Ester local anesthetics:
- Chlorprocaine with epinephrine.
- Tetracaine (topical only).
- Benzocaine (topical only).

DRUG COMBINATIONS An alternative strategy for controlling postoperative dental pain has been advocated using combinations of NSAIDs and long-acting local anesthetics. Of the later, both etidocaine and bupivacaine provide analgesia well into the post-treatment period when the anticipated pain response is greatest. A normal dose of an NSAID is taken soon after treatment and before the return of normal oral sensations. This combination of drugs has been shown to reduce the intensity of pain in the immediate post-treatment period and reduce the need for opioid medications. Pretreatment NSAIDs have also been advocated to help reduce the intensity of pain in the immediate post-treatment period, but the effects are variable.

Chronic orofacial pain

In contrast to acute pain, chronic orofacial pain is complicated by a myriad of patient and diagnostic issues. It may result from conditions that initiate acute pain, but many other causes must be considered because the etiology can be elusive.

The pattern of chronic orofacial pain, its persistent nature, and the patient's frustration with unsuccessful treatment modalities, are associated with psychologic and behavioral responses that must be considered in all management schemes.

Chronic orofacial pain can arise from:
- Inflammation or internal derangements of the temporomandibular joint.
- Myalgia associated with the oral and facial musculature.
- Lesions in the central nervous system.

The diagnosis and management of chronic orofacial pain frequently requires a multidisciplinary approach. Examples of therapy can include selected medications, restoration of occlusal disharmony with dental appliances, surgical intervention, psychologic intervention, and physiotherapy.

Management

 Drugs are used to control both the pain and associated symptoms

The NSAIDs are used for the symptomatic management of pain associated with injury or inflammatory processes. The best results are usually obtained using adequate doses to control the symptoms and regular administration for a sufficient time to evaluate responses. Longer-acting NSAIDs with once- or twice-daily dosing are generally preferred. Opioids should be limited to longer-acting drugs, used only to initiate pain control or completely avoided because of the possibility of dependence, unless the pain is due to oral cancer.

Tricyclic antidepressants (see Chapter 14) may be used to alleviate pain and symptoms such as depression and altered sleep patterns. The pain of trigeminal neuralgia responds to the anticonvulsant drugs, carbamazepine and phenytoin (see Chapter 14).

Centrally acting skeletal muscle relaxants, methocarbamol or cyclobenzaprine, are sometimes useful if myalgia or muscle spasm is present. Drugs used for chronic facial pain should not be considered as curative, but a positive response can be useful in making a more definitive diagnosis.

 Management of acute dental pain

- Match choice of drug to intensity of pain
- Nonsteroidal anti-inflammatory drugs are effective for controlling dental pain
- Use combination of long-acting local anesthetics and nonsteroidal anti-inflammatory drugs
- Consider pain referred from other orofacial tissues

Adverse effects of analgesic drugs

- *The most common adverse effects of opioids at pharmacotherapeutic doses are nausea, sedation, and dizziness*
- *The most common adverse effect of nonsteroidal anti-inflammatory drugs is gastrointestinal irritation*
- *The most common adverse effects of local anesthetics are usually psychogenic, such as syncope and anxiety*

Anxiety

A visit to the dentist is such an intimidating experience for many patients that they avoid dental care until the pain demands emergency attention. Dentists have long been portrayed as the harbingers of pain, so reinforcing the patient's anxiety. However, modern dental practice employs a variety of behavioral modifying techniques and anxiolytic drugs which has made a visit to the dentist less threatening for the majority of anxious patients.

Management

To overcome fear and anxiety, both behavioral and pharmacologic methods of pain and anxiety control have been developed. The use of anxiolytics and their cellular and molecular mechanisms of action are described in detail in Chapter 14. Sedation techniques include the use of a variety of drugs given by several routes of administration. Sedative drug selection is dependent on the degree of anxiety, the patient's medical status, the dental procedure, and the professional training of the dentist. Mild anxiety can be effectively controlled with oral doses of benzodiazepines (see Chapter 14). Examples include diazepam, triazolam, lorazepam and midazolam from the benzodiazepine group of drugs. Promethazine or hydroxyzine alone, or in combination with meperidine, is often used in sedation procedures for children. However, the quality of oral sedation is not always predictable and may be inadequate for an extremely anxious patient.

NITROUS OXIDE USE IN DENTISTRY Inhalation sedation with nitrous oxide–oxygen is an important modality for the management of fear and anxiety in dental patients. Concentrations ranging from 25% to 50% nitrous oxide in oxygen, administered by nasal mask, are commonly used to provide sedation sufficient for the mildly anxious dental patient. Patients are responsive to commands and remain conscious throughout the procedure with intact protective reflexes. Limited analgesia may be evident in some patients. The pharmacokinetics of nitrous oxide dictate the advantages of this technique including rapid onset, ease in regulation of sedation depth, and rapid recovery. Nitrous oxide–oxygen delivery systems are equipped with failsafe regulators limiting the concentration of administered nitrous oxide to 50%. Local anesthetics are used in combination with nitrous oxide conscious sedation to ensure adequate pain control. Limitations to the use of nitrous oxide sedation include uncooperative patients and upper airway obstruction. Yet, for the extremely anxious patient, this modality may not be adequate.

Nitrous oxide–oxygen dental units are equipped with scavenger systems to reduce trace concentrations of nitrous oxide in the confines of the dental operatory. This is important as chronic exposure to high levels of trace anesthetic gases have been implicated in preterm abortion and infertility. Recovery from nitrous oxide sedation is usually uneventful and only occasionally accompanied by nausea and headache. Nitrous oxide sedation is sometimes combined with orally administered anxiolytic drugs for the more anxious patient and additional doses of local anesthetic as more procedures are attempted per appointment. This requires careful attention to drug doses and patient monitoring as excessive CNS depression and toxicity can result especially in the pediatric patient.

INTRAVENOUS SEDATION is ideal for the very anxious patient and for more extensive dental procedures. Again, midazolam or diazepam alone or in combination with meperidine has been extensively employed. Other drugs suitable for i.v. administration include the rapid acting barbiturates or opioids such as fentanyl. Intravenous administration of sedative drugs allows for controlled induction and dose titration for adjustment to a desired sedation level. Parenteral sedation requires additional training and in many areas, certification, to establish qualifications for the use of this modality of sedation. Patient monitoring is paramount to ensure safe use of any sedation technique.

Acute odontogenic infections

The general principles of treatment of bacterial and viral infections are described in Chapters 9 and 8, respectively.

Dental caries, periodontal disease, acute periapical abscesses, salivary gland infections, and many other oral infections are caused by micro-organisms that are part of the normal oral flora. Other oral infections are caused by micro-organisms introduced into the oral cavity by trauma (staphylococcus) or other means (herpes).

Separate microenvironments within the oral cavity account for the growth of aerobic and both facultative and obligate anaerobic micro-organisms existing in a commensal relationship. As a result, most odontogenic bacterial infections are caused by a mix of pathogens with significant involvement of both facultative and obligate anaerobes. Aerobic streptococci and, to a lesser extent, staphylococci along with fungi (yeast) are also part of the normal oral flora and are potential pathogens.

■ *Odontogenic oral infections cause fever, malaise, swelling, pain, and pus formation*

Odontogenic oral infections can present with acute symptoms of fever, malaise, swelling, and pain. Redness and pus formation may be evident, depending on the site of the infection. Pulpal infection often expands to the periapical tissues, with involvement of alveolar bone if dental treatment is delayed. At this point, pain will usually prompt the patient to seek dental care, but the abscess may continue to spread from the alveolar bone until it opens onto a soft tissue surface as an intraoral fistula. With an avenue of drainage for the abscess, either through the tooth or soft tissue fistula, acute symptoms often abate and the infection assumes a chronic status. However, the infection may also spread diffusely in soft tissues with resulting cellulitis. Rarely, the infection will spread from a mandibular site, dissecting along the facial planes into the neck or, from a maxillary site, spreading to the cavernous sinus of the brain. These latter infections can create life-threatening situations and require aggressive treatment.

Management

Acute odontogenic infections are best managed with a combination of dental intervention and antibiotic therapy.

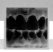

How to manage an acute dental infection

- Recognize the cardinal signs of infection
- Consider the integrity of the patient's immune system
- Know which are the potential oral pathogens
- Match the antibiotic's spectrum to the causative pathogens
- Incise and drain any abscess if possible

If an abscess is pointing, surgical incision and drainage are indicated

Drainage can also be achieved by opening into the pulp chamber of an infected tooth if soft tissue incision is not feasible.

Self-limiting infections may respond to dental treatment without the use of antibiotics.

For most dental infections, selection of an antibiotic drug is empirical

For most dental infections, antibiotic drug selection is based on the presenting symptoms, the location of the infection, a knowledge of the micro-organisms usually associated with the type of infection, and experience (Fig. 28.4) (see below). Antibiotic drugs selected for acute odontogenic infections should have a spectrum that includes streptococcal species and anaerobic bacteria. Fortunately, most micro-organisms that cause common oral infections have remained sensitive to traditional antibiotic drugs. However, laboratory culturing and sensitivity tests should be performed if the infection fails to respond as expected, when sampling without contamination can be accomplished, and in osteomyelitis. As sophisticated deoxyribonucleic acid probes become available, dentists should be able to identify causative pathogens more readily to facilitate drug selection.

Penicillin V potassium remains a drug of first choice for many acute odontogenic infections

Penicillin V potassium is bactericidal and has a spectrum that includes the streptococcal and anaerobic organisms frequently encountered in acute infections. Amoxicillin is also favored as a first choice because of its oral bioavailability and its effectiveness against some Gram-negative organisms. Penicillin G or ampicillin is preferred for parenteral administration. Erythromycin and related macrolides are used as alternative drugs for the penicillin-allergic patient and if the infection is less severe. However, clindamycin has a favorable Gram-positive and anaerobic spectrum of action and is considered by many as the alternative choice to penicillin.

Cephalosporins are seldom drugs of first choice, but are used when staphylococcal organisms are involved, for example in cases of osteomyelitis or oral trauma.

Metronidazole, which has an anaerobic spectrum, is rapidly becoming a drug of choice for selected periodontal infections. It is most often used in combination with another antibiotic with a desirable aerobic spectrum.

Tetracyclines are generally limited to infections associated with the periodontium, but are also used as an alternative to penicillin V in the treatment of actinomycosis.

The role of the quinolone antibiotics for common dental infections remains to be established. There are recent data to suggest limited use in some in oral infections where culture and sensitivity testing indicate a favorable clinical outcome.

Drug interactions of antibiotics used in dentistry are given in Fig. 28.5.

Periodontal infections

Periodontitis (infection of the periodontium) can present in several acute or chronic forms and with different etiologies. In adults it is typically chronic with symptoms limited to an erythematous-appearing gingiva that bleeds on probing or brushing. The distinguishing feature of periodontal disease is a continuing infection of the supporting tissues of the teeth, resulting in a progressive loss of gingival attachment and alveolar bone. It is the most common cause of tooth loss in adult patients.

Periodontitis often goes undetected until the patient presents with loose teeth or an acute exacerbation. People reporting bleeding gums or the presence of blood on the toothbrush should be referred for dental evaluation. In the younger age group it can present as a juvenile periodontitis.

Antibiotic drugs used for oral infections

Penicillins	Penicillin V potassium Amoxicillin Amoxicillin with clavulanate Ampicillin
Tetracyclines	Tetracycline Doxycycline Minocycline
Cephalosporins	Cephalexin Cefaclor
Macrolides	Erythromycin Azithromycin Clarithromycin
Clindamycin	
Metronidazole	

Fig. 28.4 Antibiotic drugs used for oral infections.

Adverse effects of antibiotics

- All antibiotics can cause gastrointestinal adverse effects and diarrhea
- Allergic reactions occur more frequently with the penicillins
- Anti-infectives alter the normal flora causing a risk of opportunistic candidiasis, especially in immunosuppressed patients
- Tetracycline use in children causes permanent gray–yellow mottling of teeth

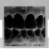

Drug interactions of antibiotics used in dentistry

All antibiotics	Reduced effectiveness of oral contraceptives Effectiveness of bactericidal drugs may be reduced when combined with bacteriostatic antibiotics
Penicillins and cephalosporins	Probenecid inhibits renal excretion and prolongs duration of action Allopurinol increases the risk of non-allergic skin rashes in patients taking ampicillin Bioavailability of atenolol may be decreased by ampicillin
Macrolides	Concurrent use with terfenadine, astemizole, or cisapride may result in serious cardiac arrhythmias (torsades de pointes syndrome) May increase serum levels of theophylline, lithium, carbamazepine, valproic acid, cyclosporine, and digoxin Compete with clindamycin for 50S ribosomal binding site in micro-organisms Increase bioavailability of triazolam enhancing the level of sedation Erythromycin may increase the effects of oral anticoagulants, therefore monitor blood clotting times
Tetracyclines	Absorption impaired when given concurrently with antacids, dairy products, or iron salts Barbiturates, phenytoin, ethanol, and carbamazepine may increase hepatic metabolism of doxycycline
Clindamycin	Increases effects of nondepolarizing neuromuscular junction blockers Absorption impaired when given with kaolin or antacids Competes with erythromycin for 50S ribosomal binding sites in micro-organisms
Metronidazole	Avoid concurrent use with ethanol, ethanol-containing products, and disulfiram May potentiate warfarin oral anticoagulants, so monitor blood clotting times Barbiturates can decrease its effectiveness Can increase serum lithium levels

Fig. 28.5 Drug interactions of antibiotics used in dentistry.

Management

◼ *Periodontal disease is controlled by reducing the number of micro-organisms infecting the periodontium*

Controlling periodontal disease involves a variety of treatment modalities, all of which are designed to reduce the numbers of micro-organisms infecting the periodontium. Earlier in this chapter, the control of plaque and gingivitis was presented as a way of reducing the numbers of supragingival micro-organisms, and bacteria in plaque contribute to the inflammatory aspect of periodontal disease. However, if there is microbial invasion of the deeper tissues of the periodontium, systemic anti-infective drugs, irrigation with anti-infectives, and surgical débridement may be required to control the disease.

Systemic anti-infective drugs should include drugs that are effective against multiple anaerobic organisms. Selection depends on the causative organisms and antibiotic sensitivity. Tetracyclines and amoxicillin alone or in combination with metronidazole or even ciprofloxacin have been used. Recently, a low dose (20 mg, twice daily) doxycycline product has been introduced. It appears that this dose has no antimicrobial activity, rather it acts by inhibition of crevicular bacterial collagenase responsible for injury to the periodontium. In addition, specialty doses forms, including a tetracycline-containing monofilament fiber, a doxycycline polymer gel, a metronidazole gel, minocycline powder, and a chlorhexidine, resorbable chip have been developed for adjunctive treatment in refractory periodontal disease. The gels, fiber, powder or chip are placed into the periodontal pocket around the tooth while the drug is slowly released over several days. Contraindications to the use of the specialty doses forms include the presence of an acute, periodontal abscess or hypersensitivity to the individual drug component.

Prophylactic use of anti-infective drugs in dentistry

The prophylactic use of antibiotics in dentistry is not generally required for routine dental treatment in patients without risk factors and with a normally functioning immune system. However, selected patients with pre-existing myocardial or valvular pathology may be at risk for endocarditis secondary to a bacteremia. Certain dental procedures, including extractions, oral and maxillofacial surgery, periodontal therapy, deep scaling, and other dental procedures are associated with a transient bacteremia that usually lasts less than 15–20 minutes. Selected oral micro-organisms have been implicated as a cause of infective endocarditis in patients at risk.

Advisory groups throughout the world have established guidelines for antibiotic prophylaxis for patients at risk. Amoxicillin, penicillin V potassium, or other suitable alternative drug (clindamycin, a macrolide or cephalosporin) is usually recommended for prophylactic use immediately prior to the dental procedure.

◼ *Prophylaxis guidelines to prevent bacterial endocarditis are not intended for other 'at risk' patients*

There is considerable debate about the risks and benefits and drug choice for patients with joint prostheses; however, prophylaxis may be considered for patients with a compromised

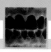

Patients 'at risk' of spreading bacterial infection and requiring antibiotic prophylaxis

Bacterial endocarditis can develop in patients with:

Prosthetic cardiac valves (bioprosthetic and homograft)
A previous history of bacterial endocarditis
Surgically constructed systemic–pulmonary shunts
Complex congenital cyanotic cardiac malformations
Rheumatic and other acquired valvular dysfunction
Hypertrophic cardiomyopathy
Mitral valve prolapse with regurgitation

Other types of infection may develop in patients with:

A compromised immune system

Need for prophylaxis and antibiotic choice made after consultation between the physician and dentist if the patient has:

Organ or tissue transplants
Traumatic orofacial wounds
Chemotherapy for cancer
Vascular grafts
A major joint prosthesis
Renal dialysis
Insulin-dependent diabetes mellitus

Fig. 28.6 Patients 'at risk' of spreading bacterial infection and requiring antibiotic prophylaxis.

immune system. Recommended guidelines cannot address every patient situation, and consultation between the physician and dentist is advised. 'At risk' patients with poor oral hygiene, extensive caries, gingivitis, or periodontitis should be placed on a dental treatment program that includes elimination and prevention of dental disease (Fig. 28.6).

Common diseases of the oral mucosa
Candida *infections*

Candida albicans is the most common cause of an oral yeast infection. The incidence of oral candidiasis has increased in recent years, and is particularly common among people with

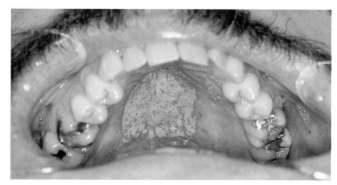

Fig. 28.7 Acute candidiasis of the palatal mucosa. The lesions produce an erythematous oral mucosa covered with white patches. (Courtesy of Dr John Wright.)

human immunodeficiency virus (HIV) infection or other causes of immunosuppression. Decreases in saliva flow associated with Sjogren's syndrome or the use of drugs that decrease salivary flow contribute to the risk of candidiasis.

The lesions of candidiasis are seen on the buccal and palatal oral mucosa and the tongue (Fig. 28.7), and can produce an angular cheilitis. Erythematous mucosal lesions appearing on a tissue-bearing surface for a denture prosthesis are typically the result of a *Candida* infection.

MANAGEMENT Antifungal drugs (see Chapter 10) used for the treatment of candidiasis include:
- The topical agents nystatin, clotrimazole, amphotericin B and chlorhexidine.
- The systemic agents fluconazole, itraconazole and ketoconazole.

Nystatin is the drug of choice for acute candidiasis

The drug of choice for acute candidiasis is nystatin, which can be used as a topical rinse, ointment, or lozenge. Chlorhexidine rinse is also effective. Candidiasis in denture wearers can also be treated with topical nystatin, but resolution of the infection can be difficult because the organism attaches to the denture base and is a potential source of re-inoculation. Soaking the denture in nystatin or chlorhexidine solutions or remaking the denture is usually required. Patient compliance for a topical regimen can become a problem. Systemic ketoconazole or fluconazole (Fig. 28.8) may be required for:
- The noncompliant patient.
- The treatment of chronic atrophic candidiasis.
- Candidiasis in the immunocompromised patient.

Oral viral infections
Viral infection and its treatment in general terms are dealt with in detail in Chapter 8.

Drug interactions with systemic antifungal drugs

Ketoconazole

Concurrent use with terfenadine, astemizole, and cisapride not indicated due to high risk of arrhythmias (torsades de pointes)

May increase serum levels of cyclosporine

Risk of hepatotoxicity with ethanol and other hepatotoxic drugs

Decreased bioavailability when given with antacids and histamine H_2 antagonists

Fluconazole

Increases effects of warfarin oral anticoagulants, so monitor blood clotting times

Increases plasma levels of phenytoin, tacrolimus, and possibly cyclosporine

Fig. 28.8 Drug interactions with systemic antifungal drugs.

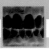

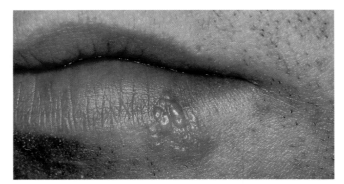

Fig. 28.9 Recurrent herpes labialis. The lesions present with multiple vesicle formation at the vermilion border of the lip extending to the skin of the face. (Courtesy of Dr John Wright.)

▪ Herpes viruses cause most oral viral infections

An initial herpes infection can manifest in an adult or child as an acute herpetic gingivostomatitis or in the adult as pharyngotonsilitis. Both are associated with fever and lymphadenopathy with significant pain and ulcerative-like acute lesions. However, the most common manifestation of herpes infection is recurrent herpes labialis (cold sore, fever blisters). It appears with a prodromal onset of tingling or burning, which is usually followed by vesicle formation and rupture, pain, and finally crusting (Fig. 28.9).

Other members of the herpes virus group such as herpes zoster, Epstein–Barr virus, and, rarely, coxsackie viruses can also produce oral lesions. Hairy leukoplakia, which is observed in patients with HIV, is associated with the Epstein–Barr virus.

MANAGEMENT of initial herpetic infections is usually symptomatic and includes topical local anesthetics, systemic analgesics, and chlorhexidine rinses. Repeated episodes of recurrent herpes labialis can sometimes be controlled with systemic acyclovir. Topical acyclovir or penciclovir applied during the early prodromal stage may reduce the pain and duration of the lesion. Valacyclovir could also be used for systemic administration.

Acute aphthous ulceration

Recurrent aphthous stomatitis (canker sores) is probably one of the most prevalent oral mucosal diseases, with a general population incidence of 20%. Minor aphthous ulcers are the most common and appear as small (5 mm diameter or less) painful ulcerative lesions covered with a gray pseudomembrane (Fig. 28.10). They are seen on the nonkeratinized oral mucosa and the lateral borders of the tongue. Major aphthous ulcers occur less frequently, but are larger (over 1 cm in diameter) and extremely painful. Herpetiform ulcers occur as clusters of ulcers on the palate but are rarely observed. Their etiology remains unknown, but emotional stress, trauma, and nutritional deficiencies have been implicated. Oral ulcers are also associated with malabsorption diseases. Ulcers that persist and fail to respond to treatment often require biopsy to rule out oral cancer.

MANAGEMENT No magical cures exist and treatment is symptomatic, usually with topical medications (Fig. 28.11). Systemic

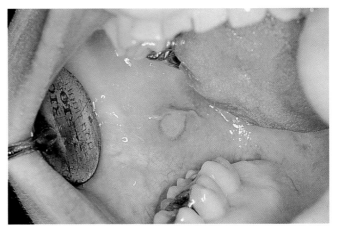

Fig. 28.10 A minor aphthous lesion on the buccal mucosa. It has a characteristic appearance with an erythematous halo surrounding the ulcer, which is covered with a gray pseudomembrane. Aphthous ulcers make it painful to eat. Minor aphthous lesions tend to heal without scarring. (Courtesy of Dr John Wright.)

 Ulceration of the oral mucosa

- Commonly due to oral tissue trauma
- If painful may be due to aphthous ulcers
- May be a manifestation of a systemic disease (e.g. HIV infection)
- May be a cancer if it fails to heal

Topical and systemic medications for aphthous ulceration

Topical medications	
Local anesthetics	Lidocaine rinse or ointment Dyclonine rinse Diphenhydramine rinse
Anti-inflammatory glucocorticosteroids	Triamcinolone ointment Fluocinonide gel
Anti-infectives	Chlorhexidine rinse Tetracycline rinse
Systemic medications	
Anti-inflammatory glucocorticosteroids	Prednisone

Fig. 28.11 Topical and systemic medications for aphthous ulceration.

glucocorticosteroids are sometimes required for frequent and repeated episodes.

Other mucosal lesions

▪ Lichen planus and benign mucous membrane pemphigoid are chronic mucocutaneous diseases

Lichen planus and benign mucous membrane pemphigoid

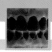

cause inflammation of the oral mucosa as well as other tissues. Pemphigoid is an autoimmune disease. Lichen planus has an immune component, but the etiology is less clear.

Lichen planus occurs in 0.5–1.5% of adults and is manifest as painful red ulcerative lesions (erosive or bullous) or as an asymptomatic nonerosive form on the buccal, palatal, gingival, or tongue mucosa. Nonerosive lesions include white striae (Wickham's striae) and a reticular pattern (Fig. 28.12). Skin lesions may or may not be present.

Pemphigoid also causes painful red ulcerative lesions along with desquamation of the mucosal epithelium, but without the striae (Fig. 28.13). Immunofluorescent staining of tissue samples is required for confirming the diagnosis.

The oral lesions of both lichen planus and pemphigoid are not always clearly defined and pemphigus, lupus erythematosus, lichenoid drug reactions, and, rarely, squamous cell carcinoma should be considered in the differential diagnosis.

Management

The acute symptoms of lichen planus are usually treated with topical anti-inflammatory glucocorticosteroids. Treatment objectives include eradicating the ulcerative lesions and control-

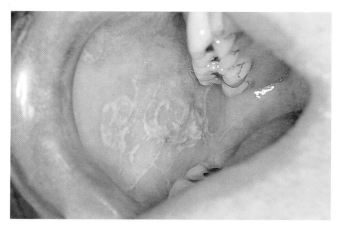

Fig. 28.12 Reticular or nonerosive lichen planus. The lesion on the buccal mucosa has a white lace-like appearance. This type of lichen planus is likely to be symptom free, unlike the ulcerative form of the disease. (Courtesy of Dr John Wright.)

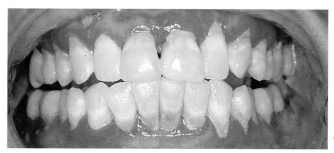

Fig. 28.13 Mucous membrane pemphigoid. This patient shows a rather diffuse presentation on the gingival mucosa with extensive desquamation of the epithelium. Antibodies attack components of the basement membrane, resulting in loss of the epithelium. This type of presentation is painful and it is difficult to maintain oral hygiene. (Courtesy of Dr John Wright.)

High-potency and highest-potency topical glucocorticosteroids
High-potency topical glucocorticosteroids
0.25% Desoximetasone 0.20% Fluocinolone 0.05% Fluocinonide
Highest-potency topical glucocorticosteroids
0.05% Betamethasone 0.05% Clobetasol 0.05% Halobetasol

Fig. 28.14 High-potency and highest-potency topical glucocorticosteroids.

ling symptomatic exacerbations. High potency topical gluco-corticosteroids (Fig. 28.14) in gel form seem to produce the most favorable response and least risk of systemic absorption. If the lesions are not responding, higher-potency topical glucocorticosteroids (see Fig. 28.14) are used and sometimes systemic prednisone is indicated. An intralesional injection of triamcinolone is sometimes given.

Pemphigoid generally responds well to topical anti-inflammatory glucocorticosteroids. However, severe refractory pemphigoid requires more aggressive treatment with a systemic glucocorticosteroid such as prednisone or the use of an immunosuppressive drug such as azathioprine. Dapsone has occasionally been used.

The long-term use of systemic glucocorticosteroids or the use of immunosuppressive drugs should be managed by a physician as the adverse effects can be more severe and need to be carefully monitored. The use of topical glucocorticosteroids for any of these lesions may suppress the immune system and lead to the development of candidiasis, which should then be treated with nystatin or chlorhexidine oral rinses.

Topical drugs used in dentistry

- *Chlorhexidine alters taste and causes easily removed staining of the teeth*
- *Local itching, burning, and erythema of the oral mucosa may occur with topical glucocorticosteroids*
- *Excessive topical local application to a large denuded surface may produce systemic toxicity*

Systemic drugs used for oral mucosal diseases

- *Suppression of adrenal cortical activity with systemic glucocorticosteroids*
- *Azathioprine can cause bone marrow depression, secondary infection, and neoplasia*
- *Dapsone has been associated with severe cutaneous reactions and hematologic defects*

Drug-induced adverse effects involving the mouth

Adverse effect	Causative drugs
Lichenoid-drug eruptions	Allopurinol, furosemide, chloroquine, chlorpropamide, gold salts, methyldopa, lithium salts, mercury, penicillamine, phenothiazines, propranolol, quinidine, spironolactone, thiazides, tetracyclines, tolbutamide
Lupus erythematosus-like eruptions	Gold salts, phenytoin, griseofulvin, isoniazid, penicillin, primidone, procainamide, thiouracil, hydralazine, streptomycin, methyldopa
Pemphigus-like drug eruptions	Penicillamine, phenobarbital, rifampin, captopril
Erythema multiforme	Antimalarials, barbiturates, carbamazepine, salicylates, chlorpropamide, sulfonamides, clindamycin, tetracyclines
Gingival hyperplasia	Phenytoin, cyclosporine, nifedipine (and other Ca^{2+} antagonists)
Xerostomia	Anorexiants, antidepressants, isotretinoin, anticholinergics, anticonvulsants, antihistamines, captopril, clonidine, prazosin, reserpine, diflunisal, piroxicam, antiparkinsonian drugs, antipsychotics, diuretics, cyclobenzaprine, opioids, albuterol

Fig. 28.15 Drug-induced adverse effects involving the mouth.

Drug-induced oral disease

Many dental patients will be taking one or more prescribed medications, which may produce adverse effects that can manifest as painful oral mucosal reactions (stomatitis). Such adverse effects include mucositis and oral ulcerations associated with cancer chemotherapy, lichenoid drug reactions, lupus erythematosus-like reactions, pemphigus-like drug reactions, and erythema multiforme (Fig. 28.15).

Contact allergic reactions may also be observed, but occur with less frequency. Angioedema has been observed with some drugs and cinnamon-based ingredients in dentifrices. Dental materials, including metals and acrylic polymers, have also been implicated in soft tissue allergic reactions.

Phenytoin, cyclosporine, and the Ca^{2+} antagonists can cause gingival hyperplasia (Fig. 28.16), which develops in approximately 40% of patients who take phenytoin. Among the Ca^{2+} antagonists, some data suggest isradipine is less likely to cause

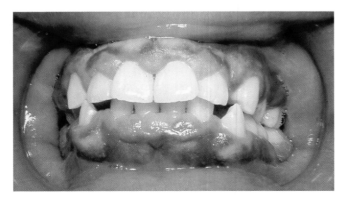

Fig. 28.16 Drug-induced gingival hyperplasia. The gingival papillae show mild hyperplasia associated with the use of phenytoin. Attention to dental hygiene and routine dental scaling to control local factors help to reduce the severity of the hyperplasia. Cyclosporine and Ca^{2+} antagonists produce a similar hyperplasia.

> **🔑 Xerostomia**
>
> - Commonly causes a 'burning tongue'
> - Carries a high risk for dental caries
> - Carries a high risk for candidiasis
> - May be caused by prescribed medications

gingival hyperplasia. The gingival mucosa begins to enlarge and cover the teeth. In severe cases the overgrowth will almost entirely cover the teeth and must be surgically reduced.

Drugs with anticholinergic effects frequently reduce salivary flow, leading to a drug-induced xerostomia. A dry mouth can also be due to systemic disease and must be considered in these cases.

Management

Management of drug-induced oral adverse effects includes:
- Identifying the suspect drug.
- Working with the physician and patient to seek an alternative drug whenever possible.

Otherwise, palliative care and efforts to improve dental hygiene and control plaque are needed. Acute inflammatory symptoms often respond to topical or systemic anti-inflammatory glucocorticosteroids. An antifungal agent such as nystatin or a chlorhexidine rinse can be used for opportunistic candidiasis. Local anesthetic rinses may be beneficial for stomatitis associated with cancer chemotherapy.

A dry mouth presents a significant challenge as there are no suitable artificial saliva substitutes, and drug-stimulated salivary flow is less than satisfactory. Oral pilocarpine may produce some benefit in patients who have a reduced salivary flow following head and neck radiation. Cevimeline, a cholinergic agonist, was recently introduced for treatment of dry mouth symptoms associated with Sjögren's syndrome.

FURTHER READING

Jastak JT, Yagiela JA, Donaldson D. *Local Anesthesia of the Oral Cavity.* Philadelphia: WB Saunders; 1995. [Excellent textbook with a comprehensive coverage of local anesthetics in dentistry.]

Lewis MAO, Lamey PJ. *Clinical Oral Medicine.* Oxford: Wright; 1993. [A comprehensive text on oral disease and oral medicine.]

Neubrun E. *Cariology.* Chicago: Quientessence; 1989. [Comprehensive textbook on caries development and prevention, and fluoride use.]

Peterson LJ. Principles of antibiotic therapy. In: Topazian RG, Goldberg MH (eds) *Oral and Maxillofacial Infections*, 3rd edn. Philadelphia: WB Saunders; 1994, pp. 160–197. [A detailed review of potential pathogenic microorganisms of the oral cavity, and antibiotic selection and use.]

Rees TD. Drugs and oral disorders. *Periodontology 2000* 1998; **18**: 21–36. [An updated review of oral manifestations of drug reactions.]

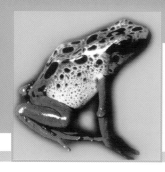

Chapter 29

Toxins and Poisons

■ *Every natural or synthetic chemical can cause injury if exposure is high enough*

Exact definitions of terms such as venom, toxin, and poison are not possible, chiefly because every chemical can cause injury if given in a high enough dose (see Fig. 29.1). Whether a chemical is considered a venom, toxin, or poison depends mainly on its source, not its actions. Thus, for practical purposes:

• Venoms are substances injected by one species into another.
• Poisons are chemicals that can injure, or impair, bodily functions. They may or may not have beneficial actions, in addition to being poisonous.
• Toxins were originally described as the poisons produced by micro-organisms, but the word is now used more broadly for other species (e.g. the ω conotoxins from coneshells).

Venoms and toxins are usually proteins or polypeptides, particularly those produced by vertebrates, whereas poisons are often small molecules. Invertebrates and plants also produce a wide diversity of toxins and poisons, many of which are alkaloids (small molecules which contain nitrogen).

■ *Venoms, toxins and poisons are potential sources of useful drugs*

As illustrated by various examples given later in this chapter, venoms, toxins and poisons have been a source of many drugs. Examples from plants include such useful drugs as atropine, tubocurarine, vinca alkaloids and eserine. Fungi have been the source of a host of antibiotics (penicillin, tetracyclines, cyclosporine) and anticancer drugs. Toxins from bacteria (streptokinase) and fractions from snake venoms (ancrod) are used to dissolve blood clots. In addition to therapeutic drugs many pharmacologic tools have been isolated from venoms, toxins and poisons.

■ *Generally, acute toxicity results from brief exposure, chronic toxicity from months or years of exposure*

Exposure to venoms involves direct contact with a venomous animal whereas ingestion is a common route of exposure to toxins and poisons. Chemicals in the air, water, and food (e.g. poisons such as pesticides, heavy metals, chlorinated hydrocarbons) lead to chronic low-level exposure. Exposure by inhalation is a common route of poisoning in the workplace. The skin is an effective barrier to most water-soluble poisons, but not to highly fat-soluble substances.

■ *Toxins and poisons can have direct and indirect mechanisms of action*

Many toxins and poisons act relatively selectively on target organs, often as the result of the particular physiologic and biochemical functions of these organs (Fig. 29.2). The kidneys are particularly vulnerable. However, metallothioneins, a unique protein class, can help protect organs by avidly binding some poisons (e.g. cadmium).

Whether poison-induced damage is reversible, or irreversible, often depends upon the repair and regenerative capabilities of the target tissue. For example, liver damage is

Potency of various poisons in terms of acute lethality	
Lethal potency in terms of average lethal dose in mg/kg body weight	Toxins, venoms and poisons
1,000,000	Water
10,000	Ethanol, other alcohols, general anesthetics
1,000	Iron salts, vitamins
100	Barbiturates
10	Morphine, some snake venoms
1	Nicotine and many plant poisons
0.1	Curare, sea snake venoms, jellyfish toxins
0.01	Tetrodotoxin
0.001	Ciguatoxin, palytoxin
<0.0001	Botulinum toxins

Fig. 29.1 The acute lethal potency of a range of poisons.

Chemicals hazardous to man

• Venoms from animals
• Toxins from animals and plants
• Poisons from natural and man-made sources

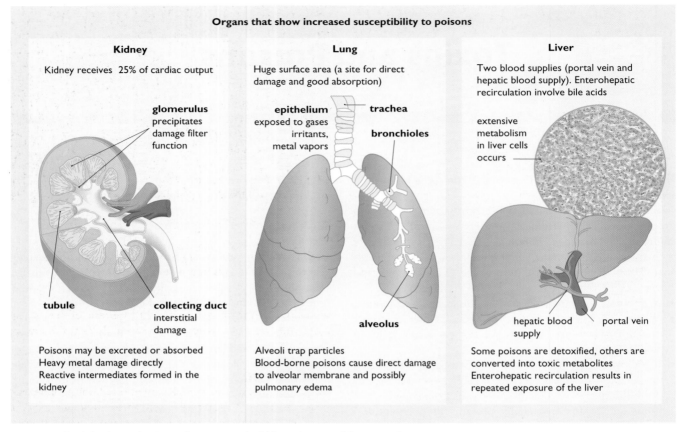

Organs that show increased susceptibility to poisons

Kidney

Kidney receives 25% of cardiac output

glomerulus
precipitates
damage filter
function

tubule

collecting duct
interstitial
damage

Poisons may be excreted or absorbed
Heavy metal damage directly
Reactive intermediates formed in the
kidney

Lung

Huge surface area (a site for direct
damage and good absorption)

epithelium
exposed to gases
irritants,
metal vapors

trachea

bronchioles

alveolus

Alveoli trap particles
Blood-borne poisons cause direct damage
to alveolar membrane and possibly
pulmonary edema

Liver

Two blood supplies (portal vein and
hepatic blood supply). Enterohepatic
recirculation involve bile acids

extensive
metabolism
in liver cells
occurs

hepatic blood
supply

portal vein

Some poisons are detoxified, others are
converted into toxic metabolites
Enterohepatic recirculation results in
repeated exposure of the liver

Fig. 29.2 Physiologic mechanisms that expose the kidney, lung, and liver to poisons.

often reversible, because the liver has a marked regenerative ability. However, damage to the central nervous system (CNS) is more likely to be irreversible because neurons do not generally regenerate under normal conditions. The axons of neurons are particularly vulnerable since they have limited metabolic functions and rely on transport, often over long distances, of materials from the cell body. Furthermore, the normal age-related loss of neurons can result in neuropoisons reducing the age at which neurologic and behavioral deficits appear (e.g. drug-induced Parkinsonism).

■ *Poisons can act indirectly*

Allergic reactions are immunologically mediated adverse reactions to repeated exposure and sensitization to allergens. Poisons can also act directly on the immune system and cause immunosuppression, rendering a person liable to infection. The activation and recruitment of phagocytic cells to sites of chemically induced injury plays a role in the progression of tissue injury.

■ *Approximately eight million people in the US suffer acute poisoning each year*

Hazards due to exposure to poisons are monitored and limited by the regulations resulting from recommendations provided by the government committees and agencies responsible for protecting the public from toxic hazards. A key measure in assessing the potential hazard to humans resulting from toxins

and poisons is the no-observed-adverse-effect level (NOAEL) of exposure. The NOAEL for a hazardous chemical is determined by dosing laboratory animals with a toxin or poison. For humans likely to be exposed to a particular poison, 1/100th of the NOAEL is considered to be the permitted maximum level of exposure. (The fraction is obtained by allowing 1/10 for individual differences, and 1/10 for species differences.) The use of such a factor is related to the fact that the Environmental Protection Agency (USA) considers a risk of one death per million individuals exposed as the maximum acceptable exposure level. In order to give this level of risk meaning in comparison with other hazards, consider that in the USA 20,000 people die each year from the effects of illicit drugs while acute toxicity due to drug or poison ingestion accounts for at least 10% of hospital admissions. Motor vehicle accidents and firearms are an even greater hazard. For interesting insight as to how hazards are viewed by the public see Fig. 6.2 in Chapter 6.

■ *Standard medical procedures and specific therapies are available in many cases of envenomation and poisoning*

The obvious first step in the treatment of envenomation or poisoning is to remove the source of the exposure (Fig. 29.3). This is followed by procedures designed to limit absorption and/or speed excretion of the venom or poison, for example by:

• Restricting dispersion of venom from the envenomation site by tourniquets and immobilization.

- Remove source of poison or victim from source (e.g. rescue)

- Remove and limit absorption of poison (e.g. fresh air, wash, emesis, limit contact)

- Supportive therapy (e.g. ventilation, external cardiac massage, saline/oxygen, drugs)

- Specific therapies
  Antivenins for animal venoms
  Antitoxins for bacterial toxins
  Chelators for heavy metals
  Gases (e.g. oxygen for carbon monoxide)

- Other drug therapies
  Ethanol for methanol
  Digoxin antibodies for digoxin
  Pyridoxine for isoniazid
  Nitrite and thiosulfate for cyanide
  N-acetylcysteine for acetaminophen

- Specific antagonists
  Atropine and oximes for organophosphate anticholinesterases
  Flumazenil for benzodiazepines
  Opioid antagonists (naloxone) for opiates
  Anticholinesterases for neuromuscular blockers

Fig. 29.3 Principles for the treatment of poisoning.

- Removing poisons from the stomach or skin.
- Acidification or alkalinization of the urine.
- Ingestion of water.

Another step is to use specific antidotes, antivenins, or antitoxins where they are available. Other steps can include hemodialysis to remove toxins by filtration, and hemoperfusion to remove toxins by circulating the blood of the victim through an activated charcoal filter.

VENOMS, TOXINS AND POISONS FROM NATURAL SOURCES

Venoms from animals

Venomous animals occur in all animal phyla (Figs 29.4, 29.5). Venoms are usually, but not always, proteins or polypeptides of various types of structures, and many different mechanisms of action. Specialized venom glands and injection apparatus are required to inject the venom. In addition fatal allergies can develop to venoms, particularly to those of bees, hornets, and

Treatment of poisoning

- Remove the source of poison
- Minimize absorption of the poison
- Supportive therapy
- Specific therapy, if available

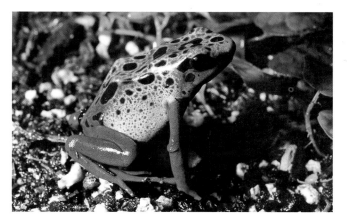

Fig. 29.4 A typical poisonous frog. Extracts from the skin of similar poisonous frogs (*Dendrobates* sp.) are painted on the tips of arrows and darts in Central and South America. Many vertebrates are capable of injecting venoms or contain poisons. (Photograph by Ron Kertesz, with permission of the Vancouver Aquarium.)

wasps, where the non-allergenic direct effects of their stings are mainly local skin reactions and are only fatal if there are many stings.

Snake venoms

Many snake venoms are complex mixtures of polypeptides and proteins; some of the latter are enzymes. Such enzymes can account for some of the systemic toxicity, and much of the local toxicity, seen following crotalid snake (rattlesnake and pit viper) bites. Crotalid venoms can affect blood coagulation and hemostasis, and cause tissue necrosis at the wound site. The enzymatic actions, which include proteolysis, lipolysis, and phospholipase activity, resulting in cell disruption and lysis.

■ Non-enzymatic polypeptides and proteins in snake venoms can have specific molecular actions

Many elapid snake (e.g. cobra, krait) venoms contain neuromuscular-blocking polypeptides. Some of these block nicotinic cholinoceptors (Chapter 20) in such a selective manner that one such polypeptide (α bungarotoxin) was first used to identify and label nicotinic receptors. The related β bungarotoxin selectively blocks the release of acetylcholine at the neuromuscular junction of skeletal muscle.

■ The lethality of snake venoms varies widely

The danger due to snake bites varies with the species and the dose of venom injected. The venom glands of many snakes contain enough venom to kill many humans but snakes rarely inject all of their venom when attacking man. The lethality of snake venoms depends upon the toxicologic actions of their various components. Of the many venomous snakes, potentially the most dangerous are probably the tropical sea snakes (Hydrophidae), which, despite having very small fangs, are able to inject lethal amounts of nicotinic cholinoceptor-blocking polypeptides. In addition, the venom also contain phospholipases which break down muscle membranes and as a result cause myoglobinuria in victims.

603

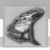

Toxin	Source	Mechanisms of action
Small molecules		
Tetrodotoxin	Puffer fish, octopus, salamander	Na^+ channel blocker
Saxitoxin	Shellfish contaminated with dinoflagellates	Na^+ channel blocker
Ciguatoxin	Large tropical fish contaminated with dinoflagellates	Actions on Na^+ channel
Cardiac glycosides	Toad skin	ATPase inhibitor
Batrachotoxin	Frog skin	Na^+ channel activator
Domoic acid	Shellfish (mussels)	CNS toxin
Palytoxin	Sea anemone	Ionophore
Proteins and polypeptides		
α Bungarotoxin	Elapid snakes (kraits)	Nicotinic receptor blocker
β Bungarotoxin	Elapid snakes (kraits)	Presynaptic cholinergic nerves
α Conotoxin	Coneshells	
μ Conotoxin	Coneshells	Skeletal muscle Na^+ channel blocker
ω Conotoxin	Coneshells	N-type Ca^{2+} antagonist
Cardiotoxin	Elapid snakes	Direct acting cardiotoxin
Phospholipases	Many snakes	Cell membrane destruction
Bacterial toxins		
Botulinum toxin	*Clostridium botulinum*	Synaptin in cholinergic nerve endings
Cholera toxin	*Cholera vibrio*	Activation of G_s protein
Pertussis toxin	*Bordetella pertussis*	Inactivates G_o/G_s protein
Endotoxin	Gram-negative bacteria	Cell membranes
Tetanus toxin	*Clostridium tetani*	Cell membrane inophore
Staphylococcal toxin	*Staphylococcus* sp.	Enterotoxin

The sources and mechanisms of action of various animal venoms and toxins

Fig. 29.5 **Sources and mechanisms of action of various animal venoms and toxins.**

Antivenins (antibodies) are produced for many snake venoms as well as for spider and scorpion venoms. Treatment with antivenins, combined with local procedures using tourniquets and immobilization, are used to limit the escape of venom from the wound site, and can be very effective in the treatment of snake bite and other types of envenomation. It is increasingly recognized that systemic effects following envenomation can be limited by reducing the spread of venom, via the lymphatics, from the site of envenomation.

■ *Studies into the actions of snake venoms have led to pharmacologic developments*

A bradykinin-potentiating polypeptide isolated from a Brazilian snake venom led to the development of captopril, the first clinically useful angiotensin converting enzyme inhibitor (see Chapter 18). Ancrod is a fibrinolytic factor from the Malayan pit viper (*Ankistrodon rhodostoma*) that breaks down fibrinogen into fragments of fibrin and thereby produces afibrinogenemia. The highly selective molecular actions of other components of snake venoms have led to their use as pharmacologic tools and potential therapeutic agents.

Other venoms

Other well-studied venoms include those from scorpions. Scorpion venoms can be lethal for children but are much less so for adults. These venoms target a variety of cellular macromolecules, including K^+ channels. Many marine animals contain venoms, including vertebrates such as fishes (e.g. stingrays, scorpion and lion fish) which have venomous spines. These venoms can inflict severe pain and injury, but are not usually lethal. Such venoms are usually mixtures of proteins and polypeptides. On the other hand, tetrodotoxin is a small molecular weight poison found in puffer fish. It is a highly selective sodium channel blocker that has been used as a local anesthetic, and as a pharmacologic tool. Interestingly, puffer fish are eaten, after very careful preparation to remove the most poisonous parts (liver and intestitine), as a delicacy (known as fugu) in Japan.

Nonvertebrate species also possess dangerous venoms:
- The venoms of jellyfish (coelenterates) and corals (Fig. 29.6) are contained within special organelles known as nematocysts. The venoms are injected via the nematocysts in limited quantities unless large areas of the skin are involved. Some of the box jellyfish found in tropical Australian waters can cause fatal stings in children, while many coastal areas around the world are subject to invasions by jellyfish such as the Portuguese man-of-war although this is not a true jellyfish but a hydroid, *Physalia* sp.
- Some species of octopus inject tetrodotoxin, a selective blocker of Na^+ channels, into their prey. In Australia such species have killed children.
- Venoms of various tropical shellfish, the coneshells, show remarkable molecular target selectivity. Depending upon the species considered (Fig. 29.7), coneshells are predators of fish, worms, or other coneshells. Coneshells inject their venoms via a specialized hollow harpoon. Each prey-specific

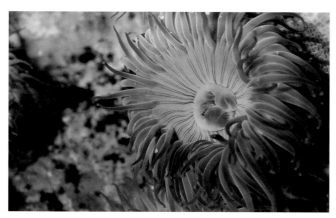

Fig. 29.6 Many marine invertebrates contain venoms and poisons. Venoms in corals, anemones, and jellyfish are contained within special cellular organelles, nematocysts. Nematocysts contain a stinging thread that penetrates the skin and injects venom. Many of these invertebrates are very attractive and children are particularly liable to be stung. (Photograph by Ron Kertesz, with permission of the Vancouver Aquarium.)

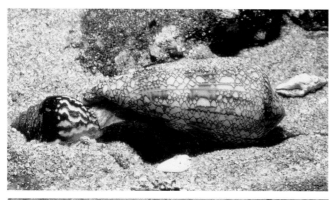

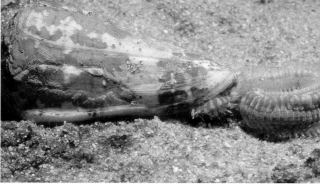

Fig. 29.7 Different coneshells have evolved venoms that are relatively specific for their prey species, whether other snails, worms or even fish. Conotoxins are often highly selective for certain ion channels. (Photographs by Alex Kerstitch.)

species of coneshell has its own special conotoxins that target, very selectively, specific molecular sites including ion channels and receptors. For example, certain conotoxins are specific blockers of neuronal (N) type calcium channels and one such conotoxin is currently being tested clinically for treatment of severe pain.

Various other phyla contain a variety of toxins whose actions relate to the role such venoms play in the ecology of the species. Examples include the stings of various insects such as bees and hornets. Other fascinating examples include ticks which produce venomous saliva which has anticoagulant, anti-inflammatory, and analgesic properties. The latter peptides help the tick avoid detection by their host for 7–10 days. Leeches are able to attach themselves to their hosts and draw blood without being detected. The leeches inject hirudin, a thrombin antagonist, to ensure a continuous flow of blood. Hirudin is used clinically (see Chapter 13) as an anticoagulant.

Toxins and poisons from animals

Vertebrate species, apart from those with venoms, contain few substances that are poisonous to other species. Invertebrates species (e.g. fungi and bacteria) often contain toxins. Bacterial toxins are produced by many species and probably serve purposes other than killing hosts. Many antibacterial polypeptides isolated from bacteria are presumably used for defense purposes. Fungi also use a large variety of complex nonprotein molecules as deterrents to competitors and predators. Many of the poisons produced by fungi have adverse effects on many species, especially bacteria. Thus, the source of most antibiotics used therapeutically is still fungi, although usually they are now given as semi-synthetic derivatives of the parent compound. On the other hand fungal contamination of foods, and the ingestion of the wrong type of fungi, are the cause of many cases of poisoning. Examples of the former include aflatoxin, a liver toxin and carcinogen, produced by Aspergillus fungi, a contaminate of peanuts. Various large poisonous fungi are often ingested in mistake for the edible species. These poisonous fungi contain a wide variety of toxic molecules which produce damage to the liver and kidneys in particular.

■ *Bacterial toxins vary in chemical nature and actions*
Botulinum toxin is one of a group of bacterial endotoxins that includes tetanus and diphtheria toxins. Botulinum toxin itself is an orally absorbed protein from *Clostridium* sp. (an anaerobe), responsible for potentially fatal botulism. Poisoning typically occurs by ingesting preformed botulinum toxin in inadequately canned foods, or via contamination of wounds with live organisms. The latter is a much rarer cause of botulism. The symptoms of botulism arise as a result of the loss of acetylcholine from cholinergic nerve endings. This results in disruption of cholinergic transmission in autonomic ganglia, as well as parasympathetic and motor neurons. The latter leads to muscle weakness, diplopia, and respiratory failure, the former to autonomic dysfunction. Therapy is supportive although the use of antitoxin may be of value. Recovery depends on repletion of nerve endings with acetylcholine. Botulinum toxin is so potent that a single molecule can deplete a single nerve ending. The mechanism appears to involve inactivation of a synaptin responsible for the exocytosis of acetylcholine. Botulinum toxin is used therapeutically to treat various dystonias involving muscle spasm such as around the eyes, in the neck, or in the anus in the presence of an anal fissure. It is even used to disperse wrinkles.

605

Cholera toxin released by the cholera vibrio causes a massive diarrhea. The molecular mechanism involves ADP ribosylation of the adenylyl cyclase stimulatory G_S protein, causing irreversible inactivation of GTPase and therefore permanent activation of G_S protein (see Chapter 3). As a result cAMP accumulates and there is salt and water hypersecretion from gut epithelium. In contrast, pertussis toxin inactivates G_i/G_o proteins. Other exotoxins released from bacteria as well as endotoxins released by bacterial breakdown are often responsible for many of the adverse consequences of bacterial infection. Complex polysaccharide endotoxins have a variety of actions including causing cardiovascular collapse (endotoxic shock) and fever.

Poisons from plants

Plants use chemicals for defense, and as a result produce many poisons, and even venoms (stinging plants), to deter or kill predators (Fig. 29.8). Plant toxins and poisons are usually small organic molecules. The diversity, availability, and ease of ingestion of plant poisons led to the discovery of the first drugs. Many drugs are still extracted from plants, or are chemical derivatives of their extracts (e.g. atropine, tubocurarine, digoxin, reserpine, morphine, caffeine, nicotine, paclitaxel, aspirin, quinidine, quinine, vincristine).

Plant poisons are particularly dangerous to domestic animals and children. Information about the nature of the common plant poisons and their treatment is readily obtained from Poison Control Centers. Not all cases of such poisoning are recognized and the physician should be aware of the possibility of plant poisoning when faced with perplexing symptoms. It should be noted that herbal concoctions can contain plant poisons. Many cases of liver and kidney damage have been caused by folklore medicines.

 Industrial poisoning

- The major industrial poisons are metals (elemental, salt, and organic forms), air pollutants and gases, aromatic and aliphatic hydrocarbons (liquid and vapor), insecticides, pesticides, and herbicides
- All produce both acute and chronic toxicity
- Mutagenic and carcinogenic actions can be difficult to detect

INDUSTRIAL POISONS

Industrial poisons are either intentional products of industry or byproducts of industrial processes (e.g. air or water pollution). Environmental poisons are those that reach the environment, cause acute or chronic poisoning and/or may be carcinogenic and/or mutagenic. While the concentration of industrial poisons can be high enough in the workplace to produce acute poisoning, concentrations in the general environment are not usually high enough to constitute an acute toxic hazard. However, low concentrations in the general environment can be sufficient to produce chronic poisoning.

Metals

Heavy metals such as mercury, cadmium, and lead are toxic, the toxicity arising from both the salts and the elemental metal, particularly vapors and dusts. The mechanism of toxicity often involves their combination with specific groups on essential macromolecules (Fig. 29.9). Heavy metals such as arsenic tend to react with the oxygen/sulfur groups on essential macro-

The sources and mechanisms of action of various plant and fungal poisons

Poison	Source	Mechanism of action
Some plant poisons		
Atropine, scopolamine	Solanaceae (jimson weed, deadly nightshade)	Muscarinic receptor antagonists
Cardiac glycosides	Digitalis, strophanthus, oleander, convallaria	ATPase inhibitors
Aconitine	Hellebores	Cardiac Na⁺ channel activator
Capsaicin	*Capsicum* sp. (peppers)	Substance P depleter
Ricin	Castor bean	Protoplasmic poison
Myristicin	Nutmeg and mace	Hallucinogenic
Emetine	*Ipecacuana* sp.	Vomiting center stimulant
Pennyroyal oil	*Mentha* sp.	Hepatotoxic and oxytoxic
Safrole	Sassafras tree	Animal carcinogen
Pyrrolizidines	Heliotropium, comfrey (herbal tea)	Hepatotoxic
Some fungal toxins		
Muscarine	Clitocybe, *Amanita* sp., *Inocybe* sp.	Muscarinic agonist
Phallotoxins, amatoxins	*Amanita* sp. (death cap, destroying angel)	Hepatotoxic
Coprine	*Coprinus* sp.	Blocks aldehyde dehydrogenase
Ibotenic acid	*Amanita* sp.	Hallucinogenic
Psilocybin	*Psilocybe* sp.	Hallucinogenic
Aflatoxins	*Aspergillus* sp.	Hepatocarcinogenic
Ergot alkaloids	*Claviceps* sp.	Multiple actions
Orelline	*Corinarius* sp.	Nephrotoxic

Fig. 29.8 Sources and mechanisms of action of various plant and fungal poisons.

Mechanisms of action of heavy metal toxicity

Metal	Site and mechanism of molecular actions	Tissue and organ target
Mercury	Direct toxicity Sulfhydryl binding and disruption of important macromolecules (enzymes, pumps, receptors) Also binds phosphoryl, amino, and other groups	Corrosive damage to lungs and gastrointestinal tract CNS, lung, and renal damage
Lead	Sulfhydryl group binding Impaired heme synthesis	CNS and peripheral nervous system, cardiovascular, blood, kidney and skin
Cadmium	Binds to macromolecules and disrupts function	Lung and renal damage
Arsenic	Sulfhydryl groups and oxidative metabolism uncoupling	Peripheral nervous system, CNS, gastrointestinal tract, liver, and cardiovascular system

Fig. 29.9 Mechanisms of action of heavy metal toxicity.

molecules, such as enzymes, to form inactive metal complexes (coordination compounds).

Mercury

Mercury is used extensively in industry, and is a common cause of accidental poisoning. Paints, mercury thermometers, and laboratories are a less common source. Toxic quantities of mercury vapor can be absorbed from the lungs, while ingestion of inorganic and organic mercurial salts is mainly responsible for oral poisoning. Methylmercury-contaminated food led to hundreds of deaths in Iraq, while its accumulation in sea food poisoned the residents of Minamata Bay in Japan.

Elemental (liquid) mercury is poorly absorbed in the gut, but the vapor is well absorbed from the lungs. Acute poisoning affects the respiratory tract, producing cough, dyspnea, and interstitial pneumonitis. Ingestion of inorganic mercury compounds results in acute corrosive damage to the gastro-intestinal tract, and renal damage. Symptoms of chronic poisoning are more insidious and are often neurologic (visual disturbances, ataxia, paresthesias, and neurasthenias) in origin. The diagnosis of mercury poisoning is based upon symptoms and history, and is associated with mercury concentrations (>40 μg/liter in blood and >5 μg/liter in urine (Fig. 29.10).

The amount of oral absorption of mercury compounds depends upon chemical type. Inorganic salts are absorbed as Hg^{2+} (approximately 10% of the ingested dose). Organic mercurial molecules are well absorbed orally and distributed fairly uniformly. Mercury readily forms covalent bonds with sulfur (as -S- bonds or -SH groups) and this bonding is the ultimate mechanism responsible for poisoning. Mercury also binds to phosphoryl, carboxyl, amide, and amine groups thereby disrupting the functioning of enzymes, receptors, and other important cellular macromolecules.

Specific treatment of elemental mercury poisoning includes the use of chelators (see page 609) such as intramuscular dimercaprol for those with severe intoxication, and oral penicillamine for less severe exposure. Oral succimer is a useful replacement for penicillamine. Dimercaprol is contraindicated for organic mercurial poisoning since it can elevate mercury

concentrations in the brain. The enterohepatic recirculation of mercury allows for the oral use of nonabsorbable polythiol resins which irreversibly bind mercury resulting in its loss in the feces. L-Cysteine, infused intra-arterially, forms a dialyzable complex with methylmercury. Organic mercurial poisoning is harder to treat since organic mercury does not chelate well.

Lead

Lead was used routinely for centuries in the manufacture of water pipes, glazes and paints. In some countries organic lead compounds are added to gasoline to prevent premature ignition (antiknock). Older paints have a lead content of up to 40% of their dry weight. For such reasons environmental and

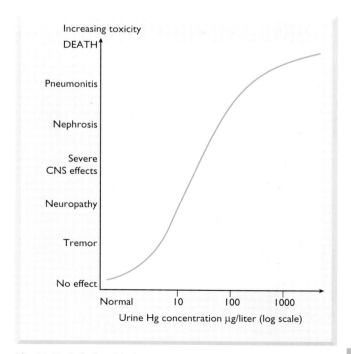

Fig. 29.10 Relationship between mercury concentrations in urine, and symptoms of mercury poisoning.

607

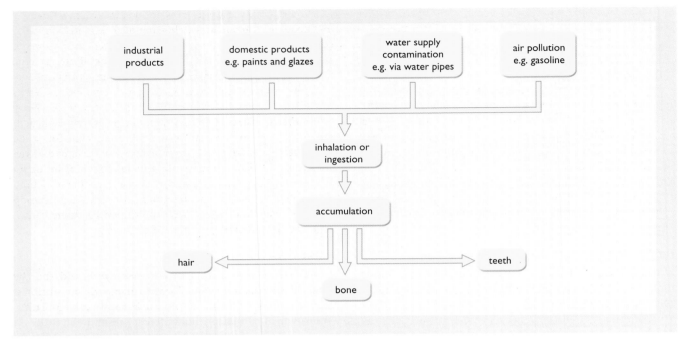

Fig. 29.11 Sources of lead and its distribution in the body.

occupational exposure used to be common, and still is in some countries. Chronic lead poisoning, particularly in urban regions, has led to government restrictions on lead use, especially in paint and gasoline (Fig. 29.11).

Acute lead poisoning, as the result of ingestion or exposure to lead vapor, is less common than chronic poisoning. The symptoms of acute poisoning include nausea, vomiting, a metallic taste, and severe abdominal pain. There can also be acute severe CNS symptoms, a hemolytic crisis, kidney damage, and shock.

Chronic poisoning (plumbism) causes gastrointestinal, neuromuscular, renal, and CNS symptoms, as well as symptoms related to other body systems. Neuromuscular and CNS symptoms usually follow severe poisoning; gastrointestinal symptoms follow less severe poisoning (Fig. 29.12). CNS symptoms are more common in children and include disturbed motor control, restlessness, and irritability. Progressive deterioration of mental function may occur in children as a result of low-level environmental exposure and is difficult to diagnose and detect.

Lead is absorbed from the gastrointestinal and respiratory tracts. Gastrointestinal absorption is greater in children. Lead is distributed throughout the body, and deposited in the bones, teeth, and hair. Chelation therapy (guided by the blood concentrations of heavy metal) is useful with, in order of priority:

- CaNa$_2$ ethylenediaminetetra-acetic acid (EDTA) (i.m. or i.v.).
- Dimercaprol (i.m.).
- D-Penicillamine (orally).
- Succimer.

Cadmium

Perhaps surprisingly, cadmium poisoning can be as common as mercury and lead poisoning. This is due in part to the wide-

spread and increasing industrial use of cadmium in plastics, paints, and batteries. Cadmium accumulates in food such as animal livers and kidneys, food grains and particularly shellfish. Exposure as a result of food contamination is important, but industrial workers can be exposed to cadmium vapors in the air.

Acute poisoning is generally due to airborne exposure and is associated with initial lung irritation followed by pneumonitis, chest pains, residual emphysema, and possibly fatal pulmonary edema. Oral ingestion causes vomiting, diarrhea,

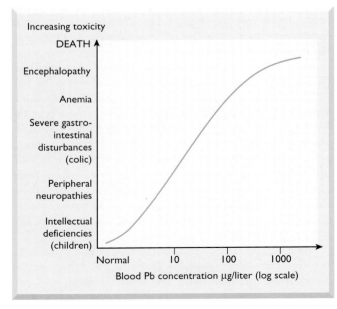

Fig. 29.12 Relationship between lead concentrations in blood, and symptoms of lead poisoning.

and abdominal cramps. The results of chronic poisoning depend upon the mode of exposure: the lung is a major target with air exposure, the kidney and lungs with ingestion. Chronic cadmium poisoning is associated with osteomalacia and carcinogenesis.

Cadmium (Cd^{2+}) is poorly absorbed from the gastrointestinal tract, and absorption from the lungs is up to four times higher. It distributes slowly around the body, but concentrates in the kidney. Kidney damage follows oral ingestion—the proximal tubules are damaged first and the glomeruli later. Lung tissue is damaged directly by an unknown mechanism. 'Itai-itai' disease in Japan was found to be due to the chronic ingestion of cadmium. There is limited specific therapy of cadmium poisoning and chelation therapy does not appear to be beneficial.

Arsenic

Arsenic has been used extensively in the past for therapeutic purposes including the treatment of syphilis and parasitic infections. Indeed, some arsenical drugs are still in use for the latter. Most arsenic poisoning arises from industrial and environmental exposure. High concentrations of arsenic are found in some water supplies, including those in the western US. Certain pesticides and herbicides are a source of arsenic (Fig. 29.13). Arsenicals are sometimes added to animal food stock to promote growth, or in excess as vermin poisons. Arsenic was commonly used in the past as a cosmetic (applied to the skin to lighten the complexion) and to commit murder.

Acute arsenical poisoning is now rare because the availability of arsenical compounds is strictly regulated. Symptoms following acute ingestion develop within 12 hours including severe gastric pain, projectile vomiting, and severe diarrhea. Renal collapse, anuria, and shock can lead to death. Neuropathies and encephalopathies are common sequelae of acute poisoning if death does not occur. Chronic poisoning causes early signs of muscle weakness and myalgias, hyperpigmentation, and hyperkeratosis. Other symptoms include sweating, stomatitis, lacrimation, excessive salivation, coryza, dermatitis, and alopecia.

The absorption of arsenic depends on the form in which it is ingested. It is stored mainly in heart, lung, liver, and kidney, but concentrates in the keratin of the hair and nails (a useful forensic fact), as well as in bones and teeth. Biochemically, arsenic uncouples oxidative metabolism by substituting for phosphate. It causes capillary leakage and myocardial damage as well as epithelial sloughing in the gastrointestinal tract and bloody feces. The renal capillaries and renal tubules are severely damaged, while damage to cerebral vessels is responsible for some neuropathies. Central necrosis and cirrhosis can occur in the liver.

Arsenic is also carcinogenic and teratogenic, inducing squamous and basal cell skin carcinomas, and possibly lung and liver cancers. Specific treatment for arsenic poisoning includes chelation therapy with intramuscular dimercaprol, followed by oral penicillamine or succimer.

Chelators

Chelators are molecules that complex with, and thereby hold, metal ions in inactive forms suitable for mobilization and excretion. Those used medically include EDTA,

Arsenical drugs and poisons	
Type of arsenic	Poison/drug
Inorganic Elemental Trivalent arsenite Pentavalent arsenate Arsine gas	Insecticides, rat poisons, fungicides (source of most arsenical poisoning via food contamination) Released by acids
Organic Antiparasitic drugs	Carbarsone, tryparsamide, melarsoprol (rarely used)

Fig. 29.13 Arsenical drugs and poisons. Arsenic is the most common cause of acute heavy metal poisoning, and is the second most common source (after lead) of chronic heavy metal poisoning.

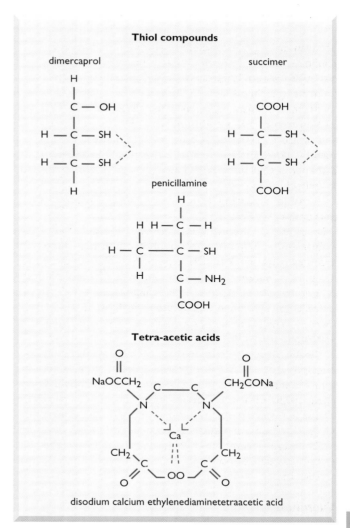

Fig. 29.14 Molecular structure of chelator drugs.

609

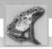

diethylenetriaminepenta-acetic acid (DTPA), dimercaprol, succimer (Fig. 29.14), penicillamine, and deferoxamine. The main use of chelators is to treat poisoning with heavy metals. However, chelators are also promoted for use in such diseases as atherosclerosis (chelation therapy), but controlled trials of such therapies have failed to show benefit.

EDTA is usually given as the calcium disodium salt and these ions are easily displaced by heavier toxic metals, manganese, zinc, and iron. Administration is by intravenous or intramuscular routes, but the latter is painful. Treatment schedules must be followed carefully since rapid infusion of EDTA in other than the calcium disodium form can cause transient hypocalcemia. However, since the body has a huge excess of calcium ions over EDTA ions, calcium concentrations quickly return to normal.

DIMERCAPROL is a dithiol analog of glycerol. Since the chelate formed with thiol groups of dimercaprol is not very stable, dimercaprol therapies are designed to maximize chelate excretion. Dimercaprol is given intramuscularly and is more effective when given early after exposure. Adverse effects include reversible hypertension, tachycardia, nausea, vomiting, burning sensations, salivation, pain, and feelings of anxiety and unrest.

SUCCIMER, a thiol derivative of succinic acid, combines with cysteine to form a mixed disulfide. It chelates arsenic, lead, and mercury, as well as other heavy metals, and is less toxic than dimercaprol.

PENICILLAMINE (D-β,β-dimethylcysteine) is another thiol-containing chelator. It is well absorbed when given orally and is metabolized slowly.

Air pollutants

Most urban air pollution is due to carbon monoxide (CO), sulfur oxides, hydrocarbons, and nitrogen oxides. These come from burning coal and its products, and gasoline. Photochemical pollution (smog) contains hydrocarbons, oxides of nitrogen, and photochemical oxidants. Airborne particles account for 10% of all air pollution (Fig. 29.15).

Airborne particles

Airborne particles >5 μm in diameter are usually deposited in the upper airways, whereas those of 1–5 μm reach the terminal airways and alveoli. A mucus blanket, propelled by cilia (the mucociliary escalator), carries larger insoluble particles upwards to the pharynx, from whence they can be expectorated or swallowed. Silica particles larger than 1 μm reach the alveoli where they are either removed, phagocytized, or absorbed into lymphatics. Pneumoconiosis is caused by inhalation of small dust particles, which are phagocytized. These subsequently form fibrotic silicotic nodules throughout the lungs. Symptomatic pneumoconiosis usually takes years to develop. As it develops it causes an increased lung susceptibility to infection. Asbestos (fibrous hydrated silicates) was widely used in

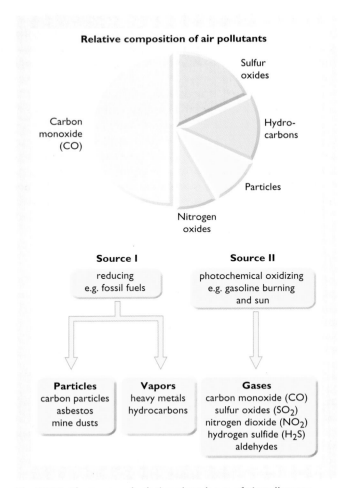

Fig. 29.15 The type and relative abundance of air pollutants.

industry, but bronchial cancer can occur 20–30 years after initial exposure to asbestos. Concomitant smoking increases the chance of developing such a cancer (see page 615). Mesoepithelioma in the pleura or peritoneum is a rapidly fatal malignancy that appears to be related to exposure to chrysolite asbestos fiber and occurs 25–40 years after initial exposure. The wave of litigation following the recognition and publicity of the carcinogenic risk of asbestos bankrupted many manufacturers and their insurance companies. It also led to a massive removal of asbestos and possibly greater exposure of the public than would have occurred if it had been left in place. The correct calculation of the toxic risk to a population is difficult to quantitate and can be severely overestimated.

Carbon monoxide

Carbon monoxide is a colorless, odorless, tasteless, non-irritating gas formed by incomplete combustion of carbon compounds, e.g. car exhaust. It is a major cause of accidental and suicidal deaths. When a fire occurs in an enclosed space, most victims die from acute CO poisoning, rather than from burns. CO binds to hemoglobin (Hb) to form carboxyhemoglobin (COHb), which bind oxygen very ineffectively. The high affinity of CO for hemoglobin (220 times that of oxygen) means that even low concentrations of CO are dangerous and give rise to hypoxia. The reduction in the oxygen-carrying capacity of blood is proportional to the amount of COHb, and the effects of poisoning are due to hypoxia. In addition to decreasing the oxygen-carrying capacity of blood ('functional anemia'), CO also impairs the capacity of Hb to deliver oxygen to the tissues. This is due to a shift in the oxygen dissociation curve to the left (Fig. 29.16). Moderate concentrations of COHb have little effect on vital functions (blood pressure, heart rate) at rest in healthy subjects owing to the considerable reserve in oxygen-carrying capacity of blood, and to the reserve in the cardiovascular system.

COHb fully dissociates and CO is excreted easily by the lungs. Treatment of CO poisoning therefore involves immediate

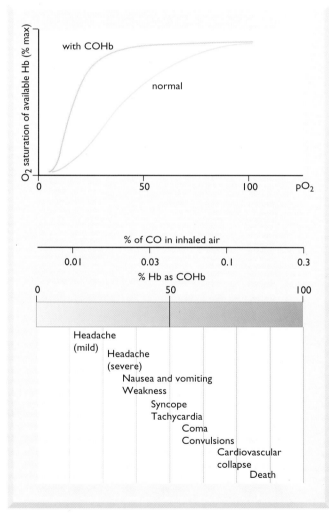

Fig. 29.16 Effects of carboxyhemoglobin (COHb) on oxygen dissociation, and symptoms associated with CO poisoning. The affinity of carbon monoxide (CO) for hemoglobin (Hb) is 220 times higher than oxygen thereby decreasing the oxygen-carrying capacity of blood. In addition, COHb shifts the oxyhemoglobin (O_2Hb)–oxygen saturation curve to the left, making oxygen release during hypoxia more difficult. This is illustrated in the upper panel which is normalized to 100% maximum. If the data were expressed as absolute oxygen content, the values in the presence of COHb would be decreased compared with normal.

transfer to fresh air, with artificial respiration if required. Rapid administration of 100% oxygen is often the only therapy required. It is important to note that certain clinically used transcutaneous oximeters cannot distinguish between carboxy- and oxyhemoglobin and thus are useless in assessing CO poisoning. The cardiovascular system, particularly the heart, is susceptible to low concentrations of CO, since the heart normally extracts a large fraction of oxygen delivered to it. Experimental and clinical studies suggest that long-term exposure to CO facilitates the development of arteriosclerosis. The fetus is especially susceptible to CO and the persistent low levels of COHb produced by smoking during pregnancy may adversely affect fetal development.

In addition to CO being formed during a fire the burning of plastic can release halogenated compounds which are acutely toxic to the lung, causing massive tissue and capillary damage resulting in death. Fires in aircraft and factories are particularly dangerous in this respect.

Other air pollutants

Other air pollutants include sulfur oxides, nitrogen oxides, and aldehydes:

- Inhaled sulfur dioxide causes a parasympathetic-dependent bronchoconstriction in normal people, but this may be very severe in asthmatics, who are sensitive to concentrations as low as 0.25 parts per million.
- Nitrogen dioxide is a lung irritant capable of causing pulmonary edema. It is a particular risk to farmers since it is formed in, and released from, silage and may cause pulmonary damage ('silo-filler's lung').
- Aldehydes are formed by sunlight acting on the products of incomplete combustion, or are released from aldehyde-containing resins. Formaldehyde irritates respiratory mucous membranes and can provoke skin reactions.
- Acrolein is more irritating than formaldehyde and is the major reason for the irritating quality of cigarette smoke and photochemical smog.

Industrial chemicals
Petroleum distillates

Gasoline and kerosene are hydrocarbon distillates containing aliphatic, aromatic, and other hydrocarbons. Most gasolines contain benzene and chronic exposure to benzene can cause leukemia. Intoxication following ingestion or inhalation of gasoline and kerosene (Figs 29.17, 29.18) resembles that due to ethanol intoxication, while inhalation of vapors can cause ventricular fibrillation or chemical pneumonitis complicated by bacterial pneumonia and pulmonary edema. Death due to hemorrhagic pulmonary edema may occur within 24 hours of inhalation. Management of such poisoning is symptomatic and supportive.

Gasoline contaminated drinking water can result in chronic gasoline exposure and possible toxicity. Higher molecular weight compounds in gasoline, like most organic solvents, depress the CNS and cause dizziness and incoordination. Neuropathy is an important toxic effect of n-hexane.

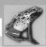

Industrial chemicals

Solvents and vapors	Poisons (varying selectivity)
Gasoline, kerosene, and their derivatives Hydrocarbons (e.g. butane, ethane) Halogenated hydrocarbons Aromatics (e.g. benzene, toluene) Alcohols (ethanol, methanol, propanol) Higher alcohols (glycols) Ethers	Pesticides (many synthetic and a few natural compounds) Insecticides (organophosphates, organochlorines, pyrethrins) Vermin poisons Many rodenticides and general fumigants Herbicides

Fig. 29.17 Dangerous industrial chemicals. Most of the above are varyingly toxic to humans. Solvents and vapors sometimes have similar CNS effects. Herbicides and insecticides, except organophosphate anticholinesterases, have relatively selective actions, but vermin poisons are not so selective. Industrial chemicals generally cause acute toxicity. There are many solvents and vapors whose chemical nature makes them ideal fuels and solvents.

Toxic solvents

Compound	Source
Acetone, esters	Glues Adhesives Dyes Nail polish remover
Hydrocarbons	Gasoline Lighter fuel Acrylic paints
Halogenated hydrocarbons	Paints Glues Rubber cement Shoe polish Spot removers

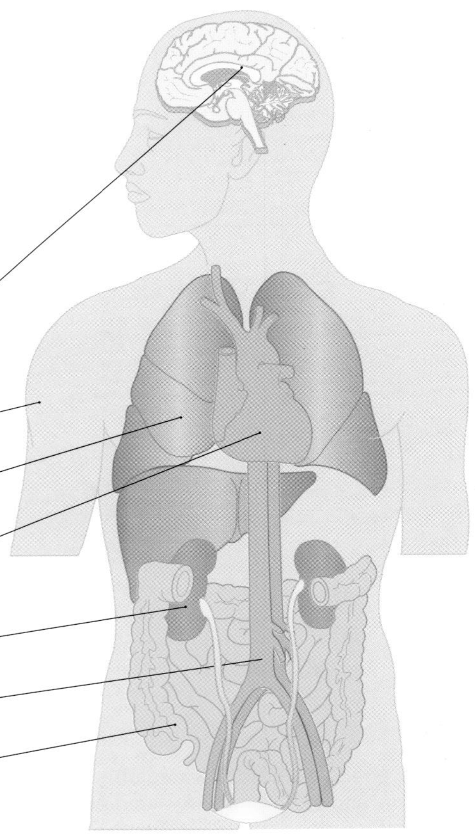

Toxicity of halogenated hydrocarbons

Toxicity to various body systems

Neurologic
drunkenness, anesthesia, coma, seizures, tremors

Skin
burns, dermatitis, eczema

Pulmonary
pulmonary effusions, pneumonitis, pulmonary edema

Cardiovascular (cardiac)
arrhythmias (including ventricular fibrillation),
myocardial necrosis

Renal
tubular necrosis, nephritis

Blood
aplastic anemia, leukemia, myeloma

Gastrointestinal
nausea, vomiting, diarrhea, mucosal inflammation

Fig. 29.18 Toxic solvents and the toxic effects of halogenated hydrocarbons on various body systems.

Halogenated hydrocarbons

Halogenated hydrocarbons are widely used as industrial solvents. Several small chlorinated hydrocarbons are formed in drinking water as a result of the chlorination of drinking water. Other halogenated hydrocarbons can contaminate water supplies. Since there are correlations (casual or causal) between water chlorination and cancer of the colon, rectum, and bladder, there is concern about the exposure of large populations to chlorinated drinking water but at the moment it seems that the benefits of chlorination outweigh the disadvantages.

Transient exposure to carbon tetrachloride vapor causes ocular and nasal irritation, nausea, vomiting, dizziness, and headache. Death may result from ventricular fibrillation, or respiratory depression. Serious and delayed toxic effects include liver and kidney damage. Hepatotoxicity is common with halogenated hydrocarbons in general, but not with the more complex halogenated hydrocarbons used as inhalational anesthetics (see Chapter 26).

Alcohols

Methanol (wood alcohol) is a common industrial solvent and in some countries is added to contaminate ethanol in order to avoid taxes on drinkable ethanol. The absorption, distribution, and metabolism of methanol and ethanol are similar, and their metabolism is by zero-order kinetics (see Chapter 4). Methanol inebriates less than ethanol, and produces headache, vertigo, vomiting, upper abdominal pain, and hyperventilation. Retinal damage may be severe and lead to blindness (see Chapter 24). The other major problem with methanol is metabolic acidosis, which may be severe.

Ethanol has a 100-fold greater affinity for alcohol dehydrogenase than methanol. As a result, a specific treatment for methanol poisoning is to maintain blood ethanol concentrations at >100 mg/100 ml thereby preventing formation of the toxic methanol metabolites, formaldehyde and formic acid (acidosis). Dialysis may be required to decrease methanol concentrations so as to avoid blindness. Maintaining appropriate ethanol concentrations in blood while conducting hemodialysis may present a pharmacokinetic challenge. Methylpyrazole (fomepizole), an alcohol dehydrogenase inhibitor, may be of benefit in the therapy of methanol poisoning.

Other alcohols (isopropanol, ethylene and ethylene glycol (anti-freeze), and propylene alcohol) are also toxic. Fomepizole is effective in the treatment of ethylene glycol poisoning.

Aromatic hydrocarbons

Benzene is an excellent solvent, but highly toxic and carcinogenic. Toxic effects following limited exposure to benzene include blurred vision, tremors, disturbed respiration, cardiac arrhythmias, paralysis, and unconsciousness. Chronic intoxication can cause aplastic anemia and leukemia. Toluene is a CNS depressant and low concentrations produce fatigue, weakness, and confusion, but it probably does not cause aplastic anemia or leukemia. 'Glue sniffers' inhale toluene vapors from glue.

PESTICIDES

Over 0.5 billion kg of pesticides are used in the US every year, 2.0 billion worldwide. Herbicides are most commonly used, followed by insecticides and fungicides.

Insecticides

The insecticide residues that contaminate food result in low-level exposures for the general population, and normally acute poisoning only results from eating heavily contaminated foods, or during agricultural spraying.

Organochlorine insecticides

CHLORINATED ETHANE DERIVATIVES such as DDT have been used extensively as insecticides. The prototype, dichlorodiphenyltrichloroethane (DDT), is highly lipid soluble and therefore only slowly eliminated from the body. It has a wide margin of safety and there are no reports of human deaths. However, adverse effects of DDT on birds high in the food chain, and other potential ecological problems, led to the banning of DDT in many countries. Unfortunately, DDT was, and is, the best insecticide for controlling malarial mosquitoes. Methoxychlor (Fig. 29.19), a replacement for DDT, stimulates the CNS by antagonizing γ aminobutyric acid (GABA) ionotropic receptors resulting in decreased Cl^- currents and reduced inhibition. Methoxychlor and similar compounds can induce convulsions before other less serious signs of toxicity.

CHLORINATED CYCLODIENES, unlike DDT, are readily absorbed from intact skin. Aldrin and dieldrin have the greatest carcinogenic potential among the insecticides and are banned in the US, while chlordane and heptachlor are banned for use on crops.

HYDROCARBONS that have been used as insecticides include the γ isomer of benzene hexachloride (BHC) and the related lindane. Poisoning with lindane causes tremors, ataxia, convulsions, and prostration. Both lindane and BHC have been implicated as a cause of aplastic anemia. Toxaphene induces tumors in mice. Other chlorinated hydrocarbon insecticides concentrate several thousandfold in the food chain.

Interestingly some plants grown in pesticide-free conditions (so-called organic vegetables) are found to contain much greater amounts of natural toxic chemicals than those grown with pesticides. This could be an evolutionary response to increased pest predation in the absence of synthetic pesticides.

Organophosphate insecticides

Organophosphate insecticides (irreversible cholinesterases) are alternatives to organochlorine insecticides. One of them, parathion, is the most frequent cause of fatal poisoning. Cholinesterase inhibition, due to phosphorylation of the enzyme, results in massive acetylcholine accumulation, excessive muscarinic (parasympathetic) receptor stimulation (hypersecretion, diarrhea, sweating), confusion, agitation, and coma. In addition, cholinesterase inhibition leads to excess accumulation of acetylcholine at neuromuscular junctions leading to

613

tetany and muscle weakness. Respiratory failure due to weakness of respiratory muscles may occur. Treatment involves use of atropine as a muscarinic receptor antagonist in the periphery and more importantly in the CNS (see Chapter 14) and artificial

ventilation to support respiration. If organophosphate poisoning is detected promptly, the drug pralidoxime may be used to reactivate the cholinesterase which has been inactivated by phosphorylation. Once reactivated, the accumulated acetylcholine can be hydrolyzed. Pralidoxime is most effective when used early after poisoning. The phosphorylated cholinesterase is thought to 'age' with time, presumably owing to conformational changes, making it less susceptible to re-activation.

Botanic insecticides

Botanic insecticides such as pyrethrin are increasingly used. The crude extract, pyrethrum, is obtained from the pyrethrum plant (related to chrysanthemums) and is considered safe in terms of direct toxicity, but can cause contact dermatitis and respiratory allergy. In the past nicotine has been used as an insecticide, but it is extremely toxic and absorbed through the skin. Rotenone, another natural product previously used in Malaysian jungle streams to catch fish for food, rarely causes human poisoning and is used to treat head lice, scabies, and other ectoparasites. Local effects include conjunctivitis, dermatitis, and rhinitis. Other insecticides are used as ectoparasiticides (e.g. lindane is used as a miticide for scabies, and malathion for nits, see Chapter 23).

General pesticides
Fumigants

Fumigants used to control insects, rodents, and soil nematodes include hydrogen cyanide (HCN), acrylonitrile, carbon disulfide, carbon tetrachloride, ethylene dibromide, ethylene oxide, and methyl bromide, all of which are very poisonous to humans.

HCN is a rapidly acting poison and kills within minutes of exposure. It is released during fires in which nitrogen-containing plastics are burnt. HCN has a high affinity for ferric iron, particularly in mitochondrial cytochrome oxidase where it inhibits cellular respiration. HCN victims die quickly, or recover fully, although chronic neurologic sequelae can occur as result of a period of CNS hypoxia. Treatment of cyanide poisoning has to be rapid. Treatment involves giving nitrites to form methemoglobin, which has a great affinity for HCN, followed by thiosulfate to form the nontoxic thiocyanate. CN salts can be equally toxic to HCN.

Rodenticides

The toxicity of rodenticides varies. For example, the anticoagulant warfarin is relatively safe to nonrodent species since toxicity depends on repeated ingestion, but sodium fluoroacetate and fluoroacetamide, which are among the most potent rodenticides, are very poisonous to man. Strychnine, a poisonous alkaloid,

---

(a) The four major types of organochlorines and their analogs

Compound	Analogs
DDT	Methoxychlor
Benzene chloride	Lindane
Cyclodienes	Aldrin Chlordane Dieldrin
Toxaphenes	Toxaphene

b Organophosphates and carbamates
All are cholinesterase inhibitors with simular structures based upon three themes: phosphates, sulfonates, and carbamates – which all target the esteratic site of acetylcholinesterase

$$\underset{\text{phosphates}}{\overset{\text{S or O}}{\underset{\overset{|}{\text{OR'}}\atop\text{or NHR}}{\overset{\overset{\text{OR}}{\text{or NHR}}}{P}}-S-R}}$$

phosphates

sulfonates

carbamates

The R/R' groups are small groups such as CH_3 or C_2H_5

Molecular target is acetylcholinesterase

Binding irreversible for phosphates but not carbamates

Anionic site   serine   Esteratic site

(c) Pyrethrins

- Pyrethrins are plant extracts, while pyrethroids are semisynthetic analogs
- Metabolized rapidly by man
- Allergenic

Fig. 29.19 Poisonous insecticides, pesticides, and herbicides.
(a) The four major types of organochlorines and their analogs all contain a heavily chlorinated hydrocarbon backbone of MW 300–550, but vary in their toxicity. They are lipid soluble and act on the CNS but are also inducers of hepatic drug-metabolizing enzymes. (b) Organophosphates and carbamates. All are cholinesterase inhibitors with related chemical structures based on phosphate, sulfonate, or carbamate moieties that target the esteratic site of acetylcholinesterase. Over 35 different organophosphates and 20 carbamates are available. (c) Pyrethrins.

is still used as a pesticide and is a source of accidental poisoning. It increases neuronal excitability, which may lead to severe seizures by selectively blocking that neuronal inhibition which is mediated by glycine. Other rodenticides include white or yellow elemental phosphorous spread onto bait. Zinc phosphide reacts with water and acid in the stomach to produce the extremely poisonous phosphine. Thallium sulfate, which is hazardous and not selective for rodents, is now strictly regulated in many countries.

Herbicides

Most herbicides have low toxicity, but they have caused human fatalities. Dioxin (plus byproducts, CDD and TCDD) is a minor impurity in herbicides, and a byproduct of manufacturing processes that use chlorine (e.g. paper making). Several epidemiologic studies of people exposed to high concentrations of dioxin suggest low toxicity, but other studies suggest that TCDD might be carcinogenic and teratogenic.

Several substituted dinitrophenols are used to kill weeds, and human poisoning with dinitro-orthocresol (DNOC) has occurred. The short-term toxicity of dinitrophenols is due to uncoupling of oxidative phosphorylation, and death or recovery occurs within 24–48 hours. Paraquat is responsible for many accidental or suicidal poisonings. It damages the lungs, liver, and kidneys. The serious nature of its delayed pulmonary toxicity makes prompt treatment mandatory. Many other herbicides have relatively low acute toxicities.

Fungicides

Fungicides are a heterogeneous group of chemical compounds, but few have been extensively investigated for toxicity. Dithiocarbamates have some teratogenic and/or carcinogenic potential.

CARCINOGENESIS AND MUTAGENESIS

Chemicals known to cause cancer in humans after prolonged exposure include vinyl chloride, benzene, and naphthylamine. Cigarette smoke contains cancer-causing chemicals, and chronic consumption of ethanol increases the risk of esophageal and liver cancer. Charcoal broiling contaminates food with carcinogenic polycyclic aromatic hydrocarbons (the hydrocarbons found in coal tars). Some foods contain carcinogens and these probably partly account for regional differences in cancer incidences.

Multiple steps are involved in chemical carcinogenesis. The nature of exposure to carcinogens is important (i.e. duration, dose, and frequency). Chemical induction of cancer involves initiation, promotion, and progression. Initiation (by initiating agents) is the conversion of normal cells into neoplastic cells via actions on DNA. However, additional events convert transformed cells to malignant cells. In animals, promoter chemicals increase the incidence of cancers, or decrease the latency to tumor growth, although they do not act on DNA directly, or produce mutations.

A mutation is an alteration in DNA sequence that may change the cellular phenotype. Spontaneous mutagenesis occurs by mostly unknown mechanisms, but this natural rate can be increased 10–1000-fold by mutagens. Mutations are more likely to cause cancer in cells with deficient DNA repair

Carcinogens, cocarcinogens, and promoters

Genotoxic agents (mutagenic)	Chemical alkylating agents Ionizing and ultraviolet (skin) radiation Nickel, cadmium Hydrocarbons (polycyclics) and polyamines (arylamines, nitrosamines)
Epigenetic agents	Hormones such as estrogens Promoters such as phorbol esters Trauma Alcohol ingestion

Fig. 29.20 Carcinogens, cocarcinogens, and promoters.

enzymes, or in which division is so rapid that DNA repair is incomplete. Many cancers are thought to begin as a routine mutation or are a hereditary trait.

Chemical carcinogens are either genotoxic or epigenetic

Genotoxic carcinogens (Fig. 29.20) react covalently with DNA to produce genetic mutations. Mutagenic potential can be detected by tests such as the Ames test for bacterial mutagenicity. Genotoxic carcinogens can be further subclassified on the basis of whether they require biotransformation before they become active. Most genotoxic agents are procarcinogens or activation-dependent genotoxic agents. Nitrosamines are typical procarcinogens.

Epigenetic agents enhance the effects of genotoxic carcinogens. They act by:

- Increasing effector concentrations of genotoxin.
- Enhancing metabolic activation of a genotoxin.
- Decreasing detoxification of a genotoxin.
- Inhibiting DNA repair.
- Increasing proliferation of DNA-damaged cells.

Tumor promoters enhance carcinogenic activity when given after a genotoxin. Phorbol esters are tumor-promoting agents that act by binding to protein kinase C. TCDD (dioxin) is also a potent tumor promoter. Immunosuppressive drugs are epigenetic agents that suppress the immune system and thereby 'allow' carcinogenesis.

Asbestos is an epigenetic carcinogen

Asbestos fibers are centers of mitotic activity and these add to tobacco smoke as a carcinogenic mechanism. Smokers have a 10-fold greater risk of developing lung cancer than nonsmokers. Asbestos increases this risk to 50-fold.

Mechanisms of action of chemical mutagens and carcinogens

- Genotoxins cause genetic damage, which may lead to cancer
- Epigenetic compounds amplify the cancer-forming actions of genotoxins
- Promoters (chemical, physical, and biologic) amplify the adverse effects of mutagens and carcinogens

615

FURTHER READING

Hay A. How to identify a carcinogen. *Nature* 1988; **332:** 782–783. [Procedures for identifying potential carcinogens.]

Klassen CD, et al. (eds) *Casarett & Doull's Toxicology: The Basic Science of Poisons*, 6th edn. New York: McGraw-Hill; 2001. [A standard toxicological reference book.]

Meier J, White J. *Handbook of Clinical Toxicology and Animal Venoms and Poisons*. Boca Raton, Fla: CRC Press; 1995. [Source of information on venoms and animal poisons with a global perspective.]

Sullivan JB, Krieger GR. *Clinical Environmental Health and Toxic Exposures*, 2nd edn. Baltimore: Lippincott Williams and Wilkins; 2001. [Source for material on toxicological hazards in the environment.]

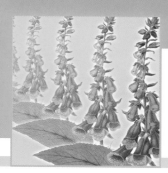

Chapter 30

Herbs

Herbs are plants, containing multiple molecules. Most of the chemicals in plants are structural, such as cellulose, or are concerned with cellular metabolism, for example, multiple enzyme systems. Plants also produce organic molecules which are involved in protection against viruses, bacteria, fungi, insects, animals or other plants that threaten the plant's survival. Many of these chemicals are biologically active in isolation. Therefore, plants are rich sources of chemicals with pharmacological activity which can be considered potential drugs. When parts of plants or extracts of plants are used for medicinal purposes they are called herbal medicines.

From antiquity to the present, plants and plant products have been used to treat disease (see Fig. 1.6). The medical use of herbs is widespread and seems to be increasing. In a multi-ethnic group of patients attending an emergency department in New York, 22% reported that they used herbal medicines; use was highest (37%) among Asians. In North America, most of the herbs are self-administered or provided by health food stores, herbalists or naturopaths. Prescription of herbal preparations by the medical profession is quite common in continental Europe and Asia. Germany and France have the highest *per capita* consumption of herbal medicines in Europe. Germans spent $37 *per capita* on herbal preparations, a total of $2.5 billion, in 1998.

The botanical name of a plant consists of its genus followed by its species designation. Fig. 30.1 shows important medicines that have been isolated and purified from plants, and illustrates several points in the complex relationship between plants and pharmacology:

- Many important drugs have been identified and purified from plants.
- Plants from quite different genuses can produce identical chemicals, e.g. *Atropa* and *Datura* spp. both produce atropine.
- Dissimilar chemicals which have pharmacologically similar actions can be produced by plants from different genuses, e.g. *Hyoscyamus* and *Atropa* each produce antimuscarinic drugs (scopolamine and atropine). Similarly, plants from both *Digitalis* and *Strophanthus* genuses manufacture cardiac glycosides (e.g. digoxin and ouabain).
- Plants from different species of the same genus can produce different chemicals, e.g. *D. purpurea* and *D. lanata* respectively produce the cardiac glycosides digitoxin and digoxin.
- Traditional uses of a plant extract might or might not predict the pharmacology and subsequent use of pure compounds isolated from that plant, e.g. vincristine and vinblastine are used as anticancer drugs owing to their capacity to inhibit

cell division. These drugs were isolated from the plant *Vinca rosa*, claimed to be an oral hypoglycemic agent. In other words, pharmacologically active substances with unexpected actions can be isolated from herbs used for unrelated purposes.

Pharmacologists in the late nineteenth and early part of the twentieth century were active in the identification of pharmacologically active principles in plants and in the standardization of herbal extracts. Their goal was to produce consistent and standardized medicines. Examples are belladonna leaf BP or digitalis leaf USP. The initials BP and USP respectively stood for British Pharmacopaiea and US Pharmacopea and indicated that the medicine had been standardized. Bioassays were extensively used because there were not adequate chemical methods for measurements, and/or the constituents or active ingredients of the herb were not known. Even with modern chemical techniques it is a formidable task to identify the dozens or larger number of potentially active chemicals in any plant. When more than one plant is used in a herbal remedy, the problem is increased greatly.

PROBLEMS SPECIAL TO HERBAL MEDICINES

What is (are) the active ingredient(s)?

Herbal medicines contain scores of chemicals and there is often no agreement as to which chemicals are therapeutically active. An example is garlic (*Allium sativa*), comprised of many sulfur compounds, several of which are candidates for possible therapeutic activity. Another is St. John's wort (*Hypericum perforatum*), which contains chemicals called hypericins, but it seems likely that these are not responsible for the antidepressant effect for which the herb is used; chemical constituents called hyperforins are currently believed to be therapeutically active.

What ensures that herbal medicines contain what is written on their label?

Herbal medicines are not required to pass any regulatory analysis to be sold as a health food supplement. In the United States, herbs are governed under the Dietary Supplement Health and Education Act (DSHEA). Under this legislation claims for treatment of disease can not be made, but herbs can be claimed to be 'Health Modifiers.' The constituents are not regulated unless there is an adverse report concerning a particular product, or sampling of a product shows it to be mislabeled or to contain substances not mentioned on the label.

Examples of drugs obtained from plants traditionally used as herbal remedies or poisons

Botanical name of plant (common name)	Herbal products	Chemicals isolated: used as medicines
Atropa belladonna (Deadly nightshade)	Belladonna leaf, belladonna tincture	Atropine, hyoscyamine
Datura stramonium (Jimson weed, thorn apple)	Stramonium, stramonium tincture	Atropine, hyoscyamine
Hyoscyamus niger (henbane)	Henbane tincture	Scopolamine (hyoscine)
Cinchona ledgeriana (cinchona tree)	Cinchona bark, jesuit bark, cardinal's bark, cortex peruanus	Quinine, quinidine
Colchicum autumnale (autumn crocus, meadow saffron)	Colchicum seed fluid extract, colchicum seed tincture	Colchicine
Digitalis purpurea (purple foxglove)	Digitalis folia (powdered leaf), tincture of digitalis	Digitoxin
Digitalis lanata (woolly foxglove)	Digitalis folia (powdered leaf), tincture of digitalis	Digoxin
Strophanthus gratus	Strophanthus seeds	Ouabain
Ephedra sinica (ma huang)	Ma huang	Ephedrine, pseudoephedrine, phenylpropanolamine
Papaver somniferum (opium poppy)	Powdered opium, laudanum (tincture of opium alkaloids)	Morphine, heroin, codeine, papaverine
Physostigma venenosum (Calabar or ordeal bean)	Whole beans	Physostigmine (eserine)
Pilocarpus jaborandi	Chewed leaves (induced sweating)	Pilocarpine
Rauwolfia serpentina	Rauwiloid, alseroxylon (raudixin)	Reserpine
Salix alba (white willow)	Extract of willow bark	Salicyclic acid
Strychnos toxifera, Chondrodendron tomentosum	Curare (arrow poison)	*d*-Tubocurarine
Vinca rosa (periwinkle)	Alleged oral hypoglycemic	Vincristine, vinblastine

Fig. 30.1 **Examples of drugs obtained from plants traditionally used as herbal remedies or poisons.**

The only regulatory requirements in Canada are that all products intended for medicinal use, including natural health products, are issued a Drug Identification Number. These numbers are not required for raw materials such as bulk herbs or herbal preparations labeled as foods or nutrition supplements.

There are many examples of herbal medicines that have been adulterated with other (more toxic) herbs, potent synthetic drugs (e.g. phenylbutazone, synthetic corticosteroids or other prescription drugs), or heavy metals (mercury or lead).

Occasionally the plant constituents are inadequately, or wrongly, named. For instance the term ginseng is applied to Siberian ginseng, but this plant is of the genus *Eleutherococcus* not *Panax* as is American or Korean ginseng. Consequently, the term ginseng by itself has little meaning. Only the botanical name, consisting of genus and species, identifies a plant.

How are herbal medicines standardized?

The chemical constituents of plants vary depending on the species, variety and part of the plant, with conditions of growth (soil, water and temperature), with the season of the year, and with the age of the plant. These complexities and variations of chemical content make standardization of active incredients in principle very important. In some cases standardization is attempted, but it is difficult and seldom accomplished. There are no regulations governing the standardization of chemical constituents for herbal medicines. Even if the label says 'Standardized' on some constituent, it usually is not known whether that constituent is the main contributor to any therapeutic effect. In other words, the potential for considerable variability from one preparation to another is a concern for pharmacologically active herbal products.

PROBLEMS COMMON TO ALL HERBS (as well as prescription drugs)

How can effectiveness be determined?

To establish the effectiveness of herbs as medicines, they should be tested in prospective, double blind, randomized, controlled clinical trials, preferably with a placebo arm (RCTs). Very few herbs have been tested in this manner, though it is the generally expected standard of regulatory agencies for prescription drugs. However, at the present time there is no legal requirement that herbal preparations be demonstrated to be effective in the treatment of disease in any country. The explanations for this apparent discrepancy in availability of herbal medicines versus prescription drugs involve complex political, social, and economic factors.

Adverse effects

There is a general belief amongst lay people that, because herbs are 'natural,' they are completely safe. This is not true, especially as these preparations generally have pharmacologic activity—that is, they are not inert. Herbs and herbal preparations can cause direct adverse effects, produce serious allergic reactions, and adverse drug interactions. An example is St. John's wort, which induces enzymes involved in the metabolism of cyclosporine leading to decreased steady-state concentrations of cyclosporine unless its dose is increased. St. John's wort also seems to increase the action of antidepressant drugs that modulate serotonin uptake, such as the SSRIs. Herbs also can interfere with laboratory tests. An example is Siberian ginseng, which produces fictitiously high concentrations of digoxin when taken concomitantly with digoxin.

Some examples of direct adverse effects of herbs are shown in Fig. 30.2.

HERBAL MEDICINES COMMONLY USED BY PATIENTS

Figure 30.3 provides a list of some common herbal medicines with their traditional indications. Current RCT evidence of effectiveness and some known adverse effects are included in the table. At the present time none of the trial-based evidence of effectiveness can be considered conclusive; trials where some benefit over placebo has been shown require confirmation with larger trials of longer duration. There is very little data available for the long-term safety of these preparations.

SUMMARY

Plants are rich sources of chemicals and potential sources of effective medicines. However, more research, regulation, and standardization are required before herbal medicines can be recommended as effective and safe therapies. At present it is 'Caveat emptor' (let the buyer beware). Health care providers should be aware that patients frequently consume herbal products and that these preparations may have powerful pharmacologic effects, and may cause adverse effects in their own right, as well as having pharmacodynamic and pharmacokinetic interactions with prescribed traditional drugs. Consequently, a careful history needs to be obtained from patients about the possible use of these preparations; this issue will likely grow in importance, as their use may continue to increase.

Some herbs and direct adverse effects

Common names (botanical name)	Adverse effects	Putative constituents responsible	Putative mechanisms responsible
Aconite (Aconitum carmichaelii) Monkshood (A. columbianum)	Cardiac arrhythmias	Aconitine	Activation of sodium channels
(Aristolochia fangchi)	Renal toxicity and carcinogenesis	Aristolochic acid	Chromosomal damage
Chaparral (Larrea tridentata)	Liver toxicity		Cholestatic hepatitis
Comfrey (Symphytum officinale)	Jaundice, ascites, cirrhosis	Pyrrolizidines	Hepatic venous occlusion
Ephedra or ma huang (Ephedra sinensis)	Cardiac arrhythmias, CNS stimulation	Ephedrine, norephedrine and related compounds	Sympathomimetic activity
Germander (Teucrium chamaedrys)	Liver toxicity		
Licorice (Glycyrrhiza glabra)	Increases sodium retention and potassium excretion	Glycyrrhizins	Inhibition of cortisol metabolism in kidney leading to aldosterone-like effects
St John's wort (Hypericum perforatum)	Skin photosensitivity, drug interactions (increases cyclosporine metabolism)	Hypericins	Induction of cytochrome P-450 enzymes

Fig. 30.2 Some herbs and direct adverse effects.

619

Some common herbal medicines—a brief summary of use and evidence of effectiveness

Common name (botanical name)	Traditional use	Therapeutic ingredients	Mechanism	Number of RCTs with placebo comparison (Result)	Adverse effects
Chamomile, German (*Chamomilla recutita*)	Tonic Mouthwash, oral mucositis	Unknown	Unknown	0 1 (=)	Allergy
Devil's claw (*Harpagophytum procumbens*)	Antirheumatic (low back pain)	Unknown		1 (=)	
Echinacea (*Echinacea purpurea*)	Immune stimulant (upper respiratory infections)	Unknown	Immune stimulant	12 (?) 3 (+) 2 (=)	Allergy
Evening primrose (*Oenothera biennis*)	Atopic dermatitis Rheumatoid arthritis Psoriatic arthritis Premenstrual syndrome Menopausal flushing Obesity Ulcerative colitis Hyperactivity attention deficit Raynaud's syndrome Sjögren's syndrome Psoriasis	Unknown	Unknown	5 (2+,3=) 3 (?) 1 (=) 2 (=) 1 (=) 1 (=) 1 (=) 2 (=) 1 (=) 1 (=) 2 (=)	
Feverfew (*Tanacetum parthenium*)	Migraine Rheumatoid arthritis	Parthenolides Unknown	Unknown	2 (+) 1 (=)	Allergy
Garlic (*Allium sativum*)	BP lowering Cholesterol lowering	Unknown Unknown	Unknown	7 (?) 13 (?)	
Ginger (*Zingiber officinale*)	Seasickness Hyperemesis gravidarum Postoperative nausea/vomiting	Unknown Unknown Unknown	Unknown	1 (=) 1 (+) 3 (2+, 1=)	
Ginkgo (Egb 761) (*Ginkgo biloba*)	Dementia progression Tinnitus	Ginkgolides, platelet activating factor (PAF) antagonists Unknown	Unknown	6 (5+, 1=) 2 (1+, 1=)	Bleeding
Ginseng, American (*Panax quinquefolius*)	Exercise performance	Ginsenosides	Unknown	1 (=)	
Ginseng, Korean (*Panax ginseng*)	Exercise performance Psychomotor performance Flu vaccine immunization response	Ginsenosides Ginsenosides Ginsenosides	Unknown	2 (=) 1 (=) 1 (+)	Gynecodynia
Ginseng, Siberian (*Eleutherococcus senticossus*)	Exercise performance	Eleutherosides		1 (=)	Interferes with measurement of digitalis in blood
PC-SPES Eight herbs	Prostate cancer	Estrogenic compounds	Anti-testosterone	0	Gynecomastia, Thrombosis

Some common herbal medicines—a brief summary of use and evidence of effectiveness (Continued)					
Common name (botanical name)	Traditional use	Therapeutic ingredients	Mechanism	Number of RCTs with placebo comparison (Result)	Adverse effects
Saint John's wort (*Hypericum perforatum*)	Antidepressant	Hyperforins, hypericins	SSRI	2 (+)	Skin photo-sensitivity, drug interactions
Saw Palmetto (Pemixon®) (*Serenoa repens*)	Prostatic hyperplasia	Unknown—antiadrenergic	Unknown	2 (+)	
Zemaphyte® Ten herbs	Atopic eczema	Unknown	Unknown	1 (+)	Liver toxicity

\+ reported benefit greater than placebo;
? reported benefit unlikely (due to design or analytical flaw);
= reported benefit same as placebo.
Many of these trials involved relatively few patients and cannot be regarded as definitive.

Fig. 30.3 **Some common herbal medicines—a brief summary of use and evidence of effectiveness.**

FURTHER READING

Ernst E, et al. *The Desktop Guide to Complementary and Alternative Medicine: An Evidence-Based Approach*. London: Mosby; 2001.

McGuffin M, Hobbs C, and Goldberg A (eds) *Botanical Safety Handbook*. Boca Raton and New York: CRC Press; 1997. [A publication of the American Herbal Products Association with extensive lists of herbs and their toxicities. The therapeutic use of herbs is also mentioned but is not backed up by evidence based on randomized, controlled trials.]

4

Self Assessment

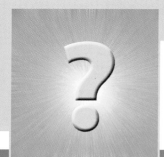

Multiple Choice Questions

Indicate which is the correct answer for each question.

2. Drug Names and Drug Classification Systems

1. A pharmacopeia Is
a) a reference book for drugs
b) a β adrenoceptor antagonist
c) a drug
d) a plant
e) a medicine

2. Drugs have been classified on the basis of all of the following, except
a) pharmacotherapeutic action
b) source
c) chemical nature
d) color
e) molecular size

3. In scientific and medical usage, drugs should be referred to by their
a) clinical name
b) generic name
c) color
d) botanic origin
e) brand name

3. General Principles of Drug Action

1. A full agonist is
a) a drug with no intrinsic activity
b) a drug with an intrinsic activity of 1
c) a drug that blocks ion channels
d) a β receptor antagonist
e) an inverse agonist

2. An inverse agonist is
a) an antagonist
b) a muscarinic receptor antagonist
c) a drug that antagonizes a symporter
d) a drug that interacts with a receptor to reduce any resting level of molecular activity
e) a drug with an intrinsic activity of 1

3. Receptor antagonists bind to
a) the nucleus
b) membrane proteins
c) lipids
d) oxygen
e) enzymes

4. G proteins are
a) part of the cellular transduction system
b) ion channels
c) found in the nucleus
d) plasma proteins
e) clotting factors

5. Tyrosine kinases are
a) ion channel proteins
b) receptors for growth factors
c) part of the Krebs cycle
d) nucleic acids
e) molecular targets for drugs

6. ion channels
a) are molecular targets for drugs
b) gate the passage of ions across nuclear membranes
c) gate the passage of ions across lipid bilayers
d) are enzymes
e) are plants

7. Glucocorticosteroids interact with
a) ion channels
b) tyrosine kinases
c) G proteins
d) intracellular receptors
e) lipids

8. β_2 Agonists bind to
a) lipids
b) nucleic acids
c) G proteins
d) seven transmembrane-spanning proteins
e) enzymes

4. Pharmacokinetic and Other Factors Influencing Drug Action

1. 600 mg of a drug is administered intravenously to a 60 kg patient. The plot of log e plasma concentration of drug versus time (t) is linear and the extrapolated concentration at t = 0 is found to be 1 μg/ml. Based only on this information, which one of the following conclusions can be drawn about the drug in question?
a) it is extensively bound to plasma proteins
b) it is largely ionized at physiologic pH
c) its apparent distribution volume approximates that of total body water
d) it is extensively accumulated in body tissue
e) it is likely to show a high first-pass effect following oral administration

2. A drug with an elimination half-life of 7 hours is given as an initial loading dose, followed by repeated maintenance doses to keep the plasma concentration within 80% of the maximal value attained with the loading dose. The maximum allowable dosing interval is
a) 1/2 hour
b) 1 hour
c) 2 hours
d) 4 hours
e) 8 hours

3. Based on the knowledge of its half-life, a drug is given as a loading dose of 100 mg followed by daily maintenance doses of 16 mg. What is the assumed half-life?
a) 2 days
b) 3 days
c) 4 days
d) 5 days
e) 6 days

4. A drug with a first-order rate constant of elimination equal to 0.3/hour is to be given as an intravenous infusion. Approximately how long would it take for the plasma concentration of this drug to reach a steady state?
a) one circulation time
b) 1.5 hours
c) 3 hours
d) 6 hours
e) 12 hours

5. The plasma concentration of a drug showing zero-order (saturation) kinetics decreases from 10 mg/liter to 8 mg/liter in 1 hour. How long would it take for the plasma concentration of this drug to fall from 10 mg/liter to 2 mg/liter assuming that zero-order kinetics still apply at this concentration?
a) 2 hours
b) 4 hours
c) 8 hours
d) 10 hours
e) none of the above

6. Which one of the following statements is incorrect?
a) conjugation (phase 2) reactions involving drugs or their metabolites are not mediated by the cytochrome P-450 system in the liver
b) metabolism of a drug usually decreases its lipid solubility
c) the extent to which a drug is bound to plasma proteins is not directly predictive of its rate of renal excretion
d) for drugs with first-order elimination kinetics, a constant amount of drug is lost per unit time
e) for drugs with zero-order elimination kinetics, the relationship between drug dosage and maximally attained plasma concentration is nonlinear

7. All the following may significantly affect the duration of a drug's effects, except
a) rate of metabolism to inactive metabolites
b) rate of absorption into the blood stream
c) rate of excretion of inactive metabolites
d) initiation of compensatory reflexes
e) extensive plasma protein binding of the drug

8. All the following may shorten the duration of a drug's effects, except
a) extensive plasma protein binding of the drug
b) compensatory reflexes
c) redistribution of the drug into skeletal muscle or adipose tissue
d) renal excretion of the drug
e) metabolism of the drug

5. Pharmacodynamics and the Measurement of Drug Action

1. Chemical groups or sites on the surface of or within the cell, with which drugs combine to produce an effect, are called
a) autacoids
b) antagonists
c) agonists
d) molecular targets (e.g. receptors)
e) placebos

2. An agent that interferes with the action of a hormone by binding to the hormone receptor is referred to as
a) an antagonist
b) an antagonist
c) an enzyme inhibitor
d) a modulator
e) a competitor

3. When the contractile response of a smooth muscle preparation to an agonist for which the receptor reserve is 1000 is recorded, all of the following are true, except
a) a competitive blocker will cause a parallel shift of the response–log dose curve, with an increase in the agonist's EC_{50} and no change in the maximum response to agonist
b) an irreversible receptor blocker will depress the maximum response to this agonist less than it blocks the maximal response to a partial agonist at the same receptor
c) an irreversible receptor blocker will shift the response–log dose curve in much the same way as a competitive blocker until dose ratios of about 100 or greater are produced
d) a noncompetitive blocker will reduce the maximum response to the agonist without changing its EC_{50}
e) the half-maximal response of the tissue will occur at a concentration of the agonist about equal to $1/1000$ (10^{-3}) of the agonist–receptor dissociation constant

4. In the absence of other drugs, pindolol increases heart rate by activating β adrenoceptors. However, when the heart rate has been increased by epinephrine, pindolol causes a dose-dependent reversible decrease in heart rate. From this information, pindolol is probably
a) a noncompetitive antagonist
b) a physiologic antagonist
c) a chemical antagonist
d) a partial agonist
e) a spare receptor agonist

5. In a test preparation, acetylcholine (ACh) is a full agonist that produces a half-maximum response at a concentration that occupies only 0.1% of the ACh receptors. The maximum response is 100 units. At a certain 'low' dose ACh produces a response of 10 units. An irreversible blocker is applied long enough to inactivate 90% of the receptors. After this treatment, responses to the 'low' dose of ACh

and the maximum response to ACh will be close to
a) 1 unit and 10 units
b) 10 units and 100 units
c) 5 units and 50 units
d) 1 unit and 100 units
e) none of the above

6. Partial agonist drugs
a) reduce the apparent potency of a full agonist acting on the same receptor
b) act at sites on the receptor remote from the agonist binding site
c) increase the apparent potency of a full agonist drug acting on the same receptor
d) are always less potent than full agonists at the same receptor
e) reduce the maximum effect produced by the combination of the partial agonist and the full agonist at the same receptor

7. Which of the following class/classes of antagonist drug produce a block that can always be overcome by increasing doses of agonist drug?
a) irreversible competitive antagonists
b) irreversible noncompetitive antagonists
c) reversible competitive antagonists
d) physiologic antagonists
e) chemical antagonists

6. Drug Safety and Pharmacovigilance

1. Anaphylaxis from penicillin ingestion is an adverse drug effect of type
a) A
b) B
c) C
d) E
e) D

2. Drug safety is the responsibility of
a) drug regulatory bodies (e.g. the Food and Drug Administration)
b) the physician
c) the pharmaceutical company manufacturing the drug
d) the American Medical Association

3. For what sort of new medicines is post-marketing surveillance essential in the public interest
a) medicines intended for widespread long-term use
b) anesthetic agents
c) all new drugs
d) drugs for sexual dysfunction

4. The following patient groups are likely to be more susceptible to the adverse effects of drugs
a) teachers
b) neonates
c) patients with liver disease
d) athletes
e) the elderly

5. Drug interactions have important clinical outcomes in
a) women taking phenobarbital who rely on oral contraceptives
b) men taking vitamin supplements who are prescribed theophylline
c) any patient prescribed lithium who is also taking a thiazide diuretic
d) any patient taking iron sulfate who is then prescribed tetracycline

7. Regulation of Drug Use

1. Regulatory agencies for drugs attempt to accomplish all of the following except
a) an evaluation of data on whether a drug is efficacious
b) an evaluation of data on whether a drug's toxicity is acceptable
c) an evaluation of preclinical data to decide whether testing a new drug in people may proceed
d) an evaluation of whether individual health care professionals are acting skilfully when administering drugs to patients

2. Controlled, randomized, double blind clinical trials
a) are biased because patients can choose which treatment to take
b) do not compare a new drug either with a placebo or with an established agent
c) are very important in phase III of drug development
d) are useful because health professionals can draw conclusions about a drug's efficacy while such trials are being conducted, since they know which therapy the experimental patients are getting

3. A parallel trial differs from a crossover trial in that
a) in a parallel trial, patients get all therapies and in a crossover trial, patients choose which therapy to take
b) a parallel trial is always controlled and a crossover trial is never controlled
c) a crossover trial uses a surrogate end-point, whereas a parallel trial uses a more definitive end-point
d) in a parallel trial, a patient receives only one regimen, whereas in a crossover trial, each patient receives several regimens

4. Which choice is true?
a) the FDA has jurisdiction to approve drugs all over the world if the drug is manufactured by an American company
b) the FDA can give advice to companies on when to initiate trials in people but can not prevent a company from doing so
c) in Europe, both the centralized and decentralized procedures for approval are more uniform among participating countries
d) the FDA, the Committee on Proprietary Medicinal Products and the Japanese Central Pharmaceutical Affairs Council must agree before a drug is approved

5. In Japan
a) the Ministry of Health and Welfare reviews data primarily for its scientific content
b) the Central Pharmaceutical Affairs Council is primarily an administrative body without scientific qualifications
c) the Central Pharmaceutical Affairs Council evaluates data and recommends a course of action to the Ministry of Health and Welfare
d) drugs are approved by the CPMP

6. Which of the following is false?
a) an end-point is an indication of a drug's effect
b) a surrogate end-point is not the real goal of therapy but is predictive of the real goal of therapy

c) 'open label' describes a clinical trial where both the health professional and patient know what agent the patient is getting

d) an end-point tells a health professional when a clinical trial is completed

8. Drugs and Viruses

1. Pharmacokinetic drug interactions are a significant concern for all of the following agents except:
   a) nevirapine
   b) ritonavir
   c) rifampin
   d) zidovudine
   e) indinavir

2. An acceptable first regimen for the treatment for symptomatic HIV infection would include any of the following except:
   a) indinavir, ritonavir, zidovudine, lamivudine
   b) stavudine, lamivudine
   c) efavirenz, didanosine, stavudine
   d) zidovudine, lamivudine, abacavir
   e) saquinavir (soft-gel capsules), stavudine, nevirapine

3. Class characteristics of nucleoside analog reverse transcriptase inhibitors (NRTIs) include which of the following:
   a) rash is a common adverse effect
   b) clearance is increased by concurrent rifampin administration
   c) single HIV-1 reverse transcriptase mutations confer resistance to the class
   d) metabolism by viral enzymes is prerequisite for antiviral activity
   e) dosing intervals reflect intracellular half-lifes of the individual agents

4. Properties of acyclovir include all the following, except:
   a) has excellent oral absorption
   b) inhibits herpes simplex virus and varicella zoster virus
   c) is eliminated largely unchanged in the urine
   d) has modest adverse effects after oral administration
   e) may cause renal tubular obstruction

5. Both amantadine and rimantadine share all the following characteristics, except:
   a) inhibit replication of influenza A virus
   b) have good oral absorption
   c) are eliminated largely unchanged in the urine
   d) are effective for the prophylaxis and treatment of influenza A virus infection
   e) are commonly associated with the development of resistance during therapy

6. Resistance to acyclovir in herpes simplex virus is likely to be resistant to all the following, except:
   a) penciclovir
   b) edoxuridine
   c) ganciclovir
   d) valacyclovir
   e) adenine-arabinoside

7. The properties of interferons include all the following, except:
   a) are cytokines
   b) have common adverse effects resembling a flu-like illness
   c) are not effective when administered orally
   d) inhibit viral replication indirectly
   e) cause renal failure at high doses

8. Treatment of a patient with HIV-1 infection with zidovudine alone for 1 year is associated with all the following, except:
   a) a sustained inhibition of HIV-1 replication
   b) anemia as the likeliest adverse effect
   c) emergence of zidovudine-resistant virus
   d) a probable improved response if lamivudine is added
   e) a probable improved response if saquinavir is added

9. Protease inhibitors of HIV-1, such as saquinavir, have all the following properties, except:
   a) inhibit HIV-1 replication by blocking uncoating of the virus during cell penetration
   b) produce an additive antiviral effect when given with zidovudine
   c) may prevent emergence of zidovudine-resistant virus when given with zidovudine
   d) are associated with the ready development of resistance if used alone
   e) have minimal adverse effects

10. Properties of zidovudine include all the following, except:
    a) undergoes phosphorylation to generate the molecule that inhibits HIV-1 replication
    b) has a narrow toxic therapeutic ration for red blood cell progenitor cells
    c) is well absorbed after oral administration
    d) crosses the blood–brain barrier
    e) does not cross the placenta

9. Drugs and Bacteria

1. Which of the following antibiotics demonstrate concentration-dependent killing of bacteria?
   a) penicillin G
   b) amoxicillin
   c) cefotaxime
   d) gentamicin
   e) vancomycin

2. The treatment of choice for serious infections due to methicillin-resistant *Staphylococcus aureus* is
   a) cloxacillin
   b) cefazolin
   c) clindamycin
   d) chloramphenicol
   e) vancomycin

3. The addition of clavulanate to amoxicillin results in activity against all the following β lactamase-producing organisms, except
   a) *Enterobacter cloacae*
   b) *Staphylococcus aureus*
   c) *Haemophilus influenzae*
   d) *Neisseria gonorrhoeae*
   e) *Bacteroides fragilis*

4. An oral drug that is effective for the treatment of urinary tract infections due to *Pseudomonas aeruginosa* is
   a) amoxicillin
   b) cefixime
   c) ciprofloxacin
   d) gentamicin
   e) ceftazidime

5. All the following statements about erythromycin are true, except
   a) it produces a relatively high incidence of gastrointestinal toxicity
   b) it is an alternative to penicillin for treating pneumococcal meningitis

c) in combination with terfenadine it can cause ventricular tachycardia
d) It is an alternative to penicillin for streptococcal pharyngitis
e) it is the drug of choice for legionnaires' disease

6. All the following antibiotics are active against *Bacteroides fragilis*, except
   a) metronidazole
   b) clindamycin
   c) amoxicillin–clavulanate
   d) trimethroprim–sulfamethoxazole
   e) imipenem

7. Tetracyclines
   a) are considered safe in pregnancy
   b) are recommended in infancy
   c) should be given with antacids
   d) are active against *Pseudomonas aeruginosa*
   e) are useful in the treatment of chlamydial infections

8. All of the following antibiotic drug combinations result in significant drug interactions, except
   a) erythromycin and astemizole
   b) clindamycin and phenytoin
   c) ciprofloxacin and theophylline
   d) rifampin and warfarin
   e) tetracycline and sucralfate

10. Drugs and Fungi

1. The following statements are correct
   a) fungi reproduce by spore formation
   b) zoophilic fungi are likely to produce less inflammation than anthropophilic species
   c) most fungi that are pathogenic to man are Fungi Imperfecti
   d) microscopy and culture of skin or tissue is the most important investigation of fungal disease
   e) Wood's light examination can help in the diagnosis and management of fungal infection

2. The following mechanisms of action are correct
   a) amidazoles and triazoles inhibit the synthesis of fungal lipids, especially ergosterol
   b) terbinafine prevents the synthesis of ergosterol by inhibiting the action of squalene epoxidase
   c) amphotericin B acts by binding to ergosterol in cell membranes
   d) amidazoles and triazoles interfere with fungal oxidative enzymes
   e) griseofulvin is thought to act by interfering with microtubule function or with nucleic acid synthesis and polymerization

3. The following statements about the metabolism of anti-fungal agents are correct
   a) amphotericin B and itraconazole are largely protein bound in the blood
   b) the azole antifungal agents are orally active and penetrate the blood–brain barrier
   c) doses of fluconazole need to be modified in renal failure
   d) terbinafine is concentrated in skin, nails, and fat
   e) blood flucytosine concentration should be monitored

4. Oral candidiasis
   a) is more common in people with diabetes mellitus
   b) is a common complication of inhaled antiasthma medication
   c) is treated with amphotericin B

d) treatment in patients with dentures includes treatment of the dentures as well as the mouth

e) suggests immunosuppression or chronic mucocutaneous candidiasis if the patient fails to respond to topical treatment

5. In cryptococcal meningitis

a) combination treatment with amphotericin B and flucytosine is the treatment of choice in non-AIDS patients

b) combination therapy delays the development of resistant organisms

c) in patients with AIDS requires long-term therapy to prevent relapse

d) fluconazole can be used to induce clinical remission

e) oral itraconazole and fluconazole suppress recurrences after induction of remission

6. The following statements about adverse effects are correct

a) headaches can be experienced with amphotericin B, griseofulvin, and itraconazole

b) thrombophlebitis can be a problem with intravenous amphotericin B and miconazole

c) amphotericin B is nephrotoxic

d) hepatotoxicity is the major adverse effect of ketoconazole

e) fluconazole and itraconazole interfere less with androgen steroid synthesis than ketoconazole

7. The following statements are correct

a) in pityriasis versicolor, shampoo preparations (e.g. ketoconazole shampoo) are a useful first-line treatment

b) *Tinea pedis* infection at swimming pools can be reduced by the use of tolnaftate powder

c) topical treatment of scalp ringworm limits spread, but systemic treatment is needed to eradicate the infection

d) cure rates and relapse rates of nail infections are better with terbinafine than with griseofulvin

e) ketoconazole can be used instead of amphotericin B for histoplasmosis and paracoccidioidomycosis of the lung

11. Drugs and Parasites

1. Which one of the following statements about metronidazole is incorrect?

a) it is extremely useful in the treatment of trichomoniasis and amebiasis

b) it has disulfiram-like effects (producing nausea and vomiting), when alcohol is consumed while the drug is still within the body

c) because of its possible mutagenic effects, its use is contraindicated in the first trimester of pregnancy unless absolutely necessary (e.g. severe life-threatening infection)

d) it is poorly absorbed from the gastrointestinal tract, and therefore has to be given parenterally

e) its mechanism of action appears to involve disruption of the structure of DNA in susceptible organisms, resulting in strand breakage and the loss of DNA's helical structure

2. Which one of the following statements about chloroquine is correct?

a) it is active against exo-red blood cell forms of malaria

b) it is used to prevent initial material infection as well as subsequent relapse

c) prolonged high-dosage therapy may cause corneal and retinal changes and optic atrophy

d) its principal sites of action are Ca^{2+} channels within the cell membranes of malarial organisms, leading to increased Ca^{2+} permeability and cell death

e) it is commonly used in the treatment of filarial worm and roundworm infections

3. Which one of the following drugs is the drug of choice for treating late African trypanosomiasis with central nervous system involvement?

a) pentamidine

b) melarsoprol

c) nifurtimox

d) suramin

e) praziquantel

4. Which of the following drugs is combined with pyrimethamine to produce an antimalarial action by sequential blockade of folic acid biosynthesis in sensitive *Plasmodium* strains?

a) chloroquine

b) primaquine

c) mefloquine

d) sulfadoxine

e) quinacrine

5. The mechanism of action of praziquantel against schistosomes is believed to be

a) alteration of Ca^{2+} handling by the schistosome

b) alteration of Na^+ handling by the schistosome

c) alteration of glucose handling by the schistosome

d) alteration of ATPases in the schistosome

e) activation of lytic enzymes in the schistosome

6. Which one of the following statements about cerebral malaria is incorrect?

a) intravenous quinine can be useful

b) derivatives of *Artemisia* can be useful

c) children are a major group affected by it

d) children are less likely to die from it than adults

e) *Plasmodium falciparum* is the major cause

12. Drugs and Neoplasms

1. All of the following drugs are correctly matched with a major adverse effect, except

a) prednisone: bone marrow suppression

b) cyclophosphamide: hemorrhagic cystitis

c) vincristine: neurologic toxicity

d) doxorubicin: cardiomyopathy

e) 5-fluorouracil: bone marrow suppression

2. All of the following drugs are correctly matched with their mechanism of action, except

a) 5-fluorouracil: antimetabolite

b) lomustine: alkylating agent

c) dactinomycin: antimetabolite

d) vincristine: antimitotic agent

e) 6-mercaptopurine: antimetabolite

3. All of the following statements regarding doxorubicin are correct, except

a) it has a narrow spectrum of antitumor activity

b) it is a natural product

c) it acts on topoisomerase II

d) it can generate free radicals

e) it can cause cardiotoxicity

4. Which one of the following statements concerning the adverse effects of anticancer drugs is false?

a) many anticancer drugs initially cause nausea and vomiting as a result of their direct gastrointestinal toxicity

b) many anticancer drugs are potential carcinogens

c) anticancer drugs can cause amenorrhea or impair spermatogenesis

d) patients undergoing chemotherapy who develop leukopenia are susceptible to opportunistic infections

e) hyperuricemia can occur when anticancer drugs produce a high tumor cell kill

13. Drugs and the Blood

1. A 73-year-old man with a history of congestive heart failure and thrombotic stroke who has been on ticlopidine is admitted for shortness of breath and atrial fibrillation. Initial laboratory evaluation shows a white blood cell count of 1.0 K (1.0×19^9/liter) and platelet count of 250 K (250×10^9/liter). What is the best treatment option?

a) continue ticlopidine since it is indicated for the prevention of thrombotic stroke

b) discontinue ticlopidine and treat with aspirin

c) discontinue ticlopidine and treat with lifelong heparin

d) discontinue ticlopidine and treat with warfarin

e) continue ticlopidine and add warfarin

2. Which of the following is a correct description of vitamin K deficiency?

a) directly inhibits synthesis of coagulation factors II, VII, IX, and X

b) commonly due to inadequate dietary intake

c) may be caused by prolonged antibiotic use

d) diagnosis is provided by prolongation of prothrombin time alone

3. Which of the following statements is incorrect regarding iron absorption?

a) absorption of iron in the gastrointestinal tract requires intrinsic factor

b) ascorbic acid facilitates iron absorption

c) many foods such as eggs interfere with iron absorption

d) an acidic environment in the intestine increases iron absorption

4. A 24-year-old woman with von Willebrand's disease has persistent bleeding following a dental procedure. In the emergency room, she has received desmopressin (DDAVP) intravenously, but she continues to bleed. Her hermoglobin level is 8 g/dl (4.96 mmol/liter). Which of the following treatment options is inappropriate?

a) repeat treatment with DDAVP until the bleeding stops

b) use a recombinant factor VIII concentrate to minimize risk of viral transmission

c) use a high purity factor since it is as good as recombinant factor VIII

d) use an intermediate purity factor VIII concentrate

5. A 54-year-old man is brought to the emergency room with an acute myocardial infarction. Two weeks ago, he was prescribed penicillin to treat a streptococcal sore throat. Which of the following treatment options is inappropriate?

a) aspirin and streptokinase

b) aspirin, heparin, and anisoylated plasminogen streptokinase activator complex (APSAC)

c) aspirin, heparin, and recombinant tissue plasminogen activator (rt-PA)

d) aspirin and APSAC

14. Drugs and the Nervous System

1. Primarily inhibitory neurotransmitters include
a) dopamine
b) glutamate
c) glycine
d) acetylcholine
e) γ-aminobutyric acid (GABA)

2. The following are examples of G protein-coupled receptors
a) GABA$_A$ receptors
b) dopamine D$_2$ receptors
c) 5-hydroxytryptamine-3 (5-HT$_3$) receptors
d) muscarinic acetylcholine receptors
e) β adrenoceptors

3. The following statements are true
a) the nucleus basalis of Meynert is the primary acetycholine-containing nucleus
b) the tuberoinfundibular dopamine tract is involved in the regulation of prolactin release
c) 5-HT is the principal neurotransmitter in the locus ceruleus
d) the amygdala has input from both noradrenergic and dopaminergic tracts
e) the raphe nuclei are the origin of most norepinephrine-containing neurons

4. Components of the limbic system include
a) mamillary bodies
b) olivary nuclei
c) cingulate gyrus
d) locus ceruleus
e) amygdala

5. In major depressive disorders
a) diurnal variation of mood and early morning awakening are common
b) cortisol concentration is sometimes raised
c) selective serotonin reuptake inhibitors are a more effective treatment than tricyclic antidepressants
d) lithium is contraindicated
e) one-third of cases relapse within 5 years

6. Characteristic symptoms of schizophrenia include
a) auditory hallucinations in the second person
b) thought withdrawal
c) mood congruent delusions
d) pressure of speech
e) 'knight's move' thinking

7. Adverse effects of typical antipsychotics include
a) cogwheel rigidity
b) hair loss
c) sedation
d) hiccoughs
e) akathisia

8. The following are true
a) patients taking monoamine oxidase inhibitors should not eat fava beans with Chianti
b) lithium can cause diabetes mellitus
c) tricyclic antidepressants can cause cardiac arrhythmias in overdose
d) the most common adverse effect of selective serotonin reuptake inhibitors is a dry mouth
e) clozapine can cause agranulocytosis

15. Drugs and the Endocrine and Metabolic Systems

1. Which of the following is the agent of choice for combined hyperlipidemia with significant elevations of both low density lipoprotein (LDL) cholesterol and triglycerides?
a) an HMG CoA reductase inhibitor
b) a bile acid sequestrant resin
c) a fibric acid derivative
d) niacin
e) levothyroxine

2. A patient with diabetes mellitus who takes a single injection of intermediate insulin each morning experiences elevated blood sugars at 7 a.m., but near-normal blood sugars at 6 p.m. Which change in therapeutic regimen would you recommend?
a) add intermediate insulin at bedtime
b) increase the dose of intermediate insulin each morning
c) add short-acting insulin each morning on waking up
d) reduce food intake in the evening
e) add an oral hypoglycemic drug

3. A 30-year-old woman experiences cessation of previously normal menses. An evaluation of hormone concentrations reveals low estradiol, low gonadotropins, elevated prolactin, normal cortisol, normal growth hormone, and normal thyroid hormone. Pituitary imaging reveals a small adenoma in the anterior pituitary. Which treatment would you recommend?
a) estrogen replacement therapy
b) a long-acting dopaminergic agonist
c) gonadotropin replacement therapy
d) octreotide therapy
e) surgery

4. A 30-year-old woman develops secondary amenorrhea. An evaluation of hormone concentrations reveals low gonadotropins, low estradiol, mildly elevated prolactin, normal growth hormone, low thyroid hormone, normal thyroid stimulating hormone, and normal cortisol. Pituitary imaging reveals a large pituitary tumor with deviation of the pituitary stalk. Which treatment would you recommend?
a) a long-acting dopaminergic agonist alone
b) a dopaminergic agonist in addition to estrogen and thyroid hormone replacement therapy
c) surgery followed by hormone replacement therapy
d) octreotide therapy
e) estrogen replacement therapy

5. Which drug treatment for diabetes mellitus improves sensitivity to the action of insulin?
a) sulfonylureas
b) biguanides
c) long-acting insulin
d) Intermediate-acting insulin
e) short-acting insulin

6. Which medication is likely to cause gynecomastia in men treated for excess mineralocorticosteroid secretion?
a) amiloride
b) spironolactone
c) triamterene
d) fludrocortisone
e) cortisol

7. A 57-year-old woman presents with rapid atrial fibrillation, a low blood pressure, exophthalmos, tremor, hyper-reflexia, and a goiter. After a blood sample for thyroid hormone has been sent to the laboratory, which of the following would you recommend?
a) a radioiodine uptake and scan of the thyroid to determine the etiology of the hyperthyroidism while awaiting the results of the hormone concentrations
b) antithyroid therapy (propylthiouracil)
c) a short-acting β adrenoceptor antagonist (e.g. esmolol) and antithyroid therapy
d) I⁻, a short-acting β adrenoceptor antagonist, and antithyroid therapy
e) I⁻ alone

8. A 60-year-old woman presents with a moon face, supraclavicular fat pads, central obesity, recent onset of noninsulin-dependent diabetes mellitus (NIDDM), and myopathy. She takes no medications other than a skin cream for psoriasis. An evaluation of hormone concentrations reveals low cortisol and adrenocorticotropic hormone (ACTH) levels.
Administration of ACTH produces a normal rise in cortisol. What is your diagnosis?
a) glucocorticosteroid deficiency (secondary)
b) Cushing's syndrome due to adrenal tumor
c) iatrogenic Cushing's syndrome
d) Cushing's disease due to a pituitary tumor
e) mineralocorticosteroid deficiency

9. All the following are correct about the combined oral contraceptive, except
a) is a mixture of a steroid and a peptide hormone
b) inhibits gonadotropin release
c) produces changes in the fallopian tube, uterus, and cervix
d) often contains ethinyl estradiol

10. The following statements about hormone replacement therapy are all correct, except
a) should consist of both estrogen and progestogen components
b) protects against cardiovascular disease
c) protects against osteoporosis
d) often contains ethinyl estradiol

11. Polycystic ovarian syndrome
a) is always associated with infertility
b) is always associated with a large number of cyst-like ovarian follicles
c) can be treated by enhancing estrogen levels using clomiphene
d) can be treated with a combined oral contraceptive

12. Disorders of the uterus (dysmenorrhea, menorrhea, endometriosis, fibroids) can be treated with all of the following, except
a) oral progestogens
b) combined oral contraceptives
c) gonadotropin preparations
d) nonsteroidal anti-inflammatory drugs

16. Drugs and the Inflammatory and Immune Response

1. The following cytokines are produced by T cells
a) Interleukin (IL)-1
b) IL-2
c) IL-3
d) IL-4
e) Interferon (IFN)-γ

2. The first choice of drug for anaphylaxis is
a) diphenhydramine
b) cromolyn sodium
c) aminophylline
d) hydrocortisone
e) epinephrine

3. Mediators responsible for anaphylaxis is/are
a) major basic protein
b) histamine
c) tumor necrosis factor (TNF)-α
d) leukotriene C4

4. The following diseases is/are mediated by IgE antibodies
a) hypersensitivity pneumonitis
b) allergic rhinitis
c) contact dermatitis
d) anaphylaxis

5. Systemic lupus erythematosus
a) is characterized by the presence of anti-DNA antibodies
b) anti-DNA antibody titer is decreased by glucocorticosteroid therapy
c) is treated with intravenous 'pulse' cyclophosphamide for lupus nephritis
d) is treated with intravenous 'pulse' cyclophosphamide because it has less urinary bladder toxicity.

6. Methotrexate is used for
a) systemic lupus erythematosus
b) polymyositis
c) rheumatoid arthritis
d) polyarteritis nodosa

7. Drugs specific for T cells include
a) cyclophosphamide
b) gold salts
c) cyclosporine
d) sulfasalazine
e) methotrexate

8. Bone marrow suppression is a major adverse effect of which of the following immunosuppressive drugs?
a) cyclosporine
b) cyclophosphamide
c) methotrexate
d) prednisone

17. Drugs and the Renal System

1. Furosemide
a) is a loop-diuretic
b) is a high-ceiling diuretic
c) produces hypokalemia
d) is sometimes administered with triamterene
e) can produce ototoxicity

2. Thiazide diuretics
a) are aldosterone antagonists
b) act on the proximal tubule
c) decrease calcium excretion
d) inhibit Na$^+$/Cl$^-$ cotransport
e) produce hyperkalemia

3. Spironolactone
a) is a potassium-sparing diuretic
b) binds to intracellular receptors
c) acts on the thick ascending loop of Henle
d) increases proton secretion
e) is used in the treatment of primary aldosteronism

4. Osmotic diuretics
a) have a direct action on renal tubule cells
b) inhibit Na$^+$ reabsorption in the distal convoluted tubule
c) increase medullary blood flow
d) are used to relieve oliguria
e) are used in the treatment of pulmonary edema

5. The following drugs are useful in the treatment of diabetes insipidus
a) insulin
b) desmopressin
c) chlorothiazide
d) mannitol
e) chlorpropamide

6. The following statements are correct
a) uricosuric drugs increase the secretion of uric acid in urine
b) the primary drug treatment of gout is either probenecid or sulfinpyrazone
c) patients treated with uricosuric drugs should maintain an alkaline diuresis
d) probenecid and sulfinpyrazone should not be given during an acute attack of gout

7. Nephrotoxicity may be anticipated following administration of
a) gentamicin
b) amphotericin B
c) cisplatin
d) cephradine
e) amoxicillin

18. Drugs and the Cardiovascular System

1. An asymptomatic female patient with mild hypertension (140/95 mmHg) should be treated with which of the following regimens of drugs?
a) guanethidine
b) nifedipine
c) hydrochlorothiazide, exercise and reduced salt intake
d) prazosin
e) clonidine

2. Drug X is used in the treatment of cardiac arrhythmias. It is not used as an anticonvulsant and is not recommended for use in asthmatic subjects because of effects on certain adrenoceptors. It is probably:
a) procainamide
b) propranolol
c) quinidine
d) disopyramide
e) lidocaine

3. In the management of cardiac arrhythmias that result from the appearance of an ectopic focus (as opposed to re-entry), the class I antiarrhythmic agents are effective because they
a) Inhibit voltage-sensitive Ca^{2+} channels
b) decrease phase 4 depolarization
c) increase atrioventricular conduction velocity
d) have negative inotropic actions
e) increase sinoatrial node automaticity

4. All of the following antiarrhythmic drugs are incorrectly matched with a statement regarding their properties and uses, except
a) amiodarone is used as an oral treatment of ventricular arrhythmias; severe adverse effects are common

b) bretylium stabilizes heart rhythm in the majority of patients with resistant ventricular fibrillation that has not responded to other treatment
c) tocainide is a new orally effective congener of lidocaine
d) acebutolol is a β$_1$ selective adrenoceptor antagonist
e) disopyramide, which is reserved by most consultants for patients not in heart failure who cannot tolerate quinidine, procainamide, or tocainide

5. All of the following antiarrhythmic drugs are correctly classified with their principal mechanism of action, except
a) quinidine: Na$^+$ channel blockade
b) verapamil: Ca^{2+} antagonism
c) bretylium: delays repolarization
d) amiodarone: Na$^+$ channel blockade
e) tocainide: Na$^+$ channel blockade

6. A frequency-dependent blockade of Na$^+$ channels is the principal mechanism of action of which of the following antiarrhythmic drugs?
a) verapamil
b) quinidine
c) propranolol
d) sotalol
e) lidocaine

7. An increase in cardiac output is associated with which one of the following drugs?
a) clonidine
b) α methyldopa
c) hydralazine
d) propranolol
e) guanethidine

8. If daily maintenance doses of digoxin are given without an initial loading dose, the maximal effect on the heart will be achieved in about
a) 7 days
b) 24 hours
c) 2 weeks
d) 5 days
e) 5 weeks

19. Drugs and the Pulmonary System

1. One of the effects of theophylline in biologic tissues is
a) stimulation of Na$^+$K$^+$ ATPase
b) inhibition of Na$^+$K$^+$ ATPase
c) inhibition of cyclic nucleotide phosphodiesterase
d) stimulation of cyclic nucleotide phosphodiesterase
e) stimulation of adenylyl cyclase

2. Cough suppression is indicated
a) if phlegm production is excessive
b) if there is severe rhinitis
c) if there is bronchiectasis
d) if the cough is induced by extrabronchial irritation

3. Prominent antitussive activity produced by therapeutic doses is characteristic of
a) morphine
b) theophylline
c) albuterol
d) dexamethasone

4. In the treatment of tuberculosis
a) up to 30% of the *Mycobacterium* cultures isolated from cases in New York City are resistant to multiple anti-microbial agents
b) oral streptomycin is effective
c) compliance in drug taking is a major problem
d) the molecular mechanisms of antibacterial resistance are well characterized

5. In treatment and prophylaxis
a) isoniazid (INH) is useful on its own for treatment of tuberculosis
b) INH is useful on its own for prophylaxis of tuberculosis
c) rifampin is useful on its own for treatment of tuberculosis
d) rifampin is useful on its own for prophylaxis of meningitis

6. Erythromycin
a) is a macrolide antibiotic
b) binds to motlin receptors
c) is useful for treating *Mycoplasma pneumoniae* infections
d) is an agent of choice for the treatment of infections due to β lactamase-producing Gram-positive staphylococci
e) first-line treatment of tuberculosis is with a combination of rifampin, INH, and pyrazinamide

7. When applied to the always of an asthmatic individual, drug X causes bronchodilation. The effect is not blocked by propanolol. Drug X does not normally have any central nervous system effect and, if it is given by mouth, has a bioavailability of less than 40%. Drug X is most likely
a) atropine
b) scopolamine
c) terbutaline
d) ipratropium
e) albuterol

8. Acute administration of the following drugs induces bronchodilation except
a) metaproterenol
b) aminophylline
c) cromolyn sodium
d) epinephrine
e) theophylline

20. Drugs and the Musculoskeletal System

1. The most effective treatment to prevent early severe postmenopausal osteoporosis is
a) Ca^{2+} alone
b) Ca^{2+} and hormone replacement therapy
c) Ca^{2+} and calcitonin
d) Ca^{2+} and bisphosphonates

2. Glucocorticosteroids have the following effects, except
a) cushingoid features
b) osteoporosis
c) inhibition of the inflammatory response
d) increased high density lipoprotein (HDL) cholesterol

3. Methotrexate has the following significant adverse effects, except
a) liver toxicity
b) bone marrow suppression
c) acute pneumonitis
d) deposition in the retina resulting in visual loss

4. Nonsteroidal anti-inflammatory drugs have the following effects, except
a) analgesia
b) antipyretic
c) anti-inflammatory
d) decrease erosions in rheumatoid arthritis

5. Appropriate treatment for acute gouty arthritis in a man with congestive heart failure and renal insufficiency might include
a) rest, ice, and simple analgesics
b) allopurinol
c) indomethacin
d) high-dose intravenous colchicine

6. A woman with longstanding well-controlled rheumatoid arthritis presents with an acute painful swollen knee and a high fever. Reasonable management would include
a) injecting the knee with intra-articular glucocorticosteroids
b) changing medication to a more effective nonsteroidal anti-inflammatory drug
c) aspirating fluid from the knee to look for crystals and for culture and starting oral colchicine
d) aspirating fluid from the knee to look for crystals and for culture and starting intravenous antibiotics

21. Drugs and the Gastrointestinal System

1. Metoclopramide is thought to act as a prokinetic drug as a result of
a) its action as an H_2 antagonist of histamine
b) its action as an inhibitor of gastrin
c) a vagolytic action caused by muscarinic blockade
d) its action as an antagonist at dopamine receptors
e) its action as an antagonist at opiate receptors

2. The drug to treat ulcerative colitis is
a) loperamide
b) sulfasalazine
c) diphenoxylate
d) carboxymethylcellulose
e) paregoric

3. An example of a drug used in the treatment of peptic ulcer disease that acts by enhancing mucosal defense mechanisms is
a) cimetidine
b) atropine
c) doxepin
d) sucralfate
e) aminosalicylate (ASA)

4. Which of the following cathartics does not itself act as a laxative?
a) mineral oil
b) phenolphthalein
c) castor oil
d) diphenyl isatin
e) bisacodyl

5. The saline cathartics such as magnesium sulfate owe much of their cathartic effect to
a) increased peristalsis due to interaction with emodin receptors of the intestinal mucosa
b) decreased reabsorption of water due to the formation of an insoluble barrier
c) a lowering of surface tension allowing water to penetrate the fecal mass
d) osmotic forces, which retain water in the digestive tract

e) formation of an emollient gel that maintains soft stools

6. All of the following statements are correct, except
a) antacids containing Mg^{2+} should be given with caution to patients with impaired renal function
b) aluminum hydroxide can decrease phosphate absorption from the gastrointestinal tract
c) stimulant (contact) cathartics (e.g. phenolphthalein) are believed to stimulate peristalsis by increasing the mucosal content of prostaglandins and 3'5'-cAMP
d) antacid mixtures are preferred to proton pump inhibitors for treating gastroesophageal reflux
e) excessive use of cathartics and laxatives may lead to functional bowel disturbances

22. Drugs and the Genitourinary System

1. Which drug has been used for the treatment of stress incontinence?
a) atropine
b) imipramine
c) oxybutynin
d) phenylpropanolamine
e) prazosin

2. Which of the following statements is correct?
a) the main excitatory transmitter of the human detrusor is norepinephrine
b) the main excitatory transmitter of the human urethra is acetylcholine
c) the main excitatory transmitter of the human detrusor is acetylcholine
d) the normal detrusor response to norepinephrine is contraction
e) the normal detrusor response to norepinephrine is relaxation

3. Which of the following statements is correct?
a) prazosin increases urethral resistance
b) the main contraction mediating-receptor in the human detrusor is not the muscarinic M_2 receptor
c) alpha-adrenoceptor antagonists are never used to treat hypertension
d) the androgen exerting the greatest influence on prostatic growth is testosterone
e) 5α-reductase inhibitors produce a rapid improvement in BPH symptoms

4. Which statement is not correct?
a) all drugs that are used to treat erectile dysfunction act peripherally
b) sildenafil acts to potentiate the nitric oxide system
c) there are several isofoms of phosphodiesterase
d) erectile dysfunction patients sometimes receive drug combinations
e) cavernosal smooth muscle contraction is dependent on calcium

5. α_1-Adrenoceptor antagonists are generally recognized as being effective in
a) acute cystitis
b) acute pyelonephritis
c) benign prostatic hyperplasia
d) stress incontinence
e) acute prostatitis

23. Drugs and the Skin

1. The following vitamins or their analogs are indicated for use in dermatology
a) vitamin A

b) vitamin B
c) vitamin C
d) vitamin D
e) vitamin E

2. The following drugs can be given orally for the treatment of chronic plaque psoriasis
a) methotrexate
b) acitretin
c) cyclosporine
d) glucocorticosteroids
e) hydroxyurea

3. In the treatment of acne
·a) isotretinoin can be given topically or orally
b) niacinamide is an anti-inflammatory non-antibiotic treatment
c) minocycline is the antibiotic of choice for an 11-year-old girl
d) *Propionibacterium acnes* resistance to antibiotics is not a problem
e) benzoyl peroxide, azelaic acid, and salicylic acid are all keratolytic

4. The following statements are correct
a) valacyclovir is a pro-drug
b) oral acyclovir, valacyclovir, or famciclovir should be prescribed for shingles
c) oral acyclovir is useful in the treatment of cold sores
d) patients with eczema herpeticum should be hospitalized for intravenous acyclovir
e) antiviral drugs are effective against cytomegalovirus

5. In the management of dermatitis
a) ketoconazole cream can be used for seborrheic dermatitis
b) systemic glucocorticosteroids may be needed to treat acute contact dermatitis
c) lithium succinate can be used for seborrheic dermatitis
d) allergy to the glucocorticosteroid molecule can be a problem
e) diapers increase the potency of topical glucocorticosteroids

24. Drugs and the Eye

1. In the eye of a normal person
a) the intraocular pressure is about 4 mmHg
b) the intraocular pressure is about 40 mmHg
c) aqueous humor is purely an ultrafiltrate of blood
d) aqueous humor production is partly controlled by the autonomic nervous system
e) the intraocular pressure falls when blood flow to the eye is reduced

2. In the normal eye, muscarinic receptor activation
a) decreases intraocular pressure
b) dilates the pupil
c) causes mydriasis
d) causes accommodation for near vision
e) causes miosis

3. In the eye of a patient with open-angle glaucoma
a) atropine will reduce intraocular pressure
b) a mixture of epinephrine and guanethidine will reduce intraocular pressure
c) the condition is often congenital
d) diagnosis is based only on increased intraocular pressure
e) timolol maleate (a β adrenoceptor antagonist) increases the intraocular pressure

4. The pupil of a normal person
a) dilates when phenylephrine hydrochloride is applied to the conjunctiva
b) contracts when light is shone into the contralateral eye
c) dilates in response to topical glucocorticosteroids
d) constricts when the person sees someone they find attractive
e) dilates in low light levels

5. In a normal person
a) the ciliary muscle is predominantly under sympathetic control
b) lidocaine is a useful local topical anesthetic for the eye
c) a pigmented iris takes longer to dilate with atropine than a non-pigmented iris
d) pilocarpine causes accommodation for near vision
e) benoxinate dilates the pupil by blocking Na+ channels

6. Which of the following drugs has a cycloplegic effect?
a) atropine
b) carbachol
c) cyclopentolate
d) epinephrine
e) tropicamide

7. In open-angle glaucoma
a) pilocarpine is given as eye drops
b) tropicamide eye drops are useful
c) β adrenoceptor antagonists lower intraocular pressure
d) carbachol eye drops lower intraocular pressure
e) YAG laser surgery is commonly used

8. In the eye of a normal person
a) the pupils constrict after instillation of a high concentration of epinephrine
b) stimulation of muscarinic receptors reduces the near point
c) phenylephrine hydrochloride eye drops dilate the pupil by a direct action on β_1 adrenoceptors
d) lidocaine can be used to produce corneal anesthesia
e) phenylephrine hydrochloride constricts the pupil

9. Increased intraocular pressure
a) may result from the topical application of glucocorticosteroids
b) may be reduced by systemic treatment with acetazolamide
c) may result from the topical application of parasympathomimetics
d) is reduced by cyclopentolate
e) may be reduced by miotics

25. Drugs and the Ear

1. Each of the following medications is ototoxic, except
a) hydrochlorothiazide
b) tobramycin
c) quinine
d) cisplatin
e) furosemide

2. A course of glucocorticosteroids is of proven benefit in the treatment of idiopathic sudden sensorineural hearing loss

a) true
b) false

3. Pharmacologic treatment of vertigo
a) aims to produce transient fluctuations in vestibular neuron activity
b) might intentionally destroy residual vestibular function
c) can promote central adaptation following loss of peripheral vestibular function
d) a) and c)
e) b) and c)

4. Treatment of Bell's palsy
a) should begin within 20 days of onset of complete facial paralysis
b) should begin within ten days of onset of partial facial paralysis
c) may include a combination of glucocorticosteroid and acycloguanosine
d) b) and c)
e) none of the above

5. Acute suppurative otitis media
a) is often due to *Streptococcus pneumoniae* or *Staphylococcus aureus*
b) can be caused by β lactamase producing organisms
c) should be treated instantly with a β lactamase-resistant antibiotic
d) b) and c)

26. Drug Use in Anesthesia and Critical Care

1. Reducing the risk of pulmonary aspiration during surgery and anesthesia includes the following therapies, except
a) preoperative fasting
b) regional anesthesia
c) laryngeal mask airway insertion
d) rapid anesthesia-intubation sequence
e) awake intubation

2. Which of the following statements is false?
a) thiopental or propofol are useful in inducing general anesthesia (GA)
b) thiopental is useful in maintaining GA
c) nitrous oxide and isoflurane are useful in maintaining GA
d) GA-induced ventilatory and cardiovascular depression is balanced against nociceptive surgical stimulation
e) morphine is useful in providing postoperative analgesia

3. With regard to pharmacokinetics and short duration of clinical drug action, which of the following combinations is true?
a) propofol: redistribution and hepatic metabolism
b) thiopental: hepatic metabolism
c) isoflurane: hepatic metabolism
d) succinylcholine: renal excretion
e) fentanyl: renal excretion

4. Neuromuscular blockers
a) do not facilitate tracheal intubation
b) do not facilitate intra-abdominal surgical exposure and wound closure
c) do not prevent reflex muscle activity during surgery and light anesthesia
d) do not prevent fractures in electroconvulsive therapy
e) require skilled airway and breathing management

5. In the treatment of morphine-induced respiratory depression in a conscious patient on the surgical ward
a) monitor the level of consciousness and respiratory rate
b) administer supplemental O_2
c) monitor oxygenation with pulse oximetry
d) withhold sedatives
e) all of the above

27. Drug Use in Disorders of Nutrition

1. Which of the following coagulation factors depends on vitamin K for synthesis by the liver?
a) prothrombin (factor II)
b) factor VIII
c) factor XII
d) factor V

2. All of the following are correct, except
a) large doses of vitamin C increase the incidence of oxalate stones in kidneys
b) absorption of vitamin B_{12} requires the presence of intrinsic factor
c) deficiency of folic acid causes megaloblastic anemia
d) the active form of vitamin A in the vision cycle is 11-cis retinal
e) osteomalacia is an expression of hypervitaminosis D in adults

3. All of the following are correct, except
a) fat-soluble vitamins require the presence of fat in the diet for proper absorption
b) body stores of vitamin B_{12} are sufficient for 3–6 months
c) storage capacity in the body is higher for fat-soluble vitamins and less for water-soluble vitamins
d) activation of vitamin D_3 occurs in the liver and kidneys
e) Wernicke's encephalopathy is associated with thiamine deficiency

4. Which one of the following vitamin D forms is synthesized by the kidneys?
a) calcitriol
b) calciferol
c) calcipotriol
d) cholecalciferol
e) ergocalciferol

5. All the following vitamins are correctly matched with the condition for which they are used pharmacotherapeutically, except
a) vitamin B_3 and pellagra
b) folic acid and peripheral neuropathy
c) vitamin C and scurvy
d) vitamin E and hemolytic anemia
e) vitamin A and acne

6. All the following terms are associated with vitamin A, except
a) retinoids
b) acne
c) rhodopsin
d) keratomalacia
e) osteomalacia

7. All the following terms are associated with vitamin D, except
a) parathyroid hormone
b) osteoclasts
c) kernicterus

d) Ca^{2+} homeostasis
e) ultraviolet light

8. All the following terms are associated with vitamin B_{12}, except
a) megaloblastic anemia
b) intrinsic factor
c) folic acid regeneration
d) hemolysis
e) transcobalamin II

9. Which of the following amino acids are non-essential?
a) leucine
b) threonine
c) glycine
d) valine
e) tyrosine

10. The following statements are correct.
a) obesity is defined as BMI ranging from 25.0 to 29.9 kg/m^2
b) obesity increases the risk of morbidity for hypertension
c) the inactive metabolites of sibutramine are termed M1 and M2
d) BMI of < 18 kg/m^2 is indicative of anorexia nervosa
e) orlistat is a pancreatic lipase inhibitor

11. Drugs currently approved for treatment of obesity are
a) fenfluramine
b) sibutramine
c) amphetamine
d) orlistat
e) ephedrine

28. Drug Use in Dentistry

1. The following drug-and-use pairs are correctly matched, except
a) chlorhexidine and gingivitis
b) fluoride and dental caries
c) carbamazepine and trigeminal neuralgia
d) nystatin and recurrent herpes labialis
e) pilocarpine and radiation-induced xerostomia

2. Select the statement that is false
a) lidocaine is an amide-type local anesthetic
b) inflammation or infection at the site of local anesthetic administration decreases the degree of regional analgesia
c) vasoconstrictors increase perfusion of tissues
d) epinephrine adverse effects can include tachycardia and palpitation
e) vasoconstrictors increase the duration of action of injected local anesthetics

3. Xerostomia is associated with all of the following classes of drugs, except
a) cholinesterase inhibitors
b) antidepressants
c) antipsychotics
d) opioids
e) antihistamines

4. Nonsteroidal anti-inflammatory drugs
a) mimic naturally occurring brain opioids
b) Inhibit prostaglandin synthesis
c) block genesis of the nerve action potential
d) interfere with the release of histamine and bradykinin
e) cause microvasculature vasoconstriction

5. Adverse effects of antibiotic drugs can include all of the following, except
a) hypersensitivity reactions including anaphylaxis
b) superinfections including candidiasis
c) antibiotic-induced diarrhea
d) tachycardia, palpitations, and a modest elevation of blood pressure
e) diarrhea with erythromycin

6. All of the following drug and oral adverse effect pairs are correctly matched, except
a) fluorides and mottled enamel
b) acyclovir and herpes labialis
c) phenytoin and gingival hyperplasia
d) allopurinol and lichenoid drug reaction
e) nifedipine and gingival hyperplasia

7. The most important reason for adding vasoconstrictors to local anesthetic solutions is
a) to increase the quality and duration of the regional analgesia
b) to overcome the patient's anxiety and fear of dental treatment
c) to prevent adverse drug reactions
d) to prevent adverse drug interactions
e) to ensure nerve conduction blockade in the presence of acute infection

8. Select the drug combination least likely to result in adverse effects
a) metronidazole and ethanol
b) sulfonamide and warfarin
c) metronidazole and penicillin V
d) erythromycin and terfenadine
e) tetracyclines and antacids

29. Toxins and Poisons

1. 2,3,7,8-Tetrachlorodibenzodioxin (TCDD) is not
a) a carcinogen in some experimental animals
b) a teratogen in some experimental animals
c) a toxic hazard
d) more potent than botulinum toxin as a lethal agent in man
e) a byproduct of manufacturing

2. Lead poisoning is not associated with
a) severe abdominal pain
b) disturbances of mood
c) peripheral neuropathy
d) red blood cell abnormalities
e) abnormal patterns of bone growth

3. A 26-year-old male presents as an emergency in a semiconscious state. He is arousable, but unable to answer questions. Investigations reveal a severe metabolic acidosis. He has most probably ingested
a) carbon tetrachloride
b) ethanol
c) methanol
d) cyanide
e) benzene

4. Which of the following statements is false?
a) parathion is an organophosphate insectide used in agriculture and horticulture
b) pyrethrins (chrysanthemic acids) are obtained by extraction from flowering plants
c) dioxin is a toxic byproduct of chlorine bleaching of wood pulp
d) dichlorodiphenyltrichloroethane (DDT) is an organophosphate insectide used in agriculture and horticulture
e) carbon monoxide is a common air pollutant

633

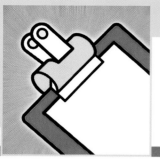

Case Studies

Make a provisional diagnosis and determine a rational pharmacologic treatment for the following hypothetical cases.

8. Drugs and Viruses

A 28-year-old man presents with multiple painful clusters of vesicles on red patches on the shaft of his penis, malaise, fever, nausea, and occasional vomiting. These symptoms began 5 days after he had sexual intercourse with a new partner. He has had a cadaveric renal transplant for 2 years for renal failure due to glomerulonephritis. His medications include prednisone and cyclosporine. His usual serum creatinine concentration is 200 mmol/l (normal 80–110).

On examination he is in some discomfort, his blood pressure is 145/85 mmHg, his pulse is 96 beats/min, and his temperature is 38.3°C. He appears slightly Cushingoid, and he has genital lesions as described above with tender bilateral inguinal lymphadenopathy.

1. What is the clinical diagnosis?
2. How would you confirm the diagnosis?
3. What is the natural history of this infection?
4. Which of the following drugs—acyclovir, foscarnet, valacyclovir, ganciclovir, adenine-arabinoside, sorivudine, idoxuridine, penciclovir, famciclovir—could theoretically be prescribed for the infection?
5. What is the drug of choice for this infection?
6. What is the preferred route for acyclovir administration?
7. Although prednisone and cyclosporine may be limiting the host response to this infection, it is decided to keep the cyclosporine dose as is, and to increase the dose of prednisone. Why are these recommendations appropriate?
8. Is knowledge of the patient's renal function critical for determining the size of the first dose? Explain why or why not.
9. Is knowledge of the patient's renal function critical for prescribing subsequent doses? Explain why or why not.

9. Drugs and Bacteria

A 4-year-old boy is brought to the emergency department of your hospital with a 2-day history of fever, lethargy, headache and poor appetite. Physical examination reveals marked nuchal rigidity, a temperature of 39.7°C, but no focal neurologic deficits.

1. Would you diagnose a viral infection and advise the parents that the illness will resolve over the next few days without intervention? Explain your answer.
2. Would you prescribe antibiotic therapy without further information? Explain your answer.
3. Would you perform a complete blood count, collect blood for culture, and cerebrospinal fluid for examinations including culture? Explain your answer.

4. If this child's cerebrospinal fluid is cloudy, would you await initial laboratory results before starting antibiotics or start antibiotic therapy at once? Explain your answer.
5. If you start antibiotic therapy at once or if the cerebrospinal fluid Gram stain shows no organisms, which antibiotic would you use?
6. Would you use the same antibiotic if the child had previously had anaphylactic reaction to amoxicillin and, if not, what would be the alternative?
7. If the cerebrospinal fluid grew *Streptococcus pneumoniae* with a high level of resistance to penicillin (MIC > 2.0 mg/ml), what would be the treatment of choice?

10. Drugs and Fungi

A 7-year-old school girl was taken to her family practitioner by her mother who was concerned about her daughter's hair loss and itchy scalp. The child's scalp was inflamed, with hair loss and scaling. Many of her school friends had reported similar symptoms over the previous few months.

1. How would you confirm whether the infection was a fungal infection?
2. What general measures would you recommend to the child's mother?
3. What drug would be most useful to treat this child?

11. Drugs and Parasites

A 49-year-old man complained of intermittent pain in his epigastrium and abdominal right upper quadrant. The pain had been present for 4 weeks. He was admitted to hospital because the right upper quadrant pain had become more severe. He had not traveled outside of Japan and had lived most of his life in Mie prefecture, a rural location. An abdominal echogram demonstrated an actively mobile worm in the gallbladder. A stool exam revealed eggs with thick mamillated shells.

1. What is the probable diagnosis?
2. What is the Latin name of the worm and to which group of helminths does it belong?
3. How might this condition have been contracted?
4. What anthelmintics would you choose to treat this condition?
5. How do these anthelmintics exert their effects?

12. Drugs and Neoplasms

A 55-year-old woman was diagnosed 3 years ago with a stage II ($T_2N_1M_0$) breast cancer. She received 4 months of adjuvant chemotherapy with cyclophosphamide and doxorubicin. She presents now with right upper gradient pain, weight loss, fevers, and jaundice. A computed tomography scan of the abdomen reveals portal hepatitis, prepancreatic, precaval, and para-aortic adenopathy.

1. Is it essential to establish a tissue diagnosis?
2. What is a differential diagnosis?

3. Why would a complete blood count be indicated?
4. Needle biopsy shows non-Hodgkin's lymphoma. What is the preferred treatment?
5. Is there anything in the patient's history which raises concerns about additional chemotherapy?

13. Drugs and the Blood

A 54-year-old man complains of excessive fatigue and unsteadiness when walking. He has a history of alcoholism. The physical examination is essentially normal except that he appears pale and vibratory sense is absent in both lower extremities.

1. Would you reassure the patient and urge him to stop drinking alcohol? Explain your answer.
2. Would you encourage better dietary intake and prescribe vitamin supplementation? Explain your answer.
3. Would you order a complete blood count and start him on an oral folate and vitamin B_{12} supplement right away? Explain your answer.
4. Would you order a complete blood count and serum folate and vitamin B_{12} levels? Explain your answer.

The patient returns the next day and his symptoms and examination remain the same. Laboratory tests show that his hemoglobin concentration is 10 g/dl (6.21 mmol/liter) and mean cell volume is 110 µm³ (110 fl).

5. Would you call a family meeting to discuss the patient's alcohol problem? Explain your answer.
6. Would you wait for serum vitamin B_{12} levels and if low, start him on oral vitamin B_{12}? Explain your answer.
7. Would you wait for the serum folate level and if low, prescribe 1 mg/day of folate? Explain your answer.
8. Would you start the patient on terrous sulfate and continue another 6 months after his hemoglobin level has normalized? Explain your answer.

14. Drugs and the Nervous System

A 27-year-old man attends the emergency room. He complains of feeling down and having suicidal thoughts for 6 months and finds it difficult to get to sleep. He also reports that other people can hear his thoughts and that words of songs on the radio refer to him. He says that he hears voices telling him he is a bad person and is responsible for a recent disaster. His friends say that he has become increasingly reclusive and has stopped attending work. When he speaks, there often seems to be little logical sequence to his thoughts and his personal hygiene is poor.

1. How would you manage this patient in the short term?
2. What are the two most likely diagnoses? List three additional features for both diagnoses that would help clarify the diagnosis.

635

3. Which drugs would you use for these two most likely diagnoses? In each case give the name of the class of drug and say which drug you would use and for how long, what the end-points of therapy are, and what adverse effects might be expected.

15. Drugs and the Endocrine and Metabolic Systems

A 32-year-old Caucasian woman has been fatigued and anorexic for several months. She lives in the tropics, spends a lot of time in the sun and eats mainly tropical fruits. She reports feeling faint on standing upright over the past three weeks, has lost 5 kg in weight, and frequently feels nauseated. She has no other medical problems. Her family history includes a sister and mother with hypothyroidism. On examination she is tanned and excessively thin. Lying blood pressure is 100/77 mmHg with a pulse of 86 bpm. Standing blood pressure is 88/-mmHg with a pulse higher than 100 bpm. Her skin is darkest over the extensor surfaces of her elbows, knees, and wrists. Her oral mucosa is hyperpigmented. Serum Na^+ is slightly low (132 mmol/liter), serum K^+ is elevated (5.6 mmol/liter), urinary Na^+ concentration is high (100 mmol/liter), and urinary K^+ concentration is low (<10 mmol/liter).

1. What would your initial approach be?
2. The patient is clinically stable. Which medications would you prescribe her?
3. What guidance do you give the patient about monitoring therapy and dose adjustment?
4. What are the adverse effects of overtreatment?

16. Drugs and the Inflammatory and Immune Response

A 23-year-old female presents with a history of facial rash, low-grade fever (up to 37.2°C), and general fatigue. On examination, the patient has facial erythema and pretibial pitting edema but is otherwise normal. Laboratory examination reveals a decreased white cell count, an increased serum creatinine, and massive proteinuria.

1. Which of the following serologic tests—antinuclear antibody, anti-DNA antibody, serum complement, anti-streptolysin O titer, rheumatoid factor—would you order to determine the diagnosis of this autoimmune disease? Explain your answer.
2. Which of the following examinations–chest radiograph, renal function tests, renal angiography, renal biopsy, muscle biopsy–would you order to determine the severity of the disease?
3. If you decided to treat this patient with drugs, what would you use? For each drug list its class, for how long it should be used, what the end-points of therapy are, and what its adverse effects are.

17. Drugs and the Renal System

An elderly male was diagnosed with mild congestive heart failure. The symptoms included breathlessness on walking and swollen ankles. The patient was prescribed bendroflumethiazide (10 mg daily) but soon after starting treatment he felt unusually fatigued and lethargic.

1. What caused the breathlessness and swollen ankles?
2. Why was a thiazide diuretic prescribed and what alternative drug treatments are available?
3. What are the possible causes of patient's fatigue and lethargy, and how might they be corrected?

18. Drugs and the Cardiovascular System

A 53-year-old man with a history of severe hypertension for at least 20 years which was generally well controlled by medication, tended to stop taking his drugs from time to time, occasionally for extended periods. Several weeks before admission he had stopped taking his medications, which included lisinopril, nifedipine, and atenolol. Several days before admission he had a headache and was noted by his wife to be confused. On admission he was obtunded with multifocal neurologic findings. His blood pressure was 240/135 mmHg, he had papilledema, and rates in both lungs, and his urine contained multiple red blood cells.

1. Is his clinical condition immediately life-threatening?
2. Which additional diagnostic tests might be indicated Immediately?
3. What properties would an ideal drug have in this setting? Give an example of such a drug.
4. What is the target goal for blood pressure?
5. After this man's blood pressure has been sufficiently lowered, what would be the long-term plan for him?

19. Drugs and the Pulmonary System

A mother reports that her 6-year-old son had a fever the previous night of 38°C and had woken periodically with coughing and wheezing. She also reported that he had been ill for 3 days with an unproductive cough. His symptoms are less severe during the day, although he has been physically less active than usual. On examination, her son has a runny nose and slightly red eardrums and throat. His respiration is not labored and his general appearance is normal. The only other signs are audible wheezing and rhonchi on auscultation that do not clear upon coughing.

1. Would you reassure the mother that all is well, and that the disease will resolve quickly without drug treatment?
2. If you decided to prescribe an antibiotic, which antibiotic would you use?
3. If you decided to prescribe an antibiotic plus a bronchodilator, which bronchodilator would you use?
4. Would you order further tests (total and differential white cell count, throat swab for bacterial culture and sensitivity)?
5. Would you prescribe anti-inflammatory drugs?
6. What is the probable diagnosis? How should this be treated?

20. Drugs and the Musculoskeletal System

A 42-year-old single mother comes to you with a 6-month history of pain and swelling in her wrists, hands, and feet. Recently she has noticed nodules over both her elbows. She reports that she has ringing in her ears because she is taking so much aspirin. She is concerned that she will be unable to run her small store. On examination the patient has synovitis affecting her wrists, metacarpophalangeal, proximal interphalangeal, and metatarsophalangeal joints as well as subcutaneous nodules.

1. Discuss appropriate management regarding the aspirin she is taking and other NSAIDs you might consider.
2. Discuss the advantages/disadvantages of starting low-dose glucocorticosteroids.
3. After being on intramuscular gold injections for 20 weeks she has had no clinical response. Discuss the available options.
4. Finally, after starting 12 weeks of methotrexate (10 mg p.o.) given weekly, she is starting to improve but her hepatocellular liver enzymes increase to twice their normal levels. Explain why.

21. Drugs and the Gastrointestinal System

A 40-year-old man was seen by his physician 12 months ago because of dyspepsia, which occurred some time after eating. The discomfort was relieved by eating a meal or taking antacids. The physician diagnosed a peptic ulcer and prescribed a proton pump inhibitor, omeprazole, which provided rapid (within 2 days) relief. The patient continued to take the drug for 1 month and had no further dyspepsia for another 6 months. However, over the next few months his symptoms grew progressively worse. Now, on a return visit to the same physician, further investigations have demonstrated the presence of a duodenal ulcer, while a culture from the ulcer shows the presence of *Helicobacter pylori*. This time the physician prescribes different drugs.

1. What drug's can be prescribed to relieve the symptoms of peptic ulcer?
2. Why did the ulcer relapse?
3. What drugs should be prescribed on the second visit?
4. If the most appropriate drugs are prescribed, what are the chances of a cure?

23. Drugs and the Skin

Carey is a 2-year-old girl with a red itchy rash in her elbow and knee flexures and on her neck. She continually scratches her skin until it bleeds, is losing a lot of sleep and is screaming at bathtime.

1. What is the likely diagnosis?
2. How often should Carey be bathed and what preparations should be used at bathtime?
3. Would you prescribe any topical treatment and if so what?
4. Would you prescribe any oral treatment and if so what?

24. Drugs and the Eye

A 52-year-old woman visited an optician for a routine eye test. On learning of a family history of glaucoma, the optician examined her eyes thoroughly and noted a slight increase in intraocular pressure and mild cupping of the optic disk with some loss of visual acuity. He advised her to go to her family practitioner.

1. What two effects are needed from drug treatment in a patient with glaucoma?
2. What is the first-line group of drugs for treating this problem?
3. Give an example of one of the above drugs and explain how it works.
4. What coexisting conditions might preclude the use of these drugs in patients with glaucoma?

25. Drugs and the Ear

A 60-year-old man complains of left ear drainage and hearing loss. He has a long history of ear infection dating back to childhood and his ear often drains, especially if he gets it wet. On examination there is purulent mucus in the ear canal and a large perforation of the eardrum. The middle ear mucosa is red and edematous. His tuning fork tests indicate a conductive hearing loss on this side.

1. Would you syringe the ear to remove the debris and tell the man to rinse it with an alcohol and vinegar solution? Explain your answer.
2. Would you prescribe an oral antibiotic alone? Explain your answer.
3. Would you prescribe a topical antibiotic? Explain your answer. Which antibiotic would you use if you did decide to prescribe one?

4. Would you take an ear swab for culture and sensitivity and while waiting for the result prescribe a topical antibiotic in combination with an oral antibiotic?

5. Two days after starting antibiotic therapy, culture and sensitivity of an ear swab reveals infection with *Pseudomonas aeruginosa* and an anaerobe. If these bacteria are not sensitive to the antibiotic therapy you have chosen, would you recall the patient to change the antibiotic, or review the patient in ten days and if the drainage persists then change the antibiotic? Explain your answer. Which antibiotic therapy would you use if you decide to change the antibiotic?

26. Drug Use in Anesthesia and Critical Care

A 23-year-old female has received extensive abdominal surgery for trauma related to a motorcycle accident. Following fluid resuscitation, her general anesthetic consisted of a rapid anesthesia intubation sequence because of the risk of aspiration of recently ingested food. Thiopental and succinylcholine were administered for induction. Oxygen, mechanical ventilation, and isoflurane were used for maintenance of anesthesia with fentanyl for analgesia and pancuronium for continued paralysis. On completion of the surgery, the anesthesiologist turns off the isoflurane and administers atropine and neostigmine intravenously to reverse the nondepolarizing neuromuscular blockade. The patient's endotracheal tube is disconnected from the ventilator and she is transferred from the operating table to the stretcher. Unexpectedly, she neither moves nor opens her eyes to command.

1. What should the immediate therapeutic approach to this unresponsive patient be?

2. Construct a differential diagnosis for 'failure to awaken and breathe' following general anesthesia.

3. How would you identify reversible causes in your differential diagnosis?

Within several minutes, the patient opens her eyes and breathes, but only on command.

4. What are the potential adverse effects of naloxone? How do these factors influence your selection of dose and rate of administration for opioid-induced respiratory depression?

5. Devise strategies to prevent complications in the immediate postanesthetic period.

27. Drug Use in Disorders of Nutrition

A 27-year-old woman is considering having another child. Her previous pregnancy ended in miscarriage because the fetus had a neural tube defect. She wants to know whether the defect is genetic and whether her next baby will have the same problem. On examination the patient looks healthy, but pale, and when asked about her eating habits she discloses she is a vegetarian.

1. Should you advise her to seek genetic advice and, if so, why?

2. Should you reassure her that there is nothing to worry about and that her next pregnancy will be fine and, if so, why?

3. As the patient is a vegetarian, should you prescribe a multivitamin preparation and reassure the patient about her next pregnancy and, if so, why?

4. Does the patient have a high risk of vitamin B_{12} deficiency and, if so, what would should you do and why?

5. In view of this patient's desire to become pregnant, which drugs would you recommend and for how long would you recommend them?

28. Drug Use in Dentistry

A 65-year-old woman reports to the clinic with a persistent dry mouth and acute pain of 4 days' duration. She is postmenopausal and has a history of hypertension, congestive heart failure, anxiety, and anemia. Current medications include clonidine, hydrochlorothiazide, digoxin, estrogen, a potassium supplement, and alprazolam. Other symptoms include malaise, a loss of appetite, and altered taste. Her temperature is not increased and she has no lymphadenopathy. Oral examination reveals a diffusely red oral mucosa with white patches and angular cheilitis. Her tongue is inflamed and has a smooth dorsal surface lacking papillae with a white coating. The coating and white patches are easily rubbed off, but the underlying oral mucosa is red and painful.

1. Would you reassure the patient and tell her that she has a local allergic reaction that can be managed with a systemic antihistamine? Explain your answer.

2. Would you prescribe a systemic antibiotic as the patient has a generalized stomatitis, which will resolve after a few days? Explain your answer.

3. Would you prescribe a topical or systemic antiviral agent for a primary viral infection? Explain your answer.

4. Would you prescribe a topical antifungal rinse, instruct her to avoid hot spicy foods and to increase her fluid intake, and reassure her that her symptoms will quickly resolve with the use of medication? Explain your answer.

5. Suppose you prescribed a topical antifungal rinse (such as nystatin oral suspension), what is the class of drug, why is it administered topically, how long should it be continued, what is the end-point of therapy, and what adverse effects/drug interactions can you anticipate?

6. Would you order laboratory tests and, if so, what and why?

7. How could this woman's drug therapy have contributed to her oral symptoms?

29. Toxins and Poisons

While on holiday in Indonesia a friend has spent the day swimming over coral reefs. The surrounding land is agricultural, and streams from fields and villages flow into the sea. Your friend leaves the sea complaining of coral cuts and has a variety of skin abrasions, cuts, and skin lesions on his lower legs. He has a shower and a snack of local hot foods and drinks. Shortly afterwards he says he feels weak and appears to have ptosis. He grows increasingly weak, but his pulse remains strong and he has no other symptoms.

1. What would you do first?

2. What supportive measures should be taken?

3. Is the probable cause of your friend's problems an octopus bite, envenomation by a snake or coneshell, botulism from contaminated food, organophosphate insecticide from run-off or food contamination, or general food poisoning?

4. What specific therapy is available?

Answers

MCQ Answers

2. Drug Names and Drug Classification Systems
1. a
2. d
3. b

3. General Principles of Drug Action
1. b
2. d
3. b
4. a
5. b
6. c
7. d
8. d

4. Pharmacokinetic and Other Factors Influencing Drug Action
1. d
2. c
3. c
4. e
5. b
6. d
7. c
8. a

5. Pharmacodynamics and the Measurement of Drug Action
1. d
2. d
3. b
4. d
5. d
6. a
7. c

6. Drug Safety and Pharmacovigilance
1. a) F, b) T, c) F, d) F, e) F
2. a) T, b) T, c) T, d) F
3. a) T, b) F, c) T, d) F
4. a) F, b) T, c) T, d) F, e) T
5. a) T, b) F, c) T, d) T

7. Regulation of Drug Use
1. d
2. c
3. d
4. c
5. c
6. d

8. Drugs and Viruses
1. d
2. b
3. e
4. a
5. c
6. e

7. c
8. a
9. a
10. e

9. Drugs and Bacteria
1. d
2. e
3. a
4. c
5. b
6. d
7. e
8. b

10. Drugs and Fungi
1. a) T, b) F, c) T, d) T, e) F
2. a) T, b) T, c) T, d) T, e) T
3. a) T, b) F, c) T, d) T, e) T
4. a) T, b) T, c) T, d) T, e) T
5. a) T, b) T, c) T, d) T, e) T
6. a) T, b) T, c) T, d) F, e) T
7. a) T, b) T, c) T, d) T, e) T

11. Drugs and Parasites
1. d
2. c
3. b
4. d
5. a
6. d

12. Drugs and Neoplasms
1. a
2. c
3. a
4. a

13. Drugs and the Blood
1. d
2. c
3. a
4. d
5. c

14. Drugs and the Nervous System
1. a) T, b) F, c) T, d) F, e) T
2. a) F, b) T, c) F, d) T, e) T
3. a) T, b) T, c) F, d) T, e) F
4. a) T, b) F, c) T, d) F, e) F
5. a) T, b) T, c) F, d) F, e) F
6. a) F, b) T, c) F, d) F, e) F
7. a) T, b) T, c) F, d) T, e) F
8. a) T, b) F, c) T, d) F, e) T

15. Drugs and the Endocrine and Metabolic Systems
1. d
2. a
3. b
4. c
5. b
6. b

7. d
8. c
9. a
10. d
11. d
12. c

16. Drugs and the Inflammatory and Immune Response
1. a) F, b) T, c) T, d) T, e) T
2. a) F, b) F, c) F, d) F, e) T
3. a) F, b) T, c) F, d) T
4. a) F, b) T, c) T, d) T
5. a) T, b) T, c) T, d) F
6. a) F, b) T, c) T, d) F
7. a) F, b) F, c) T, d) F, e) F
8. a) F, b) T, c) T, d) F

17. Drugs and the Renal System
1. a) T, b) T, c) T, d) T, e) T
2. a) F, b) F, c) T, d) T, e) F
3. a) T, b) T, c) F, d) F, e) F
4. a) F, b) F, c) T, d) T, e) F
5. a) F, b) T, c) T, d) F, e) T
6. a) F, b) F, c) T, d) T
7. a) T, b) T, c) T, d) T, e) F

18. Drugs and the Cardiovascular System
1. c
2. b
3. b
4. a
5. d
6. e
7. c
8. a

19. Drugs and the Pulmonary System
1. c
2. a
3. a
4. a
5. e
6. c
7. d
8. c

20. Drugs and the Musculoskeletal System
1. b
2. d
3. d
4. d
5. a
6. d

21. Drugs and the Gastrointestinal System
1. d
2. b

3. d
4. c
5. d
6. d

22. Drugs and the Genitourinary System
1. d
2. c
3. b
4. a
5. c

23. Drugs and the Skin
1. a) T, b) T, c) T, d) T, e) F
2. a) T, b) T, c) T, d) F, e) T
3. a) T, b) T, c) T, d) T, e) T
4. a) T, b) T, c) T, d) T, e) F
5. a) T, b) T, c) T, d) T, e) T

24. Drugs and the Eye
1. a) F, b) F, c) F, d) T, e) T
2. a) T, b) F, c) T, d) T, e) T
3. a) F, b) T, c) T, d) F, e) F
4. a) T, b) T, c) T, d) F, e) T
5. a) F, b) T, c) T, d) T, e) F
6. a) T, b) F, c) T, d) F, e) T
7. a) T, b) F, c) T, d) T, e) F
8. a) F, b) T, c) T, d) F, e) T
9. a) T, b) T, c) F, d) F, e) T

25. Drugs and the Ear
1. a
2. b
3. b
4. e
5. b

26. Drug Use in Anesthesia and Critical Care
1. c
2. b
3. a
4. e
5. e

27. Drug Use in Disorders of Nutrition
1. a
2. e
3. b
4. a
5. b
6. e
7. c
8. d
9. c, e
10. a) F, b) T, c) F, d) T, e) T
11. a) F, b) T, c) F, d) T, e) F

28. Drug Use in Dentistry
1. d
2. c

3. a		**6.** b		**29. Toxins and Poisons**	**3.** c
4. b		**7.** a		**1.** d	**4.** d
5. d		**8.** c		**2.** e	

Case Studies Answers

8. Drugs and Viruses
1. Genital herpes in an immunocompromised host.
2. Culture vesicles for herpes simplex virus, and send acute (now) and convalescent (in 2–3 weeks) serum samples to demonstrate seroconversion.
3. Slow resolution over 3 weeks.
4. All except sorivudine.
5. Acyclovir.
6. Intravenous.
7. Reducing the dose of cyclosporine may increase the risk of renal homograft rejection. Prednisone is increased to avoid the relative adrenocortical insufficiency that will occur during the stress of this severe infection.
8. No, knowledge of the patient's renal function is not critical for determining the size of the first dose. This is because only the apparent volume of distribution is critical in determining the drug concentration achieved with the first dose, and it is not expected to be markedly abnormal in a patient with mild–moderate renal insufficiency.
9. Yes, knowledge of the patient's renal function is critical for prescribing subsequent doses because acyclovir causes dose-related central nervous system toxicity and is eliminated by renal excretion.

9. Drugs and Bacteria
1. No. The presence of nuchal rigidity strongly suggests a diagnosis of meningitis and a bacterial etiology must be pursued since bacterial meningitis is usually fatal if not treated.
2. No. It is important to collect blood and spinal fluid prior to the institution of antibacterial therapy to determine the bacterial etiology and antibiotic susceptibility of the pathogen.
3. Yes. These tests confirm the diagnosis and guide therapy.
4. No. Cloudy cerebrospinal fluid (CSF) is due to a very high number of white blood cells, which occurs almost exclusively in bacterial meningitis. As bacteria multiply in the CSF approximately every 60 minutes, it is important to institute therapy as soon as the diagnosis of bacterial meningitis is probable.
5. A third-generation cephalosporin, usually cefotaxime or ceftriaxone.
6. No. Chloramphenicol is the alternative.
7. Vancomycin.

10. Drugs and Fungi
1. Scrapings of scale and plucked hairs should be sent to the laboratory for microscopy and culture.
2. The crusts should be removed and regular shampooing is recommended. The child must be kept away from school until the treatment has become established (i.e. about 1 week). If the infection is zoophilic, the child can then return to school as human-to-human transmission is limited. If the infection is arthrophilic, however, she must remain off school until repeat scrapings are negative, and the school needs to institute a screening program.
3. Griseofulvin is the drug of choice because of her age.

11. Drugs and Parasites
1. Ascariasis.
2. *Ascaris lumbricoides*, belonging to the Nematoda (roundworms).
3. By the ingestion of either mature eggs, contaminated vegetables or water.
4. Pyrantel pamoate and piperazine.
5. Pyrantel pamoate is a depolarizing neuromuscular blocking agent which inhibits cholinesterase causing slow contracture and spastic paralysis of the worm, while piperazine blocks the neuromuscular junction causing flaccid paralysis.

12. Drugs and Neoplasms
1. Yes. Treatment and prognosis is very different for different cancers.
2. Recurrent breast cancer, non-Hodgkin's lymphoma, and pancreatic cancer.
3. Although this presentation would be unusual, a similarly acute nonlymphocytic leukemia is a possibility.
4. Combination chemotherapy. The recommended treatment is CHOP (cyclophosphamide, doxorubicin, vincristine, and prednisone).
5. Yes. Previous treatment with doxorubicin. Unless provisions are made to use a cardioprotective agent or to prolong the administration of doxorubicin by infusion, there is a lifetime maximum of 450 mg/m^2 before the risk of cardiotoxicity begins to rise.

13. Drugs and the Blood
1. No. Alcohol is a direct marrow suppressant and alcoholics whose caloric intake is mainly alcohol may suffer from nutritional deficiencies such as folate. It is always a good policy to encourage moderation in intake of alcoholic beverages. This patient is probably suffering from anemia and has neurologic symptoms consistent with vitamin B$_{12}$ deficiency. It would not be appropriate to send him home without further laboratory tests to determine his complete blood count, folate and vitamin B$_{12}$ levels.
2. No. Encouraging patient to have a better life style with a balanced diet is always good clinical practice. However, vitamin B$_{12}$ deficiency is commonly due to pernicious anemia and lack of intrinsic factor. Dietary B$_{12}$ or common preparations of vitamin supplements will not contain adequate vitamin B$_{12}$ levels to treat vitamin B$_{12}$ deficiency due to pernicious anemia.
3. No. Although the patient's symptoms suggest B$_{12}$ deficiency, it would be inappropriate to start the patient on therapy with out a definitive diagnosis unless the patient is critically ill. In addition, it would be inappropriate to commit the patient to life-long treatment for pernicious anemia without an appropriate workup to confirm the diagnosis. Furthermore, by treating the patient with folate and B$_{12}$ concurrently, the clinician will lose the benefit of confirming the diagnosis when the appropriate therapy leads to clinical improvement.
4. Yes. The patient's symptoms suggest vitamin B$_{12}$ deficiency. The complete blood count will assess the severity of anemia and the blood smear may reveal macrocytosis and polysegmented neutrophils, which would be very helpful in confirming the diagnosis. Folate levels are indicated since alcoholic patients often have nutritional deficiencies including folate that may contribute to this patient's symptoms.
5. The patient's macrocytic anemia further supports the initial clinical suspicion that he may be vitamin B$_{12}$ deficient. The patient's alcoholism is probably not the only or the most immediate clinical issue.
6. No. Initial vitamin B$_{12}$ supplementation should be through the parental route although long-term treatment with large doses (1 mg) of oral B$_{12}$ has been shown to be successful despite lack of intrinsic factor needed for receptor-mediated absorption.
7. No. The patient may also be folate deficient and folate replacement may correct his anemia despite vitamin B$_{12}$ deficiency. However, if, his B$_{12}$ deficiency remains untreated, his neurologic symptoms may progress leading to irreversible damage.
8. No. Iron-deficient patients usually present with normocytic or microcytic anemia.

14. Drugs and the Nervous System
1. This man obviously has a major mental illness and is at risk of deterioration. Admission to hospital for observation is probably the most appropriate course of management. It provides the patient with a place of safety, where the risk of harm to himself and others is

minimized, and allows the healthcare team an opportunity to assess the patient more fully and gain more information about his illness. Treatment may also be started as soon as a diagnosis is made.

2. The two most likely diagnoses are acute schizophrenia (additional features required to make this diagnosis are more abnormal thought phenomena, mood incongruent delusions, and negative schizophrenic symptoms) and a major depressive disorder (any biologic symptoms of depression, a previous history of depression, and good premorbid adjustment).

3. Acute schizophrenia: any class of antipsychotic may be used. If sedation is required either a sedative antipsychotic, such as chlorpromazine, may be administered or a combination of a nonsedative antipsychotic, such as risperidone, and a short-acting benzodiazepine, such as lorazepam. There is an increasing tendency to use atypical antipsychotics, such as risperidone, sertindole, or olanzepine, as first-line treatments because they cause fewer adverse effects and therefore enhance patient compliance. Clozapine may not be used as first line. Therapy should be continued for 2–6 weeks at a therapeutic dose. If the initial medication is ineffective you may switch to another class of antipsychotic and review the diagnosis, particularly looking for an affective (mood) component. Effective therapy after a first episode should be continued for at least 6 months to 1 year. Careful monitored withdrawal may then follow. Subsequent episodes require much longer periods of maintenance but there is yet to be a clear consensus over the length of this. The adverse effects are listed in the text and are class dependent. In general, all typical neuroleptics carry a high risk of extrapyramidal adverse effects, akathisia, and tardive dyskinesias.

Major depressive disorder: any class of antidepressant may be used to treat major depressive disorder in this patient. As he is having difficulty sleeping, a sedative tricyclic such as amitriptyline may be used. If tolerance to adverse effects is an issue, an SSRI would probably be used. This would also be the class if the patient was suicidal. The drug should be used for at least 2 weeks and usually for up to 6 weeks to determine if it is effective. If the patient does not respond to the first line of therapy then either an antidepressant of a diferent class can be used or lithium can be added to 'augment' the continuing dose of antidepressant. The effective medication would usually be continued for 6–12 months before a gradual decrease, and cessation would be monitored. The adverse effects would depend on the class of drug used and the reader is referred to the relevant text.

15. Drugs and the Endocrine and Metabolic Systems

1. The patient shows clinical signs of glucocorticosteroid deficiency (nausea and weight loss) and mineralocorticosteroid deficiency (volume depletion, hyperkalemia) suggestive of adrenal failure (Addison's disease). Measurement of cortisol and aldosterone concentrations, as well as their regulatory hormones ACTH and plasma renin activity would confirm this diagnosis. A careful evaluation would exclude infection or neoplasm of the adrenals. The usual cause is autoimmune.

2. A synthetic glucocorticosteroid (e.g. hydrocortisone 10 mg p.o. at 7 a.m., 5 mg p.o. at 3 p.m.), and a synthetic mineralocorticosteroid (e.g. fludrocortisone 0.1 mg p.o. daily)

3. Patients should be aware of the symptoms of glucocorticosteroid deficiency (i.e. unexplained anorexia, nausea and fatigue) and should wear an identifying bracelet. Since an endogenous adrenal response is absent, glucocorticosteroids must be increased temporarily if the patient has a significant febrile illness or gastroenteritis or undergoes surgery. The dose of synthetic mineralocorticosteroid does not usually need adjusting.

4. Adverse effects of glucocorticosteroid therapy are osteoporosis, accelerated arteriosclerosis, glucose intolerance, obesity, myopathy, cataracts, avascular necrosis of bone, growth retardation, and infections. Adverse effects of mineralocorticosteroid therapy are hypertension and hypokalemia.

16. Drugs and Inflammatory and Immune Response

1. Antinuclear antibody, anti-DNA antibody, and serum complement. The most suspected disease from her history is systemic lupus erythematosus because the young female had facial erythema, decreased white blood cell count, and massive proteinuria. Thus, these three serological tests are necessary to make a definitive diagnosis for, and determine the disease activity of, SLE.

2. Chest radiograph, renal function tests, and renal biopsy.

3. Glucocorticosteroid (methylprednisolone) 'pulse' therapy and then high-dose prednisolone. For several weeks until clinical and serological remissions. With low-dose prednisolone, for several years. Infection, psychosis, ischemic necrosis of bone, osteoporosis, diabetes mellitus, hyperlipidemia, cataract, and glaucoma.

17. Drugs and the Renal System

1. Both symptoms are the result of edema (an increase in the volume of interstitial fluid). Edema in heart failure occurs as a consequence of elevations in capillary and venous pressures, and activation of the renin–angiotensin system that causes expansion of blood volume and a resulting reduction in the concentration of plasma proteins. Pulmonary edema creates a barrier to the diffusion of oxygen that results in breathlessness. Tissue swelling is a consequence of edema and this is most pronounced in the lower limbs, as seen in swelling of the ankles.

2. Diuretic drugs are commonly prescribed in congestive heart failure to alleviate edema. However, the most effective treatment of all grades of heart failure, in terms of relief of symptoms, exercise tolerance and reduction in mortality, is an angiotension-converting enzyme inhibitor combined with a diuretic. Thiazide diuretics are of benefit in patients with mild heart failure and normal renal function but loop diuretics are preferred in patients with poor renal function.

3. The elderly are particularly susceptible to the side effects of diuretics and a lower initial dose should have been prescribed. Fatigue and lethargy are most likely the result of thiazide-induced hypokalemia. Hypokalemia can be prevented by taking potassium supplements or combination of a thiazide diuretic with a potassium-sparing diuretic such as amiloride. In addition, potassium depletion may be reduced by taking bendroflumethiazide on alternate days. Lethargy may also result from thiazide-induced hyponatremia that, in the short term, can be treated by water restriction and oral sodium supplementation. In the longer term, a change to a loop diuretic may be required since these diuretics are less likely to produce hyponatremia.

18. Drugs and the Cardiovascular System

1. Yes.

2. Serum creatinine and electrolytes, electrocardiogram, chest radiograph.

3. Prompt lowering of blood pressure and relative ease in titrating an appropriate safe dose. Intravenous nitroprusside is commonly used in the emergency treatment of hypertension.

4. It is important to avoid lowering blood pressure too much in patients with severe long-standing hypertension to avoid decreasing cerebral blood flow. While somewhat arbitrary, an immediate goal of around 180/110 mmHg might be appropriate in this case.

5. The first goal would be to start oral drug therapy to wean the patient from the intravenous nitroprusside. The most important long-term goal should be to educate the patient about the critical need for regular medication.

19. Drugs and the Pulmonary System

1. This approach assumes an inconsequential infection and that the asthma can be ignored. It avoids drug complications, but does nothing to prevent the occurrence of possibly dangerous infections or troubling symptoms.

2. In the absence of information an antibiotic could be chosen on the basis of the probable nature of the infection (organism and prognosis), probable sensitivity to the antibiotic, and risk:benefit ratios for different antibiotics. When the identity of the organism causing the infection is not known, a best guess is based on clinical judgment. When the organism and its sensitivity are known, the choice is based upon the expected adverse effects and their frequency and importance. Since antibacterial efficacy should be high, the risk:benefit ratio depends on the adverse effects.

3. The choice of bronchodilator is based on the factors considered on pp. 422–3. The choice is between β adrenoceptor agonists for symptomatic relief, glucocorticosteroids to moderate the underlying immune processes (inflammation, release of autacoids) responsible for the asthmatic response, and aminophylline, which moderates the immune process and has some bronchodilator actions. β Adrenoceptor agonists provide good symptomatic relief, but have little effect on underlying pathology, and aerosols can be difficult to administer in children. The major adverse effects include tremor and tachycardia, and tachyphylaxis can occur.

641

4. This is a careful, but expensive, approach. The blood tests would indicate the status of the immune system with respect to infection and/or allergy, while the culture and sensitivity test would indicate whether a pathogenic bacterium is present and its sensitivity to antibiotics. Such information provides a scientific basis for planning a therapeutic strategy.

5. It is now agreed that asthma is basically an inflammatory condition and that anti-inflammatory drugs should be used early in addition to a bronchodilator. In children cromolyn is very safe and low-dose oral aminophylline reduces the inflammatory response with fewer possible adverse effects of tremor and excitement. Glucocorticosteroid given as an aerosol lacks the adverse effects seen with systemic administration.

6. The most likely diagnosis is a self-limiting viral infection, which, as a result of an allergic or other liability to asthma, has led to symptomatic bronchoconstriction. A viral infection is not treated with antibiotics, but acute symptomatic relief of the asthma can be obtained with an aerosol β adrenoceptor agonist. Since allergic asthma has an inflammatory component with hypersensitivity to bronchoconstrictor agents, topical glucocorticosteroids or oral aminophylline are more appropriate to reduce the inflammation and hypersensitivity. Aerosol glucocorticosteroids have few adverse effects, while aminophylline therapy can be titrated to known effective blood concentrations. The duration of treatment would depend upon the nature of the asthma in this patient. Most guidelines for the therapy of asthma suggest reducing medication to the lowest possible level once the patient is symptom free.

20. Drugs and the Musculoskeletal System

1. The aspirin dose can now be decreased to avoid tinnitus, but as she has not responded clinically, consider discontinuing aspirin and trying other NSAIDs, such as diclofenac or naproxen.

2. Low-dose prednisone is usually very effective in reducing the pain and morning stiffness associated with rheumatoid arthritis. Doses of prednisone at 5 mg p.o. daily (or less) are relatively well tolerated with minimal short- and long-term adverse effects. With clinical improvement, the daily dose can be tapered or an alternate-day regimen can be initiated to minimize the potential concern of glucocorticosteroid-induced osteoporosis.

3. A 20-week trial of intramuscular gold salts without clinical response requires re-evaluation of the disease-modifying agents. Considerations would be to discontinue the gold injections and start another second agent, such as methotrexate or sulfasalazine. If it was left and there were partial clinical improvement, continue the gold injections and add a second disease-modifying agent, such as antimalarials, methotrexate, or sulfasalazine.

4. Methotrexate liver toxicity is dose and time dependent. The long-term concern is the development of cirrhosis and subsequent liver failure. Liver enzymes and serum albumin should be monitored monthly. If there are persistent abnormalities then the dose can be held or reduced and the abnormalities followed. If there is concern of underlying liver disease, or the abnormalities do not resolve, the risks of proceeding to a liver biopsy can be discussed with the patient. The patient will ultimately need to decide whether to continue with methotrexate after being fully informed by the physician.

21. Drugs and the Gastrointestinal System

1. The classes of drug that will alleviate the symptoms of peptic ulcer, but not bring about a cure, are H_2 antihistamines, proton pump inhibitors, sucralfate, and antacids.

2. A relapse is liable to occur since omeprazole does not eradicate the underlying cause, which is infection with *Helicobacter pylori*.

3. The treatment would probably comprise metronidazole or amoxyllin plus clarithromycin with or without proton pump inhibitor. However, the optimum treatment for *H. pylori* infection has yet to be determined.

4. Eradication of *H. pylori* will cure a peptic ulcer, and there will be little chance of relapse provided that there is no reinfection.

23. Drugs and the Skin

1. The likely diagnosis is atopic dermatitis.

2. It is important that children with eczema are bathed daily because they have more bacteria, particularly *Staphylococcus aureus*, on their skin than children with normal skin, and there is now evidence that the staphylococcus might act as a superantigen to fuel the eczema. However, children with eczema should avoid detergents and therefore should not use soaps and bubble bath and should not have their hair

washed in the bath. Aqueous cream or some of the commercially available emollients can be used as soap substitutes. As eczematous skin has an impaired barrier to transepidermal water loss, further losses must be minimized by adding an emollient to the bath water and applying an emollient all over the body after bathing.

3. In addition to emollients, topical glucocorticosteroids (mild or moderate only in the case of a 2-year-old) need to be applied in the short term to control the allergic inflammation in the skin. The risk of adverse effects resulting from the use of glucocorticosteroids of the appropriate strength for the child's age short term is less than the risk of damage to the skin from constant scratching and secondary infection with potential systemic spread.

4. Sedative oral antihistamines have been shown to be beneficial in the treatment of eczema, probably because they help to break the itch–scratch–itch cycle. Cetirizine and ketotifen may have additional antiallergic properties.

24. Drugs and the Eye

1. Reduced production and increased drainage of aqueous humor.

2. Nonselective β adrenoceptor antagonists are the first-line therapy.

3. Levobunolol hydrochloride, carteolol hydrochloride, and timolol maleate reduce the rate of aqueous humor production by blocking β adrenoceptors on the ciliary body, thereby decreasing the effects of circulating epinephrine.

4. Asthma, obstructive airways disease, bradycardia, heart block, and heart failure.

25. Drugs and the Ear

1. No. The moisture of irrigation could make the infection worse. The ear should be kept dry.

2. No. An oral antibiotic, if given, is best used in combination with a topical antibiotic.

3. Perhaps. In mild infections, a topical antibiotic (neomycin plus polymyxin drops) alone can be effective.

4. Yes. Taking a culture initially can help to identify the etiologic agent, which may help direct further therapy if first-line treatment is not effective.

5. It would be best to review the patient in 10 days because although the cultured bacteria may not be sensitive to your choice of first-line antibiotic, the infection may settle and not need further medication. Ciprofloxacin with gentamicin or tobramycin drops given with oral ciprofloxacin would be reasonable second-line treatment if the drainage persists.

26. Drug Use in Anesthesia and Critical Care

1. The immediate goal is to ensure that brain oxygenation is taking place. The 'ABCD' mnemonic is used to organize evaluations and therapy during any critical event in anesthesia and resuscitation. In this case study, the position of the tracheal tube should be verified using auscultation and expired capnometry while oxygen is administered through bag-valve ventilation. Then, the adequacy of breathing and circulation including intravenous access should all be urgently confirmed.

2. Assuming that the ABC evaluation did not provide any concerns other than failure to awaken and breathe, your differential diagnosis should include the following: excessive anesthesia; excessive opioid administration; hypocapnia; neuromuscular blockade; hypoglycemia; and cerebral ischemic event.

3. Reversible causes in the differential diagnosis are evaluated as follows: expired inhaled anesthetic monitoring for excessive inhaled anesthetic; expired capnometry for hypocapnia; peripheral nerve stimulation for neuromuscular blockade; and blood glucometer testing for hypoglycemia.

4. Antagonism of opioid-induced respiratory depression with intravenous naloxone can be accompanied by antagonism of analgesia, sympathetic stimulation (i.e. tachycardia, hypertension, arrhythmias, pulmonary edema) and stimulation of nausea and vomiting. Since the onset of action is 1–2 minutes, intravenous naloxone should be titrated in a conscious patient to avoid the above adverse effects. Naloxone has a short duration of action (30–45 minutes) compared to most opioid agonists, so the need for additional doses of naloxone requires careful monitoring.

5. Tracheal extubation should be delayed until the patient has the cognitive and physical ability to clear her airway; this will reduce the risk of aspiration and laryngospasm. She should be in the lateral position; this will reduce the risk of upper airway obstruction from

the tongue falling back and aspiration should vomiting occur. She should receive supplemental oxygen; this will reduce the risk of hypoxemia from respiratory depression and obstructed ventilation. Pulse oximetry should be used for the early detection of hypoxemia.

27. Drug Use in Disorders of Nutrition

1. Being vegetarian, the patient has a very high risk of vitamin B_{12} deficiency. There is no need for genetic advice.
2. By no means. The patient should become aware of belonging to a high-risk group.
3. A multivitamin preparation may not be sufficient.
4. The patient does have a high risk of vitamin B_{12} deficiency with resulting folate deficiency.
5. Megaloblastic anemia due to vitamin B_{12} deficiency should be treated with vitamin B_{12}. To prevent neural tube defects, folic acid should be prescribed at least 3 months before pregnancy as well as during the first trimester.

28. Drug Use in Dentistry

1. This is not the correct approach. Although acute allergic reactions can be manifested in the mouth there should be other typical signs of an allergic reaction or a history of allergy. Antihistamines are not indicated because they would add to the drying effect and worsen the presenting symptoms.
2. This is not the correct approach. Generalized stomatitis is rarely, if ever, a symptom of a bacterial oral infection. Acute necrotizing ulcerative gingivitis can produce generalized pain and discomfort, but the oral examination should reveal significant gingival infection with necrotic tissue and not white patches. The patient should have an elevated body temperature and possibly lymphadenopathy. Antibiotic use without appropriate symptoms is inappropriate and could worsen the existing disease.
3. This is not the correct approach. Oral viral infections are associated with vesicle formation and rupture with an acute onset of pain. There should also be a fever, pain and lymphadenopathy. The symptoms do not support a diagnosis of a viral infection. Using an antiviral drug would not be effective or alleviate the painful symptoms.
4. This approach is partially correct as the presenting symptoms do appear to resemble those of acute pseudomembranous candidiasis. However, candidiasis is an opportunistic infection in the oral cavity and underlying factors can be contributory. Correcting underlying factors as far as possible is important in preventing reinfection. Advising the patient to avoid spicy or other types of foods that are irritating an already painful oral mucosa will make the patient more comfortable during the acute phase of the disease. The sore mouth may be preventing the patient from eating properly or drinking sufficient fluids. Nutritional and fluid support are always important in acute infections.
5. Nystatin is an antifungal and is not systemically absorbed. It is effective when used topically providing the patient is compliant. The drug therapy should be continued for 14 days initially. The preferable end-point of therapy is when the cultures are negative for *Candida* or,

empirically, after 14 days if there are no symptoms and signs. Because nystatin is not absorbed systemically, adverse effects are usually limited to minor gastrointestinal complaints if they occur. Allergy to this drug is very rare. Drug interactions are not reported with this drug, probably because of its lack of systemic absorption. It is therefore a first choice in patients who are already taking multiple drug therapy.

6. The identification of *Candida* species with hyphae in an oral culture is diagnostic for candidiasis. Sensitivity testing is not necessary unless the infection does not respond to the initial drug. The history does not suggest an immunocompromised patient. With a vague history of anemia, it is important to request laboratory tests that could assist in the overall evaluation. Laboratory data that could rule out anemia include ferritin, iron, folic acid, and vitamin B_{12} levels. A red blood cell count along with a microscopic inspection could help confirm or deny the presence of anemia. The smooth tongue with an absence of papillae is also seen in patients with anemia. Anemia is a contributory factor to opportunistic candidiasis.

7. This patient is taking several drugs that are associated with xerostomia, in particular the antihypertensive drugs clonidine and hydrochlorothiazide. Alprazolam is also associated with a dry mouth. This combination of drugs and the age of the patient are sufficient to reduce saliva production. Saliva contains immunoglobulins and provides protective lubrication for oral tissues. When this is impaired, tissue ageing and possible anemia present opportunistic circumstances for an oral yeast infection.

29. Toxins and Poisons

1. First, the source of poisoning should be removed and absorption minimized. Vomiting carries a high risk of aspiration due to the impaired neuromuscular reflexes. The lesions on the legs might include envenomation sites and wrapping them tightly with bandages will limit lymphatic drainage and venom absorption.
2. Respiratory failure may develop owing to severe muscle weakness and can be fatal. It is imperative that your friend is taken to the nearest hospital in case mechanical ventilation is required.
3. The absence of symptoms other than general weakness and ptosis indicates a specific neuromuscular defect. Botulism or tetrodotoxin envenomation (from an octopus) are unlikely because of their rarity and the absence of signs of parasympathetic blockade. Food poisoning and organophosphate poisoning induce an entirely different set of symptoms. Sometimes wounds from sea snake bites and coneshell stings are very small and the victim is unaware of having been bitten or stung. The probable cause of the symptoms is sea snake envenomation and the victim did not notice the bite.
4. There are antivenins for sea snake and coneshell venoms, but their availability is limited and may have to come from Australia. Specific treatments are available for the other possible causes of the victim's condition but are not relevant to this case if it is sea snake envenomation.

   Sea snake envenomation makes artificial ventilation mandatory until no longer needed. There is a risk of skeletal muscle lysis due to phospholipase activity in the venom, and myoglobinuria can damage the kidneys. The highest level of medical care is needed.

Page numbers in *italics* refer to figures and tables, those in **bold** indicate main discussions.

H

663

Drug Index

This drug index indicates differences in nomenclature of commonly used drugs in three key regions: the USA, European Union, and Japan. Only drugs mentioned in the text of this book are included in the table below.

- Drugs with minor spelling variations (e.g. cefalexin/cephalexin, cyclobendazole/ciclobendazole, dimethicone/dimeticone) are generally not included.

- The International Nonproprietary Name (INN) is generally the same as the United States Adopted Name (USAN); where it differs, it is given in the EU column.
- British Approved Names (BAN) are increasingly the same as INN; where they continue to differ, they are given in square brackets in the EU column.

USA	EU (INN) [BAN]	Japan
acetaminophen	paracetamol	acetaminophen
acyclovir	aciclovir	aciclovir
albuterol	salbutamol	salbutamol
amphetamine sulfate	amfetamine	
anthralin	dithranol	
beclomethasone dipropionate	beclometasone	beclometasone dipropionate
bendroflumethiazide	bendroflumethiazide [UK name – bendrofluazide]	bendroflumethiazide
benoxinate hydrochloride	oxybuprocaine	oxybuprocaine hydrochloride
benzocaine	benzocaine	ethyl aminobenzoate
benztropine mesylate	benzatropine	benztropine mesilate
bethanidine sulfate	betanidine [bethanidine]	betanidine sulfate
bupropion hydrochloride	amfebutamone	
calcipotriene	calcipotriol	
calcitonin	calcitonin [UK name – salcatonin]	calcitonin
calcium pantothenate	calcium pantothenate [pantothenic acid]	calcium pantothenate
	carbaril [carbaryl]	
carboprost tromethamine	[carboprost trometanol]	
chlophedianol hydrochloride	clofedanol [chlophedianol]	clofedanol hydrochloride
chloroguanide hydrochloride	proguanil	
chlorpheniramine maleate	chlorphenamine [UK name – chlorpheniramine]	chlorpheniramine
chlorthalidone	chlortalidone	chlortalidone
cholestyramine	colestyramine	colestyramine
cromolyn sodium	sodium cromoglicate	sodium cromoglicate
cyclosporine (cyclosporin A)	ciclosporin	ciclosporin
dactinomycin	[dactinomycin]	actinomycin D
danthron	dantron	
deferoxamine	deferoxamine [desferrioxamine]	deferoxamine
demeclocycline	demeclocycline	demethylchlortetracycline
dichlorphenamide	diclofenamide	diclofenamide

USA	EU (INN) [BAN]	Japan
dicyclomine hydrochloride	dicycloverine [UK name – dicyclomine]	dicycloverine hydrochloride
diethylstilbestrol diphosphate	fosfestrol	fosfestrol
dipivefrin hydrochloride	dipivefrine	dipivefrin hydrochloride
divalproex sodium	valproate semisodium [semisodium valproate]	
docusate sodium	sodium dioctyl sulfosuccinate [docusate sodium]	dioctyl disodium sulfosuccinate
echothiophate	ecothiopate	ecothiopate
epinephrine	epinephrine [UK name – adrenaline]	epinephrine hydrochloride
ergonovine maleate	ergometrine	ergometrine maleate
factor VIII (rDNA)	[octocog alfa]	
factor IX complex	[factor IX fraction]	
floxacillin	flucloxacillin	flucloxacillin sodium
flucloronide	fluclorolone acetonide	
flurandrenolide	fludroxycortide [UK name – flurandrenolone]	fludroxycortide
furosemide	furosemide [UK name – frusemide]	furosemide
gentian violet	methylrosanilinium chloride [crystal violet]	methylrosanilinium chloride
glyburide	glibenclamide	glibenclamide
glycerin	glycerol	glycerin
glycine	glycine	aminoacetic acid
halobetasol propionate	ulobetasol	
hydrogen peroxide	hydrogen peroxide	oxydol
hydroxypropyl methylcellulose	hypromellose	hydroxypropylmethylcellulose
hydroxyurea	hydroxycarbamide [UK name – hydroxyurea]	
hypromellose phthalate		hydroxypropylmethylcellulose phthalate
inamrinone	amrinone	amrinone
isopropyl alcohol		isopropanol
isoproterenol hydrochloride	isoprenaline	l-isoprenaline hydrochloride
leucovorin calcium	calcium folinate	calcium folinate
leuprolide acetate	leuprorelin	
levothyroxine sodium	levothyroxine sodium [UK name – thyroxine sodium]	levothyroxine sodium
lidocaine	lidocaine [UK name – lignocaine]	lidocaine
mannitol	mannitol	D-mannitol
mechlorethamine hydrochloride	chlormethine	nitrogen mustard N-oxide hydrochloride
meclizine	meclozine	meclizine
menthol	menthol	dl-menthol
meperidine hydrochloride	pethidine	pethidine hydrochloride
mesalamine	mesalazine	
metaproterenol	orciprenaline	orciprenaline
methamphetamine hydrochloride	metamfetamine	methamphetamine hydrochloride
methimazole	thiamazole	thiamazole
methylergonovine maleate	methylergometrine	methylergometrine maleate
mitomycin	mitomycin	mitomycin C
mitoxantrone	mitoxantrone [UK name – mitozantrone]	mitoxantrone

USA	EU (INN) [BAN]	Japan
moricizine	moracizine	
natamycin	natamycin	pimaricin
neomycin palmitate	neomycin	
neomycin sulfate		fradiomycin sulfate
niacin	nicotinic acid	nicotinic acid
niacinamide	nicotinamide	nicotinamide
norepinephrine	norepinephrine [UK name – noradrenaline]	norepinephrine
norethindrone	norethisterone	norethisterone
	ouabain	G-strophanthin
penicillin G benzathine	benzathine benzylpenicillin	benzylpenicillin benzathine
penicillin G potassium	[benzylpenicillin potassium]	benzylpenicillin potassium
penicillin G procaine	procaine benzylpenicillin [UK name – procaine penicillin]	
penicillin V	phenoxymethylpenicillin	phenoxymethylpenicillin
phytonadione	phytomenadione	phytonadione
podofilox	[podophyllotoxin]	
povidone	povidone	polyvinylpyrrolidone
prilocaine hydrochloride		propitocaine hydrochloride
proparacaine hydrochloride	proxymetacaine	
propoxyphene hydrochloride	dextropropoxyphene	
pyrilamine maleate	mepyramine	
quinacrine	mepacrine	
rifampin	rifampicin	rifampicin
salcatonin	calcitonin (salmon) [UK name – calcitonin]	calcitonin salmon (synthesis)
salsalate	salsalate	sasapyrine
scopolamine	[hyoscine]	scopolamine
somatropin	somatropin	human growth hormone
succinylcholine hydrochloride	suxamethonium chloride	suxamethonium chloride
sulbactam pivoxil	[pivsulbactam]	
sulfalene	[sulfametopyrazine]	sulfamethopyrazine
sulfamethazine	sulfadimidine	
sulfamethoxazole	sulfamethoxazole	acetylsulfamethoxazole
sulfasalazine	sulfasalazine	salazosulfapyridine
sulfisoxazole	sulfafurazole	sulfisoxazole
tetracaine	tetracaine [UK name –amethocaine]	tetracaine
theobromine calcium salicylate		theosalicin
thiabendazole	tiabendazole	tiabendazole
thioguanine	tioguanine	
trihexyphenidyl	trihexyphenidyl [UK name – benzhexol]	trihexyphenidyl
trimeprazine	alimemazine [UK name –trimeprazine]	alimemazine
valacyclovir hydrochloride	valaciclovir	
valproate sodium		sodium valproate